Tumor Markers

Tumor Markers

Physiology, Pathobiology, Technology and Clinical Applications

Editors:

Eleftherios P. Diamandis
Herbert A. Fritsche
Hans Lilja
Daniel W. Chan
Morton K. Schwartz

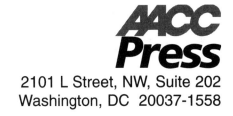

2101 L Street, NW, Suite 202
Washington, DC 20037-1558

Book Cover Legend

Upper left panel: Receiver operating characteristic (ROC) curve, indicating the diagnostic sensitivity and specificity of total PSA (PSA-T), the combination of free to total PSA ratio (PSA-F/PSA-T), and the combination of human kallikrein 2 (hK2) with total and free PSA. This figure was adapted from Chapter 16.

Upper right panel: cDNA microarray analysis of malignant ovarian tissue and normal ovarian tissue, as well as a panel of normal human tissues. The genes examined are represented in the columns. Note the significant overexpression (red) of many genes in the malignant ovarian tissue. Adapted from Chapter 34.

Lower left panel: Tissue array of 22 prostate samples containing lesions of varying histological grades. The inset A (prostate tumor of Gleason pattern 4) and B (high-grade prostate intraepithelial neoplasia) illustrate the architectural preservation of the tissue. This format allows a cell by cell analysis of the genome, the transcriptome, or the proteome of multiple samples in a parallel manner. Adapted from Chapter 32.

Lower right panel: Identification of tumor cells in peripheral blood of breast cancer patients. The staining was for cytokeratin (green) and for nucleus (purple). Adapted from Chapter 52.

©2002 American Association for Clinical Chemistry, Inc. All rights reserved. No part of this publication may be reproduced, stored in a retrieval system, or transmitted in any form by electronic, mechanical, photocopying, or any other means without written permission of the publisher.

1 2 3 4 5 6 7 8 9 0   PCP   03 02 01

Printed in the United States of America

Library of Congress Cataloging-in-Publication Data

Tumor markers : physiology, pathobiology, technology, and clinical applications / edited
Eleftherios P. Diamandis . . .[et al.].
    p. ; cm.
    Includes index.
    ISBN 1-890883-71-9 (alk. paper)
    1. Tumor markers. I. Diamandis, Eleftherios P.
    [DNLM : 1. Tumor Markers, Biological. QZ 241 T9256 2002]
RC270.3.T84 T854 2002
616.99'4075—dc21

2002066713

Contents

Preface ix
Editors xi
Contributors xiii

Part One: General Principles

1. Tumor Markers: Past, Present, and Future 3
   Eleftherios P. Diamandis

2. Tumor Markers: Introduction and General Principles 9
   Daniel W. Chan and Morton K. Schwartz

3. Clinical Evaluation Criteria for Tumor Markers 19
   Vered Stearns and Daniel F. Hayes

4. Quality Control and Standardization for Tumor Marker 25
   Elizabeth H. Hammond

5. Practice Guidelines and Recommendations for Use of Tumor Markers in the Clinic 33
   Martin Fleisher, Ann M. Dnistrian, Catharine M. Sturgeon, Rolf Lamerz, and James L. Wittliff

6. Limitations of Assay Techniques for Tumor Markers 65
   Catharine M. Sturgeon

7. Oncogenes and Tumor Suppressor Genes in Cancer 83
   Marta Sanchez-Carbayo and Carlos Cordon-Cardo

8. Proteases in Cancer: Markers of Metastatic Potential and Prognosis 99
   Michael J. Duffy

9. Circulating Cancer Cells and Cell-Free Nucleic Acids as Tumor Markers 107
   Markus Müller, Hans Krause, and Carsten Goessl

10. Autoantibodies as Circulating Cancer Markers 123
    Kwok Leung Cheung, C. Rosamund L. Graves, and John F.R. Robertson

11. Combining Multiple Biomarkers in Clinical Diagnostics—A Review of Methods and Issues 133
    Zhen Zhang

12. Elements of Study Design for Biomarker Development 141
    Margaret Sullivan Pepe, Ruth Etzioni, Ziding Feng, Gary Longton, John Potter, Mary Lou Thompson, Mark Thornquist, Marcy Winget, and Yutaka Yasui

13	Biomarkers as Therapeutic Targets: Toward Personalized Treatments in Oncology *Massimo Gion and Giampietro Gasparini*	151

Part Two: Organ-Specific Tumors Markers

14	Tumor Markers in Breast Cancer *Rafael Molina*	165
15	Prognostic and Predictive Markers for Breast Cancer *Frédérique Spyratos*	181
16	BRCA1 and BRCA2: Genes that Predispose to Breast and Ovarian Cancer *Hilmi Ozcelik and Gordon Glendon*	189
17	Adenocarcinoma of the Prostate *Alexander Haese, Charlotte Becker, Eleftherios P. Diamandis, and Hans Lilja*	193
18	Ovarian Cancer *Ie-Ming Shih, Lori J. Sokoll, and Daniel W. Chan*	239
19	Tumor Markers for Colorectal Cancer *Morton K. Schwartz*	253
20	Molecular Diagnostics of Hereditary Nonpolyposis Colorectal Cancer (HNPCC) *Michele Zysman and Bharati Bapat*	259
21	Serological Tumor Markers in Pancreatic Cancer *Matti Eskelinen and Ulf Haglund*	265
22	Tumor Markers in Primary Malignancies of the Liver *Philip J. Johnson*	269
23	Bladder Cancer and Urine Tumor Marker Tests *Herbert A. Fritsche*	281
24	Lung Cancer *Paul M. Schneider, Ralf Metzger, Jan Brabender, Sebastian Boehm, Thomas Luebke, Kourosh Zarghooni, Klaus Prenzel, Sylke Schneider, Peter H. Collet, and Arnulf H. Hoelscher*	287
25	Monoclonal Gammopathies *Ingemar Turesson*	305
26	Leukemias and Lymphomas *Joseph A. DiGiuseppe and Michael J. Borowitz*	321
27	Tumor Markers in Primary and Metastatic Brain Tumors *Susanne M. Arnold and Roy A. Patchell*	329
28	Neuroendocrine Tumors *Kjell Öberg and Mats Stridsberg*	339
29	Markers for Testicular Cancer *Ulf-Håkan Stenman and Henrik Alfthan*	351

30	Tumor Markers in Melanoma *Steven D. Trocha, Rishab K. Gupta, and Donald L. Morton*	361
31	Gastric Cancer *Sten Hammarström and Torgny Stigbrand*	375

Part Three: Genomic and Proteomic Approaches for Biomarker Discovery

32	Microarray Technology in Cancer *Paul C. Park, Ben Beheshti, and Jeremy A. Squire*	383
33	Proteomic Approaches to Tumor Marker Discovery *Darryl Palmer-Toy, Scott Kuzdzal, and Daniel W. Chan*	391
34	Tumor Marker Discovery Using Large-Scale DNA Microarray Analysis *Garret M. Hampton, John B. Welsh, and Henry F. Frierson, Jr.*	401
35	Mining the Cancer Cell's DNA Replication Apparatus for Novel Malignancy Biomarkers *Linda H. Malkus, Pamela E. Bechtel, Jennifer W. Sekowski, Lauren Schnaper, Carla R-V. Lankford, Derek J. Hoelz, Yang Liu, and Robert J. Hickey*	411

Part Four: Some Emerging Tumor Markers

36	Adhesion Molecules as Tumor Markers *Subhas Chakrabarty and Herbert A. Fritsche*	425
37	Soluble ErbB Receptors (sEGFR/sErbBs): Serum Biomarkers in Breast and Ovarian Cancer *Jacqueline M. Lafky, Tammy M. Greenwood, Andre T. Baron, Cecelia H. Boardman, Elsa M. Cora, and Nita J. Maihle*	427
38	A Multiplex Real-Time PCR Assay for the Detection of Mammaglobin and Complementary Transcribed Genes in Breast Cancer *Barbara K. Zehentner, Davin C. Dillon, Yuqiu Jiang, Jiangchun Xu, Steven G. Reed, David H. Persing, and Raymond L. Houghton*	433
39	Beta-Catenin and Maspin as Tumor Markers *Yong Wen and Mien-Chie Hung*	437
40	TIMP-1 in Colorectal Cancer *Mads Holten-Anderson, Ib Jarle Christensen, Hans Jørgen Nielsen, and Nils Brünner*	441
41	uPA and PAI-1 in Breast Cancer *Manfred Schmitt, Viktor Magdolen, Ute Reuning, and Nadia Harbeck*	445
42	Tumor-Associated Trypsin Inhibitor (TATI) *Ulf-Håkan Stenman and Annukka Paju*	449
43	Estrogen Receptor-β: Role in Breast Cancer *Michael J. Duffy*	453

44	Measurement of Tumor-Specific T Cells with MHC Tetramer Technology *Johannes Hampl and Kristine Kuus-Reichel*	457
45	A New Discovery Approach for Hormone-Responsive Genes: PC1 Prostate Cancer Gene *Cynthia French and Karen Yamamoto*	461
46	Kallikreins as Cancer Biomarkers *George M. Yousef and Eleftherios P. Diamandis*	465
47	Tumor M2-PK: A Marker of the Tumor Metabolome *Sybille Mazurek, Diana Lüftner, Hans Werner Wechsel, Joachim Schneider, and Erich Eigenbrodt*	471
48	Measurement of Hue and Chroma in Assessment of Biomarkers of Colon and Lung Cancer *Peter Horsewood, Michael Evelegh, Norman Marcon, Gerard Cox, and John Miller*	477
49	Heterogeneous Nuclear Ribonucleoprotein A2/B1 as an Early Marker of Preinvasive Lung Cancer *Jordi Tauler, Alfredo Martínez, and James L. Mulshine*	481
50	Viral Markers RAK in Early Diagnosis and Therapy of Breast, Ovarian, Uterine, and Prostate Cancers *Eva M. Rakowicz-Szulczynska*	485
51	Plasma EBV DNA as a Marker for Nasopharyngeal Carcinoma and EBV-Related Lymphomas *Philip J. Johnson*	491
52	Circulating Tumor Cells as Cancer Markers: A Sample Preparation and Analysis System *Michael Kagan, David Howard, Teresa Bendele, Chandra Rao, and Leon W.M.M. Terstappen*	495
53	Cell Dielectric Properties as Diagnostic Markers for Tumor Cell Isolation *Peter R.C. Gascoyne*	499
54	Apoptosis and Apoptosis-Related Genes in Cancer *Andreas Scorilas*	503
55	Telomerase *Evi Lianidou*	509
56	Single Nucleotide Polymorphism (SNP) Genotyping by Probe Melting Curve Analysis *Carl T. Wittwer, Philip S. Bernard, Andrew O. Crockett, Sandra D. Bohling, and Kojo S.J. Elenitoba-Johnson*	513
57	ProGRP Enables Diagnosis of Small-Cell Lung Cancer *Petra Stieber and Ken Yamaguchi*	517
	Index	523

Preface

Tumor markers were discovered many years ago and are now used for various clinical applications including cancer diagnosis, monitoring, prediction of therapeutic response, and prognosis. Although tumor marker analysis constitutes a sizeable portion of clinical laboratory activity, no major textbook exists at present. Despite great expectations in the 1960s and 1970s, tumor markers did not deliver the promised goods. It has now been clearly realized that, even though there are some notable exceptions, no true tumor markers exist; most tumor marker molecules are actually physiological compounds that occur in normal tissues.

Many clinicians do not believe that tumor marker analysis offers much in terms of patient care, unless the tumor marker alters clinical outcomes. This situation changed with the discovery of prostate-specific antigen (PSA) in the 1980s. During the past five to ten years, it has been demonstrated convincingly that this tumor marker is suitable for screening and can be used as an aid in diagnosis and as a tool for deciding further therapeutic interventions, including biopsy and initiation of anti-androgen therapy or radiotherapy in patients who relapse. This simple test has contributed enormously to the practice of urology and it is now considered an indispensable tool. More importantly, the introduction of PSA testing has altered clinical outcomes—the mortality from prostate cancer is decreasing (which may be partially due to the introduction of PSA testing). Now, metastatic prostate cancer at diagnosis is relatively rare in populations exposed to extensive PSA testing. It is very clear that tumor markers with characteristics like those of PSA could hugely impact patient outcomes in other cancers, and there is now renewed interest in discovering such molecules for other cancers.

The tumor marker field is now at a major crossroad. The completion of the Human Genome Project and the identification of all human genes have raised hopes that some of these new genes may be valuable cancer markers. Additionally, the development of miniaturized technology for studying either cDNA or protein expression in a parallel fashion (microarray technology) suggests that it may now be possible to combine many different molecules for making prognostic and diagnostic decisions instead of relying on a single molecule. These hopes become even more realistic when one considers the tremendous developments in bioinformatics, which offer the capability of intelligent combination of various markers into disease-specific algorithms. Clearly, this new trend promises to revolutionize the current status of cancer biomarkers.

In organizing this book, we have decided to separate it into four different sections.

In Part I, we review the principles of tumor markers and present other subjects of general interest. Here we have included a major chapter that deals with practice guidelines and recommendations for clinical use of tumor markers. Interestingly, these recommendations differ, depending on which organization is sponsoring them. Nevertheless, we believe that the amalgamation of all these recommendations into one chapter will allow clinicians and clinical chemists to appreciate each other's points of view. Obviously, these recommendations will likely change as new markers and new technologies evolve.

In Part II, we present organ-specific tumor markers.

In Part III, we include some important technologies that are addressing the issue of new cancer marker discovery by using powerful genomic, proteomic, and bioinformatic techniques. The power of these technologies lies in the fact that they can potentially scan the entire genome. There are hopes that some good cancer markers will be identified and evaluated further, even though we have yet to see successful tumor markers discovered with this technology. It is possible that the primary markers have already been discovered with traditional techniques and that these new technologies will contribute to discovery of second-line marker families that will be used, not as single tests but as combinations of powerful multi-parametric panels. The outcomes of these studies will be available to us over the next three to five years.

And in Part IV, the final section, we include, as a sampler, a collection of promising cancer markers that are now in a developmental stage. This is clearly a biased selection, since most of these markers were introduced at the Second Santa Barbara Tumor Marker Meeting that was held in Santa Barbara, California, on March 3–6, 2001.

We hope this book will be useful to clinicians, clinical and medical biochemists, trainees in laboratory medicine, diagnostic companies, technologists, and other allied health professionals. We welcome comments. Our hope is that this book will contribute to new developments that will ultimately lead to better clinical outcomes and, ultimately, to cancer prevention.

ACKNOWLEDGEMENTS

We would like to sincerely thank the people who have made this book possible. Foremost, we acknowledge the hard work of our

146 contributors. Without their efforts and expertise, this book could not have been completed. Four of the Editors acknowledge the leadership provided by Dr. E.P. Diamandis, who coordinated the publication of this volume during the last 18 months. Special thanks to Hassima Omar Ali, Secretary to Dr. Diamandis, who provided valuable assistance throughout this exercise. The Editors also thank AACC Press for agreeing to publish this volume, and especially Joanna Grimes, who provided valuable support and enormous help in bringing this complex effort to fruition. Last, but not least, the Editors would like to thank their families for their support and encouragement. We dedicate this book to all the scientists who have contributed, through their careers, to the new developments in this important field of investigation.

The Editors
Eleftherios P. Diamandis
Herbert A. Fritsche
Hans Lilja
Daniel W. Chan
Morton K. Schwartz

Editors

Eleftherios P. Diamandis, MD, PhD, FRCPC
Head, Section of Clinical Biochemistry
Department of Pathology and Laboratory Medicine
Mount Sinai Hospital
    and Head, Division of Clinical Biochemistry
Department of Laboratory Medicine and Pathobiology
University of Toronto
Toronto, Ontario, Canada

Herbert A. Fritsche, PhD
Professor, Department of Laboratory Medicine
Division of Pathology and Laboratory Medicine
The University of Texas, M.D. Anderson Cancer Center
Houston, Texas, USA

Hans Lilja, MD, PhD
Professor (of Clinical Chemistry), Chief Physician
Department of Laboratory Medicine, Division of
    Clinical Chemistry
Lund University, University Hospital Malmo
Malmo, Sweden

Daniel W. Chan, PhD
Director, Clinical Chemistry Division
Professor of Pathology, Oncology, Radiology and Urology
Johns Hopkins Medical Institutions
Baltimore, Maryland, USA

Morton K. Schwartz, PhD
Chairman, Department of Clinical Laboratories
Memorial Sloan Kettering Cancer Center
New York, New York, USA

Contributors

Henrik Alfthan
Department of Clinical Chemistry
Helsinki University Central Hospital
Helsinki, Finland

Susanne M. Arnold
Division of Hematology and Oncology
University of Kentucky Chandler Medical Center
and Multidisciplinary Lung Cancer Program
Markey Cancer Center
Lexington, Kentucky, USA

Bharati Bapat
Department of Pathology and Laboratory Medicine
Mount Sinai Hospital
and Department of Laboratory Medicine and Pathobiology
University of Toronto
Toronto, Ontario, Canada

Andre T. Baron
Tumor Biology Program
Mayo Clinic
Rochester, Minnesota, USA

Pamela E. Bechtel
Biochip Systems
Phoenix Research and Development Center
Motorola Inc.
Tempe, Arizona, USA

Charlotte Becker
Department of Laboratory Medicine
Division of Clinical Chemistry
Lund University, University Hospital Malmo
Malmo, Sweden

Ben Beheshti
Division of Cellular and Molecular Biology
Ontario Cancer Institute
and Department of Laboratory Medicine and Pathobiology
University of Toronto
Toronto, Ontario, Canada

Teresa Bendele
Systems Evaluation
Immunicon Corporation
Huntingdon Valley, Pennsylvania, USA

Philip S. Bernard
Department of Pathology
University of Utah School of Medicine
Salt Lake City, Utah, USA

Cecelia H. Boardman
Department of Obstetrics and Gynecology
Virginia Commonwealth University Health System
Richmond, Virginia, USA

Sebastian Boehm
Department of Visceral and Vascular Surgery
University of Cologne
Cologne, Germany

Sandra D. Bohling
Department of Pathology
University of Utah School of Medicine
Salt Lake City, Utah, USA

Michael J. Borowitz
Department of Pathology
Johns Hopkins Medical Institutions
Baltimore, Maryland, USA

Jan Brabender
Department of Visceral and Vascular Surgery
University of Cologne
Cologne, Germany

Nils Brünner
Finsen Laboratory
Rigshospitalet
Copenhagen, Denmark

Subhas Chakrabarty
Department of Molecular Pathology
Division of Pathology and Laboratory Medicine
The University of Texas, M.D. Anderson Cancer Center
Houston, Texas, USA

Daniel W. Chan
Clinical Chemistry Division
Department of Pathology
Johns Hopkins Medical Institutions
Baltimore, Maryland, USA

Kwok Leung Cheung
Professorial Unit of Surgery
City Hospital
Nottingham, United Kingdom

Ib Jarle Christensen
Finsen Laboratory
Rigshospitalet
Copenhagen, Denmark

Peter H. Collet
Department of Visceral and Vascular Surgery
University of Cologne
Cologne, Germany

Elsa M. Cora
Department of Biochemistry and Nutrition
University of Puerto Rico School of Medicine
San Juan, Puerto Rico

Carlos Cordon-Cardo
Division of Molecular Pathology
Department of Pathology
Memorial Sloan-Kettering Cancer Center
New York, New York, USA

Gerard Cox
Firestone Institute for Respiratory Medicine
St. Joseph's Healthcare
    and Department of Medicine
McMaster University
Hamilton, Ontario, Canada

Andrew O. Crockett
Department of Pathology
University of Utah School of Medicine
Salt Lake City, Utah, USA

Eleftherios P. Diamandis
Section of Clinical Biochemistry
Department of Pathology and Laboratory Medicine
Mount Sinai Hospital
    and Division of Clinical Biochemistry
Department of Laboratory Medicine and Pathobiology
University of Toronto
Toronto, Ontario, Canada

Joseph A. DiGiuseppe
Department of Pathology and Laboratory Medicine
Hartford Hospital
Hartford, Connecticut, USA
    and Clinical Laboratory Medicine
University of Connecticut School of Medicine
Farmington, Connecticut, USA

Davin C. Dillon
Molecular Biology
Corixa Corporation
Seattle, Washington, USA

Ann M. Dnistrian
Department of Clinical Laboratories
Memorial Sloan-Kettering Cancer Center
New York, New York, USA

Michael J. Duffy
Department of Nuclear Medicine
St. Vincent's University Hospital
    and Departments of Surgery
    and Conway Institute of Biomolecular and
        Biomedical Research
University College Dublin
Dublin, Ireland

Erich Eigenbrodt
Institute of Biochemistry and Endocrinology
Veterinary Faculty
University of Giessen
Giessen, Germany

Kojo S.J. Elenitoba-Johnson
Department of Pathology
University of Utah School of Medicine
Salt Lake City, Utah, USA

Matti Eskelinen
Department of Surgery
Kuopio University
Kuopio, Finland

Ruth Etzioni
Translational Outcomes Research (TOR)
Division of Public Health Sciences
Fred Hutchinson Cancer Research Center
Seattle, Washington, USA

Michael J. Evelegh
Clinical and Regulatory Affairs
IMI International Medical Innovations
    and Department of Pathology and Molecular Medicine
McMaster University Health Sciences Centre
Hamilton, Ontario, Canada

Ziding Feng
Cancer Prevention Research Program
Division of Public Health Sciences
Fred Hutchinson Cancer Research Center
Seattle, Washington, USA

Martin Fleisher
Department of Clinical Laboratories
Memorial Sloan-Kettering Cancer Center
New York, New York, USA

Cynthia K. French
Research and Development
Diogenics
Irvine, California, USA

Henry F. Frierson, Jr.
Department of Pathology
University of Virginia Health System
Charlottesville, Virginia, USA

Herbert A. Fritsche
Department of Laboratory Medicine
Division of Pathology and Laboratory Medicine
The University of Texas, M.D. Anderson Cancer Center
Houston, Texas, USA

Peter R.C. Gascoyne
Department of Molecular Pathology
The University of Texas, M.D. Anderson Cancer Center
Houston, Texas, USA

Giampietro Gasparini
Division of Medical Oncology
San Filippo Neri Hospital
Rome, Italy

Massimo Gion
Center for the Study of Biological Markers of Malignancy
General Regional Hospital
Venice, Italy

Gordon Glendon
Ontario Cancer Genetics Network
Cancer Care Ontario
Toronto, Ontario, Canada

Carsten Goessl
Oncology Business Unit
NOVARTIS
Basel, Switzerland

C. Rosamund L. Graves
Professorial Unit of Surgery
City Hospital
Nottingham, United Kingdom

Tammy M. Greenwood
Tumor Biology Program
Mayo Clinic
Rochester, Minnesota, USA

Rishab K. Gupta
Department of Protein Biochemistry and Immunodiagnosis
John Wayne Cancer Institute at Saint John's Health Center
Santa Monica, California, USA

Alexander Haese
Department of Urology
University Clinic Hamburg-Eppendorf
Hamburg, Germany

Ulf Haglund
Department of Surgery
Uppsala Academic Hospitals
    and Department of Surgery
Uppsala University
Uppsala, Sweden

Sten Hammarström
Department of Immunology
University of Umeå
Umeå, Sweden

Elizabeth H. Hammond
Department of Pathology
LDS Hospital
Salt Lake City, Utah, USA

Johannes Hampl
Research Department
Immunomics Operations
Beckman Coulter, Inc.
San Diego, California, USA

Garret M. Hampton
Department of Cell and Cancer Biology
Genomics Institute of the Novartis Research Foundation
San Diego, California, USA

Nadia Harbeck
Clinical Research Unit
Department of Obstetrics and Gynecology
Technical University of Munich
Munich, Germany

Daniel F. Hayes
Breast Oncology Program
Department of Internal Medicine
University of Michigan Comprehensive Cancer Center
Ann Arbor, Michigan, USA

Robert J. Hickey
Department of Medicine
Indiana University School of Medicine
Indianapolis, Indiana, USA

Arnulf H. Hoelscher
Department of Visceral and Vascular Surgery
University of Cologne
Cologne, Germany

Derek J. Hoelz
Department of Medicine
Indiana University School of Medicine
Indianapolis, Indiana, USA

Mads Holten-Andersen
Finsen Laboratory
Rigshospitalet
Copenhagen, Denmark

Peter Horsewood
Scientific Affairs
IMI International Medical Innovations
    and Department of Pathology and Molecular Medicine
McMaster University Health Sciences Centre
Hamilton, Ontario, Canada

Raymond L. Houghton
Molecular Biology
Corixa Corporation
Seattle, Washington, USA

David Howard
Engineering
Immunicon Corporation
Huntingdon Valley, Pennsylvania, USA

Mien-Chie Hung
Department of Molecular and Cellular Oncology
    and Breast Cancer Basic Research Program
University of Texas, M. D. Anderson Cancer Center
Houston, Texas, USA

Yuqiu Jiang
Molecular Biology
Corixa Corporation
Seattle, Washington, USA

Philip J. Johnson
Cancer Research UK Institute for Cancer Studies
University of Birmingham
Edgbaston, Birmingham, United Kingdom

Michael Kagan
Engineering
Immunicon Corporation
Huntingdon Valley, Pennsylvania, USA

Hans Krause
Department of Urology
Universitätsklinikum Benjamin Franklin
Freie Universtät Berlin
Berlin, Germany

Kristine Kuus-Reichel
Research Department
Immunomics Operations
Beckman Coulter, Inc.
San Diego, California, USA

Scott A. Kuzdzal
Serum Proteomics
Celara Genomics
Rockville, Maryland, USA

Jacqueline M. Lafky
Tumor Biology Program
Mayo Clinic
Rochester, Minnesota, USA

Rolf Lamerz
Med Klinik II
LMU-Klinikum-Grosshadern
Munich, Germany

Carla R-V. Lankford
Food and Drug Administration
U.S. Department of Health & Human Services
Bethesda, Maryland, USA

Evi Lianidou
Laboratory of Analytical Chemistry
Department of Chemistry
University of Athens
Athens, Greece

Hans Lilja
Department of Laboratory Medicine
Division of Clinical Chemistry
Lund University, University Hospital Malmo
Malmo, Sweden

Yang Liu
Department of Medicine
Indiana University School of Medicine
Indianapolis, Indiana, USA

Gary Longton
Program in Biostatistics
Division of Public Health Sciences
Fred Hutchinson Cancer Research Center
Seattle, Washington, USA

Thomas Luebke
Department of Visceral and Vascular Surgery
University of Cologne
Cologne, Germany

Diana Lüftner
Department of Internal Medicine II,
    Oncology and Hematology
University Hospital Charité
Humbold-University Berlin
Berlin, Germany

Viktor Magdolen
Clinical Research Unit
Department of Obstetrics and Gynecology
Technical University of Munich
Munich, Germany

Nita J. Maihle
Tumor Biology Program
Mayo Clinic
Rochester, Minnesota, USA

Linda H. Malkas
Department of Medicine
Indiana University School of Medicine
Cancer Research Institute
Indianapolis, Indiana, USA

Norman Marcon
Therapeutic Endoscopy Program
The Centre for Therapeutic Endoscopy and
    Endoscopic Oncology
St. Michael's Hospital
    and Department of Medicine
University of Toronto
Toronto, Ontario, Canada

Alfredo Martinez
Center for Cancer Research
National Cancer Institute
National Institutes of Health
Bethesda, Maryland, USA

Sybille Mazurek
Institute of Biochemistry and Endocrinology
Veterinary Faculty
University of Giessen
Giessen, Germany

Ralf Metzger
Department of Visceral and Vascular Surgery
University of Cologne
Cologne, Germany

John Miller
Division of Thoracic Surgery
Department of Surgery
St. Joseph's Hospital
    and Division of Thoracic Surgery
Department of Surgery
McMaster University
Hamilton, Ontario, Canada

Rafael Molina
Laboratory of Clinical Biochemistry
Unit of Cancer Research
Hospital Clinic, School of Medicine
Barcelona, Spain

Donald L. Morton
Department of Protein Biochemistry and Immunodiagnosis
John Wayne Cancer Institute at Saint John's Health Center
Santa Monica, California, USA

Markus Müller
Department of Urology
Universitätsklinikum Benjamin Franklin
Freie Universität Berlin
Berlin, Germany

James L. Mulshine
Center for Cancer Research
National Cancer Institute
National Institutes of Health
Bethesda, Maryland, USA

Hans Jorgen Nielsen
Finsen Laboratory
Hvidovre University Hospital
Copenhagen, Denmark

Kjell E. Öberg
Departments of Endocrine Oncology
    and Medical Sciences
University Hospital
Uppsala, Sweden

Hilmi Ozcelik
Department of Pathology and Laboratory Medicine
Mount Sinai Hospital
    and Department of Laboratory Medicine and
    Pathobiology
University of Toronto
Toronto, Ontario, Canada

Annuka Paju
Department of Clinical Chemistry
Helsinki University Central Hospital
Helsinki, Finland

Darryl E. Palmer-Toy
Department of Pathology
Johns Hopkins Medical Institutions
Baltimore, Maryland, USA

Paul C. Park
Division of Cellular and Molecular Biology
Ontario Cancer Institute
    and Department of Laboratory Medicine and
    Pathobiology
University of Toronto
Toronto, Ontario, Canada

Roy A. Patchell
Departments of Neurosurgery, Neurology, and
    Neuro-Oncology
University of Kentucky Chandler Medical Center
Lexington, Kentucky, USA

Margaret Sullivan Pepe
Department of Biostatistics
School of Public Health and Community Medicine
University of Washington
Seattle, Washington, USA

David H. Persing
Molecular Biology
Corixa Corporation
Seattle, Washington, USA

John Potter
Cancer Prevention Research Program
Division of Public Health Sciences
Fred Hutchinson Cancer Research Center
Seattle, Washington, USA

Klaus Prenzel
Department of Visceral and Vascular Surgery
University of Cologne
Cologne, Germany

Eva M. Rakowicz-Szulczynska
Research and Development
ViroTech LLC
    and Executive Management LLC
Daytona Beach Shores, Florida, USA

Chandra Rao
Reagent Development
Immunicon Corporation
Huntingdon Valley, Pennsylvania, USA

Steven G. Reed
Molecular Biology
Corixa Corporation
Seattle, Washington, USA

Ute Reuning
Clinical Research Unit
Department of Obstetrics and Gynecology
Technical University of Munich
Munich, Germany

John F.R. Robertson
Professorial Unit of Surgery
Nottingham City Hospital
Nottingham, United Kingdom

Marta Sanchez-Carbayo
Division of Molecular Pathology
Department of Pathology
Memorial Sloan-Kettering Cancer Center
New York, New York, USA

Manfred Schmitt
Clinical Research Unit
Department of Obstetrics and Gynecology
Technical University of Munich
Munich, Germany

Lauren Schnaper
Comprehensive Breast Care Center
Greater Baltimore Medical Center
Baltimore, Maryland, USA

Joachim Schneider
Institute and Outpatient Clinic for Occupational Medicine
    and Social Medicine
University of Giessen
Giessen, Germany

Paul M. Schneider
Department of Visceral and Vascular Surgery
University of Cologne
Cologne, Germany

Sylke Schneider
Department of Visceral and Vascular Surgery
University of Cologne
Cologne, Germany

Morton K. Schwartz
Department of Clinical Laboratories
Memorial Sloan Kettering Cancer Center
New York, New York, USA

Andreas Scorilas
National Center for Scientific Research "Demokritos"
Athens, Greece

Jennifer W. Sekowski
U.S. Army Soldier and Biological Chemical Command
Edgewood Chemical Biological Center
Aberdeen Proving Ground, Maryland, USA

Ie-Ming Shih
Gynecologic Pathology and Clinical Chemistry Division
Department of Pathology
Johns Hopkins Medical Institutions
Baltimore, Maryland, USA

Lori J. Sokoll
Clinical Chemistry Division
Department of Pathology
Johns Hopkins Medical Institutions
Baltimore, Maryland, USA

Frédérique Spyratos
Laboratoire d'Oncobiologie
Centre René Huguenin
St-Cloud, France

Jeremy A. Squire
Division of Cellular and Molecular Biology
Ontario Cancer Institute
    and Departments of Laboratory Medicine and
    Pathobiology, and Medical Biophysics
University of Toronto
Toronto, Ontario, Canada

Vered Stearns
Department of Internal Medicine
University of Michigan Comprehensive Cancer Center
Ann Arbor, Michigan, USA

Ulf-Håkan Stenman
Department of Clinical Chemistry
Helsinki University Central Hospital
Helsinki, Finland

Petra Stieber
Institute of Clinical Chemistry
University of Munich — Großhadern
Munich, Germany

Contributors

Torgny Stigbrand
Department of Immunology
University of Umeå
Umeå, Sweden

Mats Stridsberg
Departments of Endocrine Oncology
    and Clinical Chemistry
University Hospital
Uppsala, Sweden

Catharine M. Sturgeon
Department of Clinical Biochemistry
Edinburgh Royal Infirmary
Edinburgh, United Kingdom

Jordi Tauler
Center for Cancer Research
National Cancer Institute
National Institutes of Health
Bethesda, Maryland, USA

Leon W.M.M. Terstappen
Research and Development
Immunicon Corporation
Huntingdon Valley, Pennsylvania, USA

Mary Lou Thompson
Department of Biostatistics
School of Public Health and Community Medicine
University of Washington
Seattle, Washington, USA

Mark Thornquist
COMPASS
Division of Public Health Sciences
Fred Hutchinson Cancer Research Center
Seattle, Washington, USA

Steven D. Trocha
Department of Protein Biochemistry and Immunodiagnosis
John Wayne Cancer Institute at Saint John's Health Center
Santa Monica, California, USA

Ingemar Turesson
Department of Medicine
Malmo University Hospital
Malmo, Sweden

Hans Werner Wechsel
Urology Clinic
Reinhard-Nieter Hospital
Wilhelmshaven, Germany

John B. Welsh
Department of Medical Informatics
Johnson and Johnson Pharmaceutical Research Institute
San Diego, California, USA

Yong Wen
Department of Molecular and Cellular Oncology
University of Texas, M.D. Anderson Cancer Center
Houston, Texas, USA

Marcy Winget
COMPASS
Division of Public Health Sciences
Fred Hutchinson Cancer Research Center
Seattle, Washington, USA

James L. Wittliff
Hormone Receptor Laboratory
University of Louisville
    and Department of Biochemistry and Molecular Biology
    and Department of Surgery
Brown Cancer Center
Louisville, Kentucky, USA

Carl T. Wittwer
Department of Pathology
University of Utah School of Medicine
Salt Lake City, Utah, USA

Jiangchun Xu
Molecular Biology
Corixa Corporation
Seattle, Washington, USA

Ken Yamaguchi
National Cancer Center Research Institute
Tokyo, Japan

Karen K. Yamamoto
Discovery Research
Diogenics
Irvine, California, USA

Yutaka Yasui
Cancer Prevention Research Program
Division of Public Health Sciences
Fred Hutchinson Cancer Research Center
Seattle, Washington, USA

George M. Yousef
Department of Pathology and Laboratory Medicine
Mount Sinai Hospital
Toronto, Ontario, Canada

Kourosh Zarghooni
Department of Visceral and Vascular Surgery
University of Cologne
Cologne, Germany

Barbara K. Zehentner
Molecular Biology
Corixa Corporation
Seattle, Washington, USA

Zhen Zhang
Center for Biomarker Discovery
Department of Pathology
Johns Hopkins Medical Institutions
Baltimore, Maryland, USA

Michele Zysman
Department of Pathology and Laboratory Medicine,
Mount Sinai Hospital
  and Department of Laboratory Medicine and
  Pathobiology,
University of Toronto
Toronto, Ontario, Canada

Part One
General Principles

Chapter 1

Tumor Markers: Past, Present, and Future

Eleftherios P. Diamandis

If you know the past, you can understand the present and probably predict the future. In science as well as in other human activities, we tend to predict the future in too much detail. This does not always serve us well. Frequently, highly anticipated developments never materialize, perhaps due to paradigm shifts that drive "progress" in a different direction. If, on the other hand, our predictions do materialize, they arrive after decades of delay.

Over the last 20 years, however, we have probably seen many more scientific advances than we would have predicted, including the explosive growth in informatics and telecommunication, the achievement of animal cloning, and the complete sequencing of many genomes, including bacterial, plant, fly, animal, and human. Discoveries in the making, such as stem cell technology, artificial human organs, designer drugs, and gene therapy promise to eradicate all human diseases in the foreseeable future.

Despite this reasonable optimism, patients who have cancer today will likely not believe that upcoming discoveries will save their lives. In fact, the steady increase in life expectancy is accompanied by increasing prevalences of many cancers, and cancer will likely become the number one killer over the next few years. Current statistics suggest that approximately one out of every three individuals will die from cancer. This rate may increase in the future.

New approaches to identifying cancer markers (alterations in normal molecules or processes in pre-cancerous or cancerous conditions) promise to evolve truly innovative ways to investigate malignancy. Coupled with more effective treatments, these new strategies may contribute decisively to eradicating cancer as a major cause of mortality and morbidity in humans.

HELPING CANCER PATIENTS TODAY

Unfortunately, with the exception of lung cancer (which is largely due to smoking), primary prevention is not feasible for most cancers. Despite the spectacular advances of medical science, we do not as yet understand cancer pathogenesis. The best option we have now to battle cancer is early diagnosis, followed by effective (curative) treatment. The ideal scenario: a patient visits the doctor for a routine follow-up. The doctor orders blood work. The results indicate cancer. The doctor prescribes a magic cocktail that kills the cancer with no side effects.

Our role as clinical laboratory physicians and scientists is to further the treatment and eradication of cancer by participating in the discovery and evaluation of new and early diagnostics for the disease. We do this through biomarkers: tools that clinicians use to help them answer clinically relevant questions (Table 1). Other health professionals, especially those in medical imaging, may devise innovative methods to "see" cancer at an early, curable stage. As clinical laboratory scientists, we have the opportunity of identifying new biomarkers not only in serum, but also for imaging applications. In the following paragraphs, I will try to predict the future of this area of investigation by first providing a brief historical overview and then examining where we are today.

HISTORICAL BACKGROUND

In 1846, Bence-Jones described the precipitation of a protein in the acidified urine of patients with multiple myeloma. This monoclonal immunoglobulin light chain was the first identified cancer marker, and clinicians still use it today.

Many years after Bence-Jones' discovery, from about 1928 through 1963, scientists identified numerous hormones, enzymes, isoenzymes, and other proteins that, in malignancy, alter their concentration in biological fluids (1). Acid phosphatase, for example, served as a marker for prostate cancer

Table 1 Tumor markers can be used to examine clinically relevant questions

- Does a patient have cancer?
- If yes, which organ is afflicted?
- Is the cancer localized or disseminated?
- How aggressive is the cancer?
- Will the patient likely relapse or not relapse if no adjuvant therapy is given post-primary treatment?
- Will the patient respond better if one treatment type is given instead of another one?
- Can cancer relapse post-primary therapy be detected before the patient has symptoms?
- If yes, can the patient get a benefit with early treatment of relapse?

from the 1930s to the 1990s. And in 1963 and 1965 respectively, two major tumor markers for hepatoma (alpha-fetoprotein, known as AFP) and colorectal cancer (carcinoembryonic antigen, known as CEA) were discovered. These two markers are still widely used today.

In 1960, the Nobel Prize-winning discovery of radioimmunoassay, by introducing exceptional specificity and sensitivity, revolutionized the measurement of trace amounts of analytes in biological fluids. Today, most tumor markers are measured this way.

In 1975, another Nobel prize-winning technology, monoclonal antibodies, was developed. This technology facilitated the discovery of many new tumor markers, including the carbohydrate antigens CA125, CA 15.3, CA 19.9. In 1980, prostate-specific antigen (PSA), the best cancer marker, was also discovered.

In the 1970s and 1980s, new concepts—oncogenes and tumor suppressor genes—paralleled the discoveries of radioimmunoassay and monoclonal antibody technologies. In addition, recombinant DNA technology, the polymerase chain reaction (PCR), and automated sequencing and related molecular techniques facilitated easy and reliable analysis of DNA and mRNA for molecular cancer diagnostics.

Some historical milestones in the development of tumor markers appear in Table 2.

THE PRESENT

The impact of new discoveries and technologies, such as microarrays, mass spectrometry, artificial neural networks, and other bioinformatic tools, has not yet been realized. However, these technologies could raise the field of tumor biomarkers to new heights.

Literally hundreds of known tumor markers and prognostic and predictive cancer markers exist. Yet with few exceptions, their reputation among clinicians is not very good. One perception is that biomarker analysis helps diagnostic companies more than it helps cancer patients. And clinicians and clinical chemists disagree on the optimal use of tumor markers. Clinicians, for example, believe that if a marker cannot provide information that is of demonstrable benefit to the patient, then the information may not be advisable to obtain.

Table 2 Cancer biomarkers: historical overview

1846	Bence-Jones protein
1940	Acid phosphatase
1960	Immunoassay
1963	Alpha-fetoprotein (AFP)
1965	Carcinoembryonic antigen (CEA)
1975	Monoclonal antibodies
1980	CA125, PSA, Carbohydrate antigens
1970-1980	Oncogenes and Tumor Suppressor Genes
2001	Microarrays, Mass Spectrometry, Neural Networks, Multiparametric Analysis, Bioinformatics

To illustrate the point, let's say that a marker provides reliable information about patient relapse four to six weeks before clinical symptoms reappear. How will the clinician use this information? If effective treatment can work better if administered earlier, then the information is useful. But if there is no treatment for recurring disease, or if the treatment is of marginal benefit and has side effects, or if the treatment is equally effective if administered when clinical symptoms appear, then the marker is useless. In fact, knowledge that the tumor marker is present may be harmful since it shortens the disease-free survival rate and the quality of life of the patient.

Different points of view between clinicians (the users of the information) and clinical chemists (the providers of the information) are reflected in the different recommendations about the optimal use of cancer markers (see chapter 5).

Table 3 summarizes current applications of tumor markers and their limitations. (These points are developed in more detail later in this book.) The current limitations can serve as guidelines for further developments in this field.

It's important to remember that we are still viewing tumor markers largely as single tests, and that we probably won't discover any single marker that serves its intended purposes for every cancer, i.e., provides answers to the clinical questions listed in Table 1. It is also conceivable that most as yet undiscovered markers may not even be as good as the ones we already know. The future then, may look very different. That is, it may be based on multiparametric, miniaturized analysis with interpretation of data by neural networks.

Many new research fronts in biotechnology are emerging:

- The Human Genome Project and proteomics
- Nucleic acid and protein microarrays
- Miniature multi-parametric analysis
- Mass spectrometry
- Pattern recognition and artificial neural networks
- Genetic variability and cancer risk: Single nucleotide polymorphisms
- Circulating cancer cells and DNA
- From bench to bedside (clinical investigations on new cancer markers)
- Quality assurance and quality control

These research fronts were not specifically developed as pathways to cancer diagnostics but they can be utilized for this application.

The next section touches briefly on some of these issues in an effort to predict where the cancer biomarker field will likely be within the next decade. For more detail, please refer to the specific book chapters in which these issues are addressed.

CURRENT AND FUTURE KNOWLEDGE RESOURCES (2002–2010)

New knowledge resources (Table 4) will facilitate, among other developments, the discovery of new diagnostics and therapeu-

Table 3 Current applications of tumor markers and their limitations

Application	Current Usefulness	Comments
Screening for Cancer	Limited	1. For screening, you need a marker that is elevated at early disease stages, when the disease is localized and potentially curable. Most circulating cancer markers (with the exception of PSA) are elevated significantly in the late stage disease. Thus, diagnostic sensitivity is usually low for early-stage disease. 2. With the exception of PSA, most cancer markers are not specific for a particular tissue and elevations may be due to diseases of other tissues, including benign and inflammatory diseases. Thus, diagnostic specificity may be low, leading to many false positives. In screening, there is a need for a definitive diagnostic method that will separate true positives from false positives. If this procedure is invasive (e.g. surgery) and/or expensive, patients will not accept it. 3. Screening, even if effective for early cancer diagnosis, must demonstrate benefit to the screened population in terms of survival or other clinical endpoints.
Diagnosing Cancer	Limited	Same as above. Low diagnostic sensitivity and specificity. However, for selected subgroups of high-risk patients, in whom the chance of cancer is high (high prevalence), tumor marker analysis may aid the clinician in ordering more elaborate testing, e.g., imaging techniques or laparoscopic investigations.
Evaluating Cancer Prognosis	Limited	Most cancer markers have prognostic value but their accuracy is not good enough to warrant specific therapeutic interventions. For example, higher pre-operative levels of PSA are associated with capsular penetration, higher Gleason score, positive surgical margins, and positive lymph node status, but the decision to treat with two different modalities (e.g. radical prostatectomy vs. non-surgical approaches) cannot be taken based on tumor marker data alone. Same applies to many other cancers.
Prediction of Therapeutic Response	Important	Despite the importance of using biomarkers in predicting response to specific therapies, very few known markers have such predictive power. These include the steroid hormone receptors for predicting response to anti-estrogens and Her-2/neu amplification for predicting response to Herceptin in breast cancer patients. We need more predictive markers to individualize therapy and maximize clinical response.
Tumor Staging	Limited	Same comments as for prognosis. Data not good enough for accurate staging.
Detecting Tumor Recurrence or Remission	Controversial	Despite the importance of using biomarkers to detect cancer relapse, current markers are limited by the following: (a) lead time is short (weeks to a few months) and does not significantly affect outcome, even if therapy is instituted earlier; (b) therapies for treating recurrent disease are not effective at present; (c) in certain groups of patients, biomarkers are not produced and do not detect relapses; (d) sometimes biomarkers provide misleading information, e.g. clinical relapses occur without biomarker elevation, or biomarker is elevated non-specifically, without progressive disease, leading to either overtreatment or discontinuation of a current treatment protocol.
Localizing Tumor and Directing Radio-therapeutic Agents	Limited	Only a few biomarkers are available for this application and success is limited at present.
Monitoring the Effectiveness of Cancer Therapy	Important	For patients with advanced disease, who are treated with various modalities, it is important to know if therapy works. In this regard, biomarkers usually provide information that is readily interpretable and more economical, more sensitive, and safer than radiological or invasive procedures. For certain cancers, this may facilitate increased enrollment of patients into therapeutic clinical trials.

Table 4 Newly available knowledge resources (2002–2010)

- Sequence of the human genome
- All genes and splice variants (complete annotation)
- All encoded proteins in recombinant form
- Cellular localization of all proteins
- Function of proteins
- Protein structure at the 3-dimensional level
- Biochemical pathways
- Certified reagents for proteins
- Antibodies and antibody mimics
- All single nucleotide polymorphisms of human genes
- Mutational spectrum of cancer (somatic and inherited)
- High-throughput screening methods (genome-wide scans)
- Bioinformatics
- Artificial neural networks

Activity	Elapsed Time (total, years)
Discovery of the gene	0
Recombinant protein	1
Antibodies	2
Assays	2.5
Preliminary studies	3
Detailed studies	5
Clinical acceptance	7–10

Figure 2 Discovery and evaluation of a new biomarker.

tics. How can we best use these resources to identify new cancer markers?

Discovery Technologies

A number of diagnostic companies and academic institutions have adopted a general discovery strategy, outlined in Figure 1. The strategy, which resembles one used by drug companies to find new therapeutics, combines new knowledge from the human genome, microarrays, differential gene expression, and complicated bioinformatics to interpret data and suggest candidate targets. The power of this approach must be balanced by its potential pitfalls, noted below:

- Not all potential cancer markers are overexpressed in cancer. In fact, the best cancer marker we know today, PSA, is underexpressed at the mRNA and protein level in cancer (2).
- A biomarker may be widely expressed in tissues but its serum concentration may be altered in only one or in very restricted number of malignancies. For example, human kallikrein 6 is expressed in many tissues but its serum concentration increases only in ovarian cancer (3,4).
- Every potential "hit" must be further evaluated to verify that it indeed represents a novel biomarker (one possible path is shown in Figure 2). In the future, the potential bottleneck will involve following lead compounds and bring them to the clinic through preliminary and more detailed and well-designed clinical trials. It may take anywhere from two to seven years to achieve this milestone. A number of successful "genome mining" exercises have yielded many potential candidates. Examples are indicated in references 5–8 in this chapter. (See also chapter 35.)

Another discovery tool involves using mass spectrometry in combination with protein chips, two-dimensional gel electrophoresis, pattern recognition, and artificial networks. This tool aims to identify either specific proteins in cancer tissue extracts or fluids or specific cancer patterns suitable for diagnosis or monitoring (see chapter 33).

Gene Expression

It is important to remember that not all cancers of the same organ behave similarly. Efforts to classify tumors through clinical and pathological data include parameters such as age, lymph node status, grade, stage, and histological type. Recently some scientists have postulated that cancer's phenotypic heterogenicity may be due to differential gene expression, which can be captured by cDNA microarrays and artificial neural network analysis of the data. Indeed, recent reports describe more elaborate classifications based on expression profiles of a few hundred to a few thousand genes (8,9). Such classifications, based on so-called "molecular portraits" or "molecular signatures" of cancers (see also chapters 32 and 34), may bring about much better cancer subclassifications, differential diagnostics, and probably groupings that can respond better to specific treatments.

This important area of cancer research is evolving rapidly. We may soon see such "molecular classifying devices" or "mi-

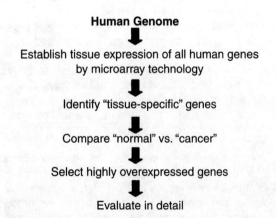

Figure 1 Generalized, genome-mining approach to discover new cancer biomarkers. For discussion, see text.

croarray pathologists" in the clinic. In these studies, every informative gene is asked to "vote" for certain classes of tumors and the counting of "votes" will declare the objective decision. Protein microarray versions could be used both for disease subclassification and for cancer diagnosis and screening. In fact, the knowledge of protein structure, protein function, and biochemical pathways could eventually lead to more rational selection of appropriate diagnostically relevant targets. Therefore, we need to identify, quantitatively and precisely, the right proteins to monitor. Perhaps future devices may be comprised of low-density protein arrays, for example, 10–100 elements suitable for disease-specific applications. Such "prostate cancer," "breast cancer," and other chips offering miniature multiparametric analysis may appear at the clinic in two to four years.

The idea of genetic predisposition to cancer has been suspected for years, but we only know of a handful of genes that definitely cause cancer. Genetic analysis of patients at risk provides valuable information, but the analysis is limited to very few patients (see chapters 16 and 20). It's possible that most cancers are due to genetic changes or genetic variability in many genes that have yet to be identified. Recently, in fact, the most prevalent genetic variability in humans, single nucleotide polymorphisms (SNPs), has been evaluated in detail, and more that 10^6 SNPs are currently known (10). Many scientists believe that possession of certain haplotypes (combinations of SNPs) may predispose to certain diseases, including cancer. Also, scientists have catalogued, in cancer, somatic mutations in many genes. The technology for identifying SNPs and other genetic changes is rapidly evolving, and it can be automated. Thousands of SNPs, for example, can be studied in hours by using methods such as microarrays or fluorescence polarization. When these "cancer risk haplotypes" are identified, genome scans will probably be useful to assess future cancer risk.

Cancer Staging and Metastasis

Scientists are divided on whether cancer is a disease that is disseminated right from the beginning, or whether it spreads after the tumor is well-established in one site. Regardless, cancer metastasis is a major cause of patient morbidity and mortality. During cancer metastasis, cancer cells move to lymph nodes through lymphatic circulation, as well as through general circulation, before they establish secondary sites at distant organs. Our ability to find such cancer cells with high sensitivity and specificity may provide opportunities for more accurate staging and even for diagnosis. Similarly, circulating DNA of tumorigenic pathogens may serve the same purpose. Important improvements in methodologies for identifying such cells, through quantitative PCR or magnetic separation and flow-cytometry, have recently occurred (see chapters 9, 38, and 52).

Given these new possibilities, we must emphasize that every new tumor marker test, single or multiparametric, must undergo rigorous evaluations to assess its clinical value. This evaluation should include pre-analytical considerations (sample collection, storage, preparation); analytical considerations (analytical sensitivity, specificity, precision, robustness, ease of use and automation); clinical considerations (diagnostic sensitivity, specificity, predictive value); and cost. Furthermore, quality assurance and quality control measures must be established, and pitfalls should be easy to identify.

Diagnostic companies and enthusiastic laboratory scientists are naturally anxious to implement new advances in tumor markers immediately. While there is no doubt that their diagnostic place will be found, it is also very likely that powerful, single tests may still remain in use for some time. Even so, we must start educating new clinical laboratory scientists about these revolutionary, emerging technologies.

SUMMARY

The current state of known tumor markers is less than desirable, although the future of cancer diagnostics looks very bright. New knowledge resources (Table 4) will likely introduce novel protein, genetic, and low-molecular-weight cancer markers, which may significantly impact cancer care. Such markers will be used in panels and on micro devices, and interpretation will be facilitated by artificial neural networks or pattern recognition. New testing modalities will be developed for fluids, cells, genetic material, or extracts. These modalities may assess predisposition to cancer (for prevention), facilitate early diagnosis, aid in differential diagnosis, or facilitate cancer subclassification for prognosis or prediction of therapeutic response. Further testing may be useful for monitoring cancer patients to assess relapse or response to treatment. Combining these technologies with imaging and new therapeutics will likely dramatically decrease cancer morbidity and mortality over the next 10–15 years.

REFERENCES

1. Chan DW, Sell S. Tumor Markers. In: Tietz textbook of clinical chemistry, 2nd ed. Burtis CA, Ashwood ER, eds. Philadelphia: Saunders, 1994:897–927.
2. Magklara A, Scorilas A, Stephan C, et al. Decreased concentrations of prostate-specific antigen and human glandular kallikrein 2 in malignant versus nonmalignant prostatic tissue. Urology 2000;56:527–532.
3. Petraki CD, Karavana VN, Skoufogiannis PT, et al. The spectrum of human kallikrein 6 (zyme/protease M/neurosin) expression in human tissues, as assessed by immunohistochemistry. J Histochem Cytochem 2001;49:1431–1442.
4. Diamandis EP, Yousef GM, Soosaipillai AR, Bunting P. Human kallikrein 6 (zyme/protease M/neurosin): a new serum biomarker of ovarian carcinoma. Clin Biochem 2000;33:579–583.
5. Welsh JB, Zarrinkar PP, Sapinoso LM, et al. Analysis of gene expression profiles in normal and neoplastic ovarian tissue samples identifies candidate molecular markers of epithelial ovarian cancer. Proc Natl Acad Sci USA 2001;98:1176–1181.

6. Welsh JB, Sapinoso LM, Su AI, et al. Analysis of gene expression identifies candidate markers and pharmacological targets in prostate cancer. Cancer Res 2001;61:5974–5978.
7. Schummer M, Ng WV, Bumgarner RE, et al. Comparative hybridization of an array of 21,500 ovarian cDNAs for the discovery of genes overexpressed in ovarian carcinomas. Gene 1999;238:375–385.
8. Khan J, Wei JS, Ringner M, et al. Classification and diagnostic prediction of cancers using gene expression profiling and artificial neural networks. Nat Med 2001;6:658–659.
9. Perou CM, Sorlie T, Eisen MB, et al. Molecular portraits of human breast tumors. Nature 2000;406:747–752.
10. Sachidanandam R, Weissman D, Schmidt SC, et al. A map of human genome sequence variation containing 1.42 million single nucleotide polymorphisms. Nature 2001;409:928–933.

Chapter 2

Tumor Markers: Introduction and General Principles

Daniel W. Chan and Morton K. Schwartz

Tumor markers, or biomarkers for cancer, represent one of the most exciting advances in the fight against cancer. The strategy for this war includes prevention, screening, early detection, and effective treatment. Our current knowledge, as well as the types of tumor markers, is limited in each of these applications.

Most tumor markers are useful for monitoring therapy, however, few of them are useful for the early detection of cancer. Even the most useful tumor marker—prostate-specific antigen (PSA)—is limited by the non-specific elevation in benign prostatic hyperplasia (BPH). Almost no tumor marker is useful for prevention.

However, we are entering the post-genomic era. Armed with the knowledge of genomics, coupled with the advances in the technology for proteomics and bioinformatics, we will be marching into the war against cancer with new weapons. These new weapons will likely be multi-analytes and much more effective than single tests. Furthermore, the knowledge that we gain from biomarkers could be used to develop prevention strategies and therapeutic targets.

In this chapter, we will first address the problem of cancer, followed by the principles of tumor markers, and end with some exciting technologies for the identifying tumor markers.

THE PROBLEM OF CANCER

In the year 2002, the estimated number of new cancer cases in the U.S. was 1.3 million. Breast cancer was the leader, followed by cancer of the prostate, lung, colon-rectum, and bladder (1).

A simple definition of cancer is "a relatively autonomous growth of tissue." Understanding the cause of autonomous growth would clearly facilitate the search for a cure. Advances in molecular genetics have provided a better understanding of the genesis of human cancer. The proliferation of normal cells is thought to be regulated by growth-promoting *oncogenes* and counterbalanced by growth-constraining *tumor suppressor genes*. The development of cancer appears to involve the activation or the altered expression of oncogenes or the loss or inactivation of tumor suppressor genes.

Early detection of cancer offers the best chance for cure. The goal is to diagnose cancer when a tumor is still small enough to be completely removed surgically. Unfortunately, most cancers do not produce symptoms until the tumors are either too large to be removed surgically or until cancerous cells have already spread to other tissues (metastasized).

CANCER STAGING

Staging is the process of dividing cancer into groups of early and late cancer. Classification is useful for prognosis and helps guide clinicians to select therapy and evaluate clinical outcomes. "TNM" is currently the most widely used system to classify cancer, and has replaced the historical system of I to IV or A to D. The TNM system describes the anatomical extent of disease in three components:

T—the extent of the primary tumor
N—the presence or absence and the extent of regional lymph node metastasis
M—the presence or absence of distant metastasis

The addition of numbers to these components indicates the extent of the disease, for example, T0, T1, T2, T3, T4; N0, N1, N2, N3; M0, M1. In general, two classifications, clinical and pathological, are described for each site. For a detailed description of the classification of malignant tumors, readers are referred to the book on TNM classification (2).

PRINCIPLES OF TUMOR MARKERS
Definition

A tumor marker is a substance present in, or produced by a tumor itself, or produced by the host in response to a tumor, that is used to differentiate a tumor from normal tissue or to determine the presence of a tumor based on the measurement in the blood or other fluids. Such a substance is found in cells, tissues, or body fluids. It is measured qualitatively or quantitatively by chemical, immunological, genomic, or proteomic methods to identify the presence of a cancer.

Morphologically, cancer tissue is recognized as resembling fetal tissue more than normal adult differentiated tissue. Tumors are graded according to their degree of differentiation as being well differentiated, poorly differentiated, or anaplastic (without form). Tumor markers are the biochemical or immunological counterparts of the differentiation state of the tumor. In general, many tumor markers represent the re-expression of substances produced normally by embryogenically related tissues (Table 1).

An ideal tumor marker should be both specific for a given type of cancer and sensitive enough to detect small tumors for early diagnosis or during screening. Unfortunately, most known tumor markers are neither specific for a single individual tumor nor sensitive enough for screening. Most are found with different tumors of the same tissue type (tumor-associated markers). They are present in higher quantities in cancer tissue or in blood from cancer patients than in benign tumors or in the blood of normal subjects. Tumor markers are most useful in determining the progression of disease status after initial therapy and in monitoring subsequent treatment modalities (3).

Potential Uses of Tumor Markers

Table 2 summarizes the potential uses of tumor markers: diagnosis, prognosis, the monitoring of therapeutic effects, and targets for localization and therapy. Ideally, a tumor marker should be produced by the tumor cells and detectable in body fluids. It should not be present in healthy people or in benign conditions. Therefore, it could be used for cancer screening to find asymptomatic individuals within a general population. Most tumor markers are present in normal, benign, and cancer tissues and are not specific enough to be used for screening of cancer. However, if the incidence of cancer is high among certain populations, screening is feasible. An example is the use of prostate-specific antigen (PSA) in conjunction with digital rectal examination for early detection of prostate cancer.

The clinical staging of cancer is aided by quantitation of the marker, that is, the serum level of the marker reflects tumor burden. The marker value at the time of diagnosis is used as a prognostic indicator for disease progression and patient survival. This is possible for an individual patient, but different levels of markers produced by different tumors do not usually allow the clinician to determine the prognosis of a tumor from the initial level. However, after successful initial treatment, such as surgery, the marker value should decrease. The rate of decrease is predicted by using the half-life of the marker. For example, the half-life of PSA is 1 to 2 days; that of chorionic gonadotropin (CG) is 12 to 20 hours; and that of alpha-fetoprotein (AFP) is 5 days. If the half-life after treatment is longer than the expected half-life, it can be assumed that the treatment has not been successful in removing the tumor. The magnitude of marker reduction may, however, reflect the degree of success of the treatment or the extent of disease involvement.

Detection of cancer recurrence facilitates treatment or therapy change. Ultrasensitive PSA assays allow earlier detection of prostate cancer after radical prostatectomy. The breast cancer marker CA 27.29 has been shown to detect recurrent disease before any clinical evidence in breast cancer patients receiving adjuvant chemotherapy appears.

Most tumor marker values correlate with the effectiveness of treatment and responses to therapy. In breast cancer, the concentration of markers such as CA 27.29 changes with the treatment and the clinical outcome of the patient (4). Marker values usually increase with progressive disease, decrease with remission, and do not change significantly with stable disease. The tumor marker kinetics in the monitoring of cancer may be more complicated. Marker values in response to treatment may show an initial delay before demonstrating the expected pattern of change.

Selection of Tumor Markers

The selection criteria for tumor markers should include clinical, biochemical, analytical, and laboratory operation parameters. Clinically, a tumor marker should be useful for a specific diagnostic application. Whether it is for screening, detection, prediction, or therapeutic monitoring, the tumor marker should exhibit high clinical sensitivity and specificity, for example, high AUC (area under the curve) in a receiver operating characteristic (ROC) curve. Biochemically, it should be well defined in protein structure, antibody-binding epitopes, and with the availability of high affinity monoclonal antibodies. Analytically, the method for measuring tumor markers should be accurate, precise, and have minimum interferences. Operationally, the assay should be automated for efficiency and rapid turnaround time. The tumor marker should receive regulatory approval by the FDA (U.S. Food and Drug Administration).

Validation of Tumor Markers

To validate tumor markers in a target population, one should start with the evaluation of published data. These could include surveys of the literature, evaluation of data submitted to the FDA, and the like, and then validating both the analytical and clinical performances.

Table 1 Production of tumor markers by various tissues

		Production of Tumor Markers by Various Tissues		
Marker	Normal producing	Embryogenically closely related	Distantly related	Unrelated
CEA	Colon	Stomach, liver, pancreas	Lung, breast	Lymphoma
AFP	Liver, yolk sac	Colon, stomach, pancreas	Lung	
Chorionic Ganodotropin	Placenta	Germinal tumors	Liver	Epidermal lung
Serotonin	Enteroendocrine carcinoid	Adrenal	Oat cell, lung	Epidermal lung

Table 2 Potential uses of tumor markers

Screening in general population
Differential diagnosis in symptomatic patients
Clinical staging of cancer
Estimating tumor volume
Prognostic indicator for disease progression
Evaluating the success of treatment
Detecting the recurrence of cancer
Monitoring responses to therapy

Analytical performance should be validated for both reagents and instrument. Clinical validation should be performed in target populations including healthy subjects, patients with appropriate benign diseases, and other patients with cancer of different types. For patients with the specific cancer being validated, different stages should be evaluated. If the tumor marker is used to monitor therapy, serial specimens should be collected and evaluated for the effectiveness of the tumor marker for this purpose. To perform such validation experiments, it is necessary to establish reference values, calculate predictive values, evaluate the distribution of marker values, and determine the role of the tumor marker values in disease management.

Reference values. Reference values of a tumor marker are obtained from a healthy population, preferably with age- and sex-matched individuals. The determination of reference values is time-consuming and requires a large healthy population (n = 120 subjects). Statistical analysis using the mean ±2 SD for a population with a Gaussian (normal) distribution is the most frequently used method. For a non-Gaussian distribution, the percentile method is probably the simplest approach.

The reference values determined using healthy subjects in this fashion are applicable to analytes with physiologically well-defined concentrations. For testing with relatively specific applications, such as the use of tumor markers in the diagnosis and management of cancer, a decision level is more appropriate than is the upper limit of the healthy population. In most cases, it is more appropriate to use patients with benign disease as the non-disease group (rather than using a healthy population). The decision level can be determined using a predictive value model.

Predictive Value Model. In the use of tumor markers it is essential to understand that sensitivity and specificity each have analytical as well as epidemiological definitions. From the analytic viewpoint, sensitivity is the lowest detection limit, and from the epidemiological view, it is the extent of false negatives. Specificity implies false positive when considered epidemiologically and method interferences by extraneous materials when considered analytically. In addition, the precision of the method (i.e., the ability to reproduce the assay value) is an essential point if the tumor marker is to be used to evaluate patients or to study populations. If positive or negative predictive values are to be considered, then an understanding of prevalence is essential. Prevalence is a difficult parameter to quantify since it is related to many factors such as age, sex, ethnicity, and race.

When screening for a disease, several factors must be taken into account. The disease must be important and common and cause substantial mortality and morbidity. There must be an understanding of the natural history of the disease to assure that early detection can play a role in reversal of the clinical course and there must be effective treatment. On the basis of these criteria, breast, prostate, ovary, and perhaps colon cancer would be most suitable for screening. There are already examples of successful screening programs for hepatocellular carcinoma (alpha-fetoprotein) and neuroblastoma (catechols) but these are relatively rare tumors in the western world. Prostate-specific antigen is now widely used to screen for prostate cancer. When deciding to apply screening techniques, particularly if biochemical or immunochemical markers are used, an understanding of analytical sensitivity (lowest detectable limit), epidemiological sensitivity (false negatives), analytical specificity (extraneous interference), and epidemiological specificity (false positives) is essential. In addition, the precision of the assay (the ability to reproduce the results) must be known and acceptable for use in large population studies.

The equation for positive predictive value (PPV+) is this:

$$PPV+ = \frac{(\text{sensitivity})(\text{prevalence})}{(\text{sensitivity})(\text{prevalence}) + (1 - \text{specificity})(1 - \text{prevalence})}$$

If a test with 95% sensitivity (5% false negatives) and 95% specificity (5% false positives) is used in a disease with a prevalence of 1% (1,000 cases/100,000), the positive predictive range would be 16%. Only 16 of 100 positive results would be true positives and 50 of the 1,000 cancers would be missed. If the prevalence is 10% (10,000/100,000), the positive predictive rate would be 68%, but we would still miss 500 cases per 100,000 screened.

An interesting exercise is to use published test data for prostate-specific antigen (PSA) and prevalence rates of prostate cancer to calculate the predictive value. A review of the literature, which included 319 patients with prostate cancer, yielded a sensitivity of 57% for PSA when the cut-off value was 4 µg/L and 20% when the cut-off was >10 µg/L. In 590 men with benign prostatic hypertrophy, the specificity was 76.2% when a cut-off value of >4 µg/L was used and 97% for cut-off values >10 µg/L. Data established at autopsy for men ages 50–70 years indicates a rate of 38% (38,000 cancer cases/100,000 screened). With this rate, the positive predictive value with the 4 µg/L cut-off would be 60%; when 10 µg/L is used, 80%.

The optimist would say that these data indicate that screening would detect 57 cancers per each 100 cases and 60% of the positive values would be true positives. However, the pessimist would point out that 43 of each 100 cases would be missed and 40% of the positive values would be false positives. When the 10 µg/L cut-off is used, only 20 cases per 100 would be detected and 80 would be missed. However, test results for only 3 persons per 100 with benign disease would be positive. This calculation was based on a prevalence rate calculated from autopsy records of men without clinically evident cancer. When one understands that most of these cancers would be latent and that only 1% of men whose autopsy demonstrated prostate cancer ever have clinically documented disease, it is difficult to recommend PSA as a general population-screening tool until methods are available to identify those individuals with potentially malignant disease. In men 55–59 years old, the clinical incidence of prostate cancer is only 0.094% (94 cases/100,000); in men >65, it is 0.739% (739 cases/100,000).

A useful approach to evaluate multiple tests for the same analyte or multiple markers for the same type of cancer is the *receiver operating characteristic* (ROC) curve. The ROC curve is constructed by plotting sensitivity vs. [1-specificity] (or alternatively, the true positive rate vs. the false positive rate). The advantage of the ROC curve is the display of performance over the entire range of decision levels. One can pinpoint the decision level where the optimal sensitivity and specificity are achieved. By superimposing the ROC curves of several markers, the most predictive marker can be selected. For example, percent of free PSA has an AUC of 0.708, which is better than total PSA with an AUC 0.582 (Figure 1).

Distribution of Marker Values. Application of the predictive value model is difficult for analytes that are not diagnostic for a single disease. Most tumor markers are elevated in more than one disease condition. When using the predictive value model, it is necessary to select a population that includes groups with and without disease.

What patients should be included in these two groups? The decision should be based on the specific clinical questions asked. If the question concerns the predictive value of carcinoembryonic antigen (CEA) for active colorectal carcinoma, the disease group should include only those patients with active colorectal carcinoma.

Selection of the non-disease group is more challenging. Should healthy individuals and those with benign conditions be included? If so, how many benign condition groups should be included? Should patients in remission be included as well because they do not have active diseases? The values calculated for sensitivity and specificity greatly depend on the types of groups included and on the number of patients in each group.

The distribution of tumor marker values is usually shown as the percentage of patients with elevated values as determined using various cut-off values in the healthy, benign, and cancerous groups. International staging criteria should be used to classify cancer patients. Diagnosis should be based on pathological findings.

Groups are selected from past experiences of similar markers. In breast cancer, normal women are used as the healthy population for comparison. The nonmalignant or benign groups are selected to include people with the most likely causes of marker elevation: benign liver and breast diseases, and pregnancy. The non-breast metastatic cancer groups are selected to show the specificity of the marker using endometrial, colon, lung, prostate, and ovarian carcinoma.

Grouping all breast cancer patients into a single category is not satisfactory because most markers are elevated in active breast cancer. The adjuvant group consists of patients who presented with no metastasis, underwent mastectomy and treatment with adjuvant chemotherapy, and have no evidence of disease. The adjuvant group should not have elevated marker values. The metastasis group includes patients in complete remission, partial remission, or with progressive breast cancer accompanied by local or distant metastases. The progressive breast cancer group should have the highest percentage of elevated marker values. The partial remission group should have an intermediate percentage of elevated marker values. The complete remission group should have the lowest percentage of elevated marker values.

Disease Management. Most tumor markers are used to monitor cancer treatment and progression. The selection of patient groups is important to illustrate the usefulness of the marker in various clinical settings. Markers are used to determine the success of the initial treatment (e.g., surgery or radiation), detect the recurrence of cancer, and to monitor the effectiveness of the treatment modality.

To determine the success of surgery, a marker level elevated prior to surgery should fall after a successful operation. The extent of the decrease in the marker value depends on the pre-treatment tumor involvement. With the recurrence of cancer after a successful initial treatment, the marker value may not fall with the normal half-life or within the normal range. It may fall to a steady level that is higher than normal, or it may fall within the reference interval of healthy individuals. A subsequent rise in the marker value suggests recurrence of the cancer. To monitor the effectiveness of cancer therapy, the marker value should increase with progression of cancer, decrease with the regression of cancer, and not change in the presence of stable disease. When evaluating candidate markers, group all the events related to the progression, stability, and regression of disease; then evaluate whether or not the marker value changes in the predicted direction in all these situations.

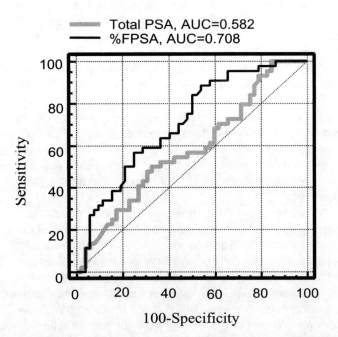

Figure 1 A receiver operating characteristic curve (ROC) for total PSA and %free PSA for total PSA between 4 to 10 ng/mL. AUC, area under the curve.

TECHNOLOGY

Specimen Collection

Specimen collection is an important aspect of tumor marker study. Although any human specimen could be used to identify tumor markers, the most useful specimens are serum, plasma, urine, cells, and tissues. Markers found in tumors or tumor-derived cell lines are usually diluted or non-existent in serum or urine.

Tissue should be harvested within 30 minutes of resection and frozen in liquid nitrogen to preserve proteins and mRNA. The tissues should be maintained thereafter at $-70°$ C. Even at dry ice temperatures, some enzymatic activity may persist. Clinical information is essential to specimen utilization. Tumors vary in type, grade, stage, treatment status, and treatment response. Markers are often easier to initially identify in tumor cells, but the real promise of early detection depends on their identification in easily accessible fluids. Linkage to genomic data permits identification of allelic variation more readily than analysis of the proteins themselves.

Tissue samples are generally obtained through gross examination and dissection of surgical specimens. Recently, laser capture microdissection (LCM) technology has been used successfully for microdissection of tumor tissues (5); see Chapter 33 for more detailed discussion.

The purification of hematopoetic tumor cells and other noncohesive tumor cells is considerably easier than the purification of solid tumor cells. Flow cytometers use a combination of specific labels to detect the cells of interest and electrostatic deflection of charged droplets for cell selection. The labels can be tagged antibodies to membrane proteins or compounds that directly interact with DNA. Labeled cells initially flow single-file in a liquid medium through a column that traverses the path of a laser beam. As the labeled cell intercepts the laser beam, light is scattered from the cell itself as well as from the labels. These signals determine whether a cell will be selected or not, based upon preselected criteria. Affinity purification is also widely used for cell sorting. The most common approach involves the covalent attachment of cell marker-specific antibodies to agarose beads, which are then packed into a column. The heterogeneous cell population is poured over the column, and non-adherent cells are washed free with a physiologic buffer. The cells of interest are subsequently eluted by washing the column with a buffer of high salt content.

Immunoassay

Immunoassay has been the most widely used technology for the measurement of tumor markers due to its high analytical sensitivity and specificity. Most clinical laboratories use automated immunoassay systems to perform tumor marker testing. Choosing an automated immunoassay system, like choosing any new instrumentation, is not an easy task (6). There are currently more than 20 immunoassay systems on the market, the majority of which are described in a review by Sokoll and Chan (7).

System evaluation should include technical, clinical, operational, and economic components. Briefly, a technical evaluation would assess within- and between-run precision; sensitivity, linearity, accuracy, including evaluation of recovery, dilutions, interferences, carryover, calibration stability, etc.; lot to lot variability; and method comparisons. A clinical evaluation would assess the diagnostic accuracy of the methods with an emphasis on reference values and disease management issues. An operational evaluation would assess system operation including data management and interface capabilities, technical service issues, and an assessment of throughput capabilities from simulation studies with the expected test mix. Finally, an economic evaluation should be performed to determine the system cost as well as the total cost of testing, including pre- and post-analytical steps, to determine the effects on labor requirements and productivity.

Technical issues such as precision, accuracy, sensitivity, and dynamic range should be considered when choosing an immunoassay analyzer. Automation has allowed for greatly improved precision of steps such as pipetting, washing, separating, and measuring such that specimens can be analyzed once, as opposed to manual assays requiring duplicate analyses. Intra- and inter-assay precision, particularly at important medical decision points, and other technical parameters, should be evaluated carefully when considering a system. It can be useful to examine proficiency survey results to determine intra- and inter-method precision as well as compare absolute values to determine whether laboratory reference ranges may be affected and need adjustment. A contributing factor to inter-assay precision, which should be minimized, is lot-to-lot variability in reagents. Sensitivity and linear range can be affected by the type of label and detection method, as well as by assay design with improvements observed with chemiluminescent signals compared to older colorimetric and fluorometric detection methods. Accuracy of results has also improved with automation due to built-in quality checks such as sensors for malfunctions. In addition, establish checks associated with pipetting of specimens and reagents and with timing of incubation and reading steps. Appropriate reagent addition as well as positive sample identification, including controls and calibrators, can be assured with bar coding. Specimen carry-over is a concern (many immunoassays have results that span a wide range). Therefore, some systems use disposable tips for specimen pipetting. Some other accuracy-associated system features include clot and short sample detection, and autodilution and autorepeat capabilities.

In order to be clinically useful, assay results need to be accurate and precise, as well as timely. Turnaround time is dependent upon how often the test is performed and how long it takes to complete the test. Random access allows tests to be performed upon receipt at the analyzer with testing time dependent upon incubation time, method of separation for heterogeneous immunoassays, and type of detection. Instrument throughput depends upon time to first result, time between results, number of assays on board the instrument, and incubation time. Incubation times are fixed in some systems while being variable in others. Specific test mix will greatly influence throughput for systems with varying incubation times, therefore, optimal throughput may not be attainable. Other system features such as wide dynamic ranges, lower dilution requirements, use of primary and secondary tubes of different sizes, reflex testing capabilities, and bar coding can also increase testing efficiency. A final clinical consideration is specimen volume. Required assay volumes and dead volumes should be as small as possible.

Quality Assurance

Quality assurance has been minimized to a large extent in an effort to find the pot of gold at the end of the rainbow—a marker useful for managing the treatment of the cancer patient. We can define quality assurance in tumor markers as the steps necessary to insure the reliability, validity, and efficacy of tumor marker data in the overall care and management of the patient. All components must be included.

The first is the pre-analytical phase: the ordering of the test; the collection of specimen from a prepared patient; the delivery of specimen to the laboratory, and its preparation and handling before analysis. The analytical phase includes choice of method, standardization, calibration and precision in performance, and calculation of the result. The post-analytical phase includes presentation of the results, their interpretation and comparison with other clinical and laboratory data, and then the use of the data in managing disease.

Proteomics

Proteomics is defined as the systematic study of global expression of proteins. Proteins can exhibit a multitude of features that become apparent after they are synthesized and released from the ribosome. This information cannot be obtained through RNA-based mining approaches, but only by analysis of the protein profile. For analytical purposes, it is assumed that the quantity and composition of the expressed genes will define the state of the cell, an assumption that will allow for the diagnosis or classification of a protein profile (see review by Rai and Chan (8), and Chapter 33).

There are actually two different types of proteomics-based approaches (9). One is *expression proteomics*, which aims to identify and catalog all the known proteins within the cell. The other is termed *cell-map proteomics*, which aims to understand the interactions of the various proteins and their involvement in signal transduction pathways. In the future, both of these proteomics-based approaches will assist in the identification of proteins that are useful as

- biomarkers for early detection, diagnosis/staging, and prognosis;
- markers to help in the understanding or monitoring disease progression, treatment, and toxicity;
- antigenic proteins for therapeutics or vaccine development; and,
- drug targets.

For more discussions, see Chapters 32, 33, 34 and 35.

The traditional method for proteomic analysis includes the use of a separation-based methodology coupled to an identification approach. By utilizing these two types of approaches sequentially, one can accurately resolve, identify, and characterize protein candidates that are differentially expressed in a particular condition.

Separation of Proteins. Two-dimensional (2D) gels provide a means for separating complex protein mixtures. Proteins are separated in the first dimension by their isoelectric points, and then in a second dimension by their molecular weight. The result is a gel which, when stained with one of a variety of protein dyes, reveals a pattern of spots. One must be aware that a single spot may correspond to more than a protein, and one protein may be found in multiple spots. A single spot may correspond to more than one protein if two proteins have similar molecular weights and isoelectric points, a phenomenon that may be exhibited with multigene families or in other cases when protein isoforms are nearly identical (e.g., tropomyosin isoforms). A single protein may be found in multiple spots if the protein can be post-translationally modified, and both forms of the protein are detectable (such as the phosphorylated and non-phosphorylated forms of a protein).

Although 2D gel electrophoresis is a commonly used approach, problems have been reported. These include issues with reproducibility, as well as the inability to separate hydrophobic proteins, which are poorly soluble. Also, it is sometimes difficult to visualize differences when comparing two gel patterns. New methodologies have proven helpful in dealing with some of these issues, and further advances will no doubt help resolve those problems that remain. Some of these advances include the use of immobilized pH gradients (IPG strips) and the use of narrow pH gradients to improve the resolution power of electrophoresis.

Identification of Proteins. After the initial separation is performed, the subsequent step is to identify the resolved proteins. Typically, this has been done using mass spectrometry (MS), the method of choice for protein identification. Information gained from MS data, usually a peptide mass fingerprint (a set of molecular weights obtained from an enzymatic digest of a protein), is compared with available information from protein databases to make positive identifications of proteins.

This fingerprint pattern is compared with that of a theoretical protein digest using the same protease, performed on all the proteins present within a database, i.e., an "in silico" digest. Because peptides and proteins fragment in a reproducible manner, this is very useful. One must be aware, however, that the mass spectrometer is subject to errors in measurements, and that peak intensity is not always correlated with protein concentration. This is because peak intensity depends on the ability of the protein or peptide to "fly down" the time-of-flight tube of the mass spectrometer. This ability further depends on protein characteristics, such as amino acid composition, hydrophobicity, and others.

The advantages of MS as a means of identifying proteins are the following: speed, simplicity, and high sensitivity. Disadvantages of this approach include these factors: a good protein database is required (not EST or genomic DNA), and the sequence of the protein of interest must be present in the database. Also, if the protein or peptide is a minor part of a complex mixture, then a more rigorous identification procedure may be necessary, such as MS/MS whereby individual peptides are further subject to an additional fragmentation. Finally, low abundance proteins or peptides may be difficult to identify if the initial mixture is of very high complexity.

By combining several approaches in tandem and obtaining several key identifying characteristics, one can increase the confidence with which a particular protein is selected. For example, by knowing the pI, molecular weight, and peptide mass fingerprint data, one can be reasonably confident when querying the proteins in a database and selecting protein candidates. Once these are obtained, the results can be analyzed. To score the data, the relevant information is compared to the likelihood that a particular match occurs by chance, i.e. a random event. Thus, one can apply standard probability techniques and established thresholds to determine the quality of the protein match. Those values that do not meet strict standards can be discarded.

ProteinChip® Technique. Although much of the work in the field of proteomics has utilized 2D gel electrophoresis, other methodologies are available. One example is the Surface-Enhanced Laser Desorption/ Ionization, or SELDI, which is marketed by Ciphergen Biosystems, Inc. (10). This technique utilizes "ProteinChip®" arrays, which are used to capture proteins of interest, coupled to a time-of-flight mass spectrometer. Biological fluids are incubated on protein chips that contain different chromatographic surfaces and utilize various chemicals or biological molecules. Proteins that are not bound are washed away before samples are subjected to time-of-flight measurements to obtain molecular weights of the corresponding peaks. Using this methodology, one can compare two different sample sets, e.g., normal and diseased, to easily perform differential expression mapping. This leads to the identification of proteins that are expressed at different levels between the two samples. The ProteinChip® analyzer also includes a software application to assist with the data interpretation. This software package utilizes multivariate analysis for pattern recognition, allowing a simple and quick analysis to identify differentially expressed proteins.

The advantages of the SELDI technique are multifold. First, sample requirements are dramatically reduced. Because SELDI employs MS for its readout, femtomolar amounts of proteins can produce a detectable signal. Reproducibility is also greater than that of 2D gels. These chips can also be used to identify proteins at extremes of pI, which is problematic under normal 2D gel electrophoresis conditions. In addition, there is a greater sensitivity and accuracy for low molecular weight proteins (<25 kD) with the SELDI technique (10). Finally, this technology acts as its own validation and diagnostic platform, thus reducing the time required to progress from start to finish. One disadvantage, however, is that 2D gels may offer better resolution as >1000 spots can be detected on a gel. Performing a fractionation prior to analysis on the ProteinChip® can circumvent this limitation.

Another methodology is multidimensional or sequential chromatography (11). This approach utilizes multiple columns that run serially in order to provide the necessary separation. The advantage of such an approach is that proteins are not precipitated and actually remain in solution during the separation procedure. As with 2D gels, this technique can be coupled to MALDI-TOF for the subsequent protein identification.

Genomics

Genomics is the study of DNA. Transcriptomics is the study of mRNA. Proteomics is the study of protein. The study of mRNA could be called functional genomics as well. Therefore, the study of genomics and functional genomics could lead to the discovery of biomarkers for cancer.

Microarray technology has been used extensively for genomics. A microarray is a device that contains a large number of well-defined capture molecules including oligonucleotides, cDNAs, clones, PCR products, or tissue sections. These molecules are immobilized on a solid support and assembled in an addressable format. Microarray is useful for simultaneous detection of large numbers of analytes in a sample. A recent survey of literature on microarray technology and its applications was recently compiled by Kricka and Fortina (12), and the analytical issues for gene expression array data was addressed by Lee (13).

Gene expression analysis is performed by using DNA microarrays that consist of oligonucleotides or cDNAs of known sequences immobilized on solid support, for example, chips. RNA from the test sample (cancer) is reverse transcribed into cDNA and labeled with a fluorescent dye. RNA is also isolated from a control sample (normal) and labeled with a different fluorescent dye. These two samples are hybridized to the arrays, and the resulting fluorescence shows the difference in the RNA transcript between the test and the control samples. This technique has been applied to classify breast cancer into different subtypes based on the differences in the expression profiles (for more details, see Chapters 32 and 34). The advantage of microarray technology is the use of small sample size to obtain extensive gene expression data. The disadvantage is that it is time consuming, expensive, has background problems, and the mRNA is not stable. Traditional formalin fixation eventually degrades RNA; therefore, frozen sections of tissues are required.

Comparative genomic hybridization (CGH) is a technique that compares differences in DNA copies between cancer and control samples. DNA is extracted from both cancer and control samples and labeled with different colored fluorescent dyes. The DNA mixtures are hybridized onto normal metaphase chromosomes. The ratio of fluorescence intensities at a given chromosome location is approximately proportional to the sequence copy. The regions with abnormalities are identified with either an increase, decrease, or no change in DNA copies. For example, an area with decreased DNA copies might be investigated for loss of heterozygosity (LOH). See Chapter 32 for details.

Single nucleotide polymorphisms (SNPs) are variations of single bases within the human genome. SNPs are the most common form of genetic variability. The identification of SNPs could lead to the discovery of disease-associated mutations. SNP microarrays have recently been developed. Sequenom, Inc., uses mass spectrometry in an automated MassARRAY™ format for the rapid analysis of SNPs. For more information on SNPs, see Chapter 56.

Bioinformatics

Bioinformatics encompasses all aspects of biological information acquisition, processing, storage, distribution, analysis, and interpretation. Therefore, bioinformatics is important in the establishment of a common database for genomics and proteomics, in the identification of potential tumor markers, and in the enhancement of the clinical usefulness of tumor markers.

The identification of a small subset of differentially expressed genes or proteins from a large volume of profiling data is a challenging task. Sophisticated bioinformatic tools are required to evaluate the complex associations between genes or proteins and the specimen phenotypes. In tumor marker discovery, the diagnoses of the patient specimens are often known beforehand. In such cases, supervised analytical methods that consider disease classification of specimens tend to be more efficient in information utilization and relevant to the desired research outcome. A basic approach would be first to construct linear or nonlinear classification functions that better separate the predefined groups of specimens. The relative importance of individual markers could then be estimated and ranked according to the way in which they contribute to the classification functions.

In the application of proteomics, for example, the Ciphergen ProteinChip® software system could be used to identify qualified peaks from the raw spectrum data by applying a threshold to peak intensities normalized against total ion current. Because more sophisticated procedures are used for the final peak selection, the initial threshold is set to capture the largest number of candidate peaks. Logarithmic transformation is applied to the data as needed to reduce peak intensity ranges. The final result is an m (peaks) by n (specimens) matrix, where an entry at Row I, Column J, presents the normalized relative abundance of proteins at mass weight corresponding to Peak I in Specimen J. Two supervised pattern classification methods, the Classification and Regression Tree (CART) (14), implemented in Biomarker Pattern Software V4.0 (BPS) (Ciphergen, CA), and the Unified Maximum Separability Analysis (UMSA) procedure (15), implemented in ProPeak (3Z Informatics, SC), were used individually and in cross-comparison to screen for peaks that contribute to the differentiation between cancer patients and the non-cancer controls.

Traditional multivariate statistical methods typically involve the use of the covariance matrix. It is difficult or impossible to obtain a stable estimate of covariance matrix from data with a very small sample size and a relatively large number of variables to be analyzed. This difficulty has forced a number of current expression data analysis approaches to evaluate the significance of individual variables (genes, proteins, or biomarkers in general), independent of other variables. The two supervised analytical methods discussed here for peak selection do not explicitly require the estimation of the covariance matrix. Both methods evaluate the significance of an individual biomarker based on its role in a multivariate effort to separate the different groups of patients. With such methods, it is possible to select biomarkers that individually may not provide good performance. However, their collective expression patterns as a whole are strongly associated with the presence or omission of a given disease condition.

For simplicity and because of the relatively small sample size of most available data, multiple biomarkers could be combined using only simple forms of logistic regression. Once these biomarkers are further validated through additional studies, it is possible to construct better predictive models using more advanced statistical and computational tools such as artificial neural networks. The CART algorithm in BPS and the nonlinear version of UMSA can also be used to construct such models. However, in the initial stages of biomarker discovery, the data sets are typically small. The direct application of overly flexible nonlinear models using a large number of variables from raw profile data could result in models that rely heavily on non-disease related artifacts to produce misleading results on the training data. For more details related to bioinformatic approaches for optimal utilization of tumor markers, please refer to Chapter 11.

THE FUTURE

The future holds great promise for the field of tumor markers. With advances in genomic and proteomic technology, human diseases will be classified based on molecular, rather than morphological, analysis. This will occur through techniques like laser capture micro-dissection for the procurement of tissues and cells, and by combining genomic and proteomic analyses. Early diagnosis of diseases will be possible using unique gene or protein profiles, consisting of multiple biomarkers. The analysis of panels of protein biomarkers may be performed by traditional ELISA or antibody-based protein chips for parallel testing. Furthermore, there will be many more diagnostic tests generated as the result of the genomic and proteomic discoveries.

In addition, many more proteins will be identified as potential drug targets. Currently, there are about 500 drugs on the market. Potentially, the repertoire of new drugs could be tenfold higher. Diagnostic and pharmaceutical companies will be merged into an industry providing integrated solutions for the health care delivery system. Biomarkers are likely to serve as surrogate end points for the assessment of drug efficacy and drug toxicity.

The biochip market, which includes both gene chips and protein chips, is fairly large. According to data provided by Frost and Sullivan, the market for biochips was $0.27 billion in 1999 and $0.53 billion in 2000; for the year 2004, it is forecasted to be $3.3 billion. The total funds raised by the initial public offering (IPO) of stocks for biotechnology companies were $8 billion in 1999 and $40 billion for the year 2000. Thus, there is a strong financial interest. According to the P-S BioPharma Fund, investors are interested in proteomics. However, they recognize that high throughput approaches to delineate protein function and disease related pathways will be important for drug discovery. The complexity of protein biochemistry and the diversity of proteomic technologies create a challenge for scientists to pick the best approaches for target validation and drug discovery.

In the future, the development of biochips will grow much faster than the rest of the diagnostics industry. These will include DNA, RNA, and protein chips, as well as those that are of the "lab-in-a-box" type. All types of specimens will be analyzed including tissue, cells, and body fluids. The diagnosis of disease will be based on the combination of genomic and proteomic methods. Integrated diagnostic tools that combine these methods with molecular imaging techniques will be used. Finally, bioinformatics will link scientific data with clinical information to provide better and more comprehensive care of the patient's health. We will witness a rapid translation of new discoveries from the laboratory to the patient's bedside. With advances in proteomics, laboratory testing and hence laboratory diagnoses will become even more important in the integrated health care delivery system.

REFERENCES

1. Jemal A, Thomas A, Murray T, Thun M. Cancer statistics, 2001. CA Cancer J Clin 2002;52:23–47.
2. Sobin LH, Wittekind Ch (eds.). TNM classification of malignant tumors, 5th ed. New York: Wiley-Liss, Inc., 1997.
3. Chan DW, Sell S. Tumor markers. In: Burtis CA, Ashwood ER (eds.). Tietz textbook of clinical chemistry, 5th ed. Philadelphia: Saunders, 2001:390–413.
4. Chan DW, Beveridge RA, Muss H, Fritsche HA, Hortobagyi G, Theriault R, et al. Use of Truquant BR radioimmunoassay for early detection of breast cancer recurrence in patients with stage II and stage III disease. J Clin Oncol 1997;15:2322–2328.
5. Palmer-Toy DE, Sarracino DA, Sgroi D, LeVangie R, Leopold PE. Direct acquisition of matrix-assisted laser desorption/ionization time-of-flight mass spectra from laser capture microdissected tissues. Clin Chem 2000;46:1513–1516.
6. Chan DW (ed.). Immunoassay automation: a practical guide. San Diego: Academic Press, 1992:1–367.
7. Sokoll LJ, Chan DW. Clinical instrumentation (immunoassay analyzers). Anal Chem 1999;71:356–362.
8. Rai AJ, Chan DW. Cancer proteomics: new developments in clinical chemistry. J Lab Med 2001;25:399–403.
9. Blackstock W. Trends in automation and mass spectrometry for proteomics. Proteomics: A Trends Guide 2000;7:12–16.
10. Fung ET, Wright GL Jr, Dalmasso EA. Proteomic strategies for biomarker identification: progress and challenges. Curr Opin Mol Ther 2000;2:643–650.
11. Washburn MP, Yates JR. New methods of proteome analysis: multidimensional chromatography and mass spectrometry, Proteomics: A Trends Guide 2000;7:27–30.
12. Kricka LJ, Fortina P. Microarray technology and applications: an all-language literature survey including books and patents. Clin Chem 2001;47:1479–1482.
13. Lee JK. Analysis issues for gene expression array data. Clin Chem 2001;47:1350–1352.
14. Breiman L, Friedman JH, Olshen RA, Stone CJ. Classification and regression trees. Monterey, CA: Wadsworths & Brooks, 1984.
15. Zhang Z, Page G, Zhang H. Applying classification separability analysis to microarray data. In: Process of critical assessment of techniques for microarray data analysis. Durham, NC: Critical assessment of microarray data analysis (CAMDA) '00. Dec. 18–19, 2000.

Chapter 3

Clinical Evaluation Criteria for Tumor Markers

Vered Stearns and Daniel F. Hayes

Diagnosis and staging of most types of cancer generally include a combination of clinical evaluation, routine laboratory tests, and radiological studies. In recent decades, oncological clinical practice has included the use of tumor markers, which are alterations in normal molecules, substances, or processes in pre-cancerous or cancerous conditions (1). Tumor markers can be measured in tissues, in exfoliated cells, or in body fluids, such as blood, urine, or sputum. Their alteration from normalcy may be qualitative or quantitative.

Tumor markers can be used to predict disease risk, to screen for disease, and to offer differential diagnosis. Tumor markers can also be used to predict prognosis, including the risk of relapse following primary therapy, or the risk of progression or death from metastasis. Serial measurements of tumor markers, most commonly in serum or plasma, are used to monitor response to treatment.

Ideally, there would be a tumor marker for every type of cancer and for every clinical use. In practice, only a few markers have entered routine use and only for a limited number of cancers and clinical settings. The roles of some tumor markers for specific diseases, such as βHCG for choriocarcinoma, are not in dispute. However, for most types of cancer there are hundreds or thousands of published investigations that assess the role of one or more markers for one or more clinical uses. Why haven't we accepted most markers for routine clinical practice?

While there are fairly strict criteria for clinical trial design for new drug investigation, tumor marker studies have not been standardized. In this chapter we will review some of the pitfalls in the published literature on tumor markers and propose a framework for standardizing and interpreting tumor marker studies.

CLINICAL UTILITY OF TUMOR MARKERS

Tumor markers represent a heterogeneous group of altered molecules, substances, or processes. A tumor marker may represent an alteration in a normal cell or in its surroundings. Thus, a tumor marker may be localized to the abnormal cell or the cell's environment, or it may be shed into blood or other bodily fluids.

A specific marker can be detected through one or more laboratory assays, reagents, or specimen sources. Due to the heterogeneity of tumor markers, it is critical to determine the utility of a specific marker for each disease and clinical use. A specific marker may play a critical role in one disease, but have no utility in another. For example, prostate specific antigen (PSA) is routinely used in prostate cancer to determine risk, diagnosis, and to monitor response to treatment (2). PSA can also be detected in normal and malignant breast tissue, and in the circulation of women with breast cancer (3,4). However, the biology, diagnostic, or monitoring importance of PSA in diseases of the breast remains unknown.

Tumor marker studies are highly variable not only in methods of marker detection, but also in study design and patient population. Most marker studies include retrospective analyses of archival tissues. Even when specimens are obtained from patients included in one prospective clinical trial, not all study participants' tissues are included in the marker study. The patients included in the marker study may have had one of many disease stages, or they may have received one of many systemic therapies, or no systemic treatment at all. Moreover, patients' outcomes are not always known. Across different studies assessing the same marker for the same disease, methods of detection may vary in the assay utilized to detect the abnormal process, reagents, cut-off levels, and specimen source or preparation.

In 1995, the American Society of Clinical Oncology convened a Tumor Marker Expert Panel to establish practice guidelines for evaluating tumor markers in breast and colon cancers (5–7). During these deliberations, panel members noted the lack of a unified methodology to assess published tumor marker studies. Subsequently, they proposed a framework for evaluation of tumor marker studies: the Tumor Marker Utility Grading System (TMUGS) (1). In this grading system, each marker is given a semi-quantitative score based on the evidence that is available to correlate the marker with the biologic process and endpoint in question (Table 1). A score of "0" signifies a marker that has been extensively investigated and has no utility for a specific use. A marker that was not investigated for a specific use is assigned a designation of "NA." When only preliminary data are available to support the clinical use of a marker, a "±" score is given. The highest designation, "3+," implies that the marker can be used independently to make clinical decisions (such as βHCG for choriocarcinoma). If a marker

Table 1 Tumor marker utility grading system (TMUGS)

Utility Grade	Explanation of Scale
0	Marker has been adequately evaluated for a specific use and the data definitively demonstrate it has *no utility*. The marker should not be ordered for that clinical use.
NA	Data are *not available* for the marker for that use because marker has not been studied for that clinical use.
±	Data suggest that the marker may correlate with biological process and/or endpoint, and preliminary data suggest that use of the marker may contribute to favorable clinical outcome, but more definitive studies are required. Thus, the marker is still considered *highly investigational* and should not be used for standard clinical practice.
+	Sufficient data are available to demonstrate that the marker correlates with the biological process and/or endpoint related to the use, and that the marker results might effect favorable clinical outcome for that use. However, the marker is still considered *investigational* and should not be used for standard clinical practice, for one of three reasons: 1) The marker correlates with another marker or test that has been established to have clinical utility, but the new marker has not been shown to clearly provide any advantage. 2) The marker may contribute independent information, but it is unclear whether that information provides clinical utility because treatment options have not been shown to change outcome. 3) Preliminary data for the marker are quite encouraging, but the level of evidence (see Table 2) to document clinical utility is lacking.
2+	Marker supplies information (not otherwise available from other measures) that is helpful to the clinician in decision making for that use, but the marker can not be used as sole criterion for decision-making. Thus, marker has clinical utility for that use, and it should be considered standard practice in *selected* situations.
3+	Marker can be used as an independent criterion for clinical decision making in that use. Thus, marker has clinical utility for that use, and it should be considered *standard* practice.

Modified with permission (1).

has clinical utility but only in the context of other data, it is assigned a score of "2+." A "1+" indicates that additional studies must be performed to establish the clinical utility of the marker.

The data used to assign these scores fall into one of five "Level of Evidence" (LOE) categories (Table 2) (1). LOE I studies carry the strongest clinical utility. These studies include prospectively performed appropriately powered clinical investigations, or a rigorous meta-analysis of studies with lower LOE designations. LOE II come from prospective studies that were set up to ask a therapeutic question, and in which specimens were collected prospectively for marker analysis. LOE III and IV derive from large and small retrospective studies respectively, and LOE V from small pilot studies.

One purpose of the development of TMUGS was to help investigators plan future tumor marker studies. Doing so requires a fundamental understanding of how tumor markers might correlate with future clinical outcomes. In this regard, tumor markers can be divided into prognostic and predictive markers (8, 9). Prognostic markers reflect the underlying tumor biology, i.e., the likelihood of a cancer to proliferate, invade, and spread. Prognostic markers may help distinguish primary cancers that have a high risk of relapse or progression from more indolent tumors. Because prognostic markers reflect the biology of a specific tumor, they are optimally evaluated in an untreated group of patients in which prognosis of a "marker-positive" group is compared to that of a "marker-negative" group. If a marker is prognostic, both marker-positive and marker-negative patients will sustain a similar proportional benefit from the same treatment (Figure 1a) (10). In contrast, predictive markers indicate relative sensitivity or resistance to specific treatment or intervention (Figure 1b). When interpreting marker studies, it is also important to note that many markers may have both prognostic and predictive properties (Figure 1c).

After determining whether a marker is prognostic and/or predictive, and weighing the evidence obtained from published data, how can one conclude if the marker is ready for clinical practice? Many marker investigations may reveal a statistically significant difference (i.e., p value < 0.05) in prognosis or response to specific treatments between marker-positive and

Table 2 Classification of level of evidence (LOE) for tumor marker studies

LOE	Type of Evidence
I	Evidence derived from prospective high-powered trial specifically addressing tumor marker utility OR Overview or meta-analysis of lower LOE studies.
II	Evidence from companion study to large clinical trial. Specimens collected prospectively and tumor marker utility determined as secondary aim of study.
III	Evidence from retrospective trials, where data about patient characteristics and treatment are often incomplete.
IV	Evidence from small retrospective studies that do not have prospectively dictated therapy.
V	Evidence from small pilot studies designed to determine or estimate distribution of marker levels in sample population.

Modified with permission (1).

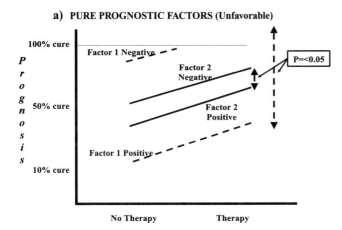

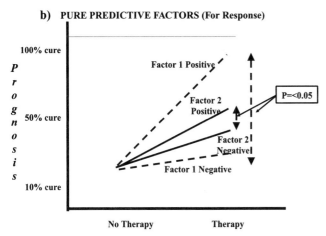

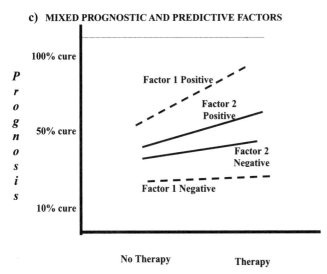

Figure 1 Schematic examples of prognostic, predictive, and mixed prognostic/predictive factors. In each schema, Factor 1 (dashed line) is a strong factor, and Factor 2 (solid line) is a weak factor [modified with permission (10)].

marker-negative groups. The clinician must be able to determine how this statistically significant difference in outcomes translates into practice. As illustrated in Figure 1, both prognostic markers 1 and 2 may reliably separate patients into groups for whom clinical outcomes will differ, with statistical analysis suggesting that the separation between "positive" and "negative" is not due to chance alone ($p < 0.05$). However, the separation between "positive" and "negative" groups for marker 1 is so great that one might treat the two groups completely differently. In contrast, marker 2 is a weak prognostic factor. Although "positive" patients have a slightly poorer outcome than "negative" patients, the separation is so small that the two groups would be treated similarly. Each marker can be assigned an arbitrary relative strength (strong, moderate, weak) that can help clinicians determine whether using that marker is justified in making treatment recommendations (11, 12). We have previously suggested that, for breast cancer, a strong prognostic marker should have a relative risk (RR) > 2.0 (Figure 2). Moderate and weak unfavorable prognostic markers will have a RR of 1.5–2.0 and less than 1.5 respectively. Based on the presence or absence of a predictive marker, treatments may vary in duration, intensity, and/or specific agent recommendations.

To illustrate these points, consider a patient with a newly diagnosed breast cancer. Several markers may be helpful in estimating her risk of relapse. The strongest marker indicating an increased risk of relapse is the presence of axillary lymph node metastases (13). Moderately strong markers include tumor grade and the presence of a lymphovascular invasion (14–17). Finally, absence of the estrogen receptor is an example of a weak, unfavorable prognostic marker.

Likewise, predictive factors can be assigned an arbitrary relative predictive strength (strong, moderate, weak). The predictive strength for individual predictive markers is best estimated from results of prospective clinical trials in which patients are randomly assigned to the therapy in question, or not (Figure 3) (10). For example, the Oxford meta-analysis of prospective randomized clinical trials of adjuvant systemic therapy demonstrated that women with ER-rich breast cancer treated with tamoxifen have a 40% reduction in risk of recurrence and death (18). In contrast, women with ER-poor cancer

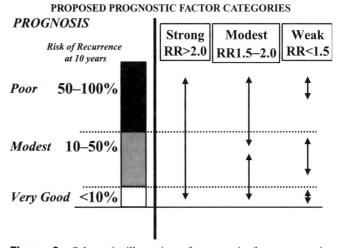

Figure 2 Schematic illustration of prognostic factor categories [modified with permission (12)]. Prognosis: odds of recurrence or death at 10 years if no systemic adjuvant therapy is administered.

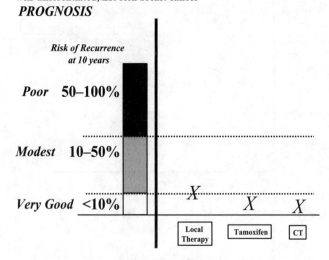

Figure 3 Determining relative strength of predictive factors [modified with permission (10)]. ER: estrogen receptor. RPV: relative predictive value. SD: standard deviation.

have a small benefit (5%). Thus, ER is a strong predictive marker for response to tamoxifen (relative predictive value of 0.4/0.05=8, Figure 3).

How can we integrate the prognostic and predictive markers to determine an individual patient's prognosis? Patient 1, for example, is a 45-year-old woman with a lymph-node-negative, well-differentiated, ER-positive, 1-cm infiltrating carcinoma of the breast. She has a 10% chance of disease recurrence over a 10-year period (Figure 4, Patient 1). The presence of the ER predicts for response to adjuvant endocrine therapy with a nearly 40% reduction in annual hazard of recurrence and death (18). Although chemotherapy decreases her relative risk by 20–30%, her prognosis is so good that only 1–2% of such patients will benefit. For this woman, the toxicity of adjuvant systemic chemotherapy probably outweighs the benefits. In contrast, patient 2 is a 45-year-old woman with two positive axillary lymph nodes, poorly differentiated, ER-negative tumor. She has a high risk of recurrence, and low chance of benefit from tamoxifen (Figure 4, Patient 2). For this woman, the benefits of adjuvant chemotherapy clearly outweigh the risks associated with the treatment. In addition, based on individual risk of recurrence, clinicians may recommend more, rather than less, therapy. A breast cancer patient with 10 positive axillary lymph nodes may benefit from a more prolonged or intense course of treatment compared to a woman with one positive lymph node.

FUTURE DIRECTIONS

Careful considerations must be applied when conducting tumor marker studies. Although LOE III studies are helpful in generating hypotheses, definitive marker studies should be hypothesis-driven, and designed prospectively, utilizing pre-specified patient populations, treatments, methods of detection, and statistical considerations. Investigators should select prospective LOE I or II studies using validated assays that can be duplicat-

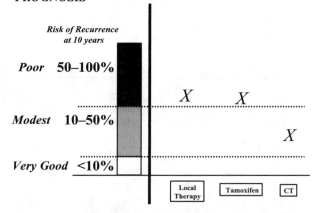

Figure 4 Illustration of treatment decision making for patients with breast cancer. CT: chemotherapy. Prognosis: odds of recurrence or death at 10 years if no systemic adjuvant therapy is administered.

ed and standardized for clinical use. In addition, results of marker studies should be presented in a consistent format, so that clinicians can assess the strength of a marker for a specific patient when discussing treatment options. Future clinical trials that evaluate tumor markers must be planned carefully and reviewed with scientific rigor. These efforts should facilitate a more rapid move from the laboratory and from hypothesis-generating studies to clinically useful results.

REFERENCES

1. Hayes DF, Bast R, Desch CE, Fritsche H, Kemeny NE, Jessup J, et al. A tumor marker utility grading system (TMUGS): a framework to evaluate clinical utility of tumor markers. J Natl Cancer Inst 1996;88:1456–1466.

2. Lilja H, Chan DW, Diamandis EP. Prostate Cancer. In: Diamandis EP, Fritche HA, Lilja H, Chan DW, Schwartz MK, eds. Tumor Markers: Physiology, pathobiology, technology, and clinical applications. Washington, DC: AACC Press, 2002.
3. Black MH, E.P. D. The diagnostic and prognostic utility of prostate-specific antigen for diseases of the breast. Breast Cancer Res Treat 2000;59:1–14.
4. Diamandis EP. Elevated serum prostate-specific antigen levels in a woman with metastatic breast cancer. N Engl J Med 2000;340:890–891.
5. ASCO Expert Panel. Clinical practice guidelines for the use of tumor markers in breast and colorectal cancer: report of the American Society of Clinical Oncology Expert Panel. J Clin Oncol 1996;14:2843–2877.
6. ASCO Expert Panel. 1997 update of recommendations for the use of tumor markers in breast and colorectal cancer. J Clin Oncol 1998;16:793–795.
7. Bast RCJ, Ravdin P, Hayes DF, Bates S, Fritsche HJ, Jessup JM, et al. 2000 update of recommendations for the use of tumor markers in breast and colorectal cancer: Clinical practice guidelines of the American Society of Clinical Oncology. J Clin Oncol 2001;19:1865–1878.
8. McGuire WL, Clark GM. Prognostic factors and treatment decisions in axillary-node-negative breast cancer. N Engl J Med 1992;326:1756–1761.
9. Gasparini G, Pozza F, Harris AL. Evaluating the potential usefulness of new prognostic and predictive indicators in node-negative breast cancer patients. J Natl Cancer Inst 1993; 85:1206–1219.
10. Hayes DF. Do we need prognostic factors in nodal-negative breast cancer? Arbiter. Eur J Cancer 2000;36:302–306.
11. Hayes DF, Trock B, Harris A. Assessing the clinical impact of prognostic factors: when is "statistically significant" clinically useful? Breast Cancer Res Treat 1998;52:305–319.
12. Isaacs C, Stearns V, Hayes DF. New prognostic factors for breast cancer recurrence. Semin Oncol 2001;28:53–67.
13. Carter CL, Allen C, Henson DE. Relation of tumor size, lymph node status, and survival in 24,740 breast cancer cases. Cancer 1989;63:181–187.
14. Neville AM, Bettelheim R, Gelber RD, Save-Soderbergh J, Davis BW, Reed R, et al. Factors predicting treatment responsiveness and prognosis in node-negative breast cancer. The International (Ludwig) Breast Cancer Study Group. J Clin Oncol 1992;10: 696–705.
15. Rosen PP, Groshen S, Saigo PE, Kinne DW, Hellman S. Pathological prognostic factors in Stage I (T1N0M0) and Stage II (T1N1M0) breast carcinoma: a study of 644 patients with median follow-up of 18 years. J Clin Oncol 1989;7:1239–1251.
16. Fisher B, Redmond C, Fisher ER, Caplan R. Relative worth of estrogen or progesterone receptor and pathologic characteristics of differentiation as indicators of prognosis in node-negative breast cancer patients: findings from National Surgical Adjuvant Breast and Bowel Project Protocol B-06. J Clin Oncol 1988;6: 1076–1087.
17. Contesso G, Mouriesse H, Friedman S, Genin J, Sarrazin D, Rouesse J. The importance of histologic grade in long-term prognosis of breast cancer: a study of 1,010 patients, uniformly treated at the Institut Gustave-Roussy. J Clin Oncol 1987;5:1378–86.
18. Early Breast Cancer Trialist's Collaborative Group. Tamoxifen for early breast cancer: an overview of the randomized trials. Lancet 1998;351:1451–1467.

Chapter 4

Quality Control and Standardization for Tumor Markers

Elizabeth H. Hammond

Nearly 20 years of advances in molecular biology culminated in the completion of the human genome project. Yet in spite of this, few tumor markers are clinically useful in predicting therapeutic responses or patient outcome, other than commonly used staging measures such as TNM and tumor histologic grade.

The American Society of Clinical Oncology (ASCO) convened a panel of experts to establish guidelines for the use of both tissue-based and circulating tumor markers in patients with breast cancer. After examining the evidence concerning all available tumor markers, the panel recommended using only estrogen receptor (ER) and progesterone receptor (PR) to determine the likelihood of benefit from endocrine therapy (1,2). The College of American Pathologists (CAP) also convened conferences in 1994 and 1999 to evaluate tumor markers and to determine which tumor markers could be recommended for clinical use in breast, prostate, and colon cancer (3,4). Pathologic staging parameters and tumor histologic grade remained as the only markers that had been validated on the basis of randomized clinical trials. Even more remarkable was the fact that the list of markers deemed clinically validated in 1999 had not significantly changed since 1994.

A useful analogy of the status of tumor marker research in the new millennium was drawn by Dr. Daniel Hayes when he compared tumor marker research to the state-of-the-art for performing therapeutic trials 30–40 years ago. At that time, to impose some order on clinical trial results, groups of investigators devised clinical trial designs (Phase I, Phase II, and Phase III) and scales for analysis (toxicity scales, performance status scales, and response criteria) that, with slight modifications and further standardization, are still in use (5). Such trials demanded a prospective hypothesis and a pre-set "protocol" that dictated the methods to be followed in conducting the study and analyzing the data. This methodology was an application of the scientific method to a clinical research setting. Even using such strict methods, meta-analyses of the results from several well-designed but relatively underpowered clinical trials would be required to determine how beneficial a specific therapy really is (6,7). Recent publications (CONSORT statement) by editors and scientists have proposed improvements in clinical trials reporting to make the results more transparent to readers and to avoid the systematic error associated with biased estimates of treatment effects. This recent effort underscores the need for continuous improvement in the way clinical trials are reported (8,9).

With certain exceptions, no consistent system to standardize tumor marker studies has been devised (10,11). Rather, most tumor marker investigations involve assays and patient populations that are readily accessible to investigators. Rarely do investigators control how patients were selected; how specimens were are collected, processed, or stored; or how the assay was performed and reported. Moreover, tumor marker studies almost never include prospective power calculations or analytical plans. While results from such studies are adequate for generating hypotheses, the results that they generate are poorly reproducible and often conflicting (12).

In the initial phases of marker development, scientists assay promising markers by a variety of methods. Serious confusion results if they do not describe the results of tumor marker studies in sufficient detail to allow others to duplicate the method and the results. Many aspects of the assay must be carefully detailed, or significant differences in results are likely. This chapter focuses on the various aspects of an immunohistochemical (IHC) tumor marker assay system and describes the conditions that must be adequately addressed if a stable, reproducible, clinically useful assay system is to be developed.

VARIABLES THAT IMPACT ASSAY PERFORMANCE

Specimen Preparation

Often investigators begin evaluating promising markers by using whatever sample type is most available to them or most applicable to the assay type they intend to use. For example, early evaluations of estrogen receptor (ER) activity in breast cancer samples were done using frozen tissue that was easily obtained for ligand-binding assays performed with radioactive ligands (13). Early studies standardized neither the conditions for freezing nor the time interval from removal of tissue to freezing of the specimen. Careful evaluations by Italo Nenci documented the detrimental effects of this variation in time at room temperature on ligand-binding assays (LBA) and estrogen receptor assay activity. He showed that estrogen receptor activity of tumor cells decreased as the estrogen receptor protein moved through various cellular compartments until it was undetectable in specimens left at room temperature for prolonged periods of time (14).

When samples of breast cancer became significantly smaller and less amenable to freezing, assaying estrogen receptor by ligand binding were replaced by immunohistochemical (IHC) assays, which could be performed on formalin-fixed tissues (15,16). Such IHC assays were conducted on samples fixed in a variety of formalin preparations for variable fixation times and after variable times between removal from the patient and fixation (17). In studies of estrogen receptor assay activity, the effects of time to fixation and type of fixation are rarely evaluated. Based on the earlier studies, it is likely that these factors continue to affect estrogen receptor assay results (18).

The purpose of tissue fixation is to preserve cellular integrity by inactivating nucleases, proteases, lipases, and saccharidases that cause cells to self-destruct after excision (19). The longer the interval between removal and fixation, the less effective any type of fixation will be on controlling these self-destructive processes. There have been no successful attempts to study these effects in any systematic way, although the National Cancer Institute has fielded and funded requests for proposals to study various aspects of tissue fixation on tumor marker values, which may ultimately provide us with answers to some of these questions.

Fixative and Fixation Timing

Another crucial aspect of specimen preparation relates to the type of fixative used and the length of time the sample is fixed prior to dehydration and paraffin embedding. An ideal fixative does not exist, but formalin is remarkably effective at maintaining structural integrity by inactivating cellular enzymes while preserving the ability to conduct immunohistochemical or molecular analysis (20). It is well known that formalin fixes tissues by cross-linking amino acids such as lysine. Cross-linking preserves secondary protein structure while destroying enzymatic activity, and masks antigenic activity because of chemical epitope modification and because antibodies used to detect antigens have difficulty penetrating cross-linked tissue. As fixation time increases, cross linking increases, which thus seriously compromises antigenicity, especially for tissues fixed longer than 24 hours (21,22). Nevertheless, studies rarely record this information.

Fixatives other than formalin are useful for some antigens and detrimental to others. If paraffin blocks are used for tumor marker studies, for example, it is impossible to determine which fixative was used and for what length of time, unless that information is specifically provided (20). Tumor marker studies that fail to detail fixative and specific conditions will definitely confound the value of the results.

Antigen Retrieval for Immunohistochemistry

Antigen retrieval methods have been developed to reduce the variation in immunohistochemical staining of tissues that results from varying fixation time and tissue-processing conditions. These methods largely rely on heating tissue in an excess of buffer at various pH. To arrive at the best method of antigen retrieval, one must evaluate the immunohistochemical reaction after a variety of antigen retrieval conditions (pH, time, temperature) to maximize staining intensity without increasing the associated non-specific background staining (17,23). Such evaluations require testing samples tissues at three heating levels and three pH levels. Samples that have been prepared in the fixatives and for the time intervals expected in normal clinical practice should be included (Table 1). Such investigations can be easily carried out on tumor tissue arrays that allow rapid assessment of multiple tissue types. (Tumor tissue arrays can be made with tumor samples of 2 mm in diameter, which allows larger areas for review [24].)

In practice, tumor marker reports rarely specify the conditions of antigen retrieval employed in a tumor marker study. This makes it difficult for others to exactly duplicate the optimal conditions found by initial investigators.

Antibody Specification

Many tumor marker assays are performed with a variety of antibody preparations, used at different concentrations, to detect the marker of interest. To determine the optimal staining protocol, it is necessary to perform a test battery (of conditions) on a slide containing the antigen of interest to determine the optimal antibody concentration and antigen retrieval conditions (25,26). This type of testing, employed routinely in large IHC laboratories, is also highly desirable for researching tumor markers (Table 1). For example, studies published about p53 protein overexpression as a prognostic tumor marker utilized at least four different antibody preparations (DO-7, CM-1, DO-1, 1801) (27). Often the antibody conditions were not clearly specified, making it difficult to compare one study with another.

If studies of a tumor marker use different antibody preparations and different test conditions, it is invalid to use the same threshold of positivity, unless this threshold is known to be similar for each preparation. Studies validating the activity of one antibody with another are rarely performed. Such validation studies are highly desirable, however, because they would allow aggregation of tumor marker data from multiple studies. This would increase to likelihood of meaningful results.

Investigators have faced other obstacles in the evaluation of various antibody preparations. One of these is the lack of standardized information provided by manufacturers concerning the antibody clone of the reagent, the concentration of the antibody in the preparation, and the expected staining characteristics of the antibody on various tissue types. These problems have recently been alleviated by the publication of guidelines for manufacturer package inserts for immunohistochemical

Table 1 Test battery approach for determining optimal antigen retrieval and antibody dilution (adapted from Hsi et al., 26)

Slide	Dilution	Antigen Retrieval	Heat*	Incubation time
1	1:10	10 mmol/L Citrate, pH 6	100 °C, 20 min	30 min
2	1:20 (optimal)	10 mmol/L Citrate, pH 6	100 °C, 20 min	30 min
3	1:40	10 mmol/L Citrate, pH 6	100 °C, 20 min	30 min
4	1:80	10 mmol/L Citrate, pH 6	100 °C, 20 min	30 min
5	1:10	1 mmol/L EDTA, pH 8	100 °C, 20 min	30 min
6	1:20	1 mmol/L EDTA, pH 8	100 °C, 20 min	30 min
7	1:40	1 mmol/L EDTA, pH 8	100 °C, 20 min	30 min
8	1:80	1 mmol/L EDTA, pH 8	100 °C, 20 min	30 min
9	1:10	Protease	RT, 8 min	30 min
10	1:20	Protease	RT, 8 min	30 min
11	1:40	Protease	RT, 8 min	30 min
12	1:80	Protease	RT, 8 min	30 min
13	1:20 (optimal)	No retrieval	RT	30 min

Table 1 illustrates the slide treatments for a battery of slides to determine the optimal protocol for a new tumor marker. Manufacturing insert suggests dilution of 1:20. All other conditions, such as staining protocol, are kept constant.

*Higher and lower temperatures or different time intervals can be tried.

Commonly used temperatures include 120 °C or 90 °C. Heating can be provided with a microwave equipped with a thermometer, a water bath (for lower temperatures), or a microwave pressure cooker. Antigen retrieval depends on the length of time the heating is maintained and the temperature achieved.

products. Since this information is readily available, all publications of tumor marker studies should provide this information in tumor marker reports (2).

Immunohistochemical Reaction and Visualization

Table 2 shows large numbers of immunohistochemical reaction, amplification, and visualization methods in common use (28). The sensitivity of the method used to detect the antigen depends on the protocol used. Often, investigators fail to specify the protocol used in their investigations, confounding the ability to duplicate the study. Since sensitivity and specificity of detection vary depending on the protocol as well as on the antibody used, this lack of information is a significant flaw in many tumor marker reports.

To evaluate whether an assay can be used clinically (as a test), one must understand these assay characteristics. Sensitivity and specificity can be determined by running the assays using samples with known marker content, or by running the assay in parallel with another assay method that has established characteristics, such as the ligand-binding assay method in the case of estrogen receptor assays. Reference materials (such as cell lines) with known ER content can also be run as positive controls to establish the assay characteristics. Using known samples, the assay characteristics (such as sensitivity, specificity, and false positive and false negative rates) can be determined (29,30). Table 3 shows a laboratory "truth table" from which these values can be determined (31).

Sensitivity and specificity can also be determined using a panel of samples with known antigen content from which a tumor tissue array has been made. The National Committee for Clinical Laboratory Standards (NCCLS) recently adopted and published a consensus guideline concerning IHC assay conditions so that laboratories could begin standardizing these procedures. Its use in reporting tumor marker assays will help to address some of the problems with assay reporting that are described (32).

Table 2 Commonly used immunohistochemical methods and detection enzymes (adapted from O'Leary, 20)

Immunohistochemical methods	Detection enzymes
Direct immunoenzyme staining	Alkaline phosphatase
Indirect immunoenzyme staining	β-Galactosidase
Antienzyme immunostaining	Glucose oxidase
Anti-enzyme immunostaining	
Enzyme-antienzyme complex immunostaining	Horseradish peroxidase
Enzyme-anti-enzyme complex immunostaining	
Enzyme conjugated avidin-biotin immunostaining	
ABC immunostaining	
Tyramide amplification immunostaining	

Table 3 Assay truth table

	Positive test	Negative test	Total samples tested
Marker present	True positive	False negative	Samples with marker present
Marker absent	False positive	True negative	Samples with marker absent
	Total positive	Total negative	Total samples

$$\text{Sensitivity of test} = \frac{\text{Samples with positive test}}{\text{Samples with marker present}}$$

$$\text{Specificity of test} = \frac{\text{Samples with negative test}}{\text{Samples with marker absent}}$$

$$\text{Positive predictive value} = \frac{\text{Number of true positive samples}}{\text{Number with positive test}}$$

$$\text{Negative predictive value} = \frac{\text{Number of false negative samples}}{\text{Number with negative test}}$$

Reference Materials and Assay Controls

Before an assay for a tumor marker can be reliably evaluated, it must be shown to be working as expected in the assay system. This requires running control samples with every assay batch to establish that

- reagents are working as expected (through the use of positive assay control specimens or cell lines with various antigenic content);
- tissue reaction is not just non-specific background (through the omission of the primary antibody on the sample to be tested); and
- tissue fixation is such that a positive reaction is possible (through the use of an internal control that should be positive if the tissue is fixed properly) (32).

It is very uncommon for such controls to be specified in publications that describe tumor marker studies, leading to the conclusion that such controls may be lacking in many of the conducted studies. For controls to be valid, they must be fixed and processed in a manner identical to that of the samples to be tested. Unfortunately, such controls have not been well defined for most tumor marker systems.

Positive control samples for various assay types are sorely needed in order to evaluate various competing assays for their value. In the 1970s, the Biological Stain Commission established a laboratory to address the standardization of chemical stains. The laboratory served as a repository of control samples and stain batches, testing reagents and issuing certificates of acceptability. This voluntary certification program greatly alleviated problems of chemical stain reagent reliability. When the BSC tried to apply this model to IHC testing, there was significant disagreement among antibody manufacturers and end users, so this program was never implemented (33–35).

Assay Reproducibility (Precision)

Another important characteristic of assay performance is the reproducibility (precision) of performance. For most tumor marker studies, reproducibility is affected by both the details of the method as well as the assay interpretation. Assay characteristics that affect reproducibility include such things as the specifics of antigen retrieval from formalin-fixed tissues, the assay detection system, and the results scoring method used by the pathologist. To assess reproducibility, the same samples must be run in replicate on multiple occasions, by identical methods, and using identical reporting criteria. The performance characteristics can then be evaluated, using inter-rater kappa statistic (36). Reproducibility is reported using the standard deviation of the measurements taken (37). This standard deviation divided by the mean of all the observations is called the coefficient of variation (CV). For a test to be considered reproducible, the CV should be <5% (31).

Assay Interpretation and Reporting Criteria

Investigators must establish a proposed scoring system for the assay, based on preliminary work, so that results from multiple laboratories or on multiple occasions can be aggregated. What constitutes a positive result? How will the results be reported (as % of positive cells, or using a scoring system with defined criteria such as 1–3+)?

Scoring specifications provide a template for reporting and data gathering. An example of the importance of this characteristic is the manner in which Gleason patterns are reported in prostate cancer. Gleason patterns are a very important prognostic factor for prostate cancer in virtually all studies that have been recently reported. A recent CAP prognostic factor conference noted that the way in which these patterns are reported vary and require further specification if the results are to be combined for meta-analyses (38). The prostate protocol for the examination of prostate cancer specimens published by the CAP was recently revised in response to these observations to clarify and specify reporting criteria (39). Thus, even established prognostic factors require periodic evaluation and modification to improve their prognostic and predictive ability.

Another timely example of the variation in reporting systems involves Her-2 protein overexpression assays. The original scoring system was devised for frozen samples used without antigen retrieval and with a protocol and antibody that were not easily applied to formalin-fixed paraffin-embedded tissue. This scoring system was directly applied to new assay systems for formalin-fixed tissue samples using different antibodies, different detection systems, and various conditions of antigen retrieval. Studies to validate the utility of these approaches in predicting clinical responses were not conducted, and the new assays have shown significant numbers of false positive results (40–44). To validate a scoring system, samples of known Her-2 content must be evaluated using the proposed system. One can then construct a laboratory truth table to evaluate this method and scoring system against other systems, as well as assess and publish the reproducibility of the scoring system to establish the value of the proposed new methods. (45).

INITIATIVES UNDERWAY TO IMPROVE THE QA OF TUMOR MARKER ASSAY SYSTEMS

As more and more tests for predicting responses to defined therapies are developed, the need for proper quality assurance of tumor marker assays becomes crucial. IHC assays for CD 20 and CD25, for example, are used to determine lymphoma therapy. Estrogen receptor assays by IHC are used to qualify patients for tamoxifen therapy. Guidelines for evaluating new tumor marker assay systems have been reported by several pathology experts and pathology organizations (4,17,20,26). These publications have served to call attention to the issue, which was a major topic of a recent CAP-sponsored conference on Her-2 testing (46).

Although these educational efforts are important first steps for trying to standardize tumor marker assay systems, other steps are needed, especially when refining a tumor marker system for use in clinical environments. It has become increasingly clear that guidelines for tumor marker development, much like those for clinical trial design, are needed to hasten the application of promising tumor markers in clinical practice where they can effectively guide therapy. The National Cancer Institute Cancer Diagnosis Program recognized this need and established a strategy group of clinicians and scientists to address these issues (Program for the Assessment of Clinical Cancer Tests, PACCT). The strategy group meets regularly to discuss ways in which tumor marker progress can be enhanced. The group unanimously agreed that producing a protocol to guide scientists through tumor marker development would be beneficial. This report has recently been submitted for publication (47). Elements in the process are provided in Table 4.

Studies must be done to establish the prevalence of the marker, the optimal patient population in which to examine utility, and the risk ratio of the marker presence on some outcome (prediction of therapeutic response or patient outcome). Then investigators must design a prospective clinical trial that can provide evidence of marker utility. The assay system must be standardized so that results are likely to provide definitive results. Such trials will not be guaranteed to illustrate the maximal benefit of the marker in question; refining the study population, assay procedure, or interpretation or endpoint of significance may require several trial iterations.

European investigators have recently succeeded in completing a prospective randomized multi-center trial using urokinase type plasminogen activator (uPA) and plasminogen activator inhibitor (PAI-1) in breast cancer patients. To conduct this trial, the investigators first established the type of patient population that should be tested and then standardized the assay method. They then conducted several trials to establish the value of the marker. Ultimately, they investigated these markers prospectively on a population of 553 node-negative breast cancer patients. In the recently published prospective trial, node-negative patients with low levels of UPA/PAI-1 were monitored but did not receive chemotherapy, while those with higher levels of UPA/PAI-1 were randomized to receive chemotherapy or observation. Patients with low levels had a 6.7% recurrence rate, compared to women with high levels whose recurrence rate was 14.6% (48).

The final step in the process of tumor marker development is the validation of a potentially useful marker so that it can be assimilated into routine clinical practice. The marker must be able to be assessed by a defined and well-characterized assay system that is routinely available and compliant with FDA guidelines. Beginning in 1976, the FDA regulated in vitro diagnostic devices (IVDs) as medical devices. Most clinically marketed tumor marker tests (like Her-2 testing) are classified as Class III devices and are generally subject to pre-market review through a pre-market application (PMA) approval process. Data that the product (test) is safe and effective must be provided. FDA review is generally directed at establishing the analytical and clinical performance expected for the intended use, which must also be clearly specified. Claims for product use will determine the types of review and the data necessary for review.

The PMA process is not the only mechanism by which a tumor marker can come into common clinical use. In 1996, the FDA introduced a new IVD called analytic-specific reagents (ASRs). The FDA recognized ASRs as the active ingredient in many tumor marker test assays, and established rules and restrictions for their use in order to insure quality and consistency of performance and to establish that the laboratory performing the testing was responsible. Thus, ASRs are restricted to laboratories designated by CLIA as high-complexity laboratories, which, according to the FDA, possess the expertise to adequately perform these tests according to CLIA 1988 regulations (49–52). The phase of maker development catalogued here and described by the NCI PACCT guideline provides the basis for performance of testing according to these established regulations.

Although these features will assure that the marker is reliable, they do not establish clinical utility or importance. For clinical utility to be established, clear understanding of marker utility in guiding or excluding therapy must be based on scientific evidence. The utility of a marker depends on <u>both</u> this magnitude of difference between marker-positive and marker-negative groups and whether the difference is unlikely to be due to chance alone (12). It must be clear which patient populations will benefit from marker assessment. Such understanding

Table 4 Optimal steps in tumor marker development (Hammond and Taube, 2002)

Steps in the process	Description
1. Discovery of promising markers	Promising markers are found and tested in small studies. Further testing justified by biologic rationale or number of positive studies suggesting benefit.
2. Development of assay system	Conditions of the assay system are established and described including types of specimens to test, population of interest, controls, conditions of assay, assay specificity, sensitivity, and precision
3. Preliminary clinical utility analysis	Using the specified assay, populations of patients are found in which to test the marker by determining the prevalence of the marker and predictive power of the marker for prognosis or for therapeutic efficacy.
4. Assay standardization	Assay conditions are refined so that the assay can be used across laboratories with standardized reagents, reporting criteria, and good inter-laboratory comparison.
5. Clinical utility assessment	Using the standardized assay system, the marker is tested on a population of patients to determine if the predicted utility of the marker holds true.
6. Validation of assay and clinical utility	If the marker predicts an effect or outcome with good statistical power and known prevalence, a prospective clinical trial is done to validate the observation.

depends on a variety of factors, including the strength of the tumor marker to predict benefit or patient outcome, and the toxicity of the proposed therapy or other negative factors, such as cost of treatment, insurance support, and availability of the tumor marker detection in the local region. Decisions to treat or not to treat a patient with a particular therapy are based on complex perceptions regarding the relative benefits, costs, and toxicities. These differ depending on the agent, the patient, the caregiver, and the society in which they exist (53). For a marker to have the highest level of scientific evidence validating its clinical utility, investigators must conduct a randomized control trial that conclusively proves its value. Such trials require sophisticated statistical input for proper design and implementation (which are beyond the scope of this review).

The European prospective randomized trial of uPA/PAI-1 is a good example of such a trial. Although these markers can select breast cancer patients who might not benefit from chemotherapy, patients may well select chemotherapy anyway, based on their assessment of the value of eliminating even the smallest risk of recurrence (54,55). Estrogen receptor activity as a predictive factor for tamoxifen therapy in breast cancer patients is another excellent example of such a prospective evaluation of a tumor marker (6).

Several tools that can help investigators assess available evidence about whether a marker under evaluation accurately predicts a therapeutic response or patient outcome and merits routine clinical use are available. The ASCO expert panel has constructed a system, TMUGS, for this purpose (see Chapter 3). The system includes a useful scale for determining the clinical utility of a marker based on the evidence that has been published about it (56). Frye and Thornbury have also published a hierarchy of study types for diagnostic tests, which is a useful scale to evaluate marker reports for their level of evidence. These tools will help to establish clinical utility (57). A group of distinguished statisticians recently submitted, for publication, a report to establish the information about a tumor marker that should appear in publications. This is another important step in helping to hasten progress in the field (58).

SUMMARY

Problems exist related to tumor marker assay quality assurance and the impact of variation in methods, interpretation, and reporting on the availability of clinically useful tumor marker tests. If guidelines and other publications on this subject are carefully followed in the future, it should be possible to improve the status of tumor marker research in this millennium.

REFERENCES

1. ASCO Expert Panel. Clinical practice guidelines for the use of tumor markers in breast and colorectal cancer: Report of the American Society of Clinical Oncology Expert Panel. J Clin Oncol 1996;14:2843–2877.
2. ASCO Expert Panel. 1997 update of recommendations for the use of tumor markers in breast and colorectal cancer. J Clin Oncol 1998;16:793–795.
3. Henson DE, Fielding LP, Grignon DJ, Page DL, Hammond EH, Nash G, Pettigrew NM, Gorstein F, Hutter RV. 1995 College of American Pathologists Conference XXVI on clinical relevance of prognostic markers in solid tumors. Arch Pathol Lab Med 1994;119:1109–1112.
4. Hammond MEH, Fitzgibbons PL, Compton CC, Grignon DJ, Page DL, Fielding LP, Bostwick D, Pajak TF. 2000 College of American Pathologists Conference XXXV: Solid tumor prognostic factors—which, how, and so what? Summary document and recommendations for implementation. Arch Pathol Lab Med 2000;124:958–965.
5. Simon, R. Design and conduct of clinical trials. In: DeVita Jr. VT, Hellman S, Rosenberg SA, eds. Cancer: principles and practice of oncology, 4th ed. Philadelphia, JB Lippincott Co, 1993:418–440.
6. Early Breast Cancer Trialist's Collaborative Group. Tamoxifen for early breast cancer: An overview of the randomized trials. Lancet 1998;351:1451–1467.
7. Early Breast Cancer Trialist's Collaborative Group. Polychemotherapy for early breast cancer: an overview of the randomized trials. Lancet 1998;352:930–942.
8. Altman DG. Better reporting of randomized controlled trials: the CONSORT statement. Br Med J 1996;313:570–571.

9. Altman DG, Schulz KF, Moher D, Egger M, Davidoff F, Elbourne D, Gotzsche PC, Lang T. CONSORT GROUP Consolidated Standards of Reporting Trials. The revised CONSORT statement for reporting randomized trials: explanation and elaboration. Ann Intern Med 2001;134:663–694.
10. Simon R, Altman DG. Statistical aspects of prognostic factor studies in oncology. Br J Cancer 1994;69:979–985.
11. McGuire, WL. Breast cancer prognostic factors: Evaluation guidelines. J Natl Cancer Inst 1991;83:154–155.
12. Hayes, DF, Trock B, Harris A. Assessing the clinical impact of prognostic factors: when is "statistically significant" clinically useful? Breast Cancer Research and Treatment 1998;52:305–319.
13. McGuire WL, Clark GM, Dressler LG, Owens MA. Role of steroid hormone receptors as prognostic factors in primary breast cancer. NCI Monogr 1986;1:19–23.
14. Nenci, I. Expression and modulation of estrogen receptors in human breast cancer. J Steroid Biochem 1985;23:1093–1096.
15. Marchetti E, Querzoli P, Moncharmont B, Parikh I, Bagni A, Marzola A, Fabris G, Nenci I. Immunocytochemical demonstration of estrogen receptors by monoclonal antibodies in human breast cancer: correlation with estrogen receptor assay by dextran-coated charcoal method. Cancer Res 1987;47:2508–2513.
16. Pertschuk LP, Eisenberg KB, Carter AC, Feldman JG. Immunohistologic localization of estrogen receptors in breast cancer with monoclonal antibodies. Correlation with biochemistry and clinical endocrine response. Cancer 1985;55:1513–1518.
17. Taylor, CR. The total test approach to standardization of immunohistochemistry. Arch Pathol Lab Med 2000;24:945–951.
18. Wick MR. Quality assurance in diagnosis immunohistochemistry. A discipline coming of age. Am J Clin Pathol 1989;92:844.
19. Pelestring RJ, Allred DC, Esther RJ, et al. Differential antigen prevention during tissue autolysis. Hum Pathol 1991;22:237–241.
20. O'Leary TF. Standardization in immunohistochemistry. Appl Immunohistochem Molec Morphol 2001;9:3–8.
21. Fox CH, Johnson FB, Whiting J, et al. Formaldehyde fixation. J Histochem Cytochem 1985;33:845–853.
22. Mason JT, O'Leary TJ. Effects of formaldehyde fixation on protein secondary structure: a calorimetric and infrared spectroscopic investigation. J Histochem Cytochem 1991;39:225–229.
23. Shi SR, Cote RJ, Taylor CR. Antigen retrieval immunohistochemistry: past, present and future. J Histochem Cytochem 1997;45:327–343.
24. Koonen J, Bubendorf L, Kalloniemi A, et al. Tissue microarrays for high-throughput molecular profiling of tumor specimens. Nat Med 1998;4:844–847.
25. Shi, SR, Cote, RJ, Chaiwun B et al. Standardization of immunohistochemistry based on antigen retrieval technique for routine formalin fixed tissue sections. Applied Immunohistochem 1998;6:89–96.
26. Hsi ED. A practical approach for evaluating new antibodies in the clinical immunohistochemistry laboratory. Arch Pathol Lab Med 2001;125:289–294.
27. Horne GM, Anderson JJ, Tiniakos DG et al. p53 protein as a prognostic indicator in breast carcinoma: a comparison of four antibodies for immunohistochemistry. Br J Cancer 1996;73:29–35.
28. Fetsch PA, Abati A. Overview of the clinical immunohistochemistry laboratory: regulations and troubleshooting guidelines. Methods Mol Biol 1999;115:405–414.
29. Rhodes A, Jasani B, Balaton AJ, Barnes DM, Miller KD. Frequency of estrogen and progesterone receptor positivity by immunohistochemical analysis in 7016 breast carcinomas: correlation with patient age, assay sensitivity, threshold value, and mammographic screening. J Clin Pathol 2000;53:688–696.
30. Leake R, Barnes D, Pinder S, Ellis I, Anderson L, Anderson T, Adamson R, Rhodes T, Miller K, Walker R. Immunohistochemical detection of steroid receptors in breast cancer: a working protocol. UK Receptor Group, UK NEQAS, The Scottish Breast Cancer Pathology Group, and The Receptor and Biomarker Study Group of the EORTC. J Clin Pathol 2000;53:634–635.
31. Griner PF, Mayewski R. Principles of test interpretation. In: Griner PF, Panzer RJ, Greenland P, eds. Clinical diagnosis and the clinical laboratory: logical strategies for common medical problems. Chicago: Year Book Medical Publishers 1986;1–16.
32. O Leary TJ, Edmonds F, Floyd AD, et al. Quality assurance for immunohistochemistry: approved guideline. Wayne, PA: NCCLS, 1999.
33. Taylor CR. FDA issues final rules for classification and reclassification of immunohistochemistry reagents and kits. Am J Clin Pathol 1999;111:443–444.
34. Elias JM, Gown AM, Nakamura RM, et al. Quality control in immunohistochemistry. Report of a workshop sponsored by the Biological Stain Commission. Am J Clin Pathol 1989;92:836–843.
35. Herman GE, Elfont EA. The taming of immunohistochemistry: the new era of quality control. Biotech Histochem 1991;66:194–199.
36. Altaye M, Donner A, Klar N. Inference procedures for assessing inter-observer agreement among multiple raters. Biometrics 2001;57:584–588.
37. Einstein AJ, Bodian CA, Gil J. The relationships among performance measures in the selection of diagnostic tests. Arch Pathol Lab Med 1997;121:611–620.
38. Bostwick DG, Grignon DJ, Hammond ME, Amin MB, Cohen M, Crawford D, Gospadarowicz M, Kaplan RS, Miller DS, Montironi R, Pajak TF, Pollack A, Srigley JR, Yarbro JW. Prognostic factors in prostate cancer. College of American Pathologists Consensus Statement 1999. Arch Pathol Lab Med 2000;124:995–1000.
39. Srigley JR, Amin MB, Bostwick DG, Grignon DJ, Hammond ME. Updated protocol for the examination of specimens from patients with carcinomas of the prostate gland: a basis for checklists. Cancer Committee. Arch Pathol Lab Med 2000;124:1034–1039.
40. Press MF, Hung G, Godolphin W, Slamon DJ. Sensitivity of Her-2/neu antibodies in archival tissue samples: potential source of error in immunohistochemical studies of oncogene expression. Cancer Res 1994;54:2771–2777.
41. Tubbs RR, Pettay JD, Roche PC, Stoler MH, Jenkins RB, Grogan TM. Discrepancies in clinical laboratory testing of eligibility of trastuzumab therapy: apparent immunohistochemical false-positives do not get the message. J Clin Oncology 2001;19:2714–2721.
42. Mitchell MS, Press MF. The role of immunohistochemistry and fluorescence in situ hybridization for Her-2/neu in assessing the prognosis of breast cancer. Semin Oncol 1999;26:108–116.
43. Jacobs TW, Gown AM, Yaziji H, et al. Specificity of HercepTest in determining HER-2/neu status of breast cancer using the United States Food and Drug Administration-approved scoring system. J Clin Oncol 1999;17:1983.
44. Ellis IO, Dowsett M, Bartlett J, et al. Recommendation for Her-2 testing in the UK. J Clin Pathol 2000;53:890–892.
45. Bloom KS. Her-2 Immunohistochemistry and FISH in Clinical Practice. Arch Pathol Lab Med 2002 (in press).

46. Tubbs RR. Accuracy and precision of clinical laboratory assays for Her-2/neu amplification: quality assurance, standardization, and proficiency testing. Arch Pathol Lab Med 2002 (in press).
47. Hammond MEH, Taube ST. A protocol for the development of clinically useful tumor markers. Seminars in Oncology 2002 (in press).
48. Prechtl A, Harbeck N, Thomssen C, Meisner C, Braun M, Untch M, Wieland M, Lisboa B, Cufer T, Graeff H, Selbmann K, Schmitt M, Janicke F. Tumor-biological factors uPA and PAI-1 as stratification criteria of a multi-center adjuvant chemotherapy trial in node-negative breast cancer. Int J Biol Markers 2000;15:73–78.
49. Medical Device Amendments of 1976. Pub L. No. 94-295, 90 Stat 539 1976.
50. Safe Medical Devices Act of 1990. Pub L No. 101-629, 104 Stat 4523 1990.
51. Medical Devices; Classification/Reclassification; Restricted Devices; Analyte-Specific Reagents, Federal Register 1997; 62225:62243–62260.
52. Gutman, S. The role of the Food and Drug Administration (FDA) in the regulation of in vitro diagnostic devices. Arch Pathol Lab Med 2002 (in press).
53. Ravdin P, Siminoff I, Harvey J. Survey of breast cancer patients concerning their knowledge and expectations of adjuvant therapy. J Clin Oncol 1998;16:515–521.
54. Janicke F, Prechtl A, Thomssen C, Harbeck N, Meisner C, Untch M, Sweep CG, Selbmann HK, Graeff H, Schmitt M. The German N0 Study Group. Randomized adjuvant chemotherapy trial in high-risk, lymph node-negative, breast cancer patients identified by urokinase-type plasminogen activator and plasminogen activator inhibitor type 1. J Natl Cancer Inst 2001;93:913–920.
55. Stephenson J. Study indicates utility for new breast cancer prognostic marker. JAMA 2002;285:3077–3078.
56. Hayes, DF, Bast R, Desch CE, Fritsche H, Kemeny NE, Jessup J, Locker GY, Macdonald J, Mennel RG, Norton L, Ravdin P, Taube S, Winn R. A tumor marker utility grading system (TMUGS): a framework to evaluate clinical utility of tumor markers. J Natl Cancer Inst 1996;88:1456–1466.
57. Fryback DG, Thornbury JR. The efficacy of diagnostic imaging. Med Decis Making.1991;112:88–94.
58. McShane L, Altman DG, Clark GM, and Sargent D. Publication guidelines for papers dealing with tumor markers. J Natl Cancer Inst 2001 (in press).

Chapter 5

Practice Guidelines and Recommendations for Use of Tumor Markers in the Clinic

Martin Fleisher, Ann M. Dnistrian, Catharine M. Sturgeon, Rolf Lamerz, and James L. Wittliff

The information represented in this chapter is based on recommendations formulated by the National Academy of Clinical Biochemistry (NACB) in the United States and by the European Group on Tumor Markers (EGTM). The U.S. recommendations were prepared at a National Academy of Clinical Biochemistry, NACB Laboratory Medicine Practice Guidelines (LMPG) Conference, and the European Recommendations EGTM Guidelines were developed independently by a group of scientists and clinicians meeting regularly in Europe.

Authors and contributors to the LMPG are: Dean Bajorin (Memorial Sloan-Kettering Cancer Center New York, NY), Robert C. Bast (MD Anderson Cancer Center, Houston, TX), George J. Bosl (Memorial Sloan-Kettering Cancer Center New York, NY), Daniel W. Chan (The Johns Hopkins Medical Institutions, Baltimore, MD), Gary M. Clark (The University of Texas Health Science Center at San Antonio, San Antonio, TX), Herbert A. Fritsche (MD Anderson Cancer Center, Houston, TX), Robert Kyle (Mayo Clinic, Rochester, MN), Nancy Kemeny (Memorial Sloan-Kettering Cancer Center, New York, NY), John S. Macdonald (St. Vincent's Comprehensive Cancer Center, New York, NY), and Morton K. Schwartz (Memorial Sloan Kettering Cancer Center, New York, NY).

Authors* and contributors to the EGTM Guidelines are: Walter Albrecht (Rudolfstiftung, Vienna), Vivian Barak (Hadassah University, Jerusalem, Israel), Peter Bialk* (Roche Diagnostics), Hans Bonfrer* (Netherlands Cancer Institute, Amsterdam, Netherlands), Arie van Dalen* (Institute of Tumor Marker & Oncology, Gouda, Netherlands), M. Joseph Duffy* (St. Vincent's Hospital, Dublin, Ireland), R. Einarsson* (AB Sangtec Medical), Massimo Gion (Azienda Hospital, Venice, Italy), Helena Goike (IDL Biotech AB), Gabriele Grunow (Brahms Diagnostica), Caj Haglund* (Helsinki University Central Hospital, Finland), Lars-Olof Hansson* (University Hospital, Uppsala, Sweden), Ute Hasholzner (Microbiology Laboratory, Munich, Germany), Ali Khalifa (Ain Shams University, Cairo, Egypt), Rainer Klapdor (Center for Clinical & Experimental Tumor Marker Diagnostics & Therapy, Hamburg, Germany), Peter Kuliffay (St. Elizabeth Cancer Institute, Bratislava, Slovakia), Jan Kulpa (Krakow Oncological Center, Poland), Ivan Malbohan (Charles University, Prague, Czech Republic), Rafael Molina* (Barcelona Hospital Clinic, Spain), Olle Nilsson (CanAg Diagnostics AB), Martina Radtke (Medac GmbH), Hans-Peter Schmid (Dept of Urology, St Gallen, Switzerland), Axel Semjonow* (Dept of Urology, University Clinic, Münster, Germany), Paul Sibley (Euro/DPC Ltd), György Sölétormos (Hillerød Hospital, Denmark), Petra Stieber* (Klinikum Grosshadern, University of Munich, Munich, Germany), Ondrej Topolcan (Charles University Medical Faculty, Pilsen, Czech Republic), Gian Carlo Torre (Azienda Ospedaliera, S. Corona-Pietra Ligure, Italy), Hugo Troonen* (Abbott GmbH), Hein van Poppel (University Hospital, Leuven, Belgium), Manfred Zwirner (University Hospital, Tübingen, Germany). [*Focus Group head or Publication Committee member]

The definition of a tumor marker has evolved considerably over the past two decades, principally as a result of advances in technology and redefinition by federal regulatory agencies. In general, a tumor marker is a naturally occurring molecule that is measured in serum, plasma, or other body fluids or in tissue extracts or paraffin-embedded tissues to identify the presence of cancer, to assess patient prognosis, or to monitor a patient's response to therapy with the overall goal of improving the clinical management of the patient. Tumor markers are found inside cells, both in the cytoplasm and nuclei, and they are associated with cell surface membranes; they circulate in blood.

Since most tumor markers are measured by immunochemical techniques, there are numerous pre- and postanalytical concerns regarding the type, handling, and storage of clinical specimens. In addition, in the United States, the Food and Drug Administration (FDA) has reclassified these molecules under the 1982 medical devices ruling (Classification Regulation 21, CFR Part 866, Subpart G) as "tumor-associated antigen immunological systems." Although numerous tumor markers have been introduced throughout the past two decades, only a few have received FDA approval, and the specific clinical applications have been limited as a matter of policy and clinical documentation. As a result, many other important clinical applications of tumor markers may be precluded in the United States. It is nevertheless the joint obligation of the clinician and the laboratory medicine specialist to thoroughly evaluate the reagents, to recommend reference intervals, and to establish clinical utility of the analyte in patient screening, diagnosis, therapeutic monitoring, or prognostic evaluation.

The use of diagnostic tests in the clinical setting is highly regulated by federal agencies, but tumor markers have been particularly identified for special consideration. Agencies that control the use of tumor markers in the United States include the FDA as mandated by the Medical Devices Amendment of 1976 and by the Clinical Laboratory Improvement Act (CLIA) of

1988 regulating clinical laboratory improvement; the Centers for Medicare and Medicaid Services (CMS) through management of Medicare reimbursement; the Joint Commission on Accreditation of Healthcare Organizations (JCAHO) via hospital accreditation; state and local regulations, which may be more stringent than those of CLIA; and insurance companies that carefully review new tests and their reimbursements. Complementing these efforts are those of professional societies and consumer groups concerned with the ethics of test performance and clinical application.

This chapter reviews consensus recommendations made by two such groups, the National Academy of Clinical Biochemistry (NACB) in the United States and the European Group on Tumor Markers (EGTM) in Europe.

NATIONAL ACADEMY OF CLINICAL BIOCHEMISTRY (NACB) WORKING GROUP

In May 1998, the National Academy of Clinical Biochemistry (NACB) sponsored a consensus conference to develop guidelines for the analytical performance and clinical utility of tumor markers (1). The guidelines, referred to as Laboratory Medicine Practice Guidelines (LMPG), presented recommendations on the analytical and clinical utility of tumor markers. These recommendations were reviewed by an expert panel comprised of clinical scientists and physicians who refined the recommendations and prepared a consensus document on the clinical use of tumor markers. The recommendations focused on pre- and postanalytical concerns, the use of reference intervals, and the manner in which tumor markers should be used clinically with specific attention to screening, diagnosis, monitoring, or prognosis.

EUROPEAN GROUP ON TUMOR MARKERS (EGTM)

In the mid-1980s, radioimmunoassays for new tumor markers including CA125, CA15-3, and CA19-9 became available. Under the initiative of Professor Rainer Klapdor, discussion of the clinical application of these tests was encouraged by bringing together German scientists and physicians from universities, hospitals, and the diagnostics industry in the annual Hamburg Symposia. These meetings soon became more international and a working group was subsequently established to consider the quality control and standardization of tumor markers. In 1993, this group published a consensus statement on the criteria for use of tumor markers with respect to clinical relevance, analytical methods, and manufacturing requirements (2). The group was more formally constituted as the European Group on Tumor Markers (EGTM) in 1997, with its constitution and bylaws accepted in 1999. Seven focus groups were formed to consider different types of cancer, and the initial conclusions of these groups were published in 1999.

OVERVIEW

The approach of both the NACB and EGTM groups has been similar, each group considering appropriate use of tumor markers for specific types of cancer. The EGTM also considered broad quality requirements relevant to all tumor markers. In this chapter we summarize the conclusions of both groups, highlighting differences in outlook where these are significant. In this context it is important to note that guidelines should evolve as knowledge increases: they should be reviewed and updated regularly. Here, the current guidelines developed by the two groups are considered as follows:

1. Quality requirements and control (EGTM)
2. Breast cancer (NACB, EGTM)
3. Gynecological cancer (NACB, EGTM)
4. Prostate cancer (NACB, EGTM)
5. Colorectal cancer (NACB, EGTM)
6. Neuroendocrine tumors (NACB)
7. Germ cell tumors (NACB, EGTM)
8. Monoclonal gammopathies (NACB)
9. Lung cancer (EGTM)

QUALITY REQUIREMENTS AND CONTROL

Once the decision to request any tumor marker measurement has been made, the quality of the result eventually reported will reflect events during the preanalytical, analytical, and postanalytical phases of analysis. Aspects of particular practical importance to those either providing or using a tumor marker laboratory service were considered by the EGTM (3) and are reviewed briefly here.

Preanalytical Requirements

Relevant preanalytical requirements identified by the EGTM are considered elsewhere in this book (see Chapter 4). It is important to note that reporting of erroneous tumor marker results (especially when they are incorrectly high) is more likely to cause undue alarm and distress to the patient than is the case for many other laboratory tests. This places a major responsibility on the laboratory to ensure correct results, as well as to provide clinicians with readily available information relevant to specific tests; e.g., avoiding measuring prostate-specific antigen (PSA) in a patient with prostatitis, or CA125 during menstruation.

Analytical Requirements

Satisfactory measurement of any analyte requires that the correct and appropriate specimen be analyzed by a method meeting defined quality requirements for both Internal Quality Control (IQC) and External Quality Assessment (EQA) (4). IQC and EQA issues including assay reproducibility, acceptance criteria, matrix effects, dynamic range, interferences, stability, target values, and interpretive exercises are addressed in Table 1.

While automated immunoassays generally achieve very good intra- and inter-assay variability (e.g., <5% and <10% respectively), this might not be possible with manually performed immunoassays. In keeping with recent international proposals (6), criteria for desirable precision performance can alternatively be based on biological variation (see also Chapter 4).

Table 1 Analytical considerations of particular relevance to the quality control of tumor marker measurements

Requirements of Internal Quality Control (IQC)	
Assessment of reproducibility	Demonstration of intra-assay variability <5% (desirable); inter-assay variability <10% (desirable). (Manual and/or research assays may be less precise.)
Established criteria for assay acceptance	Selection of appropriate criteria for acceptability of IQC, preferably based on logical criteria (5).
Specimens closely resembling authentic patient sera	In general it is inadvisable to rely exclusively on QC materials supplied with the kit, and an authentic serum matrix control from an independent source should be included.
IQC specimens of concentrations appropriate to the clinical application	Negative and low positive controls should be included for all tumor markers, but there is also a need to cover the broader concentration range, and to assess accuracy of dilution steps required for high concentration specimens.
Assessment of assay interferences	Occasionally checking for interferences (e.g., from heterophilic and other antibodies, clotting agents in blood clotting tubes) is desirable.
Requirements of External Quality Assessment (EQA)	
EQA specimens of appropriate analyte concentration	Concentrations covering the working range of assays are adequate, although occasional inclusion of higher concentrations to check behavior on dilution is desirable. Issue of normal analyte-free serum to check baseline security important for some analytes (e.g., AFP, hCG).
Assessment of assay "stability"	Assessment of the "stability" of results within a laboratory can readily be accomplished by issuing repeat specimens of the same pool and comparing results over time (e.g., 6–12 months).
Demonstrating accuracy and stability of target values	These are usually consensus means, as reference methods are not available for these analytes. The validity of the consensus means should be demonstrated by assessing their 1. Stability, by repeat distribution of the same pool. 2. Accuracy, by recovery experiments undertaken by supplementing pools with known amounts of the relevant International Standard (IS). [Such validation is possible for AFP, hCG, CEA, and PSA, for which there are currently accepted IS (BS 72/225, IS 75/537, IRP 63/601, and IS 96/670 respectively). The lack of IS for other tumor markers is currently being addressed.]
Interpretive exercises	These provide a valuable means of comparing practice (e.g., reference intervals, cumulative reporting of results) in different laboratories.

Table from the EGTM Consensus Recommendations (3). Used with permission.

The laboratory should also be aware of analytical pitfalls specific to the given analyte. These are discussed in greater detail elsewhere (Chapter 4) but three of the most important potential causes of erroneous tumor marker results are also summarized in Table 2.

Postanalytical and Reporting Requirements

Advances in automation have markedly increased the analytic reliability of the most frequently used tumor markers, allowing more time and attention to be focused on how to achieve most effective clinical use of these important tests. This requires attention to events in the postanalytical phase, as outlined in the recommendations of the EGTM (Tables 3 and 4).

Interpretive exercises and surveys undertaken through EQA schemes can have an important role in auditing the advisory service that laboratories provide for their clinical users. Participants are asked to provide clinical interpretation of results obtained for routine EQA specimens, and questions relating to other laboratory services may also be included; e.g., how results are reported to clinicians (10). Surveys carried out through the UK National External Quality Assessment Schemes have identified a need for improved consensus about the appropriate timing of tumor marker measurements, what constitutes a clinically significant change in tumor marker level, and reference ranges (11,12). Such surveys can enhance the educational value of EQA by facilitating between-laboratory comparison of practice and encouraging improved consensus. Perhaps this can also contribute to the much wider area of clinical audit.

BREAST CANCER

In 2002 it is expected that more than 203,500 new cases of breast cancer will be diagnosed in the United States and 39,600 women will die of the disease (13). The average American woman has an approximately 11% chance of developing breast cancer during her lifetime. Currently, more than one million women in the United States are living with Stage II, III, or IV

Table 2 Potential causes of erroneous tumor marker results

High-dose hook effect	Tumor marker concentrations routinely encountered range over several orders of magnitude. Protocols permitting identification of high-dose "hooking" are essential to avoid reporting misleadingly low results, particularly in patients for whom markers are being measured for the first time. [Hook effects can be minimized by using solid-phase antibodies of higher binding capacity, by assaying specimens at two dilutions, or by using sequential assays that include a wash step.]
Specimen carry-over	Potentially a problem whenever very high concentration specimens assayed, so should occasionally be checked.
Interference from heterophilic or human anti-mouse antibodies (HAMA)	Falsely high or low results may be obtained for patient specimens containing anti-immunoglobulin G (IgG) antibodies capable of reacting with antibodies used in the assay. Presence of HAMA, frequently induced in cancer patients who have undergone treatment with mouse monoclonal antibodies for imaging or therapeutic purposes, may also give erroneous results. [Such interference can be detected by re-assaying the specimen after treatment with a blocking agent (commercially available immobilized on tubes), by adding further non-immune mouse serum to the reaction mixture, or by re-assaying the specimen by a different method.]

Table from the EGTM Consensus Recommendations (3). Used with permission.

Table 3 Postanalytical requirements of particular importance to provision of a comprehensive tumor marker service

Factual requirements

Clinical information from the requesting doctor	Encouraging clinicians to provide very brief clinical information (eg "postoperative", "post-chemotherapy number 5") is essential if any interpretation is to be provided, and may help to identify occasional laboratory errors (e.g., mis-sampling on an analyzer).
Availability of appropriate reference ranges	Usually derived from an appropriately matched healthy population, reference ranges for tumor markers are usually most relevant for cancer patients before the initial treatment. Subsequently, the patient's own "baseline" provides the most important reference point for interpretation of marker results. If this is well established, increases even within the reference range may be clinically significant.
Knowledge of what constitutes a significant or clinically relevant change	Should include contributions of both biological variation and analytical variation. A confirmed increase or decrease of ± 25% is frequently considered to be of clinical significance, but further work is required in this area (7,8).
Defined protocol when changing methods	It may be helpful to the laboratory to indicate changes of method on tumor marker reports, but it is more helpful if the laboratory highlights whether any change is likely to have affected interpretation of the trend in marker result. [This may necessitate analyzing the previous specimen by the new method, for example, or requesting a further specimen to re-establish the baseline and/or confirm the trend in marker level.]
Knowledge of tumor marker half-lives	Defined as the time to 50% reduction of circulating tumor marker concentrations following complete removal of tumor tissue (i.e., distinct from definition as used in other settings). Of most relevance to interpretation of serum concentrations of certain tumor markers, e.g., AFP and hCG.
Objective comparison of tumor marker utility	The need to obtain objective clinical information about tumor marker utility remains a priority, and is being considered by a number of professional organizations (9).

Table from the EGTM Consensus Recommendations (3). Used with permission.

Table 4 Reporting requirements for provision of a comprehensive tumor marker service

Provision of fully cumulated results, since it is always the trend in marker concentration that is most informative. Minimal clinical details should appear on the report, to facilitate interpretation. Graphical representations may also be very helpful.

Recommendations as to the appropriate frequency of marker measurements.

Recommendations as to when confirmatory specimens should be requested. An apparent rise in marker concentration should always be confirmed by repeat measurement.

Good communication between laboratory and clinical staff, which facilitate appropriate use of these (and other) tests.

Table from the EGTM Consensus Recommendations (3). Used with permission.

breast cancer. Although medical science has not established a means of preventing breast cancer, advances in diagnosis and therapy can arrest the disease in many patients. Furthermore, a significant number of deaths due to breast cancer can be avoided by early detection; i.e., screening by breast self-examination, mammography, and/or clinical examination. Although tumor markers have not proven useful as screening tests, they provide clinically useful information for the management of these patients, primarily as predictive indicators for selection of certain therapies for primary breast cancer and as markers to monitor the clinical course of the disease.

The following have been used or suggested as markers for breast cancer:

- Estrogen and progestin receptors
- CA15-3
- BR27.29 (CA27.29)
- CEA
- HER-2/neu (c-erb B2) oncoprotein

Estrogen and Progestin Receptors

The main tumor markers used in breast cancer tissue are steroid receptors, p53, c-erb B2 (HER-2/neu), S phase, and ploidy. Steroid receptors are at present the only tissue markers accepted in standard practice (14–17). Although too recent to be considered by either the NACB or EGTM when originally drafting their current guidelines, assay of HER-2/neu is now mandatory in deciding which patients with metastatic breast cancer should receive treatment with the monoclonal antibody, Herceptin® (trastuzumab) (15).

Clinical utility of estrogen and progestin receptors. In addition to a number of characteristics of breast cancer, such as size, pathologic category, and axillary lymph node status, certain protein biomarkers are useful in assessing differences in growth rates and invasive and metastatic potential (18,19). Estrogen and progestin receptors have been used as predictive indicators of response to endocrine therapies such as tamoxifen, toremifene, and droloxifene ("anti-estrogens") (20,21), and to medroxyprogesterone acetate and megestrol acetate (progestin mimics) (22). As predictive factors, receptor levels have been used to assess potential for endocrine therapy response in both the adjuvant setting and for metastatic disease. In addition, sex hormone receptors are used to assess the likely clinical course of breast cancer patients; i.e., they are prognostic factors (19,22).

In general, patients with estrogen receptor-positive tumors have a better prognosis, at least in the short term, than those with estrogen receptor-negative malignancies (23). Approximately 30% of node-negative and up to 75% of node-positive breast cancer patients will relapse with metastatic disease and die within 10 years. Estrogen and progestin receptors have been employed as prognostic tests with other factors to distinguish breast cancer patients in both nodal classes at high risk for recurrence (poor prognosis) from those at low risk (good prognosis) (19,22). Levels of estrogen and progestin receptors should only be quantified in primary and metastatic breast cancers of both pre- and postmenopausal patients if the results would influence treatment decisions, in agreement with American Society of Clinical Oncology (ASCO) clinical practice guidelines (15). Immunohistochemical determinations should only be performed if the amount of the tissue biopsy precludes receptor quantification or if fresh tissue is unavailable.

Reference intervals. Ethical considerations mean that estrogen and progestin receptors are rarely determined in normal breast tissue from women without breast carcinoma, so well-documented reference ranges are not available. However, a number of biochemical studies using ligand-binding techniques or enzyme immunoassays have indicated that non-cancerous breast tissue adjacent to a carcinoma contains very low (i.e., <15 fmol/mg extract protein) or undetectable levels of the sex-hormone receptors (24). This has been confirmed in many studies in which estrogen and progestin receptors have been determined immunohistochemically using well-characterized antibodies. Values of 10 fmol/mg extract protein (by ligand binding) or 15 fmol/mg protein (by enzyme immunoassay) are generally used as cut-off levels (20,21,25). The presence of estrogen and progestin receptors in a metastasis of unknown origin at preliminary pathologic review often indicates the presence of a hormone-responsive primary breast carcinoma or other sex hormone-responsive primary tumor. Levels and distribution of estrogen and progestin receptors in biopsies of breast carcinomas are influenced by the age and menopausal status of the patient (Figure 1) (26). In general, biopsies from premenopausal patients with breast cancer contain lower levels of these receptors than do those from postmenopausal women with breast cancer. Since the response of breast cancer patients given administrative hormone therapy is related to estrogen and progestin receptor content in their tumor biopsies (19,20,22), quantification of receptor levels should be performed.

Estrogen receptor-beta and other sex-hormone receptor variants. Investigations have indicated that these regulatory proteins exhibit polymorphism (27). For example a new estrogen receptor gene, estrogen receptor-beta (ER-β), has been discovered, which shows considerable sequence homology with the widely studied estrogen receptor-alpha (ER-α) in both the DNA and ligand-binding domains (96% and 58% homology, respectively) (28,29). In addition the ligand-binding properties and biological activities of these two isoforms appear to be different. The co-expression of ER-β with ER-α and progesterone receptor (PR), as well as its association with the other indicators of low biological aggressiveness of breast cancer, suggest the ER-β-positive tumors are likely to respond to anti-estrogen therapy (30). The independent predictive value of ER-β remains to be established. Furthermore, almost 20 sex hormone-receptor variants discovered in the last decade show defects due to truncations, exon deletions, and point mutations (24). In order to investigate the clinical significance of these naturally occurring isoforms and variant receptors, new reagents and reference specimens must be developed.

Preanalytical concerns and specimen storage. Regardless of the chosen type of assay technique, proper selection and handling of breast tissue biopsies are essential for reproducible results. First, the tissue must be frozen at a temperature of −20 °C or less shortly after surgical excision and

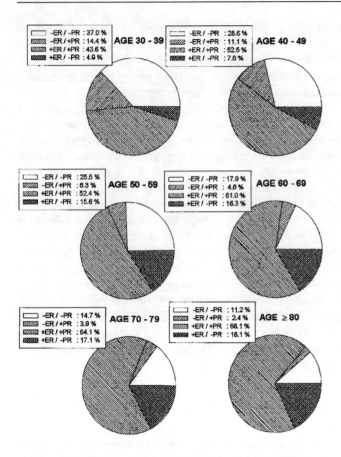

Figure 1 Distribution of sex-hormone receptor status in breast carcinoma biopsies as a function of potential for endocrine responsiveness. The four combinations of estrogen and progestin receptor status of the biopsies are given as the percentage of the total patient population examined for each age group. Reprinted with permission from Wittliff JL, Pasic R, Bland KI. Steroid and peptide hormone receptors: methods, quality control and clinical use. In: Bland KI, Copeland III EM, eds. The breast: comprehensive management of benign and malignant diseases. Philadelphia, PA: WB Saunders Co, 1998; 458–498.

transported frozen to the laboratory. Optimum cutting temperature (OCT) compound used in the preparation of frozen sections must be completely removed prior to the tissue extraction process (31). If dyes such as those of the Davidson Dye Marking Kit are present, involved tissue should be removed. Presence of large amounts of normal and hemorrhagic tissue should also be avoided.

Sex hormone receptors are unstable in tissue extracts at room temperature and lose activity at 4 °C within 2–4 hours (19). Extracts should be frozen at –70 °C immediately after assay. The stability of receptor content in these frozen extracts varies depending upon the type of tumor, involvement of hemorrhagic and normal tissue, and other factors. A fresh extract of frozen residual tissue should be prepared if the original extract is not re-analyzed within 48 hours.

Analytical concerns. The analytical precision of the currently available radioligand binding assay and enzyme immunoassay methods (which use standardized reagents and stable reference specimens) is considerably better [coefficients of variation (CVs) 4–15%] than that required for clinical decision-making (22,25). The total imprecision required to satisfy medical decision-making is 10–20% at estrogen and progestin levels of 30–50 fmol/mg extract protein (20,32). The total imprecision required at estrogen and progestin receptor levels of >100 fmol/mg protein is 30–40%.

Reporting concerns. Data on assay precision from cooperative clinical trials suggest that estrogen and progestin receptor values of less than 10–15 fmol/mg extract protein represent a clinically insignificant quantity of these analytes in human breast cancer biopsies (20–22,32). K_d values of 1 to 9 × 10^{-10} M to 1 to 9 × 10^{-11} M are indicative of high-affinity estrogen receptor-α, and K_d values of 1 to 9 × 10^{-9} M to 1 to 9 × 10^{-10} M are indicative of the presence of high-affinity progestin receptors (19). The ligand-binding characteristics of estrogen receptor-β and other variants of both sex-hormone receptors are being established. The type of assay, which determines the cut-off value, should be reported. Certain groups recommend inclusion of a receptor status distribution by decades of age since the receptor level expressed is age-related (Figure 1).

CA15-3

The CA15-3 antigen is a high-molecular-weight mucin glycoprotein termed MUC-1 (33). It has been characterized with monoclonal antibodies developed against purified extracts of a membrane fraction isolated from a human breast cancer metastasis to liver (clone DF3) (34) and against human milk fat-globule (clone 115D8). The mucin-type markers for breast cancer include BR27.29, CA-549, MCA, CA-M26, and CA-M29 (for review, see reference 35). The sensitivity and specificity of these mucins are similar and use of more than one mucin marker does not provide additional information (36,37). Only CA15-3 and BR27.29 have been approved by the FDA for following the clinical course of breast cancer patients with advanced metastatic disease.

Clinical utility. Although carcinoembryonic antigen (CEA) has been used for the detection of metastatic breast cancer (38–40), numerous recent studies have established the comparative superiority of CA15-3 (35,36). Briefly, levels of CA15-3 are elevated in 60–80% of patients with metastatic breast cancer and these levels correlate with changes in clinical status and tumor therapy response (40–45). CA15-3 also appears effective for evaluating the clinical course of patients being treated for metastatic disease. A number of studies have demonstrated that the tumor marker is useful in monitoring disease progression and regression following treatment for breast cancer (35,46,47).

The EGTM guidelines (48) suggest that by using both CA15.3 and CEA it is possible to increase the sensitivity obtained as well as the clinical utility (49,50). Some groups report that simultaneous use of both CA15-3 and CEA allows the detection of early recurrence in more patients than the use of CA15-3 alone (49,50) but there is some conflicting evidence in the literature (51). Serial determinations of markers are particularly sensitive for early detection of bone and liver metastases (49,50). Despite the ability of markers to detect recurrent disease preclinically, the long-term benefit of early detection on therapy response and patient survival has yet to be demonstrated.

It is now clear that the main use of CA15-3 is as a monitor of breast cancer activity. An objective for future work should be to provide consensus for guidelines to interpret CA15-3 sequential measurements during therapy and follow-up. There is evidence that CA15-3 monitoring of breast cancer may be more complicated than hitherto recognized (52–54). Computer simulation suggests that criteria (which must be sufficiently robust to false-positive signals) can be developed to allow rational assessment of possible recurrence and progression (55,56). However, it is clear that such criteria remain to be clinically validated.

Preanalytical concerns and specimen storage. CA15-3 measurements should be performed on specimens after prompt separation of serum from the clot. CA15-3 is stable in serum stored in plain tubes or those containing thixotropic gel when stored at 4 °C for 24 hours (35,36). Storage of serum frozen at –20 °C (short-term) and at –70 °C (long-term) is recommended to ensure stability of the analyte if the need for re-analysis occurs. For long-term storage, tubes containing thixotropic gel should not be used because of apparent instability of CA15-3.

Analytical concerns. The type, analytical precision, and reference interval of the CA15-3 assay selected should be validated within each institution to include the medical decision limits (41).

Postanalytical and reporting concerns. Additional studies should be performed to establish the influence of gender, race, age, and menopausal status on the expression of CA15-3 in normal subjects and in patients with breast carcinoma. The implications of these for quoted reference intervals should be documented.

BR27.29 (CA27.29)

BR27.29 is a newly developed member of the mucin-type breast cancer markers, which include CA15-3 (57,58). The assay was developed with antibodies against the same mucin antigen (MUC-1) using a different antibody termed B27.29. The reactive sequence of the B27.29 monoclonal antibody was shown to overlap with that recognized by the DF3 antibody used in the CA15-3 assay, using epitope mapping (34,35,57).

Clinical utility. Numerous investigations have explored the use of BR27.29 levels in the detection and diagnosis of breast carcinoma (35,58). As was concluded from CA15-3 evaluations, BR27.29 also lacks the specificity and sensitivity required for routine detection of breast cancer. Several reports suggest that BR27.29 is a more sensitive but less specific marker than CA15-3.

Collectively, many institutions have used elevations in the levels of BR27.29 to detect relapse in breast cancer patients at high risk for recurrence and to monitor disease progression in patients with advanced disease (47). These studies provide clinical evidence of the utility of BR27.29 levels in the detection of late-stage metastatic disease and suggest that elevations in the levels of this tumor marker reflect disease activity. Several studies have reported the use of BR27.29 as an aid to predict recurrent breast cancer in patients with Stage II or Stage III disease (58). Recent studies also suggest that elevations in BR27.29 levels may predict the probability of bone metastases in breast cancer patients with bone disease (40,57).

Preanalytical concerns and specimen storage. Since BR27.29 is a member of the MUC-1 family of antigens containing carbohydrate, the handling of serum or plasma samples is similar to that recommended for other tumor-associated mucin antigens. The main concern appears to be enzymatic cleavage of sequences recognized by the antibodies incorporated in the assay.

BR27.29 analysis should be performed on specimens after prompt separation of serum from the clot. Samples may be stored at 4 °C for up to 24 hours. Storage of serum frozen at –20 °C (short-term) and at –70 °C (long-term) is recommended to ensure stability of the analyte if the need for re-analysis occurs. Further research is required on the influence of freezing and thawing on the stability of BR27.29 in serum.

Analytical concerns. Each laboratory analyzing BR27.29 should ensure that the sensitivity and specificity of assays meet clinical recommendations. The type, analytical precision, and reference interval of the BR27.29 assay selected should be validated within each institution to include the medical decision limits (41).

There have been no reported interferences from common matrix effects, but further study would be desirable. A need for significant quality control is evident from studies of analytical sensitivity (35,36,41). It is strongly recommended that reference specimens of BR27.29 be developed and that proficiency surveys be implemented with the aim of improving inter-laboratory agreement of results for BR27.29.

Postanalytical and reporting concerns. It is recommended that a statement on the result report regarding the clinical utility of BR27.29 be restricted to the follow-up of breast cancer patients with advanced disease. Several institutions contributing to the NACB guidelines recommend that the laboratory report should state that the clinical utility of BR27.29 is restricted to the follow-up of breast cancer patients with advanced disease.

NACB and EGTM Recommendations for Use of Tumor Markers in Breast Cancer

1. Estrogen and progestin receptor status should be used to identify those breast cancer patients most likely to respond to hormone therapy (e.g., tamoxifen) given in the adjuvant setting. Levels of these receptors should be quantified in every primary breast cancer of both pre- and postmenopausal patients at the time of diagnosis, in agreement with ASCO Clinical Practice Guidelines. Immunohistochemical determinations should only be performed if the amount of the tissue biopsy precludes receptor quantification. Immunochemistry performed on paraffin-embedded tissue should also be the method of choice when no fresh tissue is available.

2. The total imprecision required to satisfy medical decision-making is 10–20% at estrogen and progestin receptor lev-

els of 30–50 fmol/mg of extract protein. The total imprecision required at estrogen and progestin receptor levels of >100 fmol/mg of protein is 30–40%.
3. Levels of estrogen and progestin receptors should be quantified only in those metastatic breast cancers of both pre- and postmenopausal patients if the results would aid in treatment decisions, in agreement with ASCO Clinical Practice Guidelines. Immunohistochemical determinations should be performed only if the amount of the tissue biopsy precludes receptor quantification.
4. CA15-3 or BR 27.29 determinations are useful for the early detection of breast cancer recurrences in patients previously treated for stage II and stage III carcinomas who are clinically free of disease. High CA15-3 levels in a patient with breast cancer almost certainly indicate the presence of metastatic disease.
5. Decreasing concentrations of circulating CA15-3 are indicative of successful therapeutic response, and persistent or increasing CA15-3 levels are associated with disease progression and poor response to therapy. It is therefore recommended that CA15-3 be used with caution as an aid in following the clinical course of breast cancer patients. In addition, measurement of CEA is recommended by the EGTM for the early diagnosis of distant metastases.
6. Since elevated levels of CA15-3 are observed in a number of other malignant and nonmalignant diseases, its use is precluded in screening, diagnosis, or staging of breast cancer, in agreement with the ASCO clinical practice guidelines.
7. The use of BR27.29 in the clinical setting is restricted to the follow-up of breast cancer patients with advanced disease.
8. CA15-3 should be assayed after prompt separation of serum from the clot. Samples may be stored at 4 °C for up to 24 hours. Storage of serum at –20 °C (short-term) or –70 °C (long-term) is recommended to ensure stability of the analyte if the need for re-analysis occurs. For long-term storage, tubes should not contain thixotropic gel.

Emerging Markers for Breast Cancer Management

Epidermal growth factor receptors. Epidermal growth factor (EGF) is a single polypeptide chain of MW 6000, with a high heat stability conferred by three disulfide bridges. EGF receptor protein is a complicated molecule consisting of a large extracellular domain responsible for the association with EGF, a transmembrane portion that secures the receptor in the cytoplasmic membrane, and an internal domain that contains an ATP-binding site and exhibits tyrosine kinase activity (19).

EGF receptors are present in certain breast, endometrial, and ovarian cancers, as detected by binding studies with radiolabeled EGF (59–62). As radiolabeled EGF is expensive, most investigators prefer a ligand competition assay, which measures both specific binding capacity and EGF affinity (61–64). The overexpression (i.e., increased numbers) of EGF receptors in a breast tumor biopsy appears to correlate with a shorter disease-free interval and with a decreased overall survival (63–65). In contrast to steroid hormone receptors, high levels of EGF receptors in a breast tumor biopsy appear to indicate poor prognosis. Although the ASCO clinical practice guidelines (15) did not address the use of EGF receptors, there is growing evidence of their value as prognostic factors and as predictive tests for response to new drugs targeting EGF receptor-positive breast cancer (19,63,64).

HER-2/neu (c-erb B2) oncoprotein. The *neu* oncogene, originally isolated from rat neuroblastomas, encodes a 185-kDa surface glycoprotein termed "p185 neu" and exhibits tyrosine kinase activity with a structure similar to the EGF receptor. When various molecular properties and chromosomal localization studies were conducted, it was revealed that the EGF receptor was distinct from p185 neu (19,66). The identity of the native ligand for p185 neu is the focus of research in many laboratories.

The human homologue of the *c-neu* gene, which is termed *c-erb B2*, is reportedly amplified (i.e., increased in copy number) in human breast cancer and correlates with decreased disease-free survival and lower overall survival (65,67,68). The oncogene is also called *HER-2/neu*. Furthermore, elevated levels of the HER-2/neu oncoprotein are associated with poor prognosis in breast cancer patients (69) and indicate the use of Herceptin® (trastuzumab) therapy. In 1997, the ASCO panel considered that available data were insufficient to allow recommendation of the use of *c-erb B2* (*HER-2/neu*) gene amplification or overexpression for management of breast cancer patients (15). The principal difficulties in assessing the clinical utility of this analyte are the wide variety of assays that have been used in the absence of a universally accepted reference material (61,66–68). In the ASCO 2000 update, measurements of HER-2/neu oncoprotein are recommended on every primary breast cancer either at the time of diagnosis or at the time of recurrence (15). Amplification of the *HER-2/neu* gene may also be of value (70). A recent Erratum to the ASCO 2000 update (16) contains additional recommendations relating to methods for measuring the oncoprotein and the use of results in trastuzumab therapy, and in chemotherapy selection and response. Measurements of HER-2/neu oncoprotein, either in tumor extracts or circulating extracellular domain, are not recommended for prognostic use.

Cathepsin D. Cathepsin D belongs to a class of acidic lysosomal proteases, which are found in all cells (71). The digestive pattern of cathepsin D appears to be similar in breast cancer and normal breast. This interesting protease is estrogen-induced in cultured breast cancer cells, where it is secreted as a 52-kDa precursor. Pro-cathepsin D, a phosphoglycoprotein, is cleaved to mature forms of 48-kDa, 34-kDa, and 14-kDa molecules. Monoclonal antibodies have been produced against these forms and have been assimilated into an immunoradiometric assay (IRMA) kit format (72,73). Excellent enzyme immunoassay (EIA) and enzyme-linked immunosorbent assay (ELISA) kits have also been developed for quantifying this analyte in breast cancer extracts. Evidence suggests that overexpression of cathepsin D in node-negative breast cancer correlates with shorter disease-free survival and with decreased overall survival (65,71). However, the ASCO panel concluded that there are insufficient data currently available to recommend the use of cathepsin D in the management of breast cancer patients.

Urokinase-type plasminogen activator, its receptor, and its inhibitor. The serine proteases, urokinase-type plasminogen activator (uPA), and tissue-type plasminogen activator (tPA), are known to convert plasminogen to plasmin. tPA participates mainly in intravascular thrombolysis while uPA mediates pericellular proteolysis during cell migration and tissue remodeling under physiological and pathophysiological conditions (mammary gland involution, trophoblast invasion, spermatogenesis, wound healing) (for review, see reference 74).

The enzymatically inactive form, or proenzyme of uPA (pro-uPA), is secreted by the cells and is bound to its receptor (uPAR) on the cell surface. Certain proteases (e.g., plasmin, trypsin, kallikrein, cathepsin B) convert pro-uPA (411 amino acids) to an enzymatically active, high-molecular weight form (HMW uPA, MW = 52,000), which is composed of two polypeptide chains linked by a disulfide bond [A chain (158 amino acids, MW = 32,000) and B chain (253 amino acids, MW = 20,000)]. The activated uPA subsequently converts plasminogen to plasmin. Plasmin is a broad-spectrum protease that catalyzes degradation of multiple proteins in the extracellular matrix, thus allowing invasion and metastasis. Plasminogen activator inhibitors (PAI-1 and PAI-2), which are produced by normal and tumor cells, inhibit uPA even when it is bound to its receptor (75).

uPA appears to play a role in mediating tumor cell invasion in cancer. Elevated levels of uPA, PAI-1, and PAI-2 have been demonstrated in tissue extracts of various carcinomas, including breast (75), ovary (76), uterus (77), cervix, prostate, and colon. Expression of both uPA and PAI-1 in breast carcinomas correlates with the clinical course in numerous studies (75) (for review, see ref. 74). When both are overexpressed in the same biopsy, the risk of disease recurrence and decreased overall survival is more accurately predicted (78). However, this has not been tested in a rigorous, cooperative clinical trial in North America. Two Level 1 evidence studies carried out in Europe, i.e., a prospective randomized trial (79) and a pooled analysis (78), have recently validated the prognostic value of uPA/PAI-1 in node-negative breast cancer patients (see also Chapters 8 and 41). uPA and PAI-1 are thus among the first biological prognostic factors to have their clinical value confirmed by two different Level 1 evidence studies. Advances accelerating these studies include the production of standardized ELISA kits for measuring uPA, uPAR, and PAI-1, and the availability of stable reference preparations for clinical trials.

GYNECOLOGICAL CANCER

In the Western world, gynecological cancers represent approximately 15% of all cancers in women and are responsible for approximately 10% of all cancer deaths. In terms of frequency, endometrial cancers are the most common, followed by cancers of the ovary and the uterine cervix. However, ovarian cancer has the highest mortality rates, with more women dying of ovarian cancer than from cervical and endometrial cancer combined. Annually in the United States, there are approximately 23,300 new cases with about 13,900 deaths due to the disease (80).

Ovarian Cancer

Over 90% of ovarian malignancies are epithelial tumors arising from the coelomic epithelium. Most of the remaining types are either germ cell or sex cord stromal cancers. The lack of early symptoms means that approximately 70% of patients with ovarian cancer present with advanced disease. While the overall five-year relative survival rate is on the order of 30%, the survival rate for Stage III and IV disease combined is only 10%. In contrast, a survival rate of 90% may be achieved for patients with early stage disease confined to the ovary.

At present there are no effective methods to screen for ovarian cancer in asymptomatic women. Tumor markers that would detect early ovarian cancer would be extremely useful, but available markers have not been helpful in detecting early epithelial cell cancers. The best available marker for epithelial ovarian cancer is the mucin, CA125 (81,82). Although elevated CA125 levels have been found in approximately 80% of all patients with epithelial ovarian cancer, high levels are found in only about 50% of patients with FIGO Stage 1 disease.

Use of CA 125 in screening. As a screening test, the main problems with CA125 are lack of sensitivity for early-stage disease (only about 50% of patients with Stage I have elevated levels) and lack of specificity. The EGTM guidelines state that use of CA125 cannot be recommended for general population screening to detect sporadic forms of this disease (82).

In combination with transvaginal sonography (TVS), however, CA125 may have a role in the early detection of ovarian cancer in women with a hereditary ovarian cancer syndrome. An NIH consensus statement has recommended that these women undergo at least annual rectovaginal pelvic examination and TVS, and that serum CA125 is measured (83).

Use of CA 125 in diagnosis. It is possible to make some general recommendations about interpretation of CA125 results obtained in a "case-finding" setting (84,85). Doubling of CA125 levels in serum above baseline at any interval should prompt physical examination, TVS, and abdominal computerized tomography (CT) scan. Abnormalities detected by any of these indicate the need for laparoscopy or laparotomy.

In postmenopausal women, CA125 may be useful in the differential diagnosis of benign and malignant pelvic masses. Significantly elevated values of serum CA125 (>95 U/mL) in a postmenopausal woman with a pelvic mass should prompt referral to a surgeon specializing in thorough abdominal exploration, node sampling, omentectomy, and cytoreductive operations (86).

Use of CA125 in prognosis and monitoring. The rate of decline of CA125 following initial cytoreductive surgery and during cytotoxic chemotherapy has been shown to be an independent prognostic factor in multiple trials and could be used to determine eligibility for subsequent additional chemotherapy (87,88). Following potentially curative surgery and cytotoxic chemotherapy, CA125 should be measured every three months. As above, an increase of CA125 above 35 U/mL, or a doubling of CA125 above baseline, should prompt further investigation and possible laparoscopy, if the patient is a candidate for salvage chemotherapy (89).

Doubling of an elevated CA125 value during salvage chemotherapy is associated with disease progression in more than 90% of cases and indicates failure of that particular salvage chemotherapy. However, disease can progress without a concomitant increase in CA125 and tumor deposits should be measured by physical examination or imaging whenever possible. (For reviews see ref. 90 and ref. 91).

Reference intervals. Some 95% of healthy adult women have a CA125 value of 35 U/mL or less. Postmenopausal women patients tend to have lower values (<20 U/mL in 99% of apparently healthy women). CA125 is not a specific marker for ovarian cancer and may be elevated in adenocarcinomas of the fallopian tube, endometrium, cervix, pancreas, colon, breast, and lung.

Serum CA125 levels may be elevated in benign gynecologic conditions including endometriosis, fibroids, adenomyosis, pelvic inflammatory disease, menstruation, and the first trimester of normal pregnancy. CA125 can also be elevated in plasma by benign ascites or by any condition that can inflame the peritoneum, pleura, or pericardium. Severe hepatic disease can also increase CA125 in the presence or absence of ascites. Reproducible effects of medications have not been observed.

Preanalytical concerns. Serum tumor markers containing carbohydrate generally are reasonably stable at room temperature under routine laboratory conditions. However, rapid processing of samples to minimize degradation is prudent. CA125 should be measured after prompt separation of the serum from the clot. Storage of sera at 4 °C or frozen at –20 °C (short-term) and –70 °C (long-term) is recommended to ensure stability of the analyte if the need for re-analysis occurs.

Analytical concerns. The NACB considers a CV of <15% desirable for sequential monitoring of CA125 values. At this CV, the range of 21–39 U/mL is within the 95% confidence interval for a mean value of 30 U/mL. The EGTM recommends a somewhat tighter inter-assay variability of <10% for automated tumor marker measurements (Table 1). Both biological variation and analytical imprecision should be taken into account (92).

Postanalytical and reporting concerns. Since kit reagents and formats from different manufacturers may give slightly different values, the source of the assay kit as well as the range of normal values should be indicated on the report.

NACB AND EGTM RECOMMENDATIONS FOR THE USE OF TUMOR MARKERS FOR OVARIAN CANCER

1. CA125 should not be used for screening a general asymptomatic population to detect sporadic ovarian cancer.
2. CA125 levels should be determined every six months with transvaginal sonography (TVS) performed annually as an aid in early detection of ovarian cancer in individuals with either a strong family history of breast or ovarian cancer, a demonstrated mutation in BRCA1, BRCA2, or a mismatch repair gene.
3. CA125 levels should be determined in women presenting with pelvic masses to distinguish benign from malignant lesions.
4. CA125 levels should be determined during primary therapy to predict prognosis.
5. CA125 levels may be used to document failure of salvage therapy.
6. Since loss of CA125 activity has been observed on repeated freezing and thawing, it is recommended that aliquots of sera be stored at –70 °C.

Cervical Cancer

Worldwide, cervical malignancy ranks second to breast cancer as the main cause of cancer mortality in women. In the United States, the overall five-year survival for this malignancy is approximately 70%. However, for patients diagnosed with early stage disease, the five-year survival increases to almost 90%. For squamous cell carcinomas, squamous cell carcinoma antigen (SCCA) is the marker of choice. Other markers that have been investigated in cervical cancer include carcinoembryonic antigen (CEA), human chorionic gonadotropin (hCG) beta-core fragment (hCGβcf), and cytokeratins (TPA and CYFRA 21.1), but based on currently available evidence their use for cervical cancer cannot be recommended (82).

Clinical utility of SCCA in cervical cancer. Results from SCCA determinations may be used with caution to balance prognostic variables employed to select patients in clinical trials or to identify individuals at sufficiently high risk to justify experimental adjuvant therapy. Elevated serum levels of SCCA at the time of diagnosis of stage IB or IIA cervical cancer indicate a three-fold increased risk of disease recurrence, independent of tumor diameter, grade, or the presence of lymph node metastases. Results of SCCA determinations may be used with caution to monitor disease recurrence.

Two consecutively rising SCCA values indicate progression or recurrence in 76% of cases, with false-positive elevations observed in 2.8–5%. Consequently, measurements of serum SCCA levels every three months in patients who are candidates for salvage radiotherapy or surgery may be helpful in therapy decisions, although a clinical benefit has not yet been documented.

Reference intervals for SCCA. Some 99% of apparently healthy women have an SCCA value of 1.9 µg/L or less. Values in women are higher than in men. No consistent difference has been observed between smokers and nonsmokers. SCCA is not a specific serum marker for cancer of the uterine cervix, but it is elevated in a variety of squamous cell neoplasms including cancers of the skin, lung, head and neck, esophagus, bladder, penis and anus, benign skin diseases, lung diseases, and severe renal malfunction.

Preanalytical concerns. Since large amounts of SCCA are often found in saliva, sweat, and respiratory secretions, exposure of blood to skin or saliva should be avoided.

Analytical concerns. Mean daily variations of 24% have been observed in serum levels of SCCA. Cut-off values should therefore be individualized when monitoring disease recurrence.

Postanalytical and reporting concerns. Manufacturer of kit reagents and limits of normal values should be reported. In the United States, results should be marked "for investigational use only."

Endometrial Cancer

No existing marker has the necessary sensitivity and specificity to screen for early endometrial cancer, and tumor markers contribute little to diagnosis. For monitoring patients with endometrial cancer, CA125 is the best available marker, with elevated levels found in approximately 60% of patients with recurrent endometrial cancer. However, as with SCCA in cervical cancer, there is no evidence that follow-up with serial CA125 levels enhances patient outcome. The role of CA125 in monitoring patients with uterine serous carcinoma is clinically of questionable value (93).

PROSTATE CANCER

Prostate cancer is the most common male malignancy in the United States (excluding skin cancer) and the second leading cause of male death from cancer. According to the American Cancer Society, there will be 189,100 new cases in 2002 and 30,200 men are expected to die from this disease (13). Once prostate cancer reaches an advanced stage and becomes hormone-refractory, there is no effective therapy, and prevention of the disease is not yet possible. Thus, early detection and local treatment have been advocated in an effort to influence the significant morbidity and mortality associated with the disease.

Clinical utility of prostate-specific antigen (PSA) in prostate cancer. Prostate-specific antigen (PSA) is the most important marker in the evaluation of prostate cancer and has significant application in detection and clinical management. The determination of prostatic acid phosphatase (PAP) does not add clinically useful information to PSA measurement, and is not recommended by the EGTM. PSA is associated almost exclusively with prostatic disease but is not specific for cancer and may be elevated in other conditions, including benign prostatic hyperplasia (BPH) and or prostatitis (94).

PSA in detection of prostate cancer. This lack of specificity and the inability of PSA to determine tumor aggressiveness represent the most serious limitations of PSA in the setting of prostate cancer detection. The conventional reference range for PSA is between 0 and 4 ng/mL, but there is no absolute normal cut-off value applicable to all men or all PSA assays. Approximately 25% of men with known prostate cancer exhibit normal PSA levels, whereas as many as 50% of men with benign prostatic disease will have elevated PSA levels (95). Recent data from Swiss researchers demonstrate that a significant number of prostate cancer cases are diagnosed in men with PSA values between 1 and 3 ng/mL, and the indications are that most of these tumors may be clinically significant (96).

The positive predictive value of PSA [the number of positive tests in patients with the disease divided by the total number of positive tests (true positives + false positives)] in screening populations is disturbingly low (30%). Moreover, use of certain drugs and herbal remedies that decrease serum testosterone also decrease PSA levels, confounding interpretation of results.

Reference intervals for PSA. Use of age-specific reference ranges is intended to increase sensitivity in younger men and increase specificity in older men. For younger men, using an upper reference limit of 2.5 ng/mL has been proposed to improve the early detection of organ-confined disease (97). However, this would result in an increased number of false-positive results in men without cancer. Conversely, use of higher PSA reference ranges in older men could result in the missed diagnosis of clinically significant tumors in a population that might potentially benefit from early treatment.

Although there is no consensus, some experts tend to favor using lower PSA values in younger men while using the conventional 4 ng/mL upper limit for older men. The EGTM view is that the use of age-specific reference ranges cannot be recommended yet, since only limited experience exists showing the efficacy of prostate biopsies for age-specific PSA decision points at concentrations lower than 4 ng/mL (98). In contrast, the NACB does endorse the use of age- and race-specific intervals for PSA (97,99,100). However, because of the controversy regarding the use of PSA for detecting very small tumors, the NACB does not recommend the use of a low cut-off value for PSA (2 ng/mL).

PSA in screening for prostate cancer. Despite limitations, PSA is currently the best screening modality available for the detection of early stage prostate cancer, for which there is the greatest potential for successful treatment. Apart from the use of age-specific reference ranges, there have been several attempts to increase the specificity of PSA in the detection of prostate cancer. PSA density, PSA velocity, PSA doubling time, and percent-free PSA have also been considered, but with the exception of free PSA, these strategies have not been widely used in practice. Benign disease is associated with higher levels of free PSA versus complexed PSA, and use of percent-free PSA may decrease the number of unnecessary biopsies in men with PSA concentrations in the diagnostic gray zone between 4 and 10 ng/mL (101).

Percent-free PSA may be particularly useful in identifying patients who actually have prostate cancer despite initial negative biopsy findings. In cases suspected of harboring malignant disease because the percent-free PSA indicates a high-risk profile, a cancer diagnosis may become evident with repeat biopsy (102). Some authors have reported that percent-free PSA determination also may have prognostic significance since relatively low levels of percent-free PSA have been associated with a more aggressive form of the disease (103). However reports from other authors contradict these results. The NACB and EGTM recommends the use of percent-free PSA as an aid in distinguishing prostate cancer from benign disease in highly selected subpopulations, e.g., when the total PSA level in serum is 4–10 ng/mL and digital rectal examination (DRE) is negative. This recommendation is tempered by the need to validate the medical decision limits for each combination of free and total PSA assays.

More recently, an assay has been developed to quantify the PSA complexed to alpha-1 antichymotrypsin (104,105). The measurement of this parameter results in slightly enhanced specificity as compared to total PSA (106), but no equivalence of the performance of complexed PSA to percent-free PSA has been proven yet.

Preanalytical concerns. The NACB has issued recommendations for blood drawing and handling of specimens for PSA determinations. Since a number of factors may influence PSA concentrations, it is essential that blood be drawn prior to any manipulation of the prostate, after at least 24 hours following ejaculation if free PSA is being measured (if within 24 hours, the time of last ejaculation should be noted), and several weeks after resolution of prostatitis, prostate biopsy, or transurethral resection of the prostate.

Blood should be centrifuged and serum samples refrigerated within three hours of phlebotomy. Serum may be stored at refrigerated temperatures for up to 24 hours, but samples that will not be analyzed within 24 hours of collection should be stored frozen at temperatures of at least −20 °C (preferably at least −30 °C to avoid the eutectic point). Samples requiring long-term storage should be frozen at temperatures of at least −70 °C (107,108; see ref. 109 for review). Recognizing that recommendations about specimen collection may be difficult to implement in routine practice, the EGTM has suggested that specimens be taken under preanalytical conditions as similar as possible to those used in generating the reference values of the particular assays used (98).

Analytical and reporting concerns. A statement should be appended to each report of results indicating that a single PSA measurement should not be used as a diagnostic tool for the detection and diagnosis of prostate cancer, but should be used in conjunction with a physical examination.

The report should indicate the sensitivity of the assay and the normal reference range for the test. It should include a statement saying that the results cannot be interpreted as evidence of the presence or absence of malignant disease, unless several measurements show rising PSA concentrations with a slope that cannot be explained by increases in benign prostatic tissue. The report should disclose the manufacturer of the PSA assay and state that results cannot be used interchangeably with any other method (98,110).

When monitoring patients post-treatment, a single PSA measurement should not be used as a diagnostic tool for the detection of recurrent prostate cancer. Demonstration of a rising PSA concentration is necessary.

Following radical prostatectomy, a sustained increase in PSA (based on several PSA measurements) indicates recurrence of disease. When an ultrasensitive assay is used for follow-up after radical prostatectomy (the only clinical indication for use of an ultrasensitive assay), the analytical sensitivity of the assay should be established and reported to the physician. It is essential that quality control material be available and determined at the ultrasensitive level. Within-individual biological variation may be quite high at these low concentrations, and demonstration of a sustained increase in PSA level is therefore highly desirable. The EGTM view is that clinical treatment decisions should not be made on the basis of ultrasensitive PSA assay results.

Guidelines for the early detection of prostate cancer. The American Cancer Society has issued guidelines for the early detection of prostate cancer (111). The guidelines recommend an annual screening with digital rectal examination (DRE) and serum PSA measurement beginning at the age of 50 in men at average risk with at least 10 years of life expectancy. PSA is the best biochemical test currently available for the detection of prostate cancer, but a DRE should be included whenever possible. Screening at an earlier age (45 years) would be appropriate in men at increased risk, including men of African-American descent and those with a family history. African-American men and those with one or more first-degree relatives with prostate cancer may develop prostate cancer several years earlier than other individuals and often develop a more aggressive type of cancer (112).

Individuals with a strong family history of prostate cancer involving first-degree relatives diagnosed at an early age could begin screening at 40 years of age. The recommendation for follow-up testing of these individuals would depend on the initial PSA result. Those with PSA levels less than 1 ng/mL would resume testing at 45 years of age, those with levels greater than 1 but less than 2.5 ng/mL would be tested annually, while those with levels of 2.5 ng/mL or greater would be evaluated further and considered for biopsy (113).

These guidelines are not an endorsement for mass screening for prostate cancer in men at average risk for the disease. Rather, the guidelines recommend that men be offered screening, but only after careful consideration of the benefits and limitations of prostate cancer testing. The essential difference in more recent recommendations for the detection of prostate cancer is the greater emphasis on informed decision-making by the patient. The revised guidelines emphasize that patients should be counseled concerning the risks, benefits, limitations, and potential harms associated with testing. It is important to indicate the disparity between incidence and mortality associated with prostate cancer and that many more men are diagnosed with prostate cancer than eventually die from the disease (114). It is therefore essential to put the proper emphasis on the risk and benefits associated with screening: the physician must not overestimate the possible benefits of early detection or underestimate the risks associated with early intervention. Men should also be informed that there are many uncertainties concerning treatment of early-stage disease and that the preferred treatment for clinically localized prostate cancer is not known (115).

Merits of early detection of prostate cancer. There is still considerable debate regarding the merits of early detection of prostate cancer and not all physician organizations advocate routine screening. While the American Urological Association and the NACB endorse the American Cancer Society policy statement on the early detection of prostate cancer, other organizations differ about the benefit of prostate cancer screening. Arguments against screening are based on the fact that there is no conclusive evidence that early detection and treatment influence overall mortality, while the standard treatments for organ-confined prostate cancer are associated with significant and frequently irreversible side effects. Thus, the US Preventive Task Force, the American Academy of Family Physicians, the American College of Physicians, the National Cancer Institute (NCI), and the EGTM do not recommend population-based prostate cancer screening. The overriding concern is that screening will result in over-diagnosis and over-treatment of early stage disease that may not be clinically significant (116). The view of the EGTM is that application of screening to the general population should depend on the results of prospective randomized studies showing that early detection and treatment can decrease prostate cancer mortality.

Several prospective randomized studies are already in progress to evaluate the impact of prostate cancer screening on survival from prostate cancer, but it will be several years before the controversy regarding prostate cancer screening will be resolved. The NCI and the US Public Health Service are conducting long-term, multi-center prostate cancer screening trials, and other large prospective studies are in progress in Canada and Europe (117). In the absence of definitive data from prospective randomized trials, evidence for the efficacy of testing has depended largely on demonstration of some association between prostate cancer testing and reduced prostate cancer mortality (118).

At present, there is no clear-cut evidence that screening is effective in saving lives. One study of registry data from Tyrol, Austria (where prostate cancer screening has been widely accepted), indicates a significant recent decline in the expected death rate from prostate cancer (119). This is in contrast with other parts of Austria where mortality rates have declined, but to a much lesser extent. The decrease in observed mortality was associated with a shift towards a more favorable stage at diagnosis with an increase in the proportion of organ-confined disease at presentation (120,121). The implications are that early detection and the availability of effective treatment resulted in a corresponding improvement in disease-specific survival. Trend data from the National Cancer Institute's Surveillance, Epidemiology, and End Results (SEER) program also suggest a decrease in prostate cancer mortality associated with a more favorable stage at presentation. Another indication that screening may be effective comes from a study conducted in Olmsted County, Minnesota, where a decline in the rate of advanced disease was linked with a corresponding improvement in survival (122).

Even though recent data suggest that the apparent stage shift to early disease and subsequent treatment of localized prostate cancer detected with PSA has positively influenced mortality rates, there is no conclusive irrefutable evidence that early intervention alters the natural history of the disease (123). Observed benefits may be the result of lead-time bias. The stage at diagnosis may be more dependent on the biological behavior of the tumor (aggressiveness) than on delay in presentation, and early detection may not have a significant impact on mortality. It is unlikely that the decline in prostate cancer mortality is entirely attributable to PSA testing, and more aggressive treatment of localized prostate cancer may account for some of the change in the mortality statistics (124).

PSA in patient management. Treatment decisions for early-stage disease are perplexing since there are controversies about optimal therapy. Options for patients include expectant management (watchful waiting), radical prostatectomy, or radiation therapy (external beam radiation or brachytherapy). Patients with advanced metastatic disease usually undergo some form of hormonal therapy to achieve androgen deprivation and those with hormone-refractory disease may be entered into experimental chemotherapy protocols. PSA plays a vital role in the follow-up of prostate cancer patients during different phases of management, including surveillance, determination of eligibility for treatment, estimation of prognosis, and post-therapeutic monitoring. (Free PSA has not been shown to offer clinically relevant information and should not be determined during follow-up of prostate cancer.)

Radical prostatectomy is an option only for patients with organ-confined disease, but evaluation of the extent of disease and predicting response to surgical removal of the prostate have proven difficult. Attempts have been made to use biochemical parameters in estimating the probability of organ-confined disease but PSA as a single marker is not useful in this regard (125). However, the combination of PSA, clinical stage, and Gleason score has proven informative in the prediction of pathological stage for localized prostate cancer; predictive tables incorporating these parameters have been published (126). Physicians have used these tables to estimate the probability of organ-confined disease and determine whether the patient is a candidate for radical prostatectomy.

Following successful surgery, PSA should decrease to undetectable levels, persistently elevated PSA providing evidence of residual disease. However, undetectable PSA following surgery does not necessarily mean that the disease is cured, since approximately 35 percent of these patients will exhibit a detectable PSA elevation within 10 years following surgery. A rising PSA level after radical prostatectomy is a sign of relapsing disease and may pre-date other signs of progression by years (127). Following endocrine therapy, PSA does not always reflect the behavior of the tumor. Anti-androgenic medication can lead to low PSA concentrations although prostate cancer is present.

The use and interpretation of serial PSA data for assessing outcomes and determining prognosis still present major challenges to the clinician. Not all patients with biochemical recurrence will progress to metastatic disease or symptoms of disease in their lifetimes and not all patients will need to be treated (128). Factors reported to predict the time course to the development of metastatic disease include time to biochemical recurrence, Gleason score, and PSA doubling time (129). These parameters have been incorporated into an algorithm to estimate the likelihood of patients remaining free of overt metastatic disease. Use of this diagnostic tool allows physicians to stratify patients into low-risk and high-risk categories and to make better treatment decisions.

Monitoring response after initial treatment and evaluating outcome during subsequent therapy are significant clinical applications of PSA determinations. PSA levels provide essential information about the efficacy of surgery or radiation therapy, help establish the possibility of residual disease (local or distant), signal recurrent metastatic disease before it can be detected by other conventional diagnostic procedures, and provide a useful adjunct in the evaluation of therapeutic response.

Knowledge of post-treatment PSA values can enhance quality of life when they suggest absence of residual disease. Conversely, however, increasing PSA values can lead to diminished well being in otherwise asymptomatic patients who may anticipate the clinical progress of the disease by rising PSA values months or years prior to the appearance of symptoms. The possible drawbacks of PSA determinations following treatment should always be weighed against the therapeutic means that can be offered to the patient in case of rising PSA values. However the clinical status of prostate cancer patients requires constant reassessment, and PSA can play a central role throughout the disease process.

Advances in patient management—use of nomograms incorporating PSA for treatment decisions. The development and validation of prognostic nomograms (computerized models) incorporating PSA, Gleason score, and clinical stage to assist in determining eligibility of patients for treatment and in making informed treatment decisions reflect the most recent advances in patient management. Prediction is central to strategy, and nomograms provide the most accurate predictions currently available for most clinical situations and outcomes (130). Rather than relying on physician experience or general risk assessments of patient populations with similar characteristics to determine the optimal approach, nomograms provide specific information with maximum predictive accuracy.

During initial prostate evaluation, nomograms help determine whether biopsy is indicated, whether treatment is necessary, and which treatment would offer the best prognosis. After definitive therapy, where there is uncertainty concerning efficacy of treatment, nomograms provide prognostic information by estimating risk of recurrence. For patients with biochemical recurrence (rising PSA), nomograms indicate whether the patient requires further therapy and may help guide treatment strategies.

Predictive outcomes provided by computer models are not perfect, but nomograms can be extremely useful for making treatment decisions. The difficulty arises in the selection of the appropriate device when several competing nomograms may be applicable. At present, predictive models are available for determining outcomes for patients considering radical prostatectomy, three-dimensional conformal radiation therapy, and brachytherapy. A predictive model for expectant management is under development to assist in clarifying the risks and benefits of treatment versus watchful waiting.

NACB and EGTM Recommendations for Use of PSA in Prostate Cancer

1. The NACB and the EGTM agree with the American Cancer Society recommendation that for diagnosis, PSA must not be used alone, but should be evaluated in conjunction with DRE.
2. Given the controversy regarding the use of PSA for detecting very small tumors, a low cut-off (2 ng/mL) is not recommended.
3. The use of age- and race-specific reference intervals for each PSA assay is strongly recommended by the NACB, but age-specific reference ranges are not recommended by the EGTM.
4. The use of percent-free PSA is recommended as an aid in distinguishing prostate cancer from BPH when the total PSA level in serum ranges from 4–10 ng/mL and DRE is negative. This recommendation is tempered by the need for proper validation of the medical decision limits for each combination of free and total PSA assays within each institution.
5. It is recommended that blood be drawn before any manipulation of the prostate and several weeks after resolution of prostatitis.
6. The following recommendations apply to sample handling:
   - Samples should be centrifuged and refrigerated within three hours of phlebotomy.
   - Samples may be stored at refrigerated temperatures for up to 24 hours.
   - Samples that will not be analyzed within 24 hours of collection should be stored frozen (at least at −20 °C, and preferably at −30 °C or less).
   - For long-term storage, samples should be frozen at −70 °C or less.
7. It is recommended that when an ultrasensitive assay is used for clinical purposes, the lowest reportable concentration should be determined by the laboratory and reported to physicians. Quality control at such levels should be established. The contribution of within-individual biological variation (which may be quite high at these low concentrations) should also be taken into account.
8. It is recommended that the following statements and information be appended to each report of results:
   - PSA used in conjunction with DRE.
   - The name of the assay.
   - The analytical sensitivity of the assay.
   - A valid reference range specifically generated for the assay used. (Ethnic or regional differences between reference range populations should be considered.)

COLORECTAL CANCER

Colorectal cancer is a leading cause of cancer death in the United States (representing 11% of all cancer deaths), and is second only to lung cancer. According to the American Cancer Society, there will be 148,300 new cases in 2002 and 56,600 people are expected to die from this disease (13). The five-year survival is about 90% when colorectal cancer is diagnosed at an early stage, but most cases are detected only after the cancer has spread and cure is not possible (120). Screening is key to controlling colorectal cancer since early detection and removal of adenomas that give rise to cancer have a major impact on survival (111). Tumor markers have not been useful in screening because of lack of specificity, but are a useful adjunct in predicting recurrence and assessing efficacy of treatment (15).

Guidelines for the Early Detection of Colorectal Cancer

The American Cancer Society has advocated screening for colorectal cancer for the past two decades and has issued guidelines for early detection of the disease (111). The updated guidelines for 2001 provide several options for screening patients with an average risk for colorectal cancer, as well as for screening high-risk groups (those at greater than twice the average risk). Since colorectal screening utilization among individuals is low, these guidelines allow for greater flexibility in achieving screening goals.

Most patients (75%) who develop colorectal cancer exhibit no specific risk factors for the disease and are considered to be at average risk (131). The first option for average-risk adults 50 years of age or over is annual fecal occult blood testing (FOBT), which has been shown to decrease the risk of death by about one-third when performed routinely (132). Other options for screening at intervals of five years include flexible sigmoidoscopy (with or without FOBT) or double contrast barium enema. Flexible sigmoidoscopy is considered a reliable screening test for cancer within reach of the sigmoidoscope (133,134); combined with FOBT, which screens for cancer anywhere in the colon, sigmoidoscopy is even more effective (135). Double contrast barium enema refers to a procedure that allows radiological examination of the entire colorectum; however, this method is rather insensitive for visualizing smaller neoplasms. A final option is colonoscopy, the most sensitive method (136,137), recommended once every 10 years for individuals at average risk for colorectal cancer. A shorter time interval may be desirable in certain cases.

Individuals at increased risk for colorectal cancer are those with inflammatory bowel disease, familial adenomatous polyposis, hereditary nonpolyposis colorectal cancer, or a family history of cancer (111,138). High-risk individuals are more likely to benefit from screening at an earlier age and in many cases require special screening approaches and more intense follow-up surveillance. A family history for colorectal cancer involving one first-degree relative with either colon cancer or an adenomatous polyp increases an individual's risk approximately two-fold; these individuals develop cancer approximately 10 years sooner than those of average risk. Colorectal screening guidelines therefore recommend that men and women with a family history be offered screening at 40 years of age.

Merits of Early Detection of Colorectal Cancer

Most colorectal cancers arise from precursor adenomatous polyps, lesions that may take as many as 10–12 years to progress to the malignant state (138). This long interval for cancer development offers a substantial opportunity for intervention before cancer actually develops. There is now considerable evidence to indicate that screening, diagnosis, and removal of the polyp are effective in decreasing the incidence and mortality of colorectal cancer (131).

Procedures for early detection can at the same time identify and remove precancerous adenomatous polyps, thereby preventing the development of colorectal cancer (111). In addition to prevention of colon cancer by polypectomy, screening enables the detection of early-stage cancers that can be treated with significantly less morbidity. Most importantly, screening for colorectal cancer not only results in a shift to an earlier stage of disease, but in randomized controlled trials, screening is associated with a decrease in disease-specific mortality. Unfortunately, screening rates for colorectal cancer are low, and the major challenge is to increase public awareness and implement effective colorectal cancer detection programs (131).

Clinical Utility of Carcinoembryonic Antigen (CEA) in Colorectal Cancer

A panel of the American Society of Clinical Oncology (ASCO) has developed guidelines for the use of tumor markers in colorectal cancer (15). CEA is considered the marker of choice, but CEA has no role in detection and diagnosis. Although CEA may identify the occasional patient with colorectal cancer, the high false-positive rate is unacceptable (139). Furthermore, there are no data to indicate that screening with CEA would have an effect on survival. The ASCO panel therefore does not recommend CEA testing for colorectal cancer screening. It is generally agreed that the primary role of CEA in the management of colorectal patients is as an adjunct in determining prognosis, monitoring for recurrence, and assessing response to therapy. Similar proposals have been published by the EGTM (140).

Pre- and immediately postoperative measurement of CEA. The ASCO panel recommends that CEA measurement may be requested prior to surgical intervention in patients with colorectal cancer because the test may be useful as a prognostic indicator to complement pathologic staging and surgical treatment planning (141). In a recent consensus conference, the American Joint Committee on Cancer has proposed that CEA be included in the TNM staging system for colorectal cancer (142).

The ASCO recommendation is based on the panel's conclusion that most studies indicate that abnormal preoperative CEA values are associated with a higher risk of recurrence and a worse prognosis (143). However, despite the increased risk, there is no evidence that patients benefit from adjuvant therapy solely on the basis of an abnormal preoperative CEA level. In certain studies, preoperative levels of CEA have been shown to be prognostic in patients with Dukes' B stage disease, approximately 40–50% of these patients having aggressive disease. Recent preliminary data suggest that adjuvant chemotherapy has a modest but detectable beneficial effect on the outcome of patients with Dukes' B stage disease. It has yet to be established, however, whether CEA measurement can identify the patients within this subgroup who could benefit from adjuvant chemotherapy. Consequently, the panel does not endorse the use of CEA to select patients for adjuvant therapy. An elevated postoperative CEA is also an adverse prognostic indicator (144), but this information is not clinically relevant in terms of any major outcomes. The recommendation is that the CEA test should not be used in the immediate postoperative period.

Monitoring with CEA following surgery. There is a limited role for CEA as an indicator for asymptomatic recurrence. CEA elevations frequently precede clinical evidence of disease progression by several months (145–147) and may be the first sign of a potentially curable recurrence. For identifying recurrences in patients with diagnosed colorectal cancer, CEA reportedly has a sensitivity of about 80% (range 17–89%) and a specificity of approximately 70% (range 34–91%). CEA testing was found to be most sensitive for diagnosing hepatic or retroperitoneal disease and relatively insensitive for local, peritoneal, or pulmonary involvement.

Some investigators have reported that a slowly rising CEA usually indicates locoregional recurrence, while rapidly increasing levels usually suggest hepatic metastasis. The value of CEA in detecting local recurrence was recently evaluated in a single institution prospective randomized trial (148). In this study with 207 patients, an elevated CEA value was the most frequent indicator of local recurrence without symptoms. The authors concluded that for the diagnosis of local recurrence, CEA measurement was more cost-effective than other procedures, including computerized tomography (CT). It was also suggested that intensive follow-up with CEA might be more beneficial for patients with rectal cancer than for those with colon cancer, as local recurrence is more frequent for rectal cancer.

The value of resecting recurrent cancer is controversial since early detection may not necessarily lead to a better outcome and there are no data to indicate that initiating therapy solely on the basis of an elevated CEA improves survival. However, two meta-analyses support the potential value of early detection of recurrence (149,150). The first meta-analysis, while not discriminating between the effect of follow-up intensity and CEA testing on survival, considered pooled data from various small-scale randomized and comparative cohort studies. A statistically significant difference in cumulative five-year survival was demonstrated for patients undergoing intensive follow-up, as compared to a control group not offered such follow-up. (Intensive follow-up as defined in this study included clinical history, physical examination, and CEA testing at least three times per year for at least two years.) The second meta-analysis indicated that intensive monitoring only improved five-year survival rates if CEA assays were included.

Resection of isolated hepatic metastasis, if detected early, may enhance survival and quality of life (151). The ASCO panel therefore recommends that if resection of liver metastases would be clinically indicated, CEA testing should be performed postoperatively every two to three months in patients with stage II or stage III disease for about two years after diagnosis. If an abnormal CEA is confirmed, further evaluation for metastatic disease is essential before any therapy is initiated.

Monitoring with CEA following chemotherapy and in advanced disease. Although surgery remains the most effective therapy for colorectal cancer, chemotherapy (e.g., with 5-fluorouracil and levamisole) is finding increasing use, especially in patients with advanced disease. CEA may be measured to assess response to treatment and is particularly useful in assessing metastases without easily measurable disease (152). It is important to note that transient elevations of CEA levels may occur following administration of 5-fluorouracil/levamisole (153).

CEA alone should not be used to determine the type or duration of treatment but can be used in evaluating disease status and may contribute additional information to that afforded by other clinical and diagnostic criteria (150). In the setting of metastatic disease, CEA accurately reflects disease activity and allows the physician to recognize and discontinue ineffective therapy (154). Although there is no consensus regarding the value of CEA in the management of advanced colorectal cancer, the NACB, ASCO, and EGTM all recommend the use of CEA for monitoring therapeutic response.

The ASCO panel regards CEA as the marker of choice for monitoring patients with advanced colorectal cancer but also recognizes that the serum test alone may not be sufficient for monitoring response to treatment. In evaluating response, ASCO and the EGTM recommend that CEA should be measured before the initiation of therapy and at regular intervals every two to three months thereafter, at least for the first two years after initial diagnosis.

Progressive disease may be documented with two successive CEA values that are above baseline, even in the absence of other confirmatory diagnostic criteria. This is based on the view that the predictive value of CEA is high enough to preclude the need for confirmatory testing. These recommendations represent a useful approach to the management of patients with advanced disease; but the value of this strategy in terms of clinical outcome and cost effectiveness remains to be determined.

While a clear benefit for serial CEA determination has not yet been shown in prospective randomized trials, the EGTM view is that CEA may be of use in the follow-up of certain patients with diagnosed colorectal cancer, i.e., to detect asymptomatic recurrences that can be operated on with intention to cure. Furthermore, the use of CEA in the follow-up of patients may prolong the interval between radiological examinations and may even reduce the number of these examinations required, albeit without wholly replacing them. This may help reduce cost and improve patient compliance. However, the following caveats must always be kept in mind when serially monitoring patients with diagnosed colorectal cancer:

- CEA elevations usually only occur in patients with advanced disease.
- Not all patients with recurrent colorectal cancer will exhibit increased levels.
- High levels may occur in conditions unrelated to recurrence.
- Certain cytotoxic therapies may transiently increase CEA concentrations.

NACB AND EGTM RECOMMENDATIONS FOR USE OF CEA IN COLORECTAL CANCER

1. CEA testing is not recommended for colorectal cancer screening.

2. CEA may be ordered prior to surgical intervention in patients with colorectal cancer to complement pathologic staging and treatment planning.
3. CEA should not be used in the immediate postoperative period.
4. CEA testing may be performed postoperatively if resection of liver metastases would be clinically indicated.
5. CEA may be measured during treatment to monitor response to therapy and to document progressive disease.

NEUROENDOCRINE TUMORS (PHEOCHROMOCYTOMA, NEUROBLASTOMA, CARCINOID TUMORS)

Neuroendocrine tumors arise from neural crest cells and include pheochromocytoma, neuroblastoma, medullary carcinoma of the thyroid, islet cell carcinoma, carcinoid of the gut, and Merkel cell tumors (155,156). An important clinical feature of all neuroendocrine tumors is that they produce and secrete excessive amounts of physiologically active compounds that are normally found in blood and urine, but at lower non-pathologic concentrations. In many instances, pathology is associated with elevated levels of tumor markers, and this feature may be diagnostic of the disease. Tumor markers associated with different neuroendocrine tumors are listed in Table 5.

In each cancer the tumor marker should be utilized for case finding to confirm the existence of disease. Consecutive normal levels of the tumor marker do not necessarily rule out the presence of disease. Laboratory tests, appropriately used, are important and useful adjuncts for the diagnosis of neuroendocrine tumors (157). As described in detail below, major concerns with all these tumor markers are the need for rigorous specimen collection and preservation, and the effects of iatrogenic interferences.

Catecholamines

Collection of urine for determination of catecholamines. A 24-hour urine specimen must be refrigerated immediately after collection. Sample preservation can be enhanced by maintaining an acid pH of 2–4 with the addition of 6N hydrochloric acid (HCl). The sample acidity should not be lower than pH 2 as assay interference may result. If HCl is added to the collection container prior to collection, 6 mL of 6N HCl will be satisfactory in maintaining pH for adult collections (based on urine output of 1–2 L/24-hour period). Acid preservation should be adjusted for volume in pediatric specimen collection.

Collection of plasma for determination of catecholamines. A heparinized, anti-coagulated blood specimen should be collected from the patient, who should be calm and/or in a supine position for 30 minutes prior to collection. The specimen should be chilled in ice water immediately after collection and the plasma separated as soon as possible (158). The specimen must be frozen immediately. Specimens are stable at –70 °C for 6–8 months, but the analytes are unstable at ambient temperature, or 4 °C.

Iatrogenic-related problems influencing the determination of catecholamines. Urinary catecholamines may be extremely elevated (sometimes unpredictably) as a result of medication that directly interferes with the assay or due to physiologic interference (157,159,160). Medications such as alpha-methyldopa (Aldomet) interfere with the quantitation of dopamine. Monoamine oxidase (MAO) inhibitors also affect physiologic levels of catecholamines. Plasma catecholamines cannot be quantified in patients receiving isoproterenol, isoetharine, or labetalol.

Reference ranges for catecholamines. High-performance liquid chromatography (HPLC) is the analytical method of choice for measurement of catecholamines (158,161,162). Age-related reference ranges obtained using this technique are shown in Table 6.

Vanillylmandelic Acid (VMA) and Homovanillic Acid (HVA)

Collection of urine for determination of VMA and HVA. The 24-hour collection procedure is the same as that for catecholamines. VMA and HVA can also be determined in random specimens and reported as a ratio of VMA or HVA to urinary creatinine.

Iatrogenic-related problems influencing the determination of VMA and HVA. The effects of some drugs on VMA and HVA determinations may not be predictable. Medications that may interfere are shown in Table 7. A markedly elevated total catecholamine concentration accompanied by a normal VMA suggests that the patient is taking methyldopa, which is metabolized to α-methylnorepinephrine and is not consistent with the presence of a pheochromocytoma (163).

Reference ranges for VMA and HVA. HPLC is the analytical method of choice for measurement of VMA and HVA.

Table 5 Neuroendocrine tumors and the tumor markers associated with them

Disease	Laboratory tests used in diagnosis and monitoring
Pheochromocytoma	Urinary and plasma catecholamines
	Epinephrine, norepinephrine, dopamine
	Vanillylmandelic acid (VMA), homovanillic acid (HVA)
Medullary thyroid carcinoma	Calcitonin
Islet cell carcinoma	Insulin[a] (nonspecific)
Carcinoid of the gut	Urinary 5-hydroxyindoleacetic acid (5-HIAA)

[a] Not recommended as a marker for this tumor.

Table 6 Age-related reference ranges for catecholamines (measured by HPLC)

Age (years)	Norepinephrine (µg/total volume)	Epinephrine (µg/total volume)	Dopamine (µg/total volume)
0–1	0–10	0–2.5	0–85
1–2	1–17	0–3.5	10–140
2–4	4–29	0–6.0	40–260
4–7	8–45	0.2–10	65–400
7–10	13–65	0.5–14	65–400
10–15	15–80	0.5–20	65–400

Age-related reference ranges obtained using this technique are shown in Table 8.

Hydroxyindoleacetic Acid (5-HIAA)

Measurement of the urinary excretion of 5-HIAA, the major metabolite of serotonin, has been the principal laboratory test for the diagnosis of serotonin overproduction in carcinoid tumors (164). Serotonin is one of many vasoactive substances contributing to the carcinoid syndrome of flushing, diarrhea, and cardiac valvular disease. The absence of 5-HIAA in patients suspected of having carcinoid tumor may be due to its intermittent secretion.

Collection of urine for determination of 5-HIAA. The 24-hour collection procedure is the same as that for catecholamines.

Iatrogenic and food-related problems influencing the determination of 5-HIAA. Patients should be instructed to abstain from certain foods rich in serotonin and other indoles as well as medications. Common foods and medications that should be avoided are listed in Table 9.

Reference range for 5-HIAA. HPLC is the analytical method of choice for measurement of 5-HIAA. The reference range with this method is 3–15 mg/dL.

Medullary Thyroid Carcinoma (MTC)

Medullary thyroid carcinoma (MTC) is a neoplasm of the calcitonin-secreting parafollicular or C-cells of the thyroid gland and represents approximately 10% of all thyroid cancers. While follicular cells of the thyroid gland metabolize iodine and produce and elaborate thyroid hormones (i.e., T_3 and T_4), the C-cells produce and secrete calcitonin (165).

Indications for measurement of calcitonin. Calcitonin determinations should be performed on patients who are suspected to have MTC because elevations in calcitonin levels are highly specific for the diagnosis and follow-up of MTC. In most patients with MTC, the concentration of calcitonin is sufficiently elevated to be diagnostic for the tumor. Indeed, calcitonin may be elevated prior to any clinical evidence of a tumor. There is also a positive correlation between tumor mass and circulating calcitonin concentration. After treatment of MTC by total thyroidectomy, calcitonin measurements should be used to monitor the patient for recurrent disease (166,167).

Specimen collection and handling for calcitonin. Calcitonin can be measured in serum or plasma (EDTA). Specimens should be processed immediately following collection and stored at 2–8 °C for a maximum of one day or frozen (–20 °C) for no more than 15 days. Rapid processing of specimens for calcitonin analysis is required. Specimens should be separated in a refrigerated centrifuge and serum (or plasma) should be frozen quickly in plastic tubes.

Interpretation of provocative tests for MTC. Calcitonin is the only biochemical marker that can be used to detect the

Table 7 Medications that may interfere with VMA and HVA determinations

Amphetamines and amphetamine-like compounds
Appetite suppressants
Bromocriptine
Buspirone
Caffeine
Carbidopa-levodopa (Sinemet)
Clonidine
Dexamethasone
Diuretics (in doses sufficient to deplete sodium)
Methyldopa (Aldomet)
MAO inhibitors
Nose drops
Propafenone (Rythmol)
Tricyclics
Vasodilators

Table 8 Age-related reference ranges for vanillylmandelic acid (VMA) and homovanillic acid (HVA) (measured by HPLC)

Age	VMA (µg/mg creatinine)	HMA (µg/mg creatinine)
1 day	<17	<42
3 months	<16	<39
6 months	<15	<37
9 months	<14	<35
1 year	<13	<33
1.5 years	<12	<29
2 years	<11	<26
3 years	<10	<22
4 years	<9	<19
5 years	<8	<17
6 years	<8	<14
7 years	<7	<13
8 years	<7	<12
9 years	<7	<11
10 years	<6	<10
11 years	<5	<9
18 years and adult	1.08–4.23	0.5–4.2

Table 9 Foods and medications that may interfere with the measurement of urinary 5-HIAA

Decreased 5-HIAA values	Increased 5-HIAA values	
Medications	*Medications*	
Aspirin	Acetaminophen	Methamphetamine (Desoxyn)
Chlorpromazine	(Thorazine)	Acetanilid Naproxen
Corticotropin	Caffeine	Nicotine
Dihydroxyphenylactic acid	Coumarin acid	Phenacetin
Ethanol	Ephedrine	Phenmetrazine
Gentisic acid	Fluorouracil	Phenobarbital
	Glycerol	Phentolamine
Homogenistic acid	Guaiacolate (guaifenesin)	Rauwolfia
	Melphalan (Alkeran)	Reserpine
Hydrazide derivatives	Mephenesin	Robaxin
Imipramine (Tofranil)		Valium (Diazepam)
Isocargoxazid (Marplan)		
Levodopa ← Methocarbamol		
Keto acids	*Foods*	
Monoamine oxidase (MAO) inhibitors	Avocados	
Methenamine	Bananas	
	Coffee	
Methyldopa (Aldoclor)	Eggplant	
Phenothiazine (Compazine)	Plums	
Perchlorperazine	Pineapple	
Promazine	Tomatoes	
Promethazine (Mepergan)	Walnuts	

presence of the tumor before clinical symptoms have evolved in patients with occult C-cell carcinoma or suspected familial MTC (168). As a marker for provocative testing using pentagastrin or calcium, calcitonin levels exceeding four times the upper reference limit or that of the basal values are diagnostic for MTC. In normal individuals, pentagastrin stimulation will result in calcitonin levels less than four times the upper limit of normal, with calcitonin normalization within 30 minutes. Determination of basal calcitonin levels prior to therapy is essential for interpreting the results of provocative tests.

Reference intervals for calcitonin. All U.S. laboratories are required by federal (CLIA) or state regulations to test and establish reference intervals for all assays. Whether the calcitonin assay employed is a radioimmunoassay (RIA) or a two-site immunometric assay (IMA) will influence results considerably. Immunometric methods, using monoclonal antibodies, generally give lower results than do RIA, which use polyclonal antibodies. The reference intervals for calcitonin therefore vary, reflecting differences in methodology and antibody specificity, as well as the purity of the standards employed. Generally, a basal calcitonin level useful for clinical interpretation is 5–19 pg/mL, with lower results observed for IMA.

In order to achieve the assay stability essential for diagnosis and monitoring of MTC, manufacturers should provide clinical laboratories with calcitonin reagents and standards that have minimal lot-to-lot variation. Provision to laboratories of kits with long shelf lives (e.g., by sequestering of lots) is also recommended.

Performance criteria. As both circulating calcitonin and the antisera used in the reagents for assay are heterogeneous, it is not possible to specify performance criteria that are applicable to all assay procedures. Each laboratory must determine its own performance criteria and use internal reference standards to monitor assay quality.

Determination of calcitonin should be performed on specimens from a statistically significant number of normal volunteers in the age range of 5–17, 18–30, 31–50, and over 50 years, to obtain an approximation of normal values for fasting calcitonin.

This is particularly important if calcitonin is measured after stimulation of secretion by pentagastrin and calcium. Failure to do so may lead to the reporting of totally uninterpretable clinical data.

NACB RECOMMENDATIONS FOR USE OF TUMOR MARKERS IN NEUROENDOCRINE TUMORS

1. Measurement of plasma catecholamines is useful in the diagnosis of a pheochromocytoma but extreme care must be taken in obtaining the samples for analysis. It must also be remembered that a plasma catecholamine determination represents a single point in time and does not have the advantage of the integrating effect of a timed urine collection. A urine catecholamine fractionation should be performed to assist in the diagnosis of pheochromocytoma.
2. All medications that are not absolutely required clinically should be discontinued for at least 72 hours prior to specimen collection.

3. Catecholamine fractionation should be performed. This is preferable to the use of total catecholamine levels for the diagnosis of pheochromocytoma.
4. Specimens should be stored between 2–8 °C to optimize preservation.
5. HPLC is recommended as the analytical method for catecholamine, VMA, and HVA determinations.
6. Serial determinations of 5-HIAA should be performed during an episode if practical, when the patient is symptomatic.
7. Urine specimens to be used for determination of catecholamines, VMA, HVA, and 5-HIAA should be refrigerated during the collection period. Specimens must be acidified between pH 2–4.

Germ Cell Tumors

Germ cell tumors, despite their rarity, constitute the most common cancer in males between the ages of 15 and 35 (169). This disease is highly curable, with long-term remissions being observed in more than 90% of patients following treatment, whether by surgery, radiation therapy, chemotherapy, or a combination of these (170,171).

Survival and prognosis in germ cell cancer are both highly dependent on TNM stage, vascular invasion, number and extension of visceral metastases (liver, bone, lung, brain), and the initial concentrations of the serum tumor markers α-fetoprotein (AFP), human chorionic gonadotropin (hCG) and/or its β-subunit (hCGβ), lactate dehydrogenase (LDH), and placental alkaline phosphatase (PLAP). Pre-treatment serum concentrations of these markers all influence the choice of therapy (172,173).

Germ cell tumors are divided into seminomas and nonseminomatous germ cell tumors (NSGCT). In contrast to seminoma, NSGCT can contain any combination of multiple cell types such as teratoma, embryonal cell carcinoma, choriocarcinoma, or endodermal sinus tumor. The rationale for this classification is that it correlates with clinical treatment: seminoma is highly sensitive to radiation therapy whereas NSGCT is highly radiation-resistant. The correct diagnosis is therefore critical for optimal treatment outcome (170).

Tumor Markers in the Identification and Treatment of Germ Cell Tumors

Diagnosis. The routine evaluation for patients who present with a testicular mass includes a CT scan of the abdomen, chest, and pelvis, as well as measurement of serum tumor markers including AFP, hCG, and LDH (174,175). The production of AFP is restricted to endodermal sinus tumor and embryonal carcinoma. Syncytiotrophoblastic cells produce hCG, and elevated levels of hCG can be found in patients with pure seminoma as well as patients with NSGCT histologies. Measurement of both intact hCG and hCGβ, both commonly detected by some commercial hCG tests, is essential, as some tumors may produce only hCGβ. It is important to note that not all commercially available assays for hCG recognize both these forms.

The EGTM also recommends measurement of placental alkaline phosphatase (PLAP), a heat-stable isoenzyme of alkaline phosphatase that is normally expressed by placental syncytiotrophoblasts (176,177). PLAP or PLAP-like activity occurs in normal tissue (e.g., testis, cervix, thymus, lung) as well as in malignant tissue (e.g., germ cell, ovarian, and lung tumors). Raised serum concentrations of PLAP are found in seminomas (sensitivity 51–90%) and NSGCT (sensitivity 20–36%), as well as in ovarian tumors. Measurement of serum PLAP, which has a half-life of 0.6 to 2.8 days, is advantageous as it is raised in up to 80% of testicular seminomas (Stage I and metastatic), while hCG is raised in fewer than 20%. Measurement of PLAP is not recommended in smokers, however, as serum levels are increased up to ten-fold relative to those of nonsmokers, with considerable inter-individual variation.

The serum level of LDH, and possibly its subunit LDH-1, is an independent prognostic factor in patients with advanced germ cell tumors (178). LDH has a relatively constant rate of degradation from patient to patient. Increases in the serum level are influenced primarily by tumor burden and growth rate, cell proliferation, and death. LDH is elevated in approximately 60% of NSGCT patients with advanced disease and 80% of patients with advanced seminoma. Historically, either hCG or AFP, or both, were elevated in approximately 80% of patients with advanced GCT (172). As a consequence of stage migration, hCG and AFP are each elevated in only 40% of nonseminoma patients in more recent series; hCG is also raised in 7–18% of seminomas. In contrast, an increased AFP is seen only in nonseminomatous histologies even if histopathology suggests pure seminoma.

Prognosis. The International Germ Cell Cancer Collaborative Group (IGCCCG) studied the use of serum tumor markers as prognostic variables and analyzed data from GCT trials in Europe, North America, and Australia to determine independent prognostic factors for use in a single classification system (179). This study was performed in over 5000 GCT patients and confirmed that pre-treatment levels of LDH and hCG, the site of the primary tumor (mediastinal vs. testis or retroperitoneal), and the presence of nonpulmonary visceral metastases were independent factors for survival. Due to the larger number of patients in this study, the pre-treatment level of AFP was confirmed as independently prognostic. Using tumor markers, histology, site of primary tumor, and extent of disease, patients with advanced disease were allocated to three prognostic strata (Table 10). Based on the finding that prognosis was dependent on pre-treatment serum tumor marker concentrations, GCT staging was completely revised in 1997 to include their use. Both the American Joint Committee on Cancer (AJCC) and the Union Internationale Contre le Cancer (UICC) have adopted the new system. AFP, hCG, and LDH each contribute to the (S) variable.

Post-treatment monitoring. Determination of the half-lives of AFP and hCG is recommended for monitoring treatment, with normalization of both markers (AFP half-life with-

Table 10 Contribution of serum tumor marker measurements to the prognostic classification of metastatic germ cell tumors (179)

Prognostic group[a]	Tumor marker concentration		
	AFP (ng/mL)	HCG (U/L)	LDH (Multiple of RR)[b]
Good (S1)	<1000	<5000	<1.5 × (RR)
Intermediate (S2)	≥1000 and ≤10,000	≥5000 and ≤50,000	≥1.5 × (RR) and 10 × (RR)
Poor (S3)	>10,000	>50,000	>10 × (RR)

[a] S, serum tumor marker.
[b] LDH concentrations expressed as multiples of the upper limit of the reference range (RR).

in 5 days; hCG half-life within 1–2 days) indicating favorable prognosis (180). Half-lives may be calculated using linear regression, which requires a minimum of three well-spaced measurements within a 10-day period post-orchiectomy. After two cycles of chemotherapy, patients with marker half-lives of more than seven days for AFP and/or more than three days for hCG have significantly lower survival rates than those with shorter marker half-lives (181). An abnormal serologic response, defined as failure to normalize, or a prolonged half-life by either marker can predict relapse months after chemotherapy. The majority of patients with slow marker decline will relapse despite early clinical improvement. This first experience with the rate of tumor marker decline during chemotherapy (181) has recently been confirmed to possess prognostic value independent of risk (stratified according to the classification system of the IGCCCG) (182).

By combining the prognostic criteria of the UK Medical Research Council (MRC) with analysis of marker half-lives, prognostic discrimination can be improved and three different risk groups identified. Patients in the "poor risk" category may then be selected for more aggressive chemotherapy (183).

Guidance of post-chemotherapy surgery. Cure of patients with metastatic GCT is optimized by the use of surgery after chemotherapy in selected patients (173). The role of surgery in patients with advanced GCT after chemotherapy has evolved substantially in the era of combined modality therapy. Patients with residual masses after chemotherapy should undergo post-chemotherapy surgery to remove residual carcinoma or teratoma. It is essential that only patients whose serum tumor marker levels are normal be subjected to post-chemotherapy surgery.

The large majority of patients with a persistently elevated AFP or HCG after chemotherapy will probably have surgically unresectable disease. These patients should be referred for salvage chemotherapy.

Management of germ cell tumors. Clinical research has resulted in the cure of the majority of patients presenting with GCT. A major advance in the diagnosis and treatment of GCT patients is the integration of serum tumor markers in staging and treatment. The use of serum tumor markers in GCT is unique in that:

- Serology may predominate over histology in treatment decisions; e.g., the presence of AFP in a patient with seminoma dictates that the patient is treated as an NSGCT even if the histology is seminoma.
- The extent of elevation of tumor marker levels defines the prognostic classification of metastatic germ cell tumors.
- Tumor marker normalization is required to assess response to chemotherapy.
- The potential for relapse months after chemotherapy can be predicted by the rapidity of decline in the serum AFP or hCG in the first six weeks of therapy.
- Normalization of serum tumor markers is a requirement for the integration of post-chemotherapy surgery.

NACB and EGTM Recommendations for Use of Tumor Markers in Germ Cell Tumors

1. Determine AFP, hCG, and LDH as aids in the evaluation and staging of germ cell tumors prior to orchiectomy.
2. Any patient with a seminoma and an elevated AFP should be considered to have a nonseminomatous tumor and treated accordingly.
3. These tumor markers should be determined immediately before orchiectomy and, if elevated, should then be measured serially after orchiectomy. The rate of fall should be compared with the normal rate of disappearance of AFP (half-life <7 days) and hCG (half-life <3 days). All GCT patients should be staged using the new TNMS system incorporating tumor marker results.
4. The surveillance schedule should include determinations of AFP, hCG, and LDH monthly in the first year, and alternating months during the second and third year. Clinical investigations should include physical examination, chest X-ray, and ultrasonography or CT scan of the abdomen and pelvis at 2- to 3-month intervals during the first three years after therapy.
5. Stage IIA and Stage IIB patients who do not receive chemotherapy immediately after surgery should undergo surveillance incorporating determinations of AFP, HCG, and LDH with a monthly physical exam and chest X-ray for the first year, every other month in the second year, and every third month in the third year.

MONOCLONAL GAMMOPATHIES (MYELOMA)

The monoclonal gammopathies constitute a group of disorders characterized by the proliferation of a single clone of plasma cells that produce a homogeneous, monoclonal (M) protein (184). Each M-protein consists of two heavy polypeptide chains of the same class [gamma (γ) in IgG, alpha (α) in IgA, mu (μ) in IgM, delta (δ) in IgD, and epsilon (ϵ) in IgE] and two light polypeptide chains [kappa (κ) or lambda (λ)] of the same type.

Laboratory Diagnosis and Monitoring

Preanalytical concerns. These include preference for a fasting sample in order to avoid hyperlipemia. Samples should be covered to avoid evaporation if they are stored in the refrigerator. If cryoglobulin is suspected, the specimen should be kept at 37 °C. If bacterial growth appears, the specimen must be discarded. Hemolysis should be avoided because the presence of a haptoglobin-hemoglobin complex will produce an α_2-β spike in the electrophoretic pattern. The serum should be frozen at –20 °C if it is not used immediately. An increase or decrease of 0.5 g/dL in the size of the M-spike indicates a significant change.

Sulfosalicylic acid or Exton's reagent is more reliable than dipstick tests for the detection of monoclonal light chains (Bence Jones proteins). An aliquot from a 24-hour urine specimen with no preservative is needed.

The amount of M-protein in the urine is a direct measure of the tumor mass in the patient, and thus is useful in following the clinical course.

Electrophoresis. Electrophoresis is performed on agarose gel, with high voltage applied across the electrodes and gel. After staining with Ponceau S, the preparation is dried and each pattern is visually inspected. A scanning densitometer quantitates each component after the total protein has been determined (185).

Electrophoresis is useful as a screening test and as an aid to the diagnosis of multiple myeloma (MM) or related disorders. It is also useful in monitoring the course of a patient with MM or Waldenström's macroglobulinemia (WM) because the size of the M-protein is a direct reflection of the tumor mass of the patient. Consequently, one can determine whether the patient is responding to therapy or has progressive disease (186,187).

Immunofixation or immunoelectrophoresis. Immunofixation (or immunoelectrophoresis) is necessary for determining the presence and type of the M-protein. It is particularly helpful for detecting a small M-protein in patients with primary systemic amyloidosis (AL) or in following a patient with solitary plasmacytoma or extramedullary plasmacytoma. (185,188). Immunofixation is very helpful in the recognition of biclonal or triclonal gammopathies.

Quantitation of immunoglobulins (nephelometry). Nephelometry is an excellent test for quantitation of immunoglobulins. The degree of turbidity produced by antigen-antibody interaction is measured by nephelometry in the near ultraviolet (UV) regions. This technique accurately measures 7S and 19S IgM, monomers and polymers of IgA, or aggregates of IgG accurately (189). The levels of IgM may be 1,000 to 2,000 mg/dL greater with nephelometry than expected from the size of the M-protein in the densitometer tracing. The IgG and IgA levels may also be spuriously increased. Therefore, the clinician must use the same or both techniques for following the size of an M-protein in a patient (190).

Serum viscosity. Viscosity is the property of fluid to resist flow. Signs or symptoms of hyperviscosity include oronasal bleeding, blurring or loss of vision, headache, vertigo, nystagmus, deafness, ataxia, paresthesias, diplopia, somnolence, stupor, and coma. There is segmental dilation of retinal veins and retinal hemorrhages. WM is the most common cause of hyperviscosity, but it can also be found in patients with IgA or, rarely, IgG myeloma (191). The Ostwald-100 viscometer is a satisfactory instrument for measurement of viscosity, but a Wells-Brookfield viscometer is preferred because it is more accurate, requires less serum, and can perform at different shear rates and at variable temperatures. In addition, the determinations can be made much more quickly, especially if the viscosity of the serum is high.

Cryoglobulin determination. Cryoglobulins are proteins that precipitate when cooled and dissolve when heated. They may be classified as type I (monoclonal IgM, IgG, IgA, or rarely, monoclonal light chains); type II (mixed; two or more immunoglobulins of which one is monoclonal), and type III (polyclonal in which no M-protein is found). The specimen must be collected at 37 °C and then placed in a 37 °C thermos and delivered to the laboratory. The specimens are allowed to clot at 37 °C and are then centrifuged at 37 °C. The serum is placed in a refrigerator or an ice bath and read at 24 hours. If no precipitate occurs, the specimen is kept at 0 °C for seven days. The precipitate is washed, and immunoelectrophoresis is performed with monospecific antisera to determine the type of immunoglobulin in the cryoprecipitate (192).

Capillary electrophoresis. Capillary zone electrophoresis is performed on fused silica capillary tubes with a large surface-to-volume ratio and high voltage. This produces rapid separation of the proteins. The densitometry tracings of the separation obtained with capillary and agarose gel electrophoresis produce very similar patterns. Better resolution with capillary electrophoresis allows for more accurate quantitation of the M-protein (189,193). Immunosubtraction with capillary electrophoresis for typing of the M-protein is performed by repeating electrophoresis with antisera to IgG, IgA, IgM, κ, and λ. The presence of an M-protein is detected by its removal with the appropriate heavy- and light-chain antisera. This is less labor-intensive and more economical than immunofixation. The latter is still the gold standard for the detection of a monoclonal protein. Capillary electrophoresis is not yet available for evaluation of M-proteins in the urine.

NACB Recommendations for Laboratory Testing in Multiple Gammopathies (Myeloma)

1. Electrophoretic studies should be performed whenever multiple myeloma (MM), Waldenström's macroglobulinemia (WM), or primary systemic amyloidosis (AL) is suspected.

2. It is essential to differentiate a monoclonal from a polyclonal increase in immunoglobulins. Immunofixation should be performed when a sharp peak or band is found on the agarose electrophoretogram or when MM, WM, AL, or a related disorder is suspected.
3. Quantitation of immunoglobulins by radial immunodiffusion is not recommended.
4. The specimen must be allowed to clot because fibrinogen appears as a distinct narrow band between the β and γ fractions in plasma and may be mistaken for an M-protein.
5. Analysis of urine is essential for patients with monoclonal gammopathies.
6. The serum viscosity should be performed when the IgM monoclonal protein value is >3 g/dL or the IgA or IgG protein value is >4 g/dL. It should also be performed on any patient with oronasal bleeding, blurred vision, or neurologic symptoms suggestive of a hyperviscosity syndrome.

LUNG CANCER

The generally poor prognosis of patients with lung cancer and the lack of effective therapy for recurrent disease limit the application of tumor marker determinations, especially in follow-up care. Nevertheless, measurement of tumor markers may be helpful; guideline recommendations for their proper use in differential diagnosis and in monitoring the efficacy of therapy have been proposed by EGTM (194).

Most primary lung tumors can be classified into four major histological types—squamous cell carcinoma, adenocarcinoma, large cell carcinoma, and small-cell lung cancer (SCLC). SCLC accounts for 20–25% of the cases of bronchogenic carcinoma and differs clinically and biologically from the other three histological types, which are all generally referred to as non-small-cell lung cancer (NSCLC). It is now evident that many tumors have features of more than one histological type of cancer. Thus, both SCLC and NSCLC represent heterogeneous groups in which there is considerable overlap among the major histological types of lung cancer.

Use of Tumor Markers in Lung Cancer

The tumor markers most frequently used or suggested as markers for lung cancer include neuron-specific enolase (NSE), carcinoembryonic antigen (CEA), squamous cell carcinoma antigen (SCCA), CYFRA 21-1, and pro-gastrin-releasing peptide (ProGRP). The properties of CEA and SCCA (195) are described elsewhere in this chapter.

Neuron-specific enolase (NSE). The glycolytic enzyme enolase (2-phospho-D-glycerate hydrolase, EC 4.2.1.11) exists as several dimeric isoenzymes ($\alpha\alpha$, $\alpha\beta$, $\alpha\gamma$, $\beta\beta$, and $\gamma\gamma$). The ag- and $\alpha\gamma$-enolase isoenzymes are also known as neuron-specific enolase (NSE) as they are produced in central and peripheral neurons and malignant tumors of neuroectodermal origin (e.g., SCLC, neuroblastomas, intestinal carcinoid) (196).

CYFRA 21-1. CYFRA 21-1 is a relatively new tumor marker for which the assay uses two monoclonal antibodies directed against a cytokeratin 19 fragment. Immunohistochemical studies demonstrate that cytokeratin 19 is abundant in carcinomas of the lung, thus CYFRA 21-1 is the most sensitive marker for NSCLC (197). Since CYFRA 21-1 represents only fragments of cytokeratin 19, the CYFRA 21-1 tumor marker test shows a higher specificity than that for tissue polypeptide antigen (TPA), which determines a mixture of cytokeratins 8, 18, and 19.

Pro-gastrin-releasing peptide (ProGRP). ProGRP is a relatively stable precursor of the hormone gastrin-releasing peptide (GRP). In humans, GRP is found predominantly in the gastrointestinal and respiratory tract and also in the central nervous system. Several studies suggest that GRP is released by tumor cells of small cell lung cancer and may even stimulate the growth of SCLC cells. ProGRP has not yet been incorporated in the EGTM recommendations, but is discussed in more detail in Chapter 57.

Clinical Utility of Tumor Markers in Lung Cancer

Screening and diagnosis. Their lack of sensitivity and organ- and tumor-specificity means that none of the tumor markers described above is suitable for screening for lung cancer, either in asymptomatic persons or in patients at high risk of malignancy (e.g., smokers).

The diagnosis of lung cancer generally requires medical imaging, endoscopy, intra-operative findings, and histology. Although tumor marker measurements cannot replace histological results, they can be very helpful where it is not possible to establish a final diagnosis by biopsy (approximately 20% of cases). For example, release of NSE in tissue and in serum in patients where histological evidence is absent may support a diagnosis of SCLC (198,199). Similarly a high serum level of SCCA provides a strong suspicion of NSCLC and of squamous cell carcinoma in particular (200). CYFRA 21-1 has the highest sensitivity for lung cancer in general (200–202).

Although serum CYFRA 21-1, TPA, NSE, and CEA all show a correlation with tumor burden, there is no consistent relationship between production of these markers and tumor stage. Generally, high tumor marker concentrations reflect advanced tumor stage and suggest a bad prognosis. Low or mildly increased marker concentrations never exclude malignancy or progression. Pre-treatment measurement of tumor markers at the time of primary diagnosis may be helpful (Table 11).

Table 11 Tumor markers of use in lung cancer

Histology known	Baseline marker*
Adenocarcinoma	CYFRA 21-1 and CEA
Squamous cell carcinoma	CYFRA 21-1
Large cell carcinoma	CYFRA 21-1 and CEA
Small cell carcinoma	NSE and CYFRA 21-1
Unknown	CYFRA 21-1, NSE, CEA

*Markers raised at baseline are likely to be most relevant for monitoring.

Markers raised at that time are likely to be most relevant for monitoring. The rate at which marker levels decrease after surgery can give some indication of remaining tumor burden and the effectiveness of therapy (203–205).

Prognosis. Two comprehensive reviews on the prognostic use of serum tumor markers in NSCLC (206) and SCLC (207) have recently been published.

All parameters investigated by multivariate analysis in NSCLC and SCLC patients have yielded conflicting results in different studies. Nevertheless, the use of CYFRA 21-1 in NSCLC has been most frequently evaluated and found to be a significant prognostic factor in multivariate analysis (208).

There are several reasons for the contradictory results from different studies on prognostic value:

- The heterogeneity of the study populations (tumor stage, histology, etc.).
- The parameters studied.
- The procedure by which optimized cut-off values have been chosen.
- The use of different procedures to determine cut-off values within the same study.

It is particularly important that potential new markers are compared with existing markers where appropriate. Well-designed trials are essential to verify the prognostic significance of markers such as NSE or CYFRA 21-1. The effect on therapeutic decision-making has yet to be assessed in prospective randomized intervention trials.

Post-treatment monitoring. An important indication for tumor marker determinations in lung cancer is in assessing the efficacy of therapy and post-operative follow-up care. As for tumor markers in other carcinomas, the rate of post-operative decrease of the relevant marker provides information regarding patient outcome. Decreasing levels after primary surgery are the first sign of curative resection and therefore an indication of good prognosis. Tumor marker concentrations that decrease slowly and/or do not fall to within the reference range are suggestive of residual disease or incorrect staging (e.g., due to occult metastases not identified at the time of initial staging).

The risk of recurrence in lung cancer is high (70–90%), and follow-up care with tumor markers should only be performed if treatment options are available. Where tumor markers are used for follow-up, determination of post-operative baseline levels is necessary to allow appropriate interpretation of later results, with a confirmed increase from this baseline providing the first sign of recurrent disease.

Tumor markers may also give some indication of the effectiveness of chemotherapy. For more than 10 years, it has been accepted that in patients with SCLC, serum levels of NSE reflect the response to chemotherapy (199,209,210). It should be noted that during chemotherapy, transient increases in NSE may occur 24 to 72 hours after treatment (i.e., tumor lysis syndrome) and have been interpreted as first sign of effective therapy. Where there is a good response to chemotherapy, elevated pre-treatment serum NSE levels generally decrease rapidly within a week or by the end of the first treatment cycle. In contrast, failure of therapy is associated with persistently elevated or transiently decreased levels. Increasing tumor markers generally indicate progressive disease, often weeks or months before this is evident from imaging techniques (211–213). Whether implementing treatment early (solely on the basis of an increasing tumor marker level) can prolong survival or increase the quality of life is not yet known.

Preanalytical Concerns

Samples for lung cancer markers may be stored at 4 °C (short-term) and at −70 °C (long-term). When frozen samples are thawed for cytokeratin analysis, vigorous mixing of samples should be avoided, as cytokeratins may adhere to tube walls after extreme agitation.

Specimens for NSE determination should be separated from the clot within 60 minutes of collection to avoid leaking of NSE present in normal erythrocytes, and in plasma cells. NSE should not be determined on hemolyzed specimens.

When measuring SCCA, contamination of samples with skin or saliva must be avoided, as this may lead to erroneously high results. CYFRA 21-1- and SCCA values may be significantly influenced by renal failure, a condition in which higher results may be observed.

EGTM Recommendations for Use of Tumor Markers in Lung Cancer

1. CYFRA 21-1, CEA, and NSE should not be used for screening purposes either in asymptomatic populations or in those at high risk for lung cancer (e.g., smokers).
2. Depending on histology, CYFRA 21-1, CEA, and/or NSE may be ordered in lung cancer patients prior to first therapy. Where no histology can be obtained before surgery, measurement of all three markers is necessary to identify the leading marker (usually that present in highest concentration).
3. Where inoperable lung cancer is suspected but no histology is available, raised serum NSE is suggestive of small-cell lung cancer.
4. Follow-up of asymptomatic patients after primary therapy of lung cancer is controversial. However, serial determinations of the leading marker may help assess the completeness of tumor removal and provide early indication of recurrence.
5. NSE can be measured during systemic treatment of SCLC to reflect response to therapy and to document progressive disease.
6. Careful attention to preanalytical factors is essential. Specimens for NSE determination should be separated from the clot within 60 minutes of collection, and hemolyzed samples should not be assayed. Vigorous mixing of serum samples after thawing should be avoided for cytokeratin measurements. Contamination of samples with skin or saliva must be avoided for SCCA measurements.
7. Samples may be stored at 4 °C (short-term) and at −70 °C (long-term).

Table 12 Summary of key guideline recommendations

Cancer type	NACB	ASCO	ACS	EGTM
Breast	ER / PR on all cancers CA15-3 / CA27.29 for monitoring advanced disease	Routine use of CA15-3 or CA 27.29 alone *not* recommended Increasing CA15-3 or CA27.29 may be used to suggest treatment failure Routine use of CEA not recommended Estrogen and progesterone receptors to be determined for primary lesions Steroid hormone receptors to be used to select patients for endocrine therapy HER-2/neu (c-erb B2) over-expression or amplification may be used to select patients for Herceptin® (trastuzumab) therapy	None	Steroid receptors in tissue for predicting response to hormone therapy CEA and one MUC1-gene-related protein in serum for prognosis, follow-up and monitoring of therapy HER-2/neu in tissue for predicting response to Herceptin® (trastuzumab®) in patients with advanced disease
Ovarian	CA125 as a diagnostic aid and for monitoring therapy	None	None	CA125 as an aid in diagnosis, for monitoring treatment, and early prediction of recurrence
Prostate	PSA with DRE %fPSA when PSA is between 4–10 ng/mL and DRE is negative	Guidelines under development for metastatic disease	PSA and DRE for screening and detection	tPSA with DRE for screening (studies), case finding, or prognosis. tPSA in follow-up and and monitoring of therapy if additional means of therapy can be offered in case of rising tPSA. %fPSA for differential diagnosis when tPSA is 4–10 ng/mL and DRE is negative
Germ cell	AFP, hCG, and LDH for detecting and monitoring testicular tumors AFP is diagnostic for NSGCT	None	None	AFP, hCG, LDH, and PLAP* for case-finding, staging, prognosis, follow-up, and monitoring of therapy AFP is diagnostic for non-seminomatous germ cell tumors (NSGCT)
Colon	CEA for monitoring therapy	CEA for prognosis, detecting recurrence, and monitoring therapy	None	CEA for case-finding, prognosis, follow-up, and monitoring of therapy
Neuroendocrine	Urinary catecholamines, VMA, HVA as indicators for pheochromocytoma and neuroblastoma Calcitonin for medullary thyroid carcinoma	None	None	None
Myeloma	Serum protein electrophoresis for M spike Immunofixation electrophoresis to differentiate monoclonality	None	None	None
Lung	None	None	None	NSE in differential diagnosis CYFRA 21-1, CEA, and/or NSE for follow-up and monitoring of therapy

NACB, National Academy of Clinical Biochemistry; ASCO, American Society for Clinical Oncology; ACS, American Cancer Society; EGTM, European Group on Tumor Markers; tPSA, total PSA; fPSA, free PSA.

"None" indicates that the relevant group has not yet considered this cancer type.

*Placental alkaline phosphatase (PLAP), for monitoring of seminomas in nonsmokers only.

SUMMARY

The key guidelines recommended by the NACB (LMPG), ASCO, ACS, and EGTM for the use of tumor markers are summarized in Table 12. This information is clearly still in development and should be updated periodically, perhaps every two years. As the guidelines reflect the results of clinical research, they should inevitably change with advances in technology and their adoption in clinical practice.

The single most important caveat for the use of tumor markers in a clinical setting relates to the inter-laboratory variability of tumor marker measurement, which is discussed in greater detail elsewhere in this book. An assay performed using a specific antibody or a particular instrument may give results different from those obtained with a different method. This does not necessarily reflect poor individual methods or instrumentation, but rather differences in assay reagents and procedures. It is, therefore, essential that where tumor markers are used to monitor cancer patients, information about the method is included with the assay results.

REFERENCES

1. Witliff JL, Kaplan LA, eds. Guidelines for the analytical performance and clinical utility of tumor markers. Rye Brook, NY: NACB, 1998 (Draft).
2. Van Dalen A. Quality control and standardization of tumor marker tests. Tumor Biol 1993;14:131–135.
3. Sturgeon C, Dati F, Duffy, MJ, Hasholzner U, Klapdor R, Lamerz R, et al. Quality requirements and control: EGTM recommendations. Anticancer Res 1999;19:2791–2794.
4. Seth J. Quality assurance. In: Price CP, Newman DJ, eds. Principles and practice of immunoassay, 2nd ed. London: Macmillan, 1997;209–241.
5. Westgard JO, Stein B. Automated selection of statistical quality control procedures to assure meeting clinical or analytical quality requirements. Clin Chem 1997;43:400–403.
6. Fraser CG, Hyltoft Petersen P. Analytical performance characteristics should be judged against objective quality specifications. Clin Chem 1999;45:321–323.
7. Sölétormos G, Schioler V, Nielsen D, Skovsgaard T, Dombernowsky P. Interpretation of results for tumor markers on the basis of analytical imprecision and biological variation. Clin Chem 1993;39:2077–2083.
8. Bonfrer JMG. Working group on tumor marker criteria (WGTMC). Tumor Biol 1990;11:287–288.
9. Hayes DF, Bast RC, Desch CE, Fritsche H, Kemeny ND, Jessup JM, et al. Tumor marker utility grading system: a framework to evaluate clinical utility of tumor markers. J Nat Cancer Inst 1996;88:1456–1466.
10. Sturgeon CM, Seth J, Ellis AR. Clinical interpretation of laboratory results. Proc UK NEQAS Mtg 1996;2:110–115.
11. Sturgeon CM, Seth J. Why do immunoassays for tumor markers give differing results?—a view from the UK National External Quality Assessment Schemes. Eur J Clin Chem Clin Biochem 1996;34:755–759.
12. Sturgeon CM. Tumor markers in the laboratory: closing the guideline–practice gap. Clin Biochem 2001;34:353–359.
13. Jemal A, Thomas A, Murray T, Thun M. Cancer Statistics 2002. CA Cancer J Clin 2002;52:23–47.
14. Tumor Marker Expert Panel (ASCO). Clinical practice guidelines for the use of tumor markers in breast and colorectal cancer. J Clin Oncol 1996;14:2843–2877.
15. Bast RC, Radvin P, Hayes DF, Bates S, Fritsche H, Jessup JM, et al. 2000 update of recommendations for the use of tumor markers in breast and colorectal cancer: clinical practice guidelines of the American Society of Clinical Oncology. J Clin Oncol 2001;19:1865–1878.
16. Bast RC, Ravdin P, Hayes DF, Bates S, Fritsche H, Jessup JM, et al. 2000 update of recommendations for the use of tumor markers in breast and colorectal cancer: clinical practice guidelines of the American Society of Clinical Oncology. Erratum. J Clin Oncol 2001;19:4185–4188.
17. Duffy MJ. Biochemical markers in breast cancer: which ones are clinically useful? Clin Biochem 2001;34:347–352.
18. Isaacs C, Stearns V, Hayes DF. New prognostic factors for breast cancer recurrence. Semin Oncol 2001;28:53–67.
19. Wittliff JL, Pasic R, Bland KI. Steroid and peptide hormone receptors: methods, quality control and clinical use. In: Bland KI, Copeland III EM, eds. The breast: comprehensive management of benign and malignant diseases. Philadelphia, PA: WB Saunders Co, 1998;458–498.
20. Fisher B, Redmond C, Brown A, Wickerham DL, Wolmark N, Allegra J, et al. Influence of tumor estrogen and progesterone receptor levels on the response to tamoxifen and chemotherapy in primary breast cancer. J Clin Oncol 1983;1:227–241.
21. Fisher B, Redmond C, Brown A, Womark N, Wittliff JL, Fisher ER, et al. Treatment of primary breast cancer with chemotherapy and tamoxifen. N Engl J Med 1981;305:1–6.
22. Clark GM. Prognostic and predictive factors. In: Lippman ME, Morrow M, Hellman S, eds. Diseases of the breast. Philadelphia, PA: Lippincott-Raven, 1996;461–485.
23. Duffy MJ. Biochemical markers as prognostic indices in breast cancer. Clin Chem 1990;36:188–191.
24. Wittliff JL, Raffelsberger W. Mechanisms of signal transduction: sex hormones, their receptors, and clinical utility. J Clin Ligand Assay 1995;18:211–235.
25. Pasic R, Djulbegovic B, Wittliff JL. Comparison of sex steroid receptor determinations in human breast cancer by enzyme immunoassay and radioligand binding. J Clin Lab Anal 1990;4:430–436.
26. Wittliff JL, Miseljic S, Cummins JA, Pasic R. Does menopausal status influence sex-steroid receptor content and specific binding capacity? J Clin Ligand Assay 1996;19:203–207.
27. Wittliff JL, Beatty BW, baker DT, Savlov ED, Cooper RA. Clinical significance of molecular forms of estrogen receptors in human breast cancer. In: Vermeulen A, Klopper A, Sciarra F, Jungblut P, Lerner L, eds. Research on Steroids, Vol VII. Amsterdam: Elsevier/North-Holland Biomedical Press, 1977;393–403.
28. Kuiper GG, Enmark E, Pelto-Huikko M, Nilsson S, Gustafsson JA. Cloning of a novel estrogen receptor expressed in rat prostate and ovary. Proc Natl Acad Sci 1996;93:5925–5930.
29. Mosselman S, Polman J, Dijkema R. ER beta: identification and characterization of a novel human estrogen receptor. FEBS Lett 1996;392:49–53.
30. Jarvinen TA, Pelto-Huikko M, Holli K, Isola J. Estrogen receptor beta is co-expressed with ER-alpha and PR and associated with nodal status, grade, and proliferation rate in breast cancer. Am J Pathol 2000;156:29–35.

31. Pasic R, Djulbegovic B, Wittliff JL. Influence of O.C.T. embedding compound on determinations of estrogen and progestin receptors in breast cancer. Clin Chem 1989;35:2317–2319.
32. Fisher B, Dignam J, Tan-Chiu E, Anderson S, Fisher ER, Wittliff JL, et al. Prognosis and treatment of patients with breast tumors of one centimeter or less and negative axillary lymph nodes. J Natl Cancer Inst 2001;93:112–120.
33. Gendler SJ, Spicer AP. Epithelial mucin genes. Ann Rev Physiol 1995;57:607–634.
34. Kufe D, Inghirami G, Abe M, Hayes D, Justi-Wheeler H, Schlom J. Differential reactivity of a novel monoclonal antibody (DF3) with human malignant versus benign breast tumors. Hybridoma 1984;3:223–232.
35. Duffy MJ. CA 15-3 and related mucins as circulating markers in breast cancer. Ann Clin Biochem 1999;36:579–586.
36. Bon GS, von Mensdorff-Pouilly S, Kenemans P, van Kamp GJ, Verstraeten RA, Hilgers J, et al. Clinical and technical evaluation of ACS BR serum assay of MUCI gene-derived glycoprotein in breast cancer, and comparison with CA 15-3 assay. Clin Chem 1997;43:585–593.
37. Price MR, Rye PD, Petrakou R, Murray A, Brady K, Imai S, et al. Summary report on the ISOBM TD-4 workshop: analysis of 56 monoclonal antibodies against the MUC1 mucin. Tumor Biol 1998;19(S1):1–20.
38. Hayes DF, Zurawski VR, Kufe DW. Comparison of circulating CA 15-3 and carcinoembryonic antigen levels in patients with breast cancer. J Clin Oncol 1986;1:542–550.
39. Ballesta AM, Molina R, Filella X, Jo J, Gimenez N. Carcinoembryonic antigen in staging and follow-up of patients with solid tumors. Tumor Biol 1995;16:32–41.
40. Coveney EC, Geraghty JG, Sherry F, McDermott EW, Fennelly JJ, O'Higgins NJ, et al. The clinical value of CEA and CA 15-3 in breast cancer management. Int J Biol Markers 1995;10:35–41.
41. Bon GG, Kenemans P, Verstraeten R, van Kamp GJ, Hilgers J. Serum tumor marker immunoassays in gynecologic oncology: establishment of reference values. Am J Obstet Gynecol 1996;174:107–114.
42. Robertson JF, Jaeger W, Syzmendera JJ, Selby C, Coleman R, Howell A, et al. The objective measurement of remission and progression in metastatic breast cancer by use of serum tumor markers. European Group for Serum Tumor Markers in Breast Cancer. Eur J Cancer 1999;35:47–53.
43. Sölétormos G, Nielsen D, Schioler V, Skovsgaard T, Dombernowsky P. Tumor markers cancer antigen 15.3, carcinoembryonic antigen, and tissue polypeptide antigen for monitoring metastatic breast cancer during first-line chemotherapy and follow-up. Clin Chem 1996;42:564–575.
44. Van Dalen A, Heering KJ, Barak V, Peretz T, Cremashi A, Geroni P, et al. Treatment response in metastatic breast cancer. A multicenter study comparing UICC criteria and tumor marker changes. Breast 1996;5:82–88.
45. Safi F, Kohler I, Rottinger E, Beger H. The value of tumor marker CA 15-3 in diagnosis and monitoring of breast cancer. A comparative study with carcinoembryonic antigen. Cancer 1991;68:574–582.
46. Cheung K, Graves CR, Robertson JF. Tumor marker measurements in the diagnosis and monitoring of breast cancer. Cancer Treat Rev 2000;26:91–102.
47. Shering SG, Sherry F, McDermott EW, O'Higgins NJ, Duffy MJ. Preoperative CA 15-3 concentrations predict outcome of patients with breast carcinoma. Cancer 1998;83:2521–2527.
48. Molina R, Duffy MJ, Aronsson AC, Lamerz R, Stieber P, Van Dalen A, et al. Tumor markers in breast cancer: EGTM Recommendations. Anticancer Res 1999;19:2803–2805.
49. Molina R, Zanon G, Filella X, Moreno F, Jo J, Daniels M, et al. Use of serial carcinoembryonic antigen and CA 15-3 assays in detecting relapses in breast cancer patients. Breast Cancer Res Treat 1995;36:41–48.
50. Gion M, Peloso L, Mione R, Vignati G, Fortunato A, Saracchini S, et al. Tumor markers in breast cancer monitoring should be scheduled according to initial stage and follow-up time: a prospective study on 859 patients. Cancer J 2001;7:181–190.
51. Guadagni F, Ferroni P, Carlini S, Mariotti S, Spila A, Aloe S, et al. A re-evaluation of carcinoembryonic antigen (CEA) as a serum marker for breast cancer: a prospective longitudinal study. Clin Cancer Res 2001;7:2357–2362.
52. Cotlove E, Harris EK, Williams GZ. Biological and analytical components of variation in long-term studies of serum constituents in normal subjects. III. Physiological and medical implications. Clin Chem 1970;16:1028–1038.
53. Harris EK, Yasaka T. On the calculation of a reference change for comparing two consecutive measurements. Clin Chem 1983;29:25–30.
54. Fraser CG, Hyltoft-Petersen P, Lytken-Larsen M. Setting analytical goals for random analytical error in specific clinical monitoring situations. Clin Chem 1990;36:1625–1628.
55. Sölétormos G, Hyltoft-Petersen P, Dombernowsky P. Assessment of CA 15.3, CEA, and TPA concentrations during monitoring of breast cancer. Clin Chem Lab Med 2000;38:453–463.
56. Sölétormos G, Hyltoft-Petersen P, Dombernowsky P. Progression criteria for cancer antigen 15.3 and carcinoembryonic antigen in metastatic breast cancer compared by computer simulation of marker data. Clin Chem 2000;46:939–949.
57. Dnistrian AM, Schwartz MK, Greenberg EJ, Schwartz DC. BR27.29 as a marker in breast cancer. J Tumor Marker Oncol 1995;10:91–97.
58. Chan DW, Beveridge RA, Muss H, Fritsche HA, Hortobagyi G, Theriault R, et al. Use of Truquant BR radioimmunoassay for early detection of breast cancer recurrence in patients with stage II and stage III disease. J Clin Oncol 1997;15:2322–2328.
59. Fekete M, Wittliff JL, Schally AV. Characteristics and distribution of receptors for [D-TRP6] luteinizing hormone-releasing hormone, somatostatin, epidermal growth factor, and sex steroids in 500 biopsy samples of human breast cancer. J Clin Lab Anal 1989;3:137–147.
60. Srkalovic G, Wittliff JL, Schally AV. Detection and partial characterization of receptors for [D-Trp6] luteinizing hormone-releasing hormone and epidermal growth factor in human endometrial carcinoma. Cancer Res 1990;50:1841–1846.
61. Miseljic S, Cavazos AS, Wittliff JL. Influence of menopausal status on expression of epidermal growth factor receptors, HER-2/neu oncoprotein and cathepsin D in breast cancer. J Clin Ligand Assay 1995;18:176–180.
62. Miseljic S, Yang AR, Cline VJM, Wittliff JL. Expression of epidermal growth factors receptors in human breast cancer: mass vs. ligand-binding capacity. The Breast J 1995;1:102–106.
63. Klijn JG, Berns, PM, Schmitz PI, Foekens JA. The clinical significance of epidermal growth factor receptor (EGF-R) in human breast cancer: a review on 5232 patients. Endocr Rev 1992;13:3–17.

64. Klijn JGM, Berns PM, Schmitz PI et al. Epidermal growth factor receptor (EGF-R) in clinical breast cancer: update 1993. Endocr Rev 1993;1:171–184.
65. Fleisher M. Prognostic markers other than hormone receptors in breast cancer. J Clin Ligand Assay 1998;21:1–6.
66. Tandon AK, Clark GM, Chamness GC, Ullrich A, McGuire WL. HER-2/neu oncogene protein and prognosis in breast cancer. J Clin Oncol 1989;7:1120–1128.
67. Slamon DJ, Clark GM, Wong SG, Levin WJ, Ullrich A, McGuire WL. Human breast cancer: correlation of relapse and survival with amplification of the HER-2/neu oncogene. Science 1987; 235:177–182.
68. Slamon DJ, Godolphin W, Jones LA, Holt JA, Wong SG, Keith DE, et al. Studies of the HER-2/neu proto-oncogene in human breast and ovarian cancer. Science 1989;244:707–712.
69. Paik S, Hazan R, Fisher ER, Sass RE, Fisher B, Redmond C, et al. Pathological findings from the National Surgical Adjuvant Breast and Bowel Project: prognostic significance of c-erb B2 protein overexpression in primary breast cancer. J Clin Oncol 1990;8: 103–112.
70. Simon R, Nocito A, Hübscher T, Bucher C, Torhorst J, Schraml P, et al. Patterns of HER-2/neu amplification and over-expression in primary and metastatic breast cancer. J Natl Cancer Inst 2001;93: 1141–1146.
71. Tandon AK, Clark GM, Chamness GC Chirgwin JM, McGuire WL. Cathepsin D and prognosis in breast cancer. N Engl J Med 1990;322:297–302.
72. Shaheen RM, Miseljic S. Wiehle RD, Wittliff JL. Relation between cathepsin D expression and other prognostic factors in breast carcinomas. Clin Chem 1995;41:1585–1591.
73. Shaheen RM, Miseljic S, Doering DL, Wittliff JL. Comparison of cathepsin D determinations in human carcinomas by enzyme immunoassay and immunoradiometric assay. J Clin Lab Anal 1995;9:351–358.
74. Andreasen P A, Kjoller L, Christensen L, Duffy MJ. The urokinase-type plasminogen activator system in cancer metastasis: a review. Int J Cancer 1997;72:1–22.
75. Grondahl-Hansen J, Hilsenbeck SG, Christensen IJ, Clark GM, Osborne CK, Brünner N. Prognostic significance of PAI-1 and uPA in cytosolic extracts obtained from node-positive breast cancer patients. Breast Cancer Res Treat 1997;43:153–163.
76. Tecimer C, Doering DL, Goldsmith LJ, Meyer JS, Abdulhay G, Wittliff JL. Clinical relevance of urokinase-type plasminogen activator, its receptor, and inhibitor type 1 in ovarian cancer. Int J Gynecol Cancer 2000;10:372–381.
77. Tecimer C, Doering DL, Goldsmith LJ, Meyer JS, Abdulhay G, Wittliff JL. Clinical relevance of urokinase-type plasminogen activator, its receptor, and its inhibitor type 1 in endometrial cancer. Gynecol Oncol 2001;80:48–55.
78. Look MP, van Putten WLJ, Duffy MJ, Harbeck N, Christensen IJ, Thomssen C, et al. Pooled analysis of prognostic impact of urokinase-type plasminogen activator and its inhibitor PAI-1 in 8377 breast cancer patients. J Nat Cancer Inst 2002;94: 116–128.
79. Janicke F, Prechtl F, Thomssen C, Harbeck N, Meisner C, Untch M, et al. Randomized adjuvant chemotherapy trial in high-risk lymph node-negative breast cancer patients identified by urokinase-type plasminogen activator and plasminogen activator inhibitor type 1. J Nat Cancer Inst 2001;93: 913–920.
80. Holschneider CH, Berek JS. Ovarian cancer: epidemiology, biology, and prognostic. Semin Surg Oncol 2000;19:3–10.
81. Bast RC Jr., Xu FJ, Yu YH, Barnhill S, Zhang Z, Mills GB. CA 125: The past and the future. Int J Biol Markers 1998;13: 179–187.
82. Bonfrer JMG, Duffy MJ, Radtke M, Segurado O, Torre GC, van Dalen A, et al. Tumor markers in gynecological cancers: EGTM recommendations. Anticancer Res 1999;19:2807–2810.
83. NIH Consensus Developmental Panel on Ovarian Cancer: NIH Consensus Conference. Ovarian cancer: screening, treatment and follow-up. JAMA 1995;273;491–497.
84. Petignat P, Joris F, Obrist R. How CA 125 is used in routine clinical practice. Eur J Cancer 2000;36:1933–1937.
85. Von Schlippe M, Rustin GJ. Circulating tumor markers in ovarian tumors. Forum (Genova). 2000;10:383–392.
86. Menon V, Jacobs IJ. Tumor markers and screening. In: Berek JS, Hacker NF, eds. Practical gynecologic oncology, 2nd ed. Baltimore: Williams and Wilkins, 2000:89–90.
87. Colakovic S, Lukic V, Mitrovic L, Jelic S, Susnjar S, Marinkovic J. Prognostic value of CA 125 kinetics and half-life in advanced ovarian cancer. Int J Biol Markers 2000;15:147–152.
88. Van Dalen A, Favier J, Baumgartner L, Hasholzner U, De Bruijn H, Dobbler D, et al. Serum levels of CA 125 and TPS during treatment of ovarian cancer. Anticancer Res 2000;20:5107–5108.
89. Selman AE, Copeland LJ. The roles of second-look laparotomy and cancer antigen 125 in the management of ovarian carcinoma. Curr Oncol Reports 1999;1:71–76.
90. Eagle K, Ledermann JA. Tumor markers in ovarian malignancies. Oncologist 1997;2:324–329.
91. Markman M. The role of CA-125 in the management of ovarian cancer. Oncologist 1997;2:6–9.
92. Tuxen MK, Sölétormos G, Rustin GJ, Nelstrop AE, Dombernowsky P. Biological variation and analytical imprecision of CA 125 in patients with ovarian cancer. Scand J Clin Lab Invest 2000;60:713–721.
93. Price FV, Chambers SK, Carcangiu ML, Kohorn EI, Schwartz PE, Chambers JT. CA125 may not reflect disease status in patients with uterine serous carcinoma. Cancer 1998;82: 1720–1725.
94. Duffy MJ. PSA as a marker for prostate cancer: a critical review. Ann Clin Biochem 1996;33:511–519.
95. Brawer MK. Prostate-specific antigen. Semin Surg Oncol 2000;18:3–9.
96. Recker F, Kwiatkowski MK, Huber A, Stamm B, Lehmann K, Tscholl R. Prospective detection of clinically relevant prostate cancer in the prostate-specific antigen range 1 to 3 ng/mL, combined with free to total ratio 20% or less: the Aarau experience. J Urol 2001;165:851–855.
97. Oesterling JE, Cooner WGH, Jacobsen SJ, Guess HA, Lieber MM. Influence of patient age on the serum PSA concentration. An important clinical observation. Urol Clin North Am 1993;20:671–680.
98. Semjonow A, Albrecht W, Bialk P, Gerl A, Lamerz R, Schmid HP, et al. Tumor markers in prostate cancer: EGTM recommendations. Anticancer Res 1999;19:2799–2801.
99. Morgan TO, Jacobsen SJ, McCarthy WF, Jacobsen DJ, McLeod DG, Moul JW. Age-specific reference ranges for serum prostate-specific antigen in black men. N Engl J Med 1996;335:304–310.
100. Brawer MK. Prostate-specific antigen: current status. CA Cancer J Clin 1999;49:264–281.
101. Catalona WJ, Partin AW, Slawin KM, Brawer MK, Flanigan RC, Patel A, et al. Use of the percentage of free prostate-specific antigen to enhance differentiation of prostate cancer from benign

prostatic disease: A prospective multi-center clinical trial. JAMA 1998;279:1542–1547.
102. Letran JL, Blasé AB, Loberiza FR, Meyer GE, Ransom SD, Brawer MK. Repeat ultrasound guided prostate needle biopsy: use of free-to-total prostate-specific antigen ratio in predicting prostatic carcinoma. J Urol 1998;160:426–429.
103. Carter HB, Partin AW, Luderer AA, Metter EJ, Landis P, Chan DW, et al. Percentage of free-prostate-specific antigen in sera predicts aggressiveness of prostate cancer a decade before diagnosis. Urology 1997;49:379–384.
104. Zhou Z, Ng PC, Very DL, Allard WJ, Yeung KK. Technicon Immuno 1 PSA assay measures both free and alpha-1-antichymotrypsin complexed prostate-specific antigen on an equimolar basis. J Clin Lab Anal 1996;10:155–159.
105. Allard WJ, Cheli CD, Morris DL, Goldblatt J, Pierre Y, Kish L, et al. Multi-center evaluation of the performance and clinical utility in longitudinal monitoring of the Bayer Immuno 1 complexed PSA assay. Int J Biol Markers 1999;14:73–83.
106. Brawer MK, Meyer GE, Letran JL Bankson DD, Morris DL, Yeung KK, et al. Measurement of complexed PSA improves specificity for early detection of prostate cancer. Urology 1998;52:372–348.
107. Woodrum D; French C, Shamel, LB. Stability of free prostate-specific antigen in serum samples under a variety of sample collection and sample storage conditions. Urology 1996;48;(Suppl 6A):33–39.
108. Woodrum D, York L. Two-year stability of free and total PSA in frozen serum samples. Urology 1998;52:247–251.
109. Price CP, Allard J, Davies G, Dawnay A, Duffy MJ, France M, et al. Pre- and post-analytical factors that may influence use of serum prostate-specific antigen and its isoforms in a screening program for prostate cancer. Ann Clin Biochem 2001;38:188–216.
110. Semjonow A, Brandt B, Oberpenning F, Roth S, Hertle L. Discordance of assay methods creates pitfalls for the interpretation of prostate-specific antigen values. Prostate 1996;7:3–16.
111. Smith RA, von Eschenbach AC, Wender R, Levin B, Byers T, Rothenberger D, et al. American Cancer Society guidelines for the early detection of cancer: update of early detection guidelines for prostate, colorectal, and endometrial cancers. Also: Update 2001—testing for early lung cancer detection. CA Cancer J Clin 2001;51:38–75.
112. Powell IJ. Prostate cancer in the African American: is this a different disease? Semin Urol Oncol 1998;16:221–226.
113. Smith RA, Cokkinides V, von Eschenbach AC, Levin B, Cohen C, Runowicz CD, et al. American Cancer Society Guidelines for early detection of cancer (2002). CA Cancer J Clin 2002;52:8–22.
114. Whitmore WF. Localized prostatic cancer: management and detection issues. Lancet 1994;343:1263–1267.
115. Middleton RG, Thompson IM, Austenfeld MS, Cooner WH, Correa RJ, Gibbons RP, et al. Prostate Cancer Clinical Guidelines Panel Summary report on the management of clinically localized prostate cancer. The American Urological Association. J Urol 1995;154:2144–2148.
116. Wilt TJ. Prostate cancer screening: practice what the evidence preaches. Am J Med 1998;104:602–604.
117. Zoorob R, Anderson R, Cefalu C, Sidani M. Cancer screening guidelines. Am Fam Physician 2001;63:1101–1112.
118. Gann PH. Interpreting recent trends in prostate cancer incidence and mortality. Epidemiology 1997;8:117–120.
119. Bartsch G, Horninger W, Klocker H, Reissigl A, Oberaigner W, Schonitzer D, et al. Prostate cancer mortality after introduction of prostate-specific antigen mass screening in the Federal State of Tyrol, Austria. Urology 2001;58:417–422.
120. Ries L, Eisner MP, Kosary CL. SEER cancer statistics review, 1973–1997. Bethesda, MD: National Cancer Institute, 2000.
121. Tarone RE, Chu KC, Brawley OW. Implications of stage-specific survival rates in assessing recent declines in prostate cancer mortality rates. Epidemiology 2000;11:167–170.
122. Roberts RO, Bergstrahl EJ, Katusic SK, Lieber MM, Jacobsen SJ. Decline in prostate cancer mortality from 1980 to 1997, and an update on incidence trends in Olmsted County, Minnesota. J Urol 1999;161:529–533.
123. Drachenberg DE. Treatment of prostate cancer: watchful waiting, radical prostatectomy, and cryoablation. Semin Surg Oncol 2000;18:37–44.
124. Etzioni R, Legler JM, Feuer EJ, Merrill RM, Cronin KA, Hankey BF. Cancer surveillance series: Interpreting trends in prostate cancer—Part III: Quantifying the link between population prostate-specific antigen testing and recent declines in prostate cancer mortality. J Natl Cancer Inst 1999;91:1033–1039.
125. Schwartz MK. Biochemical markers in staging clinically organ-confined prostate cancer. Molecular Urol 1997;1:129–133.
126. Partin AW, Kattan MW, Subong EN, Walsh PC, Wojno KJ, Oesterling JE, et al. Combination of prostate-specific antigen, clinical stage, and Gleason score to predict pathological stage of localized prostate cancer: A multi-institutional update. JAMA 1997;277:1445–1451.
127. Pontes JE, Chu TM, Slack N, Karr J, Murphy GP. Serum prostatic antigen measurement in localized prostatic disease: correlation with clinical course. J Urol 1982;128:1216–1218.
128. Scher HI. Management of prostate cancer after prostatectomy: treating the patient not the PSA. JAMA 1999;281:1642–1645.
129. Pound CR, Partin AW, Eisenberger MA, Chan DW, Pearson JD, Walsh PC. Natural history of progression after PSA elevation following radical prostatectomy. JAMA 1999;281:1591–1597.
130. Ross PL, Scardino PT, Kattan MW. A catalog of prostate cancer nomograms. J Urol 2001;165:1562–1568.
131. Winawer SJ. A quarter century of colorectal cancer screening: progress and prospects. J Clin Oncol 2001;19:6S–12S.
132. Mandel JS, Bond JH, Church TR, Snover DC, Bradley GM, Schuman LM, et al. Reducing mortality from colorectal cancer by screening for fecal occult blood. Minnesota Colon Cancer Control study. N Engl J Med 1993;328:1365–1371.
133. Selby JV, Friedman GD, Quesenberry CP, Weiss NS. A case-control study of screening sigmoidoscopy and mortality from colorectal cancer. N Engl J Med 1992;326:653–657.
134. Newcomb PA, Norfleet RG, Storer BE, Surawicz TS, Marcus PM. Screening sigmoidoscopy and colorectal cancer mortality. J Nat Cancer Inst 1992;84:1572–1575.
135. Winawer SJ, Flehinger BJ, Schottenfeld D, Miller DG. Screening for colorectal cancer with fecal occult blood testing and sigmoidoscopy. J Nat Cancer Inst 1993;85:1311–1318.
136. Lieberman DA, Weiss DG, Bond J, Ahnen DJ, Garewal H, Chejfec G. Use of colonoscopy to screen asymptomatic adults for colorectal cancer (Veterans Affairs Co-operative Study Group). N Engl J Med 2000;343:162–168.
137. Winawer SJ, Stewart ET, Zauber AG, Bond JH, Ansel H, Waye JD, et al. A comparison of colonoscopy and double contrast bari-

um enema for surveillance after polypectomy. N Engl J Med 2000;42:1766–1772.
138. Winawer SJ, Zauber AG, Gerdes H, O'Brien MJ, Gottlieb LS, Sternberg SS, et al. Risk of colorectal cancer in families of patients with adenomatous polyps. National Polyp Study Workgroup. N Engl J Med 1996;334:82–87.
139. Fletcher RH. Carcinoembryonic antigen. Ann Intern Med 1986; 104:66–73.
140. Klapdor R, Aronsson AC, Duffy MJ, Hansson LO, Khalifa R, Lamerz R, et al. Tumor markers in gastrointestinal cancers: EGTM recommendations. Anticancer Res 1999;19: 2811–2815.
141. Wanebo HJ, Rao B, Pinsky CM Hoffman RG, Stearns M, Schwartz MK, et al. Preoperative carcinoembryonic antigen level as a prognostic indicator in colorectal cancer. N Engl J Med 1978;299:448–451.
142. Compton C, Fenoglio-Preiser CM, Pettigrew N, Fielding LP. American Joint Committee on Cancer Prognostic Factors Consensus Conference: Colorectal Working Group. Cancer 2000;88:1739–1757.
143. Duffy MJ. Carcinoembryonic antigen as a marker for colorectal cancer: is it clinically useful? Clin Chem 2001;47:624–630.
144. Filella X, Molina R, Pique JM, Grau JJ, Garcia-Valdecasas JC, Biete A, et al. CEA as a prognostic factor in colorectal cancer. Anticancer Res 1994;14:705–708.
145. Begent RHJ. The value of carcinoembryonic antigen measurement in clinical practice. Ann Clin Biochem 1984;21:231–238.
146. MacDonald JS. Carcinoembryonic antigen screening: pros and cons. Semin Oncol 1999;26:556–560.
147. Makela JT, Laitinen SO, Kairaluoma MI. Five-year follow-up after radical surgery for colorectal cancer results of a prospective randomized trial. Arch Surg 1995;130:1062–1067.
148. Pietra N, Sarli L, Costi R, Ouchemi C, Grattarola M, Peracchia A. Role of follow-up in the management of local recurrence of colorectal cancer: a prospective, randomized study. Dis Colon Rectum 1998;41:1127–1133.
149. Rosen M, Chan L, Beart RW, Vukasin P, Anthone G. Follow-up of colorectal cancer: a meta-analysis. Dis Colon Rectum 1998;41:1116–1126.
150. Bruinvels DJ, Stiggelbout AM, Kievit J, van Houwelingen HC, Habbema JD, van de Velde JC. Follow-up of patients with colorectal cancer, a meta-analysis. Ann Surg 1994;219:174–182.
151. Niederhuber JE, Ensminger WD: Treatment of metastatic cancer to the liver. In: DeVita VT, et al., eds. Cancer: principles and practice of oncology. Philadelphia PA: Lippincott, 1993; 2201–2225.
152. Mulcahy MF, Benson AB. The role of carcinoembryonic antigen monitoring in management of colorectal cancer. Curr Oncol Rep 1999;1:168–172.
153. Moertel CG, Fleming TR, Macdonald JS, Haller DG, Laurie JA. Hepatic toxicity associated with fluorouracil plus levamisole adjuvant therapy. J Clin Oncol 1993;11:2386–2390.
154. Mitchell EP. Role of carcinoembryonic antigen in the management of advanced colorectal cancer. Semin Oncol 1998;25: 12–20.
155. Lechago J. Neuroendocrine cells of the gut and their disorders. In: Goldman H, Appelman HD, Kaufman N, eds. Gastrointestinal pathology. Baltimore, MD: Williams and Wilkins, 1990;181–219.
156. Oberg K. Advances in chemotherapy and biotherapy of endocrine tumors. Curr Opin Oncol 1998;10:58–65.
157. Gitlow SE, Bertani LM, Rausen A, Gribetz D, Dziedzic SW. Diagnosis of neuroblastoma by qualitative and quantitative determination of catecholamine metabolites in urine. Cancer 1970;25:1377–1383

158. Koch DD, Polizin GL. Effect of sample preparation and liquid chromatography column choice on selectivity and precision of plasma catecholamine determination. J Chromatogr 1987;386: 19–24.
159. Haymond RE, Knight JA, Bills AC. Normal values for urinary 3-methoxy-4-hydroxymandelic acid (VMA) in children. Clin Chem 1978;24:1853–1854.
160. Knight JA, Wu JT. Catecholamine and their metabolites: Clinical and laboratory aspects. Lab Med 1987;18:153–158.
161. Eisenhofer G, Friberg P, Pacak K, Goldstein DS, Murphy DL, Tsigos C, et al. Plasma metadrenalines: do they provide useful information about sympatho-adrenal function and catecholamine metabolism? Clin Sci (London) 1995;88:533–542.
162. Moyer TP, Jiang NS, Tyce GM, Sheps SG. Analysis for urinary catecholamines by liquid chromatography with amperometric detection: method and clinical interpretation of results. Clin Chem 1979;25:256–263.
163. Mannelli M. Diagnostic problems in pheochromocytoma. J. Endocrinol Invest 1989;12:739–757.
164. Feldman JM. Urinary serotonin in the diagnosis of carcinoid tumors. Clin Chem 1986;32:840–844.
165. Austin LA, Heath H. Calcitonin: physiology and pathophysiology. N Engl J Med 1981;304:269–278.
166. Deftos LJ. Radioimmunoassay for calcitonin in medullary thyroid carcinoma. JAMA 1974;227:403–406.
167. Heath H, Sizemore GW. Radioimmunoassay for calcitonin. Clin Chem 1982;28:1219–1226.
168. Lips CJ, Hoppener JW, Thijssen JH. Medullary thyroid carcinoma: role of genetic testing and calcitonin measurement. Ann Clin Biochem 2001;38:168–179.
169. Devesa SS, Blot WJ, Stone BJ, Miller BA, Tarone RE, Fraumeini JF. Recent cancer trends in the United States. J Natl Cancer Inst 1995;87:175–182.
170. Bosl GJ, Vogelzang NJ, Goldman A, Fraley EE, Lange PH, Levitt SH, et al. Impact of delay in diagnosis on clinical stage of testicular cancer. Lancet 1981;2:970–973.
171. Scher H, Bosl G, Gellder N, Cirrincione C, Whitmore W, Golbey R. Impact of symptomatic interval on prognosis of patients with stage III testicular cancer. Urology 1983;21:559–561.
172. Norgaard-Pedersen B, Raghavan D. Germ cell tumors: a collaborative review. Oncodev Biol Med 1980;1:327–358.
173. Bosl GJ, Motzer RJ. Testicular germ cell cancer. N Engl J Med 1997;337:242–253.
174. Doherty AP, Bower M, Christmas TJ. The role of tumor markers in the diagnosis and treatment of testicular germ cell cancers. Br J Urol 1997;79:247–252.
175. Lamerz R, Albrecht W, Bialk P, Dati F, Duffy MR, Gerl E, et al. Tumor markers in germ cell cancers: EGTM recommendations. Anticancer Res 1999;19:2795–2798.
176. Nielsen OS, Munro OJ, Duncan W, Sturgeon J, Gospodarowicz MK, Jewett MA, et al. Is placental alkaline phosphatase (PLAP) a useful marker for seminoma? Eur J Cancer 1990;26: 1049–1054.
177. Albrecht W, Bonner E, Jeschke K, Stoiber F, Schmidt P, Scheiber K, et al., and the Austrian Uro-Oncology Group. PLAP as a marker in germ cell tumors. In: Jones WG, Appleyard I, Harnden P, Joffe JK, eds. Germ cell tumors IV. London: John Libbey & Co. Ltd., 1998;105–109.
178. Von Eyben FE. A systematic review of lactate dehydrogenase isoenzyme I and germ cell tumors. Clin Biochem 2001; 34:441–454.
179. International Germ Cell Cancer Collaborative Group (IGCCCG). International germ cell consensus classification: a prognostic

factor-based staging system for metastatic germ cell cancers. J Clin Oncol 1997;15:594–603.
180. Horwich A, Peckham MJ. Serum tumor-marker regression rate following chemotherapy for malignant teratoma. Eur J Cancer Clin Oncol 1984;20:1463–1470.
181. Toner GC, Geller NL, Tan C, Nisselbaum J, Bosl GJ. Serum tumor marker half-life during chemotherapy allows early prediction of complete response and survival in non-seminomatous germ cell tumors Cancer Res 1990;50:5904–5910.
182. Mazumdar M, Bajorin DF, Bacik J, Higgins G, Motzer RJ, Bosl GJ. Predicting outcome to chemotherapy in patients with germ cell tumors: the value of the rate of decline of human chorionic gonadotrophin and alpha-fetoprotein during therapy. J Clin Oncol 2001;19:2534–2541.
183. Gerl A, Lamerz R, Clemm C, Mann K, Wilmanns W. Does serum tumor marker half-life complement pre-treatment risk stratification in metastatic non-seminomatous germ cell tumors? Clin Cancer Res 1996;2:1565–1570.
184. Kyle RA, Katzmann JA. Immunochemical characterization of immunoglobulins. In: Rose NR, Conway de Macario E, Folds JD, Lane HC, Nakamura RM, eds. Manual of Clinical Laboratory Immunology, 5th ed. Washington, DC: American Society for Microbiology, 1997;156–176.
185. Keren DF, Warren JS, Lowe JB. Strategy to diagnose monoclonal gammopathies in serum: high-resolution electrophoresis, immunofixation, and kappa/lambda quantification. Clin Chem 1988; 34:2196–2201.
186. Kyle RA, Robinson RA, Katzmann JA. The clinical aspects of biclonal gammopathies. Review of 57 cases. Am J Med 1981;71: 999–1008.
187. Whicher JT, Calvin J, Riches P, Warren C. The laboratory investigation of paraproteinemia. Ann Clin Biochem 1987;24: 119–132.
188. Kyle RA. Monoclonal gammopathy of undetermined significance and solitary plasmacytoma. Implications for progression to overt multiple myeloma. Hematol Oncol Clin North Am 1997;11: 71–87.
189. Katzmann JA, Clark R, Wiegert E, Sanders E, Oda RP, Kyle RA, et al. Identification of monoclonal proteins in serum: a quantitative comparison of acetate, agarose gel, and capillary electrophoresis. Electrophoresis 1997;18:1775–1780.
190. Riches PG, Sheldon J, Smith AM, Hobbs JR. Overestimation of monoclonal immunoglobulin by immunochemical methods. Ann Clin Biochem 1991;28:253–259.
191. Kyle RA. Sequence of testing for monoclonal gammopathies. Arch Pathol Lab Med 1999;123:114–118.
192. Kallemuchikkal U, Gorevic PD. Evaluation of cryoglobulins. Arch Pathol Lab Med 1999;123:119–125.
193. Katzman JA, Clark R, Sanders E, Landers JP, Kyle RA. Prospective study of serum protein capillary zone electrophoresis and immunotyping of monoclonal proteins by immunosubtraction. Am J Clin Pathol 1998;110:503–509.
194. Stieber P, Aronsson AC, Bialk P, Kulpa J, Lamerz R, Molina R, et al. Tumor markers in lung cancer: EGTM recommendations. Anticancer Res 1999;19:2817–2819.
195. Lamerz R. SCC (squamous cell carcinoma antigen) In: Thomas L, ed. Clinical laboratory diagnostics. Verlag Frankfurt:TH-Books, 1998;900–986.
196. Lamerz R. NSE (neuron-specific enolase) In: Thomas L, ed. Clinical laboratory diagnostics. Verlag Frankfurt:TH-Books, 1998; 979–981.
197. Stieber P. CYFRA 21-1 (Cytokeratin-19-fragments). In: Thomas L, ed. Clinical laboratory diagnostics. Verlag Frankfurt:TH-Books, 1998;966–970.
198. Paone G, De Angelis G, Munno R, Pallotta G, Bigioni D, Saltini C, et al. Discriminant analysis on small-cell lung cancer and non-small-cell lung cancer by means of NSE and CYFRA 21-1. Eur Respir J 1995;8:1136–1140.
199. Fischbach W, Schwarz-Wallrauch C, Jany B. Neuron-specific enolase and thymidine kinase as an aid to the diagnosis and treatment monitoring of small-cell lung cancer. Cancer 1989;63: 1143–1149.
200. Molina R, Agusti C, Mane JM, Filella X, Jo J, Joseph J, et al. CYFRA 21-1 in lung cancer: comparison with CEA, CA 125, SCC, and NSE serum levels. Int J Biol Markers 1994;9: 96–101.
201. Stieber P, Hasholzner U, Bodenmüller H, Nagel D, Sunder-Plassmann L, Dienemann H, et al. CYFRA 21-1—a new marker in lung cancer. Cancer 1993;72:707–713.
202. Nisman B, Lafair J, Heching N, Lyass O, Baras M, Peretz T, et al. Evaluation of tissue polypeptide specific antigen, CYFRA 21-1 and carcinoembryonic antigen, in non-small-cell lung carcinoma. Does the combined use of cytokeratin markers give any additional information? Cancer 1998;82:1850–1859.
203. Nisman B, Heching N, Barak V. Serum tumor markers in resectable and non-resectable non-small-cell lung cancer. J Tum Marker Oncol 2000;15:195–207.
204. Yoshimasu T, Maebeya S, Suzuma T, Bessho T, Tanino H, Arimoto J, et al. Disappearance curves for tumor markers after resection of intrathoracic malignancies. Int J Biol Markers 1999; 14:99–105.
205. Christofori R, Aimo G, Mengozzi G, Oliaro A, Revello F, Rapellino M. Tumor markers kinetic in malignant lung neoplasms. J Cardiovasc Surg (Torino) 1999;40:299–305.
206. Watine J. Prognostic evaluation of primary non-small-cell lung carcinoma patients using biological fluid variables. A systematic review. Scand J Clin Lab Invest 2000;60:259–273.
207. Watine J. Laboratory variables as additional staging parameters in patients with small-cell lung carcinoma. A systematic review. Clin Chem Lab Med 1999;37:931–938.
208. Pujol JL, Boher JM, Grenier J, Quantin X. Cyfra 21-1, neuron specific enolase and prognosis of non-small-cell lung cancer: prospective study in 621 patients. Lung Cancer 2001;31: 221–231.
209. Bork E, Hansen M, Urdal P, Paus E, Holst JJ, Schifter S, et al. Early detection of response in small-cell bronchogenic carcinoma by changes in serum concentrations of creatine kinase, neuron-specific enolase, calcitonin, ACTH, serotonin, and gastrin-releasing peptide. Eur J Cancer Clin Oncol 1988;24: 1033–1038.
210. Bonner JA, Sloan JA, Rowland KM Jr, Klee GG, Kugler JW, Mailliard JA, et al. Significance of neuron-specific enolase levels before and during therapy for small-cell lung cancer. Clin Cancer Res 2000;6:597–601.
211. Ebert W, Hoppe M, Muley T, Drings P. Monitoring of therapy in inoperable lung cancer patients by measurement of CYFRA 21-1, TPA, CEA, and NSE. Anticancer Res 1997;17: 2875–2878.
212. Ebert W, Muley T. CYFRA 21-1 in the follow-up of inoperable non-small-cell lung cancer patients treated with chemotherapy. Anticancer Res 1999; 19:2669–2672.
213. Hamzaoui A, Thomas P, Castelnau O, Roux N, Roux F, Kleisbauer JP. Usefulness of longitudinal evaluation of CYFRA 21-1 variations in advanced lung cancer monitoring. Lung Cancer 1997;16: 191–202.

Chapter **6**

Limitations of Assay Techniques for Tumor Markers

Catharine M. Sturgeon

Analysis of tumor markers in body fluids has contributed to the diagnosis and management of cancer patients ever since Henry Bence Jones first described, in 1847, the inappropriate presence of immunoglobulin light chains in the urine of patients with multiple myeloma (1). Early methods for detecting Bence Jones proteins involved heat treatment and precipitation of the proteins, but by the mid-twentieth century more convenient analysis using immunoelectrophoresis was possible. Similar immunological techniques were also applied to the detection of other molecules associated with malignancy, i.e., tumor markers.

The development of radioimmunoassay (RIA) techniques in the 1960s allowed more convenient quantitation of some of these markers, and by the late 1970s RIAs were well established for α-fetoprotein (AFP), carcinoembryonic antigen (CEA), and human chorionic gonadotropin (hCG). Introduction of monoclonal antibody (mAb) technology brought further progress, including the identification of new cancer-associated molecules defined solely by their immunoreactivity with specific mAbs (e.g., CA125, CA15.3, CA19.9). The subsequent development of immunometric assays, and their ready availability on automated systems, means that many more hospital laboratories now have the facilities to measure tumor markers, whereas these were previously available only in specialized laboratories. For example, the number of laboratories participating in the UK National External Quality Assessment Scheme (UK NEQAS) for CEA increased from 38 to 245 between 1988 and 2002 (2).

As the frequency of tumor marker measurement increases, improved awareness of the limitations—both analytical and clinical—of these tests is essential if the risk of their inappropriate interpretation is to be minimized. The fundamental clinical limitations of tumor marker tests, which relate to their sensitivity and specificity, are considered elsewhere (see chapters 2, 4 and 5). Generally, the preanalytical limitations of tumor marker assays are common to all tests in clinical chemistry, while their analytical limitations are shared with all immunoassays. Manufacturers very helpfully draw attention to some of these limitations in the product information supplied with kit reagents. It is very important that laboratory staff carefully note these stated limitations, which are likely to vary, depending both on the analyte and on the method. It is always essential to have appropriate internal quality control and external quality assessment protocols in place, and to act promptly if the former suggests an assay problem.

Inevitably, as the number of tumor marker tests performed worldwide increases, so does the risk of analytical discrepancies and other errors that may adversely affect clinical care. These analytical limitations perhaps have added importance for tumor marker assays, tests that are often performed for the same patient over long periods of time, sometimes in different laboratories and by different methods. In this chapter reasons for discrepancies in tumor marker analysis are considered under three broad headings:

- Comparability of tumor marker results (reflected in accuracy, calibration, imprecision, analytical specificity)
- Preanalytical factors (e.g., specimen type, specimen timing)
- Individual method robustness to potential interferences (e.g., heterophilic antibodies, "hooking")

COMPARABILITY OF TUMOR MARKER RESULTS

Automation has brought major advances in analytical performance, but the lack of comparability between results obtained using different methods remains a major limitation. It is still essential to recognize, for all tumor markers, that results obtained with different methods are usually not readily interchangeable. As most tumor markers are complex and heterogeneous analytes, often best regarded as families of molecules, this is not surprising. Even for AFP, a relatively simple molecule structurally closely related to albumin, the spread of results is considerable, as illustrated in Figure 1, a Box and Whisker plot showing the cumulative bias (or deviation) from the target value for ten AFP methods. These values range from -10% to $+7.5\%$, reflecting method-related differences in results (2).

It is useful to review briefly some of the aspects of immunoassay design that influence assay performance, in order to consider the implications of these for tumor marker measurements. The principles and designs of RIA and immunometric methods have been well described elsewhere (3,4). While early tumor marker assays were predominantly reagent-limited

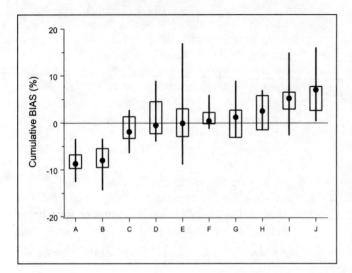

Figure 1 UK NEQAS data showing Box and Whisker plots for ten major AFP methods (A–J). Median, interquartile, and extreme ranges are shown (2).

RIAs, most laboratories now use commercially available, reagent-excess immunometric methods for tumor marker measurements. These methods generally employ nonisotopic labels, as the optical detection systems are easier to automate, shelf lives are longer, and the health hazards associated with isotopic labels are absent.

Influence of Signal Detection (Label) on Assay Performance

The reagent-limited assays originally commonly (but now rarely) used for tumor marker measurements employ radiolabels (most frequently ^{125}I-labeled antigens) or enzyme labels (most often horseradish peroxidase or alkaline phosphatase). Theoretically, analytical sensitivities should be similar with either, but in practice enzyme labels rarely achieve the analytical sensitivity of RIA. They are limited by the lower and upper limits of spectrophotometric measurement, and are also more susceptible to interference and changes in assay conditions during the signal generation stage. These difficulties can however be minimized by removing serum constituents prior to the enzymatic reaction, as is done in some methods (e.g. Bayer Immuno-1™).

Analytical sensitivity can be improved somewhat by use of enzyme amplification techniques. Further improvement by as much as an order of magnitude can be achieved by using the same enzyme labels with substrates that convert to fluorescent products. These products can be stimulated repeatedly to produce a signal in a short space of time, a reaction that is employed in a number of methods (e.g., Abbott AxSYM™). Direct fluorescence assays, in which fluorophore labels are substituted for ^{125}I-labels, are also available (e.g., Wallac DELFIA™). The Wallac method employs time-resolved rather than conventional fluorometry, significantly increasing the working range and almost eliminating the interference from background fluorescence and quenching effects that can limit sensitivity achievable by conventional methods.

Similarly, chemiluminescent reactions, which emit light during the course of a chemical reaction, and which can be initiated chemically or electrically, also avoid these problems, the latter forming the basis of the Roche ElecSys™ methods.

Sensitivities and Detection Limits

The definition of detection limit generally adopted by manufacturers is the concentration two standard deviations higher than the mean of the "zero" calibrator measurement values, representing the lowest measurable concentration of analyte that can be distinguished from zero. There are difficulties in comparing data provided by different kit manufacturers, since the composition of the "zero" calibrator (whether buffer, animal sera, etc) is relevant. Detection limits determined in buffer may give an overly optimistic impression of performance in pathological fluids, which may contain nonspecific factors (sometimes referred to as "matrix effects"). It has been suggested that a detection limit determined using assay buffer alone should be at least five-fold lower than the discrimination limit required (5). It would also be useful if the minimal quantifiable concentration (the lowest concentration for which a coefficient of variation of 20% can be achieved [6]) was also specified with the product information supplied, but these data are rarely presented. For some tumor markers, e.g., AFP, hCG, and PSA, good precision at low concentrations is essential as clinical decisions may be taken on the basis of very small increases in marker concentration. A suitable detection method and minimal nonspecific interference are therefore particularly important for these measurements.

Working Range

The serum concentrations of tumor markers can vary considerably, from undetectable in healthy persons to several millions of units per liter in those with advanced malignancy, particularly for AFP, hCG and CEA. As the highest kit calibrator concentrations for most markers are between 500 and 1000 concentration units/liter, some specimens require pre-dilution. A wide working range is therefore highly desirable, in order to minimize the number of specimens that must be diluted. Availability of sufficient and appropriately constituted diluent is essential, and automatic dilution facilities are very helpful. Experience suggests that poor skills present in some laboratories may lead to more frequent errors of dilution. (See also later discussion of hook effects.)

Imprecision

In general, the precision of automated methods is very good, but knowledge of individual method performance is always essential, as illustrated in Figure 2, which shows within-method, between-laboratory precision profiles for four major hCG methods. Clearly the precision achievable with Method D is far superior to that achievable with Method A. Users of the latter method need to be aware of its apparent imprecision, as

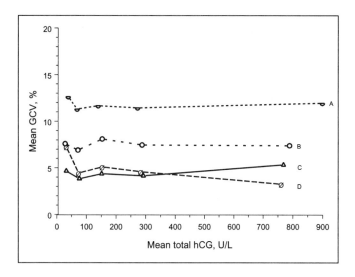

Figure 2 UK NEQAS data showing within-method between-laboratory precision profiles for four major hCG methods (A-D) (2).

this may influence the interpretation of sequential patient results obtained using the method.

This is of particular importance in determining what constitutes a significant or clinically relevant change. Clearly, contributions of both biological and analytical variation need to be considered. Both are discussed in detail elsewhere (7,8) (see also Chapter 2), and have also been discussed in relation to the use of prostate-specific antigen (PSA) in screening for prostate cancer (9) (see also Chapter 17). Briefly, what constitutes an analytically significant change in results can best be considered in terms of the reference change value (RCV) (sometimes called the critical difference), which may be calculated using the formula

$$RCV = \sqrt{2} \times Z \times (cv_a),$$

where Z is the standard normal deviation, or Z-score, and cv_a is the coefficient of (analytical) variation (i.e., analytical precision). For any analyte the cv_a can be readily calculated from routine internal quality control data; the within-run precision should be used where the samples are assayed in one run, and the between-run precision used where samples are assayed in different runs. Z-scores of 1.96 and 2.58, respectively, are used to calculate the probability that an observed change is significant (95% probability) or highly significant (99% probability) (7).

While available product information often provides very useful data about the within-run and between-run performance achievable by the particular method at different analyte concentrations, according to the National Committee for Clinical Laboratory Standards (NCCLS) protocol (10), relating such data to that provided for kits from other manufacturers is often difficult. The concentrations and number of pools for which figures are reported vary, and in some cases no indication of concentrations is provided. Minimizing lot-to-lot variability is an important responsibility of manufacturers. Relatively small changes can influence patient results, particularly for methods with very good precision. By including appropriate additional quality control checks following changes of lot and/or re-calibration, laboratories can gain some assurance of the constancy of the reagents with which they are supplied

Accuracy/Calibration

Recovery data for pools of normal serum to which known amounts of the working calibrator has been added are usually available in the product information supplied with the reagents; reported recoveries generally vary from 95 to 105%. Some manufacturers also provide data showing recoveries obtained for specimens containing known added concentrations of the relevant International Standards (Table 1). Provision of data relating kit standards to International Standards (where they exist) (i.e., "traceability") will become a requirement when the In Vitro Diagnostics Directive (IVDD) is implemented in Europe in 2003 (15). As yet, no International Standards have

Table 1 Current international standards for tumor markers[a]

Tumor marker	International Standard	Year established	Source	Reference
AFP	IS 72/225	1972	Crude cord serum (50%)	11
CEA	IRP 73/601	1973	Partially purified CEA (liver metastases)	12
HCG	IS 75/537	1975	Purified hCG, contaminated with hCGβ and nicked hCG	13
hCGβ	IRP 75/551	1975		13
PSA	IS 96/670	2000	90:10 ratio of bound:free PSA	14
Free PSA	IS 96/668	2000	Purified free PSA	14
CA125	None	—	—	—
CA15.3	None	—	—	—
CA19.9	None	—	—	—
CA72.4	None	—	—	—

[a] International Assay Standards are available from the National Institute for Biological Standards and Control [NIBSC], PO Box 1193, Blanche Lane, South Mimms, Herts EN6 3QH, UK. [e-mail: standards@nibsc.ac.uk].

been established for several important tumor markers (Table 1). However, the recent development of International Standards for PSA and Free PSA, largely as a result of the efforts of a urologist who recognized this as an important contribution towards improving assay comparability (16), will hopefully encourage similar activity for other tumor markers, particularly CA125, CA15.3, and CA19.9.

Data comparing recoveries of International Standards in different methods are sometimes available from proficiency testing (external quality assessment) schemes (17), and can provide valuable objective information about which methods are appropriately calibrated and which require attention. Where International Standards are not yet available, as for the CA antigens, it is much more difficult to compare results between methods. The difficulties are analogous to those for CEA, for which most manufacturers calibrate their methods in mass units (ng/mL). The method-specific conversion factors required to express ng/mL of CEA in terms of U/L of the International Standard for CEA (IRP 73/601) range from 11.4 to 18.6. As well as confirming that one manufacturers' "nanogram" of CEA is not necessarily the same as another's, this illustrates why reference to a common standard is generally desirable. Encouragingly, introduction of the first International Standard for PSA already appears to have contributed to improved between-method agreement for PSA (18). In one proficiency testing scheme, coefficients of variation (CVs) for individual specimens were 15–20% in the 1990s, but following introduction of the International Standard, mean CVs of <10% are now frequently observed (19). (Improved assay design, and in particular replacement of assays preferentially recognizing free PSA ["non-equimolar assays"] with "equimolar assays," has also been important.)

Linearity

Product information routinely supplied with kit reagents by some assay manufacturers provides information relating to linearity, i.e., parallelism on dilution, generally reporting linear results for experiments in which serum samples are assayed at serial dilutions. Good linearity on dilution is also regularly demonstrated for many tumor markers in different proficiency testing schemes. In routine practice, deviation from linearity for most tumor markers is generally rare and is most often attributable to interfering substances present in occasional specimens. Such nonlinear dilution, with increased recovery of the antigen, is probably most frequently observed in immunoassays for mucins (CA125, CA15.3, etc) (20), possibly due to a variety of factors, including the presence of high levels of anti-carbohydrate antibodies in serum (generating complexes), the inherent property of mucins to aggregate and disaggregate into a range of molecular species, and other matrix-related effects (3).

Method Specificity

The analytical specificity of any immunoassay is primarily determined by the antibodies employed, although method design is also important. The advent of monoclonal antibodies has facilitated the development of specific procedures for measuring tumor markers, as has been elegantly described for hCG (21), although dual antibody assays can be designed to have wider specificity. If methods are correctly calibrated in terms of a common standard, then the major factor contributing to method-related differences in results will be the differing specificities of the antibodies employed.

Recognizing this, the International Society for Oncodevelopmental Biology and Medicine (ISOBM) has initiated a series of Tissue Differentiation (TD) Workshops, with the primary aim of comparing the numerous monoclonal antibodies apparently identifying the same antigen. Workshops have been held on antibodies to AFP, CA125, CEA, hCG, PSA, MUC-1 (CA15.3, CA27-29, etc.), sialyl-Lewis[a] (CA19.9, etc.), and cytokeratins (CYFRA 21.1, tissue polypeptide specific antigen, etc.) (22–29). Results of these and similar studies may in the future facilitate development of broad recommendations about the antibody specificities and combinations likely to yield the most clinically useful immunoassays. Until such recommendations are made it is unlikely that significant improvement in between-method comparability will be achieved.

The heterogeneity of antibody specificities and affinities clearly demonstrated in the TD Workshops helps to explain the differences in tumor marker results observed for specimens issued through proficiency testing schemes. These differences are most readily seen for specimens containing known amounts of added cross-reacting substances, e.g., normal cross-reacting antigens 1 and 2 in assays for CEA. While the heterogeneity of antibodies employed in CEA assays can readily be demonstrated in this way, the clinical implications of these cross-reactions for CEA measurements in patient sera are not clear (30).

For some analytes, recognizing a spectrum of related molecules is important, although this may depend on the clinical application. Measurement of hCG provides a good example of the difficulties encountered when developing methods for the measurement of heterogeneous analytes (31). As is the case for other tumor markers, "hCG" is perhaps most appropriately regarded as a family of closely related molecules, the most important of which are intact hCG (hCG), a nicked form of hCG (hCGn), the free alpha- and beta-subunits (hCGα and hCGβ), a nicked form of hCGβ (hCGβn), and the core fragment of hCG (hCGβcf). The clinical relevance of some of these hCG-related molecules has yet to be established and also depends on the biological fluid being considered. HCGβcf, for example, is the major form of hCG present in urine but it is present only in very low concentration in plasma. In monitoring apparently normal pregnancy, determination of intact hCG alone will suffice. When using "hCG" as a tumor marker, it is well accepted that at least intact hCG and hCGβ should be measured. This can be achieved either by using a broad-spectrum method recognizing both molecules, or by using two specific methods—one recognizing the intact molecule and one its free subunit. While the latter approach is attractive, and theoretically desirable, the additional cost involved may mean it is not practicable. Whether measurement of hCGn and hCGβn is of importance in oncology has yet to be established as few clinical data are available.

There is undoubtedly a fundamental requirement for awareness not only of what molecules are being measured by a particular immunoassay, but also of which molecules it is clinically most relevant to measure. For hCG, the first requirement is currently being addressed by the International Federation of Clinical Chemistry (IFCC), under whose auspices potential International Standards for the six hCG-related molecules described above are being prepared (32). These standards will enable both manufacturers and users of assays for hCG-related molecules to better characterize what their methods measure, also hopefully improving understanding of the causes of between-method differences in results. Results of a recent ISOBM Workshop on antibodies to hCG are likely to contribute to this (25).

The poor comparability of immunoassay results for most tumor markers clearly illustrates the problems inherent in attempting to measure "mixtures," a goal that may well be regarded as "impossible" on theoretical grounds (33). Over the last ten years there have been major developments in microarray technology, which may ultimately overcome these difficulties by permitting simultaneous assay of a number of analytes (34). Multi-analyte assays are likely to become part of the routine laboratory repertoire within the next decade. This technology should bring exciting advances in the field of tumor markers, for example enabling measurement of six or more hCG-related molecules on a single chip, together with isoforms of other relevant tumor markers. These exciting prospects will bring new challenges for both quality control and data interpretation.

PREANALYTICAL FACTORS AFFECTING TUMOR MARKER RESULTS

Simple specimen handling errors in the preanalytical phase probably account for a relatively large proportion of errors for all laboratory tests (35). Predominant among such errors are (a) the use of inappropriate specimen collection tubes, and (b) specimen mix-ups, either in the requesting unit or following specimen arrival at the laboratory. While the first should be recognized and corrected (by requesting a repeat specimen in the correct tube) when the sample reaches the laboratory, the second are more frequently identified post-analysis, when results are clinically authorized. It is important to note that these errors will generally escape detection by either internal quality control (IQC) or proficiency testing (PT) procedures. While cumulative reporting of results and/or delta checking can facilitate the identification of such errors, which are a hazard with all laboratory tests, a significant proportion undoubtedly remain undetected. Some other preanalytical requirements of particular relevance to tumor marker testing are highlighted in Table 2.

Sample timing is usually not critical for most tumor marker measurements. However, sampling at an inappropriate time occasionally results in misleading and transiently elevated results, which can cause undue alarm and distress to the patient, as well as decreasing confidence in laboratory testing (36). Serum PSA levels greater than 50 μg/L, which could be consistent with prostatic malignancy, are observed in some patients with urinary tract infections or prostatitis, although these levels usually decrease to within the reference range following successful antibiotic treatment. Similarly, hCG levels may be transiently elevated if specimens are taken too soon after chemotherapy. The mild and transient increase in serum CA125 that can occur during menstruation can cause significant anxiety in patients with a family history of ovarian cancer, if screening samples are inadvertently taken when the patient is menstruating. Clinicians requesting tumor marker measurements are not always aware of these potential hazards, but the laboratory can provide cautionary reminders about these when reporting results, and can also suggest repeat testing at an appropriate time interval.

Kit manufacturers usually include instructions about specimen type (e.g., whether plasma or sera) and storage (e.g., length of time on the blood clot, whether at 4 °C or −30 °C), and these instructions should always be followed. It is unrealistic to expect clinicians to be aware of these detailed requirements, so it is the responsibility of the laboratory to keep them informed (36). Good communication between laboratory and clinical staff is a requisite.

INDIVIDUAL METHOD ROBUSTNESS TO POTENTIAL INTERFERENCES

The robustness of immunoassays refers to their ability to give accurate results in the presence of potential interferences. Interferences can be exogenous (Table 3), arising from the assay system or equipment used, or endogenous (Table 4), arising from particular properties of the sample being analyzed (37–40). Such interferences are perhaps the most serious cause of clinically misleading results for the following reasons:

- They are sporadic, varying in effect across time.
- They are not detected by internal quality control (IQC) procedures.
- They vary between methods, depending on the robustness of the assay design.

Interferences are difficult to avoid completely, but their impact can be reduced by careful design of methods, and critical awareness of the assayist.

Exogenous Interference

Discrepancies in results relating primarily to the method used are common to all immunoassays. It is important to be aware of these possible causes of error (Table 3), of which carry-over and analyzer mis-sampling are most likely to cause problems for tumor marker measurement in routine practice.

Carry-over. Where specimens are analyzed in sequence, there is a danger of contamination of each specimen by the previous one. This is most likely to occur if the same sample probe or pipette is used for different specimens and is not adequately rinsed, and is probably more likely with manual assays. Sample probes on automated systems are generally designed to minimize the risk of carry-over (e.g., by Teflon™ coating) but

Table 2 Preanalytical considerations of relevance when measuring tumor markers[a]

Timing of specimen collection	Pre-treatment specimen always desirable. No strong evidence of diurnal variation for most markers, so specimens can be taken at any time of day. Timing post-operatively (e.g., CA125 may be increased by peritoneal trauma). Prostatic biopsy/transurethral resection of the prostate (TURP), catheterization or acute painful urinary retention may markedly elevate serum PSA, but the magnitude of the increase in PSA levels is variable. Blood should be taken before any manipulation of the prostate. Prostatitis may also increase serum PSA levels. Specimens should be taken several weeks after resolution of prostatitis or urinary tract infections, and raised concentrations in patients with such infections should always be confirmed by repeat analysis post-treatment. Digital rectal examination (DRE) may transiently elevate serum PSA; best to take blood prior to DRE. May also be increased post-ejaculation (note time of ejaculation where relevant).
Effect of other treatment / medication	Immunometric methods vulnerable to interference from human anti-mouse antibody (HAMA); previous treatment with these should be noted on the request form.
Effect of renal failure / impairment	Not much documented evidence. Published reports suggest most likely to cause inappropriately elevated results for CEA, tissue polypeptide specific antigen (TPS) and other cytokeratins.
Effect of cholestasis	May markedly increase serum CA19.9 concentrations.
Contamination with saliva	May markedly increase apparent concentrations of CEA, CA19.9, and TPS.
Effect of smoking	May slightly increase apparent CEA levels in some immunoassays.
Type of specimen	Serum or plasma generally most appropriate and suited to most commercial assays, but requirements should be checked in the product information supplied. Gel tubes may not be suitable for some assays.
Stability of specimen on storage	Generally stable, although separation of serum from the clot and storage at 4 °C (short term) or –30 °C (long term) desirable as soon as possible. Heating of specimens usually undesirable (e.g., hCG, PSA). For PSA separation from the clot and storage at 4 °C (short term) or –30 °C (longer term) is desirable as soon as possible, and preferably within 3 hours especially if free PSA is measured. Samples may be stored at refrigerated temperatures for up to 24 hours, but if analysis is delayed beyond 24 hours, specimens should be stored frozen (at least at –20 °C). For longer-term storage, specimens should be stored frozen at –70 °C.

[a] Table from Recommendations of the European Group for Tumor Markers [36] and used with permission.

difficulties can still occur if the probe surface is inadvertently damaged.

The consequences of carry-over are likely to be most severe for analytes such as tumor markers with very wide concentration ranges. Given carry-over of just 0.1% for a serum specimen containing 100,000 kU/L of AFP, the erroneous result obtained for a following specimen of undetectable AFP concentration could be 100 kU/L. Identification of such errors may occur on close inspection of sequential results, for example when investigating reasons for a patient result that does not seem in accord with the clinical picture. Identification may be particularly difficult when the analyte concentration in the first sample is so high that it "hooks," giving an erroneously low result, so that carry-over is not suspected. Also difficult is a situation that may occur in random access analyzers, where the analyte that carries over is not measured for the first specimen: for example, when thyroid function tests for a pregnant patient are followed by measurement of hCG on a non-pregnant patient (38).

Contaminants affecting label detection. Nonisotopic assays are generally more susceptible than isotopic assays to this type of interference. False signals in label detection may result from contamination of sample, reagents, or plastic tubes or plastic wells with dyes, fluorophores, or particulate matter. Good laboratory practice, especially segregation of laboratory areas used for reagent preparation from those used for analytical work, will reduce the risks of such contamination.

In isotopic assays, high radioactive backgrounds are the most common cause of contamination. Regular counter monitoring of background radiation and the laboratory environment should avoid these risks. Contamination of working surfaces during preparation of nonisotopic labels can also adversely affect assay results. Particular care is required to minimize the risk of such contamination, which is more difficult to detect than for radiolabels.

Blood collection tubes and additives. The use of serum gel tubes has been shown to interfere with some immunoassays, although there is little published evidence about this for

Table 3 Exogenous interferences (arising from equipment or assay system) that can potentially yield discordant results in immunoassays for tumor markers[a]

Type of error	Comments and examples relevant to the measurement of tumor markers
Specimen carry-over	Potentially a problem whenever very high concentration specimens assayed.
Contaminants affecting label detection	Factors interfering with measurement of label, e.g., enzyme inhibitors in enzyme immunoassays, endogenous fluorophores in fluoroimmunoassays, radioactive contamination of specimens. Misleadingly high results measured for hCG in a fluorometric assay have been attributed to contamination of the microtiter plate wells by powder used on laboratory gloves. High radioactive background counts, either in the laboratory or in detector wells of γ-counters, may affect radioisotopic assays and are likely to be most serious in assays giving low count rates, e.g., immunoradiometric assays at low concentrations.
Blood collection tubes	Few published reports but differences in results between serum and EDTA or citrate plasma may be due to inhibition of complement activity by chelating agents.
Heat-treatment of sera prior to assay	Heat treatment carried out to deplete serum complement components or to inactivate HIV can result in major increases in concentrations of hCGα and hCGβ, or free PSA.
Mis-sampling by automated analyzer	Failure of mechanisms for level sensing or clot detection.

[a] Based on table in Reference 31, with permission.
EDTA—ethylenediaminetetraacetic acid

tumor markers. Whether such interference is significant is both analyte- and method-dependent and requires careful investigation. Generally the results of such studies are summarized in relevant product information, and recommendations given by manufacturers should always be followed. For many tumor markers, both serum and plasma samples are equally suitable, but this is not always the case. Again it is important to follow manufacturers' guidance. Anti-coagulating agents such as ethylenediaminetetraacetic acid (EDTA) may interfere in some detection methods, either by binding metallic ions that are constituents of labels (e.g., europium in Wallac Delfia assays) or cofactors that are required for activity of enzyme labels (e.g., zinc ions for alkaline phosphatase). Preservatives such as sodium azide, which may be present in proficiency testing specimens, can also adversely affect results by interfering with signal detection. It is always the responsibility of proficiency testing scheme organizers to ensure that specimens issued resemble physiological specimens as closely as possible and that added preservatives do not adversely affect any methods surveyed.

Effect of storage temperature on tumor marker results. Most tumor markers are reasonably stable in serum or plasma, but it is usually desirable to freeze specimens if their measurement is to be delayed for more than 24 to 48 h after receipt at the laboratory. Storage at –30 °C or –70 °C is generally preferable to storage at –20 °C, which is near the eutectic point. Heat treatment is unlikely to occur under normal circumstances, and most heavily glycosylated tumor markers (e.g., CEA) are very stable at elevated temperature. Heating dimeric hCG at 60 °C for 30 min diminishes or abolishes its immunoreactivity, and increases the concentration of hCGβ. Stability studies for hCG therefore require particular care. The stability of total and free PSA under different storage conditions is also highly relevant, particularly in the context of screening programs (9).

Mis-sampling by automated analyzers. While most analyzers have mechanisms for level sensing or clot detection, these occasionally fail to recognize a sampling error. This is most likely to occur when specimens contain unsuspected bubbles, and some laboratories routinely centrifuge all specimens immediately prior to analysis to avoid this. Of several hundred errors reported to a proficiency-testing scheme for AFP, hCG and CEA during a two-year period, only four were attributed to analyzer mis-sampling (2).

Endogenous Interference

Factors potentially most likely to cause confusion or misinterpretation of tumor marker results include the presence in the specimen of cross-reacting substances, anti-reagent antibodies, and unexpectedly high concentrations of analyte (the so-called high dose "hook" effect) (Table 4). The almost universal adoption of immunometric methods means that problems associated with heterophilic antibodies and assay hooking are now particularly important, since neither of these is likely to cause major difficulties in competitive radioimmunoassay.

Cross-reacting substances. Misleading results may be obtained when substances unexpectedly present in a sample cross-react with the antibody to the analyte. The mechanism by which this occurs depends on the specificity and homogeneity of the antibody used, and also on the type of assay. For competitive immunoassays, the availability of high-affinity, specific anti-analyte antibody is essential to minimize cross-reactivity with related molecules (e.g., human luteinizing hormone [hLH] cross-reaction in assays for hCG). Most tumor markers are now measured using two-site non-competitive immunoassays, which generally achieve high specificity because only substances with epitopes bound simultaneously by at least two antibodies are detected. However, because the capture and

Table 4 Endogenous interferences (arising from properties of the specimen) that can potentially yield discordant results in immunoassays for tumor markers[a]

Type of error	Comments and examples relevant to the measurement of tumor markers
Cross-reacting substances	hCGβ, giving different results in hCG assays depending on the extent to which the method recognizes this species; hLH, present in post-menopausal women and in patients with iatrogenic primary hypogonadism following chemotherapy, in assays for hCG. Free PSA in non-equimolar assays for total PSA. Normal cross-reacting antigens in assays for CEA.
Non-specific interference	Rarely reported; interference in an hCG assay has resulted in inappropriate chemotherapy being given to a seminoma patient (41). Decreased by minimizing ratio of specimen volume to total incubation volume, provided pipetting precision is not jeopardized.
Non-immunoreactive isoforms	Not hitherto reported for tumor markers (although have been reported for hLH); biosynthetic defects of hCG synthesis can yield false-negative hCG results, e.g. in ectopic pregnancy (42).
Anti-analyte antibodies	Anti-hCG antibodies may occur in patients treated with urinary hCG, e.g., during ovulation induction, and may interfere in assays for hCG.
Anti-reagent antibodies	Heterophilic antibodies, present in up to 40% of normal individuals, and human anti-mouse antibodies, present in up to 70% of patients who have been treated with mouse monoclonal antibodies, may bind to reagent antibodies to produce falsely high or low results (43). Inappropriate treatment may result. A particular hazard in assays for CA125, as antibodies to CA125 are frequently used for immunoscintigraphic imaging.
Rheumatoid factor	Mostly IgM autoantibodies directed against a determinant in the Fc portion of the IgG molecule in patients with rheumatoid disease; their effect on tumor marker immunoassays is uncertain, with little documented information.
Non-linear dilution	Non-linear dilution, with increased recovery of the antigen on increasing dilution, particularly in immunoassays for mucins (CA15.3, CA19.9 and CA125). Probably due to several factors including the presence of high levels of anti-carbohydrate antibodies in serum (generating complexes), the inherent property of mucins to aggregate and disaggregate into a range of molecular species, and other matrix-related effects (44).
High-dose hook effect	Failure to recognize extremely high levels of tumor markers can lead to misdiagnosis of potentially fatal but curable malignancy; of particular importance for AFP in childhood neuro- or hepatoblastoma and hCG in testicular tumors and choriocarcinoma (45).
Iatrogenic causes	Use of cannabis can transiently elevate serum hCG levels (46).
Lipids, hemoglobin, paraproteins, and other serum constituents	Tend to be more of a problem in homogeneous assays so are not of major relevance to most tumor marker immunoassays. Complement has been reported to interfere in assays for CEA (30).
Bacterial contamination	Mucins and immunoassays for these are sensitive to viral and bacterial neuraminidases, which may result in false negatives.

[a] Based on table in Reference 31, with permission.
HLH = Human luteinizing hormone; IgG = immunoglobulin G.

labeled antibodies are used at relatively high concentrations, they may react with substances with epitopes shared in common with the analyte, even though the equilibrium constant for these other substances is relatively low.

Depending on whether the cross-reactant binds to either or both capture and labeled antibodies in a two-site immunometric assay (Figure 3a), interference may be positive (Figure 3b) or negative (Figure 3c). For tumor markers, such cross-reactivity is probably most relevant for hCG (with hLH and hCG-related molecules), PSA (with free PSA and PSA-related antigens such as the kallikreins), and CEA (with normal cross-reacting antigens). CA125, CA15.3, and other mucin markers are much larger and more heterogeneous molecules (essentially high molecular mass glycoprotein aggregates) that are defined by their immunoreactivity with relevant monoclonal antibodies. Cross-reactivity with related antigens is perhaps less relevant for these markers, although carbohydrate microheterogeneity almost certainly contributes to the between-method differences in results occasionally observed for individual patient specimens.

Nonspecific interference. Causes of nonspecific interferences, sometimes termed matrix effects, are not precisely known, but they are observed as signals generated in an assay in the absence of analyte or known cross-reactants, i.e., the difference in the assay response given by zero calibrant and that by analyte-free serum. A contributory factor may be nonspecific binding of label to the assay tube or other components of the assay, but this can be minimized by adding a protein carrier (e.g., 0.5% bovine serum albumin) to the assay buffer. Nonspecific interference may be reflected in the degree of

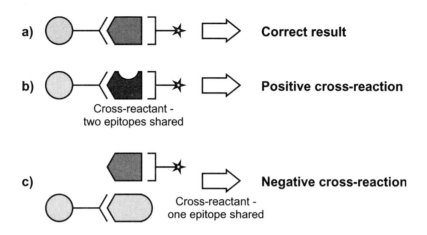

Figure 3 Cross-reactions in two-site immunometric assay. (a) antibodies bind to specific analyte—correct result obtained; (b) cross-reactant sharing two epitopes in common with analyte—positive cross-reaction; (c) cross-reactant sharing only one epitope in common with analyte—negative cross-reaction. Reproduced with permission from Seth J, Sturgeon CM. Pitfalls in immunoassays in endocrinology. Endocrinology and Metabolism In-Service Training and Continuing Education 1993;11(4):89–99. American Association for Clinical Chemistry, Inc.

imprecision observed at low analyte concentrations, and is conveniently termed "baseline security." Good baseline security is particularly important for AFP, hCG, and PSA in patients being monitored post-therapy, since further treatment may be implemented on the basis of very small increases in marker levels. Data from proficiency testing schemes confirm the excellent precision achievable at low concentration with many automated immunoassay systems (2), but laboratories should always monitor carefully their own performance. Inclusion of specimens of appropriately low concentration should be a routine part of IQC procedures.

It is important to be aware that stable low increases in serum marker levels may not represent active disease. The cases of six patients with treated germ cell tumors who had elevated serum AFP and/or hCG but no active disease, despite careful repeat evaluation, have recently been described (47). The markers were only mildly raised and remained constant or spontaneously normalized during repeat measurements. In the absence of clinical or radiographic evidence of disease, the patients were treated conservatively with physical examination, radiological tests, and repeat marker assays. It was concluded that, provided an experienced clinician has undertaken appropriate studies to exclude active disease, stable low increases in AFP and hCG may not represent active disease, and it was recommended that consideration be given to managing such cases with close surveillance to avoid unnecessary chemotherapy. No reason was identified for the minor elevations in marker levels observed for these patients.

Method-related differences in marker results at low concentrations have been demonstrated in a study of 55 patients with non-seminomatous testicular germ cell tumor patients referred to a regional clinical oncology center over a three-year period (48). Paired baseline AFP and hCG assays were undertaken using polyclonal radioimmunoassays and monoclonal fluoroimmunoassays. While no discrepancies were observed with AFP assays, serial paired measurements in four patients showed discordance on baseline assays of hCG, and the authors concluded that no single currently available assay is conclusive in all patients (48).

Anti-reagent antibodies. Some patient sera contain immunoglobulins capable of reacting with animal antibodies used in immunoassays, thereby causing interference (39,43,49). There have been a few reports of interference from anti-reagent antibodies in competitive assays, but interference is more frequently recognized in two-site immunometric assays with monoclonal antibodies (Figure 4a). Falsely high results will be obtained if the anti-reagent antibodies bind to sites other than the analyte-binding site and cross-link labeled and capture antibodies (Figure 4b). If the interfering antibody binds to and blocks only one reagent antibody, however, results will be low (Figure 4c). Presumably as a result of other steric effects, such interfering antibodies may also affect recognition by reagent antibody, as well as interfering by direct binding of reagent antibody.

Minimizing interference from anti-reagent antibodies
Assay formulation strongly influences the likelihood of anti-reagent antibody interference. Methods using only one mouse mAb (with the second antibody a polyclonal) are less prone to interference than those using two mAbs. Avoiding use in in vitro diagnostic kits of mAbs that are used in vivo for imaging is also desirable. (See section on human anti-mouse antibody (HAMA), below.) For example, on replacing the capture anti-CA125 mAb OC125 with an alternative mAb (M11) in a commercial immunoassay for CA125 that also used OC125 as the labeled mAb, interference from HAMA was markedly reduced (39). The use of chimeric human-mouse antibodies may also decrease the likelihood of anti-reagent antibody interference.

In practice, adding non-immune animal serum to the assay system will generally eliminate interference by anti-reagent antibodies (Figure 4d), and most commercial kit manufacturers adopt this approach. The serum source preferred is usually that from the same species used in the assay (most frequently mouse). Non-immune serum containing immunoglobulins

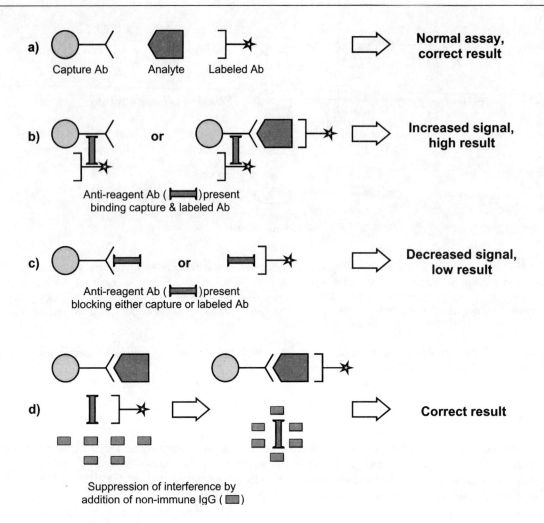

Figure 4 Interference from anti-reagent antibodies in two-site immunometric assays. (a) interfering antibodies absent—correct result obtained; (b) cross-linking of capture and labeled antibody in the presence of anti-reagent antibody—incorrectly high result (analyte may or may not be bound as well, depending on steric factors, but in either case the result will be falsely high); (c) interfering antibodies binding to either capture or labeled antibody only, reducing sandwich formation—incorrectly low result obtained; (d) effect of adding non-immune animal IgG to reduce interference—correct result obtained. Reproduced with permission from Seth J, Sturgeon CM. Pitfalls in immunoassays in endocrinology. Endocrinology and Metabolism In-Service Training and Continuing Education 1993;11(4):89–99. American Association for Clinical Chemistry, Inc.

from other species (e.g. horse, cow, goat) will also reduce the effect of interfering antibodies (37), probably reflecting similarities in the structure of immunoglobulins of these species. For several reasons, however, adding non-immune animal serum is not always effective in eliminating interference by anti-reagent antibodies:

- Individual human immune responses to animal immunoglobulins may vary considerably, both qualitatively and quantitatively, and with time.
- The designated concentration of blocking animal immunoglobulin is often chosen empirically.
- The interfering antibody may bind specific Fab epitopes on the reagent antibodies that are not present on the added animal immunoglobulin.

If anti-reagent interference is still suspected, despite use of a method already "protected" by presence of non-immune serum, alternative methods of detecting and/or removing anti-reagent interference can be used. These include:

- Prior extraction of the analyte from the sample.
- Addition of immobilized normal non-immune serum, Protein A or Protein G suspension.
- Polyethylene glycol precipitation (using 50% v/v of 16% PEG 6000).
- Heating (to 70–90 °C) in acetate buffer, pH 5.0 (only suitable for analytes such as CEA which can survive these antibody-denaturing conditions).
- Assay of the specimen at several dilutions to assess linearity on dilution, i.e., assuming that specimens containing interfering antibodies will not dilute out in parallel.

- Pre-treatment with commercially available antibody blocking tubes (obtainable, e.g., from Scantibodies Laboratory Inc. at website *www.scantibodies.com*).
- Assay of the specimen by another method, preferably utilizing a different methodology, e.g., radioimmunoassay.

Of these, the last two are probably most convenient. Pre-treatment with blocking tubes requires only incubation of the suspect specimen followed by re-assay, and assay by another method either confirms that there is interference or provides some reassurance that the original result obtained is correct. Affinity chromatographic procedures to quantitate anti-reagent antibodies have also been developed and while they are perhaps not suitable for routine use, they can provide a useful means of confirming suspected interference (50).

Identifying possible interference from anti-reagent antibodies It is often difficult to identify specimens that may be subject to anti-reagent interference, and a high index of clinical suspicion is required. Where a panel of tests is requested (e.g., a female reproductive hormone profile), interference may be more readily suspected if only one or two immunoassays are affected, thus giving results out of accord with results for the other analytes measured. In contrast, if a single test is requested, as is often the case for tumor markers, the possibility of interference is probably less likely to be considered. Severe interference is also easier to detect than mild interference. The extent of interference observed generally reflects the type of antibody causing it, as described below.

Human anti-mouse antibody (HAMA). Direct intravenous administration of mouse mAbs (frequently anti-CEA or anti-CA125) for imaging or therapeutic purposes in oncology is likely to produce anti-mouse antibodies in treated patients. A prevalence of >70% in treated patients has been reported (37), while estimates of the number of people in the general population who are positive for HAMA range from <1% to 80% (49). The variation in figures probably reflects the difficulty of measuring these antibodies, for which no universal assay is available, because the antigen causing the HAMA response in any given patient is usually unknown. The variability of the immune response is such that human anti-animal responses may be of the IgG, IgA, IgM or (rarely) the IgE class. Antibody specificity may be anti-isotype or anti-idiotype, i.e., directed against the hypervariable or constant region of the immunoglobulin molecule. While there are at least six commercially available assays for measuring HAMA, inter-method and inter-laboratory comparability of results from these is poor, probably reflecting lack of standardization and differences in calibrators (e.g., baboon anti-mouse IgG and plasma from patients infused with mAbs were two of the calibrators used) (49). Serum concentrations of HAMA tend to be high (in the μg/L to g/L range) in patients who are HAMA-positive as a result of treatment with mouse mAbs, since these HAMA are produced in response to a direct antigenic stimulus. The duration of a HAMA response is variable, but antibodies may persist in the circulation for at least 30 months after exposure to mouse immunoglobulin.

Measures that can be taken to minimize induction of the HAMA response in patients receiving treatment with mAbs include the following:

- Immunosuppressant treatment before and after antibody treatment.
- Use of Fab fragments (which are less immunogenic) rather than the whole immunoglobulin molecule for treatment.
- Use of humanized and chimeric antibodies (although IgG is still potentially antigenic).
- Pre-coating therapeutic mAbs with polyethylene glycol to decrease their immunogenicity.

While these measures all have some effect, the potential for interference remains significant, and represents a particular hazard for tumor marker assays, with which many of these patients are monitored. With the increasing use of mouse mAbs in imaging, it is also important to remember their potentially adverse effects on other immunoassays (e.g. cardiac markers, reproductive hormones, etc.) that may be undertaken for cancer patients. In a UK NEQAS distribution in 1998, a specimen containing 0.5% v/v of HAMA-containing serum from a patient who had undergone treatment with mouse mAbs was distributed, together with a specimen of the same pool without added HAMA (2). Most methods appeared to be reasonably well protected. While previously reported interference for two methods was confirmed, a third was no longer affected. AFP and CEA results for another method were affected to an extent that could be clinically misleading.

While interference from HAMA is well recognized, and numerous authors have reported the frequency of HAMA responses following administration of various mAbs (49), there are few case reports describing possible adverse clinical consequences resulting from failure to recognize HAMA interference. Two such reports are summarized below (Cases 1 and 2).

Case 1.
A 61-year-old male with a history of tumors at various sites presented with progressive growth of a tumor in his neck, at which time he had clear signs of thyrotoxicosis. Initial measurements of thyroid-stimulating hormone (TSH), α-fetoprotein (AFP), prostatic acid phosphatase (PAP), and CEA all indicated clearly raised results (26.0 mU/L, 74 μg/L, 94 μg/L, and 335 μg/L respectively). These results could have led to much unnecessary clinical investigation had the possibility of assay interference not been recognized. On repeat of the four assays in the presence of mouse serum, much lower results were obtained (0.14 mU/L, 6 μg/L, 3.7 μg/L, and 5.3 μg/L respectively). The patient had previously undergone two immunoscintigraphy studies using anti-CEA mAbs, explaining the initial spuriously high results (51).

This case clearly illustrates the potential for misinterpretation of results if HAMA is not suspected, and also the advantage in having a number of test results to consider. Without the TSH result, which clearly did not fit the clinical picture, the tumor marker results were not implausible.

Case 2.
A 39-year-old woman with a positive family history of breast cancer presented with repeatedly increased CA125 serum concentrations of 133–221 kU/L. No abnormalities of the ovaries were found on laparoscopic inspection, and peritoneal cytology was also normal. After referral for genetic studies that showed that she did not have a mutation in BRCA1 or BRCA2 breast cancer genes, repeat measurement of CA125 by a different method gave results of 3.1 and 4.3 kU/L, i.e., well within the reference range. Using an affinity chromatographic technique, the presence of HAMA IgG (but not IgM) was subsequently demonstrated in her sera (52).

Heterophilic antibodies. Similarly erroneous results may be obtained for serum specimens containing heterophilic antibodies, poorly defined antibodies developed in response to no clear immunogen, and characterized by substantial non-specificity. Heterophilic antibodies tend to be of lower concentration than HAMA and may also have lower affinity for other antibodies. There are at least two classes of heterophilic antibodies, one directed to an epitope present on rabbit immunoglobulin only and the other detecting epitopes on goat, cattle, horse, and mouse immunoglobulin, but not rabbit (43). As many as 40% of normal individuals possess these antibodies, which primarily recognize epitopes on the Fab fragment and which are capable of forming Fab-Fab interactions with reagent antibody.

Possible non-iatrogenic causes of heterophilic antibodies include close contact with animals (e.g., by handling or inhaling fur when undertaking animal house work, or caring for domestic pets), transfer of dietary antigens across the gut wall (it is generally assumed that the immunizing agent in many patients is bovine immunoglobulin absorbed from meat and milk), and certain disease states (e.g., idiopathic cardiomyopathy). Possible iatrogenic causes include exposure to diagnostic and pharmaceutical agents from animal sources, desorption of immobilized IgG during purification of recombinant proteins used therapeutically, vaccination against infectious diseases, and blood transfusion.

Assays for CEA, CA125, and hCG have all been reported to be affected by heterophilic antibodies, but it is in assays for hCG that the clinical consequences of failure to recognize such interference have been most damaging. In 1989, increased concentrations of serum hCG in a 41-year old woman led to an unnecessary laparoscopic examination (53). Serum hCG had first been measured with a radioimmunoassay using antibodies raised in rabbits. Reanalysis of the specimens with a goat antibody-based assay revealed normal concentrations of hCG in all samples. A report ten years later described the cases of twelve female patients, who were diagnosed as having trophoblastic disease on the basis of spuriously high serum hCG concentrations (ranging from 17 to 175 U/L). Most of these women were subjected to needless surgery or chemotherapy (54). The false-positive hCG results were attributed to the presence of heterophilic antibodies on the basis of lack of parallelism on dilution, although this was not conclusively demonstrated. The authors suggested that a compulsory test for hCG in urine should be included in current protocols for the diagnosis and treatment of choriocarcinoma. This would seem sensible, particularly when biochemical results do not fit the clinical picture, but in practice is not entirely straightforward, as most commercially available quantitative hCG methods are not validated for measurements of hCG in urine (55). An editorial accompanying the original paper commented that the problem of inadequate assays and lack of information relating to them is particularly relevant in countries where services for patients with trophoblastic disease have not been formally centralized (56). These countries include the United States, Germany, and Spain. Later it was also strongly suggested that better communication between clinical and laboratory staff before clinical decisions are made could reduce the risk of unnecessary clinical interventions due to false positive laboratory results (55,57,58).

More recently, in a lawsuit against the hospital in which she was treated and the major diagnostics company that manufactured the hCG assay used, a 22-year-old woman was awarded $16 million for a misdiagnosis of cancer based on spurious elevation of serum hCG levels attributable to heterophilic antibodies (Case 3).

Case 3.
A twenty-two-year old woman presented with irregular bleeding, and was found to have moderately raised serum hCG. Scans showed no sign of a tumor, but she was diagnosed as having cancer, and was immediately started on chemotherapy. This was continued for four months, during which time her hCG level remained elevated, fluctuating between 250 and 350 U/L (upper limit of the reference range 5 U/L). The patient was told a hysterectomy was necessary. This was performed, but tissue samples showed no evidence of malignancy. Although serum hCG decreased post-surgery, the level subsequently increased to the previous level. Two suspicious spots were observed on a lung scan so additional surgery was undertaken, but again no evidence of cancer was found, and her hCG level continued to be elevated. Only then were the laboratory hCG results checked using a different method, at which time heterophilic antibody interference in the first method was recognized (59).

This case serves as a salutary reminder that no single currently available immunoassay is perfect in all clinical situations, and, perhaps even more importantly, that laboratory results not in accord with the clinical picture should always be viewed with a high degree of suspicion. Clinicians should always seek confirmation using a complementary biochemical method. This is particularly desirable for tumor marker tests, which contribute to diagnosis of both primary and recurrent malignancy, diagnoses that may lead to invasive and often unpleasant treatment. It also places considerable responsibility on those providing tumor marker laboratory services to ensure that they provide a quality service that is as informative and helpful as possible. Better communication between clinical and laboratory staff might have spared the above patient the unnecessary and damaging treatment she underwent. Although for at least fifteen years there have been occasional reports in the literature describing false positive immunoassay results due to heterophilic antibodies, it is not surprising that the doctors treating this patient were unaware of them. Similarly, the product information supplied with the kits, which clearly described this potential hazard (as required by the United States Food and Drug Administration), were readily available to laboratory, but not clinical, staff.

Rheumatoid factor. Autoantibodies present in the sera from patients with rheumatoid disease may bind to multiple antigenic determinants on the Fc region of IgG (37). Called rheumatoid factors, these antibodies may be of the IgM, IgG or IgA classes and are particularly likely to cause falsely high values in assays involving turbidimetry or latex particle agglutination. Interferences caused in two site immunoassays are likely to be due to a number of mechanisms, including aggregation of antibody molecules by binding to the Fc portion of other immunoglobulins. Whether they are of high enough affinity to cause the bridging phenomenon observed with HAMA or heterophilic antibodies is not clear. Nevertheless, particular care should be taken when assaying sera from patients with rheumatoid disease, because of the high frequency of interference in these specimens.

Miscellaneous antibody interference. Spuriously high immunoassay results for hCG, AFP, CA125, cardiac troponin I, and thyrotropin were measured in sera from a patient who been treated for *Escherichia coli* septicemia (60).

Case 4.

Following *E. coli* septicemia, a 56-year-old male patient was found to have increased immunoassay results for cardiac troponin I, thyrotropin, hCG, AFP, and CA125. The patient also had a restricted IgM gamma paraprotein on immunofixation. None of the possible diagnoses associated with these results (myocardial infarction, hyperthyroidism, or occult germ cell, hepatic or other malignancy) was consistent with his state of health. (A number of other analytes were also measured; results were within normal limits.) After incubation of plasma from the patient with irrelevant murine monoclonal antibodies or the *E. coli* organism, normal immunoassay results were obtained and the IgM gamma paraprotein disappeared. It was concluded that the patient had produced a very restricted IgM gamma antibody response to the *E. coli* infection that had anti-immunoglobulin activity and was responsible for the falsely increased immunoassay values (60).

This is interesting, as it is known that microorganisms in experimental settings can induce anti-immunoglobulin antibodies. Further studies would be desirable to determine whether other patients with anti-bacterial carbohydrate responses express similar interfering activities and whether suspicion of interferences in immunometric assays should be heightened in patients with recent infections with gram-negative organisms.

The case again demonstrates the importance of awareness of the possibility of falsely increased values in two-site immunoassays. It may also provide a clue for the best "recipe" for a blocking reagent, since not all assays from the same manufacturer were affected—highlighting again the variability of the antibody interactions involved in this type of interference.

High-dose hook effect. Two-site immunoassays in which capture and labeled antibody are added simultaneously are vulnerable to the high-dose hook (or prozone) effect (Figure 5). At high analyte concentration, when amounts of both capture and labeled antibody become limiting, low results may be obtained. Under these conditions, there is competition of free analyte and analyte bound to labeled antibody for the limited number of solid-phase antibody binding sites. Binding of label to solid phase will therefore decrease rather than increase in the presence of higher concentrations of analyte. If analyte concentrations are sufficiently high and are not recognized as such, erroneously low results, which may even be within the reference range, may be reported. The risk of high results is greatest for analytes with a very wide concentration range, i.e., most tumor markers. An example of a high-dose hook effect in a CEA assay is described below (Case 5) and illustrated in Figure 6.

Case 5.

A specimen from a 65-year-old female was received at the laboratory for CEA measurement. No clinical details were on the test request form. CEA was measured by a one-step IRMA (normal range <5 μg/L) as 4.9 μg/L, but some non-parallelism was noted—the result of a 1:2 dilution was 17.6 μg/L. The result was reported as "Appears to be a normal level but fails to dilute out satisfactorily." A further confirmatory specimen was requested. The second sample was received with "Known liver metastases" noted on the form. The sample was further diluted and a result of 359,600 μg/L obtained. The correct result, confirmed in another laboratory by a different method, was in the region of 400,000 μg/L (38).

The risk of hooking may be minimized by (a) using two-step assays which include a sequential wash step, (b) using solid-phase antibodies of higher binding capacity, or (c) by assaying specimens at two dilutions. Each approach has some disadvantages. While sequential ("two-step") assays prevent hooking, they require more time, and decrease sample throughput in automated methods. Reagent costs increase if higher capacity solid-phase antibodies are used, while performing assays at two dilutions essentially doubles the cost in terms of the number of tubes required. Use of kinetic rate measurements can reduce the risk of failing to detect a hooked sample, an approach that has been adopted by some manufacturers of automated instruments (61).

Most manufacturers quote concentrations above which their methods may hook, and laboratories should be aware of these for all the tumor markers they measure. It has been recommended that laboratories institute protocols permitting identification of high-dose hooking, particularly in patients for whom markers are being measured for the first time (36). A UK NEQAS exercise demonstrated clearly the benefits of having such protocols in place. On distributing a specimen of unexpectedly high hCG concentration (700,000 U/L), almost all laboratories reported appropriate results. However, for one method, three of five users of one method reported results that were almost 100-fold less than expected (~7,000 U/L). The other two users reported appropriately high results of >10,000 U/L and 500,395 U/L, suggest-

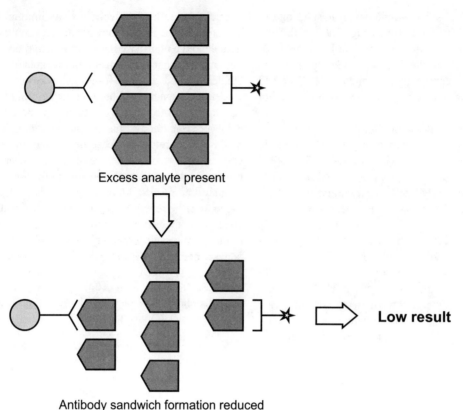

Figure 5 Mechanism of high-dose hook effect in two-site immunometric assay. As analyte concentrations increase to very high concentrations, both capture and signal antibodies become saturated with analyte, decreasing antibody sandwich formation. Reproduced with permission from Seth J, Sturgeon CM. Pitfalls in immunoassays in endocrinology. Endocrinology and Metabolism In-Service Training and Continuing Education 1993;11(4):89–99. American Association for Clinical Chemistry, Inc.

ing a protocol designed to check for hooking was in place (62). Analytically, the method was performing according to specification, as the stated hooking limit is 500,000 U/L.

Although the proportion of patients with tumor marker levels high enough to "hook" is very small, the clinical consequences of failure to recognize extremely high concentrations can be severe. This is particularly the case if the disease is potentially fatal but curable, as when measuring hCG in suspected choriocarcinoma (45), or AFP in suspected childhood hepatoblastoma. This again emphasizes the importance of understanding the limitations of assay technology.

COMMUNICATION BETWEEN LABORATORY AND CLINICAL STAFF

Good communication between laboratory and clinical staff is likely to encourage clinicians to contact the laboratory promptly when results of diagnostic tests do not fit the clinical picture. This is highly desirable, as it helps to facilitate early investigation of potential errors by the laboratory, as well as decreasing the risk of inappropriate and potentially harmful clinical decisions being made on the basis of erroneous laboratory data. Provision of very brief clinical details about the patient (e.g., "known liver metastases," "previous immunoscintigraphy," etc.) when requesting tests can help alert the laboratory to potential problems (as in Case 5 above). Similarly, provision by the laboratory of cumulative results and/or short interpretative comments when reporting tumor marker results may contribute to improving communication, as well as helping to encourage better use of these tests (62).

Clinical decisions made on the basis of tumor marker results potentially have more serious consequences for the patient than may be the case for results of other immunoassays (e.g., those for reproductive hormones). In some oncology centers, for example, chemotherapy may be instituted solely on the basis of a rising tumor marker, in the absence of other diagnostic evidence such as ultrasound. This places a major responsibility on laboratories to ensure that tumor marker results are correct, primarily for the patient's sake, but also to avoid damaging and costly litigation.

SUMMARY AND PRACTICAL APPLICATIONS

Clinical and laboratory staff must be aware of the many factors that can contribute to differences and errors in tumor marker results (Tables 3 and 4), as these can undoubtedly adversely affect patient care. However, an appreciation of the relative importance of these is also desirable, if every laboratory test is not to be regarded with suspicion. The most common

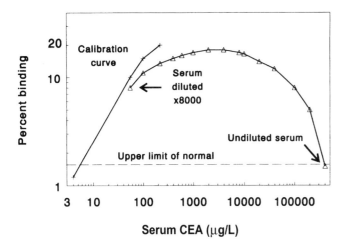

Figure 6 Example of high-dose hook effect with a serum containing very high concentrations of CEA (~400,000 µg/L) in an immunometric assay. The percent binding observed for successive dilution of sample (undiluted to 1:8000) is shown, as is part of the standard curve. Reproduced with permission from Seth J, Sturgeon CM. Pitfalls in immunoassays in endocrinology. Endocrinology and Metabolism In-Service Training and Continuing Education 1993;11(4):89–99. ©American Association for Clinical Chemistry, Inc.

reasons for discrepancies in tumor marker results are summarized in Table 5.

Method-related differences mean that tumor marker results obtained in different methods are not necessarily interchangeable. This situation is unlikely to change until broad recommendations are made about the most clinically appropriate antibody specificities. In practice, method-related differences in analytical results for any tumor marker are most relevant when a laboratory changes method or when a patient is (sometimes unknowingly) monitored by more than one method, perhaps in different laboratories. The interpretative confusion that may arise, for example, when PSA is measured for the same patient in different laboratories using different methods has been highlighted (63). It has previously been recommended that laboratories should have in place a defined protocol for changing methods (36). This may require analyzing the previous specimen by the new method, or requesting a further specimen to re-establish the baseline and/or confirm the trend in marker level. While it may benefit the laboratory to indicate changes of method on tumor marker reports, it is generally more helpful to clinicians if the laboratory highlights whether a method change is likely to affect interpretation of results.

The errors most likely to occur when providing a routine tumor marker service are probably the same preanalytical errors that are common to all laboratory tests, i.e., errors of sample identification made either before or after blood specimens arrive at the laboratory. Care and attention to detail are required to minimize the risk of these errors. Requesting repeat specimens to check high results that are likely to contribute to diagnosis is frequently desirable, especially where the result is clinically unexpected. Errors of sample transposition are much less likely to occur when primary tubes are used and specimens are bar-coded. Close scrutiny of analytical results before they are clinically authorized may help to reduce the risk of reporting incorrect results due to sample misidentification, as can "delta-checking," particularly when there are previous results from the same patient. Care taken in the post-analytical phase can also help to identify errors occasionally encountered with automated analyzers. Relevant errors reported by participants to UK NEQAS have included unintentional changes (following analyzer maintenance) of the units used for reporting (e.g., from mass units to International Units for AFP), and misinterpretation by computer software packages of results for specimens originally flagged by the analyzer as "high" results and for repeat, as low results (e.g., <5 U/L for hCG).

Awareness of the robustness of the assay used to detect interferences such as the high-dose hook effect or heterophilic

Table 5 Key points: Major causes of discrepancies in tumor marker results

Type of discrepancy	Causes	Action required to minimize adverse effects
Method-related differences	Poor calibration Lack of International Standards Imprecision Cross-reaction with related molecules Assay design Differing antibody specificities	Most relevant when a laboratory changes method or when patient is monitored in different laboratories Analysis of the specimen by the previous method may be necessary in order to "re-baseline"
Preanalytical factors	Errors of specimen identification before or after arrival at the laboratory Inappropriate specimen type Inappropriate timing of specimen	Care and attention to detail Provision of readily available advice from the laboratory regarding specimen requirements
Variable method robustness to potential interferences	High-dose hook effect Specimen carry-over Interference from anti-reagent antibodies	Protocol permitting identification of high-dose hooking, e.g., by assaying specimens at two dilutions, use of a two-step assay High degree of clinical suspicion and protocol for investigation of suspected interference, e.g., by re-assaying after treatment with blocking agents, re-assaying by a different method

antibodies is essential if reporting of erroneous results is to be avoided. In practice, a high degree of clinical suspicion is required to identify such errors, and many are probably not recognized. Minor interference is generally more difficult to identify than gross interference. The proportion of specimens of concentrations high enough to hook is generally likely to be very low, but it is extremely important not to miss high concentrations where tumor markers contribute to the diagnosis of malignancies that are potentially fatal but curable. Interference from heterophilic antibodies is likely to be a more commonly encountered problem in routine practice.

The ultimate key to avoiding laboratory errors arising from discrepancies in tumor marker results, whatever their cause, is for both clinical and laboratory staff to recognize that errors can occur in even the best-managed laboratory. Identification of these errors is often difficult, and for both parties a high index of suspicion is an essential element. Promoting regular dialogue between laboratory and clinical staff, thereby encouraging early discussion and investigation of any results that are not in accord with the clinical picture, is the most effective way to minimize the risk of unwarranted clinical intervention based on erroneous laboratory results.

REFERENCES

1. Bence Jones H. Chemical Pathology. Lancet 1847;2:88–92.
2. Seth J, Sturgeon C, Ellis AR. Annual Reviews of the UK NEQAS for Peptide Hormones and Related Substances. Edinburgh: UK NEQAS 1988–2001.
3. Wild D (ed.). The immunoassay handbook, 2nd ed. London: Nature Publishing Group, 2001.
4. Price CP, Newman DJ (eds.). Principles and practice of immunoassay, 2nd ed. Basingstoke: MacMillan Press Ltd, 1997.
5. Stenman U-H, Bidart J-M, Birken S, Mann K, Nisula B, O'Connor J. Standardization of protein immunoprocedures. Choriogonadotropin (CG). Scand J Clin Lab Invest 1993;53 Suppl 216:42–78.
6. National Committee for Clinical Laboratory Standards. Choriogonadotropin testing: nomenclature, reference preparations, assay performance, and clinical application; approved guideline. NCCLS Document I/LA10-A. Wayne, PA: NCCLS, 1996.
7. Fraser CG. Biological variation: from principles to practice. Washington, DC: AACC, 2001.
8. Sölétormos G, Schioler V, Nielsen D, Skovsgaard T, Dombernowsky P. Interpretation of results for tumor markers on the basis of analytical imprecision and biological variation. Clin Chem 1993;39:2077–2083.
9. Price CP, Allard J, Davies G, Dawnay A, Duffy MJ, France M, et al. Pre- and post-analytical factors that may influence use of serum prostate specific antigen and its isoforms in a screening program for prostate cancer. Ann Clin Biochem 2001;38: 188–216.
10. National Committee for Clinical Laboratory Standards (NCCLS). Evaluation of precision performance of clinical chemistry devices, 2nd ed. Tentative Guidelines Document EP5-T2. Wayne, PA: NCCLS, 1992.
11. Sizaret P, Anderson SG. The international reference preparation for alpha-fetoprotein. J Biol Standardization 1976;4:149.
12. Laurence DJR, Turberville C, Anderson SG, Neville AM. First British standard for carcinoembryonic antigen (CEA). Br J Cancer 1975;32:295–299.
13. Storring PL, Gaines-Das RE, Bangham DR. International reference preparation of human chorionic gonadotrophin for immunoassay: potency estimates in various bioassay and protein-binding assay systems; and international reference preparations of α and β subunits of human chorionic gonadotrophin for immunoassay. J Endocrinol 1980;84:295–310.
14. Rafferty B, Rigsby P, Rose M, Stamey T, Gaines Das R. Reference reagents for prostate specific antigen (PSA): establishment of the first international standards for free PSA and PSA (90:10). Clin Chem 2000;46:1310–1317.
15. European Community. In vitro diagnostics directive. Directive 98/79/EC. December 7, 1998.
16. Chen Z, Prestigiacomo A, Stamey TA. Purification and characterization of prostate-specific antigen (PSA) complexed to alpha 1-antichymotrypsin: potential reference material for international standardization of PSA immunoassays. Clin Chem 1995;41: 1273–1282.
17. Sturgeon CM, Seth J. Why do immunoassays for tumor markers give differing results? A view from the UK National External Quality Assessment Schemes. Eur J Clin Chem Clin Biochem 1996;34:755–759.
18. Milford Ward A, Catto JWF, Hamdy FC. Prostate-specific antigen: biology, biochemistry and available commercial assays. Ann Clin Biochem 2001;38:633–651.
19. Milford-Ward AM, White PA. UK NEQAS for PSA, Sheffield. Personal communication.
20. Milford Ward A, White PA. External quality assessment of commercial assays for CA125. Contemp Rev Obstet Gynecol 1997; 319–323.
21. Bidart J-M, Bellet D. Human chorionic gonadotropin: molecular forms, detection, and clinical implications. Trends Endocr Metab 1993;4:285–291.
22. Alpert E, Abelev GI. Summary report: epitope analysis of human alpha–fetoprotein. Tumor Biol 1998;19:290–292.
23. Nustad K, Bast RC, Jr, Brien TJ, Nilsson O, Seguin P, Suresh MR, et al. Specificity and affinity of 26 monoclonal antibodies against the CA 125 antigen: first report from the ISOBM TD–1 workshop. Tumor Biol 1996;17:196–219.
24. Nap M, Hammarstrom ML, Bormer O. Specificity and affinity of monoclonal antibodies against carcinoembryonic antigen. Cancer Res 1992;52:2329 2339.
25. Berger P, Sturgeon C, Bidart JM, Paus E, Gerth R, Niang M, et al. The ISOBM TD-7 Workshop on hCG and related molecules. An important step towards user-orientated standardization of pregnancy and tumor marker diagnosis: Assignment of epitopes to the 3D structure of diagnostically and commercially relevant monoclonal antibodies (mAbs) Tumor Biol 2002;23:1–38.
26. Rye PD, Bormer OP, Paus E (eds.). ISOBM TD-3 international workshop on monoclonal antibodies against prostate-specific antigen. Tumor Biol 1990;20:Suppl 1.
27. Price MR, Rye PD, Petrakou E, Murray A, Brady K, Imai S, et al. Summary report on the ISOBM TD–4 Workshop: analysis of 56 monoclonal antibodies against the MUC1 mucin. Tumor Biol 1998;19:1–20.
28. Rye PD, Bovin NV, Vlasova EV, Molodyk AA, Baryshnikov A, Kreutz FT, et al. Analysis of twenty monoclonal antibodies against Sialyl Lewis[a] and related antigens. Summary report on the ISOBM TD-6 Workshop. Tumor Biol 1998,19: 390–420.

29. Stigbrand T, Andres C, Bellanger L, Bishr Omary M, Bodenmuller H, Bonfrer H, et al. Epitope specificity of 30 monoclonal antibodies against cytokeratin antigens: the ISOBM TD5-1 Workshop. Tumor Biol 1998;19:132–152.
30. Børmer O. Interference of complement with the binding of carcinoembryonic antigen to solid-phase monoclonal antibodies. J Immunol Methods 1989;121:85–93.
31. Sturgeon CM, McAllister EJ. Analysis of hCG: clinical applications and assay requirements. Ann Clin Biochem 1998; 35: 460–491.
32. Sturgeon C, Stenman U-H, Bidart J-M, Birken S, Berger P, Lequin R, et al. IFCC Working Group for Standardization of hCG Measurements: Progress report. Proc UK NEQAS Meeting 1998;3:94–103.
33. Ekins R. Immunoassay standardization. Scand J Clin Lab Invest 1991;205S:33–46.
34. Price CP. Microarrays: The reincarnation of multiplexing in laboratory medicine, but now more relevant? Clin Chem 2001;47: 1345–1346.
35. Lapworth R, Teal TK. Laboratory blunders revisited. Ann Clin Biochem 1994;31:78–84.
36. European Group for Tumor Markers (EGTM): Consensus recommendations. Anticancer Res 1999;19:2785–2820. (www.med.uni-muenchen.de/egtm/index2.html).
37. Weber TH, Käpyaho KI, Tanner P. Endogenous interference in immunoassays in clinical chemistry. A review. Scand J Clin Lab Invest 1990;50:Suppl 201:77–82.
38. Seth J, Sturgeon CM. Pitfalls in immunoassays in endocrinology. AACC Endo 1993;11:89–106.
39. Selby C. Interference in immunoassay. Ann Clin Biochem 1999;36:704–721.
40. Kricka LJ. Interferences in immunoassay—still a threat. Clin Chem 2000;46:1037–1038.
41. Bulger KN, Hesketh PJ, Babayan PK. Discordant human chorionic gonadotropin results giving rise to inappropriate therapy in a case of testicular cancer. J Urol 1989;142:1574–1575.
42. Taylor RN, Padula C, Goldsmith PC. Pitfall in the diagnosis of ectopic pregnancy: immunocytochemical evaluation in a patient with false-negative serum β-hCG levels. Obstet Gynecol 1988;71: 1035–1038.
43. Boscato LM, Stuart MC. Heterophilic antibodies: a problem for all immunoassays. Clin Chem 1988;34:27–33.
44. Suresh MR. Immunoassays for cancer-associated carbohydrate antigens. Semin Cancer Biol 1991;2:367–377.
45. O'Reilly SM, Rustin GJS. Mismanagement of choriocarcinoma due to a false low hCG measurement. Int J Gynaecol Cancer 1993;3:186–188.
46. McAllister EJ, Yosef H. Misleading serum hCG concentrations in a patient with testicular teratoma. Proc ACB National Meeting 1995:172.
47. Morris MJ, Bosl GJ. Recognizing abnormal marker results that do not reflect disease in patients with germ cell tumors. J Urol 2000;163:796–801.
48. Summers J, Raggatt P, Pratt J, Williams MV. Experience of discordant beta hCG results by different assays in the management of non-seminomatous germ cell tumors of the testis. Clin Oncol 1999;11:388–392.
49. Kricka LJ. Human anti-animal antibody interferences in immunological assays. Clin Chem 1999;45:942–956.
50. Koper NP, Thomas CMG, Massuger LFAG, Segers MFG, Olthaar AJ, Verrbeek ALM. Quantitation of IgG and IgM human anti-mouse antibodies (HAMA) interference in CA125 measurements using affinity chromatography. Clin Chem Lab Med 1998; 36:23–28.
51. Janssen JA, Blankestijn PJ, Docter R, Blijenberg BG, Splinter TA, van Toor H, et al. Effects of immunoscintigraphy with monoclonal antibodies in assays of hormones and tumor markers. Br Med J 1989;298:1511–1513.
52. Koper NP, Massuger LF, Thomas CMG, Beyer C, Crooy MJ. An illustration of the clinical relevance of detecting human anti-mouse antibody interference by affinity chromatography. Eur J Obstet Gynecol Reprod Biol 1999;86:203–205.
53. Berglund L, Holmberg NG. Heterophilic antibodies against rabbit serum causing falsely elevated gonadotropin levels. Acta Obstet Gynecol Scand 1989;68:377–378.
54. Rotmensch S, Cole LA. False diagnosis and needless therapy of presumed malignant disease in women with false-positive human chorionic gonadotropin concentrations. Lancet 2000;355: 712–715.
55. Price A, Gillett G. Needless treatment for presumed malignancy. [Letter] Lancet 2000;355:1724–1725.
56. Bagshawe KD. Limitations of tests for human chorionic gonadotropin. Lancet 2000;355:671.
57. Thomas CMG, Massuger LF, Merkus HM. Needless treatment for presumed malignancy. [Letter] Lancet 2000;355:1725.
58. Dietrich CG, Stiegler H, Brandenberg VM, Riehl J. Needless treatment for presumed malignancy. [Letter] Lancet 2000; 355:1725–1726.
59. ABC News Prime Time. Cancer misdiagnosed. abcNEWS.com, posted on July 26, 2001 [Date retrieved February 28, 2002]; http://more.abcnews.go.com/sections/primetime/2020/primetime_010726_abbott_feature.html.
60. Covinsky M, Laterza O, Pfeifer JD, Farkas–Szallasi T, Scott MG. An IgM λ antibody to *Escherichia coli* produces false-positive results in multiple immunometric assays. Clin Chem 2000;46: 1157–1161.
61. Hoffmann KL, Parsons GH, Allerdt LJ. A very rapid and highly sensitive qualitative and quantitative assay for hCG. Clin Chem 1984;30:1047.
62. Sturgeon CM. Tumor markers in the laboratory: closing the guideline-practice gap. Clin Biochem 2001;34:353–359.
63. Semjonow A, Brandt B, Oberpenning F, Roth S, Hertle L. Discordance of assay methods creates pitfalls for the interpretation of prostate-specific antigen values. Prostate 1996; 7S:3–16.

Chapter 7

Oncogenes and Tumor Suppressor Genes in Cancer

Marta Sanchez-Carbayo and Carlos Cordon-Cardo

Cellular homeostasis develops and is maintained by the coordinated balance of several critical processes, including cell cycle division, differentiation, and apoptosis. In cancer, cells grow abnormally, in a pattern uncoordinated with that of normal tissue. This abnormal pattern persists even after the initial transformation event has occurred, and is due to a combination of genetic (somatic or hereditary) and epigenetic alterations that result in this neoplastic transformation.

The etiopathogenesis of neoplastic diseases is characterized by multiple causes: biological, chemical, and physical agents have been identified as initiating or promoting neoplastic mechanisms. However, neoplastic diseases, all appear to a have common molecular basis. In addition to somatic mutations, which are the most frequent abnormalities identified in human cancer, germ-line mutations associated with specific familial cancer syndromes have been reported, unveiling the underlying mutations of specific genes predisposing patients to distinct cancers. It is therefore conceivable to view cancer as fundamentally a genetic disease entailing germ-line and somatic mutations. In addition, epigenetic alterations, such as promoter methylation or protein degradation, are also considered suppressive or dominant events involved in tumorigenesis and tumor progression.

Target genes implicated in cellular transformation and tumor progression have been divided into two categories: proto-oncogenes and tumor suppressor genes (also known as growth suppressor genes). Activation of proto-oncogenes by point mutation, amplification, translocation, or even insertion of non-eukaryotic sequences, yields oncogenes that have as main characteristic a "gain" of function. They have also been described as "dominant" and "positive" phenomena. Inactivation of tumor suppressor genes occurs mainly through an allelic deletion followed by a point mutation of the contralateral allele. These events have also been described as "recessive" and "negative." Alterations in proto-oncogenes and tumor suppressor genes seem equally prevalent in human cancers.

This chapter begins by describing oncogenes and tumor suppressor genes and how they can be identified both *in vitro* and *in vivo*. The biological impact of such alterations is then described using the clinical model of bladder cancer. Given that *TP53* and the retinoblastoma (*RB*) genes are among the most common genetic alterations in human cancers, their biological roles and involvement in tumor progression are described also in the context of bladder cancer.

ONCOGENES AND TUMOR SUPPRESSOR GENES AS CELL PROLIFERATION-CONTROLLING GENES

"Cancer" describes a myriad of diseases. It is difficult to ultimately understand these disease processes at the molecular level, because they do not ascribe to "monogenic" categorization. Rather, they have multiple molecular derangements. As mentioned above, cancers develop when there is a failure in the processes that control cell division cycle and/or disrupt apoptosis (cell death). These genetic abnormalities, usually occurring over a lifetime, are called somatic mutations; however, it is now well-known that certain individuals with the genetic predisposition to cancer carry inherited genetic mutations, also referred as germ-line events.

The study of cancer in genetically predisposed individuals offers the opportunity to identify those primary mutations central to cancer's development. In addition, cancer susceptibility could be influenced by polymorphic alleles that regulate distinct aspects of cellular metabolism, response to genetic damage, immunological surveillance, and those genes related to environmental exposure and cellular stress (1).

Although oncogenic activation and tumor suppressive inactivation are both prevalent in tumorigenesis and development of the final malignant phenotype, it appears that the most common inherited events relate to the lack of functional tumor suppressor alleles. Furthermore, inherited mutations that affect the genes involved in maintaining the integrity of the genome, such as the mismatch repair genes involved in hereditary nonpolyposis colon cancer syndrome, or the nucleotide-excision-repair genes responsible for xeroderma pigmentosum, have also emerged as recessive events since it is the lack of their function that causes the pathological condition leading to tumorigenesis. See Table 1.

Table 1 Oncogenes (O) and tumor suppressor genes (TS)

Gene Name	Tumor	Alteration	Type of Gene
NF2	Vestibular schwannoma, medulloblastoma, mesothelioma	L Point mutations, allele loss	TS
PTEN	Glioblastomas, prostate, breast	Chr10 allele loss	TS
p53	Gliomas, astrocytoma, lung, adrenocortical adenoma, esophageal, gastric, hepatocelular, colon, breast, uterus, prostate	CHr17 allele loss, point mutations	TS
VHL	Hemangioblastomas, phaeochromocytoma	Chr3 allele loss, point mutations	TS
N-MYC	Neuroblastoma, breast	Amplification	O
RB1	Retinoblastoma, osteosarcoma, breast, lung, bladder, esophageal, breast	Chr13 allele loss	TS
RET	Papillary thyroid, MEN2, phaeochromocytoma	Point mutation, fusion	O
MEN1	Pituitary tumors, MEN1	Chr11 allele loss	TS
GSP	GH pituitary tumors	Point mutations	O
APC	Esophageal, colon	Loss of heterozygosity	TS
MTS1	Esophageal, biliary tract, pancreatic	Chr9 allelic loss, point mutations	O
TRP-MET	Gastric	Point mutations	O
K-RAS	Gastric, colon	Point mutations	O
C-erbB-2	Gastric, breast	Point mutations, amplifications	O
DCC	Gastric, colon	Allelic loss	TS
MLH	Gastric	Point mutations	O
P15Ink4B	Biliary tract	Point mutations	O
BRCA1	Pancreatic, breast, ovarian, prostate, stomach, fallopian tube	Point mutation	TS
BRCA2	Pancreatic, breast, ovarian	Pont mutation	TS
MCC	Colon	Point mutation	O
ATM	Breast	Point mutations	O
H-RAS	Breast, ovarian	Amplification	O
INT2	Breast	Amplification	O
WT1	Renal	Chr11 deletion, point mutation	TS
WT2	Renal	Loss of heterozygosisty	TS

ONCOGENES: STRATEGIES LEADING TO THEIR IDENTIFICATION

The convergence of cytogenetics (initially of human leukemias), studies of retroviral-induced cancers in rodents and other animals, and recombinant DNA technology have created a foundation for understanding the molecular basis of cancer and for identifying candidate genes that may function as oncogenes in human carcinogenesis.

Detection of Amplified Chromosomal Sites

Decades ago, chromosomal abnormalities were described as common events. However, the issue of cause and effect concerning these changes remained controversial for years. Some investigators argued that both loss of chromosomes and structural alterations were the consequences of cancer. Others suggested that the changes were the antecedents of the cancer.

The question was not resolved until the 1970s, when chromosome-banding techniques were developed and chromosome preparations of human cancer cells could be examined routinely. Karyotype studies revealed that certain tumor types had the same chromosome aberrations, suggesting that a non-random pattern of genetic alterations was associated with specific malignant phenotypes (2). The most striking example was that of chronic myeloid leukemia, where more than 90% of cases had a translocation affecting chromosomes 9 and 22 [t(9;22)(q34.1;q11.21)]. Before it was known that chromosome 22 was actually part of a translocation and not merely a truncated chromosome, it was called the Philadelphia (Ph) chromosome. In other leukemias, specific translocations were also observed, but not to the extent of the "Ph" chromosome in CML patients.

The association of specific chromosome abnormalities with specific cancers indicated a causal relationship. (Otherwise, it would be expected that chromosome abnormalities would be distributed randomly among all types of cancers.) However, at the time, no one knew which genes were disrupted or unregulated by the various translocations. In addition to translocations, cancer cells often have a large number of chromosome abnormalities with gains and losses of entire chromosomes or parts of chromosomes (3). Although genetic and chromosome modifications are prevalent in all tumors, it is not always known which changes are specific for certain cancers and which are merely specific of genomic instability. In this context, a group of tumor cells resembles a micro-evolutionary population, because, as genetic and chromosome mutations accumulate, the individual cells become different from one another. And, by chance, subsequent changes might occur that allow a tumor to pass from one stage to another (4).

Use of Retroviral Oncogenes

For a number of years, researchers had known that a very large number of species-specific RNA viruses (retroviruses) cause cancers in rodents, cats, chickens, and other animals (5,6). By the 1970s, samples containing cancer-causing retroviruses were shown to comprise two different forms of the same virus. One viral type was able to proliferate and rarely caused cancer. The other type could not proliferate on its own (i.e., it was defective), and it frequently induced cancers.

Molecular analyses indicated that a virus that could proliferate contained a complete set of retroviral genes. The genome of the defective form usually retained the ends of the retroviral genome, but had an internal portion that was not equivalent to the viral genomic sequence. The sources and functions of these replacement sequences (inserts) that were different in different cancer-causing retroviruses were becoming the focus of interest. Hybridization studies showed that the inserts were originally derived from the genomes of the host organisms and not from retroviral sequences. In addition, the inserts represented highly conserved sequences that were also present in humans.

Additional work established that each insert originated from a messenger RNA molecule of the host cell. As part of the virus, these sequences, after infecting a host cell, either simulated cell proliferation or prolonged the life of the host cell. The presence of wild-type retrovirus is necessary to ensure that the defective virus genomes are perpetuated (7). Moreover, during many replication cycles through repeated infections, an insert in a retroviral genome accumulates mutations and diverges from the original sequence. These mutations make the protein encoded by an insert an exceptionally efficient inducer of cancer in a host cell (8).

As part of the normal life cycle of a retrovirus, the genome acts as a template for the production of a double-strand DNA version, which is incorporated into the genome of the host cell. When the DNA version of a defective retrovirus genome is integrated into a cell's chromosome site, the protein encoded by the insert disrupts the constraints of cell proliferation and cancer develops. Parenthetically, the rare instances of cancer induction by a wild-type retrovirus result from the insertion of the viral genome into a site in the host cell genome that controls cell proliferation. Clearly, it was imperative to learn as much as possible about each human gene homolog of each retroviral insert sequence (4).

The highly divergent cancer-causing sequences in retroviral genomes were called v-oncogenes, and the host sequences that gave rise to v-oncogenes were designated proto-oncogenes. Their specific names are often three-letter abbreviations derived in part from the name of the retrovirus that carries a particular v-oncogene. Later, when human cancers were observed with mutated proto-oncogenes, these alleles were called oncogenes (8).

In situ hybridizations were carried out with cloned v-oncogenes from various sources to pinpoint the chromosome sites of the corresponding human genes. It was of more than considerable interest when the locations of some of the human homologous genes of the v-oncogenes coincided with breakpoints of translocations found in various leukemias. For example, the v-*abl* oncogene identified the homologous human *ABL* gene at chromosome 9q34.1, which is at the site involved in the "Ph" chromosome. Thus, it was likely that an alteration of the *ABL* gene contributed to CML. In this way, a number of v-oncogenes were used to determine which human genes might be involved in the formation of cancers.

The focus of cancer research then shifted from v-oncogenes to human oncogenes (9). As research progressed, in addition to the v-oncogene human homologs, oncogenes were discovered that did not exist as retroviral v-oncogenes (8).

Recombinant DNA Technology

One strategy for identifying human oncogenes involves first testing whether DNA from a human cancer alters the growth characteristics of a mouse cell line in culture. If so, then the investigator eliminates extraneous human DNA before cloning the human DNA fragment with the oncogene.

One of a number of differences between normal and cancer cells in culture is that normal cells stop growing after they form a monolayer on a "Petri" plate, whereas cancer cells continue to grow on top of each other. Normal cells in culture that acquire cancer cell attributes are said to be transformed. If a mouse cell line, for example, is transformed by DNA from a human cancer, there is a strong likelihood that a cancer-causing version of a human oncogene was integrated into the mouse genome.

In the next step, DNA is isolated from the transformed mouse cells and transfected into an untreated mouse cell line. A second round of transformed cells is selected. By repeating this process four or five times, the DNA segment carrying the oncogene is reduced to the point where it can be cloned into a vector. A library is constructed with DNA from the last transformed cell line. The clones with human DNA, which can be distinguished from clones with mouse DNA inserts by the presence of *Alu* sequences, are isolated and characterized. In this way, the oncogene from the original human cancer can be identified.

FUNCTIONS OF ONCOGENES

The oncogene family is a family of genes that act dominantly to induce or maintain cell transformation. As noted above, oncogenes were first identified in RNA tumor viruses, and further research revealed that they are derived from normal cellular genes called proto-oncogenes. These genes have a role in normal cellular growth and proliferation but, when mutated, may function as oncogenes. More than 70 oncogenes have been identified as participating in cellular proliferation, cell division cycle, apoptosis, and other related cellular processes (4).

The functions of proto-oncogenes can be classified into the following four broad groups(8):

- growth factors, which include platelet-derived growth factor, epidermal growth factor, insulin-like growth factors 1 and 2, or transforming growth factor α and β. For example, overexpression of IGF2 is a feature of many Wilms' tumors.

- growth factor receptors, which provide a link between the stimulatory effects of growth factors and the intracellular signaling pathways. Examples of these proto-oncogenes include *TRK*, *FDFr1-4*, *MET*, *RET*, and *KIT*. For instance, two transmembrane receptor tyrosine kinases, *RET* and *MET*, may be mutated in inherited cancers (multiple endocrine neoplasia type 2 (*MEN2*) and familial papillary renal cancer. *RET* and *MET* mutations result in abnormal activation of the receptor protein.
- signal transducers, which may fall into different groups:
  - membrane-associated/guanine nucleotide-binding proteins (RAS, GSP and GIP);
  - membrane-associated/cytoplasmic protein tyrosine kinases (ABL, SRC, FGR), and
  - cytoplasmic protein serine-threonine kinases (RAF1, MOS, COT). Oncogenes of the RAS family (H (Harvey)-ras-1, K (Kirsten)-ras-2 and N-ras) each encode a 21-kDa protein (p21), which shares homology with G-proteins but has sustained mutations that render them constitutively active by maintaining the proteins in the GTP-bound activated state. Activating RAS mutations are frequent in human cancers (e.g., colon, pancreas, bladder, and lung), although the particular RAS gene involved varies between cancer types. Although it seems clear that RAS has an important role in controlling cellular proliferation, the precise details of the mechanism of action are not completely known. Further complexity is provided by the discovery of GTPase-activating proteins (GAPs) which may modulate RAS activation, and the suggestion that the neurofibromatosis type 1 gene (NF1) product may be a GAP protein.
- nuclear proto-oncogenes and transcription factors, which include members of the *MYC* family (*c-MYC*, *N-MYC*, and *L-MYC*), which have been widely studied, and amplification of *MYC* genes has been found in a variety of tumor types including lung (*c-MYC*, *N-MYC*, *L-MYC*), colon (*c-MYC*), breast (*c-MYC*) and neuroblastoma (*NMYC*). The MYC protein complexes with a second protein, MAX, to form a functional heterodimer which regulates expression of target genes. Other nuclear oncoproteins include FOS and JUN, which also bind together to form a functional heterodimer.

TYPES OF ALTERATION OF ONCOGENES IN CANCER CELLS

Different kinds of genomic changes can produce oncogenic effects (10). Some oncogenes have point mutations that alter the function of the encoded protein. In other cases, the activity of an oncogene can be affected by a translocation. In some instances, the rearrangement places an active promoter region or transcription regulatory element next to an oncogene (9). Consequently, the normal control mechanisms that constrain the oncogene are undermined, the oncogene is continually expressed, and the cell proliferation mode is established. For example, the t(8;14)(q24;32) translocation for Burkitt lymphoma places the *MYC* gene under the control of the very active promoter for the heavy immunoglobulin cluster. Thus, the MYC protein is overproduced, and cell proliferation genes are expressed. In other cases, the breakpoints of a translocation occur within introns of two genes, and, after joining, a single reading frame is established with genetic information from both genes, and a fusion (hybrid, chimeric) protein is synthesized. If such a fusion protein is under the control of an active promoter, then the oncogenic protein that is part of the fusion protein is synthesized (11). For example, the translocation represented by the Ph chromosome creates a chimeric gene that specifies segments from the *BCR* and *ABL* genes and is under the control of the BCR promoter. The *ABL* portion of the chimeric gene encodes tyrosine protein kinase. Thus, as part of the fusion protein, tyrosine protein kinase activity is continuously present, the signal transduction pathway is turned on, and cell proliferation persists (4).

Overproduction of oncogenic proteins often occurs when there is repeated replication (DNA amplification) of a specific chromosome region. The mechanism that brings about localized chromosome DNA amplification is not fully understood (9). When the amplification process generates a set of repeated DNA segments that are confined to a region of a chromosome, a distinctive repetitive chromosome banding pattern, called a homogeneous staining region (HSR), is produced.

Alternatively, multiple DNA elements formed by repeated replication of a chromosome region are released into the nucleoplasm. After DNA staining, these extrachromosomal DNA components have a joined double-dot appearance and are called double minutes (DMs): a pair of circular, 1Mb DNA fragments. Since they do not have centromeres, DMs are randomly distributed to daughter cells. In human tumors, about 95% of cases of amplification are DMs and the rest are HSRs. In either instance, the end result is often an enormous increase in the number of copies of an oncogene and, as a result, the overproduction of an oncogenic protein. Amplification of an oncogene occurs in a variety of cancers (4).

In summary, proto-oncogenes may be mutated to promote cell transformation by a variety of mechanisms:

- point mutations may alter the function of the gene product and produce a transforming protein (e.g., RAS and RET);
- translocations may activate the proto-oncogene, or result in fusion genes (e.g., bcr-abl in chronic myeloid leukemia) encoding a novel product (e.g., *MYC*);
- the regulation of the gene may be impaired so that there is constitutive overproduction;
- gene amplification may lead to increased concentration of the oncoprotein (9) (see Figure 1).

TUMOR SUPPRESSOR GENES: STRATEGIES FOR THEIR IDENTIFICATION

Detecting Loss of Heterozygosity-Related Alterations

In many instances, an individual will inherit a tumor suppressor allele with an inactivating point mutation and then, in a somatic cell, the wild-type allele at the tumor suppressor gene

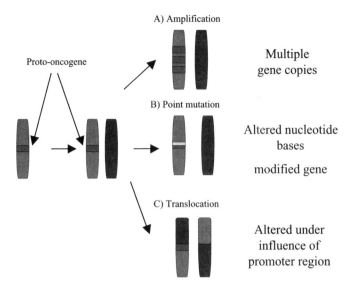

Figure 1 Mutation mechanisms of proto-oncogenes. Proto-oncogenes may promote cell transformation by a variety of mechanisms: (a) gene amplification may lead to increased concentration of the oncoprotein; (b) point mutations may alter the function of the gene product and produce a transforming protein; and (c) translocations may activate the proto-oncogene, or result in fusion genes.

locus is deleted. Such deletions are probably the consequence of faulty DNA replication or chromosome instability. The deletion of a wild-type allele in a heterozygous individual causes a loss of heterozygosity. Under these conditions, no functional tumor suppressor gene protein is produced, and the capability to prevent cancer is lost.

In addition to loss of heterozygosity at the tumor suppressor gene locus, a chromosome deletion will remove some of the neighboring alleles. If any of these flanking alleles is polymorphic, then the likelihood is high that loss of heterozygosity occurs at these loci.

The detection of loss of heterozygosity of polymorphic alleles has led to the identification of around 20 tumor suppressor genes (8). These genes have diverse functions, and many are involved in hereditary forms of cancer, such as retinoblastoma, colorectal cancer, neurofibromatosis type 1, nevoid basal cell carcinoma, or renal cell carcinoma (4).

Generally, practitioners use PCR-based short tandem repeat polymorphism (STRP) analysis of DNA from normal and cancerous cells of the same individual to direct loss of heterozygosity and localize it to a specific chromosome region. The rationale for this strategy is based on the likelihood that missing polymorphic alleles in cancer cells are closely linked to a tumor suppressor gene locus. A large panel of STRP probes is used to screen DNA from normal and cancer cells of a large number of patients with the same cancer. The losses of polymorphic marker loci are noted, and, based on STRP chromosome maps, the region with the smallest deletion is recognized. If this region does not contain a known tumor suppressor gene, then the STRP probes that delineate the smallest observed deletion are used to isolate clones from a cDNA or genomic DNA library. These clones then are analyzed for a tumor suppressor gene.

Although the loss of heterozygosity phenomenon in cancer cells commonly entails a chromosome deletion, point mutations that inactivate the functional tumor suppressor gene allele have also been noted. And, in rare instances, deletions of both alleles of a tumor suppressor gene locus have been found in some cancer cells (12). Overall, cancer is a chance phenomenon that requires various mutations in a susceptible somatic cell. However, when the alteration of a tumor suppressor gene is detected, inheritance of a mutated oncogene increases the likelihood that a cancer will form and develop (4).

Recombinant DNA Technology

That loss or inactivation was involved in oncogenesis was suggested by cell fusion experiments (13) that demonstrated that when malignant cells were fused with normal cells, the resulting hybrid cell was not malignant. The re-emergence of the malignant phenotype was correlated with the loss of chromosomes from the hybrid cells. The implication of these results was that the malignant cells had lost a normal cellular control mechanism that could be replaced by a normal cell, and that tumorigenicity behaved as a recessive genetic trait.

Weissman and Stanbridge (14) demonstrated that more than one genetic defect can cause tumurogenicity; they found that whereas hybrid cells between carcinomas remained tumorigenic, carcinoma-sarcoma and carcinoma-melanoma cell lines failed to form tumors. Further advances in knowledge about specific tumor suppressor genes have been provided by experiments in which single chromosomes (or parts of single chromosomes) have been introduced into a tumor cell line and shown to suppress tumorigenicity, e.g., Chromosome 11 in Wilms' tumor and chromosome 3 in renal cell carcinoma (15,16). In addition, the candidacy of putative tumor suppressor genes may be evaluated by transfection of wild-type gene into a "null" cancer cell line and analysis of the in-vitro and in-vivo growth (17) (See Table 2).

MODELS OF TUMOR SUPPRESSOR GENE FUNCTION

Retinoblastoma Gene Paradigm as a Reference Model

The studies of retinoblastoma have provided further evidence for the concept of tumor suppressor genes. This rare childhood tumor occurs sporadically in most cases, but a minority of children have multiple tumors or have inherited the susceptibility to retinoblastoma as a dominant trait. By analysis of the age at onset of unilateral retinoblastoma, it was observed that it could arise from two rate-limiting steps or mutations (12). A different pattern was observed for children with multiple tumors: these children were diagnosed at an earlier age and the data fit into a one-step mutation model.

Table 2 Relevant cloned candidate tumor suppressor genes

Tumor Suppressor Gene	Chromosomal Location	Possible Function
RB	13q14	Cell Cycle Regulator
TP53	17p13	Transcription Factor
p16/INK4A	9p21	Cell Cycle Regulator
ATM	11q22-23	Cell Cycle Regulator/Signal Transduction
WT1	11p13	Transcription Factor
NF1	17q11	ras GTPase Activator
NF2	22q12	Cytoskeleton-Cell Membrane Linking Protein
APC	5q21	Cell Communication
DCC	18q21	Cell Adhesion/Communication
MCC	5q21	G Protein Activation
PTP	3p21	Protein-tyrosine Phosphate
BRCA1	17q21	Transcription Factor

It was suggested that retinoblastoma was initiated by mutations at both alleles of a single locus. Children with multiple tumors were predicted to have inherited a germ line mutation of one allele so that only one somatic mutation of the other allele was necessary for retinoblastoma to develop. In unilateral sporadic tumors, both alleles were inactivated by acquired mutations. Mutations of the retinoblastoma gene are therefore recessive at the cellular level, since one normal allele can prevent tumorigenesis and tumors only developed from retinoblasts with homozygous mutations.

This model explained the earlier age at onset and occurrence of multiple tumors in patients with germline mutations. It was estimated that 80% of individuals with a germline mutation developed retinoblastoma. The retinoblastoma gene was later mapped to chromosome 13 and further evidence for the concept of the retinoblastoma gene functioning as a recessively acting tumor suppressor gene was provided by reports of chromosome 13 deletions and allele loss in tumor tissue. Several mechanisms by which the wild-type retinoblastoma gene can be mutated have been described (18). Some of these mechanisms—chromosome loss and reduplication, deletion, mitotic recombination—result in loss of heterozygosity at loci close to the retinoblastoma gene in tumor tissue when compared to normal tissue. The cloning of the retinoblastoma gene and the observation that the tumorigenicity of retinoblastoma cells can be suppressed by introducing the normal gene has confirmed the tumor suppressor gene hypothesis (19).

Studies of loss of heterozygosity have become widely used to map the location of tumor suppressor genes in a variety of cancers (20). De novo methylation of the tumor suppressor gene promoter and silencing of transcription has been identified as an important mechanism of tumor suppressor gene inactivation in familial and sporadic cancers (21,22). The use of loss of heterozygosity studies also led to the identification of replication errors (microsatellite instability) in tumors from patients with familial cancer syndromes caused by defects in mismatch repair genes, such as hereditary non-polyposis colon cancer syndrome.

Other Models of Tumor Suppressor Gene Function

The retinoblastoma model of tumorigenesis with loss of both alleles at a single locus is the paradigm for the action of a class of recessive tumor suppressor genes. Whereas many tumor suppressor genes also comply with this model, others are more complex.

In Wilms' tumors, loss of heterozygosity studies have demonstrated that allele loss can occur at two separate loci on chromosome 11. Wilms' tumor differs from retinoblastoma in that the two mutations do not necessarily occur at a single locus and a single mutation at each of the two loci can produce a tumor (23). In sporadic Wilms' tumor, the situation is complicated by the observation that there is preferential loss of alleles on the maternally inherited chromosome. Genomic imprinting has then a role in some embryonal tumors such as Wilms', rhabdomyosarcoma, and osteosarcoma.

There are further differences in the mechanisms of tumorigenesis in retinoblastoma and Wilms' tumor. In the former tumor, both germline and acquired mutations involve the same locus. In contrast, a locus for familial Wilms' has been excluded from the short arm of chromosome 11 by linkage analysis (and one locus for familial Wilms' tumor maps to chromosome 17). Although mutations in the retinoblastoma gene are recessive at the level of cellular phenotype (i.e., in the presence of one normal allele no malignant effect is observed), for other tumor suppressor genes there may be gene-dosage or dominant-negative effects (e.g., the effect of mis-sense mutations in p53 and the relationship between phenotype and position of APC gene mutation in familial polyposis coli).

TUMOR SUPPRESSOR GENES AND GENOMIC IMPRINTING

The loss of heterozygosity found on many different chromosomes in a wide variety of tumors has implicated the existence of multiple tumor suppressor genes. Under the Knudson's two-hit hypothesis of hereditary cancer, the loss of heterozygosity events is the second step in the inactivation of both alleles of a tumor suppressor gene. Thus, two genetic alteration events are required to inactivate a tumor suppressor gene (see Figure 2). To date the number of identified tumor suppressor genes that are inactivated mainly at the somatic level in cancers and are not inherited has remained disappointingly small (12,24).

Genomic imprinting is a relatively recent discovery. In this mechanism, the activity of genes may be altered epigenetically in a manner dependent on the parent of each of the two alleles. There is evidence that genomic imprinting may play a role in the pathogenesis of some embryonal tumors (25). In sporadic Wilms' tumor, embryonal rhabdomyosarcoma, and sporadic osteosarcoma (but not retinoblastoma), there is preferential retention of paternal alleles in tumor tissue (26). Under the

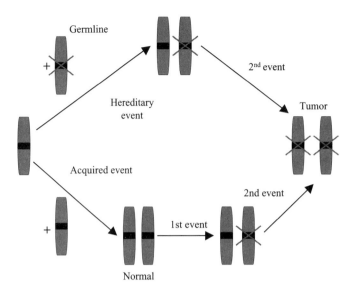

Figure 2 Tumor suppressor genes: Knudson two-hit hypothesis. The loss of heterozygosity found on many different chromosomes in a wide variety of tumors has implicated the existence of multiple tumor suppressor genes. Under the Knudson's two-hit hypothesis, the loss of heterozygosity event is the second step in the inactivation of both alleles of a tumor suppressor gene.

original Knudson two-hit hypothesis, no such bias could be expected.

At a clinical level, genomic imprinting effects are suggested by differences in expression of an inherited disease depending on the sex of the transmitting parent. For example, in familial glomus tumor the inheritance of susceptibility to glomus tumors is autosomal dominant, with expression of the tumors almost exclusively in individuals inheriting the gene from the father (27). Genomic imprinting could explain this pattern of inheritance.

MODELS OF TUMORIGENESIS: MULTI-STEP MODEL OF CANCER

There is evidence that human tumorigenesis is a multi-step process. Molecular genetic analysis of human cancers usually demonstrates multiple abnormalities, e.g., activation of two or more oncogenes and loss of tumor suppressor genes. Thus although a particular alteration may be necessary for tumorigenesis, in most cases a single event (e.g., oncogene activation) is not sufficient. Multiple mutations appear to be required to conform the malignant phenotype. Genetic instability leads to a sequence of events that creates phenotypic alterations, granting a selective advantage to specific tumor cells.

The study of multiple tumors in a given patient, as well as solitary lesions in cohorts of patients, has provided strong evidence for the multi-step nature of cancer. Metastasis is the ultimate outcome of tumor progression in this selective process. It appears that it is the accumulation rather than the order of these pleiotropic events that confers neoplastic cells the ability for tumor progression.

Statistical analysis of the age at onset of human cancers suggests that between four and six steps may be required for a diagnosable tumor to develop (28). Yet the linearity introduced by this working model is not in accord with morphologic observations and natural history of early disease in a variety of tumor types. Two distinct presentations can be generically described as early tumor lesions in most neoplasias, mainly those of epithelial origin:

- the low-grade, well differentiated (if epithelial usually papillary) tumors, which tend to recur but not to progress; and
- the high-grade, poorly differentiated (if epithelial flat) tumors with a high progression rate.

Examples of the first sort of lesions includes colonic adenomas and bladder papillomas, which are architecturally well-organized and lack cellular atypia. An archetype of the second kind would include certain carcinoma in-situ lesions (i.e., bladder Cis), which are composed of tumor cells exhibiting marked dysplastic changes. These two separate pathways are also of unequal clinical significance, as has been documented in tumors of the urinary bladder and cervix.

There is therefore a need to reconsider the linear working model as well as what we may define as primary and secondary molecular alterations in tumor progression. Various types of events can be differentiated. "Primary" chromosome aberrations are those directly related to the genesis of cancer. These are frequently found as the sole abnormality, often associated with particular tumors, and can be considered tissue-specific. Conversely, "secondary" abnormalities may be fortuitous, or may determine the biological behavior of the tumor (29).

Primary abnormalities would be expected to occur early in tumorigenesis and may have a dual nature: (1) primary events involved in the production of low-grade/well-differentiated neoplasms would destabilize cellular proliferation, but have minimal or no effect on cellular "social" interactions and differentiation; and (2) primary events leading to high-grade/poorly-differentiated tumors would disrupt growth control and have a major impact on cellular differentiation.

An example of the first type of primary event may be the *APC* gene, in which mutations produce the adenomas of the familial adenomatous polyposis coli syndrome (see below). Alterations of the *RB* gene, resulting in the intraocular retinoblastoma lesion, may serve as an illustration of the other primary events, producing a highly proliferative and undifferentiated cancer.

Some primary events may occur as secondary abnormalities. Mutations of the *TP53* gene exemplify this condition. As a primary event, *TP53* germ-line mutations appear to be the underlying molecular abnormality of tumors arising in patients affected with the Li-Fraumeni syndrome (30). However, somatic mutations of *TP53* have been reported as the most frequent genetic aberrations in human cancer (31,32), arising as secondary events related to tumor progression (30,33–35). That preneoplastic morphologic changes are preceded by molecular alterations constitutes the working hypothesis of many groups. Dinucleotide repeat assays have revealed micro-satellite abnormalities, suggesting that replication errors had occurred in these sequences (36). Furthermore, through the analysis of a cohort of patients affected with hereditary nonpolyposis colorectal cancer (HNPCC), a locus predisposing to colonic tumors has been mapped to the short arm of chromosome 2 (2p15-16) (37). This is the first of a new family of target genes or nucleotide sequences in cancer that will probably be expanded in the near future. These abnormalities, by their nature, appear to be very early alterations, and may account for the great degree of genetic instability found in cancer cells.

Colorectal and bladder cancer progression models have represented some of the relatively well-characterized models for progression in solid tumors. In the following sections we will summarize the most relevant genetic events associated with colorectal cancer. Additionally we will review how the sequential identification of the genetic alterations of bladder tumors has led to the establishment of the currently accepted model of bladder cancer progression.

MODEL OF TUMOR PROGRESSION IN COLON CANCER

For colon cancer, a specific series of genetic alterations appears to occur in the progression of benign adenoma to carcinoma (38). Under this model, mutation of the *APC* gene on chromosome 5q is an early event and is followed sequentially by mutation of the *K-ras* oncogene, and loss of *DCC* and *p53* tumor suppressor genes on chromosome 18q and 17p respectively (39).

The critical factor is the accumulation of mutations rather than the order in which they occur. Such models are compatible with the concept that the normal cell has multiple independent mechanisms to control growth and differentiation, and that aberrations in several distinct pathways or at several sites within a pathway are needed to overcome these control mechanisms. For inherited cancer syndromes caused by genes maintaining the genome integrity—e.g., *hMSH2* mutations causing hereditary non-polyposis colorectal cancer (HNPCC)—additional mutations are required before cancer can be initiated (40). Hence, mutation of the normal MSH2 allele inherited from the unaffected parent then needs to be followed by somatic mutations of both alleles of the relevant cell proliferation-controlling gene (e.g., *APC* in HNPCC-associated colorectal cancers).

BLADDER CANCER AS A MODEL OF TUMOR PROGRESSION

Through cytogenetic and molecular genetic analyses of bladder cancer, investigators have identified abnormalities in a number of chromosomes. These abnormalities appear to be involved in the development and progression of such tumors (41,42). Gibas and collaborators reported non-random chromosomal changes in transitional cell carcinomas of the urinary bladder, namely monosomy of chromosome 9 and interstitial deletions of chromosome 13 (37). Babu and co-investigators found 3p duplication, trisomy of chromosome 7, and 11p deletions as being common events in urothelial cancer (43). Loss of heterozygosity (LOH) of the short arm of chromosome 11 was reported in five out of 12 bladder tumors by Fearon et al. (44). Tsai and collaborators were the first to report allelic loss of chromosome 9q in bladder cancer (45). They examined 25 human bladder tumors and found that the greatest frequency of allelic loss was for 9q, occurring in 67% of informative cases. They also observed 17p LOH in 63% of informative cases, and 10 of these tumors had also lost chromosome 9q.

In an attempt to define the role of molecular abnormalities and altered patterns of expression of products encoded by tumor suppressor genes in the pathogenesis and progression of human bladder cancer, investigators performed an approach that combined molecular genetics and immunopathology. A cohort of 34 unselected patients affected with bladder cancer who were clinically and pathologically well characterized was studied (46). Restriction fragment length polymorphism (RFLP) analysis was directed at 5 suspected or established tumor suppressor gene regions (3p21-25, 11p15, 13q14, 17p11-3, and 18q21). Immunohistochemical assay utilizing RB-PMG3-245 monoclonal antibody to the retinoblastoma gene product (pRB) has also been used. This study demonstrated that tumor grade correlated with deletions of 3p ($p = 0.004$) and 17p ($p = 0.063$). Tumor stage was correlated with deletions of 3p ($p = 0.010$), 17p ($p = 0.015$), and altered pRB expression ($p = 0.054$). Vascular invasion correlated with deletions of 17p ($p = 0.038$). This study also demonstrated that deletions of 17p (*TP53* locus) and 18q (DCC gene locus) occur only in invasive tumors, while deletions of 3p and 11p occur in superficial and invasive tumors. Altered pRB expression was observed mainly in muscle-invasive tumors.

To test the hypothesis that genetic alterations proceed in a sequence of events that leads to bladder cancer progression, 60 paired bladder tumors and normal tissues were analyzed using polymorphic DNA markers, correlating specific allelic deletions with pathological parameters of poor clinical outcome (47). The main conclusions of this study may be summarized as follows:

- distinct genotypic patters were associated with early and late stages of bladder cancer. Deletions of 9q were observed in all superficial papillary tumors (Ta) and almost all tumors invading the lamina propria (T1), suggesting that this event associates with the genesis of superficial bladder tumors. However, 3p, 5q, and 17p deletions were absent in the Ta tumors analyzed, but were identified in invasive tumors.
- Two different genetic pathways characterize the evolution of superficial bladder tumors (Figure 3). Alterations of 9q were detected in the majority of superficial bladder tumors, but only 43% of muscle-invasive neoplasms manifested such genetic abnormalities in the present study. It has been hypothesized that certain chromosomal abnormalities play a definite role in bladder tumor development, while others correlate with pathological parameters of poor clinical outcome and should be further tested as potential prognostic markers (48).

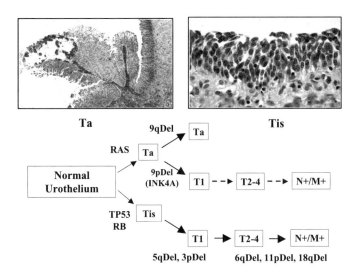

Figure 3 Genetic model of bladder cancer progression. Two different pathways have been proposed to characterize early tumorigenic events occurring in the urothelium, which may be associated in the production of papillary versus flat tumor lesions. These events are followed by secondary abnormalities that appear to be involved in tumor progression. **Color representation of figure appears on Color Plate 1.**

Two studies of allelic losses support the proposed hypothesis. Habuchi et al. have shown accumulation of deletions in the development of invasive bladder cancer. They analyzed the allelic loss of five chromosomal arms, including 9q, 11p, 17p, 13q, and 3p (49). More recently, Knowles et al. conducted an allele-typing analysis of human bladder cancer and found that the most frequent losses were apparent monosomies of chromosome 9 (9p, 51%; 9q, 57%), and that other frequent losses were on 11p, 17p, 8p, 4p, and 13q (50).

The studies summarized above have prompted pursuing two lines of investigation: analyzing alterations of the *RB* gene and its encoded product, as well as characterizing the molecular abnormalities of the *TP53* gene and corresponding patterns of expression of mutant p53 products.

In a study aimed at better defining the role of pRB in bladder cancer, the mouse monoclonal antibody RB-PMG3-245 to detect the expression of pRB in bladder tumors was used and the data was correlated with clinical outcome (51). Expression of pRB was examined by immunohistochemistry using frozen tissue sections, and computerized image analysis served to quantify the level of pRB in individual tumor cells. The overall five-year survival for this cohort of patients was 66%, with a median follow up of 42 months. Normal levels of expression, detected as a homogeneous immunoperoxidase staining in the majority of tumor cells (RB-positive group), were found in 34 patients. However, a spectrum of altered patterns of expression, from undetectable pRB levels to heterogeneous expression of pRB in less than 50% of tumor cells (RB-negative group), was observed in 14 patients. Thirteen of the 38 patients diagnosed with muscle-invasive tumors were categorized as RB negative and only one of the 10 superficial carcinomas was pRB-negative. The survival was significantly decreased in RB-negative patients compared to those with positive RB expression ($p < 0.001$). This data suggests that altered pRB expression occurs in all grades and stages of bladder cancer, but is more commonly associated with muscle-invasive tumors. Furthermore, altered patterns of the *RB* gene product may be an important prognostic variable in patients presenting with invasive bladder cancer.

Two studies have been reported that support these initial observations. Cairns et al. identified loss of heterozygosity at the *RB* locus in association with muscle invasive bladder cancers (52). Similarly, Logothetis et al. found altered expression of the retinoblastoma protein in locally advanced bladder cancer (53).

The alterations of chromosome 17 in human bladder tumors and the correlations of p53 nuclear overexpression with 17p deletions in those neoplasms were studied (47). Sixty bladder tumors were analyzed using restriction fragment length polymorphism analysis directed at five different loci on chromosome 17. The same tumors were studied with a panel of mouse monoclonal antibodies (PAb1801, PAb240, and PAb1620) to mutant and wild-type p53 proteins using immunohistochemistry. Deletion of 17p correlated with grade ($p = 0.039$), stage ($p = 0.004$), and the presence of vascular invasion ($p = 0.056$). None of the pathologic parameters correlated with 17q deletions; p53 nuclear overexpression correlated with grade ($p = 0.027$), stage ($p = 0.008$), vascular invasion ($p = 0.021$), and the presence of nodal metastases ($p = 0.007$). In superficial (Ta) lesions, 17p was not deleted, while 55% of T1 and T2–T4 tumors showed loss of heterozygosity. Mutations of *TP53* as detected by immunohistochemistry were seen in superficial as well as invasive tumors, whereas loss of heterozygosity was seen only in invasive tumors. There was a strong correlation between the presence of mutation and loss of heterozygosity of the remaining allele ($p = 0.0003$).

The hypothesis that altered patterns of p53 expression correlated with tumor progression in patients with early invasive disease (T1 bladder cancer) was then investigated (54). Detection of p53 nuclear overexpression was evaluated in tumors of 43 patients with T1 bladder cancer by immunohistochemistry, using the mouse monoclonal antibody PAb1801 on deparaffinized tissue sections. Patients with T1 bladder tumors could be stratified into two groups. Eighteen patients (42%) had no or less than 20% tumor cells with positive nuclear staining (group A), while the remaining 25 patients (58%) had more than 20% tumor cells with nuclear immunoreactivity (group B). Patients in group B had a significantly lower progression-free interval ($p < 0.001$). These results suggest that T1 bladder cancers exhibiting p53 nuclear overexpression have a higher rate of disease progression. This study also suggests that p53 overexpression is an important prognostic factor in these patients, and may be useful in selecting appropriate therapy.

The prevalence and clinical relevance of p53 nuclear overexpression in 54 patients with pathologically confirmed Ta bladder carcinomas, who did not receive any prior adjuvant therapy, was then studied (54). The median follow-up was 110 months. Using the same threshold for the scoring of IHC as above, patients were stratified into two groups: Group A ($<$ 20% positive tumor cells) (n = 42); and Group B ($>$ 20% positive tumor cells) (n = 12). Tumor progression was observed in five patients in Group A and in seven patients in Group B (p = 0.002). Nuclear overexpression of p53 was the only independent variable associated with death due to bladder cancer (p = 0.04).

Following a similar strategy, the analysis of p53 nuclear overexpression in 33 patients affected with carcinoma in situ of the urinary bladder was performed (55). Like the groups discussed above, those patients did not receive prior adjuvant therapy. The median follow-up for this cohort of patients was 124 months, and 16 patients' disease progressed during that period. Disease progression occurred in 3 of 18 patients with p53-negative phenotype, while 13 of 15 p53-positive patients progressed (p < 0.001, Cox's regression analysis). Moreover, death specifically due to bladder cancer was also associated with altered pattern of p53 expression (p = 0.01, Fisher's exact test).

Additional studies supporting this data have been reported by Lipponen (56) and others (57). Lipponen used 252 unselected bladder tumors and 20% positive nuclear staining as the cut-off value. Overexpression of p53 nuclear oncoprotein was associated with decreased survival in the cohort of patients analyzed (58). Esrig et al. analyzed 243 patients affected by transitional cell carcinoma of the bladder treated by radical cystectomy. Detection of nuclear p53 was associated with increased risk of recurrence (p < 0.001) and decreased overall survival (p < 0.001) (59).

A next series of studies had the objectives of better defining the deleted regions of the chromosome 9 in bladder tumors, as well as evaluating the frequency of micro-satellite alterations affecting certain loci on this chromosome in urothelial neoplasms (60,61). Orlow et al. studied 73 primary bladder tumors with a set of highly polymorphic markers, and results were correlated with pathological parameters associated with poor clinical outcome. Overall, 77% of the tumors showed either loss of heterozygosity (LOH) for one or more chromosome 9 markers and/or micro-satellite abnormalities at chromosome 9 loci. Detailed analyses showed that two regions, one on 9p at the IFN cluster (9p21), and the other on 9q associated with the q34.1-2 bands, had the highest frequencies of allelic losses. Furthermore, Ta lesions appeared to present mainly with 9q abnormalities, while T1 tumors displayed a mixture of aberrant 9p and 9q genotypes. These observations indicated that LOH of 9p may be associated with the development of superficial tumors with a more aggressive biological behavior or, alternatively, they may be related to early disease progression. This study was followed by an in-depth analysis of p16/INK4A/MTS1 and p15/INK4B/MTS2, the two candidate tumor suppressor genes identified in 9p21, in a cohort of 110 primary bladder tumors (61). The overall frequency of deletions and rearrangements for the p16 and p15 genes in bladder cancer was 19% and 18%, respectively. Moreover, this study revealed that p16 and p15 alterations were associated with low-stage, low-grade bladder tumors. It should be emphasized that only Ta and T1, but not Tis, lesions showed deletions of either p16 or p15. Since p16 alterations occur independently of p53 mutations (62), and p53 mutations are frequent events in Tis bladder tumors (63,64), data from that report further support the hypothesis that bladder carcinogenesis may develop through two distinct molecular pathways. Taken together, the results suggest that p16 and p15 alterations confer selective growth advantage to urothelial tumor cells, but mutations in other genes are required to produce an overt malignant phenotype.

RB/p53 Pathways as a Model of the Involvement of Cell Proliferation-Controlling Gene Alterations in Cancer

p53/*RB1* pathways are the most frequent altered cell proliferation-controlling genes in cancer. Thus, in this chapter, we will primarily focus on these two prototype tumor suppressor genes, *RB* and *TP53*, and how their mutations relate to tumorigenesis and tumor progression in clinical settings. The following sections will address data showing evidence of their involvement in cell transformation, their biological characteristics, and the impact of detecting these tumor suppressor gene alterations in the areas of early diagnosis, prognosis, and treatment planning.

Evidence of the Inactivation of p53 and *RB* Tumor Suppressor Genes in Tumor Cells Transformation

Besides the evidence revealed by clinical observations and molecular epidemiology studies, two other lines of investigation support the concept of tumor suppressor gene inactivation as being intimately involved in cellular transformation. First, due to efforts in establishing biological systems to study the nature of certain tumor suppressor genes, targeted gene disruption or knockout murine models have been developed and characterized. Germline mutations in p53 and *RB* each predispose mice to cancer. Animals homozygous for an *RB* mutation die in utero with defects in fetal hematopoiesis and widespread neuronal cell death (65,66). However, p53 homozygous mice, as well as *RB* heterozygous and p53 heterozygous mice, are viable but develop a variety of tumors. The most common neoplasms after p53 disruption are sarcomas and lymphomas (67), while pinealoblastomas and medullary thyroid carcinomas are usually found in heterozygous *RB* mice (68). It should be emphasized that germline homozygosity for p53 mutation causes pronounced cancer susceptibility, since 90% of the p53-deficient animals develop one or more tumors by 6 months of age. In a recent study, the cooperative tumorigenic effects of germline mutations in p53 and *RB* have been established. Heterozygous mice mutant for both genes have reduced viability and exhibit increased tumor burden and metastatic spread (68). Taken together, these observations parallel those observed in the clinical setting of inherited cancer traits.

Another line of evidence supporting the concept that inactivation of suppressor gene encoded products leads to cellular transformation has resulted from studies dealing with oncoviruses. Several viral and cellular proteins have been shown to interact with p53 and/or pRB, altering their functions. The SV40 large T antigen, the adenovirus E1B-55 kDa protein, and the human papilloma virus (HPV) E6 protein each bind to p53 and inactivate its transcriptional activity (69–71). Similarly, underphosphorylated pRB molecules may form complexes with viral transforming proteins, including the SV40 large T antigen, the adenovirus E1A protein, and the papilloma virus E7 protein (72–74). Complex formation with these proteins inactivates pRB function and leads to cellular immortalization. It is believed that the growth deregulation produced by pRB inhibition is counteracted by apoptotic cell death orchestrated by normal p53 function. Therefore, the loss of one tumor suppressor gene is compensated by the activity of the other, serving as a safeguard mechanism to protect against the emergence of neoplastic cell growth. Without both pRB and p53, it appears that E2F activation stimulates cell proliferation permitting tumor formation (see below) (75). High transformation strains of tumor viruses encode proteins that bind and inactivate both p53 and pRB, revealing the crucial role of these molecules and their close interaction. A clinical archetype that illustrates this phenomenon is the high incidence of cervical carcinomas that develop in women affected with certain subtypes of papilloma viruses, such as the HPV 16 and 18 (76).

Biological Properties of the *TP53/RB* Pathway Tumor Suppressor Genes: Impact on Cell Cycle Control

TP53 gene. Findings from several lines of investigation suggest that p53 controls a cell cycle checkpoint responsible for maintaining the integrity of the genome. It has been shown that wild-type p53 mediates arrest of the cell cycle in the G1 phase after sublethal DNA damage (77). In addition, p53 appears to be involved in transcriptional control (78). Like most of the well-characterized transcription factors, p53 proteins possess a nuclear localization signal and a sequence-specific DNA-binding domain. Very recently, the crystal structure of the p53 fragment that extends from amino acid residue 94 to 312, containing the critical site-specific DNA-binding core domain (residues 102 to 292), has been resolved (79). Analysis of the structure has revealed that the conserved regions of the core domain are the sites of the majority of *TP53* mutations identified in human primary tumors, further supporting the hypothesis that DNA binding is critical for the biological activity of p53. These studies provide a framework for our understanding of how mutations inactivate p53 functions.

The *RB* gene. The retinoblastoma gene encodes an approximately 105-kDa nuclear phosphoprotein (80–82). While the amount of pRB does not change during progression of the cell cycle, the phosphorylation state of pRB is cell-cycle dependent, and is a target for the enzymatic activity of cyclin-Cdk complexes (83–85). pRB is in the underphosphorylated form in G1, and as cells progress into late G1 and early S phase, pRB becomes highly phosphorylated and remains phosphorylated in G2. The underphosphorylated form of pRB is believed to be the functionally active form of pRB in G0/middle G1; pRB does not appear to possess sequence-specific DNA-binding activity, and the underphosphorylated form of pRB most likely exerts its negative regulatory effect on gene expression through complex formation with DNA-binding proteins. A colinear segment comprised of more than 350 amino acids, located within the carboxyl two-thirds of pRB, has been identified as a functional internal protein receptor and is designated the "pocket" domain (86). pRB can complex stably by the interaction of this region with cellular proteins, including members of the E2F family (87,88). E2F is a 60-kDa transcription factor originally identified through its role in transcriptional activation of the adenovirus E2 promoter. Unbound E2F transcription factors could stimulate transcription of cellular genes. E2F sites are present in genes implicated in induction of S phase, such as thymidine kinase, Myc, Myb, dihydrofolate reductase, and DNA polymerase-α (89). This suggests that E2F family members may be responsible for transversing the G1/S restriction point of the cell cycle. It may then be concluded that pRB functions by sequestering other cellular proteins with growth-promoting activities. The fact that the operative "pocket" region is the target for viral oncoproteins that inhibit pRB, as well as a common site for *RB* mutations, provides insight into how specific alterations inactivate pRB.

Cyclin-dependent kinase inhibitory genes. A relatively new family of negative cell cycle regulators, which function as Cdk-inhibitory molecules, has been identified, and the genes that encode these proteins designated *CKI* genes. The mechanism whereby they achieve their function appears to be the formation of stable complexes that inactivate the catalytically operative units composed of a cyclin and a cyclin-dependent kinases (Cdk). The first and probably best-characterized member of this family is p21, which inactivates cyclin E-cdk2, cyclin A-cdk2, and cyclins D1-, D2- and D3-cdk4 complexes (90,91). These are components of the regulatory kinases that target pRB for phosphorylation. The p21/WAF1 gene maps to 6p21.1 and encodes a 164-amino acid protein of relative molecular mass (Mr) 18,107. Another member of the CKI group is p16, which encodes a 148-amino acid protein of Mr 15,845 (92). Unlike p21, p16 forms binary complexes specifically with Cdk4 and Cdk6, inhibiting their activity and, by doing so, also inhibits pRB phosphorylation. However, p16 does not interact with Cdc2 or Cdk2. The entire p16 sequence is composed of four repeats of an ankyrin consensus motif. Based upon the biochemical properties described, p16 was designated INK4 (**in**hibitor of Cd**k4**) (92). The p15/INK4B gene has been reported, which encodes a protein of 137-amino acid with Mr 14,700, and shown to be a potential effector of TGFβ-induced cell cycle arrest (93). P15 has substantial homology to p16, and its protein sequence can be also divided into four ankyrin repeats; p15 has the ability to form binary complexes, to bind and inactivate Cdk4 and Cdk6, inhibiting pRB phosphorylation. These two genes map to the short arm of chromosome 9 (9p21), a region that accounts for loss of heterozygosity and homozygous deletions in various human tumor cell lines. Since these genes are also mutated in primary tumors, they are likely to be relevant candidate tumor suppressor genes. To this rapidly growing group of Cdk-inhibitors other members have been added, including p27/Kip1 (94,95) and p18 (96).

Clinical Implications of Molecular Alterations of *TP53/RB* Tumor Suppressor Genes

Early diagnosis and risk assessment. Some individuals, because they carry mutations in specific genes, have an increased likelihood of suffering from a specific cancer or group of cancers during their lifetime compared to the general population. Although individuals who have well-defined cancer family syndromes account for a small minority (approximately 0.1% of all people who have cancer), those belonging to families with cancer where heredity plays some role may account for 5–10% (97). The inheritance of a disease-causing gene can be determined either indirectly, by studying the segregation of DNA markers closely linked to the mutant allele, or by direct identification of a disease-causing mutation carried by an individual subject. This latter approach can now be applied to a series of conditions, since the affected genes are being identified and advances in technology are providing the basis for genetic diagnosis.

The results of direct analysis of the presence of a disease-causing mutation are more applicable in the study of diseases such as retinoblastoma, which are characterized by high rates of new germline mutations. In view of recent advances in cancer treatment for retinoblastoma patients, the identification of *RB* mutations is increasingly important with respect to early treatment intervention. Moreover, children affected with the hereditary form of retinoblastoma often develop a second malignancy several years after successful treatment of their primary tumor (98). In contrast, secondary tumors are uncommon in patients with the sporadic form of the disease. In addition to molecular diagnosis, identification of tumorigenic point mutations in the *RB* gene have been utilized and considered of value in risk estimation and genetic counseling (99).

Similar to the *RB* gene, germline mutations of the *TP53* gene are detected in patients with the Li-Fraumeni syndrome, a rare autosomal dominant trait (69,100). These patients are susceptible to a variety of cancers, such as sarcomas, leukemias, and breast carcinomas. More recently, *TP53* germline mutations were also detected in patients with no apparent family history (32), as well as a subset of patients presenting with a second primary neoplasm (31).

Biological behavior and prognosis. Loss of heterozygosity of chromosome 17 at the *TP53* locus (17p13.1) and somatic mutations of *TP53* are the most common genetic alterations reported to date in human cancer. These molecular aberrations have been associated with the development and progression of a large number of human tumors (101,102). Striking significant correlations between *TP53* mutations and/or altered patterns of p53 expression and poor survival of cancer patients have been independently documented by different groups studying common human neoplasms (103–105). Moreover, the majority of the tumor-associated mutations are found at or near the DNA-binding domain at the so-called "hot" spots (79). Two classes of mutations have been characterized; those that involved residues that contact the DNA (functional mutants), and mutations altering residues important for the structural integrity of the core domain, in particular the DNA-binding surface of the wt p53 protein (structural mutants) (79). The resolution of the crystal structure of p53 solidified the hypothesis that DNA-binding and transactivation are the critical activities of p53 required for tumor suppression and confirms the relationship between basic and clinical findings. On the basis of these observations, it has been postulated that detection of these abnormalities may become important adjuncts to the main factors associated with outcome in patients with particular neoplastic lesions. This prognostic tool may also be useful in determining whether a more aggressive therapeutic intervention should be used. It is crucial to develop assays that will assess biological activities of altered p53 proteins found in clinical specimens. This in turn will allow us to distinguish those probably irrelevant or silent mutations that are acquired by the malignant cell versus those that truly contribute to the malignant phenotype.

RB mutations and altered patterns of pRB have been detected in a wide variety of human primary tumors (52,53,106–110). These changes have also been associated with aggressive behavior and poor clinical outcome in specific tumor types, including bladder and lung carcinomas (52,53,110). However, analysis of other neoplastic processes, such as sarcomas, suggests that *RB* alterations are primary events involved in tumorigenesis or early phases of tumor progression (111). An important limitation in the characterization of *RB* mutations is the lack of "hot" spots, as those described for *TP53*. Even though some alterations are found in the "pocket" domain, the pattern of deletions and point mutations for *RB* is more random than that of *TP53*. This phenomenon, together with the complexity of the *RB* gene, offers a challenge for the analysis of molecular aberrations that occur in primary tumors.

For all of these reasons, it will be crucial to conduct in-depth studies of *RB* alterations. Analyses comparing *RB* and other tumor suppressor gene abnormalities, utilizing well-characterized groups of patients with long-term follow-up, will allow the evaluation of their critical role as potential tumor markers and possibly aid in the stratification of patients into prognostic categories.

Treatment planning and response to therapy. To date there is not a reliable marker or panel of markers to accurately predict clinical outcome and to properly design therapeutic intervention in a given cancer case. Due to the physiological role of p53 in recognizing DNA damage, arresting cells in the G1 phase of cell cycle, and subsequently inducing apoptosis if errors that cannot be repaired, it has been postulated that molecular alterations affecting p53 may abrogate such biological properties. These mutations not only would grant selective growth advantage, but also produce neoplastic clones that would be unresponsive to specific chemotherapeutic agents. This issue was initially explored in genetically engineered animal models of tumors expressing or devoid of p53 (112). Tumors expressing wild-type p53 contained a high proportion of apoptotic cells and typically regressed after treatment with gamma radiation or adriamycin. In contrast, p53-deficient tumors treated with the same regimens continued to enlarge and contained few apoptotic cells. Furthermore, acquired mutations in p53 were associated with both treatment failure and tumor relapse and progression. These studies suggested that p53 status might be an important determinant of tumor response to therapy.

Different studies have been designed to evaluate the potential clinical implications summarized above regarding the involvement of *TP53* mutations in the lack of response to certain treatments by neoplastic cells. Multi-modality approaches to the treatment of muscle-invasive bladder cancer have evolved in recent years based on the observation that, despite radical cystectomy, 50% of patients will relapse and die of bladder cancer. The M-VAC neoadjuvant trials confirm that a complete pathological response occurs in about 20–30% of patients. Therefore, modeling based on patient and tumor characteristics would be appropriate to restrict this form of therapy to the subset of patients most likely to benefit. In order to address this important issue, the hypothesis that p53 alterations may be an independent prognostic marker for survival and an indicator of treatment failure in patients with invasive bladder cancer treated with neoadjuvant M-VAC therapy was tested. Using a previously generated database and tissue blocks available for ninety patients that were prospectively treated with this regimen and followed-up with for a median period of 5.8 years, a multivariate analysis revealed that p53 overexpression had independent significance for survival ($p = 0.001$, relative risk ratio = 3.1). The impact of p53 overexpression was predominantly in T2 and T3a tumors. Investigators concluded that p53 nuclear overexpression provided an independent prognostic value for survival in patients with invasive bladder cancer treated with neoadjuvant chemotherapy and may become an important indicator of lack of response to such regimen (113).

Other studies supporting this concept have been recently published. Aberrant p53 expression was found to predict clinical resistance to Cisplatin-based chemotherapy in locally advanced non-small cell lung cancer (114). Another important contribution backing this hypothesis was a study reporting that adjuvant systemic therapy, especially with tamoxifen, along with radiotherapy, was of less value to p53-mutated breast cancer patients (115).

FINAL COMMENTS

The understanding of the biology of cancer has improved considerably over the past decade. The identification of the involvement of tumor suppressor genes and oncogenes in cancer progression has been critical. The development of high-throughput technologies such as DNA microarrays will enhance the number of identified gene candidates for displaying an oncogene or a tumor suppressor function. Translating these novel biological discoveries into therapies or strategies to manage patients suspected of or who have been diagnosed with bladder cancer will always be the ultimate goal.

REFERENCES

1. Varmus HE. The molecular genetics of cellular oncogenes. Ann Rev Genet 1984;18:553–612.
2. Rabbitts TH. Chromosomal translocation master genes, mouse models, and experimental therapeutics. Oncogene 2001;20: 5763–5777.
3. Kinzler KW, Vogelstein B. Gatekeepers and caretakers. Nature, 1997;386:761–762.
4. Pasternak JJ. Molecular genetics of cancer syndromes. In: Pasternak JJ, ed. An introduction to human molecular genetics: mechanisms of inherited diseases. Bethesda, MD: Fitzgerald Science Press, 1999.
5. Varmus HE. Viruses, genes, and cancer. I. The discovery of cellular oncogenes and their role in neoplasia. Cancer 1985;55: 2324–2328.
6. Varmus HE. Retroviruses. Science, 1988;240:1427–1435.
7. Fisher GH, Orsulic S, Holland E, Hively WP, Li Y, Lewis BC, Williams BO, Varmus HE. Development of a flexible and specific gene delivery system for production of murine tumor models. Oncogene 1999;18:5253–5260.
8. Hodgson SV, Maher ER. A practical guide to human cancer genetics. Cambridge, UK: Cambridge University Press, 1997.
9. Rabbitts TH. The clinical significance of fusion oncogenes in cancer. N Engl J Med 1998;338:192–194.
10. Tabin CJ, Bradley SM, Bargmann CI, Weinberg RA, Papageorge AG, Scolnick EM, Dhar R, Lowy DR, Chang EH. Mechanism of activation of a human oncogene. Nature 1982;300:143–149.
11. Rubie H, Hartmann O, Michon J, et al. N-Myc gene amplification is a major prognostic factor in localized neuroblastoma results of the French NBL 90 study. Neuroblastoma Study Group of the Societe Francaise d'Oncolgie Pediatrique. J Clin Oncol 1997;15: 1171–1182.
12. Knudson AG. Mutation and cancer: statistical study of retinoblastoma. Proc Natl Acad Sci 1971;68:820–823.
13. Harris H, Miller OJ, Klein G, Worst P, Tachibam T. Suppression of malignancy by cell infusion. Nature,1969;223:363–368.
14. Weissman BE, Standbridge EJ Complementation of the tumorigenic phenotype in human cell hybrids. J Natl Cancer Inst;1983; 70:667–672.
15. Weissman BE, Saxon PJ, Pasquale SR, Jones GR, Geiser AG, Stanbridge EJ. Introduction of a normal chromosome 11 into a Wilms' tumor cell line controls its tumorigenic expression. Science 1987;236:175–180.
16. Shimizu M, Yokota J, Mori N. Introduction of normal chromosome-3P modulates the tumorigenicity of a human renal-cell carcinoma cell line Ycr. Oncogene 1990;5:185–194.
17. Haber D, Harlow E. Tumor-suppressor genes: evolving definitions in the genomic age. Nat Genet 1997;16:320–322.
18. Cavanee WK, Dryja TP, Phillips RA. Expression of recessive alleles by chromosomal mechanism in retinoblastoma. Nature 1983;305:779–784.
19. Huang HS, Yeo J, Shaw Y. Suppression of neoplastic phenotype by replacement of the *RB* gene in human cancer cells. Science 1988;242:1563–1566.

20. Cavanee WK. The Beckwith-Wiedemann syndrome: lessons for developmental oncology. In: Brandi ML, White R, eds. Hereditary tumors. New York: Raven Press, 1991.
21. Versteeg, R. Aberrant methylation in cancer. Am J Hum Genet 1997;60:751–754.
22. Prowse AH, Webster AR, Richards FM, et al. Somatic inactivation of the VHL gene in von Hippel-Lindau disease tumors. Am J Hum Genet 1997;60:765–771.
23. Henry I, Jeanpierre M, Couillin P. Molecular definition of the 11p15.5 region involved in Beckwith-Wiedemann syndrome and probably in predisposition to adrenocortical carcinoma. Hum Genet 1989;81:273–277.
24. Devilee P, Cleton-Jansen AM, Cornelisse CJ. Ever since Knudson. Trends Genet 2001;17:569–573.
25. Ferguson-Smith AC, Reik W, Surani MA. Genomic imprinting and cancer. Cancer Surv 1990;9:487–503.
26. Scrable H, Cavanee C, Ghavimi F, Lovell M, Morgan K, Sapienza C. A model for embryonal rhabdomyosarcoma tumorigenesis that involves genome imprinting. Proc Natl Acad Sci 1989;86:7480–7484.
27. van der May AGL, Maaswinkel-Mooy PD, Cornelisse CJ, Schmidt PH, van de Kamp JJP. Genomic imprinting in hereditary tumors: evidence for a new genetic theory. Lancet 1898;2:1291–1294.
28. Peto R, Roe FJC, Lee PN, Levy L, Clack J. Cancer and aging in mice and men. Br J Cancer, 1975;32:411–426.
29. Esrig D, Elmajian D, Groshen S, Freeman JA, Stein JP, Chen S-C, Nichols PW, Skinner DG, Jones PA, Cote RJ. Accumulation of nuclear p53 and tumor progression in bladder cancer. New Engl J Med 1994;331:1259–1264.
30. Li FP, Fraumeni JF Jr. Rhabdomyosarcoma in children: epidemiologic study and identification of a familial cancer syndrome. J Natl Cancer Inst 1969;43:1365–1373.
31. Malkin D, Jolly RW, Barbier N, Look AT, Friend SH, Gebhardt MC, Andersen TI, Borresen AL, Li FP, Garber J, Strong LC. Germline mutations of the p53 tumor-suppressor gene in children and young adults with second malignant neoplasms. New Engl J Med 1992;326:1309–1315.
32. Toguchida J, Yamaguchi T, Dayton S, Beauchamp RL, Herrera GE, Ishizaki K, Yamamuro T, Meyers PA, Little JB, Sasaki MS, Weichselbaum RR, Yandell DW. Prevalence and spectrum of germline mutations of the p53 gene among patients with sarcoma. N Eng J Med 1992;326:1301–1308.
33. Eaton DF, Ford D, Bishop DT, and The Breast Cancer Linkage Consortium. Breast and ovarian cancer incidence in BRCA1 mutation carriers. Am J Hum Genet 1995;56:265–71.
34. Sarkis AS, Zhang Z-F, Cordon-Cardo C, Melamed J, Dalbagni G, Sheinfeld J, Fair WR, Herr HW, Reuter VE. p53 nuclear overexpression and disease progression in Ta bladder carcinoma. Int J Oncol 1993;3:355–360.
35. Muleris M, Salmon RJ, Zafrani B. Consistent deficiencies of chromosome 18 and of the short arm of chromosome 17 in eleven cases of human large bowel cancer. Ann Genet 1985;28:206–213.
36. Cleaver JE. It was a very good year for DNA repair. Cell 1994;76:1–4.
37. Gibas Z, Prout GR, Connolly JG, Pontes JE, Sandberg AA. Nonrandom chromosomal changes in transitional cell carcinoma of the bladder. Cancer Res 1984;44:1257–1264.
38. Fearon ER, Vogelstein B. A generic model for colorectal tumorigenesis. Cell 1990;61:759–767.
39. Baker SJ, Markowitz S, Fearon ER, Willson JK, Vogelstein B. Suppression of human colorectal carcinoma cell growth by wild-type p53. Science 1990;249:912–915.
40. Boland CR, Sato J, Appelman HD, Bresalier RS, Feinberg AP. Microallelotyping defines the sequence and tempo of allelic losses at tumor suppressor gene loci during colorectal cancer progression. Nat Med 1995;1:902–909.
41. Smeets W, Pauwels R, Laarakkers L, Debruyne F, Geraedts J. Chromosomal analysis of bladder cancer. III. Nonrandom Alterations. Cancer Genet Cytogenet 1987;29:29–41.
42. Atkin NB, Baker MC. Cytogenetic study of ten carcinomas of the bladder: Involvement of chromosomes 1 and 11. Cancer Genet Cytogenet 1985;15:253–268.
43. Babu VR, Lutz MD, Miles BJ, Farah RN, Weiss L, Van DD. Tumor behavior in transitional cell carcinoma of the bladder in relation to chromosomal markers and histopathology. Cancer Res 1987;47:6800–6805.
44. Fearon ER, Feinberg AP, Hamilton SH, Vogelstein B. Loss of genes on the short arm of chromosome 11 in bladder cancer. Nature 1985;318:377–380.
45. Tsai YC, Nichols PW, Hiti AL, Williams Z, Skinner DG, Jones PA. Allelic losses of chromosomes 9, 11, and 17 in human bladder cancer. Cancer Res 1990;50:44–47.
46. Presti JC, Reuter VE, Galan T, Fair WR, Cordon-Cardo C. Molecular genetic alterations in superficial and locally advanced human bladder cancer. Cancer Res 1991;51:5405–5409.
47. Dalbagni G, Presti J, Reuter VE, Fair WR, Cordon-Cardo C. Genetic alterations in bladder cancer. Lancet 1993;324:581–582.
48. Cordon-Cardo C, Dalbagni G, Sarkis AS, Reuter VE. Genetic alterations associated with bladder cancer. In: DeVita VT, Hellman S, Rosenberg SA (eds.). Important Advances in Oncology. Philadelphia: JB Lippincott, 1994:71–84.
49. Habuchi T, Ogawa O, Kakehi Y, et al. Accumulated allelic losses in the development of invasive urothelial cancer. Int J Cancer 1993;53:579–584.
50. Knowles MA, Elder PA, Williamson M, Cairns JP, Shaw ME, Law, MG. Allelotype of human bladder cancer. Cancer Res 1994;54:531–538.
51. Cordon-Cardo C, Wartinger D, Petrylak D, Dalbagni G, Fair WR, Fuks Z, Reuter VE. Altered expression of the retinoblastoma gene product: Prognostic indicator in bladder cancer. J Natl Cancer Inst 1992;84:1251–1256.
52. Cairns P, Shaw ME, Knowles MA. Initiation of bladder cancer may involve deletion of a tumor-suppressor gene on chromosome 9. Oncogene 1993;8:1083–1085.
53. Logothetis CJ, Xu H-J, Ro JY, Hu SX, Sahin A, Ordonez N, Benedict WF. Altered expression of retinoblastoma protein and known prognostic variables in locally advanced bladder cancer. J Natl Cancer Inst 1992;84:1256–1261.
54. Sarkis AS, Dalbagni G, Cordon-Cardo C, Zhang ZF, Sheinfeld J, Fair WR, Herr HW, Reuter VE. Nuclear overexpression of p53 protein in transitional cell bladder carcinoma: a marker for disease progression. J Natl Cancer Inst 1993;85:53–59.
55. Sarkis AS, Dalbagni G, Cordon-Cardo C, Melamed J, Zhang Z-F, Sheinfeld J, Fair WR, Herr HW, Reuter VE. Association of p53 nuclear overexpression and tumor progression in carcinoma in situ of the bladder. J Urol 1994;152:388–392.
56. Lipponen PK. Over-expression of p53 nuclear oncoprotein in transitional-cell bladder cancer and its prognostic value. Int J Cancer 1993;53:365–370.
57. Bochner BH, Esrig D, Groshen S, Dickinson M, Weidner N, Nichols PW, Skinner DG, Cote RJ. Relationship of tumor angio-

genesis and nuclear p53 accumulation in invasive bladder cancer. Clin Cancer Res 1997;3:1615–1622.
58. Lipponen P, Aaltomaa S, Eskelinen M, Ala-Opas M, Kosma VM. Expression of p21(waf1/cip1) protein in transitional cell bladder tumors and its prognostic value. Eur Urol 1998;34:237–243.
59. Esrig D, Freeman JA, Stein JP, Skinner DG. Early cystectomy for clinical stage T1 transitional cell carcinoma of the bladder. Semin Urol Oncol 1997;15:154–1560.
60. Orlow I, Lianes P, Lacombe L, Dalbagni G, Reuter VE, Cordon-Cardo C. Chromosome 9 deletions and microsatellite alterations in human bladder tumors. Cancer Res 1994;54:2848–2851.
61. Orlow I, Lacombe L, Hannon GJ, et al. Deletion of the p16 and p15 genes in human bladder tumors. J Natl Cancer Inst 1995;87: 1524–1528.
62. Gruis NA, Weaver-Feldhaus J, Liu Q, et al. Genetic evidence in melanoma and bladder cancers that p16 and p53 function in separate pathways of tumor suppression. Am J Pathol 1995;146: 1199–1205.
63. Fradet Y, Lacombe L. Can biological markers predict recurrence and progression of superficial bladder cancer? Curr Opin Urol 2000;10:441–445.
64. Ozen H, Hall MC. Bladder cancer. Curr Opin Oncol 2000;12: 255–259.
65. Lee E, Chang C-Y, Hu N, Wang YC, Lai CC, Herrup K, Lee WH, Bradley A. Mice deficient for *RB* are nonviable and show defects in neurogenesis and hematopoiesis. Nature 1992;359:270–271.
66. Jacks T, Fazeli A, Schmitt EM, Bronson RT, Goodell MA, Weinberg RA. Effects of an *RB* mutation in the mouse. Nature 1992;359:295–300.
67. Donehower LA, Harvey M, Slagle BL, McArthur MJ, Montgomery CA Jr, Butel JS, Bradley A. Mice deficient for p53 are developmentally normal but susceptible to spontaneous tumors. Nature 1992;356:215–221.
68. Williams BO, Remington L, Albert DM, Mukai S, Bronson RT, Jacks T. Cooperative tumorigenic effects of germline mutations in *RB* and p53. Nature Genet 1994;7:480–484.
69. Linzer DI, Levine AJ. Characterization of 54K dalton cellular SV40 tumor antigen present in SV40-transformed cells and uninfected embryonal carcinoma cells. Cell 1979;17:43–52.
70. Sarnow P, Ho YS, Williams J, Levine AJ. Adenovirus E1b-58kd tumor antigen and SV40 large tumor antigen are physically associated with the same 54 kd cellular protein in transformed cells. Cell 1982;28:387–394.
71. Werness BA, Levine AJ, Howley PM. Association of human papillomavirus types 16 and 18 E6 proteins with p53. Science 1990;248:76–79.
72. DeCaprio JA, Ludlow JW, Figge J, Shew JY, Huang CM, Lee WH, Marsilio E, Paucha E, Livingston DM. SV40 large tumor antigen forms a specific complex with the product of the retinoblastoma susceptibility gene. Cell 1988;54:275–283.
73. Whyte P, Buchkovich KJ, Horowitz JM, Friend SH, Raybuck M, Weinberg RA, Harlow E. Association between an oncogene and an anti-oncogene: the adenovirus E1A proteins bind to the retinoblastoma gene product. Nature 1988; 334:124–129.
74. Dyson H, Howley PM, Munger K, Harlow E. The human papilloma virus-16 E7 oncoprotein is able to bind to the retinoblastoma gene product. Science 1989;243:934–937.
75. Morgenbesser SD, Williams BO, Jacks T, DePinho RA. p53-dependent apoptosis produced by *RB* deficiency in the developing mouse lens. Nature 1994;371:72–74.
76. de Villiers EM. Human pathogenic papillomavirus types: An update. In: zur Hausen H, ed. Human Pathogenic Papillomaviruses. Heidelberg: Springer Verlag, 1994:1–12.
77. Kastan MB, Onkyekwere O, Sidransky D, Vogelstein B, Craig RW. Participation of p53 protein in the cellular response to DNA damage. Cancer Res 1991;51:6304–6311.
78. Zambetti G, Bargonetti J, Walker K, Prives C, Levine AJ. Wild-type p53 mediates positive regulation of gene expression through a specific DNA sequence element. Genes Dev 1992;6: 1143–1152.
79. Cho Y, Gorina S, Jeffrey PD, Pavletich NP. Crystal structure of a p53 tumor suppressor-DNA complex: understanding tumorigenic mutations. Science 1994;265:346–355.
80. Friend SH, Horowitz JM, Gerber MR, Wang XF, Bogenmann E, Li FP, Weinberg RA. Deletions of a DNA sequence in retinoblastomas and mesenchymal tumors: organization of the sequence and its encoded protein. Proc Natl Acad Sci 1987;84:9059–9063.
81. Lee W-H, Shew J-Y, Hong FD, Sery TW, Donoso LA, Young LJ, Bookstein R, Lee EY. The retinoblastoma susceptibility gene encodes a nuclear phosphoprotein associated with DNA binding activity. Nature 1987;329:642–645.
82. Fung Y-K, Murphree AL, T'Ang A, Qian J, Hinrichs SH, Benedict WF. Structural evidence for the authenticity of the human retinoblastoma gene. Science 1987;236:1657–1661.
83. DeCaprio JA, Ludlow JW, Lynch D, Furukawa Y, Griffin J, Piwnica-Worms H, Huang CM, Livingston DM. The product of the retinoblastoma susceptibility gene has properties of a cell cycle regulatory element. Cell 1989;58:1085–1095.
84. Buchkovich K, Duffy LA, Harlow E. The retinoblastoma protein is phosphorylated during specific phases of the cell cycle. Cell 1989;58:1097–1105.
85. Chen PL, Scully P, Shew J-Y, Wang JY, Lee WH. Phosphorylation of the retinoblastoma gene product is modulated during the cell cycle and cellular differentiation. Cell 1989; 58:1193–1198.
86. Kaelin WG Jr, Pallas DC, DeCaprio JA, Kaye FL, Livingston DM. Identification of cellular proteins that can interact specifically with the T/E1A-binding region of the retinoblastoma gene product. Cell 1991;64:521–532.
87. DeFeo-Jones D, Huang PS, Jones RE, Haskell KM, Vuocolo GA, Hanobik MG, Huber HE, Oliff A. Cloning of cDNAs for cellular proteins that bind to the retinoblastoma gene product. Nature 1991;352:251–254.
88. Chellappan SP, Hiebert S, Mudryj M, Horowitz JM, Nevins JR. The E2F transcription factor is a cellular target for the RB protein. Cell 1991;65:1053–1061.
89. Johnson DJ, Schwarz JK, Cress WD, Nevins JR. Expression of transcription factor E2F1 induces quiescent cells to enter S phase. Nature 1993;365:349–352.
90. Harper JW, Adami GR, Wei N, Keyomarsi K, Elledge SJ. The p21 cdk-interacting protein Cip1 is a potent inhibitor of G1 cyclin-dependent kinases. Cell 1993;75:805–816.
91. El-Deiry WS, Tokino T, Velculescu VE, Levy DB, Parsons R, Trent JM, Lin D, Mercer WE, Kinzler KW, Vogelstein B. WAF1, a potential mediator of p53 tumor suppression. Cell 1993;75: 817–825.
92. Serrano M, Hannon GJ, Beach D. A new regulatory motif in cell-cycle control causing specific inhibition of cyclin D/CDK4. Nature 1993;366:704–707.
93. Hannon GJ, Beach D. p15^{INK4B} is a potential effector of TGF-β-induced cell cycle arrest. Nature 1994;371:257–261.

94. Polyak K, Kato J-Y, Solomon MJ, Sherr CJ, Massague J, Roberts JM, Koff A. p27^{Kip1}, a cyclin-Cdk inhibitor, links transforming growth factor-β and contact inhibition to cell cycle arrest. Genes Dev 1994;8:9–22.
95. Toyoshima H, Hunter T. p27, a novel inhibitor of G1 cyclin-cdk protein kinase activity, is related to p21. Cell 1994;78:67–74.
96. Guan K-L, Jenkins CW, Li Y, Nichols MA, Wu X, O'Keefe CL, Matera AG, Xiong Y. Growth suppression by p18, a p16$^{INK4/MTS1}$- and p14$^{INK4B/MTS2}$-related CDK6 inhibitor, correlates with wild-type pRB function. Genes Develop 1994;8:2939–2952.
97. Eaton D, Peto J. The contribution of inherited predisposition to cancer incidence. Cancer Surveys 1990;9:395–415.
98. Eng C, Li FP, Abramson DH, Ellsworth RM, Wong FL, Goldman MB, Seddon J, Tarbell N, Boice JD. Mortality from second tumors among long-term survivors of retinoblastoma. J Natl Cancer Inst 1993;85:1121–1128.
99. Yandell DW, Campbell TA, Dayton SH, Petersen R, Walton D, Little JB, Buckley EG, Dryja TP. Oncogenic point mutations in the human retinoblastoma gene: their application to genetic counseling. N Engl J Med 1989;321:1689–1695.
100. Malkin D, Li FP, Strong LC, Fraumeni JF Jr, Nelson CE, Kim DH, Kassel J, Gryka MA, Bischoff FZ, Tainsky MA, Friend SH. Germ line p53 mutations in a familial syndrome of breast cancer, sarcomas, and other neoplasms. Science 1990;250:1233–1238.
101. Drobnjak M, Latres E, Pollack D, Karpeh M, Dudas M, Woodruff JM, Brennan MF, Cordon-Cardo C. Prognostic implications of p53 nuclear overexpression and high proliferation index of Ki-67 in adult soft tissue sarcomas. J Natl Cancer Inst 1994;86: 549–554.
102. Thor AD, Moore DH II, Edgerton SM, Kawasaki ES, Reihsaus E, Lynch HT, Marcus JN, Schwartz L, Chen L-C, Mayall BH, Smith HS. Accumulation of p53 tumor suppressor gene protein: an independent marker of prognosis in breast cancers. J Natl Cancer Inst 1992;84:845–855.
103. Allred DC, Clark GM, Elledge R, Fuqua SAW, Brown RW, Chamness GC, Osborne CK, McGuire WL. Association of p53 protein expression with tumor cell proliferation rate and clinical outcome in node-negative breast cancer. J Natl Cancer Inst 1993; 85:200–206.
104. Mitsudomi T, Oyama T, Kusano T, Osaki T, Nakanishi R, Shirakusa T. Mutations of the p53 gene as a predictor of poor prognosis in patients with non-small cell lung cancer. J Natl Cancer Inst 1993;85:2018–2023.
105. Zeng Z-S, Sarkis AS, Zhang Z-F, Klimstra DS, Charytonowicz E, Guillem JG, Cordon-Cardo C, Cohen AM. p53 nuclear overexpression: an independent predictor of survival in lymph node-positive colorectal cancer patients. J Clin Oncol 1994;12: 2043–2050.
106. Cance WG, Brennan MR, Dudas ME, Huang CM, Cordon-Cardo C. Altered expression of the retinoblastoma gene product in human sarcomas. N Engl J Med 1990;323:1457–1462.
107. Wunder JS, Czitrom AA, Kandel R, Andrulis IL. Analysis of alterations in the retinoblastoma gene and tumor grade in bone and soft-tissue sarcomas. J Natl Cancer Inst 1991;83:194–200.
108. Phillips SMA, Barton CM, Lee SJ, Morton DG, Wallace DMA, Lemoine NR, Neoptolemos JP. Loss of the retinoblastoma susceptibility gene (RB1) is a frequent and early event in prostatic tumorigenesis. Br J Cancer 1994;70:1252–1256.
109. Kornblau SM, Xu H-J, del Giglio A, Hu S-X, Zhang W, Calvert L, Beran M, Estey E, Andreeff M, Trujillo J, Cork MA, Smith TL, Benedict WF, Deisseroth AB. Clinical implications of decreased retinoblastoma protein expression in acute myelogenous leukemia. Cancer Res 1992;52:4587–4590.
110. Xu H-J, Quinlan DC, Davidson AG, Hu S-X, Summers CL, Li J, Benedict WF. Altered retinoblastoma protein expression and prognosis in early-stage non-small-cell lung carcinoma. J Natl Cancer Inst 1994;86:695–699.
111. Benedict WF, Xu H-J, Hu S-X, Takahashi R. Role of the retinoblastoma gene in the initiation and progression of human cancer. J Clin Invest 1990;85:988–993.
112. Lowe SW, Bodis S, McClatchey A, Remington L, Ruley HE, Fisher DE, Housman DE, Jacks T. p53 status and the efficacy of cancer therapy in vivo. Science 1994;266:807–810.
113. Sarkis AS, Bajorin DF, Reuter VE, Herr HW, Netto G, Zhang Z, Schultz PK, Cordon-Cardo C, Scher HI. The prognostic value of p53 nuclear overexpression in patients with invasive bladder cancer treated with neoadjuvant M-VAC. J Clin Oncol 1995;13: 1384–1390.
114. Rush V, Klimstra D, Venkatraman E, Oliver J, Martini N, Gralla R, Kris M, Dmitrovsky E. Aberrant p53 expression predicts clinical resistance to Cisplatin-based chemotherapy in locally advanced non-small-cell lung cancer. Cancer Res 1995;55: 5083–5042.
115. Berg J, Norber T, Sjogren S, Lindgren A, Holmberg L. Complete sequencing of the p53 gene provides prognostic information in breast cancer patients, particularly in relation to adjuvant systemic therapy and radiotherapy. Nature Med 1995;1:1029–1034.

Chapter 8

Proteases in Cancer: Markers of Metastatic Potential and Prognosis

Michael J. Duffy

Clinicians who want to optimally manage the care of patients with cancer must determine their accurate prognosis. Prognostic factors (such as tumor size, tumor grade, and local lymph node status) are therefore required to avoid overtreating indolent disease and undertreating aggressive disease (1). Although these parameters are widely used, they are not ideal for predicting patient outcome. Table 1 lists some of the limitations of these classical factors when applied to breast cancer.

The primary determinant of outcome in patients with cancer is the formation of distant metastasis. Metastasis is a multi-step event involving local invasion of the extracellular matrix (ECM), angiogenesis (growth of new blood vessels from pre-existing vessels), invasion of the blood vessel wall, survival of malignant cells in the vascular system, extravasation, and establishment of a secondary growth (see Figure 1) (2). Once dissemination to distant sites has occurred, most cancers are unresponsive to therapy.

A number of steps involve the degradation of natural barriers that normally prevent the spread of cancer. It is now widely believed that the breakdown of these barriers is catalyzed by proteolytic enzymes released from the invading tumor (for review, see reference 3). The enzymes involved include, but are not limited to, urokinase plasminogen activator (uPA), cathepsins such as cathepsin B (CB), and cathepsin D (CD) and spe-

Table 1 Traditional prognostic factors for breast cancer and their limitations

Factor	Limitations
Tumor size	Size may be more related to chronological age of the tumor than aggressiveness.
Tumor grade	Poor inter-observer variability, lack of standardization.
Nodal status	(a) Requires major surgery. (b) No good prognostic index exists for node-negative patients.
Estrogen receptor	A weak prognostic factor. Its prognostic impact disappears with medium- and long-term follow-up.

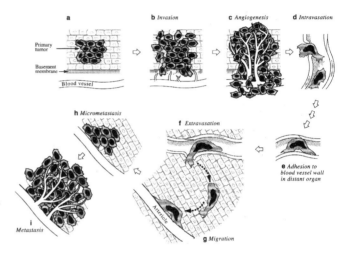

Figure 1. Main steps in cancer invasion and metastasis. Reproduced with permission from the Annual Review of Medicine, Volume 49, 1998, by Annual Reviews.

cific matrix metalloproteinases (MMPs) (Table 2). These proteases appear to function as a cascade that mediates dissolution of the ECM (4).

As proteases are causally involved in cancer spread, their activities or concentrations in primary cancers might be expected to correlate with metastatic potential and thus with patient prognosis (5). Over the past 10–15 years multiple investigations have tested this hypothesis. These studies have shown that certain matrix-degrading proteases are among the most powerful biological prognostic factors for cancer described to date.

This chapter reviews the chemistry, biology, and clinical value of the most widely studied proteases. In addition, the assay of these proteases will be briefly discussed.

UROKINASE PLASMINOGEN ACTIVATOR

Structure and Function

uPA is a 53 kDa serine protease initially synthesised as a catalytically inactive single chain peptide (6). Conversion to the active form involves cleavage at a lysine-isoleucine bond

Table 2 Key proteases implicated in cancer invasion and metastasis

Protease	Type	Gene Location	Main Substrate	Inhibitors
uPA	Serine	10q24	Plasminogen	PAI-1, PAI-2
Cathepsin B	Thiol	8p22	Multiple	Stefins, cystatins
Cathepsin D	Aspartyl	11p15.5	Multiple	NF
MMP-2**	Metallo	16q13	Collagen IV	TIMP-1,2,3,4
MMP-9	Metallo	20q11.1-q13.1	Collagen IV	TIMP-1,2,3,4

*NF, none found, at least in mammalian cells.
**MMP, matrix metalloproteinase.

(K158-I159). In vitro, activation can be induced by a number of proteases, including plasmin, cathepsin B, cathepsin L, and human kallikrein type 2 (6). Although the physiological activator of pro uPA remains to be determined, a glandular kallikrein (mGk-6) was recently shown to promote conversion in plasminogen-deficient mice (7).

The active form of uPA consists of a 2-chain molecule in which the amino terminal A-chain is linked to the B-chain by a single disulfide bond. The A-chain (amino acids 1–158) contains a growth factor-like domain (amino acids 1–49) that links uPA to a membrane-bound receptor (uPAR) while the B-chain possesses the catalytic site (6).

The best-known reaction of uPA is catalyzing the conversion of inactive plasminogen to active plasmin. Plasmin, in contrast to uPA, has multiple substrates (6):

- It can promote degradation of the ECM, a necessary step for cancer invasion and metastasis.
- It can activate the precursor forms of certain matrix metalloproteinases (MMPs) such as MMP-3, MMP-9, MMP-12, and MMM-13 (formation of the active MMPs allows further degradation of the ECM).
- It can activate or release specific growth factors such as FGF2 and TGFb (8). These pleitrophic growth factors can enhance tumor progression by stimulating cell proliferation, migration, and adhesion (6,8).

Originally, it was believed that uPA promoted cancer spread by catalyzing ECM degradation, thereby allowing malignant cells to invade local sites, and eventually disseminate to distant sites. It is now clear however, that uPA can promote cancer metastasis by a number of different mechanisms. For example, recent findings suggest that uPA can also stimulate angiogenesis, cell proliferation, and cell migration (6). All of these processes are necessary for primary cancers to spread to a distant site.

In vivo, uPA catalytic activity can be controlled by two endogenous inhibitors: PAI-1 and PAI-2 (6). Although PAI-1 and PAI-2 were originally identified as protease inhibitors, it is now clear that both these proteins are multifunctional. PAI-1, in particular plays a role in angiogenesis, cell adhesion, and cell migration (6). Furthermore, both PAI-1 and PAI-2 have been shown to inhibit apoptosis (9,10).

uPA AS A PROGNOSTIC MARKER IN BREAST CANCER[1]

uPA was the first protease, implicated in experimental metastasis, to be evaluated for possible prognostic value in human cancer. In 1988, Duffy et al. (11) reported that patients with breast cancers containing high activities of uPA in their primary tumor had a worse disease-free pattern than those patients with low activity levels. In the intervening years, these results have been confirmed by at least 20 independent groups worldwide (12). Most investigators find that the prognostic impact of uPA is independent of traditionally used markers such as axillary node status, tumor size, tumor grade, and estrogen receptor (ER) status (12). In most studies with short-term follow-up, uPA is a more potent predictor of disease-free and overall survival than tumor size, tumor grade, or ER status, and a predictor of similar strength to nodal status (12).

The subgroup of patients with breast cancer for whom new prognostic factors are most urgently required are those with axillary node-negative disease. With the advent of screening mammography, approximately two-thirds of newly diagnosed breast cancer patients present without histological evidence of metastasis in their local lymph nodes. The long-term survival of these patients, with local therapy alone, should be 70–80%. Thus, if all node-negative patients are given adjuvant chemotherapy, the majority will derive no benefit. If however, the patients who are cured by local treatment could be identified, they could be spared the costs and side effects of the adjuvant therapy while more intensive treatment could be given to those at highest risk.

At least eight different groups have shown that that high levels of uPA predict adverse outcome in node-negative breast cancer patients (12). Measuring uPA should thus help in differentiating between the majority of node-negative patients who are cured by surgery from the minority with aggressive disease and who might benefit from systemic treatment.

Paradoxically, high levels of the uPA inhibitor, PAI-1, have also been correlated with aggressive disease in breast cancer, including the subgroup with node-negative disease (12). The reasons why high levels of PA-1 predict adverse outcome are not clear, but they may relate to the involvement of this inhibitor in angiogenesis (12).

[1] See also chapter 41 for further discussion

Because of multiple and consistent reports linking high levels of both uPA and PAI-1 with adverse prognosis in breast cancer, the findings that both these proteins are independent prognostic indicators, and particularly because the levels of both correlate with outcome in node-negative patients, these markers are now potential candidates for routine application in the management of patients with breast cancer. However, before entering clinical use, their prognostic value should be confirmed by Level 1 Evidence Studies. Level 1 evidence may be obtained either by a large prospective randomized trial when evaluation of the marker is the primary end point, or by a meta-analysis/pooled analysis of small-scale retrospective and prospective studies (13).

Both types of studies have recently been performed to validate the prognostic value of uPA/PAI-1 in breast cancer. The prospective study was a multi-center trial involving 674 node-negative breast cancer patients. In this study, patients with high concentrations of uPA and/or PAI-1 were randomized to receive either six cycles of adjuvant CMF or to be observed. Patients with low levels of uPA and PAI-1 were not given any adjuvant systemic treatment. After a median follow-up of 32 months, women with high levels of uPA and or/PAI-1 had a significantly shorter disease-free interval than those with low levels of both proteins (14). In a multivariate analysis, which included factors such as tumor size, tumor grade, hormone receptor status, and type of surgery, uPA/PAI-1 was a strong and independent prognostic indicator (relative risk, 2.8, $p = 0.008$).

The pooled analysis for uPA and PAI-1 included over 8,000 patients from 18 different data sets with a median patient follow-up of 79 months (15). Multivariate analysis showed both uPA and PAI-1 to be independent prognostic factors. The prognostic benefit of both proteins was also confirmed in patients with node-negative disease, including the subgroup of these patients who did not receive adjuvant therapy (15).

To the author's knowledge, uPA and PAI-1 are the first tumor markers to have their clinical value validated using two different types of Level 1 Evidence Studies. When combined with analytical validations of assays for uPA and PAI-1 (see below), these findings should now allow these factors to enter routine clinical use. In the clinic, the main application of these two markers is likely to be selecting the indolent node-negative breast cancer patients who do not need adjuvant chemotherapy.

uPA As a Prognostic Marker in Gastrointestinal Cancers

Although not as extensively investigated as in breast cancer, multiple studies have reported a correlation between high levels of uPA and poor prognosis in patients with colorectal cancer (12). In one of these studies, the ratio of cancer tissue to normal mucosa for uPA was independent of tumor stage in predicting overall survival (16), while in another, uPA was found to be a marker of disease outcome in patients with Dukes' B disease (17). Dukes' B is perhaps the subgroup of colorectal cancer patients for whom new prognostic markers are most urgently required. Whether uPA will be able to detect the subgroup of aggressive Dukes' B patients who might benefit from adjuvant chemotherapy remains to be shown. High levels of uPA were also found to correlate with aggressive disease in patients with both gastric and esophageal cancers (12).

uPA As a Prognostic Marker in Other Cancers

In preliminary studies uPA has been shown to be a prognostic indicator in a variety of other cancers: ovarian, renal, hepatocellular, pancreatic, gliomas, urinary bladder, adenocarcinoma of the lung, and cervical cancer of the uterus (12). uPA thus appears to be a generalized prognostic marker.

Assay of uPA

Although the original assay that showed a prognostic value for uPA utilized a catalytic activity assay (11), most of the subsequent studies used ELISA. Several research and commercially available ELISA kits have now been described for the measurement of uPA concentration (18). A number of the commercially available kits have been subjected to detailed evaluation (18). The main conclusions to emerge from this study were these:

- All the kits developed for measuring uPA in tissue extracts had a sensitivity < 32 pg of uPA per ml and thus had adequate sensitivity for detecting uPA in breast cancer extracts.
- Within-assay precision for all assays investigated was satisfactory.
- All assays displayed an acceptable degree of parallelism following dilution of tissue extracts.
- In general, although the absolute level of uPA measured varied depending on the method used, good correlations were found between the various assays.
- One of the kits (American Diagnostica, Greenwich, CT) was subsequently investigated in external quality assurance studies and shown to perform in a satisfactory manner (19).

Unlike the serum-based markers discussed in this book, assay of the proteases described in this chapter are usually carried out on tumor tissue. To obtain optimal prognostic information with uPA, it appears necessary to extract tissue with Triton X-100 (20). Extraction with this detergent may allow scientists to measure a greater proportion of receptor-bound uPA than is found in the cytosol.

While most studies showing a prognostic value for uPA have measured the protease using an ELISA, a minority used immunohistochemistry (21,22). Compared to ELISA, immunohistochemistry is subjective and only-semi-quantitative. However, immunohistochemistry is simpler to perform and requires less tissue. Furthermore, with immunohistochemistry, the identity of the cell type containing the marker of interest can be identified. Despite these potential advantages, the use of immunohistochemistry for the detection of uPA has not to-date undergone rigorous evaluation. ELISA therefore remains the method of choice for measuring uPA in tumor tissue.

CATHEPSIN B (CB)
Structure and Function

CB is a thiol-dependent protease normally found in lysosomes (for review, see ref. 23). In tissue, CB can exist as either a single chain or as both a single and double chain. Like all known proteases, CB is initially synthesised as a high-molecular-weight inactive precursor (Mr, 37000). Activation can be induced by other proteases such as CD-like enzyme or by an MMP. In turn, CB can activate the precursor form of uPA as well as certain MMPs (23).

While in normal tissue CB is predominantly a lysosomal enzyme, in tumor cells it can either be attached to the cell membrane or secreted (23). This altered trafficking in malignant cells appears to be due to a deficiency of the mannose-6-phosphate receptor (23). Secretion or cell membrane-attachment enables CB to degrade substrates in the ECM. Among the proteins hydrolyzed by CB are fibronectin, laminin, and collagen IV. As well as degrading certain ECM proteins, CB may indirectly contribute to metastasis by activating the precursor form of uPA (6).

CB As a Prognostic Marker

Although not as widely investigated as uPA, high levels of CB have been found to correlate with aggressive disease in multiple types of malignancies, including cancer of the breast (24–27), colorectum (28), and lung (29). All of these studies are retrospective and with one exception, contain relatively low numbers of patients. In the only large study (n = 1500 patients), CB was shown to be an independent prognostic marker for both relapse-free and overall survival in patients with breast cancer (25). As a predictor of outcome in breast cancer, CB however, is not as strong a prognostic factor as uPA (26).

Assay of CB

The early assays for measuring CB activity used chromogenic substrates containing the Arg-Arg sequence (30). The most frequently used leaving groups were 2-naphthylamide and 7-amino-4-methylcoumarin. Because CB has an acidic optimum pH, assays were carried out at pH 6.0. These catalytic activity assays lacked specificity and furthermore are likely to have been subjected to interference by endogenous inhibitors (e.g., cystatins and stefins). More recently, commercially available ELISAs have been described for CB (24,25). These ELISAs seem to give different absolute values for CB and to date, no comparison has been made between them. A number of different antibodies have been utilized for the immunohistochemical detection of the cathepsin (27,28) but none appear to have been subjected to detailed evaluation.

CATHEPSIN D (CD)
Structure and Function

Cathepsin D (CD), like CB, is also a lysosomal protease with an acidic optimum pH (31,32). However, unlike CB, CD belongs to the aspartyl group of proteases. CD, as produced by breast cancer cells in vitro, can exist in multiple molecular weight forms. It is initially synthesized as a 52 kD, a protein. This precursor protein is transported to lysosomes where it is processed to an intermediate 48 kDa protein. The 48 kDa form is later converted into mature forms with molecular weights of 34000 and 14000 (31,32). CD processing appears to be slower in cancer cells than in normal cells (31). As a result, cancer cells accumulate greater proportions of the 52 and 48 kDa forms than do non-malignant cells (31).

CD can potentially promote metastasis by several different mechanisms. These include direct degradation of the ECM, indirect dissolution of the ECM, via activation of proCB or degradation of cystatins, liberation of growth factors such as FGF2 from the ECM or inactivation of growth inhibitors, e.g., IGF-binding protein 3 (31). It is unclear which of these mechanisms predominate in cancer dissemination.

CD As a Prognostic Marker

Almost all the published data relating to the prognostic value for CD has focussed on breast cancer. Two main types of assays have been used to measure CD, i.e., quantitative immunoassay such as immunoradiometric assay (IRMA) and immunohistochemistry. With a specific commercially available IRMA (Cis Bio International, Gif-sur-Yvette, France), almost all investigators found a significant correlation between high levels of CD and poor prognosis (31,32). In a large study containing approximately 3000 patients, CD was found to be an independent prognostic factor in the total population as well as in the node-negative patients (33).

Recently, the prognostic impact of CD was confirmed in a meta-analysis of 11 published studies containing 2690 patients (34). In this meta-analysis, high levels of CD also predicted an adverse outcome in patients free of nodal metastasis.

In contrast to the IRMA, the application of immunohistochemistry to detect CD has led to conflicting results regarding the prognostic value of CD (31,32). Although some investigators reported a significant association between immunohistochemically determined CD and a poor outcome, others found no relationship. Possible reasons for the conflicting data include differences in the specificity of the antibodies used, different scoring systems to quantify CD staining levels, different cut-off points for discriminating high from low values, and different types of tissue, i.e., fresh versus formalin-fixed and paraffin-embedded (31,32).

Assay of CD

As mentioned above, the majority of studies that showed a correlation between high levels of CD and aggressive disease have used a specific commercially available IRMA. This assay, which detects total CD including proCD, the intermediate form (48 kDa) and mature forms (34 kDa and 14 kDa) can be carried out on the same cytosols that are used to detect steroid hormone receptors. The analytical performance of this assay has been evaluated in both internal quality control and external quality assurance programs (35,36). In these studies, the between-assay variation ranged from 4.6–13.6%, while the between-laboratory variation was always < 24%.

Other assays that have been used to assay CD include activity assays, Western blotting, and immunohistochemistry. None of these methodologies have been optimized or subjected to detailed investigations. Further work is particularly required to ascertain the reasons for the conflicting results with immunohistochemistry.

MATRIX METALLOPROTEASES

Structure and Function

Currently, more than 20 different MMPs have been described in mammalian systems (Table 3). The main characteristics of these proteases follow:

- All MMPs possess specific domains that are conserved between different members.
- Catalytic activity depends on the presence of zinc ions at the catalytic active site.
- Most are synthesized and secreted in a zymogen form.
- Activation is usually accompanied by loss of a 10 kDa amino terminal domain.
- Most cleave at least one component of the ECM.
- Proteolytic activity is inhibited by tissue inhibitors known as TIMPs (37,38).

Based on in vitro substrate specificity and domain structure, the MMPs have traditionally been divided into 4 main subgroups, i.e., the interstitial collagenases, gelatinases, stromelysins, and membrane MMPs (37,38). The collagenases comprise interstitial collagenase (MMP-1), neutrophil collagenase (MMP-8), and collagenase 3 (MMP-13). These MMPs catalyze degradation of fibrillar forms of collagen, i.e., types I, II, and III. MMP-1 shows a preference for the type III form, MMP-8 preferentially degrades type I collagen, while MMP-13 has highest affinity for type II collagen.

The gelatinases, which are also known as type IV collagenases, degrade gelatin (denatured collagen) and types IV, V, VII, IX and X collagen. Type IV collagen is particularly abundant in basement membranes. Degradation of type IV collagen by the gelatinases occurs within the triple helical regions. This subgroup has two distinct members, known as gelatinase A (MMP-2) and gelatinase B (MMP-9). Generally, these two gelatinases are thought to have similar substrate specificity with respect to ECM substrates, but they may have different specificity toward growth factor receptors (38).

The third subgroup of the MMPs are the stromelysins, i.e., stromelysin 1 (MMP-3), stromelysin 2 (MMP-10), stromelysin 3 (MMP-11 or ST-3), and matrilysin (MMP-7). MMP-3, -7, and -10 have relatively broad substrate specificity, catalyzing the degradation of many different ECM substrates. The substrates include proteoglycans (core protein), non-collagenous proteins such as laminin, fibronectin, and the non-helical regions of collagen IV. ST-3, on the other hand, has not yet been found to degrade any matrix protein, but has been shown to hydrolyze the serine proteinase inhibitor, α1-proteinase inhibitor (37).

The fourth subgroup consists of the membrane-type or MT-MMPs, as these proteinases possess a transmembrane domain. Five members of this group have been described, the best-characterized species being MT1-MMP. This MMP has been shown to catalyze activation of progelatinase A and to degrade a variety of ECM substrates.

While at least 20 different MMPs have been described to date, only some appear to be directly involved in cancer invasion and metastasis. The latter include the two gelatinases (MMP-2, MMP-9) (37,38). Other MMPs, such as ST-1 and ST-3, may play a role in either cancer initiation or the early steps of cancer progression (37,38).

Prognostic Value of MMPs

Most of the work relating MMPs to prognosis has been carried out with gastrointestinal cancers. Thus, high levels of MMP-2, MMP-9, and MT-MMP-1 have all been shown to predict adverse outcome in patients with gastric cancers (37) while high concentrations of both MMP-1 and MMP-9 were related to poor prognosis in colorectal cancer (37). These studies contained relatively low numbers of patients, were retrospective in design, and did not use validated assays. Paradoxically high levels of 2 of the MMP inhibitors, i.e., TIMP-1 and TIMP-2, have also been shown to correlate with poor prognosis, at least in breast cancer (39,40).

Assay of MMPs

The most commonly used method for detecting MMPs is gelatin zymography, which measures MMP-2 and MMP-9 activities (41). This technique involves polyacrylamide gel electrophoresis in the presence of SDS. Following electrophoresis, the SDS is

Table 3 List of matrix metalloproteinases (MMPs) and their main substrates

MMP	Other Name	Preferred Substrate
MMP-1	interstitial collagenase	fibrillar collagen
MMP-2	gelatinase A	gelatin, collagen IV
MMP-3	stromelysin-1	proteoglycans, collagen IV
MMP-7	matrilysin	proteoglycan, collagen IV
MMP-8	neutrophil collegenase	fibrillar collagen
MMP-9	gelatinase B	gelatin, collagen IV
MMP-10	stromelysin-2	pnoteoglycan, collagen IV
MMP-11	stromelysin-3	No ECM substrate identified
MMP-12	metalloelastase	elastin
MMP-13	collagenase-3	fibrillar collagen
MMP-14	membrane-type MMP-1	proMMP-2, fibrillar collagen
MMP-15	membrane-type MMP-2	?
MMP-16	membrane-type MMP-3	proMMP-2
MMP-17	membrane-type MMP-4	?

removed. This results in refolding the MMPs (at least partially), which then digests gelatin at the location of the separated MMP. Although this technique is tedious, it has the advantage of being able to differentiate between the precursor and active forms of these MMPs. Gelatin zymography however, is of little use for the measurement of MMPs other than MMP-2 and MMP-9 as these other MMPs lack hydrolytic activity against this substrate.

In recent years antibodies specific for different MMPs have been described and are being utilized in both ELISA and immunohistochemistry. Commercial kits are available for the detection of some MMPs by ELISA but these assays have not been validated for use in tissue extracts.

SUMMARY

As matrix-degrading proteases are causally involved in cancer dissemination, they should be good candidates for evaluation as prognostic factors in this disease. As discussed above, there is now substantial evidence associating high levels of these proteases with adverse outcome in multiple types of cancer. The protease investigated in greatest detail is uPA (in breast cancer). At least 20 independent groups have now confirmed the prognostic value of this protease in breast cancer and these findings have also been validated in two different types of Level 1 Evidence Studies. In addition, specific assays for uPA have been evaluated in External Quality Assurance Studies and shown to perform satisfactorily. uPA should thus be now ready for routine clinical use. As a cancer marker, its main value is likely to be in selecting the subgroups of node-negative breast cancer that are unlikely to benefit from adjuvant chemotherapy. Paradoxically, high levels of the uPA inhibitor, PAI-1, also predict an adverse outcome in patients with breast cancer and, as with uPA, the prognostic value of the inhibitor has also been confirmed in Level 1 Evidence Studies. With a widely used quantitative immunoassay, CD also appears to be a strong and independent prognostic marker in breast cancer.

However, as mentioned above, use of immunohistochemistry to detect CD has produced conflicting findings. Further work is necessary to confirm the preliminary findings currently available for CB and MMPs. In addition to being prognostic, proteases may also be predictive. MMP inhibitors are currently undergoing trials as anti-invasive, anti-metastatic, and anti-angiogenic agents. Inhibitors of uPA and specific cathepsins are likely in the future to be used as anti-cancer therapies. The patients most likely to respond to these treatments should be those whose tumors contain high levels of the target protease.

A number of other proteases and inhibitors, not within the scope of this chapter, are described elsewhere in this book (see Chapters 39, 40, 41, and 46).

REFERENCES

1. Elston CW, Ellis IO. Pinder SE. Pathological prognostic factors in breast cancer. Crit Rev Oncol Hematol 1999;31:209–223.
2. Zetter B. Angiogenesis and tumor metastasis. Ann Rev Med 1998;49:407–414.
3. Duffy MJ. The role of proteolytic enzymes in cancer invasion and metastasis. Clin Exp Met 1992;10:145–155.
4. Duffy MJ. The biochemistry of metastasis. Adv Clin Chem 1996;32:135–166.
5. Duffy MJ. Do proteases play a role in cancer invasion and metastasis? Eur J Cancer Clin Oncol 1987;23:583–589.
6. Andreasen PA, Kjoller L, Christiansen L, Duffy MJ. The urokinase-type plasminogen activation system in cancer metastasis. Int J Cancer 1997;72:1–22.
7. List K, Jensen ON, Bugge TH, Lund LR, Plough M, Dano K et al. Plasminogen-independent initiation of the prourokinase activation cascade in vivo. Activation of prourokinase by glandular kallikrein (mGK–6) in plasminogen-deficient mice. Biochemistry 2000;39:508–515.
8. Rifkin DB. Cross-talk among proteases and matrix in the control of growth factor action. Fibrinol Proteolysis 1997;11:3–9.
9. Kwaan HC, Wang J, Svoboda K, Declerck PJ. Plasminogen activator inhibitor 1 may promote tumor growth through inhibition of apoptosis. Br J Cancer 2000;82:1702–1708.
10. Kumar S, Baglioni C. Protection from tumor necrosis factor-mediated cytolysis by overexpression of plasminogen activator inhibitor type-2. J Biol Chem 1991;266:20960–20964.
11. Duffy MJ, O'Grady P, Devaney D, O'Siorain L, Fennelly JJ, Lijnen RJ. Urokinase-plasminogen activator, a marker for aggressive breast cancer. Preliminary report. Cancer 1988;62:531–533.
12. Duffy MJ, Maguire T, McDermott EW, O'Higgins N. rokinase plasminogen activator: a prognostic marker in multiple types of cancer. J Surg Oncol 1999;71;130–135.
13. Hayes D, Bast RC, Desch CE, Fritsche H, Kemeny NE, Jessup JM, et al. Tumor marker utility grading system (TMUGS): a framework to evaluate clinical utility of tumor markers. J Natl Cancer Inst 1996;88:1456–1466.
14. Janicke F, Prechtl A, Thomssen C, Harbeck N, Meisner C, Sweep F, et al. For the German Chemo N_0 Study Group. Randomized adjuvant chemotherapy trial in node-negative breast cancer patients identified by urokinase-type plasminogen activator and plasminogen activator inhibitor type 1. J Natl Cancer Inst 2001;93:913–920.
15. Harbeck N, Look M P, Ulm K, Duffy MJ on behalf of the Pooled Analysis Study of the EORTC Receptor and Biomarker Group (RBG). Proceedings of the ASCO Annual Meeting, 2001;20:Abstract 1646.
16. Skelly M, Troy A, Duffy MJ, Mulcahy H, Duggan C, Connell T, et al. Urokinase-type plasminogen activator in colorectal cancer: relationship with clinicopathological features and patient outcome. Clin Cancer Res 1997;3:1837–1840.
17. Mulcahy H, Duffy MJ, Gibbons D, McCarthy P, Parfrey N, O'-Donoghue D, et al. Urokinase-type plasminogen activator and outcome in Duke's B colorectal cancer. Lancet 1994;344:583–584.
18. Benraad TH, Geurts-Moespot J, Grondahl-Hansen J, Schmitt M, Heuvel J, De Witte JH, et al. Immunoassays (ELISA) of urokinase-type plasminogen activator (uPA): report of an EORTC/BIOMED-1 Workshop. Eur J Cancer 1996;32:1371–1381.
19. Sweep CGJ, Geurts-Moespot J, Grebenschikov N, De Witt JH, Heuvel J, Schmitt M, et al. External quality assessment of trans-European multi-center antigen determination (enzyme-linked immunosorbent assay) of urokinase plasminogen activator (uPA) and its type-1 inhibitor (PAI-1) in human breast cancer extracts. Br J Cancer 1998;78:1434-1441.
20. Janicke F, Pache L, Schmitt M, Ulm K, Thomssen C, Prechtl A, et al. Both cytosols and detergent extracts of breast cancer tissue s are suitable to evaluate the prognostic impact of urokinase-type

plasminogen activator and its inhibitor, plasminogen activator inhibitor type 1. Cancer Res 1994;54:2527–2530.
21. Umeda T, Eguchi Y, Okino K, et al. Cellular localization of urokinase-type plasminogen activator, its inhibitors and their mRNA in breast cancer tissue. J Pathol 1997; 183:388–397.
22. Dublin E, Hanby A, Patel NK, Liebman R, Barnes D. Immunohistochemical expression of uPA, uPAR, and PAI–1 in breast carcinoma. Am J Pathol 2000;157:1219–1227.
23. Koblinski JE, Ahram M, Sloane BF. Unraveling the role of proteases in cancer. Clin Chim Acta 2000;291:113–135.
24. Thomssen C, Schmitt M, Goretzki L, Oppelt P, Pache L, Dettmar P, et al. Prognostic value of cysteine proteases cathepsin B and cathepsin L in human breast cancer. Clin Cancer Res 1995;1:741–746.
25. Foekens JA, Kos J, Peters HA, Krasovec M, Look MP, Cimerman N, et al.
Prognostic significance of cathepsin B and L in primary human breast cancer. J Clin Oncol 1998;16:1013–1021.
26. Maguire TM, Shering SG, Duggan C, McDermott E, O'Higgins NJ, Duffy MJ. High levels of cathepsin B predict poor outcome in patients with breast cancer. Int J Biol Markers 1998;13:139–144.
27. Lah T, Cercek M, Blejec A, Kos J, Gorodetsky E, Somers R, et al. Cathepsin B, a prognostic indicator in lymph node-negative breast carcinoma patients: comparison with cathepsin D, cathepsin L, and other clinical indicators. Clin Cancer Res 2000;6:578–584.
28. Campo E, Munoz J, Miquel R, Palacin A, Cardesa A, Sloane BF, et al. Cathepsin D expression in colorectal carcinomas correlate with tumor progression and shortened survival. Am J Path 1994;145:301–309.
29. Sukoh N, Abe S, Ogura S, Isobe H, Takekawa H, Inoue K, et al. Immunohistochemical study of cathepsin B, prognostic significance in human lung cancer. Cancer 1994;74:46–51.
30. Barrett AJ, Kirschke H. Cathepsin B, cathepsin H, and cathepsin L. Methods Enzymol 1981;80:535–561.
31. Rochefort H. Cathepsin D in breast cancer: a tissue marker associated with metastasis. Eur J Cancer 1992;28A:1780–1783.
32. Westley B, May FEB. Cathepsin D and breast cancer. Eur J Cancer 1996;32A:15–24.
33. Foekens JA, Look M, Bolt-de Vries Meijer-van Gelder ME, van Putten WLJ, Klijn JGM. Cathepsin-D in primary breast cancer: prognostic evaluation involving 2810 patients. Br J Cancer 1999;79:300–307.
34. Ferrandina G, Scambia G, Bardell F, Benedetti P, Mancuso S, Messori A. Relationship between cathepsin-D content and disease-free survival in node-negative breast cancer patients: a meta-analysis. Br J Cancer 1997;76:661–666.
35. Benraad TJ, Geurts-Moespot A, Sala M, Pigganelli A, Ross A, Foekens J. Quality control of cathepsin D measurements by the EORTC Receptor Study Group. Eur J Cancer 1992;28:72–75.
36. Shaheen RM, Miseljic S, Wiehle RD, Wittliff JL. Relationship between cathepsin D expression and other prognostic factors in breast carcinomas. Clin Chem 1995;41:1585–1591.
37. Duffy MJ, McCarthy K. Matrix metalloproteinases in cancer: prognostic markers and targets for therapy. Int J Oncol 1998;12:1343–1348.
38. Nelson AR, Fingleton B, Rothenberg ML, Matrisian LM. Matrix metalloproteinases: biological and clinical implications. J Clin Oncol 2000;18:1135–1149.
39. McCarthy K, Maguire T, McGrael G, McDermott E, O'Higgins N, Duffy MJ. High levels of tissue inhibitor of metalloproteinase-1 predicts poor outcome in patients with breast cancer. Int J Cancer. 1999;84:44–48.
40. Remackle A, McCarthy K, Noel A, Maguire T, McDermott E, O'Higgins N, et al. High levels of TIMP-2 correlate with adverse prognosis in breast cancer. Int J Cancer 2000;89: 118–121.
41. Woessner J. Quantification of matrix metalloproteinases in tissue samples. Methods Enzymol 1995;248:510–528.

Chapter **9**

Circulating Cancer Cells and Cell-Free Nucleic Acids as Tumor Markers

Markus Müller, Hans Krause, and Carsten Goessl

In 1869, Wilhelm Waldeyer postulated the currently accepted concept that malignant tumors arise from epithelial cells which have undergone neoplastic change, and that these can metastasize through both the blood and the lymphatic system (1). Circulating tumor cells (CTC) were first identified in animal studies and recognized as an early step in the process of tumor cell invasion (2). Recent data (3) have confirmed that about 0.01% of CTC are capable of initiating metastasis. CTC in peripheral blood is an early process in the cascade of events that lead to metastasis. CTC may remain dormant for variable periods of time or grow into clinically detectable metastases.

Ashworth identified, in 1869, cells derived post-mortem from the blood of a cancer patient that appeared to be identical to those of the primary tumor (4). About a century later, investigators used light microscopy to analyze circulating tumor cells obtained from patients with various forms of malignancies to see if they could be used as tumor markers (5). Depending on the type of tumor and stage, immunomagnetic separation techniques have produced detection rates ranging from < 10% in colorectal carcinoma (6) to 32% in renal cell carcinoma (7). Reports in the literature state that the number of CTC in peripheral blood range from 1 to nearly 1,000 cells per milliliter of whole blood (6,7). Despite immunocytologic detection techniques, sensitivity and specificity of the methods remain inadequate (8), and light microscopic determination of CTC could not establish itself as a standard modality in tumor detection.

Since the late 1980s, it has been possible to detect circulating tumor cells in blood and in bone marrow micrometastases in oncologic patients using methods based on polymerase chain reaction (PCR) (9,10). However, because of the invasive nature of obtaining biopsy material, the detection and prognostic importance of micrometastases in the bone marrow (11) will not be addressed in this chapter.

In most cases, the molecular detection of tumor cells utilizes mRNA, using the reverse transcriptase polymerase chain reaction (RT-PCR). It is assumed that benign epithelial cells do not appear in whole blood and that any transcripts of epithelial origin identified are surrogates indicating the existence of CTC in the blood. The suitability of this technique as a tumor marker in the initial work-up and prognosis of various malignancies has undergone intense scrutiny (8,12), most recently in regard to quantitative aspects (13,14) and to its efficacy in detecting recurrent disease as part of the follow-up of treated patients (15).

Beginning in the early 1990s, cell-free tumor DNA (16,17), cell-free viral DNA (18), and cell-free circulating tumor RNA (19) have been studied both qualitatively and quantitatively in oncologic patients (18). The data concerning cell-free circulating tumor mRNA are limited (19,20) and, for malignant melanoma at least, the detection of cell-free circulating tumor mRNA is less reliable than the detection of CTC (21).

The present chapter is restricted to discussing molecular detection techniques for CTC and circulating cell-free DNA in patients who have solid tumors. The chapter describes potential applications as a nucleic acid-based tumor marker (22). For more discussion on cell-free nucleic acid analysis in cancer patients, please see Chapter 51.

DETECTION OF CIRCULATING TUMOR CELLS (CTC): METHODICAL CONSIDERATIONS

Historically, the first attempts to detect CTC involved cytological approaches that used light microscopy. However, investigators soon realized that these techniques showed limited sensitivity and were associated with a high rate of false-positive results.

Immunocytochemical analyses of peripheral blood smears taken from cancer patients have also been used to identify CTC. This approach, too, has poor sensitivity, due to the loss of antigen expression in poorly differentiated tumors, as well as the reported presence of cytokeratin and epithelial membrane antigen in non-epithelial cells (12).

Continuous developments in flow cytometry, magnetic activated cell sorting (MACS), and immunomagnetic methods in combination with the continued arrival of new antibodies recognizing epithelial type, cell type (PSA), or tumor type (erb-B2) specific antigens will challenge the role of the nucleic acid based detection of CTC, which is the main focus of this chapter.

The major strategy for detecting occult tumor cells is to detect either tumor or organ/tissue-specific alterations in the DNA or mRNA of these cells (Figure 1). Tumor-specific

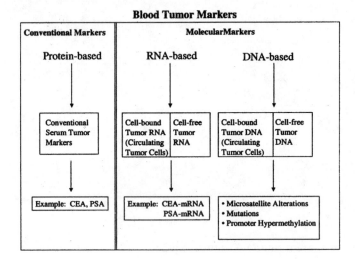

Figure 1 Conventional and nucleic-acid-based tumor markers.

translocations, for example, can be detected at the DNA level using primers that hybridize to the regions flanking the translocation (9) and will therefore amplify the expected PCR fragment only when the translocation is present.

Hybrid mRNAs may similarly be detected by RT-PCR. Most solid tumors of non-hematopoietic origin do not display such specific alterations. Therefore, the basis of tissue-specific CTC detection rests in the ability of malignant cells to continue to express markers of the tissue from which the tumor originated. Consequently, the mere detection of transcripts of such cells in areas of the body distant from the tissue of origin implies tumor spread. A good example for "illegitimate" organ/tissue-specific expression at unusual sites is the detection of prostate-specific antigen (PSA) transcripts in lymph nodes or bone marrow (23,24).

The reverse transcriptase polymerase chain reaction (RT-PCR) is the most widely used method for detecting CTC, due to its ultra-high sensitivity when applied on the basis of optimized protocols. In addition, RNA is highly unstable outside cells—therefore its detection by RT-PCR clearly indicates the presence of intact cells in the tissue examined. Some groups report the detection of one malignant cell among up to 10^7 normal cells (25).

However, RT-PCR-based tests have yet to become routine. Compared to the above-mentioned immunological techniques, they require laborious optimization for each of the isolation, enrichment, and detection steps involved, as well as the inclusion of many sample and assay controls for each experiment performed (Figure 2). This is one of the main reasons that results obtained from different laboratories show such wide disparity. A recent report of the EORTC Melanoma Group described the most common causes of disparities, highlighted the pitfalls, and advised a streamlined protocol for this particular tumor entity (26). In addition, PCR-based methods require a specifically designed workspace and special precautions to avoid carry-over contaminations.

Despite these obstacles, the high sensitivity of PCR-based methodology and its application to body fluids that are easy to get from cancer patients will be the preferred option for detecting minimal residual disease. An overview of older and currently applied variations of RT-PCR detection methods is given in Figure 3. Improvements in instrumentation and automatic sample handling, particularly the introduction of real-time PCR with its potential for streamlined quantification, warrants hopes for better standardization and inter-laboratory data comparison.

CTC detection by RT-PCR involves several steps (see discussion, below). Peripheral blood samples are also specifically discussed; however, the basic technology can be adapted to bone marrow, lymph nodes, and surgical margins.

SAMPLE COLLECTION

Peripheral blood samples can be collected using heparin or EDTA as anticoagulant agents. Many groups, including ours, prefer EDTA, since heparin is known to inhibit Taq polymerase. Reports of the volume of blood obtained vary; 3–5 mL is the minimum amount. Berteau et al. (27) extensively studied the influence of blood storage and sample processing on the detection of CTC by RT-PCR. They demonstrated an important loss in RNA recovery within six hours when samples are stored at room temperature. Results will stay stable for at least six days when samples are immediately stored at 4 °C.

ISOLATION OF NUCLEATED CELLS

Although few, if any, systematic reports exist, most researchers agree that the method of obtaining nucleated cells (or their nucleic acids directly) from the remaining blood is the limiting step in the whole procedure of RT-PCR-based detection of CTC (28). If CTC are lost or if RNA is degraded due to inadequate handling within this step, the sensitivity of the entire assay will be reduced, despite optimized performance in subsequent steps.

Some researchers avoid particular isolation steps and opt for *direct RNA isolation* using commercially available kits mainly based on hypotonic lysis and removal of erythrocytes. Reported decreases in test sensitivity are probably due to adhesion of hemoglobin to nucleic acids, and to partial inhibition of Taq polymerase. *Density gradient centrifugation* of blood samples and subsequent careful transfer of PBS-washed nucleated cells to immediate RNA isolation seems to be the most efficient procedure for isolating CTC. There are several gradient media available and it is advisable to perform reconstruction experiments with metabolically labeled tumor cells (appropriate cell lines) spiked into blood samples to calculate the percentage of recovery after the centrifugation step.

RNA ISOLATION

Many quick and easy-to-handle reagents exist for the isolation of total RNA. Most protocols are derivatives of the guanidinium-isothiocyanate-phenol-chloroform isolation method first described by Chomczynski and Sacchi (29). Depending on the skill of laboratory personnel, RNA preparations obtained by these techniques may be affected by a certain degree of DNA contamination. In our experience, using commercially available

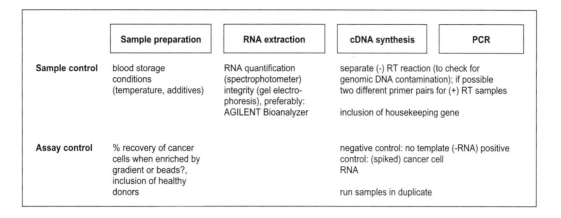

Figure 2 Recommended controls for RT-PCR-based detection of circulating tumor cells. Adapted from Eur J Cancer, 34 Suppl 3, Keilholz U, New prognostic factors in melanoma: mRNA tumor markers, S37–S41, 1998, with permission from Elsevier Science.

kits based on ion exchange columns, including DNase-treatment, resulted in superior RNA quality although smaller amounts of RNA were recovered. Most laboratories agree that the use of purified mRNA improves cDNA synthesis in comparison to total RNA preparations. Including this additional step, however, complicates the whole procedure and may be avoided if possible. Accompanying quality (absence of degradation, presence of shorter RNAs, agarose gel electrophoresis), quantity, and purity (spectrophotometry) controls are prerequisites for every RNA sample. Capillary gel electrophoresis instruments are available. These instruments conveniently combine various above-mentioned controls and use minimal amounts (1 µl) of sample (AGILENT Bioanalyzer).

cDNA SYNTHESIS

Target mRNA, whose expression is restricted to particular organs or tissues or, better yet, to certain tumor specimens, must be converted into DNA to be accessible to PCR amplification. Although one-step RT-PCR kits are available from certain manufacturers, the majority of published protocols use separate reactions for cDNA synthesis and PCR amplification. The major advantage of this two-step protocol is the generation of surplus cDNA, which is suitable for additional assays. cDNA synthesis using gene-specific primers (gsp) is very efficient, but it prevents additional cDNA testing with primer pairs for other specifically expressed genes. Conversely, random hexam-

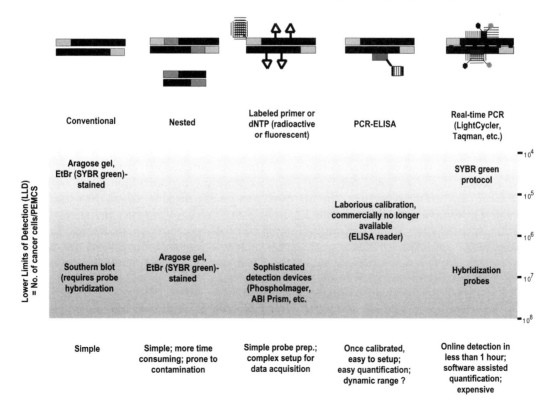

Figure 3 Schematic overview of currently used variations of RT-PCR for the detection of circulating tumor cells.

er- or oligo d(T)-primed cDNA synthesis converts all present mRNAs into single-stranded cDNA. Depending on the enzyme used, cDNA lengths in excess of 1000 bases can be readily achieved, although they are not mandatory for most primer combinations during PCR (see below). Reverse transcriptases specifically engineered for synthesis of longer cDNA products require additional RNaseH treatment. When using oligo d(T) priming for cDNA synthesis, one should avoid placing PCR primers into the very 5′ end of the gene, since synthesis starts at the opposite 3′ end—and amplification may fail, due to insufficient cDNA length. Commercially available cDNA synthesis kits provide suitable (in-vitro transcribed) RNA for assay validation (see also reference 5).

Three interdependent parameters are of critical importance for the outcome (i.e., "positivity" or threshold) of the assay and comparability to results obtained by other groups: the amount of blood processed, the volume used to re-suspend the RNA, and the amount of RNA used for cDNA synthesis. These findings, combined with data obtained from reconstruction experiments (see above), will give a rough estimate of the "lower limit of detection" (LLD) for the assay in question. Since the expression level of a particular gene in the spiked cells and the CTC cells are not accurately known, these estimates may still vary in orders of magnitude. Most protocols use 1 μg of total RNA for cDNA synthesis.

PCR-BASED AMPLIFICATION OF cDNA

Successful detection of CTC is certainly influenced by the choice of PCR parameters and, in particular, by the choice of primers. With regard to desired inter-laboratory comparability of results and standardization, one should seriously consider the use of previously published primer pairs. Adhering to this (simple) proposal, however, may prove difficult, as is implied by the more than 20 published primer combinations for prostate-specific antigen (PSA) alone (30).

Primers should usually span an intron-exon boundary to prevent (or at least to detect) amplification from contaminating DNA. However, unwanted amplification of pseudogenes, derived from illegitimate reverse transcription, cannot be circumvented by primer selection alone. Using RNA preparations directly in PCR amplification ("– RT reaction") can easily unmask DNA contamination and, if known for the gene in question, pseudogenes. Most protocols also use internal control primer sets for ubiquitous expressed genes known to show little or no expression variation. For many commonly used "housekeeping" genes (β-actin, GAPDH, etc.) expression variation and pseudogenes have been described. Our favorites include 18S rRNA and porphyrobilinogen deaminase (PBGD); they are used by leading manufacturers of commercially available kits. Failure to amplify housekeeping genes points to more profound errors during the assay (e.g., massive RNA degradation, pipetting errors, etc.). To check the integrity of the assay itself, a negative assay control (water instead of cDNA) as well as positive controls (e.g., cDNA from spiking experiments and the control RNA provided with the cDNA synthesis kit) should also be included in PCR amplification reactions.

Setting up successful PCR reactions for detection of CTC follows the general rules for optimizing PCR conditions (primer design, product length, magnesium concentration, cycle number, duration of each cycle, etc.) and is outside the scope of this chapter. Needless to say, the pipetting order of the various reagents also influences the outcome of a particular assay. Putting the water control at the very beginning does not make sense for unmasking "carry-overs." The use of "master mixes" is highly recommended to reduce interassay variation, and all probes should be analyzed in at least two independent assays.

Specific PCR product detection methods (see below), especially those based on real-time PCR equipment, require the addition of further reagents. For example, detection of PCR products by the hybridization probe protocol on the LightCycler instrument, or using TaqMan technology, requires additional primer(s), whose location on the target needs to be optimized by appropriate software provided by the vendor. Insist on high-purity reagents.

DETECTION OF PCR-AMPLIFIED PRODUCTS

Figure 2 summarizes the various techniques for sensitive detection of RT-PCR products. Basically, they can be divided into two groups: those that still need gel separation for the final detection, and those using special instruments for the "readout." Among the more common improvements for the detection of tiny amounts of PCR product is the use of SYBR Green instead of ethidium bromide in gel stainings. Radioactive detection methods (either by incorporation of labeling into the PCR reaction or Southern blotting of the probes in question) are also commonly used techniques but are not always available (and recommended) for routine clinical practice. Before the introduction of real-time PCR equipment in our laboratory, we used fluorescence-labeled primers in combination with GeneScan analysis software on an ABI 377 automatic sequencer for semi-quantitative detection of PCR products. Many laboratories have opted for nested PCR. In this case, take additional measures to prevent carry-over contamination.

The future of RT-PCR-based detection of CTC will lie in automated real-time PCR (for which there are several instruments on the market). Despite the ability to accurately quantify the amount of a target and assess user-friendliness, these instruments cannot estimate the actual number of tumor cells present in a sample, because the transcription rate (i.e., the actual amount of target mRNA) varies between individual samples.

INTERNAL STANDARDS

The advent of automated real-time PCR made the use of internal standards (IS) customary. Commercially available kits usually provide in-vitro transcribed RNA in fixed copy numbers made from cloned genes. Software provided with the instrument allows easy preparation of internal or external calibration curves for quantification purposes. To be an "ideal" IS, the products of the target sequence and the IS should be of similar size, although not of the same length (e.g., a difference of 20 bp). They should also share the same sequence, so that they can be co-amplified with the same primers. Figure 4 outlines the generation of a recombinant RNA standard that fulfills the above-mentioned criteria and can be easily cloned into run-off transcription vectors.

TUMORS: GENERAL OBSERVATIONS

Epithelial tumors are the most frequently encountered type of cancer and, therefore, responsible for the majority of cancer-related deaths. Mortality in patients with malignant disease depends primarily on the extent of the disease at the time of initial diagnosis. Localized malignancies confined to certain organs may be amenable to curative surgical treatment. In certain patients, currently available conventional diagnostic imaging techniques such as ultrasound, computed tomography (CT), magnetic resonance imaging (MRI), or bone scanning may return findings negative for advanced disease spread; because of disseminated tumor cells, however, these patients may experience early disease recurrence. These disseminated tumor cells, which evade detection with conventional methods, characterize minimal residual disease (MRD).

The molecular detection of CTC offers new perspectives in the search for these occult tumor cells. Two points are of particular interest in quantifying their clinical importance and application to routine clinical practice.

First, it must be demonstrated that the subsequent clinical course in patients with confirmed CTC actually leads to recurrent malignant disease, which would support their prognostic relevance. Second, adjuvant therapeutic methods, such as chemotherapy or hormone therapy, must be available for the malignancy in question, facilitating early treatment with possible prevention of tumor recurrence.

In recent years, a large number of epithelial tumors have been studied for occult tumor cells using various molecular targets. The molecular targets used should be tumor specific or, at least, organ specific. The results of these investigations, of course, depend directly on the quality of the detection techniques and the sensitivity and specificity of the molecular target itself. Recently, PCR technology for detection of mRNA using RT-PCR has established itself as a sort of quasi-standard. Samples for RT-PCR can be derived from blood, bone marrow, or lymph nodes. Because of its non-invasive nature, the use of blood samples is of particular interest. Targets for the tumors most frequently studied to date are given in Table 1.

PROSTATE CANCER

Carcinoma of the prostate is the most common urologic tumor. In Western industrial societies, carcinoma of the prostate ranks high among the leading causes of cancer-related mortality. Peak age is between the seventh and eighth decades). Epidemiological data indicate an increase in deaths related to prostate carcinoma due to generally increased life expectancies.

The diagnosis of carcinoma of the prostate is usually made on the basis of digital rectal examination (DRE) and serum levels of the tumor marker prostate-specific antigen (PSA). Depending on the exact constellation of findings, the positive predictive value ranges up to 70% (32). Diagnosis is confirmed by transrectal biopsy of tissue taken from the prostate. Current practice includes six to ten systematic, ultrasound-guided transrectal punch biopsies. Prostatic carcinoma shows quite variable biologic growth patterns. At present, the only generally accepted prognostic factors are the tumor stage and degree of differentiation (grading and/or Gleason score).

In general, carcinoma of the prostate has a good prognosis provided it is recognized early, i.e., limited to the organ itself. When still confined to the prostate (T2), radical prostatectomy represents the primary curative therapy. An alternative in high-risk patients is radiation treatment. At the time of first diagnosis, however, often disease has already progressed past the prostatic capsule with corresponding worsening of patient prognosis. Unequivocal clinical differentiation between prostatic carcinoma limited to the organ (T2) and carcinoma that has

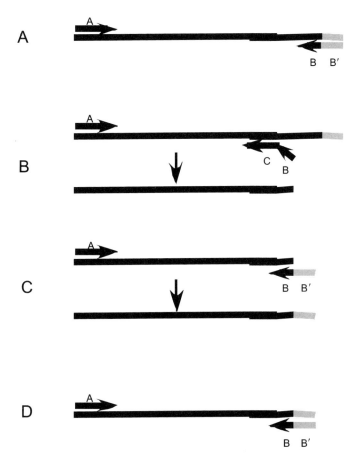

Figure 4 Recommended strategy for generating internal standard RNA from any given mRNA template. Starting from the original mRNA, a PCR fragment is amplified using primer pair A/BB′ (A). In a first re-amplification with primer pair A/CB, a fragment is amplified where sequence B is artificially attached to sequence C (B). Using the original primers (A/BB′) in a second amplification, a shortened fragment is amplified (C) that can be used as template for in vitro transcription of internal standard RNA molecules (D).

Table 1 Important targets for CTC of carcinomas of the breast and prostate and malignant melanoma (mRNA)

Prostate cancer	PSA, prostate-specific antigen
	PSMA, prostate-specific membrane antigen
Breast carcinoma	Cytokeratin 19 mRNA
	CEA, carcinoembryonic antigen
	MUC1
	Human mammaglobin (hMAM)
Melanoma	Tyrosinase
	MART1
	MAGE3
	GAGE

progressed beyond the capsule but remains locally delineated (T3) remains impossible. Evidence of CTC in peripheral blood could provide important data and possibly affect disease management, assuming a correlation between the detection of these CTC and patients' subsequent clinical course. In addition, detection of CTC could provide early evidence of disease recurrence during follow-up. The predominant therapeutic measure in systemic spread of prostatic carcinoma is hormone ablation.

The most useful molecular targets for detecting circulating prostatic carcinoma cells in peripheral blood are the respective mRNA of either prostate-specific antigen (PSA) or prostate-specific membrane antigen (PSMA) using RT-PCR. While neither PSA nor PSMA are completely tumor specific for prostatic carcinoma, they are practically organ specific for detecting cells of prostatic origin.

The first report describing the detection of the mRNA of PSA in peripheral blood using RT-PCR was published in 1994 by Buttyan's group (33). In that study, CTC were detected in 25 of 65 patients (38%) with locally limited prostatic carcinoma and in 14 of 18 patients (78%) with metastatic prostatic carcinoma. Later in the same year, the first report describing the detection of mRNA of PSMA in peripheral blood using nested RT-PCR was published (34). Using PSMA, CTC were identified in 13 of 18 patients (72%) with locally limited disease and in 16 of 24 patients (67%) with metastatic disease. In addition, PSMA detection results were compared to corresponding results for PSA. With PSA, CTC were found in 0 of 18 patients (0%) with locally limited prostatic carcinoma and in six of 24 patients (25%) with metastatic disease.

Both of these early studies showed promising results, pointing to potential new applications. They were, however, inadequate for evaluating the clinical relevance of the method, which would require larger studies examining patients' long-term clinical course. Since these two first publications, there have been a number of corresponding but also contradictory findings. Both the prediction of pathologic tumor stage (33,35–37) and the prognostic relevance of detecting the mRNA of PSA and/or PSMA in peripheral blood using RT-PCR remain controversial (35,38–41). Particularly for PSMA, which is present in both normal and malignant prostatic tissue, though in differing amounts (42), results have been contradictory (43,44).

Based on the available results, routine clinical detection of the mRNA of PSA and/or PSMA in peripheral blood using RT-PCR cannot be recommended. The exact clinical meaning of a "positive" PCR as evidence of CTC in prostatic carcinoma remains unclear. Major problems include the absence of standardization for primers, the wide variation in conditions under which PCR is performed, and the fact that detection of the target markers by PCR has been qualitative or only semi-quantitative. The specificity of non-quantitative RT-PCR of PSA mRNA and PSMA mRNA seems to be especially problematic (44,45).

Recently introduced real-time online PCR techniques, which, for the first time, permit "real" quantification, offer new perspectives. Calculation of cut-off levels is also possible now. The first experiences with their use in the detection of CTC in prostatic carcinoma using mRNA of PSA appear to be very promising, showing a significantly higher number of tumor cells in peripheral blood in patients with advanced tumors in comparison to those with disease limited to the organ or normal subjects (14). Large-scale clinical validation of these methods, however, also remains unavailable so far. Additional information on this subject is provided in Chapter 17.

BREAST CANCER

Carcinoma of the breast is the most common malignant disease affecting women. Its incidence has increased steadily over the past 20 years. Because of the relative improvement in treatment results, however, the associated mortality has not increased to a corresponding degree. Peak incidence lies between the fourth and sixth decades of life.

Tumors of the breast are most commonly discovered by self-examination by the woman herself and/or by mammography. Suspected mammary carcinoma is confirmed by the histologic examination of material obtained at biopsy, sample excision, or from the tumor extirpated in its entirety. Like prostatic carcinoma, carcinoma of the breast is a very heterogeneous tumor entity showing great variation in patients' clinical course. Classical prognostic factors include tumor stage and status of the axillary nodes, in addition to the respective histologic type and hormone receptor status. An elevation in tumor markers CEA and CA 15-3 is found in 20–30% of patients with primary mammary carcinoma and is also considered an unfavorable prognostic factor.

Despite very effective localized treatment measures, including surgery and radiation, minimal residual disease (MRD) in the sense of occult metastasis quite often results in recurrence and distant metastasis of the disease. Micrometastases are probably present in about two-thirds of patients. It is hoped that detection of CTC might result in the earlier recognition of such occult metastases. Systemic therapeutic options include chemotherapy and hormone therapy in those who are suited for that treatment.

The central problem related to the detection of CTC in mammary carcinoma was the lack of known specific molecular targets. The main molecular targets used to date are carcinoembryonic antigen (CEA) and the epithelial markers cytokeratin 19 and MUC 1, none of which is tumor specific or even organ specific. Thus, the conventional, non-quantitative examinations using RT-PCR returned false-positive results in healthy patients in a high percentage of cases, with associated low specificity for the method (46). Poor specificity is particularly problematic for routine clinical applications, because a large number of patients would undergo unnecessary adjuvant therapy.

Improved specificity is promised by the introduction of a quantitative RT-PCR for detection of the mRNA of cytokeratin 19 (47). The use of new real-time online PCR techniques for detecting cytokeratin 19 reduced the proportion of false-positive findings to under 10% in the first published study (48). Large-scale clinical validation, however, is not yet available.

Another possible new marker is the detection of human mammaglobin (hMAM). The hMAM gene, which resides on chromosome 11q12.3-13.1, was first discovered by Watson and Fleming in 1996 (49). As far as is currently known, mammaglobin is specific to the adult mammary gland and is often overexpressed in primary mammary carcinomas (49–51). The first studies investigating the detection of the mRNA of mammaglobin in peripheral blood show very good specificity (52). The improved specificity is particularly striking when compared directly with cytokeratin 19. In this comparison, hMAM was not detected in any sample obtained from the control group, compared with a false-positive rate of 39% for cytokeratin 19 (53).

The detection of CTC in peripheral blood is breaking new ground by determining the activity of the enzyme telomerase. In one early study, there was no detectable telomerase activity in blood samples taken from nine healthy subjects. In samples obtained from 25 women with advanced, stage IV mammary carcinoma, however, telomerase activity was found in 84% of cases (54).

To date, no large-scale clinical validation of any of these methods is available. Thus, the routine clinical application of the detection of CTC in carcinoma of the breast cannot yet be recommended. For more information on this subject, please refer to Chapters 14 and 38.

MALIGNANT MELANOMA

Malignant melanoma (MM) is one of the few epithelial neoplasms with a continuously increasing incidence. The life-time risk of developing the disease currently stands at one in 74 (55). Major risk factors include both endogenous traits, such as skin type and heredity, and exogenous factors such as exposure to ultraviolet light, many of which can be avoided. While MM's chances of cure are excellent in patients undergoing surgery at early disease stages, the prognosis in more advanced cases is extremely poor due both to the high metastatic potential of the tumor (lymph nodes, lung, brain) and to the current lack of adequate chemo- and immunotherapeutic options.

The diagnosis of MM is made on the basis of clinical inspection and pathohistologic confirmation of the findings. When surgery is possible, adequate margins are selected based on the vertical extent of the tumor. Elective lymph node dissection in clinical stage I is being increasingly abandoned, primarily because of side effects such as lymphedema, in favor of sentinel lymphadenectomy using lymphoscintigraphy and/or vital dye techniques (56,57). Lymph node involvement has traditionally been evaluated using histopathologic methods. In this case, molecular diagnosis using RT-PCR for tyrosinase mRNA is superior: more than 50% of negative biopsies at histopathologic examination were found positive by RT-PCR (58). These findings also correlated significantly with the probability of disease recurrence and overall survival. Immunohistochemistry, which, in comparison to conventional histopathologic diagnostics, detects about 12% more involved lymph nodes, is less effective than the molecular detection of lymph node involvement using RT-PCR either for tyrosinase mRNA alone (59) or with further targets such as MAGE-3 and MART-1 (60).

Since no suitable tumor markers exist for MM in routine clinical diagnostics, the usefulness of CTC as tumor markers for MM has been under study, beginning with Smith et al. in 1991 (10). Transcripts of the enzyme tyrosinase, a key enzyme in melanin biosynthesis, were primarily used as a molecular target. Most authors report the absence of false positive findings in controls, which represents a specificity of 100% (61). Sensitivity, which is expressed as the rate of positive RT-PCR findings in patients with confirmed MM, however, varies between reports. Even in the stage of distant metastasis, and despite the use of tyrosinase mRNA as a uniform molecular target, sensitivities between 0% and 100% —0 out of 6 patients (62); 29 out of 29 patients (63)—are reported. Such differences, which cast doubt on the clinical application of the method, may be due to methodological error, pointing to contamination (rates too high) or suboptimal conditions in the isolation of mRNA and the subsequent RT-PCR (rates too low). Another reason for this variability in findings is the possibility that biological phenomena associated with a non-constant release of tumor cells into the blood circulation may be at work (15). A review by Ghossein and Bhattacharya (8) suggests that, in AJCC (American Joint Committee on Cancer) stages I–II (locally confined), the average sensitivity of the method is 24%; in stage III (lymph node involvement), 32%; and in stage IV (metastatic spread), 44%. In a meta-analysis that included 23 corresponding studies, Tsao et al. (61) found a similar correlation between AJCC stage and the rate of positive RT-PCR findings in MM. However, at least with the use of GAGE mRNA as the target, there is a report of absence of stage dependency in the detection of CTC (64).

Several authors have found a statistically significant prognostic value in the detection of CTC in relation to disease-free and overall survival in patients with MM (8,65). With detection of CTC and the associated potentially increased risk of recurrence and metastasis, it was possible to identify melanomas in patients who, even in the absence of evidence of residual tumor, would have been referred for adjuvant therapy. Despite promising experimental findings (66,67), however, there is no adjuvant therapy option with an acceptable effect/side effect ratio. Currently, therefore, the detection of CTC alone is not routinely considered an indication for beginning chemo- or immunotherapy. Long-term follow-up of patients who have locally limited stages of MM (AJCC I-II) and evidence of CTC is necessary for a more definitive evaluation of the prognostic value of the method (61).

Interlaboratory evaluation (31,68) and methodical improvements in the collection of CTC by immunobead enrichment (69), and of RT-PCR by multimarker RT-PCR (65,70) and by quantitative RT-PCR (13), will bring the value of CTC in MM into sharper focus. Despite method optimization, current data showing continued unsatisfactory sensitivity in the use of CTC in both the initial diagnosis (13,69) and follow-up of MM (15) indicate that the method is not ready for clinical application.

OTHER NEOPLASMS

The usefulness of CTC detection has also been studied in other neoplasms to determine whether positive findings indicate the existence of a subclinical metastatic state. The recognition of minimal residual disease could serve to identify patients who, after local therapy of a primary tumor, might benefit from existing or future adjuvant forms of therapy. This aspect is of particular interest in those types of malignancy that, despite successful local surgery, show a high metastatic potential. In longitudinal analyses, it is possible to determine whether the detection of CTC can result in earlier recognition of recurrent disease during follow-up in treated patients (71). In addition to MM and mammary carcinoma, the following tumors have a high metastatic potential: pancreatic carcinoma, bronchial carcinoma, hepatocellular carcinoma, and follicular thyroid carcinoma. Only occasionally have CTC been identified through characteristic DNA alterations such as the k-ras mutations (72,73) and p53 mutations (74,75). Usually, detection of mRNA transcripts (Table 2) serves to identify CTC.

Although many studies do not describe the occurrence of the respective transcripts in whole blood obtained from controls, most of the molecular targets mentioned occur in individual patients with benign diseases and even in healthy controls (Table 2). Albumin mRNA, which has been used as a molecular target for detection of CTC in hepatocellular carcinoma (76,77), has been found in 50% of healthy controls by Wong et al. (78). In fact, Matsumura et al. (79) found albumin mRNA in 100% of patients with hepatocellular carcinoma, in 100% of patients with benign liver disease, and in 100% of healthy controls.

The inadequate specificity of these and other mRNA markers, such as AFP and PSA (80), CK 19 (81), thyroglobulin (82), and CEA (83), militates against the broad application of analysis of CTC as a basis for clinical and therapeutic decision-making. One possible explanation for obtaining false positive RT-PCR findings in healthy controls includes methodical problems (e.g., contamination) during the highly sensitive RT-PCR assays. Another explanation includes the phenomenon of illegitimate transcription (84,85), i.e., the synthesis, under conditions of stimulation in patients with inflammatory disease of mRNA not typical for the cell. These factors may account for at least some of the reported false-positives.

Despite the proven prognostic value of this method in many different malignancies (71,86), its associated poor sensitivity and/or specificity means that CTC today, in solid tumors at least, is not associated with any clinical or therapeutic consequences.

CIRCULATING CELL-FREE DNA AS A TUMOR MARKER

Besides the search for circulating tumor cells (CTC), studies have focused on cell-free circulating tumor DNA as a marker for solid tumors. Initial reports described increased levels of circulating DNA in malignant diseases (115), but definite identification as tumor DNA has only been possible within the last 10 years (16,17). Target alterations in circulating tumor DNA obtained from cancer patients have included tumor-specific gene mutations (17), microsatellite alterations (16), and, more frequently, gene promoter hypermethylation (116,117). Although the number of studies published to date has been limited, it has been shown that the analysis of circulating tumor DNA may be of prognostic value in predicting patients' subsequent clinical course after therapy (118) and, in some malignancies at least, may be suitable for detecting recurrent disease during follow-up (119–121). The specific case of lung cancer studies also demonstrated a general suitability of the method for identifying at-risk patients who, subsequently, did develop tumors of the lung (122).

The following table presents an overview of the most important malignancies for which circulating tumor DNA in plasma/serum has been described.

When will the detection of CTC or circulating free nucleic acids in peripheral blood become clinically relevant, and therefore routine? It will happen when and if clinicians, using these techniques, can diagnose malignant disease in its earliest stages or recognize recurrent disease more promptly during treatment follow-up. At the same time, the accuracy of these new methods must at least equal, or, better yet, exceed, currently available techniques, such as clinical diagnostics, diagnostic imaging methods, and conventional tumor markers. The proof has yet to be delivered. Most problematic is the poor specificity of these markers, since false positive findings create unnecessary, expensive and, for the patient, troubling, examinations and procedures. Because of their superior

Table 2 Circulating tumor cells in solid tumors other than prostate cancer, breast cancer, and malignant melanoma (at initial diagnosis; selection)

Entity	Marker	Reference	Detection rate in tumor patients (all stages)	Detection rate benign diseases	Detection rate in healthy controls	Prognostic value[a]
Colorectal carcinoma	CK 8,19,20	(87)	52	0	0	n.d.
	CEA	(88, 89)	41	56	0	No
	CK 20	(90)	13	n.d.	n.d.	n.d.
	CK 20, CEA	(91)	74	n.d.	4	n.d.
	CK 19,20 MUC 1,2	(92)	20	12	0	Yes
	EGFR	(93)	73	n.d.	11	n.d.
	CEA	(71)	69	n.d.	0	Yes
Gastric cancer	CK 19,20	(94)	10	n.d.	7	n.d
	CEA	(95)	24	n.d.	n.d.	No
Hepatocellular carcinoma	AFP	(79)	52	13	0	n.d.
	Albumin		100	100	100	
	AFP	(96)	42[b]	3[b]	2[b]	n.d.
Pancreatic cancer	CEA	(97)	33	0	0	n.d.
	CK 19	(98)	5	n.d.	0	n.d.
Lung cancer	CEA	(99)	50	0	0	n.d.
	CK 19	(100)	36	2	0	Yes
	HLM	(101)	50	n.d.	0	n.d.
	Telomerase activity	(102)	73	n.d.	0	n.d.
Thyroid carcinoma	CK 20	(103)	26	0	0	n.d.
	TG	(82)	69–85[c]	25–71[c]	18–82[c]	No
Oral cancer	CK 20	(104)	58	n.d.	n.d.	n.d.
Endometrial cancer	CK 20	(105)	35	n.d	0	No
Cervical cancer	HPV 16	(106)	92	n.d.	0	n.d.
	HPV 16, 18	(107)1999	51	n.d.	0	Yes
	SCC	(108)	40	13	0	Yes
Ovarian cancer	CK 19	(81)	84	71	60	n.d.
Urothelial carcinoma	CK 20	(109)	24	n.d.	0	n.d.
	UP 2	(110)	27	n.d.	0	Yes
Kidney cancer	MN/CA9	(111)	49	n.d.	2	n.d.
	VHL[d]	(112)	12	n.d.	0	n.d.
Testicular cancer	AFP, βHCG	(113)	33	n.d.	0	n.d.
Ewing sarcoma	EWS-FLI	(114)	30	n.d.	n.d.	n.d.

[a] Prognostic value refers to disease-free survival, overall survival, and/or recurrence from disease as endpoint markers.
[b] Meta-analysis from 9 studies.
[c] Depending on cycle number (30–40).
[d] Mutation-specific RT-PCR
mRNA Markers: AFP, alpha-fetoprotein; HCG, human chorionic gonadotropin; CEA, carcinoembryonic antigen; CK, cytokeratin; EGFR, epidermal growth factor receptor; EWS-FLI, Ewing´s sarcoma / Friend leukemia virus integration site; HPV, human papilloma virus; SCC, squamous-cell carcinoma antigen; TG, thyroglobulin; UP, uroplakin; VHL, von Hippel-Lindau gene transcript.

specificity, the detection of DNA-based markers offers definite advantages over the use of mRNA. Further, clinical application is only then sensible when adjuvant therapeutic methods are available for the malignancy in question, which make prompt therapy or prevention of further disease recurrence possible. Recent experimental evidence has shown that CTC do have a slight, but nevertheless observable, rate of metastasis formation (3). The role of circulating DNA in metastasis formation, however, has yet to be proven (143).

On the basis of current knowledge, the detection of circulating tumor cells (CTC) or circulating free nucleic acids in peripheral blood remains an experimental application. Use of these methods in a routine clinical setting cannot be recommended at this time.

Table 3 Malignancies with circulating tumor DNA in plasma/serum

	Neoplasm	Patients N =	Markers N =	Alterations inn serum/ plasma (%)	Specificity (%)	Reference
Microsatellite alterations						
LOH, MIN	Neck/head tumors	21	12	29	100	(123)
LOH, MIN	Small-cell bronchial Ca	21	3	71	100	(16)
LOH, MIN	Non-small-cell bronchial Ca	22	4	28	n. d.	(124)
LOH, MIN	Colorectal carcinoma	44	8	0	n. d.	(125)
LOH, MIN	Clear cell renal cell Ca	40	4	65	100	(126)
LOH, MIN	Melanoma	40	10	58	100	(127)
LOH, MIN	Non-small-cell bronchial Ca	87	2	40	100	(121)
LOH, MIN	Mammary carcinoma	21	7	48	100	(128)
LOH, MIN	Mammary carcinoma	62	6	61	100	(129)
LOH, MIN	Mammary carcinoma	57	2	30	100	(130)
Gene mutations						
N-ras	Hematologic neoplasms	10	1	50	n. d.	(131)
IgChain DNA	B-cell leukemia	110	1	86	100	(119)
K-ras	Colorectal carcinoma	31	1	39	100	(132)
K-ras	Colorectal carcinoma	14	1	50	100	(133)
K-ras	Colorectal carcinoma	14	1	50	100	(134)
K-ras, p53	Colorectal carcinoma	44	1, Seq.	23	n. d.	(125)
p53	Colorectal carcinoma	17	Seq.	29	100	(135)
K-ras	Pancreatic carcinoma	21	1	81	100	(118)
K-ras	Pancreatic carcinoma	44	1	27	95	(136)
p53	Mammary carcinoma	62	Seq.	5	100	(129)
p53	Small-cell bronchial Ca	35	Seq.	14	100	(120)
p53	Hepatocellular Ca	20	1	30	100	(137)
Promoter hypermethylation						
p16, MGMT, GSTP1, DAP kinase	Non-small-cell bronchial carcinoma	22	4	52	n. d.	(116)
p16	Hepatocellular Ca	22	1	73	100	(73)
p15	Hepatocellular Ca	25	1	16	100	(138)
p16	Mammary carcinoma	43	1	14	100	(139)
p16, MGMT, GSTP1, DAP kinase	Neck/head tumors	50	4	42	100	(140)
APC	Esophageal carcinoma	84	1	18	100	(141)
GSTP1	Prostatic carcinoma	32	1	72	100	(117)
hMLH1	Colorectal carcinoma	9	1	33	100	(142)

REFERENCES

1. Gallucci BB. Selected concepts of cancer as a disease: from the Greeks to 1900. Oncol Nurs Forum 1985;12:67–71.
2. Schirrmacher V. Cancer metastasis: experimental approaches, theoretical concepts, and impacts for treatment strategies. Adv Cancer Res 1985;43:1–73.
3. Luzzi KJ, MacDonald IC, Schmidt EE, Kerkvliet N, Morris VL, Chambers AF, Groom AC. Multi-step nature of metastatic inefficiency: dormancy of solitary cells after successful extravasation and limited survival of early micrometastases. Am J Pathol 1998;153:865–873.
4. Ashworth TR. A case of cancer in which cells similar to those in the tumors were seen in the blood after death. Australian Med J. 1869;14:146.
5. Christopherson W. Cancer cells in the peripheral blood: a second look. Acta Cytol 1965;9:169–174.
6. Leather AJ, Gallegos NC, Kocjan G, Savage F, Smales CS, Hu W et al. Detection and enumeration of circulating tumor cells in colorectal cancer. Br J Surg 1993;80:777–780.
7. Bilkenroth U, Taubert H, Riemann D, Rebmann U, Heynemann H, Meye A. Detection and enrichment of disseminated renal carcinoma cells from peripheral blood by immunomagnetic cell separation. Int J Cancer 2001;92:577–582.
8. Ghossein RA, Bhattacharya S. Molecular detection and characterization of circulating tumor cells and micrometastases in solid tumors. Eur J Cancer 2000;36:1681–1694.
9. Lee MS, Chang KS, Cabanillas F, Freireich EJ, Trujillo JM, Stass SA. Detection of minimal residual cells carrying the t(14;18) by DNA sequence amplification. Science 1987;237:175–178.

10. Smith B, Selby P, Southgate J, Pittman K, Bradley C, Blair GE. Detection of melanoma cells in peripheral blood by means of reverse transcriptase and polymerase chain reaction. Lancet 1991;338:1227–1229.
11. Pantel K, Izbicki J, Passlick B, Angstwurm M, Haussinger K, Thetter O, Riethmuller G. Frequency and prognostic significance of isolated tumor cells in bone marrow of patients with non-small-cell lung cancer without overt metastases. Lancet 1996;347:649–653.
12. Ghossein RA, Bhattacharya S, Rosai J. Molecular detection of micrometastases and circulating tumor cells in solid tumors. Clin Cancer Res 1999;5:1950–1960.
13. Stoitchkov K, Letellier S, Garnier JP, Toneva M, Naumova E, Peytcheva E, et al. Evaluation of standard tyrosinase RT-PCR in melanoma patients by the use of the LightCycler system. Clin Chim Acta 2001;306:133–138.
14. Straub B, Müller M, Krause H, Schrader M, Goessl C, Heicappell R, et al. Detection of prostate-specific antigen RNA before and after radical retropubic prostatectomy and TUR-P using LightCycler-based quantitative real-time PCR. Urology 2001 (in press).
15. Brownbridge GG, Gold J, Edward M, MacKie RM. Evaluation of the use of tyrosinase-specific and melanA/MART-1-specific reverse transcriptase-coupled-polymerase chain reaction to detect melanoma cells in peripheral blood samples from 299 patients with malignant melanoma. Br J Dermatol 2001;144:279–287.
16. Chen XQ, Stroun M, Magnenat JL, Nicod LP, Kurt AM, Lyautey J, et al. Microsatellite alterations in plasma DNA of small-cell lung cancer patients. Nat Med 1996;2:1033–1035.
17. Sorenson GD, Pribish DM, Valone FH, Memoli VA, Bzik DJ, Yao SL. Soluble normal and mutated DNA sequences from single-copy genes in human blood. Cancer Epidemiol Biomarkers Prev 1994;3:67–71.
18. Lo YM, Chan LY, Lo KW, Leung SF, Zhang J, Chan AT, et al. Quantitative analysis of cell-free Epstein-Barr virus DNA in plasma of patients with nasopharyngeal carcinoma. Cancer Res 1999;59:1188–1191.
19. Kopreski MS, Benko FA, Kwak LW, Gocke CD. Detection of tumor messenger RNA in the serum of patients with malignant melanoma. Clin Cancer Res 1999;5:1961–1965.
20. Chen XQ, Bonnefoi H, Pelte MF, Lyautey J, Lederrey C, Movarekhi S, et al. Telomerase RNA as a detection marker in the serum of breast cancer patients. Clin Cancer Res 2000;6:3823–3826.
21. Hasselmann DO, Rappl G, Rossler M, Ugurel S, Tilgen W, Reinhold U. Detection of tumor-associated circulating mRNA in serum, plasma, and blood cells from patients with disseminated malignant melanoma. Oncol Rep 2001;8:115–118.
22. Sidransky D. Nucleic acid-based methods for the detection of cancer. Science 1997;278:1054–1059.
23. Deguchi T, Doi T, Ehara H, Ito S, Takahashi Y, Nishino Y, et al. Detection of micrometastatic prostate cancer cells in lymph nodes by reverse transcriptase-polymerase chain reaction. Cancer Res 1993;53:5350–5354.
24. Gao CL, Dean RC, Pinto A, Mooneyhan R, Connelly RR, McLeod DG, et al. Detection of circulating prostate-specific antigen expressing prostatic cells in the bone marrow of radical prostatectomy patients by sensitive reverse transcriptase-polymerase chain reaction. J Urol 1999;161:1070–1076.
25. Johnson PW, Burchill SA, Selby PJ. The molecular detection of circulating tumor cells. Br J Cancer 1995;72:268–276.
26. Keilholz U, Willhauck M, Rimoldi D, Brasseur F, Dummer W, Rass K, et al. Reliability of reverse transcription-polymerase chain reaction (RT-PCR)-based assays for the detection of circulating tumor cells: a quality-assurance initiative of the EORTC Melanoma Cooperative Group. Eur J Cancer 1998;34:750–753.
27. Berteau P, Dumas F, Gala JL, Eschwege P, Lacour B, Philippe M, Loric S. Influence of blood storage and sample processing on molecular detection of circulating prostate cells in cancer. Clin Chem 1998;44:677–679.
28. Berteau P, Dumas F, Gala JL, Eschwege P, Lacour B, Philippe M, Loric S. Molecular detection of circulating prostate cells in cancer II: Comparison of prostate epithelial cells isolation procedures. Clin Chem 1998;44:1750–1753.
29. Chomczynski P, Sacchi N. Single-step method of RNA isolation by acid guanidinium thiocyanate-phenol-chloroform extraction. Anal Biochem 1987;162:156–159.
30. Corey E, Corey MJ. Detection of disseminated prostate cells by reverse transcription-polymerase chain reaction (RT-PCR): technical and clinical aspects. Int J Cancer 1998;77:655–673.
31. Keilholz U. New prognostic factors in melanoma: mRNA tumor markers. Eur J Cancer 1998;34 Suppl 3:S37–S41.
32. Catalona WJ, Richie JP, Ahmann FR, Hudson MA, Scardino PT, Flanigan RC, et al. Comparison of digital rectal examination and serum prostate-specific antigen in the early detection of prostate cancer: results of a multi-center clinical trial of 6,630 men [see comments]. J Urol 1994;151:1283–1290.
33. Katz AE, Olsson CA, Raffo AJ, Cama C, Perlman H, Seaman E, et al. Molecular staging of prostate cancer with the use of an enhanced reverse transcriptase-PCR assay. Urology 1994;43:765–775.
34. Israeli RS, Miller WH, Jr., Su SL, Powell CT, Fair WR, Samadi DS, et al. Sensitive nested reverse transcription polymerase chain reaction detection of circulating prostatic tumor cells: comparison of prostate-specific membrane antigen and prostate-specific antigen-based assays. Cancer Res 1994;54:6306–6310.
35. Gao CL, Maheshwari S, Dean RC, Tatum L, Mooneyhan R, Connelly RR, et al. Blinded evaluation of reverse transcriptase-polymerase chain reaction prostate-specific antigen peripheral blood assay for molecular staging of prostate cancer. Urology 1999;53:714–721.
36. Grasso YZ, Gupta MK, Levin HS, Zippe CD, Klein EA. Combined nested RT-PCR assay for prostate-specific antigen and prostate-specific membrane antigen in prostate cancer patients: correlation with pathological stage. Cancer Res 1998;58:1456–1459.
37. Sokoloff MH, Tso CL, Kaboo R, Nelson S, Ko J, Dorey F et al. Quantitative polymerase chain reaction does not improve preoperative prostate cancer staging: a clinicopathological molecular analysis of 121 patients. J Urol 1996;156:1560–1566.
38. De La Taille A, Olsson CA, Buttyan R, Benson MC, Bagiella E, Cao Y, et al. Blood-based reverse transcriptase polymerase chain reaction assays for prostatic specific antigen: long-term follow-up confirms the potential utility of this assay in identifying patients more likely to have biochemical recurrence (rising PSA) following radical prostatectomy. Int J Cancer 1999;84:360–364.
39. Ghossein RA, Rosai J, Scher HI, Seiden M, Zhang ZF, Sun M, et al. Prognostic significance of detection of prostate-specific antigen transcripts in the peripheral blood of patients with metastatic androgen-independent prostatic carcinoma. Urology 1997;50:100–105.
40. Okegawa T, Nutahara K, Higashihara E. Pre-operative nested reverse transcription-polymerase chain reaction for prostate-spe-

cific membrane antigen predicts biochemical recurrence after radical prostatectomy. BJU Int 1999;84:112–117.
41. Olsson CA, de Vries GM, Raffo AJ, Benson MC, O'Toole K, Cao Y, et al. Pre-operative reverse transcriptase-polymerase chain reaction for prostate-specific antigen predicts treatment failure following radical prostatectomy. J Urol 1996;155:1557–1562.
42. Elgamal AA, Holmes EH, Su SL, Tino WT, Simmons SJ, Peterson M, et al. Prostate-specific membrane antigen (PSMA): current benefits and future value. Semin Surg Oncol 2000;18:10–16.
43. Ghossein RA, Osman I, Bhattacharya S, Ferrara J, Fazzari M, Cordon-Cardo C, Scher HI. Detection of prostatic-specific membrane antigen messenger RNA using immunobead reverse transcriptase-polymerase chain reaction. Diagn Mol Pathol 1999;8:59–65.
44. Lintula S, Stenman UH. The expression of prostate-specific membrane antigen in peripheral blood leukocytes. J Urol 1997;157:1969–1972.
45. Henke W, Jung M, Jung K, Lein M, Schlechte H, Berndt C, et al. Increased analytical sensitivity of RT-PCR of PSA mRNA decreases diagnostic specificity of detection of prostatic cells in blood. Int J Cancer 1997;70:52–56.
46. Bostick PJ, Chatterjee S, Chi DD, Huynh KT, Giuliano AE, Cote R, Hoon DS. Limitations of specific reverse-transcriptase polymerase chain reaction markers in the detection of metastases in the lymph nodes and blood of breast cancer patients. J Clin Oncol 1998;16:2632–2640.
47. Slade MJ, Smith BM, Sinnett HD, Cross NC, Coombes RC. Quantitative polymerase chain reaction for the detection of micrometastases in patients with breast cancer. J Clin Oncol 1999;17:870–879.
48. Aerts J, Wynendaele W, Paridaens R, Christiaens MR, van den BW, van Oosterom AT, Vandekerckhove F. A real-time quantitative reverse transcriptase polymerase chain reaction (RT-PCR) to detect breast carcinoma cells in peripheral blood. Ann Oncol 2001;12:39–46.
49. Watson MA, Fleming TP. Mammaglobin, a mammary-specific member of the uteroglobin gene family, is overexpressed in human breast cancer. Cancer Res 1996;56:860–865.
50. Becker RM, Darrow C, Zimonjic DB, Popescu NC, Watson MA, Fleming TP. Identification of mammaglobin B, a novel member of the uteroglobin gene family. Genomics 1998;54:70–78.
51. Watson MA, Dintzis S, Darrow CM, Voss LE, DiPersio J, Jensen R, Fleming TP. Mammaglobin expression in primary, metastatic, and occult breast cancer. Cancer Res 1999;59:3028–3031.
52. Zach O, Kasparu H, Krieger O, Hehenwarter W, Girschikofsky M, Lutz D. Detection of circulating mammary carcinoma cells in the peripheral blood of breast cancer patients via a nested reverse transcriptase polymerase chain reaction assay for mammaglobin mRNA. J Clin Oncol 1999;17:2015–2019.
53. Grunewald K, Haun M, Urbanek M, Fiegl M, Muller-Holzner E, Gunsilius E, et al. Mammaglobin gene expression: a superior marker of breast cancer cells in peripheral blood in comparison to epidermal-growth-factor receptor and cytokeratin-19. Lab Invest 2000;80:1071–1077.
54. Soria JC, Gauthier LR, Raymond E, Granotier C, Morat L, Armand JP, et al. Molecular detection of telomerase-positive circulating epithelial cells in metastatic breast cancer patients. Clin Cancer Res 1999;5:971–975.
55. Rigel DS, Carucci JA. Malignant melanoma: prevention, early detection, and treatment in the 21st century. CA Cancer J Clin 2000;50:215–236.
56. Cochran AJ, Balda BR, Starz H, Bachter D, Krag DN, Cruse CW, et al. The Augsburg Consensus. Techniques of lymphatic mapping, sentinel lymphadenectomy, and completion lymphadenectomy in cutaneous malignancies. Cancer 2000;89:236–241.
57. Morton DL, Wen DR, Wong JH, Economou JS, Cagle LA, Storm FK, et al. Technical details of intraoperative lymphatic mapping for early stage melanoma. Arch Surg 1992;127:392–399.
58. Shivers SC, Wang X, Li W, Joseph E, Messina J, Glass LF, et al. Molecular staging of malignant melanoma: correlation with clinical outcome. JAMA 1998;280:1410–1415.
59. Blaheta HJ, Schittek B, Breuninger H, Sotlar K, Ellwanger U, Thelen MH, et al. Detection of melanoma micrometastasis in sentinel nodes by reverse transcription-polymerase chain reaction correlates with tumor thickness and is predictive of micrometastatic disease in the lymph node basin. Am J Surg Pathol 1999;23:822–828.
60. Bostick PJ, Morton DL, Turner RR, Huynh KT, Wang HJ, Elashoff R, et al. Prognostic significance of occult metastases detected by sentinel lymphadenectomy and reverse transcriptase-polymerase chain reaction in early-stage melanoma patients. J Clin Oncol 1999;17:3238–3244.
61. Tsao H, Nadiminti U, Sober AJ, Bigby M. A meta-analysis of reverse transcriptase-polymerase chain reaction for tyrosinase mRNA as a marker for circulating tumor cells in cutaneous melanoma. Arch Dermatol 2001;137:325–330.
62. Foss AJ, Guille MJ, Occleston NL, Hykin PG, Hungerford JL, Lightman S. The detection of melanoma cells in peripheral blood by reverse transcription-polymerase chain reaction. Br J Cancer 1995;72:155–159.
63. Brossart P, Keilholz U, Willhauck M, Scheibenbogen C, Mohler T, Hunstein W. Hematogenous spread of malignant melanoma cells in different stages of disease. J Invest Dermatol 1993;101:887–889.
64. Cheung IY, Cheung NK, Ghossein RA, Satagopan JM, Bhattacharya S, Coit DG. Association between molecular detection of GAGE and survival in patients with malignant melanoma: a retrospective cohort study. Clin Cancer Res 1999;5:2042–2047.
65. Palmieri G, Strazzullo M, Ascierto PA, Satriano SM, Daponte A, Castello G. Polymerase chain reaction-based detection of circulating melanoma cells as an effective marker of tumor progression. Melanoma Cooperative Group. J Clin Oncol 1999;17:304–311.
66. Nestle FO, Alijagic S, Gilliet M, Sun Y, Grabbe S, Dummer R, et al. Vaccination of melanoma patients with pep. Nat Med 1998;4:328–332.
67. Palmer K, Moore J, Everard M, Harris JD, Rodgers S, Rees RC, et al. Gene therapy with autologous, interleukin 2-secreting tumor cells in patients with malignant melanoma. Hum Gene Ther 1999;10:1261–1268.
68. Reinhold U, Berkin C, Bosserhoff AK, Deutschmann A, Garbe C, Glaser R, et al. Interlaboratory evaluation of a new reverse transcriptase polymerase chain reaction-based enzyme-linked immunosorbent assay for the detection of circulating melanoma cells: a multi-center study of the Dermatologic Cooperative Oncology Group. J Clin Oncol 2001;19:1723–1727.
69. Fodstad O, Faye R, Hoifodt HK, Skovlund E, Aamdal S. Immunobead-based detection and characterization of circulating tumor cells in melanoma patients. Recent Results Cancer Res 2001;158:40–50.
70. Hoon DS, Bostick P, Kuo C, Okamoto T, Wang HJ, Elashoff R, Morton DL. Molecular markers in blood as surrogate prognostic

indicators of melanoma recurrence. Cancer Res 2000; 60:2253–2257.
71. Guadagni F, Kantor J, Aloe S, Carone MD, Spila A, D'Alessandro R, et al. Detection of blood-borne cells in colorectal cancer patients by nested reverse transcription-polymerase chain reaction for carcinoembryonic antigen messenger RNA: longitudinal analyses and demonstration of its potential importance as an adjunct to multiple serum markers. Cancer Res 2001;61:2523–2532.
72. Tada M, Omata M, Kawai S, Saisho H, Ohto M, Saiki RK, Sninsky JJ. Detection of ras gene mutations in pancreatic juice and peripheral blood of patients with pancreatic adenocarcinoma. Cancer Res 1993;53:2472–2474.
73. Wong IH, Lo YM, Zhang J, Liew CT, Ng MH, Wong N, et al. Detection of aberrant p16 methylation in the plasma and serum of liver cancer patients. Cancer Res 1999;59:71–73.
74. Iinuma H, Okinaga K, Adachi M, Suda K, Sekine T, Sakagawa K et al. Detection of tumor cells in blood using CD45 magnetic cell separation followed by nested mutant allele-specific amplification of p53 and K-ras genes in patients with colorectal cancer. Int J Cancer 2000;89:337–344.
75. Khan ZA, Jonas SK, Le Marer N, Patel H, Wharton RQ, Tarragona A, et al. P53 mutations in primary and metastatic tumors and circulating tumor cells from colorectal carcinoma patients. Clin Cancer Res 2000;6:3499–3504.
76. Barbu V, Bonnand AM, Hillaire S, Coste T, Chazouilleres O, Gugenheim J et al. Circulating albumin messenger RNA in hepatocellular carcinoma: results of a multi-center prospective study. Hepatology 1997;26:1171–1175.
77. Hillaire S, Barbu V, Boucher E, Moukhtar M, Poupon R. Albumin messenger RNA as a marker of circulating hepatocytes in hepatocellular carcinoma. Gastroenterology 1994;106:239–242.
78. Wong IH, Leung T, Ho S, Lau WY, Chan M, Johnson PJ. Semiquantification of circulating hepatocellular carcinoma cells by reverse transcriptase polymerase chain reaction. Br J Cancer 1997;76:628–633.
79. Matsumura M, Niwa Y, Kato N, Komatsu Y, Shiina S, Kawabe T, et al. Detection of alpha-fetoprotein mRNA, an indicator of hematogenous spreading hepatocellular carcinoma, in the circulation: a possible predictor of metastatic hepatocellular carcinoma. Hepatology 1994;20:1418–1425.
80. Ishikawa T, Kashiwagi H, Iwakami Y, Hirai M, Kawamura T, Aiyoshi Y, et al. Expression of alpha-fetoprotein and prostate-specific antigen genes in several tissues and detection of mRNAs in normal circulating blood by reverse transcriptase-polymerase chain reaction. Jpn J Clin Oncol 1998;28:723–728.
81. Takano H, Okamoto A, Fukushima K, Ochiai K, Tanaka T. Low specificity of cytokeratin 19 mRNA expression in the peripheral blood cells from patients with ovarian tumors. Oncol Rep 2000;7:1023–1025.
82. Bojunga J, Roddiger S, Stanisch M, Kusterer K, Kurek R, Renneberg H, et al. Molecular detection of thyroglobulin mRNA transcripts in peripheral blood of patients with thyroid disease by RT-PCR. Br J Cancer 2000;82:1650–1655.
83. Wong IH, Yeo W, Chan AT, Johnson PJ. Quantitative relationship of the circulating tumor burden assessed by reverse transcription-polymerase chain reaction for cytokeratin 19 mRNA in peripheral blood of colorectal cancer patients with Dukes' stage, serum carcinoembryonic antigen level and tumor progression. Cancer Lett 2001;162:65–73.
84. Chelly J, Concordet JP, Kaplan JC, Kahn A. Illegitimate transcription: transcription of any gene in any cell type. Proc Natl Acad Sci U S A 1989;86:2617–2621.

85. Jung R, Kruger W, Hosch S, Holweg M, Kroger N, Gutensohn K, et al. Specificity of reverse transcriptase-polymerase chain reaction assays designed for the detection of circulating cancer cells is influenced by cytokines in vivo and in vitro. Br J Cancer 1998;78:1194–1198.
86. Taniguchi T, Makino M, Suzuki K, Kaibara N. Prognostic significance of reverse transcriptase-polymerase chain reaction measurement of carcinoembryonic antigen mRNA levels in tumor drainage blood and peripheral blood of patients with colorectal carcinoma. Cancer 2000;89:970–976.
87. Denis MG, Lipart C, Leborgne J, LeHur PA, Galmiche JP, Denis M, et al. Detection of disseminated tumor cells in peripheral blood of colorectal cancer patients. Int J Cancer 1997;74:540–544.
88. Bessa X, Elizalde JI, Boix L, Pinol V, Lacy AM, Salo J, et al. Lack of prognostic influence of circulating tumor cells in peripheral blood of patients with colorectal cancer. Gastroenterology 2001;120:1084–1092.
89. Castells A, Boix L, Bessa X, Gargallo L, Pique JM. Detection of colonic cells in peripheral blood of colorectal cancer patients by means of reverse transcriptase and polymerase chain reaction. Br J Cancer 1998;78:1368–1372.
90. Weitz J, Kienle P, Magener A, Koch M, Schrodel A, Willeke F, et al. Detection of disseminated colorectal cancer cells in lymph nodes, blood, and bone marrow. Clin Cancer Res 1999;5:1830–1836.
91. Wharton RQ, Jonas SK, Glover C, Khan ZA, Klokouzas A, Quinn H et al. Increased detection of circulating tumor cells in the blood of colorectal carcinoma patients using two reverse transcription-PCR assays and multiple blood samples. Clin Cancer Res 1999;5:4158–4163.
92. Hardingham JE, Hewett PJ, Sage RE, Finch JL, Nuttall JD, Kotasek D, Dobrovic A. Molecular detection of blood-borne epithelial cells in colorectal cancer patients and in patients with benign bowel disease. Int J Cancer 2000;89:8–13.
93. De Luca A, Pignata S, Casamassimi A, D'Antonio A, Gridelli C, Rossi A, et al. Detection of circulating tumor cells in carcinoma patients by a novel epidermal growth factor receptor reverse transcription-PCR assay. Clin Cancer Res 2000;6:1439–1444.
94. Majima T, Ichikura T, Takayama E, Chochi K, Mochizuki H. Detecting circulating cancer cells using reverse transcriptase-polymerase chain reaction for cytokeratin mRNA in peripheral blood from patients with gastric cancer. Jpn J Clin Oncol 2000;30:499–503.
95. Noh YH, Kim JA, Lim GR, Ro YT, Koo JH, Lee YS, et al. Detection of circulating tumor cells in patients with gastrointestinal tract cancer using RT-PCR and its clinical implications. Exp Mol Med 2001;33:8–14.
96. Paterlini-Brechot P, Vona G, Brechot C. Circulating tumorous cells in patients with hepatocellular carcinoma. Clinical impact and future directions. Semin Cancer Biol 2000;10:241–249.
97. Funaki NO, Tanaka J, Kasamatsu T, Ohshio G, Hosotani R, Okino T, Imamura M. Identification of carcinoembryonic antigen mRNA in circulating peripheral blood of pancreatic carcinoma and gastric carcinoma patients. Life Sci 1996;59:2187–2199.
98. Aihara T, Noguchi S, Ishikawa O, Furukawa H, Hiratsuka M, Ohigashi H et al. Detection of pancreatic and gastric cancer cells in peripheral and portal blood by amplification of keratin 19 mRNA with reverse transcriptase-polymerase chain reaction. Int J Cancer 1997;72:408–411.
99. Castaldo G, Tomaiuolo R, Sanduzzi A, Bocchino ML, Ponticiello A, Barra E, et al. Lung cancer metastatic cells detected in blood

by reverse transcriptase-polymerase chain reaction and dot-blot analysis. J Clin Oncol 1997;15:3388–3393.

100. Peck K, Sher YP, Shih JY, Roffler SR, Wu CW, Yang PC. Detection and quantitation of circulating cancer cells in the peripheral blood of lung cancer patients. Cancer Res 1998;58:2761–2765.

101. Fournier MV, Guimaraes dC, Paschoal ME, Ronco LV, Carvalho MG, Pardee AB. Identification of a gene encoding a human oxysterol-binding protein-homologue: a potential general molecular marker for blood dissemination of solid tumors. Cancer Res 1999;59:3748–3753.

102. Gauthier LR, Granotier C, Soria JC, Faivre S, Boige V, Raymond E, Boussin FD. Detection of circulating carcinoma cells by telomerase activity. Br J Cancer 2001;84:631–635.

103. Weber T, Lacroix J, Weitz J, Amnan K, Magener A, Holting T, et al. Expression of cytokeratin 20 in thyroid carcinomas and peripheral blood detected by reverse transcription polymerase chain reaction. Br J Cancer 2000;82:157–160.

104. Kawamata H, Uchida D, Nakashiro K, Hino S, Omotehara F, Yoshida H, Sato M. Haematogenous cytokeratin 20 mRNA as a predictive marker for recurrence in oral cancer patients. Br J Cancer 1999;80:448–452.

105. Klein A, Fishman A, Zemer R, Zimlichman S, Altaras MM. Detection of tumor circulating cells by cytokeratin 20 in the blood of patients with endometrial carcinoma. Gynecol Oncol 2000;78:352–355.

106. Pao CC, Hor JJ, Yang FP, Lin CY, Tseng CJ. Detection of human papillomavirus mRNA and cervical cancer cells in peripheral blood of cervical cancer patients with metastasis. J Clin Oncol 1997;15:1008–1012.

107. Tseng CJ, Pao CC, Lin JD, Soong YK, Hong JH, Hsueh S. Detection of human papillomavirus types 16 and 18 mRNA in peripheral blood of advanced cervical cancer patients and its association with prognosis. J Clin Oncol 1999;17:1391–1396.

108. Stenman J, Lintula S, Hotakainen K, Vartiainen J, Lehvaslaiho H, Stenman UH. Detection of squamous-cell carcinoma antigen-expressing tumor cells in blood by reverse transcriptase-polymerase chain reaction in cancer of the uterine cervix. Int J Cancer 1997;74:75–80.

109. Gudemann CJ, Weitz J, Kienle P, Lacroix J, Wiesel MJ, Soder M, et al. Detection of hematogenous micrometastasis in patients with transitional cell carcinoma. J Urol 2000;164:532–536.

110. Lu JJ, Kakehi Y, Takahashi T, Wu XX, Yuasa T, Yoshiki T, et al. Detection of circulating cancer cells by reverse transcription-polymerase chain reaction for uroplakin II in peripheral blood of patients with urothelial cancer. Clin Cancer Res 2000;6:3166–3171.

111. McKiernan JM, Buttyan R, Bander NH, de la TA, Stifelman MD, Emanuel ER, et al. The detection of renal carcinoma cells in the peripheral blood with an enhanced reverse transcriptase-polymerase chain reaction assay for MN/CA9. Cancer 1999;86:492–497.

112. Ashida S, Okuda H, Chikazawa M, Tanimura M, Sugita O, Yamamoto Y, et al. Detection of circulating cancer cells with von hippel-lindau gene mutation in peripheral blood of patients with renal cell carcinoma. Clin Cancer Res 2000;6:3817–3822.

113. Hautkappe AL, Lu M, Mueller H, Bex A, Harstrick A, Roggendorf M, Ruebben H. Detection of germ-cell tumor cells in the peripheral blood by nested reverse transcription polymerase chain reaction for alpha-fetoprotein-messenger RNA and beta human chorionic gonadotropin-messenger RNA. Cancer Res 2000;60:3170–3174.

114. West DC, Grier HE, Swallow MM, Demetri GD, Granowetter L, Sklar J. Detection of circulating tumor cells in patients with Ewing's sarcoma and peripheral primitive neuroectodermal tumor. J Clin Oncol 1997;15:583–588.

115. Leon SA, Shapiro B, Sklaroff DM, Yaros MJ. Free DNA in the serum of cancer patients and the effect of therapy. Cancer Res 1977;37:646–650.

116. Esteller M, Sanchez-Cespedes M, Rosell R, Sidransky D, Baylin SB, Herman JG. Detection of aberrant promoter hypermethylation of tumor suppressor genes in serum DNA from non-small-cell lung cancer patients. Cancer Res 1999;59:67–70.

117. Goessl C, Krause H, Muller M, Heicapell R, Schrader M, Sachsinger J, Miller K. Fluorescent methylation-specific polymerase chain reaction for DNA-based detection of prostate cancer in bodily fluids. Cancer Res 2000;60:5941–5945.

118. Mulcahy HE, Lyautey J, Lederrey C, qi C, X, Anker P, Alstead EM, et al. A prospective study of K-ras mutations in the plasma of pancreatic cancer patients. Clin Cancer Res 1998;4:271–275.

119. Frickhofen N, Muller E, Sandherr M, Binder T, Bangerter M, Wiest C et al. Rearranged Ig heavy chain DNA is detectable in cell-free blood samples of patients with B-cell neoplasia. Blood 1997;90:4953–4960.

120. Gonzalez R, Silva JM, Sanchez A, Dominguez G, Garcia JM, Chen XQ, et al. Microsatellite alterations and TP53 mutations in plasma DNA of small-cell lung cancer patients: follow-up study and prognostic significance. Ann Oncol 2000;11:1097–1104.

121. Sozzi G, Musso K, Ratcliffe C, Goldstraw P, Pierotti MA, Pastorino U. Detection of microsatellite alterations in plasma DNA of non-small-cell lung cancer patients: a prospect for early diagnosis. Clin Cancer Res 1999;5:2689–2692.

122. Allan JM, Hardie LJ, Briggs JA, Davidson LA, Watson JP, Pearson SB, et al. Genetic alterations in bronchial mucosa and plasma DNA from individuals at high risk of lung cancer. Int J Cancer 2001;91:359–365.

123. Nawroz H, Koch W, Anker P, Stroun M, Sidransky D. Microsatellite alterations in serum DNA of head and neck cancer patients. Nat Med 1996;2:1035–1037.

124. Sanchez-Cespedes M, Monzo M, Rosell R, Pifarre A, Calvo R, Lopez-Cabrerizo MP, Astudillo J. Detection of chromosome 3p alterations in serum DNA of non-small-cell lung cancer patients. Ann Oncol 1998;9:113–116.

125. Hibi K, Robinson CR, Booker S, Wu L, Hamilton SR, Sidransky D, Jen J. Molecular detection of genetic alterations in the serum of colorectal cancer patients. Cancer Res 1998;58:1405–1407.

126. Goessl C, Heicappell R, Munker R, Anker P, Stroun M, Krause H, et al. Microsatellite analysis of plasma DNA from patients with clear cell renal carcinoma. Cancer Res 1998;58:4728–4732.

127. Fujiwara Y, Chi DD, Wang H, Keleman P, Morton DL, Turner R, Hoon DS. Plasma DNA microsatellites as tumor-specific markers and indicators of tumor progression in melanoma patients. Cancer Res 1999;59:1567–1571.

128. Chen X, Bonnefoi H, Diebold-Berger S, Lyautey J, Lederrey C, Faltin-Traub E, et al. Detecting tumor-related alterations in plasma or serum DNA of patients diagnosed with breast cancer. Clin Cancer Res 1999;5:2297–2303.

129. Silva JM, Dominguez G, Garcia JM, Gonzalez R, Villanueva MJ, Navarro F, et al. Presence of tumor DNA in plasma of breast cancer patients: clinicopathological correlations. Cancer Res 1999;59:3251–3256.

130. Shaw JA, Smith BM, Walsh T, Johnson S, Primrose L, Slade MJ, et al. Microsatellite alterations plasma DNA of primary breast cancer patients. Clin Cancer Res 2000;6:1119–1124.

131. Vasioukhin V, Anker P, Maurice P, Lyautey J, Lederrey C, Stroun M. Point mutations of the N-ras gene in the blood plasma DNA of patients with myelodysplastic syndrome or acute myelogenous leukaemia. Br J Haematol 1994;86:774–779.
132. Kopreski MS, Benko FA, Kwee C, Leitzel KE, Eskander E, Lipton A, Gocke CD. Detection of mutant K-ras DNA in plasma or serum of patients with colorectal cancer. Br J Cancer 1997;76:1293–1299.
133. Anker P, Lefort F, Vasioukhin V, Lyautey J, Lederrey C, Chen XQ, et al. K-ras mutations are found in DNA extracted from the plasma of patients with colorectal cancer. Gastroenterology 1997;112:1114–1120.
134. de Kok JB, van Solinge WW, Ruers TJ, Roelofs RW, van Muijen GN, Willems JL, Swinkels DW. Detection of tumor DNA in serum of colorectal cancer patients. Scand J Clin Lab Invest 1997;57:601–614.
135. Mayall F, Jacobson G, Wilkins R, Chang B. Mutations of p53 gene can be detected in the plasma of patients with large bowel carcinoma. J Clin Pathol 1998;51:611–613.
136. Castells A, Puig P, Mora J, Boadas J, Boix L, Urgell E, et al. K-ras mutations in DNA extracted from the plasma of patients with pancreatic carcinoma: diagnostic utility and prognostic significance. J Clin Oncol 1999;17:578–584.
137. Jackson PE, Qian GS, Friesen MD, Zhu YR, Lu P, Wang JB et al. Specific p53 mutations detected in plasma and tumors of hepatocellular carcinoma patients by electrospray ionization mass spectrometry. Cancer Res 2001;61:33–35.
138. Wong IH, Lo YM, Yeo W, Lau WY, Johnson PJ. Frequent p15 promoter methylation in tumor and peripheral blood from hepatocellular carcinoma patients. Clin Cancer Res 2000;6:3516–3521.
139. Silva JM, Dominguez G, Villanueva MJ, Gonzalez R, Garcia JM, Corbacho C, et al. Aberrant DNA methylation of the p16INK4a gene in plasma DNA of breast cancer patients. Br J Cancer 1999;80:1262–1264.
140. Sanchez-Cespedes M, Esteller M, Wu L, Nawroz-Danish H, Yoo GH, Koch WM, et al. Gene promoter hypermethylation in tumors and serum of head and neck cancer patients. Cancer Res 2000;60:892–895.
141. Kawakami K, Brabender J, Lord RV, Groshen S, Greenwald BD, Krasna MJ, et al. Hypermethylated APC DNA in plasma and prognosis of patients with esophageal adenocarcinoma. J Natl Cancer Inst 2000;92:1805–1811.
142. Grady WM, Rajput A, Lutterbaugh JD, Markowitz SD. Detection of aberrantly methylated hMLH1 promoter DNA in the serum of patients with microsatellite unstable colon cancer. Cancer Res 2001;61:900–902.
143. Garcia-Olmo D, Garcia-Olmo DC, Ontanon J, Martinez E, Vallejo M. Tumor DNA circulating in the plasma might play a role in metastasis: the hypothesis of the genometastasis. Histol Histopathol 1999;14:1159–1164.

Chapter 10

Autoantibodies as Circulating Cancer Markers

Kwok Leung Cheung, C. Rosamund L. Graves, and John F.R. Robertson

Tumor markers indicate the presence of an underlying neoplasm. In broad terms, they comprise all features that characterize neoplasia; in fact, all biochemical alterations that distinguish neoplastic from normal tissues could be called tumor markers. Detected in the tumor tissue itself or in secretions, as well as in circulation where their related products are shed, they may serve as diagnostic and prognostic indicators and as a means for monitoring and targeting therapy.

Circulating (or blood) tumor markers have been known for decades. In contrast to markers in tumor tissue, circulating markers reflect a dynamic situation, and their measurements can be repeated as required. The appearance of detectable tumor markers in the circulation generally represents tumor burden, which normally corresponds to the extent of disease. This is why, with a few exceptions—e.g., prostate-specific antigen (PSA) in screening prostate cancer, alpha-fetoprotein (AFP) in diagnosing hepatocellular carcinoma, and β human chorionic gonadotropin (HCG) in choriocarcinoma—the use of blood tumor markers is most established in the diagnosis and monitoring of symptomatic metastatic disease. The role of blood tumor markers in screening, early diagnosis, and treatment of most solid malignancies remains to be elucidated. One important reason is the low sensitivity of existing assays that measure circulating tumor-related antigens, e.g., MUC1 mucin.

In contrast, autoantibodies produced against tumor-related antigens as part of an immune response may provide an in vivo amplification of an early carcinogenesis signal (Figure 1). Measuring autoantibodies may give rise to a higher sensitivity, which would make screening and earlier diagnosis a tantalizing possibility.

This chapter compares antigen-based tumor marker assays with autoantibody assays. It also discusses various aspects of autoantibody assays and their potential use as circulating cancer markers.

AUTOANTIBODY ASSAYS

Characteristics

Circulating autoantibodies are detected by immunoassay, predominantly the Enzyme Linked Immnoadsorbent Assay (ELISA). Various ways to improve the sensitivity of such assays have been explored, including preparation of an antigen purified from the serum of patients with metastases from the respective cancer (such as MUC1 antigen purified from the serum of women with metastatic breast cancer). This antigen is clearly a more appropriate target for screening patient serum than a synthetic or "normal" MUC1 mucin material. Assays for detecting autoantibodies to oncoproteins (e.g., c-erbB-2, p53) may be designed using various recombinant protein forms produced with or without any one of numerous tags. Such tags offer the possibility of non-constrained attachments of the protein to the plate, while more traditional attachment methods rely on antibody capture (thus holding the protein in a constrained format and masking at least one epitope site).

Although an ELISA is the predominant autoantibody assay, protocols vary from one assay to another, and these may

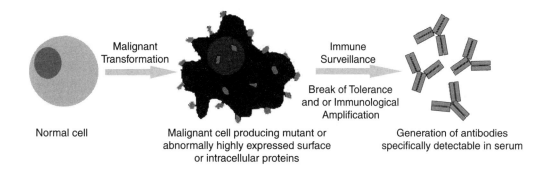

Figure 1 Serological diagnosis of cancer.

seriously affect the ability to discriminate between normal and cancer samples. For instance, an assay using time-resolved fluorometry may be superior to radioactive labeled techniques (1). Furthermore, using different control populations to define cut-off values and differing definitions of normality also significantly impact an assay's specificity.

Despite these possible variations, autoantibody assays appear to demonstrate profound temporal stability. For example, the titre of p53 antibodies detected in a series of patients with mesothelioma remained stable throughout the course of their illness (2). Unpublished data from our group also showed minimal fluctuation of autoantibody levels in women at risk of breast cancer. These data have suggested the promising prospect of sequentially testing autoantibody levels, since there are no random fluctuations within individuals. However, whether the autoantibody detection rate can be maintained after long-term storage of samples (e.g., after years) to allow for retrospective studies remains uncertain, although some studies have shown p53 autoantibodies, for example, to remain stable under cryopreservation (3).

Specificity of Autoantibody Assays

Most autoantibody assays thus far developed are qualitative: i.e., either positive or negative depending on cut-off criteria. As immunoassays continue to be refined, different patterns of changes for use in monitoring disease—such as those seen in antigen-based cancer marker assays in which the biochemical index score is calculated using cancer antigen 15.3 (CA15.3), carcinoembryonic antigen (CEA), and erythrocyte sedimentation rate (ESR) for metastatic breast cancer (4)—can be defined quantitatively.

Circulating autoantibodies develop as a result of a humoral response to cancer-related antigens (in vivo amplification of a signal of carcinogenesis). It would therefore be apparent that cancer patients have a considerably higher level of autoantibodies than do individuals who are cancer-free. Using measurements obtained for the cancer-free population allows us to set a "cut-off" point above which no "normal" values should lie. Thus samples with autoantibody levels above this point can be deemed positive for cancer. The results of autoantibody detection can hence be obtained using a 100% confidence limit, and if the normal range was obtained from an appropriately large number of "normals" and if none of the "normal" samples was positive, then the specificity of the assay is 100% for the detection of the respective cancer.

On the other hand, as in cancer-antigen-based assays, an increase in specificity is often obtained at the expense of a decrease in sensitivity. Therefore, when using an autoantibody assay, one may consider setting the "normal" cut-off value at a confidence level of 95% rather than 100% to allow some degree of false positive detection. This may be useful in the concept of autoantibody production as an early signal of carcinogenesis, since it is logical to assume that some apparently normal individuals may harbor circulating autoantibodies indicative of such signals.

Figure 2 illustrates the difference in autoantibody detection rates using 100% and 95% confidence intervals for an unpublished series of measurements for breast cancer from our group.

Owing to the concept of in vivo amplification, an autoantibody assay has great potential to be used for cancer screening compared to conventional antigen-based assays. As mentioned above, setting the normal cut-offs at a confidence interval of 95% allows for the fact that some individuals in the normal population could be "harboring" an occult cancer (i.e., their autoantibody levels would be elevated). However it depends on how one chooses a normal control population. If members of this group have been evaluated (including taking a history), examined, investigated (some of them), and biopsied (some of them), and if the possibility of cancer has been excluded as much as possible, taking a cut-off value using 100% confidence interval may seem more realistic (i.e., not 5% of these individuals will be harboring an occult cancer). This could be even more important if autoantibody assays were exploited for cancer screening in an "at-risk" population. Increasing cut-off values improves the specificity of the assays, because specificity is considered more important than sensitivity in a group of "at-risk" individuals, especially when considering possible preventive or therapeutic intervention if positive autoantibodies are detected.

Carcinogenesis is a process. There may be little distinction between its different phases (e.g., from benign to pre-invasive). When using the above-mentioned normal cut-off values, individuals with the relevant benign conditions may have positive autoantibodies (i.e., benign breast diseases such as fibroadenoma if the assay is used for screening early invasive breast carcinoma). Autoantibody-based tumor marker assays for cancer screening is a new concept. It would be useful to explore various results by also using "non-malignant" cut-offs (i.e., amalgamating the normal and benign controls to calculate cut-off values). Such an approach may have the advantage of further increasing assay specificity for this specific "at risk" group. The same approach has previously been reported in antigen-based markers (4).

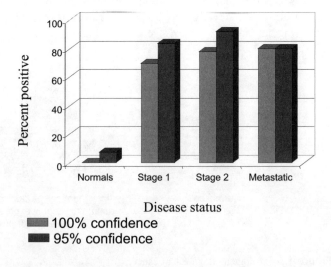

Figure 2 Autoantibody detection rates in breast cancer

Sensitivity of Autoantibody Assays

Many cancers (e.g., breast cancer) are heterogeneous. From early studies it was clear that no single antigen-based circulating cancer marker would suffice for diagnosing and/or monitoring most advanced cancers. But the sensitivity of antigen-based circulating markers can be increased by using a combination of markers, as in a panel (5). For example, the sensitivity of tumor marker measurements for detecting metastatic breast cancer can be increased to over 80% when both CA15.3 and CEA are used.

Using the same concept, autoantibody detection is likely to be increased by employing a panel of assays. Unpublished data from our group (for a series of patients with primary breast cancer) have shown that increasing the number of autoantibody assays in a panel increases sensitivity (Table 1).

The choice of individual markers against which their autoantibodies are measured depends on individual cancers. Molecular biology has increased the understanding of early tumorigenesis and thereby identified potential new markers that might be useful for screening and early diagnosis, a difficult area in which most antigen-based cancer markers have virtually no role. These new markers are based on the understanding of genetic abnormalities associated with the respective cancers and on the role of growth factors, cellular transcription factors, and the cell cycle. Autoantibodies to markers of early carcinogenesis such as MUC1 (differentiation marker), c-erbB-2 (a poor prognostic factor in most cancers), and p53 (the commonest mutation seen in human neoplasia) may be included in most assay panels. Autoantibodies to more specific antigens may then be added to further improve sensitivity for individual cancers (for example, BRCA1 and BRCA2 for breast cancer, PSA for prostate cancer, *ras* for colorectal cancer).

Effects on Autoantibody Assays

A recently published review reported that patients with cancers could develop autoimmune phenomena and rheumatic diseases as a result of generating autoantibodies (7). Anti-oncoprotein and anti-tumor suppression gene antigens were detected, for example, before the diagnosis of the cancer or in the early stages of the cancer. This suggests a potential role in cancer screening, as mentioned earlier.

Unpublished data from our group have suggested good discrimination in terms of autoantibody detection between patients with autoimmune disease and those with early primary breast cancer. Therefore, although autoimmune phenomena can occur in malignancies, the detection of circulating autoantibodies remains useful as a potential tool for cancer screening and early diagnosis, provided that the previously described cut-off based criteria are followed.

The effects of different cancer therapies on autoantibody detection have not been widely studied. Poeze et al. suggested that a persistent humoral response could be due to a long-term effect of radiotherapy, which had been found to be associated with increased expression of p53 in the normal breast tissue (8). In this instance autoantibodies could be detected in the circulation even many years after radiotherapy. This discovery is especially relevant for patients treated by breast-conserving surgery and intact breast irradiation. Caution must therefore be taken in interpreting the autoantibody assay results during patient follow-up. Unpublished, pilot, retrospective data from our group showed that previous use of chemotherapy (as adjuvant therapy after initial surgery for primary breast cancer) did not compromise the subsequent formation of autoantibodies—i.e., prior chemotherapy did not seem to affect autoantibody detection. This appears encouraging, especially when using autoantibody assays for follow-up of cancer patients, since it has become increasingly common to use neoadjuvant/adjuvant chemotherapy in addition to surgical treatment for most solid cancers. However, pilot data need to be confirmed by larger prospective studies.

Correlation with Cancer Antigen Expression

The correlation between the expression of a cancer antigen in the tumor tissue and the appearance of the respective autoantibody in the circulation depends on the mechanisms that elicit the humoral response and how the antigen expression is measured. We have shown a significant correlation between tissue staining and autoantibody detection for MUC1 in a series of primary breast cancer (Table 2). However there were still differences between different types of tissue (e.g., cytoplasmic, apical membranes) and the presence of circulating MUC1 autoantibodies. This may be due to a variation in glycosylation and the presence of various epitopes in the MUC1 molecule.

Detection by immunohistochemistry of the over-expression of c-erbB-2 tissue gives different sensitivity when compared with detection by fluorescent *in situ* hybridization

Table 1 Sensitivities of autoantibody assays

	% primary breast cancer positive
Single assay*	35–47
Double assay*	51–60
Triple assay*	63–76
Quadruple assay*	82

* Assay to detect one or more of four autoantibodies (to MUC1, c-erbB2, c-myc, p53).

Table 2 Correlation between MUC1 tissue staining and circulating autoantibodies to MUC1

MUC1—staining for apical membranes (intracytoplasmic lumina formation)	MUC1 AAb negative	MUC1 AAb positive	Total (N)
Negative	50	38	88
Positive	10	19	29
Total (N)	60	57	117

p = 0.03
AAb = Autoantibodies
[Unpublished data from Nottingham]

(FISH). This will in turn lead to different correlations between tissue expression and circulating autoantibody detection. Similarly, p53 can be measured by immunohistochemistry or by sequencing for mutations. It has been reported that p53 mutations (as detected by currently available means) may not be mandatory for eliciting the humoral response that leads to production of autoantibodies. For instance, p53 autoantibodies could be found not only in the presence of p53 mutations but also in their absence (9).

CLINICAL APPLICATIONS

The use of autoantibodies as potential cancer markers is a new concept. In contrast to antigen-based cancer markers, they represent a humoral response to cancer antigen and as a result, may be more sensitive in their detection—a minute amount of antigen is capable of inducing a humoral immune response that leads to the production of a vast amount of circulating autoantibodies. This has great potential for screening and early cancer diagnosis compared to existing conventional antigen-based cancer markers. Whether autoantibodies play significant clinical roles in providing prognostic information, follow-up information after treatment (e.g., surgery), and guidance for monitoring cancer therapy remains to be seen.

Screening and Early Diagnosis

Mutations of the p53 tumor suppresser gene are the most frequent abnormalities in human neoplasia and as a result p53 autoantibodies have been the most widely studied. Accumulation of mutant p53 in tumor cells may lead to a humoral immune response: the development of p53 autoantibodies. Autoantibodies to p53 have been reported to be present in 9–48% of patients with primary breast cancer (10–13), and have been noted to be more frequently observed in those patients with over-expression of the oncoprotein in the tumor tissue (10). Autoantibodies to p53 have been detected in 11–62% of patients with lung cancer (14–17). In a study of 134 patients with primary lung cancer, autoantibodies to p53 were more frequently detected in non-small cell carcinoma than in their small cell counterparts (13/99 vs. 4/35) (16). p53 autoantibodies were also detected in hepatocellular carcinoma (18), oral cancer (15), esophageal carcinoma (19), gastric cancer (15), colorectal cancer (15,20), bladder cancer (21,22), gynecological malignancies (23–26), and lymphoma (27).

Abnormally glycosylated MUC1 mucins (CA15.3, CA27.29) are already of clinical value in advanced breast cancer, but despite numerous clinical studies none has proven MUC1 mucin assays to be of value in the diagnosis of primary breast cancer. This finding is also true for other assays that detect tumor-associated antigens such as CEA or c-erbB2. The lack of clinical value in the primary breast cancer is due to the insensitivity of current assays. It has been reported that only 10–25% of patients with primary breast cancer express antibodies to MUC1 mucins (28,29). Antibodies to MUC1 mucin were found in patients' blood either as free antibodies, or complexed to the mucin molecule. Our group has also reported the identification of MUC1 in immune complexes isolated from the sera of breast cancer patients (30). These papers suggest that an antibody response occurs before the level of MUC1 mucin itself is elevated in the serum, thus giving anti-MUC1 autoantibodies the potential to be a useful diagnostic blood marker in early disease.

Antibodies to c-erbB-2 oncoproteins had been found in breast cancer tissue that over-expressed c-erbB-2 (31,32). A large study involving 1,200 histology samples from patients who had primary breast cancer found a discordant result with better prognosis in patients who were node-negative, lymphoplasma cell-infiltration-positive (generally a good prognostic factor) and in patients who were c-erbB-2 oncoprotein-positive (generally a poor prognostic factor) (32). These results suggested the presence of an antibody response specifically directed against the p185 oncoprotein. On the other hand, detection of circulating c-erbB-2 autoantibodies had not been very successful, although it has been reported that they were found in 55% of patients who had c-erbB-2 over-expression in the primary breast cancer tissue (Note: Tissue c-erbB-2 over-expression is seen in about 30% of primary breast cancer).

Other autoantibodies have also been identified in various kinds of malignancies. An early study found that significantly more patients with colorectal cancer had circulating c-myc autoantibodies when compared to controls (25/44 vs. 8/46), suggesting a potential use in the diagnosis of the cancer (33). Antibodies to the 27-kDa-heat shock protein were found in 41% of a recent series of 96 women with gynecologic cancers, while the detection rates in the normal and benign controls were 3.4% and 4.3% respectively (35).

The finding of reasonable sensitivity to autoantibody detection in patients with various cancers, and the hypothesis that the production of autoantibodies represents a signal of early carcinogenesis, suggest that autoantibodies can be detected in the pre-malignant phase of the disease, rendering their use in cancer screening feasible. Clinical studies have supported this concept. Heavy smokers, for example, were found to develop squamous carcinoma of the lung 5–15 months after detection of serum p53 autoantibodies (15,36). Other studies have demonstrated circulating autoantibodies in individuals with pre-malignant or high-risk lesions. Regele et al. reported that p53 autoantibodies were found in 11.6% (5/43) of patients who had ductal carcinoma *in situ* (DCIS) of the breast (37). In a recently reported small series, nine out of 13 patients suffering from pre-malignant oral lesions had detectable p53 autoantibodies (38). Another report found high p53 autoantibody detection rates in patients with idiopathic pulmonary fibrosis (57% and 53% in cases with and without lung cancer respectively), an entity known to be associated with increased risk of lung cancer (17). Our group has preliminary, unpublished data showing positive autoantibodies to a panel of cancer-related antigens in a proportion of women at risk of breast cancer. This includes not only individuals with family histories of breast cancer but also those with high-risk pathology (e.g., atypical ductal hyperplasia, or ADH).

These results support the hypothesis that the production of autoantibodies seems to signal carcinogenesis. Circulating autoantibodies are not only present at the time of diagnosis of early primary invasive cancer or pre-invasive cancer but are also found *prior* to the diagnosis (by clinical presentation and/or by radiological investigations such as mammography for breast cancer) in a population known to be at a significantly higher risk of developing the respective cancer. Based on the hypothesis that production of autoantibodies is a signal of early carcinogenesis, it is expected that autoantibodies will become detectable in the circulation at some point prior to the development of diagnosable (e.g., by radiology) early primary cancer. Longer-term longitudinal studies are required to ascertain the duration from the time of the first appearance of circulating autoantibodies to the time of such 'anatomical' diagnosis (i.e., the "lead time"). Both Soussi's report (36) and our unpublished data suggested a lead time of at least five to six months. Such a period (which in fact suggests a much longer "lead time") means that some form of prophylactic (or "therapeutic" in the real sense, because the presence of autoantibodies should imply an ongoing process of carcinogenesis) intervention may be feasible. Furthermore, exploiting the same concept of using a panel of tumor marker assays, including additional markers may prove useful for increasing assay sensitivity in the high-risk group, especially in the subgroup with genetic mutations that are often the focus of research today.

A panel of different markers may prove to be more useful in the future. In breast cancer, for example, autoantibodies to c-erbB-2 could be used. Other potential markers would include the detection of autoantibodies to the other gene products (e.g., BRCA1, BRCA2).

These studies and the resulting data indicate that autoantibody assays may have initial clinical applicability in the following areas.

- *At-risk populations*: Current clinical strategies often involve regular follow-up and imaging techniques (e.g., mammography) of individuals at risk of a certain cancer (such as breast cancer due to strong family history). First, this strategy involves the detection of cancers once they have developed. Second, current treatment strategies aiming at prevention in these individuals are based on risk assessment, since most of them will never develop the cancer. Therefore, while an individual may be at statistical risk because of a family history, few are truly at biological risk. Tumor marker assays that measure autoantibodies may be able to provide better biological information on which to base clinical advice and decisions. Health care systems stand to accrue substantial benefit in a number of areas if current screening and surveillance are superseded by serum tumor markers. Current methods do, however, have their weaknesses:
    1. Current care is based on risk assessment. The strongest of these (family history) does not take biological data into account.
    2. Imaging detects cancers when they have become established.
    3. Imaging may be uninformative. For instance, mammography is not sensitive in the majority of younger women due to their dense breast tissue. Most women with a strong family history suggestive of BRCA1 or BRCA2 mutation are, however, at highest risk of developing breast cancer before the age of 50 years.
    4. The investigations lack sensitivity in measuring the extent of disease.
    5. Some tests (e.g., ultrasonography) are operator dependent and therefore reproducibility is variable.
    6. The investigations are time consuming and costly.

- *Early diagnosis:* Potential benefits of using circulating autoantibodies as markers to detect early cancer occur in the following areas:
    1. Clinicians will be able to detect disease earlier. The panel of markers could be used to alert clinicians to biopsy small lesions that, in imaging techniques, do not appear suspicious radiographically (e.g., on mammography for breast cancer, or on ultrasound scan for hepatocellular carcinoma). The panel could also be used to carry out an early repeat test or to order alternative tests (e.g., MRI or CT scan). The marker measurements themselves should be more objective and reproducible within the limits of variation of the assays compared to current imaging tests.
    2. Patients receive direct benefits, especially from the use of serum markers. Today, patients must wait days to a few weeks for the results of some tests. Serum tumor markers could be measured on the same day. With an automated system results could even be available to the patients at the same clinic visit. Standardizing follow-up for at-risk individuals using a panel of reproducible assays should reduce variation between centers.
    3. Health care providers will be able to plan the cost of regular, standardized follow-up of at-risk individuals and cancer patients. The potential cost benefit of serum markers over radiological imaging in advanced breast cancer has already been estimated (38). The cost of sequential measurements of serum tumor markers should also be much less than the costs for imaging tests currently used to follow patients who have primary disease or of individuals attending the family history/"at-risk" clinics. Furthermore, once proven valuable, such a method of follow-up by serum markers could be carried out by the primary care physician with individuals being referred back to specialists when markers become elevated. Such a system offers potentially large cost savings.

Prognostic Value

The prognostic value of circulating autoantibodies appears controversial. Studies often involve only small series of patients. Prognostic value varies depending on which series is used, which cancers are involved, and which autoantibodies are measured (12,13,16,20–23,26,29,40–47, unpublished data from Nottingham) (Table 3).

Despite these controversial results, more recent series and our own data for the most widely studied p53 autoantibody consistently showed a poor prognostic role (16,21,26,42, unpublished data from Nottingham). These data appear to suggest that circulating autoantibodies can provide prognostic information independent of the status of the tumor-related antigens. The reason for this finding remains unclear. One possibility is that the production of autoantibodies is the consequence of the stimulation of a humoral response from overexpression of the respective tumor-related antigen at a distant metastatic site. The site may be undetectable at the primary cancer diagnosis stage but its presence indicates the systemic nature of the disease, hence resulting in a poor survival rate despite adequate treatment of the primary cancer (e.g., by surgery with or without radiotherapy). However its presence could be evident from the presence of autoantibodies, since theoretically a minute amount of antigen can elicit a significant humoral response (in vivo amplication of a carcinogenesis signal). If this is true an autoantibody assay will be much more useful in providing prognostic information to guide adjuvant systemic therapy than all the conventionally employed prognostic factors (such as size, nodal status, histological grade). These are proven independent prognostic factors that help clinicians decide if a certain patient will benefit from adjuvant systemic therapy to improve survival. However they are based on assessing the risk of dying from the disease in the future. In contrast, the detection of autoantibodies, like other blood tumor markers (e.g., CA15.3) offers a dynamic "snapshot" of carcinogenesis. As postulated above, the presence of circulating autoantibodies may already indicate the presence of micrometastases at a distant site. (Note: Post-operative measurement of circulating autoantibodies may reflect this better than pre-operative samples, as employed in most studies). Any therapeutic intervention given at this stage (as compared to the traditional administration of adjuvant systemic therapy) would have a definite value—especially in allowing the clinician to target such therapies to those patients at highest risk of developing distant recurrence and dying of the respective cancer.

Monitoring

Using circulating autoantibodies as cancer markers for clinical application is a new concept, and extensive studies are sparse. Results from studies on the potential use of autoantibody detection to monitor or follow up patients after initial treatment of their cancer have been controversial.

p53 autoantibodies remain the focus of the studies. Of 14 patients who were seropositive for p53 autoantibodies prior to surgery for superficial esophageal squamous cell carcinoma, 12 turned seronegative after resection, suggesting a potential for the monitoring of residual tumor cells post-operatively (48). In the same study, autoantibodies to p53 were found to be more sensitive than other antigen-based markers such as CEA and squamous cell carcinoma antigen. In another study of similar scale, 27 (96%) of 28 patients with colorectal cancer and positive pre-operative p53 autoantibodies became seronegative for the autoantibodies after resection of the tumor (49). Autoantibodies to p53 remained negative after 7–26 months with no evidence of recurrence detected. In another study involving ovarian and breast cancer, serial measurements of p53 autoantibodies show similar patterns with CA 125 (Figure 3) (20). Autoantibody titers seemed to reflect tumor volume since they decreased after surgery and increased after relapse.

As indicated earlier, the use of autoantibody detection to monitor disease recurrence offers potential advantages in terms of sensitivity and therefore improved lead time. Aberrant proteins expressed by the primary tumor are likely to be present in both locally recurring tumors as well as distant metastases. The re-appearance of any aberrant proteins that elicited a primary immune response in the patient will act as a re-presentation of antigen, leading to a rapid secondary immune response. Thus the presence of minimal amounts of tumor bearing the antigen will be amplified many-fold by the resultant autoantibody production. As mentioned above, pilot data on sequential serum samples from a small number of patients with recurrent and non-recurrent disease support this concept. The benefits of

Table 3 Prognostic role of circulating autoantibodies

Cancer	Autoantibody	Favorable series	Unfavorable series	Series showing limited prognostic role
Breast	Membrane, cytoplasmic antigens			(40)
	MUC1	(29)	(Unpublished)	
	p53	(41)	(12,42, unpublished)	(12,13,43,44)
	c-erbB2		(Unpublished)	
Lung (non-small cell)	Anti-neural, nuclear	(45)		
	p53		(16)	
Colorectal	p53			(20)
	Tropomyosin	(46)		
	dsDNA	(47)		
Bladder	p53		(21)	(22)
Ovarian	p53		(26)	(23)

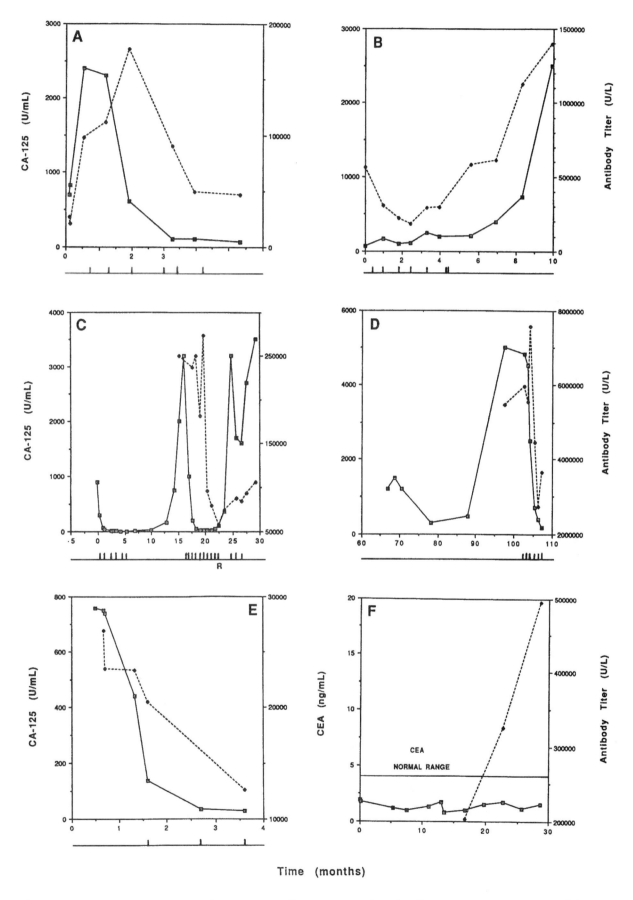

Figure 3 Monitoring five ovarian cancer patients (a–e) and a breast cancer patient (f) with CA-125 (a–e) or CEA (f) (solid lines) and with the p53-antibody test (broken lines). Surgery was performed at time 0 in all cases; laparoscopy was performed for patient e. Adjuvant chemotherapy was administered repeatedly, as shown by vertical lines below the X-axis. R 5 radiation therapy. Reprinted with permission (20)

monitoring disease recurrence using autoantibody production include the following:

- Earlier detection of recurrent disease will allow treatment regimes (local or systemic) to be initiated or altered earlier in the course of the disease. Already pilot data show that such an early intervention strategy based on established antigen-based markers of tumor bulk (e.g., CA15.3) could lead to a longer metastasis-free interval for patients who have breast cancer (50,51).
- Improved quality of life and potentially improved patient survival of the magnitude seen with adjuvant systemic therapy.
- Standardization of cancer follow-up investigations. (Currently this varies from clinical examination alone to rigorous imaging assessment.)
- Objectivity and reproducibility of the tests would be valuable compared to that characteristic of imaging tests.
- When metastatic disease is diagnosed too late, there may be time to try only one systemic therapy, which may or may not be effective. Earlier diagnosis of recurrence would allow clinicians more time to identify and deliver an effective regimen.
- Follow-up assays could be performed routinely in the primary setting, thus decreasing the number of hospital consultations required. Again, such a system of follow-up offers the potential of large cost savings.

Limitations. In a study involving 109 patients with head and neck cancer, 21 had positive p53 autoantibodies (52). Correlation between detection of autoantibodies and the clinical course of the disease was observed only in five of these 21 patients after a follow-up period of at least three years. The investigators concluded that the clinical value of using p53 autoantibodies for follow-up of head and neck cancer patients was limited.

Similarly, in a recent study of 1,006 patients with primary breast cancer (with median follow-up duration of four years), serial measurements of p53 autoantibodies did not seem to offer any informative value for detecting relapse during follow-up (53). Patients with positive p53 autoantibodies in the earlier period tended to remain positive for the autoantibodies; those without tended to remain negative throughout the follow-up period. Unpublished data from our group using historical sequential serum samples to detect autoantibodies during the follow-up of patients with primary breast cancer showed similar findings.

It is understandable that for patients in whom autoantibodies had not been detected initially, the autoantibodies tended to stay negative throughout, since a humoral response had never been successfully induced. However it remains uncertain why autoantibodies, once produced by a positive humoral response, may remain positive even after removal of the primary tumor. One possibility is that the persistently positive autoantibodies may represent a persistent antigenic stimulation from a distant micrometastasis present in the majority of patients with primary cancer (except for those with an excellent prognosis who can be considered to have been cured by surgery alone). No matter how much time has elapsed since the initial primary treatment, these patients eventually develop overt metastatic disease and die from it. Since even a minute stimulus is enough to cause a humoral response of a reasonably large magnitude, the detection of autoantibodies *per se* may not be useful to distinguish between different recurrence patterns (e.g., early aggressive recurrence vs. very late recurrence). Moreover, evidence suggests that a persistent humoral response can be due to the long-term effect of radiotherapy (8). In this instance autoantibodies can be detectable even many years after radiotherapy. This is especially relevant in patients who received post-operative radiotherapy after surgical treatment of their cancer.

While the use of antigen-based markers to monitor therapeutic response in metastatic breast cancer, for instance, is established, circulating autoantibodies have not been tested in this setting. Nonetheless some data suggest that the presence of autoantibodies (e.g., to the heat shock protein 90 [Hsp 90]) might predict a better response to neoadjuvant chemotherapy for patients with osteosarcoma (54).

SUMMARY AND FUTURE DIRECTIONS

The use of circulating cancer markers to identify symptomatic metastatic disease for most cancers is an extensively studied and well-established area of knowledge. The potential role of circulating autoantibodies as cancer markers has been reviewed especially in the difficult areas in screening and early diagnosis, where most current markers either have virtually no role or have not been exploited.

Currently, tumor marker antigen-based assays (e.g., MUC1 detected as CA15.3) have little to offer in screening and early diagnosis because of their lack of sensitivity. These markers appear to reflect the total tumor burden in the body and are therefore significantly elevated mainly in metastatic disease.

Detection of circulating autoantibodies exploits the concept of *in vivo* amplification of an early carcinogenesis signal in the form of a humoral immune response. Studies to date have shown that autoantibodies can be detectable in individuals at risk of cancer (e.g., women with family history of breast cancer and/or with ADH, individuals with idiopathic pulmonary fibrosis, chronic smokers, etc.). Autoantibodies may be found in premalignant lesions and in individuals who subsequently develop cancer. This has suggested that autoantibody production, being a humoral immune response to a carcinogenesis signal, could occur well before the clinical/radiological diagnosis of the disease, especially in high-risk groups. These findings support the hypothesis that autoantibody production implies an early carcinogenesis signal.

Longer follow-up of the at-risk individuals will confirm this hypothesis and further elucidate the lead time and change patterns of autoantibody levels prior to the diagnosis of the respective cancer. (Note: The autoantibody assay has remained virtually qualitative at this stage in most studies.) Refinement of available assays (including better definition of cut-off-based criteria) will be helpful to further improve the ability to discriminate this group from individuals who have benign conditions. Including other markers (such as autoantibodies to BRCA1 or

BRCA2 mutation products) in the panel may also improve the sensitivity of the assays in selected groups of individuals.

Cancer diagnosis and treatment have improved over the past decades. Screening has facilitated early detection (as with mammography and the cervical smear); surgeries such as breast conservation, limb-saving surgery, and sphincter-preserving surgery have reduced its mutilating effect; and adjuvant/neoadjuvant therapy has improved locoregional control and survival. Yet the majority of these approaches are based on an anatomical diagnosis (i.e., a radiological abnormality) and/or a risk estimation (e.g., a prognostic factor) to predict the benefit of a potential therapy. Similarly, potential preventive measures (e.g., tamoxifen, prophylactic mastectomy, colectomy, oophorectomy) may be undertaken as a result of a statistical risk calculation (e.g., family history, genetic mutations). The prognostic value of circulating autoantibodies remains controversial. However, it is also true that the production of autoantibodies may be due to stimulation by cancer-related antigens present at a distant site, and if so, autoantibodies may provide better dynamic and biological prognostic information than conventional prognostic factors. Future work will require that they be compared with established prognostic factors.

The positive detection of a humoral immune response in the form of circulating autoantibodies in at-risk individuals and patients with pre-malignant lesions (as mentioned above) has opened a new avenue for targeted treatment. If such immune response represented an early signal for carcinogenesis, any form of intervention would be truly therapeutic and could be instituted at a much earlier stage, based on a biological rather than an anatomical diagnosis. For instance, at-risk individuals with positive autoantibodies would be able to receive therapeutic (currently called prophylactic) interventions such as mastectomy and "chemoprevention." Therapeutic (currently called adjuvant) systemic treatment could be offered at the time of diagnosis, and potentially toxic treatments could be avoided. Therapy may therefore be better targeted, resulting in better survival and quality of life.

The studies described suggest that the use of autoantibody assays has not been particularly informative when following patients after treatment of their primary cancer, although further work is ongoing. In contrast, conventional tumor marker measurements (e.g., CA15.3 and CEA for breast cancer) have been shown to have definite potential value in this area as well as in early therapeutic intervention. It seems, therefore, that judicious measurement of circulating cancer markers (using a panel of conventional antigen-based assays as well as autoantibody assays) offers great promise for extending their current use from metastatic disease to screening, diagnosis, prognosis, follow-up, and treatment of early cancer. To establish their use and to implement them in clinical practice, manufacturers will need to further refine new assays (e.g., to improve stability, sensitivity, and specificity; to quantify for sequential measurements; to compress for rapid measurement; and to select the appropriate panel for different cancer types and population groups). Investigators will need to perform longer-term follow-up and larger randomized studies.

REFERENCES

1. Hassapoglidou S, Diamandis EP. Antibodies to p53 tumor suppressor gene product quantified in cancer patient serum with a time-resolved immunofluorometric technique. Clin Biochem 1992;25:445–449.
2. Creaney J, McLaren BM, Stevenson S, et al. p53 autoantibodies in patients with malignant mesothelioma: stability through disease progression. Br J Cancer 2001;84:52–56.
3. Metcalfe S, Wheeler TK, Picken S, et al. p53 autoantibodies in 1006 patients followed up for breast cancer. Breast Cancer Res 2000;2:438–443.
4. Robertson JFR, Pearson D, Price MR, et al. Objective measurement of therapeutic response in breast cancer using tumor markers. Br J Cancer 1991;64:757–763.
5. Robertson JFR. New criteria in response to treatment in advanced breast cancer. Doctor of Medicine Thesis, University of Glasgow 1989.
6. Cheung KL, Graves CRL, Robertson JFR. Tumor marker measurements in the diagnosis and monitoring of breast cancer. Cancer Treat Rev 2000;26:91–102.
7. Abu-Shakra M, Buskila D, Ehrenfeld M, et al. Cancer and autoimmunity: autoimmune and rheumatic features in patients with malignancies. Ann Rheumatic Dis 2001;60:433–441.
8. Poeze M, von Meyenfeldt MF, Peterse JL, et al. Increased proliferative activity and p53 expression in normal glandular breast tissue after radiation therapy. J Pathol 1998;185:32–37.
9. Soussi T. Screening and early detection of primary breast cancer: p53 autoantibodies. Presented in 5th Specialist Workshop on Blood Tumor Markers in Breast Cancer preceding the 6th Nottingham International Breast Cancer Conference. Nottingham. September 1999.
10. Green JA, Mudenda B, Jenkins J, et al. Serum p53 auto-antibodies: incidence in familial breast cancer. Eur J Cancer 1994;30A:580–584.
11. Mudenda B, Green JA, Green B, et al. The relationship between serum p53 autoantibodies and characteristics of human breast cancer. Br J Cancer 1994;69:1115–1119.
12. Huober J, Sprenger H, Costa SD, et al. Prognostic significance of p53 autoantibodies in serum of patients with breast carcinoma. Zentralblatt fur Gynakologie 1996;118:560–564.
13. Willsher PC, Pinder SE, Robertson L, et al. The significance of p53 autoantibodies in the serum of patients with breast cancer. Anticancer Res 1996;16:927–930.
14. Lubin R, Zalcman G, Bouchet L, et al. Serum p53 antibodies as early markers of lung cancer. Nature Med 1995;1:701–702.
15. Soussi T. p53 antibodies in the sera of patients with various types of cancer: a review. Cancer Res 2000;60:1777–1788.
16. Mack U, Ukena D, Montenarh M, et al. Serum anti-p53 antibodies in patients with lung cancer. Oncol Reports 2000;7:669–674.
17. Oshikawa K, Sugiyama Y, et al. Serum anti-p53 autoantibodies from patients with idiopathic pulmonary fibrosis associated with lung cancer. Respiratory Med 2000;94:1085–1091.
18. Raedle J, Roth WK, Oremek G, et al. Alpha-fetoprotein and p53 autoantibodies in patients with chronic hepatitis C. Digest Dis Sciences 1995;40:2587–2594.
19. Ralhan R, Arora S, Chattopadhyay TK, et al. Circulating p53 antibodies, p53 gene mutational profile, and product accumulation in esophageal squamous cell carcinoma in India. Int J Cancer 2000;85:791–795.

20. Angelopoulou K, Stratis M, Diamandis EP. Humoral immune response against p53 protein in patients with colorectal carcinoma. Int J Cancer 1997;70:46–51.
21. Sanchez-Carbayo M, Chulia MT, Niveiro M, et al. Autoantibodies against p53 protein in patients with transitional cell carcinoma of the bladder. Anticancer Res 1999;19:3531–3537.
22. Morita T, Tachikawa N, Kumamaru T, et al. Serum anti-p53 antibodies and p53 protein status in the sera and tumors from bladder cancer patients. Eur Urol 2000;37:79–84.
23. Angelopoulou K, Rosen B, Stratis M, et al. Circulating antibodies against p53 protein in patients with ovarian carcinoma. Correlation with clinicopathologic features and survival. Cancer 1996;78:2146–2152.
24. Angelopoulou K, Diamandis EP. Detection of the TP53 tumor suppressor gene product and p53 auto-antibodies in the ascites of women with ovarian cancer. Eur J Cancer 1997;33:115–121.
25. Gadducci A, Ferdeghini M, Buttitta F, et al. Serum anti-p53 antibodies in the follow-up of patients with advanced ovarian carcinoma. Anticancer Res 1998;18:3763–3765.
26. Vogl FD, Frey M, Kreienberg R, et al. Autoimmunity against p53 predicts invasive cancer with poor survival in patients with an ovarian mass. Br J Cancer 2000;83:1338–1343.
27. Jezersek B, Rudolf Z, Novakovic S, et al. The circulating autoantibodies to p53 protein in the follow-up of lymphoma patients. Oncol Reports 2001;8:77–81.
28. Kotera, Y, Fontenot, JD, Pecher G, et al. Humoral immunity against a tandem repeat epitope of human mucin MUC1 in sera from breast, pancreatic, and colon cancer patients. Cancer Res 1994;54:2856–2860.
29. Gourevitch MM, von Mensdorff-Pouilly S, Livinov SV, et al. Polymorphic epithelial mucin (MUC1) containing circulating immune complexes in carcinoma patients. Br J Cancer 1995;72:943–948.
30. Croche MV, Price MR, Segal-Eiras A. Expression of monoclonal antibody-defined antigens in fractions isolated from human breast carcinomas and patients serum. Cancer Immunol & Immunotherapy 1995;40:132–137.
31. Pupa SM, Ménard S, Andreola S, et al. Antibody response against the c-erbB-2 oncoprotein in breast carcinoma patients. Cancer Res 1993;53:5864–5866.
32. Disis ML, Bernhard H, Gralow JR, et al. Immunity to the HER-2/Neu oncogenic protein. Ciba Foundation Symposia 1994;187:198–211.
33. Colnaghi MI. Prognostic value of and antibody response to c-erbB-2 oncoprotein in breast carcinoma patients. Mastolo Breast Dis 1995;31:319–323.
34. Ben-Mahrez K, Sorokine I, Thierry D, et al. Circulating antibodies against c-myc oncogene product in sera of colorectal cancer patients. Int J Cancer 1990;46:35–38.
35. Korneeva I, Bongiovanni AM, Girotra M, et al. Serum antibodies to the 27-kd heat shock protein in women with gynecologic cancers. Am J Obs Gynecol 2000;183:18–21.
36. Soussi T. The humoral response to the tumor-suppressor gene product p53 in human cancer: implications for diagnosis and therapy. Immunol Today 1996;17:354–356.
37. Regele S, Kohlberger P, Vogl FD, et al. Serum p53 autoantibodies in patients with minimal lesions of ductal carcinoma in situ of the breast. Br J Cancer 1999;81:702–704.
38. Castelli M, Cianfriglia F, Manieri A, et al. Anti-p53 and anti-heat shock proteins antibodies in patients with malignant or pre-malignant lesions of the oral cavity. Anticancer Res 2001;21:753–758.
39. Robertson JFR, Whynes DK, Dixon A, et al. Potential for cost economies in guiding therapy in patients with metastatic breast cancer. Br J Cancer 1995;72:174–177.
40. Lee YT, Sheikh KM, Quismorio FR Jr, et al. Circulating anti-tumor and autoantibodies in breast carcinoma: relationship to stage and prognosis. Breast Cancer Res Treat 1985;6:57–65.
41. Porzsolt F, Schmid M, Hoher D, et al. Biologic relevance of autoantibodies against p53 in patients with metastatic breast cancer. Onkologie 1994;17:402–408.
42. Lenner P, Wiklund F, Emdin SO, et al. Serum antibodies against p53 in relation to cancer risk and prognosis in breast cancer: a population-based epidemiological study. Br J Cancer 1999;79:927–932.
43. Regidor PA, Regidor M, Callies R, et al. Detection of p53 autoantibodies in the sera of breast cancer patients with a new recurrence using an ELISA assay. Does a correlation with the recurrence free interval exist? Eur J Gynaecol Oncol 1996;17:192–199.
44. Dalifard I, Daver A, Larra F. Cytosolic p53 autoantibody evaluation in breast cancer. Comparison with prognostic factors. Anticancer Res 1999;19:5015–5022.
45. Blaes F, Klotz M, Huwer H, et al. Antineural and antinuclear autoantibodies are of prognostic relevance in non-small-cell lung cancer. Ann Thoracic Surg 2000;69:254–258.
46. Syrigos KN, Charalampopoulos A, Pliarchopoulou K, et al. Prognostic significance of autoantibodies against tropomyosin in patients with colorectal adenocarcinoma. Hybridoma 1999;18:543–546.
47. Syrigos KN, Charalampopoulos A, Pliarchopoulou K, et al. The prognostic significance of autoantibodies against dsDNA in patients with colorectal adenocarcinoma. Anticancer Res 2000;20:4351–4353.
48. Shimada H, Takeda A, Arima M, et al. Serum p53 antibody is a useful tumor marker in superficial esophageal squamous cell carcinoma. Cancer 2000;89:1677–1683.
49. Takeda A, Shimada H, Nakajima K, et al. Monitoring of p53 autoantibodies after resection of colorectal cancer: relationship to operative curability. Eur J Surg 2001;167:50–53.
50. Jäger W, Merkle E, Lang N. Increasing serum tumor markers as decision criteria for hormone therapy of metastatic breast cancer. Tumor Biol 1994;12:60–66.
51. Nicolini A, Anselmi L, Michelassi C, et al. Prolonged survival by "early" salvage treatment of breast cancer patients: A retrospective 6-year study. Br J Cancer 1997;76:1106–1111.
52. Gottschlich S, Maune S, Maass JD et al. Serum p53 autoantibodies in the follow-up of head and neck cancer patients. Oncology 2000;59:31–35.
53. Metcalfe S, Wheeler TK, Picken S, et al. p53 autoantibodies in 1006 patients followed up for breast cancer. Breast Cancer Res 2000;2:438–443.
54. Trieb K, Gerth R, Holzer G, et al. Antibodies to heat shock protein 90 in osteosarcoma patients correlate with response to neoadjuvnat chemotherapy. Br J Cancer 2000;82:85–87.

Chapter 11

Combining Multiple Biomarkers in Clinical Diagnostics—A Review of Methods and Issues

Zhen Zhang

Recent advances in genomic and proteomics research have opened a new era for the discovery and utilization of biomarkers for clinical diagnosis, staging and prognosis, and disease management. It is well understood now that what used to be considered a single diagnosis may actually consist of a number of different phenotypes with distinct disease pathways and varying genomic and proteomics expression patterns. On the other hand, molecular biomarkers discovered for a particular disease are often found in additional studies to be implicated in other disease processes.

The growing number of new biomarkers and the possible many-to-many associations between these markers and different diseases make it difficult for a practicing physician to consistently and objectively interpret, in a clinical setting, a large number of test results with often seemingly contradicting indications. It has become increasingly necessary for us to rely on computational approaches and pattern recognition techniques to derive algorithms that combine multiple clinical inputs into single-valued diagnostic indices for easy interpretation and validation.

Traditionally, the evaluation and combination of multiple variables are performed using statistical multivariate analysis methods, such as multivariate logistic regression. More recently, however, complex nonlinear models and techniques typically found in fields such as signal/image processing, pattern recognition, and machine learning have been deployed. These models and techniques all possess unique characteristics that make them more suitable than others for some problems and vice versa for others. It is important for us to know the pros and cons of these methods and understand that there is not a single method that outperforms other methods all the time. The performance of a particular method is largely determined by how well the method's underlying assumptions match the actual distributions of data.

This chapter briefly reviews some of the popular multivariate models and examples of clinical diagnostic applications that have been reported in the literature. The review is accompanied by a series of simple figures using a two-variable example (for easy visualization) to illustrate how each of these methods arrives at its decision functions. Artificial neural networks (ANNs) have been increasingly accepted as a nonlinear modeling tool for clinical diagnostic applications. A significant portion of this review is devoted to discussing the basic operations of ANNs and issues in the development of ANN models for clinical diagnostics. These issues are not typically discussed in reports on ANN clinical applications.

In the following sections, for each of the methods reviewed, one or two reports on its applications to clinical diagnostic problems are listed as examples.

A BRIEF REVIEW OF MULTIVARIATE MODELS

For clinical diagnostic applications, most computational and statistical models are derived using the so-called "supervised" learning (training) methods. In a supervised approach, one or more data sets of patients with clinical input values paired with known clinical designations are used as the training data. The models, through the learning process, extract the information and knowledge implicitly coded in the training data. The derived models will then be subjected to various test and validation processes to confirm their ability to *generalize* on new data.

The term "model" as used in this discussion in the context of clinical diagnostic applications, refers mainly to the classification decision functions resulting from such a learning process. The output of a model could be a simple "yes" or "no" answer coded numerically (e.g., 0 or 1), or in most cases, a continuous numerical value for which a cut-off value will have to be applied. Generally, such values do not directly correspond to a particular probability. However, with a sufficient sample size, it is possible to reformulate them into statistically meaningful numbers.

The simplest approach to multivariate models for clinical diagnostics is to use a "voting" panel. In such a model, each of the multiple clinical inputs individually uses its own cut-off value to produce a positive or negative result. The results from individual inputs are then combined using a mixture of logic "AND" or "OR" operators. In Figure 1a, the shaded area indicates the joint region in which both test A ***and*** test B are positive. In comparison, the shaded area in Figure 1b corresponds to the region where either test A *or* test B *or* both are positive (1). For problems with several inputs, a frequently used voting scheme is to assign a patient positive if at least m out of n tests are positive (2).

It is easy to show that such a scheme can be equivalently expressed as a mixture of AND/OR combinations. In general, the use of AND operators improves specificity at the expense of sensitivity while the use of OR operators improves sensitivity at the expense of specificity. It should be noted that the simple voting panel approach results in nonlinear decision functions. The Classification and Regression Tree (CART) analysis described later in this section is closely related to the voting panel approach (Figure 4).

Multivariate logistic regression is probably the most commonly used statistical model for combining multiple clinical inputs into a single-valued output (2–4). The decision boundary derived from logistic regression is defined by a linear function (i.e., a weighted sum plus a constant term) of individual inputs (Figure 2a). In practice, second-order terms could be introduced into the logistic regression function to explain interactions between input variables. In that case, the decision boundary is defined by a quadratic function of the inputs (Figure 2b). Fisher's linear discriminant analysis (LDA), developed in the 1920s (5), has also been widely used to derive linear or quadratic decision functions (6).

One of the most noticeable advantages of multivariate logistic regression is that the resultant model is easy to interpret. The effect of individual inputs and the interactions among them are clearly quantifiable. Statistically, using the Bayes decision rule (7), we can prove that for two classes of data (both with *normal distributions*), if they have similar distribution patterns (the two distributions have similar covariance matrices), the optimal classifier to separate the two classes is of the linear function form; otherwise, the optimal decision function would be of the quadratic form. For this same reason, the effectiveness of multivariate logistic regression could degrade noticeably when the actual data distribution deviates significantly from the normality assumptions.

A multivariate model does not have to use all different biomarkers. It could also be based on multiple measurements of the same markers at sequential time intervals. There are different ways to capture the longitudinal information in time series data. As a relatively straightforward approach, a linear regression line could be individually fitted for each patient using the multiple measurements (Figure 3a). The intercept and slope of the fitted line summarize the baseline and rate of chance of the single marker measured at time intervals. A second level multivariate logistic regression would then be used to derive a classification decision function using each sample's computed intercept and slope as its new inputs (Figure 3b) (8). Using the same approach, one could also alter the form of the regression function in the first step to extract information of more complex temporal changes. The usefulness of such longitudinal models, however, is significantly affected by a number of factors, among which are the degree of non-disease-related biological variance of the single biomarker assay and whether the duration of early-stage disease development is long enough to allow for a positive identification of the disease before it is too late.

Decision trees derive nonlinear decision boundaries by recursively partitioning the training data set so that each partition consists of mostly one class of data. A special form of decision tree is the Classification and Regression Tree (CART) method (9). The process starts with a root node representing all

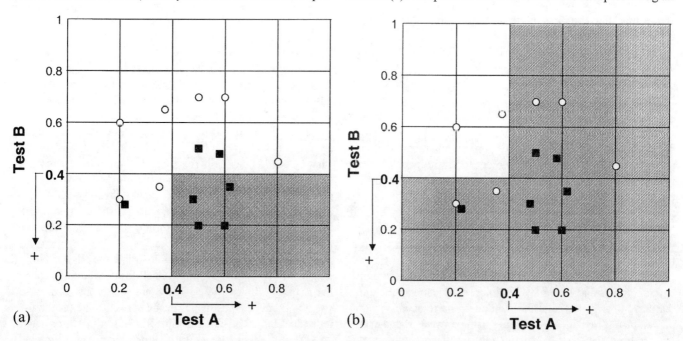

Figure 1 Combined use of multiple biomarkers with logic "AND" and "OR" operators on a fabricated data set. ■: positive cases; ○: negative cases. The shaded area indicates positive classification by the decision function. (a) A sample is positive if both test A AND test B are positive; (b) A sample is positive if either test A OR test B is positive.

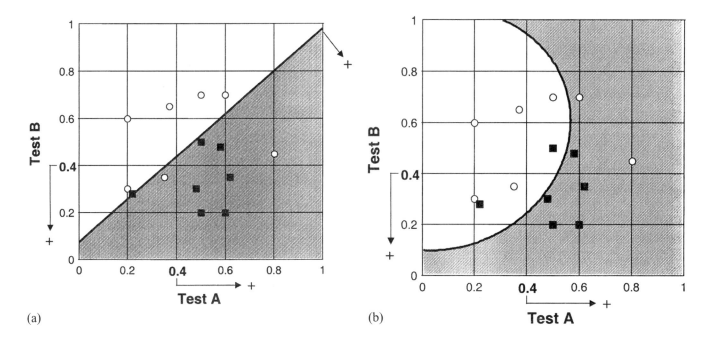

Figure 2 Results of multivariate logistic regression on a fabricated data set. (a) Linear classification function; (b) Quadratic classification function.
■: positive cases; ○: negative cases. The shaded area indicates positive classification by the decision function.

the training data. It then selects one of the variables along with a particular cut-off value that best separates the training data into two subsets such that each of the samples has more uniform class memberships. The newly formed subsets are child nodes to their parent node (in this case, the root).

The same variable selection and data partition process are repeated recursively to these child nodes. The recursive process stops when some global criteria are met. Typically, a cost function that balances improvement in classification accuracy and the number of nodes (partitions) controls the "growth" of the CART model. Due to the nature of the data-partitioning process, decision boundaries derived using CART typically have the "city-block" type of zigzag shape (Figure 4).

CART is a training data-driven approach. Unlike logistic regression, the model does not assume any particular form for its decision boundary. This makes it a powerful tool for developing nonlinear classification models. However, it suffers the same drawback of many other data-driven approaches; i.e., without proper control, the model could form boundaries between classes of data based on a few and possibly erroneously labeled training samples. Finally, it should be noted that the voting panels described earlier have similar forms of decision boundaries as the ones from CART. A human expert-derived multivariate voting scheme could be viewed as a "handmade" decision tree while a CART, once its learning algorithm has determined the selection of variables and cut-off values,

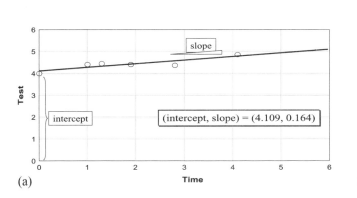
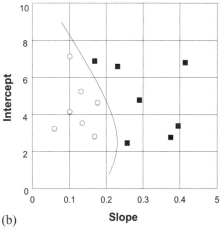

Figure 3 Longitudinal analysis of biomarkers. (a) Stage one: using linear regression to fit longitudinal data of individual patients and estimate the intercept and slope of the regression line; (b) Stage two: results of a two-variable logistic regression using intercept and slope as its input variables.

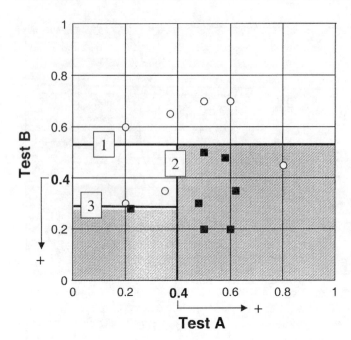

Figure 4 Results from CART analysis on the made-up data set. ■: positive cases; ○: negative cases. The shaded area indicates positive classification by the decision function.

can always be expressed as a mixture of AND/OR operations among the input variables.

Artificial neural network (ANN) has been steadily gaining acceptance as a nonlinear modeling tool among researchers in clinical diagnostics (10–12). At the conceptual level, an ANN is a collection of simple information-processing elements (artificial neurons) arranged in a particular interconnection pattern. There are many different types of ANNs with unique interconnection patterns. Multi-layer Perceptron (MLP) (13–14), however, is still the most widely used ANN architecture for clinical diagnostic applications. MLP is characterized by multiple layers of artificial neurons connected in a feed-forward fashion (Figure 5). In an MLP, a neuron receives outputs from all neurons in the layer before it, in the form of a weighted sum (including a constant term). Within the neuron, the total input passes through a sigmoid-shaped activation function that serves as a soft-shoulder switch (Figure 6). The neuron in turn sends its output to each and every neuron in the layer immediately

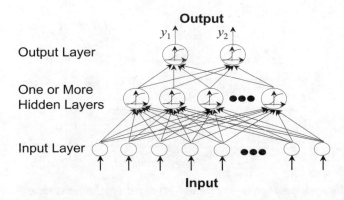

Figure 5 The generic architecture of Multi-Layer Perceptron.

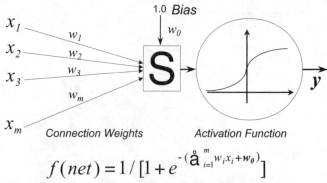

$$f(net) = 1/[1 + e^{-(\sum_{i=1}^{m} w_i x_i + w_0)}]$$

Figure 6 A single neuron and its activation function.

after it. There are no lateral connections among neurons within the same layer.

Because of this interconnection pattern, MLP is also referred to as feed-forward network. In an MLP, the first layer receives inputs from outside and the last layer produces the final output. The layers in between are called *hidden layers* and the neurons in them are termed *hidden neurons*. In most cases, the number of neurons in the input and output layers is determined by the number of inputs and the way target output values are coded. The number of hidden layers and the number of hidden neurons defines to a large degree the modeling "capacity" of an MLP. By comparison, the ANN learning algorithm has some control over the "amount" of capacity actually being used. In deriving an MLP model, the functional form of the decision boundary need not be defined beforehand. It has been proven that with a sufficient number of hidden neurons, an MLP can be used to model any functional form to an arbitrary precision (15). The difficult tasks are the selection of an appropriate ANN design with the right modeling capacity and the control of the learning process.

Support vector machine (SVM) is another supervised method that has been recently applied to derive nonlinear models for biomedical applications (16–18). Conceptually, one may imagine that the original data are first mapped using some selected nonlinear functions (kernels) to a new space with a much higher dimension than the original space. In this new space, two hyperplanes locked in parallel positions are inserted between the two classes of data to separate them (Figure 7). The data points are assigned a certain level of "softness" so that overlapping points may be (imaginatively) pushed back with resistance to allow for the insertion of the parallel hyperplanes. Through an optimization procedure, the hyperplanes eventually settle down to positions in which the resistance forces from the pushed-back data points are balanced and the distance (margin) between the two parallel hyperplanes is maximized. The hyperplane at the midpoint between the two parallel hyperplanes defines a linear classifier in the new space (an optimal soft margin hyperplane classifier). Since the functions used to map the data from the original space to the new space are nonlinear, the linear classifier in the new space corresponds to a nonlinear classifier back in the original space.

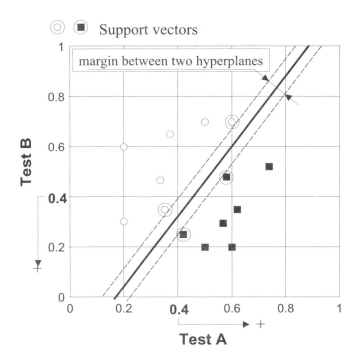

Figure 7 The optimal margin classifier that forms the basis of Support Vector Machine.

The typical SVM has several uniquely favorable qualities. Its learning process often involves only a straightforward solution to a quadratic optimization problem. It does not suffer from the possibility of being trapped in local minima during training. The SVM learning algorithm itself has built-in controls over modeling capacity, which makes over-fitting less of a problem.

However, the fundamental difficulties associated with nonlinear modeling do not disappear. The effectiveness of SVM is limited by the choice and parameterization of the nonlinear mapping function (kernels), which by no means are straightforward. In addition, the SVM classification decision function is determined by only the boundary points in the training data (the so-called support vectors). For small training data sets, the SVM solution could be very sensitive to data class labeling errors, which happens quite often in clinical diagnostic data (for example, the non-disease controls are typically assumed healthy donors—some of them may actually have the disease—or tissue samples collected from patients may be contaminated by normal tissues).

DEMYSTIFYING THE MLP NEURAL NETWORK

Artificial neural networks are sometimes criticized as being a "black box." In fact, the nonlinear classification function of an ANN can be explained in a fairly straightforward manner. Figure 6 shows the inner workings of a typical single artificial neuron. The weighted sum of its total inputs plus a bias term passes through an "activation" function to produce the neuron's output. The numerical function it implements has the equivalent form of a multivariate linear logistic regression function. It defines a linear classification function (Figure 8). In an MLP, there are no lateral connections among neurons in the same layer. Each neuron in the hidden layer, therefore, independently implements a linear classification function, which corresponds to the straight lines in Figure 9. The output neuron superimposes these multiple linear classification functions together to form the final nonlinear classification function, depicted as the curved lines between the two classes of data in Figure 9 (adopted from ref. 19) for the fabricated data in this paper).

ISSUES IN DEVELOPING ANN-BASED MODELS FOR CLINICAL DIAGNOSES

The universal modeling capacity of ANN makes it possible to capture complex relations between clinical inputs and diagnoses. This flexibility also makes it easy for an ANN to inadvertently learn from non-disease-related artifacts in the training data and then result in over-fitted models with poor predictive power on future data. There have been several review papers discussing the basic concept of ANN, the training process, and the construction of basic measures that will help avoid over-fitting (11). However, there are still a number of important issues that have not been seriously discussed in the context of developing clinical diagnostic ANN models.

Computer analysis for clinical diagnostics is often an ill-posed problem in the sense that the clinical variables available as model inputs may not provide the necessary information to account for all the variations in the diagnostic results. For a particular clinical diagnostic problem and a given training data set of a sufficient size, there is a *theoretically achievable minimum error rate* (7), determined mostly by the type of information carried in the input variables. Model over-fitting typically occurs when one does not realize the limitation of the collected clinical variables and tries to push the ANN training process to reach an error rate below what is possible. For nonlinear classification problems, there is no simple way to know this minimum error rate beforehand. A useful indication that the input variables might not be carrying enough information for the problem is that the ANN training sessions tend to flip-flop easily between not training well and performing poorly on the test data.

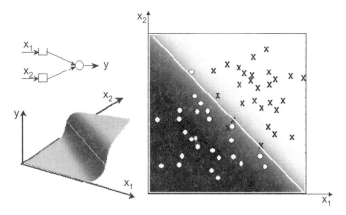

Figure 8 A neural network with two inputs and a single neuron implements a linear classifier.

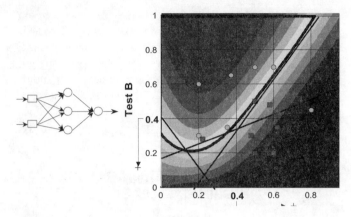

Figure 9 An MLP with two inputs, three hidden neurons, and a single output neuron. The three hidden neurons individually and independently implement three linear classifiers shown as three straight white lines. The output neuron superimposes the output from the three hidden neurons to form a nonlinear classifier shown as the black curve line. **Color representation of figure appears on Color Plate 1.**

Clinical data for ANN development are often intrinsically biased. Data sets collected from different sites, under different protocols, and with slightly different definitions of diagnoses in practice, contain non-disease-related artifacts that do not generalize from one data set to another. In order to eliminate some of the biases and to have consistent data (independently and identically distributed, or i.i.d. as termed in statistics), a common practice is to pool the data sets together and, through random selection, to divide the data into training sets and independent test sets. Doing it this way allows the model being derived to capture all possible data variations from different sites.

It must be understood, however, that by doing so, the test data and training data are artificially made to have the same distribution. When the original data are from a *limited number of sites*, the model performance estimated from such split test data tends to appear better than what the model will do when it is placed in actual "field use." In recent publications, statistical re-sampling methods, such as bootstrap, are used to obtain more stable estimation of the diagnostic performance of ANN models. However, due to the intrinsic site-to-site differences in clinical data, to validate whether an ANN model has captured the real essence of the disease process, there is no substitute for new independent test sets from sites unrelated to the those involved in the training process.

The main advantage of ANN is that the models do not rely on a predefined functional form for the decision functions. With a sufficient number of hidden neurons, an ANN is capable of forming decision functions of any given shape. However, ANN may not always be the most effective way of deriving classification decision functions. For example, when the data from two diagnostic groups all have normal distributions, the traditional logistic regression will result in the optimal results. A neural network, even though theoretically capable of forming the same type of decision functions with no sacrifice in performance, requires a much more involved training process.

For the same reason, the oft-mentioned argument about the general superiority of multivariate logistic regression or ANN is not very meaningful. The variables and interaction terms included in a regression model define the basic shape of the classification decision boundary. If the lines bordering the actual data distributions of the diagnostic groups have a similar shape, the regression approach would definitely work well and would also be the easiest. On the other hand, for a problem of a large number of input variables with scattered and interwoven distribution patterns, the selection of terms to be included in the logistic regression function could be difficult. Deriving an ANN model might be well worth the trouble.

To repeat a previous statement, there is no single method that works well for all problems. The selection of the best model requires knowledge about the problem to be solved and understanding of the characteristics of individual methods.

SUMMARY

Practicing clinicians intuitively apply the aggregation of information from multiple clinical variables. With the addition of each new piece of information, such as the result of a laboratory test, the clinician, based on his or her *individual experience*, modifies the estimated probabilities of a patient having one or more possible disease conditions. Although it will be true for a long time to come that no computational models will be able to replace this important involvement of human intelligence in clinical decision-making, the reliance on pure individual experience to analyze the ever-increasing amount of clinical information does have its limitations. The efficacy of a clinical diagnostic test is evaluated on the results of well-designed clinical studies. Those studies (and the manufacturers' product labels) usually do not provide any information about how such a test should be combined with other tests in practice. The fact that multiple tests, targeted for the same disease, often carry a considerable yet undefined amount of redundant information makes such combinations very difficult.

The multivariate models reviewed in this paper are only a small selection from a vast collection of computational models. These models have been successfully applied in other fields such as voice recognition, military target identification, and oil and gas exploration. They will certainly play a similarly important role in the new era of clinical diagnostic research.

REFERENCES

1. Woolas RP, Xu FJ, Jacobs IJ, Yu YH, Daly L, Berchuck A, Soper JT, Clarke-Pearson DL, Oram DH, Bast RC Jr. Elevation of multiple serum markers in patients with stage I ovarian cancer. J Natl Cancer Inst 1993;85:1748–1751.
2. Woolas RP, Conaway MR, Xu F, Jacobs IJ, Yu Y, Daly L, Davies AP, O'Briant K, Berchuck A, Soper JT, et al. Combinations of multiple serum markers are superior to individual assays for discriminating malignant from benign pelvic masses. Gynecol Oncol 1995;59:111–116.

3. Hosmer DW, Lemeshow S. Applied logistic regression. New York: Wiley, 1989.
4. Lette J, Colletti BW, Cerino M, McNamara D, Eybalin MC, Levasseur A, Nattel S. Artificial intelligence versus logistic regression statistical modeling to predict cardiac complications after non-cardiac surgery. Clin Cardiol 1994;17:609–614.
5. Fisher A. The mathematical theory of probabilities, vol. 1. New York, NY: Macmillan, 1923.
6. Lahousen M, Stettner H, Pickel H, Urdl W, Purstner P. The predictive value of a combination of tumor markers in monitoring patients with ovarian cancer. Cancer 1987;60:2228–2232.
7. Fukunaga K. Introduction to statistical pattern recognition, 2nd ed. Boston: Academic Press, 1990.
8. Skates SJ, Xu FJ, Yu YH, Sjovall K, Einhorn N, Chang Y, Bast RC Jr, Knapp RC. Toward an optimal algorithm for ovarian cancer screening with longitudinal tumor markers. Cancer 1995;76: 2004–2010.
9. Breiman L, Friedman JH. Estimating optimal transformations for multiple regression and correlation. J Amer Statist Assoc 1985; 80:580.
10. Wei JT, Zhang Z, Barnhill SD, Madyastha KR, Zhang H, Oesterling JE. Understanding artificial neural networks and exploring their potential applications for the practicing urologist. Urology 1998;52:161–172.
11. Rodvold DM, McLeod DG, Brandt JM, Snow PB, Murphy GP. Introduction to artificial neural networks for physicians: taking the lid off the black box. Prostate 2001;46:39–44.
12. Babaian RJ, Zhang Z. Computer-assisted diagnostics: application to prostate cancer. Mol Urol 2001;5:175–180.
13. Rumelhart DE, McCelland JL, eds. Parallel distributed processing: explorations in the microstructure of cognition, vol 1. Cambridge, MA: MIT Press, 1986.
14. Rumelhart DE, Hinton GE, Williams RJ. Learning representations by back-propagating errors. Nature 1986;323:533–536.
15. de Figueiredo RJP. Implications and applications of Kolmogorov's superposition theorem. J Math Anal Appl 1980;38:1227.
16. Vapnik VN. Statistical learning theory. New York: John Wiley & Sons, 1998:401–441.
17. Burges CJC. A tutorial on support vector machines for pattern recognition. Data Mining and Knowledge Discovery 1998;2: 121–167.
18. Chow ML, Moler EJ, Mian IS. Identifying marker genes in transcription profiling data using a mixture of feature relevance experts. Physiol Genomics 2001;5:99–111.
19. Penny WD, Roberts SJ. Bayesian neural networks for classification: how useful is the evidence framework? Neural Networks 1999;12: 877–892.

Chapter **12**

Elements of Study Design for Biomarker Development

Margaret Sullivan Pepe, Ruth Etzioni, Ziding Feng, Gary Longton, John Potter, Mary Lou Thompson, Mark Thornquist, Marcy Winget, and Yutaka Yasui

Early detection of cancer offers the greatest chance of cure. Thus, effective population screening programs are sought because they have the potential for cost-effective cancer control. Recent developments in areas such as expression microarrays, proteomics, and immunology offer new approaches to cancer screening (1). The surge in research to develop cancer-screening biomarkers prompted the establishment of the Early Detection Research Network (EDRN) by the National Cancer Institute (2). The purpose of the EDRN is to coordinate research among biomarker-development laboratories, biomarker-validation laboratories, clinical repositories, and population-screening programs. By coordinating research efforts the hope is to facilitate collaboration, and to promote efficiency and rigor in research.

With the goals of the EDRN in mind, we have recently defined a formal structure to guide the process of biomarker development (3). The development is categorized into five phases through which a biomarker must pass in order to produce a useful population-screening tool. The phases are generally ordered by the strength of evidence that each provides in favor of the biomarker. In addition, the results of earlier phases are generally necessary to design later phases. They range from the earliest exploratory laboratory-based phase to the final population-based efficacy phase. In this chapter we discuss objectives, ideal study designs, and appropriate evaluation for each phase. We refer to a forthcoming statistical monograph for sample size calculations (4).

Therapeutic drug development has had a phased structure in place for some time (5). This effort has been documented by the International Committee on Harmonization that is comprised of regulatory agencies across three continents. The clinical phases of testing a new cancer drug are as follows:

- phase 1, determinations of toxicity, pharmacokinetics, and optimal dose levels;
- phase 2, determinations of biological efficacy; and
- phase 3, definitive controlled trials of effects on clinical endpoints.

For each phase, guidelines exist for subject selection, outcome measures, relevant comparisons for evaluating study results, and so forth. Although deviations are common, the basic structure facilitates coherent, thorough, and efficient development of new therapies. A phased approach has also been proposed for prevention trials (6,7).

In a similar vein, we believe that our guidelines, or some related construct, will facilitate the development of biomarker-based screening tools for early detection of cancer. Although in specific applications deviations from these guidelines may be necessary, our proposal at a minimum provides a checklist of issues that should be addressed at each phase of development before proceeding to the next.

OBJECTIVES OF POPULATION SCREENING

The term "cancer" covers a diverse range of diseases. It is generally accepted that there are multiple affected sites and multiple subtypes of tumors. The process by which normal cells become cancerous involves numerous steps, many of which involve genetic and epigenetic changes to DNA (Figure 1).

In cancer screening, the goal is to detect tumors at a stage early enough that treatment is likely to be successful. Moreover, the mode of screening must be noninvasive and inexpensive in order to qualify for widespread application given limited healthcare resources. A substance secreted by tumor tissue, not secreted by non-tumor tissue, and easily detected in serum or urine is therefore an ideal biomarker, because the cancer is detected accurately at an early stage with a noninvasive screening test. Biomarkers, however, may be more complicated than this, and may involve measures of immune response to a developing tumor, hormonal changes induced by a tumor, or protein profiles of serum.

We use the term "biomarker" for cancer detection in a broad sense here. Biomarkers are used in other contexts that are not relevant to our discussion. For example, they may be used as indicators of risk, as surrogates for treatment effect, and as markers for precancerous lesions. Note that here we are concerned only with biomarkers for detecting existing cancer, although the development of biomarkers for detecting precancerous lesions follows a similar course and will be discussed later in the chapter.

Since most cancers have multiple subtypes, it is likely that most will require identification of several biomarkers that are

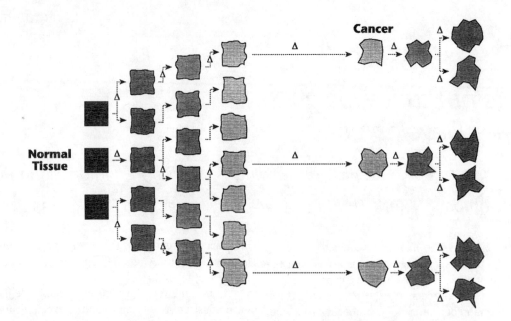

Figure 1 Multiple pathways to cancer. Δ denotes a persistent cellular change. Some pathways lead to cancer.

subtype-specific; that is, it is not likely that a single biomarker will detect a particular organ-specific cancer with high sensitivity and specificity. Indeed, biomarkers such as prostate-specific antigen (PSA) that purport to have high sensitivity, tend to have low specificity because they do not detect cancer *per se* but rather a more general process. We note that maintaining high specificity (low false-positive rates) is a priority for population screening of apparently healthy subjects. Even a small false-positive rate translates into a large number of people subjected to unnecessary costly diagnostic procedures and unnecessary psychological stress. High sensitivity, on the other hand, is important when screening subjects at high risk of disease. For example, a new biomarker for prostate cancer that is to be used in subjects that are positive for PSA should detect all subjects with cancer, while hopefully eliminating a large portion of those without. These considerations suggest, then, that several highly specific or sensitive biomarkers will be necessary for an overall sensitive and specific screening program for detecting cancer.

FIVE PHASES

Biomarker development is conceptualized as occurring in five consecutive phases (Figure 2). Each phase may be comprised of several studies to achieve different but related specific aims. In this section, we outline the basic objectives of each phase in order to provide a picture of the overall scheme.

Phase 1: Preclinical Exploratory Studies

The first step in the search for biomarkers often begins with preclinical studies, comparing tumor tissue with non-tumor tissue. These are exploratory studies to identify characteristics unique to tumor tissue that might lead to ideas for clinical tests for detecting cancer.

Immunohistochemistry and Western blotting techniques have been used for this purpose for a long time. More recent technology includes gene expression profiles based on microarrays that yield information regarding expression for thousands of genes (8), protein expression profiles based on mass spectroscopy (9), and circulating antibody levels to thousands of cancer antigens. The objective of a phase 1 gene-expression or proteomics study is to identify genes or clusters of genes (or proteins) that appear to be over- or underexpressed in tumor tissue relative to control tissue. Organ tissue, however, cannot usually be used for clinical screening purposes because its procurement is too invasive. Thus clinical assay development based on serum levels of proteins expressed by the identified genes, or on serum antibody level to those proteins, would be the task of the next phase. The basic purpose of phase 1 is to determine promising directions for further development based on knowledge gained about the biology of tumor vs. non-tumor tissue.

Phase 2: Clinical Assays with Concurrent Disease

A clinical assay based on a specimen that can be obtained non-invasively is developed in phase 2. Immune response to a protein uniquely expressed by tumor and measured with serum antibodies would be an example of such a biomarker (10). The clinical assay must be shown to discriminate subjects with cancer from those without cancer in order to be considered promising for screening. However, since the cases in a phase 2 study have established disease, with clinical assay results that are concurrent with their clinical disease, this phase does not determine if disease can be detected early with a given biomarker. That is the purpose of the next phase.

Phase 3: Retrospective Longitudinal Clinical Repository Studies

Repositories of clinical specimens collected and stored from a cohort of apparently healthy subjects who are then mon-

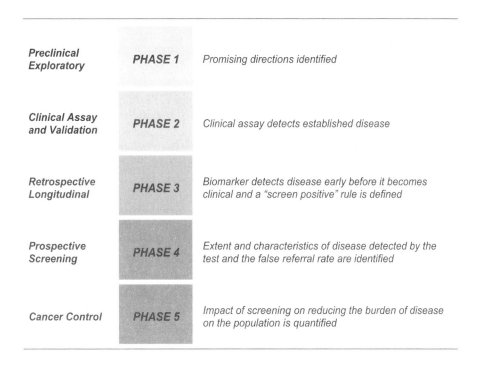

Figure 2 Phases of biomarker development.

itored for development of cancer are used in phase 3. Persons who develop cancer are identified, as are a set of appropriate controls from the cohort. Biomarker assay results on specimens collected from cases prior to their clinical diagnosis, compared with controls, provide evidence as to the capacity of the biomarker for detecting preclinical disease. If the levels of the biomarker only deviate from those of controls when the disease is close to the time of clinical diagnosis, then it will have little promise for screening. If, on the other hand, levels distinctly deviate from controls months or years before clinical symptoms appear, then the potential of using the marker for early detection is increased. In that case, criteria for "positive" screening result are defined and these will be used for prospective screening.

Phase 4: Prospective Screening Studies

The retrospective study determines if tumors can be detected early in real time, but does not establish the stage or nature of the cancer at the time it would have been detected. In a prospective screening study, the screen is applied to individuals, and definitive diagnostic procedures are applied to those who screen positive. Thus, the number and nature of cases detected with the screen are determined, as are the number of false referrals for work-up.

Phase 5: Cancer Control Studies

The final phase determines if screening reduces the burden of cancer on the population. Even if the biomarker detects disease early, there are several reasons why it might not have a substantial positive impact on the screened population. These include ineffective treatments for screen-detected tumors, poor compliance with the screening program or difficulties with implementing the program in community practice, prohibitive costs of screening and associated work-up of subjects with false-positive screening test results, and the overdiagnosis of cases that in the absence of a screening program would not be detected and would regress (11). Studies to evaluate the net impact of the biomarker-based screening are undertaken in phase 5. There should be no doubt about the net benefit in order to justify population screening. Unfortunately, for some of the screening tests currently in place, we do not yet know, with certainty, about this net benefit. Prostate cancer screening is a case in point (12,13).

Not all biomarkers will need to progress through the five phases consecutively. For example, protein mass spectrometry of serum as a biomarker might begin in phase 2. A clinical assay that potentially detects only early-stage cancer might skip phase 2 in favor of phase 3. Moreover, insights provided by studies in later phases might prompt development of an alternative biomarker that would, again, need the kind of evaluation that is done in the early phases. Although the process is not necessarily linear, the conceptual structure provided by the five phases facilitates thinking about the developmental progression. We now consider study design for each of the phases, detailing key design components for the primary objective, and listing some secondary objectives.

PHASE 1

Specific aims. Phase 1 is intended to

- identify leads for potentially useful biomarkers and
- prioritize identified leads.

Specimen selection. In phase 1, organ-specific tumor tissue and non-tumor tissue specimens are examined. Because cancer screening seeks to detect tumors that are treatable at an early stage but ultimately serious if left untreated, only such tumors are reasonable candidates for biomarker development. Tumor tissue should be obtained at diagnosis prior to treatment because treatment may interfere with biomarker behavior. It seems appropriate that a wide spectrum of tumors be evaluated in this exploratory phase (14) with attention to variability in patient demographics, histology, prognosis, stage, and mode of detection. There may be particular interest in tumors that become clinically evident only at a late stage since earlier detection of such tumors is clearly warranted. Tumors successfully detected by existing screening methods at early stages (e.g., cervical cancers) may be of lesser interest.

Non-tumor specimens are derived from various sources: non-cancerous organ tissue from the cancer patient, normal organ tissue from patients without cancer, and abnormal but non-cancerous tissue from patients without cancer (such as inflamed tissue or benign growth tissue) are all useful controls in phase 1 studies. Ideally, a biomarker will be evident in tumor tissue but not in non-tumor tissue of the cases, nor in organ tissue from non-cancer patients. In some ways, normal organ tissue from a cancer patient is the best control because differences can be attributed solely to the cancer. However, such normal tissue is not always available, or such tissue may not be truly normal if microscopic metastases are present or if cancer is preceded by widespread field changes in normal-appearing tissue. Hence, organ tissue from unaffected individuals should also be used as controls.

Matching controls with cases seems desirable in phase 1 because factors other than cancer might affect the biomarker and confound associations if such factors differ between cases and controls. In a small study, we cannot rely on random selection to yield balance. Indeed, if there are multiple factors involved, it is likely that cases and controls will differ in relation to *some* factor, due to random variability. Therefore controls should be matched to cases in regard to important factors. Normal tissue from a cancer case is, by definition, a perfectly matched control for all patient-related factors. Non-cancer control subjects should be selected so that factors potentially influencing the biomarker, other than the cancer itself, are tightly matched to those of the cancer cases. These factors might include age, sex, race, and possibly lifestyle-related characteristics such as smoking habits that might affect the biomarker and cancer risk.

Primary outcome measures. The outcome measures, or primary data items, for analysis in phase 1 are the values of the biomarkers. In a gene expression study, these might entail several hundred (or even thousands) of over- or underexpressed mRNAs. The assays to assess the primary outcome measures should be reliable and reproducible. The reliability and reproducibility should be determined before the phase 1 study is undertaken. Variability in assays or in tissue from the same subject can obscure the value of biomarkers that are otherwise promising.

Evaluation of study results. For each biomarker under consideration, one needs to ascertain how well it distinguishes between cases and controls. If a biomarker is measured on a binary scale (positive vs. negative), the true-positive rate (TPR, the proportion of cases that are biomarker positive) and false-positive rate (FPR, the proportion of controls that are biomarker positive) summarize its discrimination.

Sensitivity and specificity are commonly used terms for TPR and FPR. If a biomarker result can take many values, with larger values being more indicative of disease, a receiver operating characteristic (ROC) curve is used (15–17). Figure 3 shows data on a pancreatic cancer marker (18). The ROC curve offers these advantages over simple frequencies and summary statistics for the raw biomarker data:

- It does not depend on the scale of raw data measurements, which greatly facilitates comparison of the discriminatory capacities of different biomarkers.

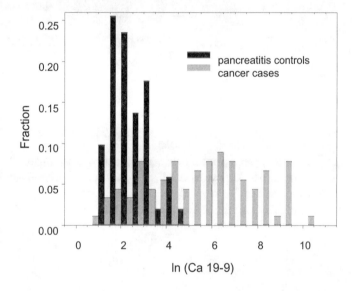

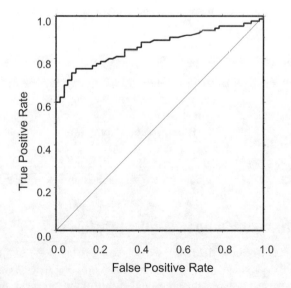

Figure 3 Histograms and ROC curve for CA 19-9 as a biomarker for pancreatic cancer (see ref. 16).

- It displays true- and false-positive rates, quantities more relevant for screening purposes than the raw biomarker values themselves.

Since low false-positive rates are of interest for screening healthy populations, that portion of the ROC curve relating to low FPRs should be the focus of data analysis for such biomarkers. On the other hand, if high sensitivity is the driving force, the focus should be on the region of the ROC curve corresponding to high TPRs.

The development of statistical algorithms for selecting promising biomarkers from a large pool of biomarkers is an active area of research (19). One simple approach is to rank the biomarkers on the basis of a summary statistic (such as the area under the ROC curve or under a portion of the ROC curve pertaining to low FPRs or high TPRs) and to select those that rank highest.

Exploratory data analysis is an integral part of phase 1. However, spurious results due to random variation occur in exploratory data analysis. If many biomarkers are under evaluation, one or more will appear to have good discrimination by chance alone. Thus, it is prudent to perform a well-controlled confirmatory study in phase 1 using a new set of tissue specimens. New outcome measures might be chosen at the confirmatory stage, such as protein expression, in a study that follows initial investigation at the mRNA level, for example.

Sample sizes. How many specimens should be tested in phase 1? This depends on the objective and extent of variability in the study. When the objective is to select a subset of biomarkers from a pool, the following factors contribute to variability: the number and relative prevalence of the cancer subtypes among the study samples; the discriminatory capacities of the biomarkers for the different cancer subtypes; the number of biomarkers under study; the number of cases and the number of controls; and the statistical algorithm used to select promising biomarkers. Simple recommendations for sample sizes, therefore, are not feasible. We suggest that computer simulations guide the choice of sample sizes; that is, simulation studies of hypothetical study data should be performed with guidance from investigators on biologically plausible models to generate data. By varying the numbers of cases and controls, one can assess which sample sizes will yield a reasonable proportion of promising biomarkers to be selected for further study.

PHASE 2

Primary aim. The primary aim of Phase 2 is to determine the TPR and FPR or ROC curve for the clinical biomarker assay in discriminating subjects with cancer from controls.

Secondary aims. These include the following:

- Optimizing procedures for performing the assay and assessing the reproducibility of the assay within and between laboratories. The assay should be reasonably simple and robust if it is to be used for widespread screening. In preparation for phase 3, the assay should also work well on stored clinical specimens.
- Correlating tissue assay results with clinical assay results for the same patients, in order to confirm that the observations in phase 2 pertain to the same source or pathway as that identified in phase 1.
- Assessing factors associated with the biomarker in controls such as sex, age, smoking behavior, etc. If such factors affect the biomarker, thresholds for screen positivity may need to be defined separately for specific subpopulations in order to keep the FPR at a low level within each screening subpopulation.
- Assessing factors associated with the biomarker in cancer cases. Similar to the preceding bullet point, thresholds may need to depend on subject characteristics in order to maintain high TPRs in subpopulations. In addition one should determine if in cancer cases disease characteristics such as stage, histology, and prognosis affect biomarker levels. Understanding the type of cancer that is detected with the biomarker is a key issue.
- Identifying combinations of markers that might work well together. If single biomarkers do not appear promising on their own, then combinations may be necessary in order to detect cancer with acceptable true- and false-positive rates. Using leads from phase 1, such combinations can be assessed in a preliminary fashion here.

Specimen selection. The same principles described for phase 1 case and control selections apply also to phase 2. The population from which cases and normal controls are selected needs careful consideration. Ideally cases and controls would be representative of those from a target screening population. However, cases and benign growth controls are often identified from a surgical clinic having been referred for biopsy or surgery on the basis of suspicious clinical findings. Normal controls from such clinics may not be representative of normal controls in the population because they, too, have been referred for some reason to the clinic. Normal control samples from a blood bank might be used but again, these may differ systematically from the target screening population. We suggest that, although selection based on convenience may be appropriate early in phase 2, final conclusions should be based on population-based studies, if possible.

Primary outcome measure. The result of the clinical biomarker assay is the primary data unit for analysis.

Evaluation of study results. Estimates of (TPR, FPR) or the ROC curve should be calculated. Note that these will likely be optimistic compared with the accuracy of the biomarker in screening for early stage cancer, because cases in phase 2 studies have clinically apparent disease.

Ideally, some target values for minimally acceptable TPR and FPR (TPR_0, FPR_0) should be decided before evaluating the data. One can then evaluate, statistically, the joint null hypothesis H_0: $TPR \leq TPR_0$ or $FPR \geq FPR_0$ using simple tests of proportions if the biomarker assay yields a binary result. The null hypothesis is that the TPR of the biomarker is too low or that the FPR is too high.

For biomarkers measured on continuous scales, the corresponding null hypothesis is H_0: ROC (FPR_0) $\leq TPR_0$ or equivalently $FPR_0 \geq ROC^{-1}(TPR_0)$ where ROC (f) denotes the true positive rate (ROC value) at a false-positive rate f. This can be tested on the basis of calculating confidence intervals for ROC (FPR_0) and for ROC^{-1} (TPR_0). For details, we refer to a forthcoming statistical textbook on the statistical evaluation of biomarkers and diagnostic tests (4).

Adjustments for multiple comparisons will be necessary if cases are to be compared against multiple control groups. Moreover, frequency matching of cases and controls, if it distorts the distribution of covariates from those in the target population, might warrant a statistical reweighting in estimating the target population's true- and false-positive rates.

Sample sizes. The sample sizes will be determined by how precisely one needs to estimate TPR, FPR, or ROC (FPR_0). One should specify desirable values for the true- and false-positive rates (TPR_1, FPR_1) and design the study so that despite random variation, a biomarker with this level of discrimination will have a high chance, $1-\beta$, of rejecting the null hypothesis, H_0, that operating characteristics are below target values. Again we refer to Chapter 8 of reference 4 for a complete discussion, along with some illustrations of sample size calculations.

PHASE 3

Primary aims. Phase 3 aims to

- evaluate as a function of time prior to clinical diagnosis the capacity of the biomarker for detecting preclinical disease; and
- define criteria for a positive screening test in preparation for phase 4.

Secondary aims. Among the secondary aims of this phase are these:

- Exploring the impact of covariates on the discriminatory properties of the biomarker prior to clinical diagnosis, including demographics, disease-related characteristics, and concomitant information on other biomarkers. If the biomarker appears to discriminate well only in certain subpopulations, this information might be used to select certain populations for prospective screening.
- Comparing markers with a view to selecting the most promising ones.
- Developing algorithms for screen positivity based on combinations of markers. Although earlier phases might suggest that particular combinations of markers work well together, formal algorithms for combining biomarker results can be developed only in phase 3 where the relative behaviors of biomarkers over the preclinical interval are established.
- Determining a screening interval for phase 4 if repeated screening is of interest.

Specimen selection. Repositories of clinical specimens collected and stored from a cohort of apparently healthy subjects who are monitored for development of cancer are used in phase 3. Subjects that develop cancer are identified, as are a set of appropriate controls from the cohort. The composition of the study cohort should reflect the target population for screening in relation to cancer and biomarker processes. Moreover, it is important that a well-defined and appropriate protocol be used for collecting, storing, and processing specimens.

The specimen collection should provide samples representative of cases and controls in the target population. In addition, the collection and processing should be those intended for general use in the population if the biomarker proceeds to large-scale application. Note that interventions may interfere with inference about the behavior of the biomarker. Therefore, cohorts in which interventions are undertaken need to be used with caution. Interventions may alter the cancer or biomarker processes, or both. Screening practices can also interfere with inference about a biomarker. For example, screening that is more intensive than is usual for the target population will affect the nature of cancer that is detected clinically, and will also affect the estimated lead time attained by the new biomarker. Simply being in a research study may alter the lifestyle and healthcare of individuals and render results about the biomarker more difficult to generalize with respect to other populations of interest.

Cases may be identified within the study or by linkage to cancer registries. The same criteria as in earlier phases might be used for selecting cases. Although multiple sequential samples are not necessary for addressing the primary aims, subjects with more specimens and a longer history of prediagnostic specimens may be preferable because they provide more information about the prediagnosis trajectory of the biomarker within individuals. However, this could also bias the case group towards slow-growing cancers such that random selection of cases should also be considered. Controls are individuals who have not developed cancer during a sufficiently long follow-up time. Matching on enrollment date and on compliance to the specimen-collection protocol might be done in a phase 3 study, in addition to matching for subject-related characteristics.

Primary outcome measure. The result of the biomarker assay again constitutes the primary outcome.

Evaluation of study results. We recently analyzed prostate cancer data from a phase 3 case-control study (20) nested in the Beta Carotene and Retinol Trial (21). The ROC curves of Figure 4 address the key question pertaining to the primary aim first. For both serum PSA markers, discrimination decreases as the time interval between specimen collection and diagnosis increases. At an FPR of 5%, the TPR for total PSA is roughly 80% at diagnosis, 60% at two years prior to diagnosis, and 40% at four years prior to diagnosis. Thus 60% of cancers could have been detected two years prior to their clinical diagnosis using total PSA as a biomarker and allowing for a 5% false-positive rate. Statistical methodology to make inferences about such time-dependent ROC curves has been described (4,20).

Consideration of the FPR is the natural starting point for choosing a threshold that will be applied for defining screen positivity in phase 4. With FPR_0 denoting the largest acceptable FPR, the corresponding threshold can be determined using data from controls. The time-dependent ROC curves determine corresponding TPRs at time lags prior to clinical diagnosis. The threshold chosen will be one that achieves an acceptable tradeoff between the time-dependent TPRs and the FPR.

Sample sizes. There are three sample sizes to consider: the number of cases; the number of controls; and the number of clinical specimens per subject. The sample sizes should ensure that,

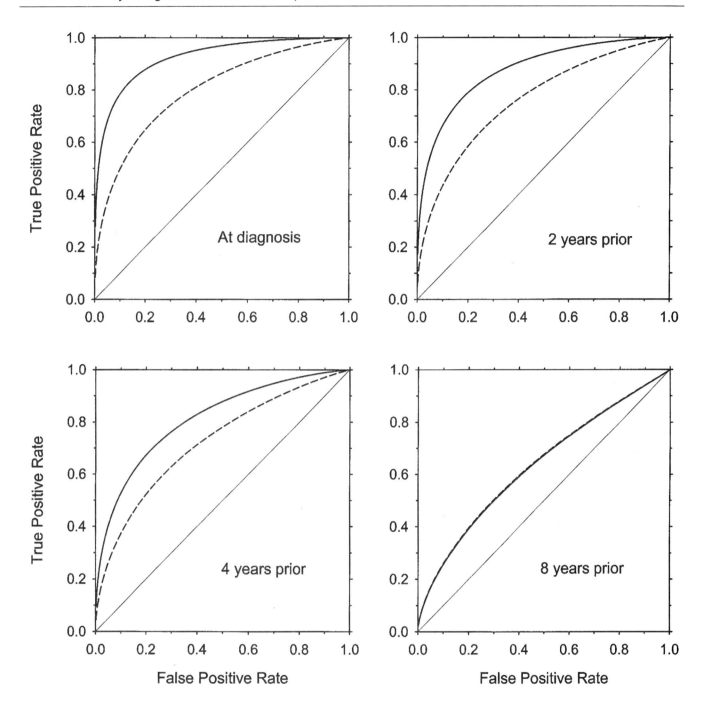

Figure 4 ROC curves for total PSA and ratio of free to total PSA at various times prior to diagnosis, calculated using a retrospective longitudinal case-control study nested in the CARET study.
——— = total PSA; ------- = PSA ratio.

for each preclinical time lag of interest (e.g., one year, two years, four years) there are enough specimens from controls and from cases close to that time such that biomarker accuracy can be estimated with sufficient precision as described for phase 2.

Although the ROC analyses of Figure 4 do not require longitudinal data, we suggest that a series of biomarker values over time from the same subjects is preferable to larger numbers of subjects each contributing only a few measurements. The longitudinal data will allow assessment of within-subject variability and more powerful comparisons of time-specific ROC curves, thereby providing better statistical evaluation of time trends in discrimination prior to clinical diagnosis.

PHASE 4

Phase 4 involves the screening and treatment of people rather than retrospective analyses of specimens. Ethical considerations, therefore, play a greater role. Moreover, since disease prevalence is low, cohort studies entail large sample sizes.

Adequate planning and piloting of studies is very important in phase 4.

Screening can be implemented as a one-time event (prevalence screen) or repeatedly at intervals over time. Although repeated screening over time may yield the best benefit, for simplicity, we focus on prevalence screening here.

Primary aim. Phase 4 aims to determine the operating characteristics of the biomarker-based screening test in a relevant population by determining the detection rate and the false referral rate.

Secondary aims. These include the following:

- Describing the characteristics of tumor detected with the screen, in particular, with regard to their potential for cure with and without treatment.
- Assessing the feasibility of screening and compliance with work-up and with treatment. Understanding factors that can result in poor compliance, for example, can lead to improvements in the screening program.
- Making preliminary assessments of the effects of screening on costs and mortality associated with cancer.
- Monitoring tumors that occur clinically but are not detected by the screening protocol.
- Comparing biomarker-based screening tests.

Subject selection. The screening cohort should be from a population that might be targeted for a screening program. One might impose additional inclusion/exclusion criteria based on disease risk, compliance potential, and characteristics identified as being related to improved test performance in phase 3. Such constraints serve to provide a setting where a useful test has the best chance of showing itself to be so, albeit at the expense of some generalizability. This seems prudent since a negative conclusion in this phase is unlikely to be expanded upon with further studies, whereas a positive conclusion will stimulate further research. An unscreened control arm should be considered in phase 4 (secondary aim 3).

Primary outcome measure. Ideally, along with the screening test result, a definitive test for cancer presence would be available for all study subjects so that true- and false-positive rates of the screening tests could be calculated. However, procedures for definitive testing, such as surgical biopsy, are invasive and can only be undertaken ethically for subjects that screen positive. Thus, negative screens are not identified as true or false negatives, which means that neither the disease prevalence nor the true- and false-positive rates are identifiable from phase 4 studies. The primary outcome measure for phase 4, which we call "the detection outcome," is one of three categories: screen positive and disease detected; screen positive and not diseased; and screen negative. This yields detection rates and false-referral rates that are defined formally below.

Secondary outcome measures. These include at least the following: tumors that occur clinically but are not detected with the screening protocol; tumor characteristics; treatment outcome; and costs of screening, work-up, and treatment.

Evaluation of study results. The detection rate is the proportion of screened subjects that test positive and are diseased, and the false-referral rate is the proportion that test positive but do not have disease. Standard statistical methods can be used to make inferences about detection rates and false referral rates. We refer to Chapter 7 of reference 4. In particular, statistical techniques for binomial proportions yield confidence intervals for these parameters. Binary regression methods are used to evaluate factors affecting the rates. Finally, methods for comparing screening tests while adjusting for concomitant factors and methods for pooling data across multiple study sites have been described (22).

Sample size. The size of the study cohort will be driven by how precisely the detection rate and the false-referral rate are to be estimated. In a comparative study, a hypothesis regarding relative performance can drive the sample size. Sample size formulas have been described for both equivalence and superiority studies (18,27).

PHASE 5

In this phase, the net impact of screening is evaluated.

Primary aim. The most important aim of this phase is to determine the reductions in cancer mortality afforded by the screening test. There should be no doubt about this net benefit in order to justify population screening. Unfortunately, for some of the screening tests currently in place, we do not yet know, with certainty, about this net benefit.

Secondary aims. These include the following:

- Determining information about the costs of screening and treatment and the cost per life saved. Health care resources are limited. Understanding costs and cost effectiveness will provide necessary information for making decisions regarding resource allocation.
- Evaluating compliance with screening and work-up in a diverse range of settings.
- Comparing variations on the screening and treatment protocols.

Subject selection. Subjects should be randomly selected from populations in which the screening program will be implemented if it is found to be successful. A standard parallel arm randomized clinical trial is ideally undertaken in phase 5 with one arm enrolling subjects to the screening protocol and the other being an unscreened control arm.

Primary outcome measure. In a randomized trial, time from entry into the study until death is the key outcome measured. In some studies, mortality only from the specific screened cancer is considered of primary relevance.

Evaluation of study results. Censored data survival analysis methods are used to compare the study arms of a randomized trial in regard to overall mortality and cause specific mortality (24). More recently methods for comparing costs and quality of life have been developed (25).

Sample size. To detect a 20% reduction in cause-specific mortality with 80% power at the .05 two-sided significance level, standard calculations indicate that 650 deaths would need to be observed in a randomized trial. Such studies in this phase are therefore huge undertakings, since the population incidence of death from a specific cancer is extremely low over reasonable study periods. Few such studies have actually been undertaken (26,27).

Computer modeling methods can be used as a preliminary step for assessing the necessity, desirability, and composition of phase 5 studies (28,29). Such models synthesize what is known about the natural history of the cancer and biomarker, treatment effects on tumor and survival, cost information, and population behavior. Screening practices are then superimposed on the model to assess the potential benefits and costs associated with screening. These models necessarily use information gained from phases 2, 3, and 4 in their construction and might be considered as an intermediate phase 4.5, between phases 4 and 5. The approach of Etzioni et al. (30), which explicitly models PSA in healthy men and in prostate cancer cases, uses estimates of sensitivity and specificity from Phase 3 studies and cancer detection rates from phase 4 studies to compare annual and biannual PSA testing. Although such phase 4.5 modeling strategies can provide insight, only a randomized phase 5 study can provide conclusive evidence on the actual impact of screening.

Case-control studies are often implemented when ethical or political considerations preclude the conduct of a randomized trial. Although not ideal, these studies, when performed carefully, can provide convincing evidence for a net benefit of screening. We refer to (31) and (32) for further discussion.

DETECTION OF PRECANCEROUS LESIONS

Biomarkers are also sought as noninvasive means of detecting precancerous lesions. For example, a serum or urine test that indicates colon polyps would greatly reduce the numbers of people requiring colonoscopy. The motivation for detecting precancerous lesions is that subjects with precancerous lesions are at high risk of developing cancer, and prevention strategies can be targeted towards these subjects in order to reduce the incidence of serious disease. Prevention strategies might include pharmacologic or behavioral interventions or more intense disease-screening practices.

Phases of development of a biomarker for precancerous lesions follow a similar path to those for cancerous lesions. Indeed, phases 1 and 2 are essentially the same except that precancerous lesions, rather than cancerous lesions, are compared with normal controls. In contrast to cancer screening, where early detection is the focus, early detection of precancerous lesions is not usually of particular interest. The purpose is simply to identify as many high-risk subjects as possible in the population. Thus phase 3 has less relevance for the high-risk biomarker than it has for the cancer biomarker. Phase 4 is simply a prevalence screen to determine detection rates and is performed without follow-up and without a control arm.

The phase 5 study for a biomarker of precancer seeks to determine if both identification of high-risk subjects and application of a preventive intervention reduce the incidence of cancer. Again, this is analogous to phase 5 for the cancer biomarker, detection of cancer being replaced with detection of precancerous lesions in this setting; cancer treatment being replaced with preventive intervention; and cancer incidence rather than mortality being the ultimate endpoint of interest. It would be natural to compare different approaches to prevention in the identified high-risk subjects during this phase.

SUMMARY

The five phases that we have described for developing biomarkers that can detect cancer are meant to provide guidance on the development process. However, these are not intended as a rigorous structure to parallel that in existence for therapeutics. Indeed, it is not clear that the same considerations apply, particularly in early phases where therapeutic studies involve patient care, whereas biomarker studies do not. The involvement of government regulatory agencies for biomarker development may not need to occur until phase 4.

Nevertheless, research groups and funding agencies do need to develop formal guidelines for biomarker development. The schema presented here may be helpful in this regard. One additional important step is to formulate criteria for when a biomarker can reasonably progress from one phase of development to another. With limited funding and specimen resources (phase 3 repositories for rare cancers are particularly precious), the research community should agree upon such criteria so that resources can be allocated in a sensible and fair fashion. These criteria include specification of minimally acceptable true- and false-positive rates for population screening tests. Acceptable rates will vary greatly with the cancer and the context in which the biomarker is to be applied and will undoubtedly require multidisciplinary panels of experts for their definition.

Such recommendations will greatly facilitate study design. Our exposition has identified additional issues to be addressed for the design of biomarker studies. Choices of cases and controls, for example, are complex and need careful consideration. Statistical methodology needs development. Indeed, the statistical issues are quite different from more classic fields for biostatistics, namely, therapeutic and epidemiologic studies. For example, new methodologies for sample-size calculations must be implemented, and algorithms for combining the results of multiple biomarkers for detecting disease should be developed.

Our discussion has focused on studies with the direct goal of developing a cancer-detection biomarker. Many studies of biomarkers are geared toward gaining an understanding of biological processes rather than being tightly bound to the ultimate objective of screening populations for cancer. We have not built in such research into the basic five-phase structure because we believe that the direct goal of detecting cancer should drive the process of identifying a biomarker. Nevertheless, studies aimed at understanding biology will naturally be included as companion studies during all phases of biomarker development. Indeed, insights gained are likely to alter the course of research and may even lead to a return to earlier phases with new ideas. As previously stated, the process is not strictly linear.

Acknowledgments

We wish to acknowledge funding provided by NIH grants GM54438–05 and CA86368–01. Our thanks also go to Pete Mesling and Noelle Noble, who helped prepare this chapter.

REFERENCES

1. Henson DE, Srivastava S, Kramer BS. Molecular and genetic targets in early detection. Curr Opin Oncol 1999;11:419–425.
2. Srivastava S, Kramer BS. Early detection cancer research network. Lab Invest 2000;80:1147–1148.
3. Pepe, MS, Etzioni R, Feng Z, Potter JD, Thompson M, Thornquist M, Winget M, Yasui Y. Phases of biomarker development for early detection of cancer. J Natl Cancer Inst 2001;93:1054–1061.
4. Pepe MS. Statistical evaluation of diagnostic tests and biomarkers. Oxford: Oxford University Press, 2003.
5. ICH E9 Expert Working Group. Statistical principles for clinical trials: ICH harmonized tripartite guideline. Stats Med 1999;18:1905–1942.
6. Greenwald P. New directions in cancer control. Johns Hopkins Med J 1982;151:209–213.
7. Greenwald P. Epidemiology: a step forward in the scientific approach to preventing cancer through chemoprevention. Public Health Rep 1984;99:259–264.
8. Schummer M, Ng WV, Bumgarner RE, Nelson PS, Schummer B. Comparative hybridization of an array of 21,500 ovarian cDNAs for the discovery of genes overexpressed in ovarian carcinomas. Gene 1999;238:375–385.
9. Merchant M, Weinberger SR. Recent advancements in surface-enhanced laser desorption/ionization time-of-flight mass spectrometry. Electrophoresis 2000;21:1164–1177.
10. Sahin U, Tureci O, Schmitt H, Cochlovius B, Johannes T, Schmits R, et al. Human neoplasms elicit multiple specific immune responses in the autologous host. Proc Natl Acad Sci USA 1995;92:11810–11813.
11. Woods WG, Tuchman M, Robison LL, Bernstein M, Leclerc JM, Brisson LC, et al. A population-based study of the usefulness of screening for neuroblastoma. Lancet 1996;348:1682–1687.
12. Guyatt GH, Tugwell PX, Feeny, DH, Haynes, RB, Drummond M. A framework for clinical evaluation of diagnostic technologies. Can Med Assoc J 1986;134:587–594.
13. Swets JA, Pickett RM. Evaluation of diagnostic systems: methods from signal detection theory. New York: Academy Press, 1982.
14. Baker SG. Identifying combinations of cancer markers for further study as triggers of early intervention. Biometrics 2000;56:1082–1087.
15. Pepe M. Receiver operating characteristic methodology. J Amer Stats Assoc 2000;95:308–311.
16. Wieand S, Gail MH, James BR and James KL. A family of nonparametric statistics for comparing diagnostic markers with paired or unpaired data. Biometrika 1989;76:585–592.
17. Dudoit S, Fridlyand J, Speed T. Comparison of discrimination methods for the classification of tumors using gene expression data. Technical Report #576, Dept of Statistics, University of California Berkeley, 2000.
18. Etzioni, R, Pepe MS, Longton G, Hu C, Goodman G. Incorporating the time dimension in receiver operating characteristic curves: a prostate cancer case study. Med Decis Making 1999;19:242–251.
19. Thornquist MD, Omenn GS, Goodman GE, et al. Statistical design and monitoring of the carotene and retinol efficacy trial. Control Clin Trials 1993;14:308–324.
20. Pepe MS, Alonzo TA. Comparing disease-screening tests when true disease status is ascertained only for screen positives. Biostatistics 2 2001;3:249–260.
21. Kramer BS, Gohagan JK, Prorok PC. Is screening for prostate cancer the current gold standard? Eur J Cancer 1997;33:348–353.
22. The International Prostate Screening Trial Evaluation Group. Rationale for randomized trials of prostate cancer screening. Eur J Cancer 1999;35:262–271.
23. Alonzo T, Pepe MS, Moskowitz CS. Design of studies to compare accuracy of tests for detecting presence of disease. Stats Med 2002;21(6):835–852.
24. Collett D. Modeling survival data in medical research. London: Chapman and Hall/CRC, 1994.
25. Lin DY, Feuer EJ, Etzioni R, Wax Y. Estimating medical costs from incomplete follow-up data. Biometrics. 1997;53:419–434.
26. Kramer BS, Gohagan J, Prorok PC, Smart C. A National Cancer Institute-sponsored screening trial for prostatic, lung, colon, and ovarian cancers. Cancer 1993;71:589–593.
27. Gohagan JK, Prorok PC, Kramer BS, Cornett JE. Prostate cancer screening in the prostate, lung, colorectal, and ovarian cancer screening trial of the National Cancer Institute. J Urol 1994;152:1905–1909.
28. Ross KS, Carter HB, Pearson JD, Guess HA. Comparative efficiency of prostate-specific antigen screening strategies for the prostate cancer detection. JAMA 2000;284:1399–1405.
29. Urban N, Drescher C, Etzioni R, Colby C. Use of a stochastic simulation model to identify an efficient protocol for ovarian cancer screening. Control Clin Trials 1997;18:251–270.
30. Etzioni E, Cha R, Cowen M. Serial prostate-specific antigen screening for prostate cancer: a computer model evaluates competing strategies. J Urol 1999;162:741–748.
31. Weiss N. Case-control studies of the efficacy of screening for cancer: can we earn them some respect? J Med Screen 1997;4:57–49.
32. Selby J, Friedman CQ Jr, Weiss N. A case-control study of screening sigmoidoscopy and mortality from colorectal cancer. New Eng J Med 1992;326:653–657.

Chapter 13

Biomarkers as Therapeutic Targets: Toward Personalized Treatments in Oncology

Massimo Gion and Giampietro Gasparini

It has been well established that cytotoxic agents are only partially effective in solid tumors for at least three reasons:

1. the available cytotoxic and hormone treatments have a suboptimal efficacy, as shown by the low rate of complete response obtained in advanced disease;
2. tumors are capable of developing resistance to chemotherapy (1); and
3. most of the standard treatments currently used in oncology have been evaluated in prospective, controlled Phase III studies, in which homogeneous groups of patients are randomized to receive different therapeutic options. Although this strategy has achieved meaningful results in the treatment of acute leukemia and lymphomas, it presents intrinsic drawbacks for the cure of solid tumors.

The case of adjuvant therapy for invasive breast cancer is a paradigmatic example, considering that only 30% of patients experience clinical benefit from treatment (2). The wide variability of the efficacy of cytotoxic therapy in solid tumors is partly related to the outdated concept of homogeneity with reference to the clinico-pathological stage, which does not take into account the heterogeneity of human malignancies. In fact, patients with similar clinical and pathologic features may harbor malignancies with different biological characteristics (3).

While the reasons for tumor heterogeneity are complex and poorly understood, genetic polymorphism certainly plays a pivotal role. Most invasive solid tumors are characterized by genomic instability (4) such that all types of human malignancies are ultimately comprised of several cell clones that synergistically contribute to tumor growth and metastatic progression (5). In addition, the stromal cell components and the microenvironment in which the malignancy is harbored actively contribute to tumor growth (6). Genomic instability, cell heterogeneity, and microenvironmental factors (7,8) give every tumor an exquisite biological individuality.

THE SCENARIO: TOWARD A NEW VISION OF CANCER

The understanding of this growing complexity and the awareness of its relationship with the clinical outcome prompt the need to move away from the classical classification of cancer patients according to pathological stage and toward a molecular characterization of each individual patient.

A molecular classification of human acute leukemia according to gene expression using DNA microassays has been proposed and successfully applied for therapeutic decisions by Golub et al. (5). Also, Caldas (9) showed that the genetic profile of both the patient and the malignancy were effective in predicting clinical outcome and responsiveness to different treatments. A new discipline focused on the study of the relationship between the genetic pattern of patient tissues and the response to diverse agents under investigation (pharmacogenomics) has been developed (10). Basic and translational research studies are therefore moving toward a re-classification of tumors on the basis of their molecular characteristics and, ultimately toward an individually tailored anti-cancer therapy (11–13).

This new vision of cancer as a complex and heterogeneous group of diseases risks considering cancer cells as an anarchic biological machinery and, of major concern, of going toward deregulated, arbitrary therapeutic approaches. Therefore, some common alterations and pathways of progression should be identified (14).

Recently, Hanahan and Weinberg (14) suggested grouping alterations of cell physiology related to cancer development in six principal categories (Table 1). This seems a valuable starting point for a new systematized vision of a "constellation" of diseases commonly called cancer.

BIOMARKERS: PROMISES AND PITFALLS OF AN OLD PLAYER IN A NEW GAME

Tumor-associated biomarkers have been studied and used for more than 30 years as a tool for monitoring cancer patients. In

Table 1 Major biological mechanisms responsible for cancer development and progression

Mechanism	Molecular pathways involved
Self-autonomy in growth signals	- Oncogene activation or overexpression - Altered cell-to-cell growth signaling - Altered parenchymal-stromal relationship
Insensitivity to anti-growth signals	- Downregulation of oncosuppressor genes - Lack of soluble growth inhibitors
Resistance to apoptosis	- Altered balance between sensor and effectors of the apoptotic machinery - Mutation of the tumor suppressor *p53* gene
Limitless of the replicative potential	- Genetic alterations with telomere maintenance
Altered and sustained angiogenesis	- Altered balance of angiogenesis inducers and naturally occurring inhibitors
Tissue invasion and metastasis	- Cascade of complex genetic and biochemical alterations involving tumor cell, stromal cell and extacellular matrix

Modified from reference (14).

general, they have been considered coarse indicators of tumor extension. In the last few years, several biomarkers that are associated with well-known mechanisms of the cancer cell machinery have been identified; these new biomarkers seem to be the ideal candidate for linking the biological mechanism to a given clinical behavior and may lead the way to the development of dedicated and specific therapeutic agents.

However, the timely implementation of biomarkers in clinical practice is limited by the poor consensus on their potential clinical usefulness, since clinical studies on biomarkers frequently report conflicting results. Discrepancies among different studies may be due to several problems. First of all, the complexity of cell biology is too often oversimplified for practical reasons by relating only few biomarkers to a given biological mechanism. Secondly, a poor standardization of laboratory procedures, including both analytical and preanalytical phases, may be responsible for spurious variability of results. Third, decision levels are frequently arbitrarily chosen on the basis of conventional or "historical" criteria and are not properly validated.

The Complexity of Cancer Cells: How Many Biomarkers?

The role of the estrogen receptor (ER) in breast cancer is a prime example of the risk of biases due to the underlying biological complexity when using a biomarker in therapeutic decision-making. For more than 30 years, the determination of ER in tumor tissue has been used as the sole, valuable tool for submitting breast cancer patients to hormone therapy. Even in light of this simple approach, the biological complexity of ER machinery has progressively become apparent. Two different ERs have been identified (ERα and ERβ), which are diversely expressed in different tissues and may operate synergistically or independently (15), and several ER variants with impaired or modified functions have been described (16). Moreover, the biological actions of estrogens have been shown to be modulated by nuclear proteins that may enhance (co-activators) or prevent (co-repressors) ER-induced transcription (17). In addition, different ligand-independent activation mechanisms have been shown (18,19). This growing bulk of evidence is the basis for the development of new agents aimed at selective ER modulation (SERM) suitable for both cancer treatment and chemoprevention (20).

The Analytical Phase: Need for Continuous Standardization

Biomarkers may be determined using different approaches, i.e., gene expression, mRNA transcription, protein concentration, or biological activity. The choice of different analytical options may be a significant source of variability when comparing results from different investigations. Studies on HER-2/neu determination using either immunohistochemistry (IHC) or fluorescent *in situ* hybridization (FISH) represent a typical example of this problem (21). For the majority of cancer biomarkers the reference method has not yet been established. Therefore, the choice of the method is frequently based on the scenario in which the biomarker will be used; for instance, IHC may be the candidate method for a routine use, while more sophisticated biochemical approaches might be indicated for basic investigational purposes.

In addition, intrinsic potential causes of variability may occur within every individual analytical method type due to diverse factors, such as assay architecture, reagent type, etc. The IHC detection of HER-2/neu provides a meaningful example of this. Press et al. (22), reviewing the results obtained using 28 different antibodies for HER-2/neu immunochemistry, showed that 18 of them detected HER-2/neu expression when the oncogene was amplified five-fold or more, while only 12 of these 18 still provided a positive staining when the antigen was amplified only two- to five-fold.

The molecular complexity of biomarkers may introduce unexpected biases in assay results, even using the same method and the same reagents, when the molecular structure of the antigen changes in different functional statuses. Dittadi et al. (23) found that ER concentrations obtained with a commercially available, standardized enzyme-immunoassay, were consistently different in the same tissue sample when buffers with different ionic strength were used for cytosol preparation. This was due to the different reactivity of one the monoclonal antibodies used in the kit for the different functional statuses of ER. It is worth noting that these latter causes of variability may be responsible for discrepancies that can be ignored, since they occur using a method that is expected to provide reproducible results.

The use of molecular biology techniques for the detection of biomarkers is sharply growing in basic and clinical laboratories (24) and is expected to play a pivotal role in the near future. Promising results obtained to date, and their exciting potential clinical applications, should be considered with caution and mitigated by the awareness of the low level of standardization of the analytical methods. Several possible sources of variability must be taken into account, strictly standardized and monitored, such as the organization of working spaces (25), the quality and stability of reagents used (26), the choice of probes, stringency conditions, and so forth. The detection of circulating tumor cells by reverse transcriptase (RT) PCR provides a meaningful example of the problems that may occur using nonstandardized strategies. Neumaier et al. (27), reviewing the results of a number of investigations on circulating mRNA of PSA published over eight years, concluded: " . . . positive PSA RT-PCR results range from 25% to 80% for metastatic patients. Definitive conclusions about the clinical relevance of this new molecular tool have not yet been established. The heterogeneity of both preanalytical and analytical steps of PCR protocols may explain the discrepancies observed between studies. . . . " These conclusions may be applied to the majority of studies on cancer biomarkers performed so far with molecular biology techniques.

Preanalytical Phase: Pitfalls of an Apparently Simple Procedure

The procedures for sample collection, handling, storage, and preparation require standardization in order to guarantee comparable results among samples either from different patients or collected from the same patient over time. The importance of the preanalytical phase is perceived differently for tissue and blood specimens. It is well known that several preanalytical variables may significantly affect IHC results; therefore, reliable laboratories should standardize the type of fixative, time of fixation, inclusion method, time of paraffin embedding, thickness of the sections, storage of unstained slides, and the methods for antigen retrieval. Standardization is also a goal when applying biochemical methods to tissue extracts. Since 1979, the Receptor & Biomarker Group of EORTC set up the standardized procedure for sample preparation (28) that is currently used for ER and progesterone receptor determination by both enzyme immunoassay and radioligand binding assay. This strategy permitted a widespread use of the standardized protocol for tissue preparation that has been advantageously used for the evaluation of other cytosol biomarkers in breast cancer, such as UPA/PAI-1, leading to meaningful clinical results in a relatively short time (29).

Problems with standardization of the preanalytical phase are not restricted to the determination of biomarkers in the tissue. The assay of circulating vascular endothelial growth factor (VEGF) provides a clear example of the potential biases related to the lack of standardization of blood collection. Several investigators showed quite different VEGF concentrations in different blood derivatives, including serum, plasma collected with different procedures, and whole blood hemolysate (30). In addition, Dittadi et al. recently showed that the release of VEGF in serum during the clotting process increases over time up to a plateau, in a significant manner that is reached generally within two to four hours (30). This is not surprising since VEGF is present and released by both platelets and nucleated blood cells. However, in spite of these findings, several investigators studied serum VEGF in various malignancies and published promising results on serum VEGF as a cancer biomarker, without providing any information concerning the standardization of sample preparation. Unfortunately, the problem of sample standardization for the determination of circulating VEGF has not been considered even in a very recent review article in which the potential clinical role of the marker is extensively discussed (31).

A number of biomarkers related to molecular mechanisms of cell growth and control are measurable in biological fluids using commercially available methods. Adhesion molecules, markers of apoptosis, products of oncogenes and oncosuppressor genes, and angiogenic factors are among the most promising ones and allow for the investigation of intricate biochemical mechanism through a relatively simple laboratory approach. This prompts an increasing use of several markers prior to valuable laboratory validation. When scrutinizing published studies on clinical evaluation of biomarkers, it is quite infrequent to find international criteria of analytical validation (i.e., NCCLS) either applied or even quoted (32). The uncritical use of laboratory data obtained with nonstandardized approaches risks increasing the confusion on the actual biological role and clinical usefulness of new biomarkers.

Commercially available assay kits, in which all procedures are indicated by the manufacturer, should not be intended as fully standardized methods. Both preanalytical and analytical phases should be further validated through stringent protocols before using the biomarker for clinical purposes. During the preclinical validation of a biomarker, the centralization of assays in a few laboratories may be helpful. Thereafter, when a wider clinical evaluation is carried out, the adherence to standardization should be continuously monitored and both internal and external quality assurance programs be performed.

Decision Criteria: A Critical Area of Investigation

The results of biomarker determination are usually expressed as positive or negative with reference to a conventional cut-off value for both routine use and clinical investigations. These criteria have been used for both practical and historical reasons. However, the dichotomous use of a biomarker categorized according to a cut-off point relies on the assumption that it has a yes/no relationship with clinical outcome. This conventional oversimplification does not reflect cancer biology; considering that many biological phenomena occur in a continuous rather than a discrete manner, one should expect that biomarkers correlate with prognosis or prediction of response to therapy as continuous variables. Actually, several investigators showed that biomarkers elicit continuous (either monotonic or not monotonic) relationships with clinical outcome. In addition, biomarkers may interact with each other in a complex manner, thus modifying the clinical information they provide when individually considered. The use of a dichotomic decision criterion may reduce the value of the biomarker when continuous monotonic relationships occur, since cases with a variable degree of association with prognosis are artifactually combined. Toi et al. (33) found that increasing values of p53 protein concentration in breast cancer cytosol are associated with a continuously increasing risk of relapse. Also, Gion et al. showed a continuous relationship between increasing cytosol levels of the cytokeratin-associated marker TPA (Tissue Polypeptide Antigen) and a better prognosis in patients with node-negative breast cancer (34). Coradini et al. recently reported a continuous relationship between ER and prognosis when the biomarker was examined over a long follow-up period (35).

The occurrence of nonmonotonous relationships may cause even more meaningful biases when using a positive/negative cut-off point. In patients with node-negative breast cancer, Gasparini et al. (36) found that increasing levels of VEGF in tumor cytosol were associated with a worse prognosis up to a VEGF concentration of about 900 pg/mL; unexpectedly, for further increasing VEGF concentrations, the marker was associated with a better prognosis. Cases with opposite prognosis would have been included in the same group using a positive/negative cut-off point, thus probably obscuring the true prognostic value of the biomarker. A nonmonotonous association between cytosol HER-2/neu and prognosis was also shown in node-negative breast cancer patients by Dittadi et al. (37). Very low and very high HER-2/neu levels were poor prognostic indicators, while intermediate values were associated with a more favorable outcome. Complex interactions between biomarkers and clinical outcome have been reported by several investigators (38–41). Dittadi et al. (38) found that high cathepsin D cytosol levels could elicit opposite predictive values if the interaction with pS2 was considered: high cathepsin D was associated with a favorable outcome if pS2 concentration was low, while prognosis was very poor when both markers were elevated. The same value of cathepsin D provided opposite prognostic indication when the interaction with pS2 was considered.

The use of positive/negative cut-off points is certainly an advantageous approach for routine use, since it allows for an easy application and interpretation of the biomarker. However it presents several pitfalls, a situation excellently reviewed by Altman (42). Dichotomous criteria may be eventually used for practical reasons after a preliminary evaluation of the biomarker analyzed on the original measurement scale, that in many instances (always in biochemical methods) is a continuous variable. This allows for a thorough exploration of the relationships between the biomarker and clinical outcome, possibly maximizing the knowledge of the underlying biological complexity (43).

In spite of both published evidence and recommendations of statisticians, the majority of published studies still categorize biomarkers with reference to cut-off points (44). We reviewed 57 studies focused on evaluation of the prognostic/predictive value of ER on more than 51,000 patients, published from 1996 to 1999, and selected studies that

- evaluated more than 100 patients,
- measured ER with biochemical assays, and
- performed multivariate analysis.

Overall, ER was categorized using a conventional cut-off point in 47 out of 57 studies; seven studies used two to four cut-off levels; and only three studies (5%) evaluated ER on its original continuous scale of measurement. Therefore, irrespective of general agreement on the complexity of the relationship between biomarkers and clinical outcome, most of the published investigations are still performed using a simple dichotomous classification.

Standardization for Biomarker-Based Studies: An Emerging Need

The continuous improvement of investigations on new therapeutic agents and/or modalities is a strategic issue in clinical oncology. Not surprisingly, several initiatives aimed at standardizing the methodology for planning, performing, and reporting clinical trials and the criteria for peer-reviewed clinical studies have been endorsed by the editors of different international journals (45,46). On the contrary, efforts to standardize the use of biomarkers in clinical studies have been only anecdotally considered (47,48). Study protocols of clinical trials are therefore comprehensive regarding patient inclusion, treatment modalities, response evaluation, and side effects while they are often weak when dealing with biological evaluations.

The use of classical biomarkers mainly related to tumor extension has not critically affected the clinical outcome of pharmacological trials. This may in part justify the poor care that has been so far dedicated to the laboratory side of clinical trials. However, the scenario is rapidly changing with the advent of new molecular-targeted anti-cancer agents that call for a reliable and optimized use of specific biomarkers for their cost-effective clinical use. In this new setting, unrecognized analytical biases may ultimately impair the identification of the real effectiveness of therapeutic agents. Keeping in mind the criteria used in pharmacological trials, we recently prepared a three-phase approach for translating a biomarker "from the idea to the cure" (49) and proposed tentative criteria to choose, standardize, and use biomarkers in clinical trials (50). This approach is summarized in Tables 2–4. A similar approach has been developed by Pepe et al. for the evaluation of biomarkers in early cancer diagnosis (51).

MOLECULAR-TARGETED AGENTS: REALLY A NEW ANTI-CANCER TOOL?

The anti-cancer therapy based on molecular-targeted agents relies on different biological principles than cytotoxic chemotherapy (Table 5). The action of most molecular-targeted agents is cytostatic, while chemotherapy is mainly cytotoxic.

Table 2 Protocol for evaluation of predictive surrogate markers to be tested in clinical trials

	Phase I: Basic preclinical standardization
General requirements	– Centralization of evaluation in one laboratory (mandatory)
Choice of the biomarker(s)	– Relationship with the biological mechanism of interest
	– Non-redundancy with other biomarkers already available and evaluated
Choice of the method	– Reliability
	– Robustness (stability of assay performances)
	– Feasibility for possible routine setting
Standardization of the method	– Identification, optimization, and standardization of the analytical steps
	– Evaluation of analytical performances
Standardization of the pre-analytical phase (sample handling and preparation and storage)	– Identification of the analyte distribution in different compartments (tissue components and sub-fractions, different blood derivatives, i.e. serum, EDTA-plasma, citrate-plasma, etc) (when appropriate)
	– Optimization and standardization of sample collection
	– Optimization and standardization of procedures for sample preparation
	– Evaluation of analyte stability for a different time length and at different storage conditions
Design of a quality assurance program	– Choice and preparation of the appropriate biological material
	– Design of the program

Modified from reference (50).

The ultimate goal of these new agents is the control of tumor growth, as opposed to the tumor-cell-killing mechanism of cytotoxic drugs. Anti-angiogenic agents are a good example; as shown by Holmgren et al. (52), the inhibition of neovascularization induces tumor dormancy and enhances apoptosis. The different mechanism of action is the basis of synergy with conventional anti-cancer treatments. Anti-angiogenic agents (53), humanized antibodies to HER-2/neu (54), inhibitors of epidermal growth factor receptor (EGFR) (55), and farnesyl transferase inhibitors (FTase) (56) potentiate the efficacy of chemotherapy in some experimental models both in vitro and in vivo (57).

The synergistic anti-tumoral activity of combined anti-angiogenic and anti-proliferative agents or radiation therapy may be explained by the hypothesis of the double-targeting effect. The different therapeutic agents elicit their activity respectively against the parenchymal and the stromal components of the malignancy, thus impairing reciprocal paracrine stimulatory action (58). A further postulated difference between cytotoxic chemotherapy and molecular-targeted agents is the lower probability of the latter to develop drug resistance (59). All these characteristics stand for favorable toxicological profiles; if these preliminary results are confirmed in the clinical setting, these new agents will allow for a more effective chronic administration, such as that required in adjuvant treatment, maintenance setting, and chemoprevention programs. Such new anti-cancer agents are therefore expected to enhance the curative potential of conventional existing anti-cancer therapy rather than replace them.

MULTIPLE ROLES OF BIOMARKERS

The molecular pathways to which molecular-targeted specific treatments are presently under extensive research and clinical development are shown in Table 6. Biomarkers may have two principal roles in the clinical application of new molecular-targeted agents:

Table 3 Protocol for evaluation of predictive surrogate markers to be tested in clinical trials

	Phase II: Baseline clinical evaluation
General requirements	– Centralization in one laboratory (recommended)
	– Sample collection from different institutions is admitted
	– Retrospective evaluation pending the validation of standardization of the pre-analytical phase
Preliminary clinical evaluation	– Evaluation of the biomarker in healthy controls/normal tissue
	– Relationship of the marker with basic demographic characteristics of the patients (age, sex, lifestyle, menstrual history, etc.)
	– Relationship of the marker with basic characteristics of the tumor (stage, histological type and grade, other established biomarkers, etc.)
Standardization of the pre-analytical phase (clinical)	– Identification of causes of spurious results (demographic, clinical, pharmacological, etc.)
Choice of decision levels	– Identification of tentative decision levels in the group of patients of interest (trial group)

Modified from reference (50).

Table 4 Protocol for evaluation of predictive surrogate markers to be tested in clinical trials

	Phase III: Evaluation of clinical utility
General requirements	– Multi-center prospective enrollment of patients (and collection of samples) is usually necessary for the study size to be adequate for reliable conclusions – A dedicated external quality assurance program is mandatory – Study design appropriate to clinical goal(s)
Training of the staff(s) of participating institutions	– Survey facilities and expertise of laboratories of participating institutions – Preparation of detailed protocols with standardized procedures for both pre-analytical and analytical phases – Preliminary educational programs addressed to laboratory aspects for participating institutions – Preliminary to clinical studies, check the analytical reliability on a panel of samples sent to participating laboratories (ring trial)
Data collection	– Preparation and distribution of a database to be used in all the participating institutions
Validation of decision levels	– Validation of decision levels in different groups of patients with comparable characteristics (testing group) (when appropriate)
Quality assurance and monitoring	– Distribution of quality control material – Monitoring quality assurance results – Periodical survey of the adherence to the protocol in each participating institution

Modified from reference (50).

1. the prediction of the probability of responsiveness to a given agent and
2. the early prediction of response or failure to a given agent in long-term treatment plans.

In the former case they are *predictive biomarkers* for the selection of the patients to treat; in the latter they are *surrogate biomarkers* of the clinical outcome.

Predictive Biomarkers

The classification of malignancies using biomarkers is the basis for the development of molecular-targeted treatments and may eventually lead to individually tailored anti-cancer therapy (9–13). The ideal biomarker should select patients who have a high likelihood of gaining benefit from the specific agent targeting the biologic pathway to be pharmacologically modulated. ER expression in tumors has been used for more than 30 years as a predictive factor for hormone therapy in breast cancer, the first molecular-targeted treatment in cancer therapy. In spite of this consolidated practice, biomarkers are often used in a nonstandardized manner or not applied at all when testing new molecular-targeted agents. This point of weakness of clinical research should be amended quickly, given the foreseeable scenario of cancer therapy. Indeed, more than 400 new molecular-targeted anti-cancer agents are presently under investigation and some of them are being applied in clinical trials. A chimerical antibody (trastuzumab) against the extracellular domain of HER-2/neu, a member of type I growth factor receptor gene family, was approved by the US Food and Drug Administration (FDA) in 1998 for the treatment of patients with metastatic breast cancer overexpressing HER-2/neu in the primary tumor (60).

A proper evaluation of predictive biomarkers will allow for multi-target strategies as different molecular mechanisms are discovered to converge in tumor growth and progression. Several experimental models showed the association between angiogenesis and other biological pathways related to cell growth control. Some well-documented examples are:

- Tumor suppressor genes (p53/p21, Von Hippel-Lindau);
- Oncogenes (ras, fos, HER-2/neu);
- Adhesion molecules and enzymes involved in tumor invasiveness and metastasis (integrins, metalloproteinases);
- Apoptosis (Braf, TNF-α);
- The immune system (59);
- Hypoxia (61); and,
- Nitric oxide and a variety of hypoxia-induced genes (plasminogen activator inhibitor-1, insulin-like growth factor-binding protein 3, migration-inhibitory factor).

Cross-communication between different cell-signaling systems involves EGFR transactivation by G-protein-coupled receptors

Table 5 Major differences between cytotoxic chemotherapy and molecular-targeted anticancer agents

	Chemotherapy	Molecular targeted agents
Biological mechanism	Cytotoxic	Cytostatic
Expected anticancer effect	Cell killing	Growth control
Drug resistance	Frequent	Not frequent
Toxicity profile	Poor	Good
Clinical end-point	Short–medium term cancer cell eradication	Medium–long term cancer control

Table 6 Molecular-targeted anti-cancer therapeutic options: some examples of pathways and related biomarkers

Molecular target	Molecular-targeted therapy	Markers	Body compartment	Potential role
Signal transduction	Specific blocking agents	- Ras FTase - Prostaglandins	- Tumor tissue - Blood	- Predictive - Surrogate
Tumor growth factors	Neutralizing antibodies or agents	- Expression of specific growth factors (HER2/*neu*; EGFR; etc.)	- Tumor tissue - Blood	- Predictive - Surrogate
Apoptosis	Apoptosis inducers	- Bcl-2/Bax/Bcl-x - p53-mediated pathways; - TUNEL assay	- Tumor tissue	- Predictive
Angiogenesis	Inhibitors of angiogenesis	- Angiogenic factors	- Tumor tissue/blood	- Predictive/surrogate
		- Endogenous inhibitors	- Tumor tissue/blood	- Predictive/surrogate
		- Tumor vascularization	- Tumor tissue	- Predictive
Gene therapy	Several options	- Altered gene and its products	- Tumor tissue	- Predictive
Active immuno therapy	Dendritic cells; tumor-specific killer T-cells	- Markers of immune cellular activation	- Tumor tissue/blood	- Predictive/surrogate

and metalloproteinase cleavage (62), p53, mdm2, checkpoint kinases, apoptosis, DNA damage (63,64), and telomerase (65).

The identification of integrated molecular pathways may be relevant for therapeutic purposes and may eventually lead to multi-parametric predictive indexes suitable for a multi-target therapeutic approach. Possible target candidates for this strategy are

- surrogate markers of tyrosine kinases (inhibitors of different tyrosine kinases include anti-VEGF/flk-1 antagonists, trastuzumab, anti-EGFR compounds, CDK-2, and MET inhibitors);
- apoptosis (connected with angiogenesis, type I-growth factor receptor family, immune system, and others);
- angiogenesis; and
- telomerase.

For all these biological pathways, specific and sensitive modulating agents are available or under preclinical development.

In addition to the prediction of responsiveness to a given agent before starting the therapy, biomarkers could identify possible changes in the target associated with the development of drug resistance. This represents an emerging area of investigation for new biomarkers.

Surrogate Biomarkers

The concept of surrogate biomarker suits the definition first proposed by Temple (66) for surrogate end-point of clinical trial, that is, "a laboratory measurement or a physical sign used as a substitute for a clinically meaningful end-point that measures directly how a patient feels, functions or survives." Prospective clinical trials require hundreds of patients. It often takes years to assess the effectiveness of a new agent on end-points reflecting benefit to the patients (the so-called true end-point). This pitfall is certainly of major concern when using molecular-targeted agents that are expected to elicit cytostatic rather that cytotoxic action; this bears two consequences that impair the classical criteria of evaluation of clinical response: first, the efficacy of a drug may not necessarily be reflected by objective response; second, these agents must be administered for long periods of time. Surrogate markers should therefore be considered a very promising tool to shorten clinical evaluation. However, the identification of a correlation between the intervention and both the biomarker and the true outcome does not allow one to define *per se* the biomarker as a surrogate end-point. Fleming and DeMets (67) defined the basic requirements that a biomarker must meet to be considered a surrogate end-point and pointed out the possible divergences between a spurious concordance and the real prediction of the final outcome of the therapeutic intervention (68). A proper approach to defining a biomarker as a surrogate end-point needs extensive basic knowledge of the biological relationship linking the biomarker to the effects of the intervention and the application of both appropriate statistical approaches and stringent study design (69).

Recent studies showed that Prostate-Specific Antigen (PSA) fulfills the requirement of a surrogate marker for the assessment of failure to respond to endocrine therapy in advanced prostate cancer (70). Also, Rustin et al. showed that the mucin marker CA125 may be used as a surrogate marker in the evaluation of new chemotherapy regimens in patients with ovarian cancer (71). Considering that both PSA and CA125 are classical biomarkers associated with tumor extension, these findings seem very promising and call for the urgent and rigorous evaluation of new biomarkers related to well-known biological machineries.

TOWARD NEW RULES FOR THERAPEUTIC TRIALS: FROM DISEASE-ORIENTED TO BIOMARKER-ORIENTED TRIALS

Cancer therapy based on molecular-targeted agents requires new study strategies that consider innovative aspects with respect to traditional cytotoxic chemotherapy. First of all, they should be used only in target patients; in other words, predictive biomarkers should be identified and systematically used to select only patients bearing a particular molecular target. Moreover, as reported above and schematically summarized in Table 5, both biological and clinical end-points are different from those of cytotoxic agents. For this reason, most of these new agents are to be administered over a long period of time; and additive or synergistic effects are expected when they are combined with conventional anti-cancer drugs. In addition, most of these agents present lower toxicity and fewer side effects than chemotherapy, due to their biological selectivity. Therefore, the classical Phase I–III rules for designing clinical pharmacological trials should be in part modified.

We summarize a suggested study protocol recently developed on the basis of our long-term collaboration on the evaluation of biomarkers aimed at the identification of subgroups of patients with defined biomolecular characteristics (50).

Phase I Trials

The objectives of a Phase I trial for cytotoxics are:

- to define the initial dose level of administration;
- to determine pharmacokinetic parameters in humans;
- to establish the maximum tolerated dose (MTD) and the optimal and safe dose for Phase II trials.

At least four variables influence the results of a traditional Phase I trial: the starting dose, the number of patients evaluated per dose level, the planned dose escalation, and how many previous treatments each patient received. The feasibility and ethical aspects of novel methods for Phase I studies, such as the accelerated titration design (ATD) proposed by NCI (71), are presently under debate.

Regarding molecular-targeted agents, the proposed study design (50) differs on the following points:

- the optimal starting dose of administration should be identified on the results of the range of biological active doses from experimental models;
- pharmacokinetics parameters and pharmacodynamic activity should be defined through surrogate biomarkers related to the biological target of the compound;
- MTD should be replaced by the definition of the "range of biologically active doses" capable of modulating the functions of the target; and
- in order to limit the number of patients receiving low and possibly subtherapeutic doses of the new agent, more rapid dose escalation level procedures should be applied, assuming shallower dose-response curves using the ATD method (72); alternatively, the modified continual reassessment method (mCRM) developed at the San Antonio University (73) could be applied.

Phase II Trials

Conventional Phase II trials on cytotoxic agents foresee disease-oriented strategies using objective response rate as the common surrogate end-point for clinical activity and the criterion for go/not go adopting Gehan's two-step procedure (74).

New guidelines for response evaluation criteria in the treatment of solid tumors (RECIST) have also been proposed for conventional Phase II trials and are currently under debate (73–75). RECIST guidelines differ from standard World Health Organization (WHO) criteria with respect to the definition of measurability of lesions at baseline, objective response, and duration of response by the use of unidimensional measurements and different criteria for progressive disease (73).

Given the putative mechanism of action of molecular-targeted agents, objective response should not be an effective surrogate end-point, as disease-oriented screening does not seem to be the proper strategy for patient selection.

We therefore proposed two different surrogate end-points:

- the evaluation of the modulation of the target measuring soluble or tissue-based surrogate biomarkers and/or using in vivo dynamic imaging techniques (MRI, PET) and
- considering time to progression, which reflects the sum of minor response and stable disease; these minor effects should be realistically expected as the results of the administration of molecular-targeted compounds to patients with advanced disease, in which tumor stasis rather than tumor regression frequently occurs (11).

The most relevant question is whether in the development of molecular-targeted agents a traditional Phase II trial is still necessary on the hypothesis to replace disease-oriented studies with the selection strategy of patients based on the biological characteristics of their tumors. Once a new molecular-targeted agent has been evaluated in a Phase I trial, it could not be subsequently tested by traditional Phase II trials but rather by Phase IIb pilot randomized studies evaluating, for example, the activity of the novel compound alone versus its combination with those cytotoxic agents that may possess potential additive or synergistic anti-tumor activity.

Phase III Trials

Phase III controlled, prospective studies carried out with cytotoxic agents are designed to compare therapy versus placebo, or two or more different treatments randomly assigned to homogeneous groups of patients. Retrospective or prospective stratifications of the variables that potentially may influence the results among the arms of the study are advocated. Most Phase III trials on cytotoxic agents are disease- and stage-oriented studies.

Phase III studies are the most relevant step in evaluating new molecular-targeted treatments. Depending upon the antitumoral activity of each single biological compound, at least two study design strategies may be suggested:

1. Molecular-targeted compound alone versus combination with cytotoxic agent(s). This study requires a good level of anti-tumor activity of the testing compound in patients selected on the basis of the predictive surrogate marker (e.g., gene therapy with wild-type p53 in lung cancer).

2. Molecular-targeted compound combined with cytotoxic(s) versus cytotoxic(s) alone. This strategy is suggested for those tumor types in which conventional therapy gives satisfactory results and/or when the biological agent alone demonstrates only a weak-moderate anti-tumor activity, but a clinically relevant potentiation of, or synergistic combination with, cytotoxics may be expected (e.g., trastuzumab in advanced breast cancer).

In both options, the criteria of patients' eligibility should be the expression of biomarker(s) predictive of response and the end-points should be these:

- monitoring the biological effects through surrogate biomarker(s);
- time to progression, overall survival, and quality of life and the above defined concept of "overall clinical benefit" in advanced stages; relapse-free survival, quality of life, and overall survival for early stage diseases, in the adjuvant/neoadjuvant setting.

The proposed comprehensive clinical strategy for the development of molecular-targeted anti-cancer agents is summarized in Table 7 (50).

This strategy is applicable to compounds given by systemic administration. Specific study designs should be planned for locoregional treatments or gene therapy. In addition, special approaches, such as concurrent versus sequential schedules of therapy, adjuvant versus neoadjuvant therapy, and/or concurrent multi-target treatments versus sequential multi-target treatments, may require dedicated changes of the study design. Moreover, specific adjustments of the study design should be performed for investigations aimed at prospectively evaluating the predictive value of different biomarkers.

SUMMARY

The continual advancement of both basic research and technology is expected to have an extraordinary impact on the knowledge of cancer biology and to expand therapeutic options in the area of molecular-targeted agents. This will greatly expand the utility of molecular pathology and pharmacogenomic applications, possibly leading to individually tailored anti-cancer treatments based on the identification of specific molecular targets. Molecular epidemiology is also expected to address specific chemoprevention programs to subjects at high risk.

However, in spite of the fact that the biological and clinical rationale underlying these new agents and chemotherapy

Table 7 Suggested study design for molecular-targeted agents

		Classical scheme	Proposed changes
Phase I	Baseline single agent evaluation	- Define the starting dose-level of administration - Establish the maximum tolerated dose (MTD) - Establish the optimal and safe dose for Phase II trials - Assessment of pharmacokinetic parameters, toxicity, and side effectss	- Identification of predictive and surrogate biomarker/s and method validation - Definition of the optimal biological range of doses - Study of the relationship between biomarkers and pharmacokinetic
Phase II	Pilot single agent clinical evaluation based on the biologic characteristic of the tumor	- Definition of clinical response (complete and objective response criteria)	- Selection of the patients on the basis of predictive biomarker(s). - Definition of activity in terms of modulation of surrogate biomarkers and time to progression
Phase II/IIb	Pilot combination of the agent with cytotoxics/radiation therapy/hormone therapy	- Not performed	- Selection of the patients on the basis of predictive biomarker(s). - Validation of surrogate biomarker(s) - Optimization of the schedule and assessment of its feasibility and tolerability - Evaluation of the response using surrogate biomarkers and cytostatic-related clinical end-points (see text for details)
Phase III	Large randomized, prospective, controlled clinical studies to assess the efficacy of the new agent alone versus compound + cytotoxic agent/s	- Definition of clinical response (complete and objective response criteria)	- Evaluation of the response using surrogate biomarkers and cytostatic related clinical end-points (see text for details)

Modified from reference (50).

are different, the clinical efficacy of the latter is still assessed according to the conventional Phase I–III protocol. In 1996 Gasparini et al. (76) commented on the published results of a conventional Phase I trial on an anti-angiogenic agent and suggested the need for identifying proper biomarkers as intermediate surrogate end-points of activity. Nevertheless, very few studies including appropriate clinical biological monitoring of anti-angiogenic agents have been published since then. Of major concern, inhibitors of farnesyl transferase have been mainly investigated through traditional Phase I study designs. These trials did not consider the potential role of specific molecular targets for patient selection, thus probably preventing the identification of the most appropriate schedule of administration (77).

A gap between laboratory research and clinical applications still exists and may hinder the appropriate evaluation of new agents, eventually obscuring their actual usefulness. Therefore, in order to highlight the therapeutic potential of these novel molecular-targeted compounds, it is urgent to develop a consensus on a specific and comprehensive methodological approach, that also takes into consideration the biological background, the identification of predictive and/or surrogate markers, the development of proper laboratory methods, and the criteria of interpretation adequate to consider the biological complexity of pathological processes.

REFERENCES

1. Braverman AS. Chemotherapeutic failure: resistance or insensitivity? Ann Intern Med 1993;118:630–632.
2. Early Breast Cancer Trialists' Collaborative Group. Polychemotherapy for early breast cancer: an overview of the randomized trials. Lancet 1998;352:930–942.
3. Leonart ME, Martin-Duque P, Sanchez-Prieto R, et al. Tumor heterogeneity: morphological, molecular and clinical implications. Histol Histopathol 2000;15:881–898.
4. Lengauer C, Kinzler KW, Volgestein B. Genetic instabilities in human cancers. Nature 1998;396:643–649.
5. Golub TR, Slonim DK, Tamayo P, et al. Molecular classification of cancer: class discovery and class prediction by gene expression monitoring. Science 1999;286:531–537.
6. Liotta LA, Kohn EC. The microenvironment of the tumor-host interface. Nature 2001;411:375–379.
7. Shoemaker RH. Genetic and epigenetic factors in anti-cancer drug resistance. J Natl Cancer Inst 2000;92:4–5.
8. Denko N, Schindler C, Koong A, et al. Epigenetic regulation of gene expression in cervical cancer cells by the tumor microenvironment. Clin Cancer Res 2000;6:480–487.
9. Caldas C. Molecular assessment of cancer. Br Med J 1998;316:1360–1363.
10. Kleyn PW and Vesell ES. Genetic variation as a guide to drug development. Science 1998;281:1820–1821.
11. Gelmon KA, Eisenhauer EA, Harris AL, et al. Anti-cancer agents targeting signaling molecules and cancer cell environment: challenges for drug development? J Nat Cancer Inst 1999;91:1281–1287.
12. Bartelink H, Begg AC, Martin JC, et al. Translational research offers individually tailored treatments for cancer patients. Cancer J Sci Am 2000;6:2–10.
13. Frankel AE, Kreitman RJ, Sausville EA. Targeted toxins. Clin Cancer Res 2000;6:326–334.
14. Hanahan D, Weinberg RA. The hallmarks of cancer. Cell 2000;100:57–70.
15. Mosselman S, Polman J, Dijkema R. ERβ: identification and characterization of a novel human estrogen receptor. FEBS Lett 1996;392:49–53.
16. Pfeffer U, Fecarotta E, Vidali G. Co-expression of multiple estrogen receptor variant messenger RNAs in normal and neoplastic breast tissues and in MCF-7 cells. Cancer Res 1995;55:2158–2165.
17. Horowitz KB, Jackson TA, Bain DL, Richer JK, Takimoto GS, Tung L. Nuclear receptor co-activators and co-repressor. Mol Endocrinol 1996;10:1167–1177.
18. Kato S, Endoh H, Masuhiro Y, et al. Activation of the estrogen receptor through phosphorylation by mitogen-activated protein kinase. Science 1995;270:1491–1494.
19. Zwijsen RM, Buckle RS, Hijmans EM, et al. Ligand-independent recruitment of steroid receptor co-activators to estrogen receptor by cyclin D1. Genes Dev 1998;12:3488–3498.
20. Levenson AS, Jordan VC. Selective oestrogen receptor modulation: molecular pharmacology for the millennium. Eur J Cancer 1999;35:1628–1639.
21. Dowsett M, Cooke T, Ellis I, et al. Assessment of HER-2 status in breast cancer: why, when, and how? Eur J Cancer 2000;36:170–176.
22. Press MF, Hung G, Godolphin W, Slamon DJ. Sensitivity of HER-2/neu antibodies in archival tissue samples: potential source of error in immunohistochemical studies of oncogene expression. Cancer Res 1994;54:2771–2777.
23. Dittadi R, Meo S, Amoroso B, Gion M. Detection of different estrogen receptor forms in breast cancer cytosol by enzyme immunoassay. Cancer Res 1997;57:1066–1072.
24. Kiechle FL. DNA technology, the clinical laboratory, and the future. Arch Pathol Lab Med 2001;125:72–76.
25. Commission on Laboratory Accreditation. Molecular pathology inspection checklist. Northfield, IL: College of American Pathologists, 1993.
26. Bolufer-Gilabert P, Barragan-Gonzalez E, Lopez-Guerrero JA. Could the water used in polymerase chain reaction be the cause of false positive results? Eur J Clin Chem Clin Biochem 1996;34:845.
27. Neumaier M, Braun A, Wagener C, et al. Fundamentals of quality assessment of molecular amplification methods in clinical diagnostics. Clin Chem 1998;44:12–26.
28. EORTC Breast Cooperative Group. Revision of the standards for the assessment of hormone receptors in human breast cancer; report of the second EORTC Workshop, held on 16–17 March 1979, in the Netherlands Cancer Institute. Eur J Cancer 1980;16:1513–1535.
29. Janicke F, Prechtl A, Thomssen C, et al. Randomized adjuvant chemotherapy trial in high-risk, lymph node negative breast cancer patients identified by urinokinase-type plasminogen activator and plasminogen activator inhibitor type 1. J Natl Cancer Inst 2001;93:913–920.
30. Dittadi R, Meo S, Fabris F, et al. Validation of blood collection procedures for the determination of circulating vascular endothelial growth factor (VEGF) in different blood compartments. Int J Biol Markers 2001;2:87–96.

31. Tung-Ping Poon R, Fan ST, Wong J. Clinical implications of circulating angiogenic factors in cancer patients. J Clin Oncol 2001; 19:1207–1225.
32. National Committee for Clinical Laboratory Standards (NCCLS). Clinical evaluation of immunoassays: proposed guideline. NCCLS document I/LA21–P. Villanova, PA: NCCLS, 1999.
33. Toi M, Gion M, Biganzoli E, et al. Co-determination of the angiogenic factors thymidine phosphorylase and vascular endothelial growth factor in node-negative breast cancer: prognostic implications. Angiogenesis 1997;1:71–83.
34. Gion M, Boracchi P, Dittadi R, et al. Quantitative measurement of soluble cytokeratin fragments in tissue cytosol of 599 node negative breast cancer patients: a prognostic marker possibly associated with apoptosis. Breast Cancer Res Treat 2000;59: 211–221.
35. Coradini D, Daidone MG, Boracchi P, et al. Time-dependent relevance of steroid receptors in breast cancer. J Clin Oncol 2000;18:2702–2709.
36. Gasparini G, Toi M, Gion M, et al. Prognostic significance of vascular endothelial growth factor protein in node-negative breast carcinoma. J Natl Cancer Inst 1997;89:139–147.
37. Dittadi R, Gion M. More about: prognostic importance of low c-erbB-2 expression in breast tumors. J Natl Cancer Inst 2000; 92:1443.
38. Dittadi R, Biganzoli E, Boracchi P, et al. Impact of steroid receptors, pS2, and cathepsin D on the outcome of N+ postmenopausal breast cancer patient treated wit tamoxifen. Int J Biol Markers 1998;13:30–41.
39. Coradini D, Biganzoli E, Boracchi P, et al. Effect of steroid receptors, pS2, and cathepsin D on the outcome of elderly breast cancer patients: an exploratory investigation. Int J Cancer 1998; 79:305–311.
40. Bouchet C, Hacene K, Martin PM, et al. Dissemination risk index based on plasminogen activator system components in primary breast cancer. J Clin Oncol 1999;17:3048–3057.
41. Gasparini G, Toi M, Miceli R, et al. Clinical relevance of vascular endothelial growth factor and thymidine phosphorylase in patients with node-positive breast cancer treated with either adjuvant chemotherapy or hormone therapy. Cancer J Sci Am 1999;5: 101–111.
42. Altman DG, Lausen B, Sauerbrei W, Schumacher M. Dangers of using ''optimal'' cut-points in the evaluation of prognostic factors. J Nat Cancer Inst 1994;86:829–835.
43. Biganzoli E, Boracchi P, Daidone MG, et al. Flexible modeling in survival analysis. Structuring biological complexity from the information provided by tumor markers. Int J Biol Markers 1998; 13:107–123.
44. Altman DG, De Stavola BL, Love SB, Stepniewska KA. Review of survival analyses published in cancer journals. Br J Cancer 1995;72:511–518.
45. Moher D. CONSORT: an evolving tool to help improve the quality of reports of randomized trials. JAMA 1998;279:1489–1491.
46. Horton R. Medical editors trial amnesty: unreported trial registration form. Lancet 1997;350:756–757.
47. Hayes DF, Bast RC, Desch CE, et al. Tumor marker utility grading system: A framework to evaluate clinical utility of tumor markers. J Natl Cancer Inst 1996;88:1456–1466.
48. Gion M, Boracchi P, Biganzoli E, Daidone MG. A guide for reviewing submitted manuscripts and indications for the design of translational research studies on biomarkers. Int J Biol Markers 1999;13:123–133.
49. Chabner BA, Boral AL, Multani P. Translational research: walking the bridge between idea and cure. Seventeenth Bruce F. Cain memorial award lecture. Cancer Res 1998;58:4211–4216.
50. Gasparini G, Gion M. Molecular-targeted anti-cancer therapy: challenges related to study design and choice of proper endpoints. Cancer J Sci Am 2000;6:117–131.
51. Pepe SM, Etzioni R, Feng Z, et al. Phases of Biomarker Development for Early Detection of Cancer. J Natl Cancer Inst 2001;93:1054–1061.
52. Holmgren L, O'Reilly MS, Folkman J. Dormancy of micrometastases: Balanced proliferation and apoptosis in the presence of angiogenesis suppression. Nat Med 1995;1:149–53.
53. Kakeji Y, Teicher BA. Preclinical studies of the combination of angiogenic inhibitors with cytotoxic agents. Invest New Drugs 1997;15:39–48.
54. Baselga J, Norton L, Albanell J, et al. Recombinant humanized anti-HER-2 antibody (Herceptin™) enhances the anti-tumor activity of paclitaxel and doxorubicin against HER-2/neu overexpressing human breast cancer xenografts. Cancer Res 1998;58: 2825–2831.
55. Baselga J, Cooper MR, Cohen R, et al. Phase I studies of anti-epidermal growth factor receptor chimeric antibody C225 alone and in combination with cisplatin. J Clin Oncol. 2000;18: 904–914.
56. Rowinsky E, Windle JJ, Von Hoff DD. Ras protein farnesyl transferase: a strategic target for anti-cancer therapeutic development. J Clin Oncology 1999;17:3631–3652.
57. Shak S. Overview of the trastuzumab (Herceptin) anti-HER-2 monoclonal antibody clinical program in HER-2-overexpressing metastatic breast cancer. Sem Oncol. 1999;26:71–77.
58. Gasparini G, Harris AL. Does improved control of tumor growth require an anti-cancer therapy targeting both neoplastic and intratumoral endothelial cells? Eur J Cancer 1994;30A:201–206.
59. Gasparini G. The rationale and future potential of angiogenesis inhibitors in neoplasia. Drugs 1999;58:17–38.
60. Pegram MD, Lipton A, Hayes D, et al. Phase II study of receptor-enhanced chemosensitivity using recombinant humanized anti-p185$^{HER-2/neu}$ monoclonal antibody plus cisplatin in patients with HER-2/neu-overexpressing metastatic breast cancer refractory to chemotherapy treatment. J Clin Oncol 1998;16: 2659–2671.
61. Koong AC, Denko NC, Hudson KM, et al. Candidate genes for the hypoxic tumor phenotype. Cancer Res 2000;60:883–887.
62. Prenzel N, Zwick E, Daub H, et al. EGF receptor transactivation by G-protein-coupled receptors requires metalloproteinase cleavage of proHB-EGF. Nature 1999;402:884–888.
63. Sanchez Y, Bachant J, Wang H, et al. Control of the DNA damage checkpoint by Chk1 and Rad53 protein kinases through distinct mechanisms. Science 1999;286:1166–1171.
64. Hirao A, Kong Y-Y, Matsuoka S, et al. DNA damage-induced activation of p53 by the checkpoint kinase Chk2. Science 2000; 287:1824–1827.
65. de Lange T, Jacks T. For better or worse? Telomerase inhibition and cancer. Cell 1999;98:273–275.
66. Temple RJ. A regulatory authority's opinion about surrogate endpoints. In: Nimmo WS, Tucker GT (eds.). Clinical measurement in drug evaluation. New York: J Wiley,1995.
67. Fleming TR, DeMets DL. Surrogate end-points in clinical trials: are we being misled? Ann Intern Med 1996;125:605–613.
68. Prentice RL. Surrogate end-points in clinical trials: definition and operational criteria. Statistics in Medicine 1989;8:431–440.

69. Lin DY, Fleming TR, De Gruttola V. Estimating the proportion of treatment effect explained by a surrogate marker. Statistics in Medicine 1997;16:1515–1527.
70. Vollmer RT, Dawson NA, Vogelzang NJ. The dynamics of prostate-specific antigen in hormone refractory prostate carcinoma. Cancer 1998;83:1989–1994.
71. Rustin GJS. CA125: a surrogate marker for the selection of active agents for ovarian cancer? J Clin Oncol 2000;18:1733.
72. Simon R, Freidlin B, Rubinstein L, et al. Accelerated titration designs for phase I clinical trials in oncology. J Natl Cancer Inst 1997;89:1138–1147.
73. Therasse P, Arbuck SG, Elisenhauer EA, et al. New guidelines to evaluate the response to treatment in solid tumors. J Natl Cancer Inst 2000;92:205–216.
74. Gehan E, Tefft MC. Will there be resistance to the RECIST (response evaluation criteria in solid tumors)? J Natl Cancer Inst 2000;92:179–181.
75. Mariani L, Marubini E. Content and quality of currently published phase II cancer trials. J Clin Oncol 2000;18:429–436.
76. Gasparini G, Presta M. Clinical studies with angiogenesis inhibitors: biological rationale and challenges for their evaluation. Ann Oncol 1996;7:441–444.
77. Zujewski, J, Horak ID, Bol CJ,, et al. Phase I and Pharmacokinetic study of farnesyl protein transferase inhibitor R115777 in advanced cancer. J Clin Oncol 2000;18:927–941.

Part Two
Organ-Specific Tumor Markers

Chapter 14

Tumor Markers in Breast Cancer

Rafael Molina

Breast cancer remains a primary cause of death for women in Western countries, with a 12.2% lifetime risk of developing this malignancy and a 3.6% lifetime risk of death (1,2). Multiple factors are associated with an increase in breast cancer risk. These include genetic and familial factors; hormonal factors (early menarche, late menopause, and late first pregnancy); diet; benign breast diseases (mainly associated with atypical hyperplasia); and environmental factors (3).

Within the past decade, several trials using systemic treatment (chemotherapy or hormone therapy) after primary surgery have shown a significant improvement in survival for treated patients compared to controls (3). In order to rationally administer systemic therapy to patients who have local disease, it is necessary to know which patients are at risk of recurrence. The main prognostic factors for both disease-free survival (DFS) and overall survival (OS) are nodal involvement, tumor size, lymphatic and vascular invasion, histological grade, nuclear grade, and sex steroid receptors (3). Clinicians use these factors to help select patients with aggressive disease who may benefit from adjuvant therapy and to avoid over-treatment of patients with indolent disease.

Despite increased incidence of breast cancer, the mortality rate remains relatively constant. This may be because of earlier detection via screening programs, leading to improved outcome, and advances in treatment. Treatment of primary breast cancer usually includes surgery and/or radiotherapy. Following surgery, clinicians increasingly use adjuvant therapies (e.g., either tamoxifen or chemotherapy). Treatment for distant metastases involves chemotherapy, hormone therapy, and radiotherapy. About 30–50% of patients with breast cancer relapse within the first ten years after diagnosis.

Patients who have metastatic breast cancer cannot be cured with conventional therapy. It is currently believed that many patients presenting with apparently local disease may have micro-metastasis, because it appears that the proportion of distant metastases is not altered even by aggressive local therapies.

TUMOR MARKERS

A large number of markers signal breast cancer. These include MUC-1 (e.g., CA15-3), CEA, oncoproteins, milk proteins, glycolytic enzymes, oncoproteins, and cytokeratins (4–8). Compared to "normal" patients and patients with benign breast diseases, patients who have breast cancer also have many breast antigens circulating at elevated levels in their plasma and/or serum. However, only a few assays for circulating antigens are sufficiently specific and sensitive to have any clinical utility as tumor markers (4–8). Of these, CEA and CA15.3 are the most commonly used.

The sensitivity and specificity of other members of the MUC-1-gene family such as MCA, CA549, BR 27-29 and BRMA are similar to that of CA15.3 (9–13). Yet using several mucins simultaneously does not provide additional information compared to that obtained using only one (14,15). For this reason, EGTM guidelines recommend using CEA and one mucin as serum markers in patients with breast cancer (6).

Other markers such as cytokeratins (e.g., TPA, TPS, and CYFRA 21.1) and soluble oncoproteins (e.g., c-erbB-2) are promising, but are still under evaluation (6,8,14,16,17). In this chapter we will evaluate the possible clinical utility and value of the most commonly used tumor markers in the different stages of breast cancer.

USEFULNESS OF CLINICAL APPLICATIONS OF TUMOR MARKER SERUM LEVELS

Diagnosis

Most patients with breast cancer are diagnosed in a locoregional stage, and surgery is the most frequently used treatment. Pretreatment evaluation of the breast cancer patient should determine the clinical stage of the disease and identify contraindications to breast-conserving therapy or immediate breast reconstruction. The utility of tumor markers in this disease stage may be in the diagnosis, differential diagnosis with other pathologies, prognosis, or as a predictive parameter.

Tumor marker sensitivity in patients with early breast cancer is low (15–35%). In patients with advanced disease, this sensitivity increases to 50–75%. Table 1 shows the before-treatment sensitivity measured in 496 patients with primary locoregional breast cancer who were studied in the hospital clinic. Abnormal CEA (>5 ng/mL), CA 15.3 (>30 U/mL), and c-erbB-2 (>15 ng/mL) were found in 12%, 12.7%, and 7% of the patients, respectively. A wide range of sensitivities, between 10–50%, has been described in locoregional breast cancer (18). Discrepancies may be related to patient characteristics (as will

Table 1 CEA, CA 15.3, and c-erbB-2 sensitivity obtained in patients with primary untreated locoregional breast cancer, according to the most important prognostic factors in breast cancer

		CA 15.3			CEA			c-erbB-2		
	Number of patients	Percent positive	Mean ± SD U/mL	P value	Percent positive	Mean ± SD ng/mL	P value	Percent positive	Mean ± SD ng/mL	P value
Total	496	12.7	22 ± 34		12	3.5 ± 10		7	8.6 ± 7.5	
T1	140	6.4	17 ± 9	0.003	5	2.1 ± 1.5	0.023	8.6	8.7 ± 6.6	n.s.s.[a]
T2	214	9.8	19 ± 16		10.7	3.4 ± 13		8.9	9.2 ± 8.3	
T3	48	8.3	19 ± 12		10.4	2.7 ± 2.9		4.2	7 ± 4	
T4	91	31.9	41 ± 72		27.5	6.3 ± 11		5.5	8 ± 11	
Node negative	256	7.4	19 ± 29		8.4	3 ± 12		7	8.5 ± 7	
<4 nodes	151	17.2	22 ± 22		11.3	3.2 ± 4.8		9.3	8.4 ± 7.2	
≥4 nodes	79	20.2	32 ± 60		22.8	5.2 ± 10		7.6	10 ± 12	
T size[b]										
<1 cm	42	2.3	17 ± 8	0.002	4.8	2 ± 1.5	0.001	7.1	8.8 ± 3.7	0.009
1–2 cm	78	6.4	16 ± 8		2.6	1.9 ± 1.3		5.1	3.5 ± 3.7	
2–3 cm	93	9.7	18 ± 9		7.5	2.2 ± 1.5		2.2	9.5 ± 7.7	
3–5 cm	49	14.3	26 ± 31		12.2	6.5 ± 27		12.2	9.3 ± 7	
>5 cm	58	29.3	39 ± 70		24.1	6.6 ± 12		5.2	7.1 ± 5.6	
IDC[c]	431	11.6	23 ± 34	n.s.s	10	3.5 ± 10		6.2	8.6 ± 8.5	
Others	26	7.6	26 ± 55		19	5.4 ± 13		11.4	9.4 ± 4.6	
Lobular	25	8	19 ± 13		4	2.2 ± 1.5		8	8.7 ± 4.2	
H. Grade I	58	6.8	17 ± 7.7		8.5	2.3 ± 1.8		6.8	8.7 ± 3.7	n.s.s.
Grade II	134	7	21 ± 40		9.1	4.4 ± 17		9.1	9.2 ± 6.7	
Grade III	116	13.5	21 ± 14		11.7	2.7 ± 3.6		5.4	8.8 ± 9.8	
ER +	336	12.5	21 ± 23	n.s.s.	11.6	3.6 ± 11	0.075	7.4	8.7 ± 8.6	n.s.s.
ER −	155	13.5	25 ± 51		13	3.2 ± 6		7.7	8.5 ± 6.9	
PgR +	267	13.9	21 ± 18	n.s.s.	10.1	3.6 ± 12	n.s.s.	7.2	8.2 ± 6.1	n.s.s.
PgR −	224	11.6	24 ± 47		14.3	3.3 ± 6.7		8	9.3 ± 10	
Pre-menopausal	149	8.5	21 ± 38	n.s.s.	7.4	2.3 ± 2.5	0.019	5.4	7.7 ± 6	n.s.s.
Post-menopausal	347	14.7	23 ± 33		14.2	4 ± 12		8.4	9 ± 8.8	
P53 +	69	8.7	17 ± 9	n.s.s.	8.7	2.3 ± 1.6	n.s.s.	0	8 ± 2.6	0.033
P53 −	160	10.6	19 ± 13		13.1	4 ± 15.4		7.5	9 ± 7	
c-erbB-2 +	80	8.8	17 ± 10	n.s.s.	13.8	5 ± 21.4	0.015	15	12.6 ± 14	0.001
c-erbB-2 −	188	11.2	20 ± 19		12.2	2.9 ± 4.2		4.8	6.2	

[a] n.s.s, not statistically significant.
[b] T, tumor size.
[c] IDC, infiltrating ductal carcinoma.

be shown later); the cut-off used; different methodologies; etc. However, all these results are alike in that sensitivity clearly indicates that tumor markers are not useful for diagnostic purposes (8–19). Low levels of markers in patients suspected of having breast cancer do not exclude the presence of malignancy at either a primary or metastatic breast site. On the other hand, high levels of a marker in patients with breast cancer almost certainly indicate the presence of metastatic disease, i.e., distant metastasis.

Few patients have primary locoregional breast cancer and abnormal levels of this marker. This sensitivity seems to indicate that tumor markers are not useful for indicating early disease stages. However, it is important to know the significance of abnormal tumor marker levels. Only if we study the factors that influence the serum levels of these markers, will we be able to correctly interpret the results.

Table 1 shows the relationship among tumor markers and the most commonly used prognostic factors in this malignancy. (This information was obtained in a prospective evaluation in 496 patients with primary locoregional breast cancer at diagnosis.) Serum levels of CEA and CA 15.3 are clearly related to tumor size and nodal involvement. Most studies published suggest this correlation but some do not agree (9,12,20–26). These results are logical if we consider that tumor markers are synthesized by malignant cells, thus, the higher the number of malignant cells, the higher the tumor marker levels in serum. Likewise, nodal involvement also increases the possibility of arrival to the blood, using the lymph nodes to arrive to the lymph. In summary, tumor markers reflect the number of malignant cells as well as tumor extension, either locally (nodal involvement) or distant (metastases) (18,22,27).

According to the data shown in Table 1, c-erbB-2 is the only marker not related to tumor size or nodal involvement; it is only related to oncogene overexpression in tissue. Fehm et al. (18) obtained similar results in 211 node-positive patients. These results are not surprising if we consider that only 25–35% of breast tumors overexpress this oncogene.

Table 2 shows that c-erbB-2 serum levels are related to tumor size and nodal involvement only in the tumors with overexpression in tissue. In contrast, there was no correlation among prognostic factors and c-erbB-2 serum levels in patients without overexpression. Logically speaking, if a tumor overexpresses c-erbB-2, this marker will migrate to the circulation and we will be able to detect it.

This relationship between overexpression in tissue and serum has been confirmed by other authors, although it remains controversial. Differences in results may be related to the method used to evaluate c-erbB-2 or to the variability observed with immunohistochemistry (different antibodies, different dilutions) (19). Interestingly, as occurs in tissue, there is a relationship between c-erbB-2 serum levels and steroid receptors, with significantly higher levels in patients with ER or PgR-negative tumors (11,16,18).

In short, serum levels of CEA, CA15.3, or other MUC-1 products are not useful for diagnostic purposes but do provide information about tumor stage. Abnormal levels of CEA or CA 15.3 indicate, with a high probability (65% and 70% respectively), nodal invasion.

Prognosis

Prognosis is a key issue in the current management of primary breast cancer. First, prognostics are particularly important in identifying patients whose prognosis is so favorable that adjuvant treatment is unnecessary. Second, prognostic factors are useful in identifying patients whose prognosis is so poor with conventional treatment that adjuvant treatment is necessary to improve their outcome.

The most commonly used prognostic factors in breast cancer include the number of positive axillary lymph nodes, tumor size, lymphatic and vascular invasion, histologic tumor type, and sex steroid receptors. Other pathologic prognostic factors include histologic grade and nuclear grade, although there appears to be considerable interobserver variation. Many other prognostic factors are being studied but their value has not been well established since the relevant clinical data are preliminary or contradictory or standardization is weak or lacking. This last group of prognostic factors includes oncogene products (c-erbB2, p53, BCL-2); ploidy; and proliferative indexes (S phase fraction, Ki67) (28–33).

Serum levels of CEA, CA15.3, or other MUC-1 products are correlated to the well-known prognostic factors in breast cancer, such as tumor size or nodal involvement. This relationship suggests a possible prognostic value for these markers. Several studies have shown a shorter disease-free survival (DFS) and overall survival (OS) rate in patients whose values of these markers are high, but others report conflicting data (8–10,12,16,20–23,25,34,35).

Table 3 shows our experience in the prospective evaluation and follow-up (mean 151 months) of 496 patients with untreated locoregional breast cancer. We used the following prognostic factors: TNM, tumor size, histological grade, ER, PgR, adjuvant treatment, CEA, and CA 15.3. Patients with abnormal CEA had a mean DFS of 90 months, and a mean OS of 96 months, in contrast to patients with normal presurgical levels (mean of 156 DFS and 163 OS). Similar results were obtained with CA 15.3. In patients with abnormal serum levels of CA 15.3, the DFS was 99 months and the OS, 118 months; in patients with normal levels, the DFS was 154 months and the

Table 2 c-erbB-2 serum levels in relation to c-erbB-2 in tissue

	c-erbB-2 + by Immunohistochemistry			c-erbB-2 ± by Immunohistochemistry	
	Percent positive	Mean ± SD ng/mL	P value	Percent positive	Mean ± SD ng/mL
T1–2	7/62 (11.2%)	11.7 ± 11,1	n.s.s.	9/146 (6.2%)	8.5 ± 6.7
T3–4	5/18 (27.8%)	15.6 ± 21		0/42 (0%)	6.3 ± 3.3
Node negative	3/42 (7.2%)	11.48 ± 11,8	n.s.s.	5/95 (5.5%)	8 ± 6.4
Node positive	9/38 (23.4%)	13.8 ± 16.2		3/59 (5.1%)	7.8 ± 4.9
T size <2cm	1/24 (4.2%)	8.6 ± 2.3	0.049	2/37 (5.4%)	8.9 ± 3.5
2–5	5/40 (12.5%)	12 ± 10		3/87 (3.3%)	7.6 ± 4
ER +	8/53 (13.7%)	13 ± 15	n.s.s.	8/132 (6.4%)	8.3 ± 7.1
ER –	4/26 (15.4%)	12.2 ± 12		1/56 (1.8%)	7.6 ± 3.1
PgR +	4/37 (10.8%)	10.8 ± 7.4	0.032	7/104 (7%)	8 ± 6
PgR –	8/42 (19.2%)	14.4 ± 18		2/84 (2.4%)	8.1 ± 6.4
Pre-menopausal	2/27 (7.4%)	10.2 ± 8.5	n.s.s.	1/59 (2%)	7 ± 3.6
Post-menopausal	10/53 (18.9%)	13.8 ± 16		8/129 (6.4%)	8.5 ± 7
P53 +	0/17 (0%)	8.7 ± 2.6	0.092	0/48 (0%)	8 ± 2.6
P53 –	5/45 (11.1%)	11.8 ± 11		6/99 (6%)	7.9 ± 4.6

n.s.s., not statistically significant.

Table 3 Prognostic parameters in 496 patients with untreated locoregional breast cancer

	DFS univariate	DFS multivariate	OS univariate	OS multivariate
TNM	0.0001	n.s.s.	0.0001	n.s.s.
Nodes	0.00001	0.00001	0.00001	0.00001
Age	n.s.s.	n.s.s.	0.023	0.022
T size	0.001	n.s.s.	0.0001	n.s.s.
Grade	0.0004	n.s.s.	0.012	n.s.s.
Histology	n.s.s	n.s.s.	0.001	n.s.s.
ER	0.009	0.01	0.007	0.0016
PgR	0.056	n.s.s.	0.085	n.s.s.
CEA	0.002	0.025	0.0027	0.048
15.3	0.009	n.s.s.	n.s.s.	n.s.s.
Adjuvant treatment	0.001	n.s.s.	0.035	n.s.s.

n.s.s, not statistically significant.

OS, 158 months. Though these prospective results seem to indicate that tumor markers are prognostic factors, CEA and CA 15.3 are quantitative parameters and theoretically, in relation to prognosis, a patient with a CEA of 5.1 ng/mL is not the same as another patient with 15 ng/mL.

On follow-up, 10 out of 11 patients with CEA levels higher than 15 ng/mL had recurrence. Figure 1 shows the prognostic value of CEA in the 230 node-positive patients studied upon subdividing the patients into three groups: those with normal values, those with only slightly high values, and those whose CEA levels exceeded 7.5 ng/mL. These data seem to clearly indicate a subset of patients with micrometastases unknown at diagnosis.

Several authors (36,37) have suggested that the prognostic value of CA 15.3 may be related to the fact that MUC1 overexpression favors invasion and metastatic dissemination by interfering with cell adhesion and by protecting tumor cells from destruction by the cellular arm of the immune system.

Most studies to date had addressed only single prognostic risk factors. This is a major problem in estimating disease risk and recurrence, because we don't know enough about how risk factors interact. To be proven useful, a prognostic factor must be an independent variable (when other well-known prognostic factors are considered) and must be prospectively validated in a large patient population. Moreover, multivariate evaluation of tumor marker prognostic value has only been studied in the last six years.

Duffy et al. (38) reported that in relation to DFS, pre-operative CA 15.3 is a stronger prognostic indicator than tumor size, and in relation to OS, stronger than tumor size and nodal involvement. Multivariate analysis of 368 patients showed that CA 15.3 was an independent prognostic indicator in both DFS and OS. Ebeling et al. (39) evaluated prognostic parameters in 550 patients with breast cancer and found, on univariate analysis, the following factors significant in relation to DFS and OS: tumor size; lymph nodes; histological grading; age (only in DFS); hormone receptors; pre-operative value of CEA (cut-off 2 ng/mL); and CA 15.3 (cut-off 25 U/mL). Multivariate analysis found that both CEA and CA 15.3 were strong independent prognostic factors, as were tumor size, nodal involvement, and histological grading for DFS and OS in breast cancer patients.

There are fewer articles evaluating c-erbB-2 serum levels as a prognostic factor. Our group previously studied 186 patients with breast cancer, with a mean follow-up of 5 years, and found that CEA and c-erbB-2 were independent prognostic factors (16). The risk of disease recurrence in patients with abnormal presurgical c-erbB-2 serum levels was 3.3-fold higher than in patients with normal levels. Similar results were obtained by Jäger et al. (40) in 211 node-positive patients treated with adjuvant chemotherapy. However, our current experience, which involves a larger number of patients and a longer follow-up, indicates that c-erbB-2 is not a prognostic factor in breast cancer (see Table 3). In contrast, CEA has always been a prognostic factor in our evaluations. Other studies are required to clarify the prognostic value of c-erbB-2 in serum, in the group as a whole as well as in the tumors with overexpression in tissue.

In short, most studies that involve large numbers of patients and long follow-up demonstrate that tumor markers are prognostic factors in breast cancer. It is still not clear whether these serum markers are independent prognostic factors, although increasing evidence supports this. Likewise, tumor markers have all the requisites for being prognostic factors:

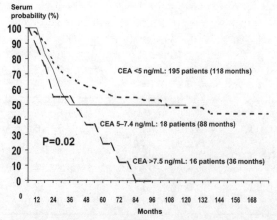

Figure 1 OS in 230 node-positive breast cancer patients, subdivided according to presurgical CEA serum levels.

- they can be identified with standard methods,
- methods are subjected to quality control,
- methods are easy to perform and inexpensive, and
- patient morbidity is low.

Early Diagnosis of Recurrence

Follow-up after treatment of primary breast cancer has two main goals: (1) to screen for new primary or locally recurrent cancers that may be cured by early intervention and (2) to diagnose metastatic breast cancer. It is impossible to achieve the first goal using tumor markers, as was clearly shown by their sensitivity in early disease stages. By contrast, serial CEA and CA15.3 serum determinations are useful tools for achieving the second goal: the early diagnosis of recurrence in patients with breast cancer and no evidence of disease (NED) after radical treatment.

We studied serial measurements of CEA and CA 15.3 every three months in 1,032 and 533 NED breast cancer patients. During follow-up, 246 patients were diagnosed with recurrent disease. CEA was the first sign of recurrence, appearing before clinical symptoms or analysis by other diagnostic tools in 40% (98/246). CA 15.3 appeared in 41% (37/91) of patients with recurrence (41). One tumor marker or another was the first sign of relapse in 56% of the patients. Other authors have described similar results, showing that CEA and CA 15.3 detect 40–60% of relapses before clinical or radiological evidence of disease (e.g., by chest X-ray, liver ultrasonography, bone scans) with a lead time of between 2 and 18 months (mean 5.2 months) (41–46).

Tumor marker sensitivity in the early diagnosis of recurrence is clearly related to recurrence site. CEA and CA15.3 are not useful in the early diagnosis of loco-regional recurrence (sensitivity <30%); clinical examination is the best detection method for these sites. In contrast, abnormal CEA and CA15.3 serum levels are found in 40–60% and 50–75%, respectively, of patients with distant metastases (41). Thus, the simultaneous use of both markers allows early diagnosis of metastases in 60–80% of patients with breast cancer.

Serial measurement of markers is particularly sensitive for the early detection of bone (65–75%) and liver metastases (85–90%). The use of markers in these situations may decrease the frequency of both isotope scans and radiological procedures. Chest X-rays should be carried out for detecting lung metastases as markers lack sensitivity for this organ.

The specificity of markers for the detection of recurrence in the follow-up of NED patients is high, but is related to the marker cut-off points used (41–47). In one study, the proportion of false positive results (abnormal values without recurrence) was 5% for CEA and 6.5% for CA 15.3 using cut-off values of 5 μg/L and 35 u/mL, respectively. When two different criteria, i.e., higher cut-off points (CEA, 10 μg/L: CA15.3, 60 u/mL) and confirmation by at least two serial increases (>15%) were used, specificity increased to 99.3% (41).

Other authors have suggested the inclusion of additional markers to increase sensitivity in the early diagnosis of recurrence. Vizcarra et al. (47) studied the utility of TPA, CEA, and CA 15.3 and found CA 15.3 to be more sensitive as an early indicator of relapse than CEA or TPA. Likewise, simultaneous determination of other markers does not necessarily add to the value of the information obtained by CA 15.3 alone. Pectasides et al. (48) studied CA 15.3, CEA, MCA, TPA, and TPS in 209 patients and 68 (32.5%) developed metastases during follow-up. The sensitivity of tumor markers was as follows: CA 15-3, 68.2%; CEA, 34.1%; MCA, 72.7%; and TPA, 72.7%. The combination of CA 15-3 with TPA or MCA with TPA showed a trend toward improved sensitivity of both markers ($p = 0.06$), with no loss of specificity ($p = 0.11$). The addition of CEA to CA 15-3 or MCA does not provide additional information for clinical evaluation.

One problem in using several tumor markers in early diagnosis is that sensitivity is increased but specificity is lost. This is an important problem when using cytokeratins, markers that express abnormally high levels in other benign and malignant diseases. Marker selection could be influenced according to proposed objectives. If tumor markers, for example, are used to select high-risk patients, and other diagnostic tools are used to make the diagnosis, then sensitivity is more important than specificity, and obtaining 5–10% false positive results is not important. However, if tumor markers are used as diagnostic tools, and we can treat patients according to tumor marker concentration, specificity is very important and a false positive rate of 5–10% is unacceptable.

C-erbB-2 is another marker that can be used in the early diagnosis of recurrence, but few studies have been performed. Our group studied CEA, CA 15.3, and c-erbB-2 in 200 NED breast cancer patients. C-erbB-2 was the first sign of recurrence in 29% of the patients, with recurrence during follow-up. Likewise, using c-erbB-2 it was possible to increase the sensitivity of CEA and CA 15.3 in the early diagnosis in 11.2% of the patients with the same specificity (49). To increase the efficiency of tumor markers in detecting disease, c-erbB-2 results were subdivided according to c-erbB-2 overexpression in tissue. Eighty-five percent of patients with c-erbB-2 overexpression in tissue had abnormal serum levels before the diagnosis of recurrence. By contrast, only 9% of patients without overexpression in tissue had abnormal c-erbB-2 levels at diagnosis of recurrence. These results suggest that we may use c-erbB-2 serum levels for early diagnosis in the small subset of patients with c-erbB-2 overexpression in tissue, in which the efficiency is high. The advantage of using c-erbB-2 in relation to other markers is its specificity. Abnormal levels of this oncoprotein are scarce in the absence of malignancy and only a few malignancies release this marker (50).

Early detection of metastasis takes two different approaches: (1) diagnostic utility and (2) the possibility of initiating systemic treatment earlier. Controversy exists as to whether intensive screening incurs extra expenses and/or increases anxiety unnecessarily, and its value is uncertain regarding ultimate outcome (51). Diagnostic tools such as chest radiography, bone scans, and liver ultrasonograms are useful in diagnosis but do not seem to increase survival. A prospective randomized trial involving more than 1,300 patients showed that no differences were observed in DFS or OS in patients with intensive screening or in the control group (52). Moreover, most patients want to be in contact with the clinician and have a physical examination, usually every three to six months for the first two or three years after the end of primary therapy. Tumor markers are sensitive and important for predicting the appearance of metastatic disease in nearly 70% of the patients before these other diagnostic parameters. Likewise, tumor markers assays are easy to perform and inexpensive, with a low morbidity for the patient. The use of tumor markers may be an intermediate system for carrying out appropriate follow-up in these patients and thereby decreasing the cost of health care.

The second goal in achieving an early diagnosis of recurrence is earlier treatment. Earlier treatment (when tumors are theoretically smaller) increases tumor response to systemic treatment, which is the basis of adjuvant treatment. In using tumor markers, we do not select high-risk patients; we select patients with subclinical metastases. The ASCO guidelines (22) indicate that there is no evidence that serial tumor marker measurement in the early detection of recurrence increases the DFS or OS, and this is true. Moreover, tumor markers are diagnostic tools and cannot improve these parameters without treatment.

Few studies evaluate tumor marker utility in selecting patients for systemic treatment. Jäger et al. (42,53) have shown that treatment of patients with abnormal tumor marker levels and no signs of recurrence results in a higher DFS than in those without treatment. We attempted a similar study, randomizing the patients according to the steroid receptor status. Randomization only occurred after extensive search for recurrence by imaging methods. Therefore, this study was impossible to perform because no patients consented to be included in this portion of the study without treatment.

In short, tumor markers are useful tools in the early diagnosis of metastases, because they have a higher sensitivity than other diagnostic methods in more than 70% of patients. Despite the ability of markers to detect recurrent disease pre-clinically, the long-term benefits of early detection in therapy response and patient survival remain to be defined.

Patients with Metastasis

Conventional therapy cannot cure patients who have metastatic breast cancer. Yet in some patients the disease can be controlled for many years and still result in a good quality of life. Assessing prognosis and devising options for disease management require knowledge of the metastatic sites and the extent of metastatic involvement.

The site of metastases is related to survival. Patients whose disease has metastasized to soft tissues tend to have a better prognosis and a better response to therapy than those whose major involvement is in bone, and those with visceral metastases have the worst prognosis (54). The number of sites of involvement is also an important prognostic marker, with the best prognosis for those whose disease has involved the smallest amount of organ systems (55). Most patients who present with metastatic disease have only one or two organ systems involved. As the disease progresses over time, multiple sites usually succumb to the disease, and at autopsy, metastases may be found in nearly every organ of the body (56).

The possible clinical application of tumor markers in advanced disease may be: diagnosis, prognosis, monitoring of therapy, and as a predictive factor of systemic treatment.

Diagnosis (differential). Tumor marker sensitivity in patients with advanced disease is significantly higher than in those with loco-regional disease (6,8,12–23). Table 4 shows the sensitivity of CEA and CA 15.3 obtained in 761 patients with advanced disease at diagnosis. CA 15.3 sensitivity is higher than CEA, 64% versus 50%, respectively. Similar and wide-ranging results have been reported by other authors (18,57,58). These discrepancies may be related to the number of patients studied, the number of sites involved, and the site of recurrence. Tumor marker sensitivity is clearly related to the site of recurrence, with the lowest sensitivity of both markers in patients with locoregional recurrence and the highest in patients with liver metastases (Table 4) (18,57,58). It is interesting to point out that CA 15.3 sensitivity in lung recurrence is significantly higher than CEA, and in contrast, CEA sensitivity in brain metastases is higher than CA 15.3. Moreover in both situations, lung and brain recurrence, tumor marker serum levels were significantly lower than in patients with bone, pleural, or liver metastases. Tomlissson et al. (59) indicated that CA 15.3 is useful in the diagnosis and follow-up of patients with bone metastases: sensitivity 70%, specificity 96%, predictive value 86%. It is interesting to point out that all patients with a positive bone scan and increased CA 15-3 levels were subsequently confirmed to have had bone metastases; no patient with normal bone scan and normal CA15-3 developed metastatic disease (to the date of follow-up). Likewise, CA15-3 levels frequently increased before otherwise detectable distant metastases were identified.

Other tumor markers may be useful in the differential diagnosis of metastases. Jager et al. (60) retrospectively studied CA 125 in 250 metastatic breast cancer patients and provided evidence that the increase in CA 125 serum levels in these patients was caused by lung metastases or pleural effusions. Seven patients with lung metastases and pleural involvement had elevated CA 125 levels, while four patients with lung metastases but without pleural effusions had normal CA 125 levels. In patients with bone or liver metastases CA 125 levels were usually not elevated.

Tumor markers are produced by malignant cells, and serum levels indirectly reflect tumor size. The number of metastases is another important point in relation to tumor marker sensitivity and serum levels. Tables 4 and 5 show that significantly higher CEA and CA 15.3 serum levels were found in patients with more than one organ involved than in those with only one site of recurrence ($p < 0.001$). Likewise, patients with more than one tissue involved, but without liver metastases, had significantly lower concentrations than those patients with more than one tissue involved including liver metastases ($p < 0.001$).

There is no tumor marker with sufficient sensitivity to be used alone in diagnosing breast cancer. CA 15.3 sensitivity is

Table 4 CEA and CA 15.3 concentrations in 761 patients with advanced disease at diagnosis of recurrence

	CEA sensitivity	Mean ± SD ng/mL	Range	CA 15.3 sensitivity	Mean ± SD U/mL	Range
Total	384/761 (50.5%)	54 ± 503	0.5–13396	487/761 (64%)	193 ± 551	2–9066
Loco-regional	21/130 (16%)	2 ± 5.8	0.5–36	34/130 (26%)	19.5 ± 38	5–276
Bone	179/315 (57%)	28 ± 104	0.5–1500	215/315 (68%)	167 ± 402	6–5567
Lung	32/83 (39%)	12 ± 28	1–210	57/83 (69%)	95 ± 112	6–560
Pleural	25/37 (68%)	68 ± 213	0.9–1178	29/37 (78%)	228 ± 380	6–1512
Brain	6/10 (60%)	20 ± 39	1–129	5/10 (50%)	70 ± 83	7–250
Liver	47/62 (76%)	93 ± 226	0.6–1590	50/62 (81%)	429 ± 837	12–4789
Others	2/5 (40%)	17 ± 21	1–43	4/5 (80%)	49 ± 21	15–65
Multiple sites (no liver)	32/65 (49%)	22 ± 74	0.5–557	47/65 (72,3%)	269 ± 453	2–2020
Multiple sites (liver)	40/54 (74%)	390 ± 1828	1–13396	46/54 (85%)	538 ± 1396	14–9066

higher than CEA, but by using both it is possible to increase the sensitivity for metastatic breast cancer.

Several authors have suggested that including CEA in a follow-up protocol of patients with advanced disease is not useful. Table 5 shows that by using CEA, it is possible to increase the sensitivity obtained with CA 15.3 from 7% to 20%. In our experience, 83 of 274 (30%) patients with normal CA 15.3 had abnormal CEA concentrations. This proportion increased to 42% (74/178) when only patients with metastases were considered (excluding locoregional recurrences). Likewise, in 15% (74/487) of patients with abnormal CA 15.3 and metastases, CEA concentrations were significantly higher than CA 15.3. These results clearly indicate that on accepting CA 15.3 as the most useful tumor marker in breast cancer, the inclusion of CEA allows us to better monitor patient follow-up. Likewise, when using both tumor markers simultaneously, results indicate that one tumor marker or another is abnormal in 75% of patients with recurrence in 83.5% (527/631) of the patients with metastases at diagnosis.

Other tumor markers for metastatic breast cancer, such as cytokeratins or oncoproteins (8,61–64), have been suggested. Using more tumor markers makes it possible to increase the sensitivity in the follow-up of metastatic breast cancer. Murray et al. (62) suggested that cytokeratins had a better sensitivity than CEA and CA 15.3, and a better correlation with the follow-up. However, including more tumor markers decreases specificity. The advantages to using them are not clear, nor are we clear about the best combination of tumor markers (6,61,65–67). This is, in part, due to the great heterogeneity in patient selection, treatments, and methods used to determine tumor markers, and to the cut-off used.

C-erbB2 is another tumor marker suggested for use in diagnosing metastatic breast cancer. Moreover, the sensitivity of c-erbB-2 in patients with metastatic breast cancer is lower than that obtained with other tumor markers. In previous studies our group reported abnormal values of this tumor marker in 39% of the patients. Leitzel et al. (68) reported abnormal c-erbB-2 results in 19% of 300 patients with metastases. Reasons for these discrepancies may be related to the cut-off used: 15 ng/mL in our studies and 30 ng/mL by Leitzel et al. (68). In our last evaluation of tumor markers in 746 patients with breast cancer, c-erbB-2 was evaluated in 282 patients. Abnormal levels of this marker were found in 39.7% of the cases. When 30 ng/mL was used as the cut-point, abnormal levels of this marker were found in only 18.9% of the patients.

Table 6 shows the relationship of c-erbB-2 to the most important prognostic factors in advanced breast cancer. Similar to all tumor markers, c-erbB-2 is related to the site of recurrence. It is highest in visceral metastases, mainly liver metastases, and lowest in locoregional recurrence. Likewise, c-erbB-2 is related to the number of organs involved; patients who have more than one organ involved register significantly higher values. The

Table 5 Tumor marker sensitivity alone or in combination in relation to the site of recurrence

	Both positive	CA 15.3 1 CEA2	CA 15.3 2 CEA1	Both negative
Total	301 (40%)	186 (24%)	83 (11%)	191 (25%)
Local	12 (9%)	22 (17%)	9 (7%)	87 (67%)
Lung	24 (29%)	33 (40%)	8 (9.6%)	18 (22%)
Pleural	18 (48.6%)	11 (30%)	7 (19%)	1 (2.7%)
Bone	141 (44.8%)	74 (23.5%)	38 (12%)	62 (19.7%)
Brain	4 (40%)	1 (10%)	2 (20%)	3 (30%)
Liver	37 (59.8%)	13 (21%)	10 (16%)	2 (3.2%)
Others	2 (40%)	2 (40%)	0	1 (20%)
Multiple not liver	27 (41.5%)	20 (30.8%)	5 (7.7%)	13 (20%)
Multiple liver	36 (66.7%)	10 (18.5%)	4 (7.4%)	4 (7.4%)

Table 6 c-erbB-2 serum levels in patients with recurrent breast cancer, according to the site of recurrence or other prognostic factors

Parameter	Number of patients	Percent >15 ng/mL	Mean ± SD ng/mL	Range	P value
Total	282	39.7%	76 ± 364	1–4.400	
Locoregional	33	15%	10.4 ± 10.8	1–59	0.001
Bone	134	42%	28 ± 55	1–411	
Lung	27	26%	37 ± 86	3–400	
Pleural	18	44%	32 ± 41	5–135	
Liver	21	48%	180 ± 601	3–2760	
Others	5	20%	189 ± 400	1–900	
Multiple no liver	22	45%	24 ± 27	4–92	
Multiple liver	22	68%	471 ± 1071	4–4400	
ER+	166	36%	65 ± 317	1–2760	0.065
ER −	75	45%	115 ± 521	3–4400	
PgR +	139	34%	50 ± 257	1–2600	0.016
PgR −	102	46%	122 ± 521	1–4400	
c-erbB-2 + IHC	40	75%	190 ± 507	1–2760	0.0001
c-erbB-2 − IHC	84	21%	11 ± 6	3–28	
CEA +	149	49%	126 ± 494	1–4400	0.0001
CEA-	133	29%	20 ± 39	1–411	
CA 15.3 +	190	45%	103 ± 440	1–4400	0.003
CA 15.3 −	92	28%	21 ± 46	1–411	

IHC, immunohistochemistry.

highest c-erbB-2 concentrations were found in patients whose cancer involved more than one tissue and in those with liver metastases.

Tumor markers are synthesized by malignant cells, and a correlation between tumor marker expression in tissue and in serum may exist. Table 6 shows that significantly higher c-erbB-2 concentrations were found in patients with overexpression in tissue determined by immunohistochemistry than in patients without overexpression (p < 0.0001). Seventy-five percent of patients with overexpression in tissue had abnormal c-erbB-2 values in serum.

These results are similar to those previously reported by our group in patients with metastases at diagnosis (49). Slightly high c-erbB-2 serum levels were found in patients without overexpression in tissue, and none had levels higher than 30 ng/mL. The positivity of c-erbB-2 in patients without overexpression may be related to the fact that immunohistochemistry was performed in the primary tumor and the metastases may have another biological profile. Another explanation may be that some of these patients (20%) had liver metastases and, as was previously indicated, c-erbB-2 catabolism may be related to the liver (50). Excluding liver metastases and multiple-site recurrence, only 3 patients (3.5%) had c-erbB-2 levels higher than 20 ng/mL.

It is interesting to point out that c-erbB-2 serum levels were related to steroid receptor status, as occurs in tissue, and significantly higher serum levels were found in patients with ER- or PgR- tumors (69). Likewise, significantly higher concentrations of this marker were found in patients with abnormal CEA and/or CA 15.3 serum levels than in those with normal values of these two tumor markers. These differences may be due to the fact that all tumor markers are clearly related to the site of recurrence and the number of organs involved. Moreover, this correlation was the same when patients with locoregional recurrence and patients with liver or multiple metastases were excluded. The reason for this correlation among the different tumor markers requires further investigation.

Monitoring therapy. The main clinical application of tumor markers in advanced disease is to monitor therapy. In contrast to markers in tissue, blood tumor markers reflect a dynamic situation and their measurements can be repeated as required. There is concordance in most of the published articles on the utility of tumor markers in disease monitoring. Patients with disease regression usually show decreased levels while patients with progressive disease generally have increased levels (70–76).

However, studies investgating the role of tumor markers in monitoring metastatic disease according to UICC criteria are few and heterogeneous in terms of criteria for marker assessment and disease status of the patients enrolled (70,71,77–80). In 98 patients with metastases, Iwase et al. (81) demonstrated that a 20% change in tumor marker concentration from the preceding assay correlated significantly with clinical findings. A significant elevation was predictive of new recurrence or tumor regrowth after complete remission, especially in patients with bone metastasis. Van Dalen et al. (78,82) considered tumor marker decrease of more than 50% and increases of more than 25% as significant indicators of tumor marker modification. Using these criteria, investigators found a good correlation between tumor marker levels and clinical outcome in 129 patients. Using three markers, CA 15.3, CEA, and TPS, investigators found a sensitivity of 95%, mainly in patients with progressive disease.

Söletornos et al. (77) evaluated tumor marker utility in monitoring metastatic breast cancer using 3,989 serum samples from 204 patients who were receiving first-line chemotherapy. The efficiency for identifying progression and nonprogression was 94% during therapy and 85% during follow-up, with no false-positive results for progressive disease. In clinically progressive disease, the median positive lead time was 35 days during therapy and 76 days during follow-up. Discordant information was observed in four patients with CEA and CA 15.3. The false-positive signals appeared within the first treatment cycles.

Other authors had previously indicated the possibility of false positive results during the early phase of therapy, synchronously with tumor regression (78,82–84). Yasasever et al. (85) found that serum CEA and CA 15.3 levels in patients with metastases displayed a transient, but significant, elevation at days 15 and 30, respectively, after commencing systemic treatment, which returned to pretreatment levels on the 60th day. In our opinion this transitory increase, which has been termed "spiking," is a rather short-term phenomenon that is hardly ever observed after an observation period of one month and that may be related to tumor cell destruction by treatment. The spiking effect observed in tumor marker levels should be carefully evaluated, and not misdiagnosed as disease progression.

Robertson et al. have (86) demonstrated the usefulness of a biochemical index score, derived from a combination of three serum tumor markers: CEA, CA 15.3, and erythrocyte sedimentation rate (ESR). This score is 0 when the markers are normal, −2 when there is a decrease of more than 10%, +1 when results are included in a variation of 10%, and +2 when tumor markers show increases higher than 10%. Robertson et al. (86) indicated a better relationship existed between the score obtained with tumor markers and tumor response than when using UICC criteria alone.

The utility of tumor markers in patient follow-up is clear in patients whose tumor marker levels are abnormal. Several authors have suggested the inclusion of more markers, not only CEA and CA 15.3, to increase utility. Soletornos et al. (77) suggested the use of CEA, CA 15.3, and TPA because these marker combinations may enhance the diagnostic ability by supplying more true-positive information about progression and more true-negative information about non-progression than do single markers. Additionally, the number of false-positive signals (in terms of progression) may be diminished or eliminated by combining information from more markers. Similar results were reported by van Dalen et al. (78) showing that the combination of the classical tumor markers—CEA, CA 15.3, and TPS—increases the sensitivity and allows a better follow-up.

Ritzke et al. (87) evaluated tumor markers and alkaline phosphatase isoenzymes in 637 patients with bone and liver metastases. They reported that the determination of alkaline phosphatase isoenzymes is a non-invasive, inexpensive, reproducible, and rapid method to detect progressive disease in breast cancer, especially in combination with the tumor markers CA 15.3 and CEA.

Robertson et al. (88,89) used their previously reported biochemical index including c-erbB-2 for prospectively monitoring therapy in patients with metastatic breast cancer in a multicenter study that included 67 patients. c-erbB-2 serum levels were positive in 12/20 (60%). One marker or another was abnormal at diagnosis of metastases in 84% of the patients, but during therapy elevated markers rose to 96%. Changes in the markers were in line with and often pre-dated therapeutic outcome as assessed by the UICC criteria for both remission and progression. The three patients in whom markers were at no time significantly elevated remained in remission. However, combining the index with serum c-erbB-2 did not improve the predictability in the small group of patients studied. Moreover, not all publications have the same conclusions. Volas et al. (17) reported no relationship between c-erbB-2 and the tumor response in a study of 300 patients treated with a second-line hormonotherapy.

Some organizations, such as the British Association of Surgical Oncology, recommend tumor marker measurement as a method for monitoring therapy (90). Similar criteria have been suggested by the working group on tumor markers criteria of the International Society of Oncodevelopmental Biology and Medicine and by the European Working Group on Tumor Markers (6,91).

In short, tumor markers, mainly CEA and CA 15.3, provide an objective method for guiding therapy in patients who have metastatic breast cancer. Monitoring therapy with markers has been shown to be superior to monitoring by conventional criteria laid down by the UICC (92,93). Likewise, biochemical assessment may result in a cost saving of at least 50% when compared with assessment by clinical/radiological criteria, which often require expensive imaging techniques such as CT scans (94). Biochemical indication of response or progression occurs earlier than clinical/radiological response or progression, thus allowing more effective palliation, which is especially important in patients who have advanced breast cancer. Early discontinuation of ineffective therapy, early change of treatment for non-responders, and further continuation of effective treatment are thus feasible. However, whether this monitoring leads to enhanced survival or better quality of life remains to be determined.

Prognosis. Tumor marker serum levels are related to the main prognostic factors in metastatic breast cancer: site of metastases, number of tissues involved, and response to treatment. This relationship suggests their possible prognostic value.

In the previously mentioned study of 761 patients with breast cancer recurrence, we found a significantly shorter OS in patients with abnormal CEA, CA 15.3, or c-erbB2 serum levels (Table 7). Moreover, this prognostic value disappears on exclusion of patients with locoregional recurrence (Table 7). Likewise, tumor markers were not independent prognostic factors in the multivariate analysis.

Results reported by other authors do not coincide. Berruti et al. (95) found that patients with CA 15.3 values <30 U/mL at the time of first recurrence survived significantly longer than those with concentrations greater than this cut-off. On multivariate analysis, CA 15.3 and visceral metastases but not patient age, performance status, and bone metastasis of soft tissue

Table 7 OS in patients with recurrent breast cancer

Parameter	Number of patients	Mean OS	Median OS	P value
Total CEA −	321	112	90	P < 0.0001
Total CEA +	296	84	66	
Metastases CEA −	224	90	69	n.s.s.
Metastases CEA +	277	84	66	
Total CA 15.3 −	242	105	84	n.s.s.
Total CA 15.3 +	375	93	72	
Metastases CA 15.3 −	156	79	63	n.s.s.
Metastases CA 15.3 +	345	89	72	
Total c-erbB2 −	137	90	84	0.02
Total c-erbB2 +	85	78	55	
Metastases c-erbB2 −	113	82	65	n.s.s.
Metastases c-erbB2 +	81	76	55	

n.s.s, not statistically significant

metastases were found to be independent prognostic factors. However, in a more recent and larger study, the same group confirmed CA 15.3 as a prognostic factor in univariate but not multivariate analysis (96).

Hayes et al. (69) reported that abnormal c-erbB-2 serum levels were related to OS in 242 patients with metastatic breast cancer, in univariate but not in multivariate analysis.

In summary, the prognostic value of tumor markers in patients with advanced disease is not clear and new prospective studies evaluating all factors related to prognosis are necessary.

Predictive value. Predictive factors imply relative sensitivity or resistance to specific treatments or agents. It is not easy to differentiate the prognostic and predictive value of a tumor marker. To assess the predictive role of a marker, in regard to relative differences in time to progression, DFS, or OS, outcome data must come from studies in which one group of patients received the specific treatment and the other group did not. This point is difficult to determine in primary locoregional breast cancer because of the lack of tumor marker sensitivity. Likewise, metastatic breast cancer trials also present problems because non-treatment control arms cannot be included for ethical considerations.

The literature suggests that c-erbB-2 amplification and/or overexpression may be useful in predicting therapeutic response (97). Several studies have evaluated the correlation between c-erbB-2 status and response to adjuvant endocrine therapy for primary breast cancer and suggest that c-erbB-2 positive patients may be resistant to adjuvant endocrine therapy (98,99). Moreover, there are contradictory results in relation to this point in patients with metastases (99). Published and reported data consistently support the conclusion that women whose tumors overexpress c-erbB-2 are relatively, but not absolutely, resistant to alkaline agent-based therapy in the adjuvant setting (100). In a review on this issue, Yamauchi et al. (99) recommended adjuvant antracycline-based therapy to patients with c-erbB-2 positive breast cancers. Likewise, preliminary results suggest a better response to taxanes in patients with c-erbB-2 overexpression in tissue, but these results should be confirmed (99,101).

c-erbB-2 overexpression is habitually determined in the primary tumor, while treatment is habitually used in patients with metastases. Likewise, there is a correlation between c-erbB-2 overexpression in tissue and in serum, and most patients with abnormal serum levels have overexpression in tissue. The evaluation of c-erbB-2 in serum may be better than in tissue, in theory, to select treatment, because it is determined when we need the result—i.e., before treatment, when metastases are diagnosed.

Results comparing c-erbB-2 serum levels and response to hormonotherapy are controversial. Leitzel (68) evaluated the relationship between c-erbB-2 overexpression in serum and the response to hormone therapy in 300 metastatic breast cancer patients. Patients randomized to receive second-line hormone therapy with either megestrol acetate or fadrozole were evaluated. The response rate to endocrine therapy was 40.9% in 242 patients with low serum c-erbB-2 levels and only 20.7% in 58 patients with elevated serum c-erbB-2 levels (P = 0.004). The median duration of treatment response was longer in the group with low serum c-erbB-2 levels (15.5 months) compared with the group with elevated serum c-erbB-2 levels (11.6 months). Survival was also significantly shorter in patients with elevated serum c-erbB-2 levels (P .0001). Yamauchi et al. (102) studied the correlation of circulating c-erbB-2 levels and response to droloxifene as first-line endocrine therapy in 96 patients with metastatic breast cancer. The response rate to endocrine therapy was only 9% (3/32) in patients with abnormal c-erbB-2 serum levels and 56% in patients with normal levels of this marker. Furthermore, patients with normal c-erbB-2 levels had a significantly longer time to progression and OS than those patients with abnormal levels even when adjusted for other known predictive factors, such as ER, PgR, site of disease, DFS, and prior adjuvant chemotherapy.

Willsher et al. (103) studied 77 breast cancer patients in stage III or IV treated with first-line tamoxifen therapy. No significant correlation was observed according to pretreatment c-erbB-2 serum levels. In addition, no correlation was observed between this marker and response rates in subgroups of ER-positive or ER-negative patients. Hayes et al. (69) reported abnormal c-erbB-2 serum levels (>10.5 ng/mL) in 37% of 242 patients with metastases and the relationship between tumor markers and tumor burden, progesterone receptor levels, and the presence of visceral metastases. In univariate but not multivariate analysis, among patients treated with endocrine therapy (megestrol acetate), elevated initial HER-2 serum levels were associated with worse OS compared to non-elevated patients. This correlation was not found in patients treated with anthracycline-containing regimens. Likewise, Hayes et al. (69) did not find a relationship between pretreatment levels and rates of response to either endocrine therapy or chemotherapy. Other authors (104) reported similar results.

The relationship between c-erbB-2 serum levels and chemotherapy response is not clear. Harris et al. (105) studied the relationship between c-erbB-2 serum levels and tumor response in 191 women who received either doxorubicin or CMF-based therapy. Although patients with negative c-erbB-2 responded to either regimen equally, patients with abnormal c-erbB-2 serum levels had a higher probability of response to doxorubicin-containing regimen and a trend toward a longer median response duration. Similar results were reported by Collan et al. (106) on evaluating serum c-erbB-2 in 280 patients with metastases treated with paclitaxel (n = 109), combination paclitaxel and doxorubicin (n = 107), or sequential doxorubicin followed by paclitaxel (n = 64). There was no association between pretreatment serum c-erbB-2 levels and objective response rates, either overall or when analyzed by treatment.

A weekly schedule of humanized anti-c-erbB-2 antibodies (Herceptin) is a new therapeutic option for the treatment of c-erbB-2 -positive, advanced breast cancer. Luftner et al. (107) compared the clinical course of the disease using the UICC criteria and c-erbB-2 serum levels in 35 patients with metastatic breast cancer who were treated with Herceptin. Abnormal serum levels of this oncoprotein were found in 28.5% of the patients. While the overall response rate in this study was 36%, the response rate among c-erbB-2 positive patients was 62%, indicating a high sensitivity of c-erbB-2 positive patients to dose-intense paclitaxel treatment. In all responders, the c-erbB-2 serum levels decreased below the detection limit either before the clinical diagnosis of response or by the end of the next cycle. However, similar results were obtained in patients with stable or progressive disease and abnormal c-erbB-2 serum levels. Lüftner et al. (107) suggested that the decrease in the serum oncoprotein might indicate a regression of the c-erbB-2 positive tumor fraction, while the c-erbB-2 negative part of the tumor progressed. Another possibility is that c-erbB-2 in serum might complex with this antibody, creating immune complexes that are rapidly cleared by the reticulo-endothelial system. This clearance might decrease activity and possibly even enhance toxicity or false monitoring results. The possible relationship between c-erbB-2 serum levels and clinical outcome in patients treated with trastuzumab are controversial. Several studies reported that c-erbB-2 serum levels failed to demonstrate any association of this marker in trastuzumab treatment, alone or associated with chemotherapy (99,108). However other studies have shown a clear correlation between c-erbB-2 levels and clinical outcome (109).

Other tumor markers that may be useful as predictive factors in the future are the mucins. MUC1 is a self-antigen that undergoes changes in its carbohydrate composition during carcinogenesis. These changes lead to exposure on the cryptic peptide molecule and/or carbohydrate epitopic sequences. This altered molecule gains access to the circulation in cancer patients and elicits immune response that could be beneficial to the patient by restricting tumor growth and dissemination (110). Immune responses to MUC1 can also be induced by MUC1-based vaccines (111). Many of these vaccines have already been applied in phase I clinical trials. The MUC1 peptide vaccines tested to date differ in vectors, carrier proteins, and adjuvants, but are similar in showing low toxicity (112,113). To our knowledge, no clear tumor responses have been observed in these phase I trials. The clinical value of these immunotherapeutic approaches to the treatment of carcinomas still remains to be proven.

In summary, the predictive value of tumor markers has not been proven, but some studies have suggested their possible application, mainly c-erbB-2 . Further studies are required to confirm this issue, especially comparing different treatment modalities.

Tumor Markers in Tissue

A logical first step in tumor marker study is tumor tissue evaluation. A tumor without presence of tumor markers in tissue, cannot, in theory, increase the serum levels of this marker. This hypothesis has been confirmed with c-erbB-2 as previously indicated in this chapter (11,13,16,49,64,89), but not with other tumor markers used in breast cancer. Several studies have evaluated CEA in tissue, mainly using immunohistochemistry or tissue homogenate (cytosol). These studies report CEA positivity in 66–85% of patients with primary breast cancer (114–118). We determined (115) the CEA concentrations in the cytoplasmic membrane (pellet) and cytosol prospectively in 298 mammary tissue samples (30 benign, 242 primary breast cancer, and 26 metastatic breast cancer). We found that CEA levels in tissue are significantly higher in pellet than in cytosol, as has been reported by immunohistochemistry. Likewise, CEA synthesis by the malignant breast cell seems to be an intrinsic characteristic of the tumor in relationship with cell differentiation (ER presence) but not with the parameters used in the evaluation of tumor spread (tumor size, nodal involvement, presence of metastases). Similar results in tissue have been described by most authors (116–118).

A clear relationship was found between CEA in pellet and in serum in both patients with primarily locoregional cancer and in patients with metastases (11,115). Gion et al. (118) found no correlation between CEA in cytosol and in serum. In our experience this correlation is found mainly in pellet, but not in cytosol. Other studies using immunohistochemistry reported no relationship between CEA positivity and serum (116,117). Differences may be related to the method used.

The correlation between tissue and serum has improved the clinical applications, allowing clinicians to select patients whose serum CEA will be useful in the prognosis and in early diagnosis of recurrence. Several studies have reported the prognostic value of serum CEA in patients with primary breast cancer (16,19,23,115–117), but tumors with and without CEA positivity in tissue were evaluated. When we excluded breast tumors without CEA in tissue in the prognostic evaluation of serum CEA, the application of this marker improved. Eighty-five percent of the tumors with high CEA levels in pellet, but with negativity in serum, were free of disease (regardless of nodal involvement), versus only 22% of patients with high CEA values in tissue and serum. Logically, CEA in serum did not have prognostic interest in the tumors with low CEA in pellet. Likewise, in this study we found that serum CEA is an independent prognostic factor in patients with breast cancer, in both DFS or OS.

The simultaneous determination of CEA in tissue and serum may open up other possibilities for clinical application. CEA is useful in the early diagnosis of recurrence with a high specificity but low sensitivity (40%). CEA was the first sign of recurrence in 73% of patients with recurrence—the CEA in pellet exceeded 10 ng/mg of protein, in contrast with the 9% found in patients with low CEA concentrations in pellet. These results indicate that CEA evaluation in tissue allows us to know in which patients serial CEA determinations would be useful for early diagnosis of relapse (those with CEA positivity in pellet), improving the sensitivity and efficacy of CEA (11,115,119).

MCA concentrations in tissue were retrospectively evaluated in 221 of the patients used in CEA evaluations (11, 64, 119). The results obtained were similar to those with CEA, with higher concentrations in pellet than in cytosol, and no relationship to the prognostic factors of breast cancer (tumor size, nodal involvement), excluding ER and PgR. The higher concentration in pellet than in cytosol is concordant with the fact that this antigen is mainly found in the cytoplasmic membrane by immunohistochemistry (120). There was also a clear relationship between tissue and serum MCA or CA 15.3 values.

In short, simultaneous evaluation of tumor markers in tissue and serum seems to provide knowledge as to which factors are related to its release and presence in serum. The study of tumor markers in tissue, mainly in pellet, improves the clinical application of tumor markers by making it possible to select the patients in whom serum tumor markers are useful in the prognosis, the early diagnosis of recurrence, and in the follow-up.

SUMMARY

MUC-1 antigen and CEA are the most useful serum markers in patients with breast cancer. Serial determinations of these markers are useful in assessing prognosis, detecting early relapse (metastasis), and monitoring therapy. Steroid receptors are the only tissue-based markers accepted in clinical practice, having an established role in predicting hormone sensitivity, and a lesser role in prognosis. Certain new markers such as c-erbB-2, p53, and uPA/PAI-1 look promising as prognostic and predictive factors but further research is necessary before their clinical utility is established.

REFERENCES

1. Madigan M, Ziegler R, Benichon C, et al. Proportion of breast cancer cases in the United States explained by well established risk factors. J NCI 1995;87:1681–1691.
2. Harris J, Lippman M, Morrow M, et al. Diseases of the breast. Philadelphia: Lippincott-Raven, 1996.
3. Harris J, Morrow M, Norton l. Malignant tumors of the breast. In: DeVita VT, Hellman S, Rosengberg SA, (eds.). Cancer Principles and Practice of Oncology, vol 2. Philadelphia, PA: Lippincott-Raven Publishers, 1997:1557–1616.
4. Eissa S. Tumor markers in breast neoplasms. In: Eissa S, Shoman S (eds). Tumor markers. London: Chapman and Hall, 1998: 262–273.
5. Clayton F, Ordoñez NG, Hassen GM, Hasen H. Immunoperoxidase localization of lactoalbumin in malignant breast neoplasms. Arch Pathol Lab Med 1982;106:268–270.
6. Molina R, Duffy MJ, Aronsson AC, et al. Tumor markers in breast cancer. EGTM recommendations. Anticancer Res 1999;19: 2803–2805.
7. Sharpin C, Lachard A, Pourreau-Schneider N, Jacquemier J, et al. Localization of lactoferrin and nonspecific cross-reacting antigen in human breast carcinoma: an immunohistochemical study using the ABC method. Cancer 1985;55:2612–2617.
8. Van Dalen A. Significance of cytokeratin markers TPA, TPA (cyk), TPS and CYFRA 21.1 in metastatic disease. Anticancer Res 1996;16:2345–2350.
9. Bieglmayer C, Szepesi T, Kopp B, et al. CA15.3, MCA, CAM26, CAM29 are members of a polymorphic family of mucin-like glycoproteins. Tumor Biol 1991;12:138–148.
10. Price MR, Rye PD, Petrakou R, et al. Summary report on the ISOBM TD–4 workshop: analysis of 56 monoclonal antibodies against the MUC1 mucin. Tumor Biol 1998;19:1–20.
11. Molina R, Ballesta AM. Evaluation of several tumor markers (MCA, CA 15.3, BCM, and CA 549) in tissue and serum of patients with breast cancer. In: Ceriani RL (ed). Breast epithelial antigens: molecular biology to clinical applications. New York, NY: Plenum Press, 1991:161–163.
12. Dnistrian AM, Schwartz MK, Greenberg EJ, Smith CA, Schwartz DC. Evaluation of CAM26, CAM29, CA15.3, and CEA as circulating tumor markers in breast cancer patients. Tumor Biol 1991; 12:1282–1290.
13. Hayes DF, Tondini C, Kufe DW. CA 15.3 . In: Ballesta AM, Torre GC, Bombardieri E, Gion M, Molina R (eds). Up Dating on tumor markers in tissues and in biological fluids. Basic aspects and clinical applications. Torino, Italy: Edizini Minerva Medica, 1993:525–532.
14. Devine PL, Duroux MA, Quin RJ, et al. CA15-3, CASA, MSA, and TPS as diagnostic serum markers in breast cancer. Breast Cancer Res Treat 1995;34:245–251.
15. Depres-Brummer P, Itzhaki M, Bakker PJ, Hoek FJ, Veenhof KH, de Wit H. The usefulness of CA15.3, mucin-like carcinoma-associated antigen and carcinoembryonic antigen in determining the clinical course in patients with metastatic breast cancer. J Cancer Res Clin Oncol 1995;121:419–422.
16. Molina R, Jo J, Filella X, et al. c-erbB-2 oncoprotein in the sera and tissue of patients with breast cancer: utility in prognosis. Anticancer Res 1996;16:2295–300.
17. Volas GH, Leitzel K, Teramoto Y, Grossberg H, Demers L, Lipton A. Serial serum c-erbB-2 levels in patients with breast carcinoma. Cancer 1996;15;78:267–272.
18. Fehm T, Maimonis P, Weitz S, Teramoto Y, Katalinic A, Jager W. Influence of circulating c-erbB-2 serum protein on response to adjuvant chemotherapy in node-positive breast cancer patients. Br Cancer Res Treat 1997;43:87–95.
19. Hayes DF. Serum (circulating) tumor markers for breast cancer. Recent Results in Cancer Res 1996;140:101–113.
20. Kuhajda FP, Offutt LE, Mendelson G. The distribution of carcinoembryonic antigen in breast carcinoma: diagnostic and prognostic implications. Cancer 1983;52:1257–1264.
21. Gion M, Mione R, Nascimben O, Valsecchi M, et al. The tumor-associated antigen CA15.3 in primary breast cancer: evaluation of 667 cases. Br J Cancer 1991; 63:809–813.
22. Bast RC, Bates S, Bredt AB, et al. Clinical practice guidelines for the use of tumor markers in breast and colorectal cancer. J Clin Oncol 1996;14:2843–2877.

23. Molina R, Filella X, Mengual P, et al. MCA in patients with breast cancer: correlation with CEA and CA 15.3 Int. J Biol Markers 1990;5:14–21.
24. O' Hanlon DM, Kerin MJ, Koent P, Maher D, Grimes H, Given HF. An evaluation of pre-operative CA15.3 measurement in primary breast carcinoma. Br J Cancer 1995; 71:1288–1291.
25. Van Dalen A. Pre-operative tumor marker levels in patients with breast cancer and their prognosis. Tumor Biol 1990;11:189–195.
26. Molina R, Jo J, Filella X, et al. C-erbB-2 oncoprotein, CEA, and CA 15.3 in patients with breast cancer: prognostic value. Br Cancer Res Treat 1998;51:109–119.
27. Gozdz SS, Kowaiska MM, Sluszniak JT, et al. Pretreatment concentrations of breast carcinoma antigen (CA 15.3) and mucin-like carcinoma-associated antigen in patients with carcinoma of the breast. Tumor Biol 1989;10:103–108.
28. Foekens JA, van Putten WLJ, Portengen H, et al. Prognostic value of pS2 and cathepsin D in 710 human primary breast tumors: multivariate analysis. J Clin Oncol 1993;11:899–908.
29. Janicke F, Schmitt M, Pache L, et al. Urokinase (uPA) and its inhibitor PAI-1 are strong and independent prognostic factors in node-negative breast cancer. Breast Cancer Res Treat 1993;24:195–209.
30. Ewers SB, Attewell R, Baldetorp B, et al. Prognostic significance of flow cytometric DNA analysis and estrogen receptor content in breast carcinomas: a 10-year survival study. Breast Cancer Res Treat 1992;24:115–126.
31. Allred DC, Clark GM, Tandon AK, et al. HER-2/neu in node-negative breast cancer: prognostic significance of over-expression influenced by the presence of in situ carcinoma. J Clin Oncology 1992;10:599–605.
32. Silvestrini R, Veronesi S, Benini E, et al. Expression of p53, glutathione S-transferase pi and Bcl-2 proteins and benefit from adjuvant radiotherapy in breast cancer. J Nat Cancer Inst 1997;89:639–645.
33. Allred DC, Clark GM, Molina R, et al. Over-expression of HER-2/neu and its relationship with other prognostic factors change during the progression of in-situ to invasive breast cancer. Human Pathol 1992;23:974–979.
34. Theriault RL, Hortobagyi GN, Fritsche HA, Frye D, Martinez R, Buzdar AU. The role of serum CEA as a prognostic indicator in Stage II and III breast cancer patients treated with adjuvant chemotherapy. Cancer 1989;63:828–835.
35. McLauglin R, McGrath J, Grimes H, Given HF. The prognostic value of the tumor marker CA 15.3 at initial diagnosis of patients with breast cancer. Int J Biol Markers 2000;15:340–342.
36. Ligtenberg MJL, Buijs F, Vos HL, Hilkens J. Supression of cellular aggregation by high levels of episialin. Cancer Res 1992;52:2318–2324.
37. Von Mensdorff-Pouilly S, Gourevitch MM, Kenemans P, et al. Humoral immune response to polymorphic epithelial mucin (MUC-1) in patients with benign and malignant breast tumors. Eur J Cancer 1996;32:1325–1331.
38. Duffy MJ, Shering S, Sherry F, McDermott E, O'Higgins N. CA 15.3: a prognostic marker in breast cancer. Int J Biol. Markers 2000;15:330–333.
39. Ebeling FC, Schmitt UM, Untch M, et al. Tumor markers CEA and CA 15.3 as prognostic factors in breast cancer. Univariate and multivariate analysis. Anticancer Res 1999;19:2545–2550.
40. Fehm T, Jager W. Clinical value of c-erbB-2 serum protein in primary and metastatic breast cancer. In: Molina R, Ballesta AM. (eds). Biologia y Utilidad Clinica de los marcadores Tumorales. Barcelona: Grafiques Sant Quirze, 1999:119–123.
41. Molina R, Zanon G, Filella X, et al. Use of serial carcinoembryonic antigen and CA 15.3 assays in detecting relapses in breast cancer patients. Br Cancer Res Treat 1995; 36:41–48.
42. Jäger W, Merkle E, Lang N. Increasing serum tumor markers as decision criteria for hormone therapy of metastatic breast cancer. Tumor Biol 1994;12: 60–66.
43. Safi F, Kohler I, Rottinger E, Beger HG. The value of the tumor marker CA15.3 in diagnosing and monitoring breast cancer. Cancer 1991;68:574–582.
44. Chang DW, Beveridge RA, Muss H, et al. Use of Truquant BR radioimmunoassay for early detection of breast cancer recurrence in patients with Stage II and Stage III disease. J Clin Oncol 1997;15:2322–2328.
45. Soletormos G, Nielsen D, Schioler V, et al. A novel method for monitoring high-risk breast cancer with tumor markers: CA15.3 compared to CEA and TPA. Ann Oncol 1993; 4:861–869.
46. Loomer L, Brockshmidt JK, Muss HB, Saylor G. Post-operative follow-up of patients with early breast cancer. Patterns of care among clinical oncologists and a review of the literature. Cancer 1991;67:55–60.
47. Vizcarra E, Lluch A, Cibrian R, Jarque F, Garcia-Conde J . CA 15.3, CEA, and TPA tumor markers in the early diagnosis of breast cancer relapse. Oncology 1994;51:491–496.
48. Pectasides D, Pavlidis N, Gogou L, Antoniou F, Nicolaides C, Tsikalakis D . Clinical value of CA 15.3, mucin-like carcinoma-associated antigen, tumor polypeptide antigen, and carcinoembryonic antigen in monitoring early breast cancer patients. Am J Clin Oncol 1996;19:459–464.
49. Molina R, Jo J, Zanon G, et al. Utility of c-erbB-2 in tissue and in serum in the early diagnosis of recurrence in breast cancer patients: comparison with carcinoembryonic antigen and CA15.3. Br J Cancer 1996;74:1126–1131.
50. Molina R, Jo J, Filella X, et al. Serum levels of c-erbB-2 (HER-2/neu) in patients with malignant and non-malignant diseases. Tumor Biol 1997;18:188–196.
51. Holli K, Hakama M. Effectiveness of routine and spontaneous follow-up visits for breast cancer. Eur J. Cancer Clin Oncol 1989:25:251–258.
52. Ghezzi P, Magnanini S, Rinaldi M, et al. Impact of follow-up testing on survival and health-related quality of life in breast cancer patients: a multicenter randomized controlled trial. JAMA 1994;271:1581–1591.
53. Jaeger W, Merkle E, Lang N. Breast cancer and clinical utility of CA 15.3 and CEA. Scand J Clin Lab Invest 1995;55:87–92.
54. Leone B, Romero A, Rabinovich M, et al. Stage IV breast cancer: clinical course and survival of patients with osseous versus extraosseous metastases at initial diagnosis. Am J Clin Oncol 1988;11:618–624.
55. Howell A, Defriend D, Robertson J, et al. Response to a specific antioestrogen (ICI 182780) in tamoxifen-resistant breast cancer. Lancet 1995;345:29.
56. Amer M. Chemotherapy and pattern of metastases in breast cancer patients. J Surg Oncol 1982;19:101–108.
57. Colomer R, Ruibal A, Genolla J, Salvador L. Circulating tumor marker levels in advanced breast carcinoma correlate with the extent of metastatic disease. Cancer 1989;64:106–112.
58. Hayes DF, Zurawski VR, Kufe DW. Comparison of circulating CA 15.3 and carcinoembryonic antigen levels in patients with breast cancer. J Clin Oncol 1986; 4:1542–1550.
59. Tomlinson IP, Whyman A, Barrett JA, Kremer JK. Tumour marker CA15-3: possible uses in the routine management of breast cancer. Eur J Cancer 1995;31:899–902.

60. Jager W, Kissing A, Ciladi S, Melsheimer R, Lang N. Is an increase in CA 125 in breast cancer patients an indicator of pleural metastases? Br J Cancer 1994;70:493.495.
61. Aydiner A, Topuz E, Disci R, Yasasever V, Dincer M, Dincol K, Bilge N .Serum tumor markers for detection of bone metastasis in breast cancer patients. Acta Oncol 1994;33:181–186.
62. Murray A, Clinton O, Earl H, Price M, Moore A. Assessment of five serum marker assays in patients with advanced breast cancer treated with medroxyprogesterone acetate. Eur J Cancer 1995;31:1605–1610.
63. Molina R, Agusti C, Filella X, et al. Study of a new tumor marker, CYFRA 21–1, in malignant and nonmalignant diseases. Tumor Biol 1994;15:318–325.
64. Molina R, Jo J, Filella X, et al. Mucin-like carcinoma-associated antigen (MCA) in tissue and serum of patients with breast cancer: clinical applications in prognosis and disease monitoring. Int J Biol Markers 1993;8:113–123.
65. Vibert HG, Houston AS, Wilkins GP, Kemp PM, Macleod MA. CA549 and TPS patterns in the diagnosis and staging of patients with breast carcinoma. Int J Biol Markers 1996;11:198–202.
66. Schuurman JJ, Bong SB, Einarsson R. Determination of serum tumor markers TPS and CA 15.3 during monitoring of treatment in metastatic breast cancer patients. Anticancer Res 1996;16:2169–2172.
67. Willsher PC, Beaver J, Blamey RW, Robertson JF. Serum tissue polypeptide specific antigen (TPS) in breast cancer patients: comparison with CA 15.3 and CEA. Anticancer Res 1995;15:1609–1611.
68. Leitzel K, Teramoto Y, Konrad K, et al. Elevated serum c-erbB-2 antigen levels and decreased response to hormone therapy of breast cancer. J Clin Oncol 1995;13:1129–1135.
69. Hayes DF, Yamauchi H, Broadwater G, et al. Cancer and Leukemia Group B. Circulating HER-2/erbB-2/c-neu (HER-2) extracellular domain as a prognostic factor in patients with metastatic breast cancer: Cancer and Leukemia Group B Study 8662. Clinical Cancer Res 2001;7:2703–2711.
70. Robertson JFR, Pearson D, Price MR, Selby C, Blamey RW, Howell A. Objective measurement of therapeutic response in breast cancer using tumor markers. Br J Cancer 1991;64:757–763.
71. Tondini C, Hayes DF, Gelman R, Henderson IC, Kufe DW. Comparison of CA15.3 and carcinoembryonic antigen in monitoring the clinical course of patients with metastatic breast cancer. Cancer Res 1998;48:4107–4112.
72. Lamerz R, Leonhards A, Ehrhardt H, von Lieven H. Serial carcinoembryonic antigen (CEA) determinations in the management or metastatic breast cancer. Oncodev Biol Med 1980;1:123–135.
73. Gion M. Serum markers in breast cancer management. The Breast 1992;1:173–178.
74. Palazzo S, Liguori V, Molinari B. Is the carcinoembryonic antigen test a valid predictor of response to medical therapy in disseminated breast cancer? Tumor 1986;72:515–518.
75. Williams MR, Turkes A, Pearson D, Twining P, Griffiths K, Blamey RW. The use of serum carcinoembryonic antigen to assess therapeutic response in locally advanced and metastatic breast cancer: a prospective study with external review. Eur J Surg Oncol 1998;14:417–422.
76. van Dalen A. TPS in breast cancer: a comparative study with carcinoembryonic antigen and CA 15.3. Tumor Biol 1992;13:10–17.
77. Soletornos G, Nielsen D, Schioler V, Skovsgaard T, Dombernowsky P. Tumor markers cancer antigen 15.3, carcinoembryonic antigen, and tissue polypeptide antigen for monitoring metastatic breast cancer during first-line chemotherapy and follow-up. Clin Chem 1996;42:564–575.
78. Van Dalen A, Heering KJ, Barak V, et al. Treatment response in metastatic breast cancer: a multi-center study comparing UICC criteria and tumor marker changes. The Breast 1996;5:82–88.
79. Dnistrian AM, Schwartz MK, Greenberg EJ, Smith CA, Schwartz DC. CA 15.3, carcinoembryonic antigen in the clinical evaluation of breast cancer. Clin Chim Acta 1991;200:81–94.
80. Loprinzi CL, Tormey DC, Rasmussen P, et al. Prospective evaluation of carcinoembryonic antigen levels and alternating chemotherapeutic regimens in metastatic breast cancer. J Clin Oncol 1986;4:46–56.
81. Iwase H, Kobayashi S, Itoh Y, et al. Evaluation of serum tumor markers in patients with advanced or recurrent breast cancer. Br C Res Treat 1995;33:83–88.
82. Van Dalen A, Barak V, Cremaschi A, et al. Increasing marker levels in breast cancer patients with clinically complete remission or stable disease: results of a multi-center study. 10th International Meeting of Gynaecological Oncology (Coimbra, Portugal) 1997:339–345.
83. Quayle JB. Tumor lysis as a factor affecting blood levels of CEA. Br J Cancer 1982; 46:213–219.
84. Kiang DT, Greenberg LJ, Kennedy BJ. Tumor marker kinetics in the monitoring of breast cancer. Cancer 1990;65:193–199.
85. Yasasever V, Dincer M, Camlica H, Karaloglu D, Dalay N. Utility of CA 15.3 and CEA in monitoring breast cancer patients with bone metastases: special emphasis on "spiking" phenomena. Clin Biochem 1997;30:53–56.
86. Robertson JFR, Pearson D, Price MR, Selby C, Blamey RW, Howell A. Objective measurement of therapeutic response in breast cancer using tumor markers. Br J Cancer 1991;64: 757–761.
87. Ritzke C, Stieber P, Untch M, Nagel D, Eirmann W, Fateh-Moghadam A. Alkaline phosphatase isoenzymes in detection and follow-up of breast cancer metastases. Anticancer Res 1998; 18:1243–1249.
88. Robertson JF, Jaeger W, Syzmendera JJ, et al. The objective measurement of remission and progression in metastatic breast cancer by use of serum tumor markers. European Group for Serum Tumor Markers in Breast Cancer. European J Cancer 1999; 35:47–53.
89. Cheung KL, Pinder SE, Paish C, et al. The role of blood tumor marker measurement (using a biochemical index score and c-erbB-2) in directing chemotherapy in metastatic breast cancer. Int J Biol. Markers, 2000;15:203–209.
90. Breast Specialty Group of the British Association of Surgical Oncology. The guidelines for the management of metastatic bone disease in breast cancer in the United Kingdom. Eur J Surg Oncol 1999;25:3–23.
91. Bonfrer JMG. Working group on tumor marker criteria (WGTMC). Tumor Biol 1990;11:287–288.
92. Dixon AR, Jackson L, Chan SY, Badley RA, Blamey RW. Continuous chemotherapy in responsive metastatic breast cancer: a role for tumor markers? Br J Cancer 1993;9:181–185.
93. van Dalen A, van der Linde DL, Heering KJ, van Oudalblas AB. How can treatment response be measured in breast cancer patients? Anticancer Res 1993;13:1901–1904.
94. Robertson JFR, Whynes DK, Dixon A, Blamey RW. Potential for cost economics in guiding therapy in patients with metastatic breast cancer. Br J Cancer 1995;72:174–177.
95. Berruti A, Tampellini M, Torta M, Buniva T, Gorzegno G, Dogliotti L. Prognostic value in predicting overall survival of two

mucinous markers: CA 15.3 and CA 125 in breast cancer patients at first relapse of disease. Eur J Cancer 1994;30:2082–2084.
96. Tampellini M, Berrutti A, Gerbino A, et al. Relationship between CA 15.3 serum levels and disease extent in predicting overall survival of breast cancer patients newly diagnosed metastatic disease. Br J Cancer 1997;75:698–702.
97. Wright C, Cairns J, Cantwell BJ, et al. Response to mitoxantrone in advanced breast cancer: correlation with expression of c-erbB-2 protein and glutathione S-transferases. Br J Cancer 1992;65:271–274.
98. Carlomagno C, Perrone F, Gallo C, et al. C-erbB-2 over-expression decreases the benefit of adjuvant tamoxifen in early-stage breast cancer without axillary lymph node metastases. J Clin Oncol 1998;16:1340–1349.
99. Yamuchi H, Stearns V, Hayes DF. When is a tumor marker ready for prime time? A case study of c-erbB-2 as a predictive factor in breast cancer. J Clin Oncol 2001;19:2334–2356.
100. Miles DW, Harris WH, Gillett CE, et al. Effect of c-erbB-2 and estrogen receptor status on survival of women with primary breast cancer treated with adjuvant cyclophosphamide/methotrexate/fluorouracil. Int J Cancer 1999, 84:354–359.
101. Baselga J, Seidman AD, Rosen PP, Norton L. HER-2 over-expression and paclitaxel sensitivity in breast cancer: therapeutic implications. Oncology 1997;11:43–48.
102. Yamauchi H, O'Neill A, Gelman R, et al. Prediction of response to anti-estrogen therapy in advanced breast cancer patients by pretreatment circulating levels of extracellular domain of the HER-2/c-neu protein. J Clin Oncol 1997;15:2518–2525.
103. Willsher PC, Beaver J, Pinder S, et al. Prognostic significance of serum c-erbB-2 protein in breast cancer patients. Breast Cancer Res Treat 1996;40:251–255.
104. Harris L, Luftner D, Jager W, Robertson JF. C-erbB-2 in serum of patients with breast cancer. Int J. Biol Markers 1999;14:8–15.
105. Harris LN, Trock B, Berris M, et al. The role of ERBB2 extracellular domain in predicting response to chemotherapy in breast cancer patients. Proc Am Soc Clin Oncol 1996;15:108[a].
106. Collan J, Sjostrom J, von Boguslawski K, et al. Predictive value of c-erbB-2 expression for response to docetaxel or methotrexate-fluoruracil in advanced breast cancer. Breast Cancer Res Treat 1999;57–64.
107. Lüftner D, Schnabel S, Possinger K. C-erbB-2 in serum of patients receiving fractionated paclitaxel chemotherapy. Int J Biol Markers 1999;14:55–59.
108. Slamon D, Leyland-Jones B, Shak S, et al. Addition of Herceptin (humanized anti-HER-2 antibody) to first-line chemotherapy for HER-2 over-expressing metastatic breast cancer (HER-2l/MBC) markedly increases anticancer activity: a randomized multinational controlled phase III trial. Proc Am Soc Clin Oncol 1998;17:98[a].
109. Yeung k, Grupta R, Haidak d, et al. Weekly herceptin and one-hour taxol infusion regimen for human epidermal growth factor receptor-2 overexpressed metastatic breast cancer. Proc Am Soc Clin Oncol 2000;19:142[a].
110. Ioannides CG, Fisk B, Jerome KR, Irimura T, Wharton JT, Finn OJ. Cytotoxic T cells from ovarian malignant tumors can recognize polymorphic epithelial mucin core peptides. J Immunol 1993;151:3693–3703.
111. Von Mensdorff-Poully S, Snijdewint FGM, Verstraeten AA, Verheijen RHM, Kenemans P. Human MUC1 mucin: a multifaceted glycoprotein. Int J Biol Markers 2000;15:343–356.
112. Goygos JS, Elder E, Whiteside TL, Finn OJ, Lotze MT. A phase I trial of a synthetic mucin peptide vaccine. J Surg Res 1996;63:298–304.
113. Reddish MA, MacLean GD, Koganty RR, et al. Anti-MUC1 class I restricted CTLs in metastatic breast cancer patients immunized with a synthetic MUC1 peptide. Int J Cancer 1998;76:817–823.
114. Horowitz JD, Au FC, Tang CK, Stein B, Campana TJ. Tissue carcinoembryonic antigen levels in benign and malignant diseases of the breast. J Surg Oncol 1989;40:248–254.
115. Molina R, Farrus B, Filella X, et al. Carcinoembryonic antigen in tissue and serum from Breast Cancer patients: Relationship with steroid receptors and clinical applications in the prognosis and early diagnosis of recurrence. Anticancer Res 1999;19:2557–2562.
116. Mansour EG, Hastert M, Park CH, Koehler KA, Petrelli M. Tissue and plasma carcinoembryonic antigen in early breast cancer: a prognostic factor. Cancer 1983;51:1243–1248.
117. Shousha J, Lyssiotis T, Godfrey V, et al: Carcinoembryonic antigen in breast cancer tissue, a useful prognostic indicator Br Med J 1989; 1:777–779.
118. Gion M, Mione R, Dittadi R, et al. Carcinoembryonic antigen, ferritin and tissue polypeptide antigen in serum and tissue. Relationship with receptor content in breast carcinoma. Cancer 1986;57:917–922.
119. Molina R. Tumor markers in serum and tissue of patients with breast cancer: correlationship with steroid receptors, clinical applications. In: Ballesta AM, Torre GC, Bombardieri E, Gion M, Molina R (eds). Torino, Italy: Edizioni Minerva Medica, 1993: 713–724.
120. Zenklusen HR, Stahli C, Gudat F, Ovebeck J, Rolink J, Heitz PhU. The immunohistochemical reactivity of a new antiepithelial monoclonal antibody (b-12) against breast carcinoma and other normal and neoplastic human tissues. Virchows Arch A Pathol Anat 1988;413:3–10.

Chapter 15

Prognostic and Predictive Markers for Breast Cancer

Frédérique Spyratos

Breast cancer is the most common type of cancer among women in western countries (1,2). The incidence rate is 80 to 90 new cases among every 100,000 women. More than 180,000 women are diagnosed with breast cancer each year in the U.S., and 25,000 each year in France. If current breast cancer rates remain constant, a woman born today has a one-in-ten chance of developing breast cancer.

The exact causes of breast cancer are not known. However, studies show that the risk of breast cancer increases as a woman ages (this disease is very uncommon in women under the age of 35). Most breast cancers occur in women over the age of 50, and the risk is especially high for women over age 60. Also, breast cancer occurs more often in Caucasian women than in African American or Asian women. The following conditions increase a woman's chances of getting breast cancer (1,2):

- Women who have had cancer in one breast face an increased risk of getting it in their other breast.
- A diagnosis of atypical hyperplasia or lobular carcinoma in situ (LCIS) may increase a woman's risk for developing cancer.
- Family history of breast cancer indicates a possible genetic contribution to breast cancer risk.
- Formal studies of families (linkage analysis) have subsequently proven the existence of an autosomal dominant form of breast cancer, and have led to the identification of several highly penetrant genes (BRCA1, BRCA2) of major effect as the cause of inherited cancer risk in many cancer-prone families (3,4). These mutations are rare and are estimated to account for no more than 5% to 10% of breast cancer cases overall.

Other factors may be associated with an increased risk for breast cancer. For example, evidence suggests that the longer a woman is exposed to estrogen (estrogen made by the body, taken as a drug, or delivered by a patch), the more likely she is to develop breast cancer (5). The risk is somewhat increased among women who began menstruation at an early age (before age 12), experienced menopause late (after age 55), never had children, or took hormone replacement therapy for long periods of time. Each of these factors increases the amount of time a woman's body is exposed to estrogen. Women who have their first child late (after about age 30) have a greater chance of developing breast cancer than women who have a child at a younger age. Most women who develop breast cancer have none of the risk factors listed above, other than the risk that comes with growing older.

A screening mammogram and clinical breast exams performed by health professionals are the best tools available for finding breast cancer early, before symptoms appear (2). Mammograms can often detect a breast lump before it is large enough to be discovered in a physical examination. Also, a mammogram can show small deposits of calcium in the breast. Although most calcium deposits are benign, a cluster of very tiny specks of calcium (called microcalcifications) may be an early sign of cancer.

Although mammograms are the best way to find breast abnormalities early, they do have some limitations. A mammogram may miss some cancers that are present (false negative) or may find things that turn out not to be cancer (false positive). If an area of the breast looks suspicious on the screening mammogram, additional (diagnostic) mammograms may be needed. Depending on the results, fluid or tissue must be removed from the breast to make a cytological (fine-needle aspiration or cytopuncture) or histological (needle or surgical biopsy) diagnosis.

Conventional clinical and histopathological tumor characteristics provide some guide to risk of relapse after surgery. Tumor-Node-Metastases (TNM) stage, axillary node status, and tumor size have long been recognized as the most powerful predictors of breast cancer recurrence (1). In addition, age, histological tumor type, standardized pathologic grade, presence of lymphatic or vascular invasion, and hormone receptor status are accepted prognostic factors (6). Sentinel lymph node biopsy is now proposed as a potential alternative to axillary dissection for staging breast cancer (7).

It is important to identify those patients at risk of relapse despite good classical prognostic indices. For example, axillary-lymph-node-negative patients with tumors less than 1 cm in diameter, of low pathological grade, and with no vascular invasion have a very low probability of relapse after surgery, but these indices are not absolutely predictive. Biological prognostic and predictive factors could be used to adjust adjuvant treatment to individual tumor characteristics. A series of biological markers has been tested for their predictive value regarding survival or treatment responses in breast cancer (8,9). In the light of the advances in molecular biology and the many reports on prognostic and/or predictive factors, the scarcity of data showing the clinical value of such factors is disappointing. A recent update of the American Society of Clinical Oncology guidelines on the use of tissue tumor markers in the management of breast cancer patients recommended measuring only estrogen receptor (ER) and progesterone receptor (PR), which has been clinical practice in many centers for more than 20 years (10). The Tumor Marker Utility Grading System (TMUGS) (11) was developed as a means to objectively evaluate the clinical utility of individual prognostic factors. In the medical management of individual patients, TMUGS can be used to determine whether sufficient evidence exists to use information derived from a specific tumor marker. In this system, specific tumor markers or factors are evaluated and assigned a semi-quantitative score ranging from 0 to 3+. Published studies proposed using relevant "levels of evidence" (see Chapter 3): LOE I gives the strongest support based on evidence derived from prospective high-powered trials while LOE III is the weakest. The data from LOE III studies are the most useful for generating hypotheses, but they require confirmation in either LOE I or II studies. Unfortunately, most of the available evidence regarding prognostic or predictive markers is based on LOE III studies.

Because research into new treatment methods continues, women with invasive breast cancer now have more treatment options and a better chance of long-term survival than ever before (12). However, the clinical progression of breast cancer remains very variable. Adjuvant medical therapies enhance the life expectancy of those who are not cured by surgery, presumably because the micrometastatic disease is eradicated or at least prevented from progressing. It remains a challenge to define which patients are surgically curable and therefore do not require adjuvant treatment (chemotherapy and hormone therapy). In addition to these systemic therapies, radiotherapy is used in selected cases as a local adjuvant treatment.

The selection of systemic adjuvant therapy is based on prognostic and predictive factors. Markers of prognostic factors predict patient outcome, irrespective of treatment given. Prognostic factors are measurements available at diagnosis or time of surgery, that in the absence of adjuvant therapy are associated with recurrence rate, death rate, or other clinical outcome. Predictive factors are measurements associated with the degree of response to a specific therapy. However, it is not uncommon for factors to be both prognostic and predictive. For example, the estrogen receptor (ER) content in breast cancer tissue is both a weakly favorable prognostic factor and more significantly a strong predictive factor of response to hormonal therapy.

HORMONE RECEPTOR STATUS

Estrogen receptors (ER) and progesterone receptors (PR) were among the first biological markers routinely used in the clinical setting to manage breast cancer, and they are now important factors in the treatment of breast cancer (13,14). Initially, ER levels were measured in tumor cytosols prepared from metastatic lesions. They were used to predict the response to hormone therapy. Subsequently, investigators showed that assays on primary tumors could also be used to predict the likelihood of early relapse, making ER a prognostic as well as a predictive indicator.

For more than 20 years, ER and PR were mainly assayed with cytosol-based dextran-coated charcoal (DCC) methods with regular quality controls (15). The availability of antibodies to ER and PR later permitted immunohistochemical assays on frozen sections, with acceptable concordance rates with DCC-based methods (16). Enzyme immunoassays (EIA) for use on tumor cytosols also became available (14). In the 1990s, the advent of heat-mediated antigen retrieval, together with the emergence of new antibodies, markedly changed the situation. Increasing numbers of pathology laboratories started to measure ER and PR by immunohistochemistry (IHC) on paraffin sections. Quality control programs are now developed in pathology laboratories (17).

When hormone receptor status is considered (positive versus negative), concordance between biochemical methods and IHC occurs in about 80% of cases. Discordant results between EIA and IHC were frequent when cellularity was low, as in lobular and mucinous carcinomas with large stromal components. Some cases were negative in EIA and positive in IHC when the level of cytosolic protein was low. A highly IHC-positive intraductal carcinoma or normal breast component with an IHC-negative invasive carcinoma component (14,18), explains some IHC-negative/EIA-positive cases.

It is important for quality assurance purposes to be able to control reagent stability over time. It is also important to ensure that the percentage of positive cases varies within acceptable limits over time (assuming that patient recruitment is stable) and that correlation between ER/PR status and classical variables is maintained. This systematic verification was proposed for EIA several years ago (19), as part of quality assurance programs.

The initial assumption that hormone treatment based on the amount of hormone receptors would be beneficial (20) has not been applied in practice, and clinical decisions have been based solely on qualitative information, whatever the assay method used. Though quantitative information available from biochemical methods is still of interest, it has been under-used. Consequently, improvement in the reproducibility of a quantitative use of immunohistochemistry appears particularly important to achieve (17).

Until 1996, only one estrogen receptor had been identified. Another member of that nuclear family has since been identified and cloned in rodent and human tissues (21). It is designated ERβ because of its strong homology with the classical ER, which is now named ERα. ERα is localized to chromosome 6 and ERβ to chromosome 14. Both ER subtypes can mediate gene transcription in two ways: via a classical estrogen-responsive element and via an activator protein AP1 enhancer element. When ER signaling mechanisms from an AP-1 response element are considered, this may have important implications for anti-estrogen resistance, as the two ER subtypes signal in opposite directions (22). The role of ERβ in normal and malignant breast is still unclear (23) (see also Chapter 43); all data regarding the clinical interest of ER were obtained on the basis of studies involving ERα. Studying both ER subtypes opens an opportunity to develop new drugs with selective estrogen actions and to better understand how estrogens mediate proliferative effects in breast cancer cells.

Nuclear receptor function is modulated by transcriptional co-regulators, which either enhance or repress receptor activity (24). Tumor sensitivity to mixed antagonists may be governed by a complex set of transcription factors, which we are only now beginning to understand (25).

A large body of evidence now supports the expression of variants and mutant ERα and ERβ mRNA species (26). The clinical significance of these variants is currently under study.

The goal of hormonal therapy is to prevent breast cancer cells from receiving stimulation from estrogen. Such stimulation occurs primarily in tumors that contain hormone receptor protein. Estrogen deprivation can be achieved by

- blocking the receptor through the use of drugs, such as tamoxifen;
- suppression of estrogen synthesis through the administration of aromatase inhibitors in postmenopausal women or LHRH agonists in premenopausal women; or
- destruction of the ovaries through surgery or external beam radiation therapy. The administration of cytotoxic chemotherapy may indirectly accomplish this same effect by damaging estrogen-producing cells in the ovaries.

The last published meta-analysis on adjuvant tamoxifen trials worldwide indicated that tamoxifen was of benefit in delaying recurrences in women with ERα-positive tumors, whatever their age, menopausal status, or nodal status (27). These results have stimulated interest in using ER to select treatment. Hormonal adjuvant therapy should not be recommended to women whose breast cancers do not express hormone receptor protein. Randomized clinical trials have not yet shown that such treatment substantially reduces the likelihood of recurrence or, in the case of tamoxifen, diminishes the likelihood of contralateral breast cancer.

The availability of anti-aromatase agents, both reversible (nonsteroidal) and irreversible (steroidal), provides clinicians with additional hormonal treatment options. Anti-aromatase agents have demonstrated efficacy in patients who have failed multiple hormonal therapies (28); they are also tested in neoadjuvant and adjuvant setting.

MARKERS OF PROLIFERATION

High tumor proliferation is an adverse prognostic factor in surgically treated breast cancers, particularly in node-negative patients, in whom it can be used to discriminate those with the highest risk of metastasis (8). Some studies have also suggested that high proliferation rates also influence the response to chemotherapy in neoadjuvant, adjuvant, and metastatic settings (29,30).

Several approaches have been developed to study tumor proliferation, including labeling index (31), immunohistochemical detection of proliferation-associated antigens (32), and thymidine kinase assay (33). However, the most widely studied technique is S-phase fraction (SPF) measurement by flow cytometry, which simultaneously provides DNA ploidy (34).

In 1992 the DNA Cytometry Consensus Conference, supported by the National Cancer Institute, concluded that the literature clearly showed a link between high SPF values and an increased risk of breast cancer recurrence and proposed technical guidelines (35). These conclusions were confirmed in 1999 by the College of American Pathologists (CAP) Consensus Statement (6) and in 2000 by the American Society of Clinical Oncology Tumor Marker Panel (10). All these reports underlined limitations on the extensive use of flow cytometry DNA measurement in clinical practice, mainly owing to the lack of standardized procedures to prepare and analyze samples, and to interpret histograms. However, many advances in technology have occurred as instruments and software programs have become more efficient, and agreement among laboratories can be improved by following recommendations on software use (36).

According to the College of American Pathologists Consensus Statement (6), clinicians should routinely assessment cell proliferation when evaluating breast cancers. Mitotic figure counts, which are a component of histologic grading systems, should be conducted in all cases. Assessment of other proliferation markers is considered optional. However, contrary to results from investigations of steroid hormone receptors or HER-2, there is no consensus on the immunohistochemical approach of proliferation indices.

One way of incorporating proliferation markers in standard clinical practice is to discuss the rationale of chemotherapy for patients who have a good prognosis and slowly proliferating tumors, which may be reassessed in terms of the likely risk-benefit ratio. This was recently noted (33,36), following the same lines of data from the San Antonio SPORE breast cancer database (34) or those of Bryant (37) in patients with node-negative ER-positive tumors. Randomized, well-controlled studies of homogeneous chemotherapy protocols are required to settle the issue.

HER-2

The proto-oncogene HER-2/neu oncogene has been localized to chromosome 17q and encodes a 185-kd transmembrane tyrosine kinase growth factor receptor. The HER-2/neu protein belongs to the family of four closely related growth factor receptors including: epithelial growth factor receptor (EGFR) or HER-1 (erb-B1); HER-2 (erb-B2); HER-3 (erb-B3); and HER-4 (erb-B4). In most cases, overexpression of HER-2 protein results from HER-2 gene amplification. HER-2 amplification and overexpression have been correlated with more aggressive disease and shortened survival of breast cancer patients (38). Amplification of the gene and/or overexpression of the protein occurs in approximately 30% of breast cancers. According to the available data, HER-2 appears to be

- a weak to moderate negative pure prognostic factor, particularly in node-positive patients, but likely a much stronger predictive factor of responsiveness to specific therapies (39,40);
- a weak to moderate negative predictive factor for response to endocrine therapy;
- a moderate negative predictive factor for response to alkylating agents; and
- a moderate positive predictive factor for response to anthracyclines. (The data regarding response to taxanes or radiotherapy are not sufficient to make recommendations regarding treatment decisions.); and
- a strong predictive factor for response to trastuzumab (41).

Pre-clinical pharmacology studies indicate that antibodies to HER-2 possess potent anti-tumor activity. Antibodies may antagonize the function of the growth-signaling properties of the HER-2 system and directly inhibit the growth of cancer cells. They also may enlist immune cells to attack and kill the tumor target and/or augment chemotherapy-induced cytotoxicity. Based on these data, the recombinant humanized anti-HER-2 monoclonal antibody trastuzumab (Herceptin, Genentech, Inc, South San Francisco, CA, USA) was evaluated in human clinical trials for efficacy and safety as a new treatment option for women with metastatic breast cancer whose tumors overexpress HER-2 (41).

The techniques used to evaluate HER-2 status in breast cancer have included gene-based assays such as Southern and slot-dot blotting, polymerase chain reactions methods, and in situ hybridization featuring both fluorescent and non-fluorescent techniques (39). Qualitative and quantitative Her-2/neu protein measurements have been performed by IHC on frozen and archival tissue, western blotting, and enzyme immunoassays (ELISA). Expression at the mRNA level can be measured by quantitative real-time RT-PCR (42). The two most common assay systems use FISH and IHC. Numerous commercial reagents have been used for each system with variable results (43). The results of breast cancer outcome studies have not been uniform and a significant discordance between HER-2 abnormality detection methods has been described. Commercial kits for FISH and IHC have been approved by the Food and Drug Administration and are commercially available. However, a large proportion of HER-2 testing uses non-standardized in-house methods and various commercial agents. In spite of 1998 Food and Drug Administration approval of Herceptin for treating breast cancer patients with HER-2 positive tumors, there is still a controversy about the method of choice to determine whether a tumor is HER-2 positive. According to recent recommendations, tumors with a cutoff point of 3+ with a membranous staining are considered positive by IHC, and intermediate cases warrant confirmatory testing using another method (6).

Other inhibitors that target the EGF receptor tyrosine kinases are moving into clinical trials (44).

MARKERS REGULATING CELL CYCLE AND CELL DEATH
P53

P53 is a tumor–suppressor gene with pleiotropic functions located on chromosome 17 (45). The p53-encoded nuclear protein is important in regulating transcription of many other genes. In response to cell damage or crisis, wild-type p53 can induce cell cycle arrest in G1. If repair mechanisms are not sufficient, p53 also serves as a critical regulator of cellular entry into the apoptotic pathway.

Mutations of the tumor suppressor gene p53 are the most frequent known genetic alterations in all human cancers. The p53 gene is mutated or deleted in up to 50% of breast carcinomas (46). Most biologically significant mutations hinder the participation of p53 in maintaining genomic stability. P53 gene alterations and accumulation of p53 protein detected mainly by immunohistochemistry are generally related to shorter disease-free survival. Mutations normally increase the half-life of the protein product and cause mutant p53 protein to accumulate in the nucleus. Methodological differences and variability in immunohistochemical assays may explain discordant results regarding the prognostic significance of p53 accumulation in breast cancer (47). Several investigators have found discrepancies between p53 protein expression and mutation status, with large numbers of false positive and false-negative results; negative results cannot rule out mutations, and positive results must be confirmed by sequencing. The interpretation of p53 protein accumulation in a tumor is difficult and prognostic data obtained by gene sequencing are certainly more reliable. The value of IHC assays could be restricted to screening for p53 mutations. Incorporating the detection of p53 abnormalities into clinical practice is generally not recommended (8,10). Recent advances in BRCA1 research stress the pivotal role TP53 may play in BRCA1-associated carcinogenesis (48).

Bcl-2 Family and Apoptosis

The apoptotic pathway is a tightly regulated mechanism for eliminating damaged and unnecessary cells. Perturbations that cause resistance to apoptosis represent one way that cancer may be formed, and both chemotherapy and hormone therapy are thought to exert their effects at least partly by the induction of apoptosis. The list of important effectors of this pathway continues to grow and the determination of whether a given cell will die in response to an apoptotic stimulus depends on the complex interaction of positive and negative regulator factors (See also Chapter 54).

The bcl-2 gene was first identified from the t(14;18) chromosomal translocation observed in follicular lymphoma and is an inhibitor of apoptosis (49). Its role in breast cancer biology is being explored (50). It was initially hypothesized that bl-2 expression, and inhibition of cell death, would be associated with inferior response to treatment and adverse prognosis. On the contrary, most studies suggest that Bcl-2 overexpression is considered a marker of good prognosis and of response to tamoxifen (50). Moreover, no convincing correlation was found between altered apoptotic activity and expression of the protein, reflecting the complexity of this pathway, in which many other regulators interact with bcl-2 to affect cell death.

Other members of the bcl-2 family include bax, a promoter of apoptosis; and bclx, which encodes $bclx_S$, a promoter of apoptosis, and $bclx_L$, an inhibitor of apoptosis. In theory, prognosis should be reflected by a balance of bax and bcl-2 family (51), but only limited data are available. Further data are needed to assess the prognostic role of bcl-2 and other mitochondrial proteins in breast cancer.

Markers of Angiogenesis

Tumor growth and metastasis are critically dependent on tumor angiogenesis, i.e., growth of new blood vessels adjacent to the tumor. This process is a highly regulated multi-step system involving a delicate balance between angiogenic and antiangiogenic factors, eventually leading to an increase in intra-tumoral microvessels (52).

The dependence of tumor growth on angiogenesis has led to numerous studies investigating the relationship between tumor angiogenesis and prognosis. The most commonly used measure of angiogenesis is light-microscopy counting of intra-tumoral blood vessels stained with anti-factor VIII-related-antigen or anti-CD31 or CD34. One of the difficulties is the great variability in density between different areas of tumors, and among observers. In addition to counting microvessel density, investigators have examined the association between patient outcome and angiogenic factors like VEGF (53). Most data are related to small retrospective studies and assessment of angiogenesis is not recommended for clinical standard care (6,10).

Markers of Invasion and Metastasis

The process of cancer invasion and metastases is complex. In order to metastasize, tumor cells need to invade, degrade extracellular matrix, intravasate, survive and migrate in vessels, and extravasate and grow. Different proteases such as serine, cysteine, and aspartyl proteases and metalloproteases are important in these processes (54,55) (see also Chapter 8). Protease systems can interact but could also be involved in different kinds of metastatic processes. Identification of markers that are related to the process of adhesion, invasion, and metastasis might therefore be very valuable, especially in women whose primary tumor has not spread to regional nodes.

Accumulated data from pre-clinical and clinical studies strongly suggest that the urokinase-type plasminogen activator system plays a central role in the processes leading to metastasis (see also Chapter 41). The urokinase-type plasminogen activator (uPA) and its inhibitor PAI-1 play a key role in tumor invasion and metastasis. In primary breast cancer, many studies have consistently associated high tumor levels of either or both factors with poor prognosis (56,57). In order to validate the clinical relevance of uPA and PAI-1 in primary breast cancer, a pooled analysis was performed on 18 data sets (n = 8,377) provided by members of the EORTC Receptor and Biomarker Group (58). uPA and PAI-1 were determined in primary tumor tissue extracts (cytosols prepared for hormone receptors assay) using ELISAs and a quality control program (59). UPA and PAI-1 appeared to be one of the strongest prognostic markers so far described in breast cancer as informative as nodal status, in spite of differences in extraction buffers, uPA standards and antibodies, and a lack of uniform cutpoints.

These results led a German group to initiate a clinical trial in node-negative patients (60): node-negative patients stratified on their tumor uPA and PAI-1 levels have been randomized between chemotherapy and observation. Using uPA and PAI-1, about half of the patients with lymph node-negative breast cancer were classified as low risk and therefore adjuvant chemotherapy could be avoided; half were classified as high risk and appeared to benefit from adjuvant chemotherapy. This trial is one example of clinical trials designed to validate the prognostic and predictive power of biological factors. According to the Tumor Marker Utility Grading System (11), uPA and PAI-1 reached the highest level of evidence (LOE1) for clinical application; they are among the very few biological factors included at a decisional level in clinical trials (60), but they are not widely used. This is mainly due to the growing abandonment of classical biochemical methods for hormone receptor determination and other biological factors. There is thus a need to validate new sensitive, quantitative methods such as real-time quantitative RT-PCR that permit a multiparametric approach of gene expression and are easily applied in small samples if the comparison between gene expression at the protein and at the mRNA level gives acceptable results.

In addition to PAI-1, another inhibitor of uPA, PAI-2 has been identified (54). Only a few studies identified the prognostic role of PAI-2 in breast cancer. High levels of PAI-2 have been shown to be associated with improved outcome. A dissemination risk index that takes into account the proteolytic activity of uPA and the two inhibitors has been proposed (61).

Data presented in the literature regarding the prognostic role of cathepsin D reviewed in a recent meta-analysis confirm a statistically significant association between high cathepsin-D values and poor disease-free survival in node-negative breast cancer patients (62).

SUMMARY

It is essential that the value of predictive and prognostic factors be evaluated in well-designed clinical studies that are based on standardized protocols and have sufficient statistical power. Because these standards are infrequently met, very few new prognostic or predictive factors have been validated in the last 10 years, and future progress will depend on greater attention to these standards (6,10). Promising pilot studies should be followed by a validation phase, during which alternative assays for the biomarker are evaluated and prognostic/predictive value is studied. The ideal trial should be performed in a prospective fashion and be specifically designed to address the clinical utility of the prognostic factor. An example is the German randomized trial using uPA and PAI-1 at a decisional level (60) with quality control programs (59). Future research should also incorporate rigorous analytic methods for the candidate prognostic and predictive markers.

Significant changes in the range and type of therapeutic options available for patients with breast cancer highlight the increasing importance of prognostic and predictive factors in the management of patients (63–65). Hormone receptors were the first example of predictive factor in breast cancer. Now, herceptin has been shown to prolong survival in patients with metastatic breast cancer that over-expresses HER-2. A better understanding of the biology of breast cancer is providing novel treatment approaches (65); novel biologic therapies interfere with signal transduction pathways, metastasis process and angiogenesis (23,28,33,44,48,51,52,56). The majority of breast cancers have such a multitude of molecular changes that it is difficult to distinguish between those that are critical to tumor progression and those that are epiphenomena of genetic instability and abnormalities in DNA repair. It is hoped that genomics and proteomics will take us forward. This involves the application of a number of new technologies to facilitate the profiling of individual tumors (66,67), including laser-guided microdissection of microscopic lesions, real-time quantitative RT-PCR, comparative genomic hybridization, loss of heterozygosity, analysis of DNA using microarray technology to study DNA and RNA, and protein profiling using 2D gel mass spectroscopy.

The challenge for the next decade will be to integrate the new promising therapeutic agents into the targeted management of metastatic and primary breast cancer, and to develop methods adapted to the small size of the tumors now observed with the widespread use of breast cancer screening campaigns.

REFERENCES

1. Harris JR Ed. Diseases of the Breast, 2nd ed. Philadelphia: Linpincott, Williams and Wilkins, 2000:1152.
2. Alberg AJ, Singh S, May JW, Helzlsouer KJ. Epidemiology, prevention, and early detection of breast cancer. Curr Opin Oncol 2000;12:515–520.
3. Nathanson KN, Wooster R, Weber BL. Breast cancer genetics: what we know and what we need. Nat Med 2001;7:552–556.
4. Welcsh PL, King MC. BRCA1 and BRCA2 and the genetics of breast and ovarian cancer. Hum Mol Genet 2001;10:705–713.
5. Clemons M, Goss P. Estrogen and the risk of breast cancer. N Engl J Med 2001;344:276–285.
6. Fitzgibbons PL, Page DL, Weaver D, Thor AD, Allred DC, Clark GM, et al. Prognostic factors in breast cancer. College of American Pathologists Consensus Statement 1999. Arch Pathol Lab Med 2000;124:966–967.
7. Van Diest PJ, Torrenga H, Meijer S, Meijer CJ. Pathologic analysis of sentinel lymph nodes. Semin Surg Oncol 2001;20:238–245.
8. Isaacs C, Stearns V, Hayes DF. New prognostic factors for breast cancer recurrence. Semin Oncol 2001;28:53–67.
9. Eisen A, Weber BL. Recent advances in breast cancer biology. Curr Opin Oncol 1998;10:486–491.
10. Bast RC Jr, Ravdin P, Hayes DF, Bates S, Fritsche H Jr, Jessup JM, et al. American Society of Clinical Oncology Tumor Markers Expert Panel. 2000 update of recommendations for the use of tumor markers in breast and colorectal cancer: clinical practice guidelines of the American Society of Clinical Oncology. J Clin Oncol 2001;19:1865–1867.
11. Hayes DF, Bast RC, Desch CE, Fritsche H Jr, Kemeny NE, Jessup JM, et al. Tumor marker utility grading system: a framework to evaluate clinical utility of tumor markers. J Natl Cancer Inst 1996;88:1456–1466.
12. Gianni L, Valagussa P, Zambetti M, Moliterni A, Capri G, Bonadonna G. Adjuvant and neoadjuvant treatment of breast cancer. Semin Oncol 2001;28:13–29.
13. Osborne CK. Steroid hormone receptors in breast cancer management. Breast Cancer Res Treat 1998;51:227–238.
14. Elledge RM, Fuqua SAW. Estrogen and progesterone receptors. In: Harris JR, (ed.). Diseases of the breast, 2nd ed. Philadelphia: Lippincott Williams and Wilkins; 2000:471–488.
15. European Organization for Research and Treatment of Cancer (EORTC): Breast cancer cooperative group. Revision of the standards for the assessment of hormone receptors in human breast cancer. Eur J Cancer 1980;16:1513–1515.
16. Alberts SR, Ingle JN, Roche PR, Cha SS, Wold LE, Farr GH Jr, et al. Comparison of estrogen receptor determinations by a biochemical ligand-binding assay and immunohistochemical staining with monoclonal antibody ER1D5 in females with lymph-node-positive breast carcinoma entered on two prospective clinical trials. Cancer 1996;78:764–772.
17. Group for Evaluation of Prognostic Factors using Immunohistochemistry in Breast Cancer (GEFPICS–FNCLCC). Recommendations for the immunohistochemistry of the hormonal receptors on paraffin sections in breast cancer. Update 1999[in French]. Ann Pathol 1999;19:336–343.
18. Ferrero-Pous M, Trassard M, Le Doussal V, Hacene K, Tubiana-Hulin M, Spyratos F. Comparison of enzyme immunoassay and immunohistochemical measurements of estrogen and progesterone receptors in breast cancer patients. Appl Immunohistochem Mol Morphol 2001;9:267–275.
19. Romain, S., Spyratos, F., Goussard, J., Formento, J.L., Magdelenat, H. Improvement of quality control for steroid receptor measurements: analysis of distribution in more than 40,000 primary breast cancers. French Study Group on Tissue and Molecular Biopathology. Breast Cancer Res Treat 1996;41: 131–139.
20. Godolphin W, Elwood JM, Spinelli JJ. Estrogen receptor quantitation and staging as complementary prognostic indicators in breast cancer: a study of 583 patients. Int J Cancer 1981;28:677–683.
21. Kuiper GG, Enmark E, Pelto-Huikko M, Nilsson S, Gustafsson JA. Cloning of a novel receptor expressed in rat prostate and ovary. Proc Natl Acad Sci U S A 1996;11:5925–5930.
22. Paech K, Webb P, Kuiper GG, Nilsson S, Gustafsson J, Kushner PJ, Scanlan TS. Differential ligand activation of estrogen receptors ERalpha and ERbeta at AP1 sites. Science 1997;277: 1508–1510.
23. Gustafsson JA, Warner M. Estrogen receptor beta in the breast: role in estrogen responsiveness and development of breast cancer. J Steroid Biochem Mol Biol 2000;74:245–248.
24. McKenna NJ, O'Malley BW. From ligand to response: generating diversity in nuclear receptor coregulator function. J Steroid Biochem Mol Biol 2000;74:351–356.
25. Katzenellenbogen BS, Katzenellenbogen JA. Estrogen receptor transcription and transactivation: estrogen receptor alpha and

estrogen receptor beta: regulation by selective estrogen receptor modulators and importance in breast cancer. Breast Cancer Res 2000;2:335–344.
26. Murphy LC, Dotzlaw H, Leygue E, Coutts A, Watson P. The pathophysiological role of estrogen receptor variants in human breast cancer. J Steroid Biochem Mol Biol 1998;65:175–180.
27. Tamoxifen for early breast cancer: an overview of the randomized trials. Early Breast Cancer Trialists' Collaborative Group. Lancet 1998;351:1451–1467.
28. Buzdar A, Howell A. Advances in aromatase inhibition: clinical efficacy and tolerability in the treatment of breast cancer. Clin Cancer Res 2001;7:2620–2635.
29. Spyratos F, Briffod M, Tubiana-Hulin M, Pallud C, Mayras C, Filleul A, Rouëssé. Sequential cytopunctures during preoperative chemotherapy for primary breast carcinoma. II. DNA flow cytometry changes during chemotherapy, tumor regression, and short-term follow-up. Cancer 1992;69:470–475.
30. Remvikos Y, Bcuzeboc P, Zadjela A, Voillemot N, Magdelénat H, Pouillart P. Pretreatment proliferative activity of breast cancer correlates with the response to cytotoxic chemotherapy. J Natl Cancer Inst 1898;81:1383–1387.
31. Silvestrini R, Daidone MG, Luisi A, Mastore M, Leutner M, Salvadori B. Cell proliferation in 3,800 node-negative breast cancers: consistency over time of biological and clinical information provided by 3H-thymidine labeling index. Int. J. Cancer 1997;74:122–127.
32. Thor AD, Liu S, Moore DH 2nd, Edgerton SM. Comparison of mitotic index, in vitro bromodeoxyuridine labeling, and MIB-1 assays to quantitate proliferation in breast cancer. J Clin Oncol 1999;17:470–477.
33. Broet P, Romain S, Daver A, Ricolleau G, Quillien V, Rallet A, et al. Thymidine kinase as a proliferative marker: clinical relevance in 1,692 primary breast cancer patients. J Clin Oncol 2001;19:2778–2787.
34. Wenger CR and Clark GM. S-phase fraction and breast cancer—a decade of experience. Breast Cancer Res Treat 1998;51:255–265.
35. Hedley DW, Clark GM, Cornelisse CJ, Killander D, Kute T, Merkel D. Consensus review of the clinical utility of DNA cytometry in carcinoma of the breast. Cytometry 1993;14:482–485.
36. Chassevent A, Jourdan ML, Romain S, Descotes F, Colonna M, Martin PM, et al. S-phase fraction and DNA ploidy in 633 T1T2 breast cancers: a standardized flow cytometric study. Clin Cancer Res 2001;7:909–917.
37. Bryant J, Fisher B, Gunduz N, Costantino JP, Emir B. S-phase fraction combined with other patient and tumor characteristics for the prognosis of node-negative, estrogen-receptor-positive breast cancer. Breast Cancer Res Treat 1998;51:239–253.
38. Yamauchi H, Stearns V, Hayes DF. When is a tumor marker ready for prime time? A case study of c-erbB-2 as a predictive factor in breast cancer. J Clin Oncol 2001;19:2334–2356.
39. Révillon F, Bonneterre J, Peyrat JP. ERBB2 oncogene in human breast cancer and its clinical significance. Eur. J. Cancer 1998; 34:791–808.
40. Ross JS, Fletcher JA. The HER-2/neu oncogene in breast cancer: prognostic factor, predictive factor, and target for therapy. The Oncologist 1998;3:237–252.
41. Mass R. The role of HER-2 expression in predicting response to therapy in breast cancer. Semin Oncol 2000;27:46–52.
42. Bièche I, Onody P, Laurendeau I, Olivi M, Vidaud D, Lidereau R, Vidaud M. Real-time transcription PCR assay for future management of ERBB2-based clinical applications. Clin Chem 1999;45:1148–1156.
43. Press MF, Hung G, Godolphin W, Slamon DJ. Sensitivity of HER-2/neu antibodies in archival tissue samples: potential source of error in immunohistochemical studies of oncogene expression. Cancer Res 1994;54:2771–2777.
44. Stern DF. Tyrosine kinase signaling in breast cancer: ErbB family receptor tyrosine kinases. Breast Cancer Res 2000;2: 176–183.
45. Phillips HA. The role of the p53 tumor suppressor gene in human breast cancer. Clin Oncol (R Coll Radiol) 1999;11:148–155.
46. Bergh J. Clinical studies of p53 in treatment and benefit of breast cancer patients. Endocr Relat Cancer 1999;6:51–59.
47. Pharoah PD, Day NE, Caldas C. Somatic mutations in the p53 gene and prognosis in breast cancer: a meta-analysis. Br J Cancer 1999;80:1968–1973.
48. Schuyer M, Berns EM. Is TP53 dysfunction required for BRCA1-associated carcinogenesis? Mol Cell Endocrinol 1999;155: 143–152.
49. Kroemer G. The proto-oncogene Bcl-2 and its role in regulating apoptosis. Nat Med 1997;3:614–620.
50. Elledge RM, Green S, Howes L, Clark GM, Berardo M, Allred DC, et al. Bcl-2, p53, and response to tamoxifen in estrogen receptor-positive metastatic breast cancer: a Southwest Oncology Group study. J Clin Oncol 1997;15:1916–1922.
51. Kumar R, Vadlamudi RK, Adam L. Apoptosis in mammary gland and cancer. Endocr Relat Cancer 2000;7:257–269.
52. Saaristo A, Karpanen T, Alitalo K. Mechanisms of angiogenesis and their use in the inhibition of tumor growth and metastasis. Oncogene 2000;19:6122–6129.
53. Gasparini G. Clinical significance of determination of surrogate markers of angiogenesis in breast cancer. Crit Rev Oncol Hematol 2001;37:97–114.
54. Andreasen PA, Kioller L, Christensen L, Duffy MJ. The urokinase-type plasminogen activator system in cancer metastasis: a review. Int J Cancer 1997;72:1–22.
55. Stamenkovic, I. Matrix metalloproteinases in tumor invasion and metastasis. Semin Cancer Biol 2000;10:415–433.
56. Look MP, Foekens JA. Clinical relevance of the urokinase plasminogen activator system in breast cancer. APMIS 1999;107: 150–159.
57. Duffy MJ. Proteases as prognostic markers in cancer. Clin Cancer Res 1996;2:613–618.
58. Harbeck N, Look MP, Ulm K, Duffy MJ, on behalf of the EORTC Receptor and Biomarker Study Group. UPA and PAI-1 ready for routine testing in primary breast cancer: Pooled analysis (n+8,377) provides Level I Evidence for clinical relevance. ASCO Meeting 2001;1646.
59. Sweep CG, Geurts-Moespot J, Grebenschikov N, de Witte JH, Heuvel JJ, Schmitt M, et al. External quality assessment of trans-European multi-center antigen determinations (enzyme-linked immunosorbent assay) of urokinase-type plasminogen activator (uPA) and its type 1 inhibitor (PAI-1) in human breast cancer tissue extracts. Br J Cancer 1998;78:1434–1441.
60. Janicke F, Prechtl A, Thomssen C, Harbeck N, Meisner C, Untch M, et al. The German N0 Study Group. Randomized adjuvant chemotherapy trial in high-risk, lymph node-negative breast cancer patients identified by urokinase-type plasminogen activator and plasminogen activator inhibitor type 1. J Natl Cancer Inst 2001;93:913–920.
61. Bouchet C, Hacène K, Martin PM, Becette V, Tubiana-Hulin M, Lasry S, et al. A dissemination risk index based on plasminogen activator system components in primary breast cancer. J Clin Oncol1999;17:3048–3057.

62. Ferrandina G, Scambia G, Bardelli F, Benedetti Panici P, Mancuso S, Messori A. Relationship between cathepsin-D content and disease-free survival in node-negative breast cancer patients: a meta-analysis. Br J Cancer 1997;76:661–666.
63. Goldhirsch A, Glick JH, Gelber RD, Coates AS, Senn HJ. Meeting highlights: International Consensus Panel on the Treatment of Primary Breast Cancer. Seventh International Conference on Adjuvant Therapy of Primary Breast Cancer. J Clin Oncol 2001;19:3817–3827.
64. Bange J, Zwick E, Ullrich A. Molecular targets for breast cancer therapy and prevention. Nat Med 2001;7:548–552.
65. Esteva FJ, Valero V, Pusztai L, Boehnke-Michaud L, Buzdar AU, Hortobagyi GN. Chemotherapy of metastatic breast cancer: what to expect in 2001 and beyond. Oncologist 2001;6:133–46.
66. Bartelink H, Begg AC, Martin JC, van Dijk M, Moonen L, van't Veer LJ, Van de Vaart P, Verheij M. Translational research offers individually tailored treatments for cancer patients. Cancer J Sci Am 2000;6:2–10.
67. Cooper CS. Applications of microarray technology in breast cancer research. Breast Cancer Res 2001;3:158–175.

Chapter **16**

BRCA1 and BRCA2: Genes that Predispose to Breast and Ovarian Cancer

Hilmi Ozcelik and Gordon Glendon

Breast cancer is one of the most common malignancies in females. The average lifetime risk of breast cancer in the general North American population is approximately 10% at age 80 with most cases being diagnosed when the woman is older than 60. Risk factors for the disease include gender (female), advancing age, hormonal status (early menarche, late menopause), reproductive history (parity, age at first birth), and a family history of the disease. Of women with breast cancer, approximately 20% have some degree of family history of breast and/or ovarian cancer. The incidence of breast cancer in many of these families may be due to chance clustering and/or to the presence of mutations in cancer-susceptibility genes. In fact, approximately 5% of breast cancers are known to result from mutations in either of the genes predisposed breast and ovarian cancer predisposition genes: BRCA1 and BRCA2. These genes are being utilized in genetic testing to identify those who are at increased risk for cancer, and are an active research target for familial cancer risk.

IDENTIFICATION

Studies of high-risk families with multiple cases of breast cancer led to the linkage of BRCA1 to chromosome 17q21 in 1990. BRCA1 was identified by positional cloning in 1994, and mutations in this gene were shown to segregate with the disease in families with high risk of breast and ovarian cancer. The BRCA1 gene spans approximately 100kb of genomic DNA, with a coding region of approximately 5592 nucleotides. It is comprised of 24 exons, of which 22 encode a protein of 1863 amino acids (220 kDa). In studies of families exhibiting both male and female breast cancers, the second major breast and ovarian cancer predisposition gene, BRCA2, was linked to 13q12 in 1994. It was identified by positional cloning in 1995. BRCA2 spans approximately 70kb of genomic DNA with a coding region of 10,254 nucleotides. It is comprised of 27 exons and encodes for a protein of 3418 amino acids (348 kDa) (1,2).

MOLECULAR AND FUNCTIONAL CHARACTERIZATION

The BRCA1 and BRCA2 proteins have been shown to have several similarities with respect to expression patterns and function:

- They are both nuclear proteins with an expression pattern regulated by cell cycle.
- The highest level of expression of both proteins has been detected in the adult testes, thymus, breast, and ovaries.
- Both genes contain a putative transcriptional activation domain, and act as co-regulators through direct interaction with sequence-specific transcription factors and with components of the transcriptional machinery.
- There is strong evidence that both genes are involved in the DNA repair pathway through control of homologous recombination and double-strand break repair in response to DNA damage. This evidence comes from the studies showing the co-localization and interaction of both proteins with human RAD51 protein, which mediates strand exchange and homologous DNA repair (3,4).

TUMOR SUPPRESSOR FUNCTION

According to the "two hit" mechanism described by Knudson in 1971, both BRCA1 and BRCA2 qualify as tumor-suppressor genes. Evidence comes from studies of the breast tumors from germline mutation carriers. The germline mutation (first-hit) is accompanied by the loss of the second copy of the gene (second-hit) in greater than 90% of breast tumors. Therefore BRCA1 and BRCA2 carriers, who are born with the first-hit, are at a greater than average risk for cancer since they need only one additional hit in any cell for uncontrolled growth to commence.

In contrast to other tumor suppressor genes, somatic mutations of BRCA1 and BRCA2 are very rare in sporadic breast and ovarian tumors, suggesting that mutational events in these genes are less likely to drive sporadic tumorigenesis. However, it has been suggested that mechanisms other than mutations may inactivate BRCA1 and BRCA2 in sporadic cases. Several studies suggest the methylation of BRCA1 and BRCA2 regulatory regions, which affects the expression patterns of these genes, may play a role in sporadic tumorigenesis (3,4).

GENETIC ALTERATIONS

The majority of the mutations identified in BRCA1 and BRCA2 are protein truncation mutations, consisting mainly of small deletions, small insertions, nonsense codons, and splicing errors. Truncating mutations also have been shown to result from large genomic deletions at the BRCA1 and BRCA2 chromosomal locations. These genetic alterations are considered to be deleterious because they lead to truncated versions of the BRCA1 and BRCA2 proteins. In addition, these genes occasionally demonstrate single base substitutions that lead to single amino acid changes referred to as missense mutations. The Breast Cancer Information Core (BIC) database has been established to accumulate data on all types of BRCA1 and BRCA2 mutations and is available to the public on the World Wide Web (http://www.nhgri.nih.gov/Intramural_research/ Lab_transfer/Bic).

The mutations identified to date are distributed throughout the entire coding region of BRCA1 and BRCA2, lacking any clustering or mutational "hot spots." However, mutational data from around the world have shown population-specific patterns due primarily to genetic founder effect. The extensively studied Ashkenazi Jewish population is a good example of founder mutations in BRCA1 and BRCA2. Two mutations in BRCA1 (185delAG, 5382insC) and one in BRCA2 (6174delT) account for the majority of the familial breast cancer cases in this population. In Iceland a single mutation in the BRCA2 gene (999del5) accounts for the majority of families at high-risk of breast and/or ovarian cancer. BRCA1 and BRCA2 founder mutations also have been reported in French-Canadian, German, Swedish, Dutch, Norwegian, and African-American populations.

GENETIC TESTING

Genetic testing of BRCA1 and BRCA2 involves identifying germline genetic alterations in these genes. This analysis typically utilizes DNA and RNA derived from the white blood cells of a blood sample and is conducted in academic, hospital-based, and commercial laboratory settings.

When covering the entire coding region of BRCA1 and BRCA2, the direct sequencing method is a very powerful technique for detecting mutations. Except for large genomic deletions, this method is very sensitive in detecting all types of point mutations in the coding region and splice junctions of these genes. Since this method is costly and labor-intensive, pre-screening methods that identify mutations are often used before sequencing to identify gene regions with potential mutations. Pre-screening methods include the protein truncation test (PTT), single nucleotide polymorphism conformation (SSCP), denaturing high-pressure liquid chromatography (DHPLC), and enzymatic cleavage. These techniques vary in terms of cost effectiveness, labor intensity, and sensitivity to mutation detection. For example, the PTT method is commonly used because of its efficient applicability to large genes and its high sensitivity in detecting protein truncation mutations of any nature, including large genomic deletions. Support for the application of this method comes from the fact that the majority of mutations with known clinical relevance in BRCA1 and BRCA2 are protein-truncating mutations. This method does not detect missense variations; however, it can be complemented with partial sequencing to increase its sensitivity in detecting such mutations. A complete analysis of the entire length of both genes may not be necessary in specific populations where the spectrum of BRCA1 and BRCA2 mutations is small. Targeted analysis for population-specific mutations may be all that is required. The best examples—the Ashkenazi Jewish and Icelandic populations—have been described above.

Discriminating between the clinically significant mutations and the naturally occurring polymorphisms in BRCA1 and BRCA2 is still a challenging problem. The majority of truncation mutations are considered to be deleterious, since they truncate the BRCA1 and BRCA2 proteins. Interpretation of the clinical significance of missense mutations remains difficult because a laboratory-based functional test for the BRCA1 and BRCA2 proteins is lacking. Clues about the clinical impact of a particular missense mutation may come from examining whether or not the alteration segregates with the disease in the family, or determining if the alteration is in an important protein domain, such as the RING finger domain of BRCA1.

In the laboratory setting, BRCA1 and BRCA2 genetic testing fails to detect a mutation in a large proportion of families with histories of breast and/or ovarian cancer. One possible explanation is the presence of mutations in areas of the BRCA1 and BRCA2 genes that are not routinely tested due to the present state of knowledge. These undetected mutations may reside in regulatory regions that control how the genes are expressed or intronic regions that are not well described due to their large size. In addition, these families may carry mutations in other, yet to be discovered, genes that predispose to breast and/or ovarian cancer.

CLINICAL SIGNIFICANCE

Germline mutations in BRCA1 and BRCA2 confer an increased risk for the development of breast and ovarian cancer. Most pathologic sub-types have been identified in BRCA1- and BRCA2-associated breast cancers; however, ductal and lobular epithelial tumors are by far the most commonly found. Although it is not understood how the BRCA1 and BRCA2 tumorigenic pathways differ from each other and from sporadic breast cancer, there is growing evidence that the histologic features of their associated breast cancers are different. Estrogen receptor positivity is lower in BRCA1-associated breast cancer than in either BRCA2 or sporadic cancers. In addition, progesterone receptor status appears to be lower in BRCA1 associated breast cancer. Early evidence indicates that BRCA1-associated breast cancers are mostly high-grade tumors (grade III) attributable to high mitotic activity. BRCA1 and BRCA2 mutations predispose to ovarian cancers of the non-mucinous type, the vast majority of which are of serous histology. Neither of these genes has demonstrated a predisposition to the development of borderline ovarian tumors.

Although BRCA1 and BRCA2 mutations confer an increased risk for the development of breast, ovarian, and possibly other cancers, not every carrier will have a diagnosis in his or her lifetime. Published lifetime risks (birth to age 70) for breast cancer are similar for both BRCA1 and BRCA2 mutations. In women, these risks range from a low of 38% to a high of 86%. Male carriers of BRCA2 mutations were shown to have an approximate 6% lifetime risk (in one study of two large families). The estimates of lifetime risk for ovarian cancer have also varied considerably between studies. Estimates of lifetime risk for ovarian cancer ranging between 10% and 60% for BRCA1 mutation carriers have been published. Most studies to date have estimated the risk for BRCA2 carriers to be less than for BRCA1, with estimates ranging between 10% and 16%. The lifetime risk for prostate cancer had been estimated as high as 16% for BRCA1 and BRCA2 carriers. Excess melanoma and cancers of the pancreas, fallopian tube, colon, and lung have been reported in various studies and will require additional research to determine the genes' involvement in these cancers.

The variation in the published estimates of risk for BRCA1 and BRCA2 mutations may reflect true differences between various study populations, between specific mutations identified within each gene, or the presence of other modifiers of cancer risk. However, this variation may also be due to the large methodological differences within the literature. Differences in molecular approaches that preferentially identify only a small proportion, or specific type, of mutation may affect risk estimates. Differences in study participant ascertainment schemes that include primarily high-risk (multiple-case) families will also yield higher estimates of risk than studies that are more population-based.

The average age of breast cancer incidence in families with BRCA1 mutations is younger than that of the general population, and the increase in risk commences in the thirties. Although the average age of breast cancer onset in BRCA2 families is younger than that of the general population, this gene appears to contribute to fewer cases than BRCA1 among young women.

The clinical presentation of families with BRCA1 or BRCA2 mutations varies considerably with respect to the age of onset, number, and type of cancers present. Many investigators have attempted to determine probabilities of carrying a BRCA1 and BRCA2 mutation based on these characteristics. Studies that have included families with early onset (< 40 years of age) breast cancer, families in which multiple family members were affected with breast and/or ovarian cancer, and those including the presence of ovarian cancer at any age have yielded the highest prevalence of BRCA1 and BRCA2 mutations. For example a study investigating families with four or more cases of breast and/or ovarian cancer appearing before the age of sixty found more than 60% of families to carry a BRCA1 or BRCA2 mutation. In contrast, studies utilizing population-based approaches have, as expected, identified a smaller proportion of BRCA1 and BRCA2 mutation carriers. A recent population-based study of women with breast cancer, not selected based on the presence or absence of family history, found 5.9% of women diagnosed under 35 and 4.1% of those diagnosed between 36 and 45 years of age to carry BRCA1 and BRCA2 mutations. The estimation of the probability of the presence of BRCA1 and BRCA2 mutations must rely on both the family's cancer history and the impact of founder effect and genetic drift in different populations. For instance, the Ashkenazi Jewish population, unselected for cancer, has a carrier rate of approximately 2%, which is approximately five times higher than that of the general North American population. BRCA1 and BRCA2 carrier rates as high as 40% have been documented for Ashkenazi women diagnosed with ovarian cancer unselected for family history compared to less than 10% in the general population (5–8).

GENETIC COUNSELING

The BRCA1 and BRCA2 genes are presently being used as predictive biomarkers for the identification of breast and ovarian cancer risk in the clinical setting. As with most other genetic tests, it is provided in conjunction with genetic counseling in either a research or clinical service setting. Most genetic testing programs specifically target those who have an increased risk of carrying a BRCA1 or BRCA2 mutation due to their strong personal or family history of the disease (see above).

Genetic counseling involves the shepherding of the patient through the complicated process of genetic testing. A pre-test genetic counseling session involves taking a full family history with pathologic confirmation of relevant family members' cancer diagnoses, the explanation of the genetic nature of breast cancer, and a thorough exploration of pros and cons of determining their BRCA1 and BRCA2 mutational status within the context of their particular personal and family situation. Another session(s) is required to deliver the genetic testing results and to determine a risk management protocol that is appropriate for their risk level. The setting is often multidisciplinary due to the overlap between the genetic, oncological, and psychological issues that arise with this test (9).

CLINICAL MANAGEMENT

The main options for management of breast and ovarian cancer risk in BRCA1 and BRCA2 mutation carriers include surveillance, risk reduction surgery, and chemoprevention. There are no specific gene therapies yet available. Since there is little evidence-based data regarding the effectiveness of these techniques, management decisions are often based on both the physician's opinion and the patient's comfort with the various strategies. To aid in these risk management decisions, a number of groups have published risk management guidelines.

Breast cancer surveillance options for BRCA1 and BRCA2 mutation carriers include a combination of clinical breast exam, breast self-exam, and mammography, each of which may start at an earlier-than-average age and be performed at more frequent intervals. Magnetic resonance imaging (MRI) and ultrasound are now being investigated for use in this setting. Risk reduction surgery involves total or skin-sparing mastectomy with or without reconstruction. Data from observational studies of women at increased risk for breast cancer indicate that the magnitude of risk reduction may be greater than 90%, although direct evidence in BRCA1 and BRCA2 mutation carriers is not yet available. The selective estrogen receptor modulation (SERM) drug Tamoxifen has been used as a chemopreventative agent in BRCA1 and BRCA2 mutation carriers after it was shown to substantially reduce the risk of breast cancer in a large study of at-risk women. The SERM Raloxifene is presently being compared to Tamoxifen in a randomized study (STAR trial) to determine its effectiveness in cancer risk reduction. Raloxifene is considered an attractive replacement for Tamoxifen in this setting because it does not increase the risk for endometrial cancer as Tamoxifen does.

Ovarian cancer surveillance options for BRCA1 and BRCA2 mutation carriers include a combination of pelvic examination, transvaginal ultrasound (with or without color Doppler enhancement), and a blood test for the tumor marker CA125. The ultrasound and CA125 blood test are often provided in combination, although no strong data is yet available as to their efficacy in BRCA1 and BRCA2 mutation carriers. Ophorectomy, with or without hysterectomy, is available as a risk reduction method. The degree of risk reduction this surgery provides is difficult to determine, due to several cases of post-surgical peritoneal cancer, indistinguishable from ovarian metastases. Decisions regarding surgery must also take into consideration the effects of surgically induced menopause for mutation carriers who are younger. Some investigators have suggested that the oral contraceptive pill may reduce ovarian cancer risk in BRCA1 and BRCA2 mutation carriers since it has a large risk reduction effect in the general population. More study will be necessary to determine its effectiveness in this population, especially since there is concern over a possible increase in risk of breast cancer associated with the birth control pill (10).

FUTURE DIRECTIONS

Additional molecular characterization of the BRCA1 and BRCA2 genes is necessary to determine the full spectrum and prevalence of deleterious mutations in different populations. This issue relates directly to the further refinement of lifetime risk estimates that may differ between populations and between those who carry mutations in the BRCA1 and BRCA2 genes. Many questions remain unanswered with respect to the function of the BRCA1 and BRCA2 proteins. Additional research detailing the precise molecular role that the proteins play within the cell may allow for the development of targeted therapeutics. Additional long-term studies will also be necessary to understand the effectiveness of various risk management strategies to reduce the burden of cancer in this population.

Acknowledgement

We would like to acknowledge the Ontario Cancer Genetics Network of Cancer Care Ontario for their support.

REFERENCES

1. Borg A. Molecular and pathological characterization of inherited breast cancer. Seminars in Cancer Biology 2001;11:375–385.
2. Ford D, Easton DF, Stratton M, Narod S, Goldgar D, Devilee P, et al., and The Breast Cancer Linkage Consortium. Genetic heterogeneity and penetrance analysis of the BRCA1 and BRCA2 genes in breast cancer families. Am J Human Gen 1998;62:676–689.
3. Goodwin PJ. Management of familial breast cancer risk. Breast Cancer Res Treat 2000;62:19–33.
4. Loman N, Johannsson O, Kristoffersson U, Olsson H, Borg A. Family history of breast and ovarian cancers and BRCA1 and BRCA2 mutations in a population-based series of early-onset breast cancer. J Natl Cancer Inst 2001;93:1215–1223.
5. Lynch HT, Watson P, Tinley S, Snyder C, Durham C, Lynch J, et al. An update on DNA-based BRCA1/BRCA2 genetic counseling in hereditary breast cancer. Cancer Gen Cytogen 1999;109:91–98.
6. Miki Y, Swensen J, Shattuck-Eidens D, Futreal PA, Harshman K, Tavtigian S, et al. A strong candidate for the breast and ovarian cancer susceptibility gene BRCA1. Science 1994;266:66–71.
7. Peto J, Collins N, Barfoot R, Seal S, Warren W, Rahman N, et al. Prevalence of BRCA1 and BRCA2 gene mutations in patients with early-onset breast cancer. J Natl Cancer Inst 1999;91: 943–949.
8. Risch HA, McLaughlin JR, Cole DE, Rosen B, Bradley L, Kwan E, et al. Prevalence and penetrance of germline BRCA1 and BRCA2 mutations in a population series of 649 women with ovarian cancer. Am J Human Gen 2001;68:700–710.
9. Welcsh PL, King MC. BRCA1 and BRCA2 and the genetics of breast and ovarian cancer. Human Molecular Genetics 2001; 10:705–13.
10. Wooster R, Bignell G, Lancaster J, Swift S, Seal S, Mangion J, et al. Identification of the breast cancer susceptibility gene BRCA2. Nature 1995;378:789–792.

Chapter 17

Adenocarcinoma of the Prostate

Alexander Haese, Charlotte Becker, Eleftherios P. Diamandis, and Hans Lilja

BACKGROUND: THE HUMAN PROSTATE GLAND

Macroscopic Anatomy

The human prostate is part of the male reproductive system and accessory male genital glands, along with the seminal vesicles and Cowper's glands. In the mature young male, the prostate has the size and shape of a chestnut and weights about 18–20 grams. The prostate is divided into the apex, the base, an anterior, a posterior, and two lateral surfaces. A capsule of collagenous and elastic fibers and smooth muscle tissue encloses the prostate, except at the apex. Based on palpation, we know that the prostate has two lateral lobes, separated by a central sulcus and a middle lobe that is not palpable unless enlarged. This designation is useful for size and shape estimation and for the description of pathologic findings on rectal palpation, but does not reflect the defined histological zones of the prostate described below.

The prostate is located in the true pelvic space, immediately below and with its base firmly adherent to the bladder neck and circumferentially around the proximal urethra. Ventrally, preprostatic adipose tissue, an extensive venous plexus, and the pubic symphysis mark the boundaries of the prostate. Dorsally, the prostate borders the rectum, from which Denonvillier's fascia separates the prostate gland. Bilaterally, a neurovascular bundle is adjacent to the prostatic capsule. These bundles carry veins of the prostatic capsule and nerves responsible for the autonomous innervation of the cavernous muscle, i.e., erectile function. Distally, the apex of the prostate is continuous with the striated urethral sphincter and is in contact to the superior fascia of the urogenital diaphragm.

The urethra runs through the prostate. Approximately halfway, a turn marks two distinct parts of the prostatic urethra. The proximal prostatic urethra is encircled by smooth muscle fibers that form the involuntary internal sphincter. This sphincter closes the urethra to prevent urinary passage during the filling phase of the bladder, and prevent retrograde passage during ejaculation. The openings of the ejaculatory ducts are located at the verumontaneum in the distal prostatic urethra. Distally, the membranous urethra is the continuum of the prostatic urethra.

The five prostate lobes (anterior, posterior, median, and two lateral lobes) do not reflect true anatomic reality: Based on anatomic studies of McNeal et al. (1), it is accepted that the prostate is separated into two main parts—the *peripheral zone*, which is the origin of up to 90% of all prostatic carcinomas (PCAs) (2) and the *central zone*, which circumvents the ejaculatory ducts toward the base of the prostate and bladder neck. Fewer than 5% of all PCAs arise in the central zone (2). Peripheral and central zones contribute about 95% of the total prostate volume. The remainder constitutes the paired *transition zone* (Figure 1). In the young, the transition zone comprises 5% of the prostatic volume. However, it is the major origin of benign tissue enlargement (3,4), gaining in volume with age and being responsible for benign prostatic hyperplasia (BPH) and associated bladder outlet obstruction. The transition zone is the origin of 15–25% of PCAs (2). Finally, the *anterior part* of the prostate is primarily composed of fibromuscular tissue, whereas glandular ducts predominate in other parts.

The seminal vesicles are paired outpouchings of the deferent ducts located posterior to the bladder and dorsocranially of the posterior surface of the prostate (Figure 1). They have an approximate size of 5 cm and an estimated volume of 3–4 mL. Their secretory epithelium contributes the majority of volume to the ejaculate. Seminal vesicles are not palpable, unless infiltrated by PCAs or inflammatory processes.

Microscopic Anatomy

The prostate contains fibromuscular (about 30%) and glandular (about 70%) components. The histological structure is that of branched ductal glands consisting of epithelial cells surrounded by stromal tissue. Prostatic epithelium consists of three types of cells: columnar secretory epithelial cells, basal cells, and neuroendocrine cells.

The cytoplasm of the secretory cells contains secretory granules filled with prostate-specific antigen (PSA), human glandular kallikrein 2 (hK2), acid phosphatase (PAP), and other enzymes. According to the life cycle of a cell, prostatic epithelial cells are separated into basal cells, immature nonsecretory glandular cells, mature secretory glandular cells, nonsecretory predegenerative glandular cells, and the degenerating glandular cells (5).

Basal cells are smaller, border the basal membrane, and contain cytokeratin, but do not stain for PSA, androgen receptor, or PAP. More than 80% of proliferating cells are found in the basal layer. The basal layer is proposed to contain epithelial stem cells for secretory cells that give rise to an intermediate amplifying cell population, the progeny of which differentiate

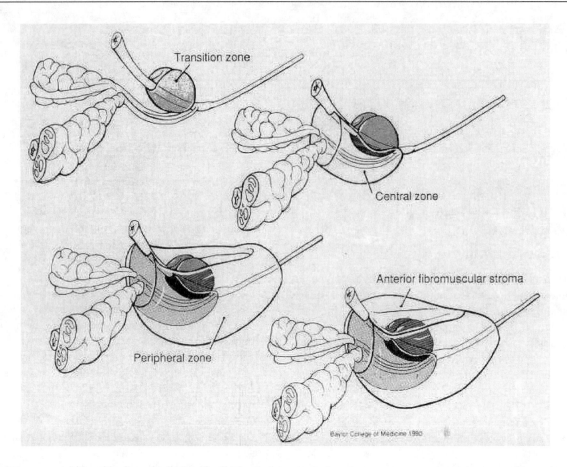

Figure 1 Zonal distribution of the prostate. Reprinted with permission from Walsh PC, Retick AB, Stamey TA, Vaughan ED, eds. Campbell's urology. Philadelphia: WB Saunders, 1992;1:344.

into luminar secretory cells. The presence of basal cells is important with regard to histological diagnosis of prostate cancer because prostate cancer acini lack basal cells, which contrast with hyperplastic or normal cells. Neuroendocrine cells, scattered among secretory cells, contain somatostatin, calcitonin, and possibly thyroid-stimulating hormone. Their origin is unclear, and it has been suggested that they act in a paracrine fashion, possibly regulating activity and growth of secretory cells in collaboration with cells of the prostatic stroma, and contribute intraluminar secretion of peptides to the ejaculate and modify sperm function. Some authors hypothesize a common stem cell as precursor of all glandular cells including neuroendocrine cells. Others propose a dual-stem cell model, suggesting that neuroendocrine cells are derived from the neural crest and suggest a second prostatic stem cell lineage that is different from the urogenital sinus lineage, which forms other prostatic cell types.

Stromal cells consist of lymphatic, smooth muscle, endothelial, and neuroendocrine cells, and fibroblasts, and axons. Stromal cells have malignant potential but lymphomas, sarcomas, or exclusively neuroendocrine prostate cancers contribute to a minute fraction of the malignant prostatic tumors and are difficult to detect at an early stage, as they do not produce PSA. Stromal cells serve as a matrix for the epithelium, and contribute a variety of growth factors that regulate secretion, proliferation, differentiation, and apoptosis. Many effects believed to be due to action of sex steroids are actually caused by growth factors, although their synthesis may require sex hormones.

Physiology and Normal Prostate Function

Prostatic secretory function is regulated by androgens. Castration prior to puberty, mutations of the Androgen Receptor (AR) (6), or 5-α-reductase deficiency (7) can impair prostatic development. Most physiologic and pathologic processes depend on androgen supply, as shown by Huggins and Hodges (8,9). Today, 60 years later, androgen manipulation maintains an undisputed central role in the management of benign and malignant prostatic disease.

The hypothalamic-pituitary-gonadal (HPG) axis (Figure 2). This is the hormonal complex that generates and regulates production of gonadal androgens for sexual maturation, maintenance of male phenotype, and fertility.

The hypothalamus. This gland is the integrating structure of the HPG axis. Information from the central nervous system and feedback from circulating testosterone and androstenedione are processed in the hypothalamus. Gonadotropin-releasing hormone (GnRH), also called luteinizing hormone-releasing hormone (LHRH), is produced in the hypothalamus (10). GnRH has a half-life of only 2–5 minutes and is released in a pulsatile manner every 65 to 90 minutes (11). These characteristics are key to the efficacy of GnRH-analogues, used for palliative treat-

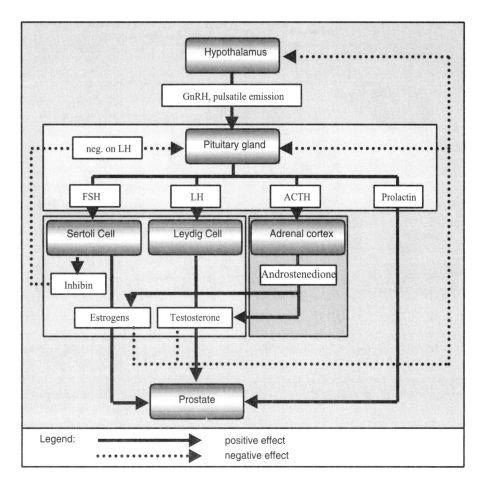

Figure 2 Positive and negative feedback regulation of the hypothalamic-pituitary-gonadal (HPG) axis.

ment of advanced PCA. GnRH-analogues contribute continuous high GnRH-levels, overriding the pulsatile GnRH secretion from the hypothalamus. This "biochemical castration" desensitizes the pituitary gland for GnRH, shuts down pituitary release of luteinizing hormone (LH) and follicle-stimulating hormone (FSH), and decreases testosterone production.

Multiple pathways regulate GnRH secretion. Norepinephrine contributes the primary stimulus for GnRH secretion (12) while testosterone and androstenedione provide feedback inhibition (13). The action of other neurotransmitters, found in cells providing input to the hypothalamus (GABA, dopamine, serotonin, and opiates), is unclear.

The pituitary gland. The anterior part of the pituitary gland secretes LH and FSH in response to the pulsatile stimulus from GnRH (10). Androgens provide a negative feedback mechanism for LH and FSH. This is evident from the LH- and FSH-surge after orchiectomy (14,15). Estrogens contribute equally strong feedback inhibition for LH and FSH secretion (16) that has been used for hormonal manipulation of PCA growth. Inhibin, a peptide synthesized by the Sertoli cells, also provides negative feedback to LH (17).

Prolactin increases prostatic growth, though elevated prolactin levels suppress LH secretion (18) that in turn reduces testosterone production. Adrenocorticotrophic hormone (ACTH) exerts positive action on the cytochrome P450 system in the adrenal cortex that results in increased production of adrenal androgens (19). Inhibition of the cytochrome P450 system is the main therapeutic action of ketoconazole, an antifungal agent used to block adrenal androgen synthesis as second-line therapy for hormone-refractory prostate cancer (20,21).

The testes. Spermatogenesis and production of testicular androgens takes place in the testes. Leydig cells are clustered in the testicular parenchyma and produce androgens. The testes account for more than 95% of the production of testosterone, while adrenals contribute less than 5% of androstenedione, peripherally converted to testosterone.

Homeostasis of Testosterone in Blood

Testosterone levels in plasma remain stable over a 24-hour cycle (13). The normal plasma concentration in healthy human males of 700 ng/mL represents a steady state of biosynthesis, binding to transport proteins and metabolic pathways (22). Testosterone has a high plasma concentration and androgenic potency. Dihydrotestosterone (DHT) has lower plasma concentration (8%) but is 1.5- to 2-fold more potent than testosterone. Testosterone is bound to sex hormone-binding globulin (57%), albumin (40%), or corticosteriod-binding protein (<1%) (23). Only 2–3% of testosterone is biologically active. Major metabolic pathways for testosterone are shown in Figure 3. The pathways are summarized briefly below:

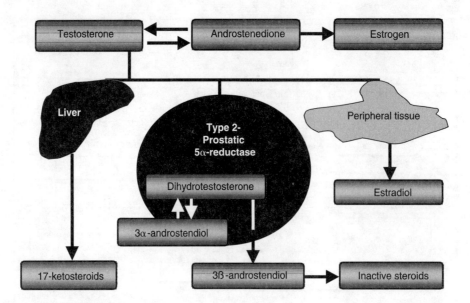

Figure 3 Metabolic pathways of testosterone.

1. Hepatic conversion of testosterone to 17-ketosteroids with minimal androgen potency.
2. Intracellular conversion of testosterone to DHT, catalyzed irreversibly by 5-α-reductase in the prostate, seminal vesicles, liver, or adrenal gland. This enzyme is a target for 5-α-reductase-inhibitors, such as finasteride, that decrease intraprostatic DHT concentration by 90% (24) and serve as drugs for symptomatic treatment of BPH (25).
3. Aromatase converts testosterone to estradiol in peripheral adipose tissue, and androstendione is converted to estrogen by this enzyme. Peripheral conversion contributes 75–90% of estrogen in men.

Regulation of Prostatic Epithelial Function

Normal prostate function depends on androgen binding that activates the androgen receptor (AR), which results in transcription of target androgen-responsive genes. Androgen deprivation massively decreases the number of secretory glandular cells (decrease of 90%) and tissue volume (decrease of 80%) (26). The effect on stromal cells is much less profound.

Intracellular androgens, the androgen receptor, and control of gene synthesis. After uptake and intracellular 5α-reductase-catalyzed conversion of testosterone to DHT, the primary target for DHT and testosterone is cytosolic-nuclear AR. AR (Figure 4) is a member of a superfamily of ligand-responsive transcription factors (27). The AR gene is located on the X chromosome (Xq11-12) and is approximately 90 kilobases in length. The protein is comprised of 917 amino acids and has a molecular mass of approximately 100 kDa. The gene is composed of eight exons that encode for three distinct functional domains (Figure 4). There is a steroid-binding domain at the C-terminus, a DNA-binding domain, which is responsible for binding to androgen response elements (AREs) of target genes, and a transactivation domain at the N-terminus (28). DHT is more potent than testosterone due to its higher affinity to AR, and at equimolar concentration, testosterone activity is only 30% of DHT (29). Upon binding to the AR, a conformational change occurs that facilitates receptor homodimerization, nuclear transport, and interaction with DNA. The binding of the AR to AREs present in the promoter of target genes results in the regulation of their transcriptional activity. Additional transcription factors form a stable transcription initiation complex. This results in transcription of target genes (e.g., PSA) into mRNA that is translated into proteins.

Recent data show that AR can be activated in absence of androgen by ligand-independent mechanisms. Several classes of substances induce androgen-independent AR activation (shown by increased PSA expression), such as butyrate (30,31), phenylacetate (32), vasoactive intestinal peptide (33), vitamin D (34), retinoic acid (35), interleukin-6 (36), neuropeptides, insulin-like growth factor 1 (IGF-1) (37), keratinocyte growth factor (KGF) (37), transforming growth factor-beta (TGF-β) (38), and epidermal growth factor (EGF).

Clinically, this translates into hormone refractory PCA. Initially, the vast majority of PCA cases respond to anti-androgen treatment. However, androgen-independent growth of PCA develops due to ligand-independent activation of PCA cells.

Regulation of Prostatic Stromal Function

The scaffolding-like fibromuscular stroma of the prostate is vital in terms of proliferation and phenotype of epithelial cells due to numerous endogenous stromal-produced factors. Apocrine and paracrine secretions of both stroma and epithelium influence surrounding cells. Androgens control the expression of these growth factors that are mediators for cellular secretion, proliferation, differentiation, and apoptosis.

Growth factors. Insulin-like growth factor 1 (IGF-1) and insulin-like growth factor 2 (IGF-2) are two peptides of 70 amino acids and 67 amino acids, respectively, with structural homology to insulin. They have mitogenic and anti-apoptotic properties due to their ability to transfer cells from G1 to the S phase of the cell cycle (39). Their biological functions are

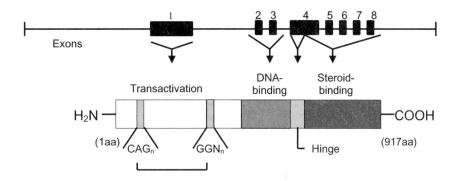

Figure 4 The androgen receptor and its three domains.

better explained in the context of an axis that includes the IGFs, IGF binding proteins, IGF proteases, and membrane-associated receptors. Most circulating IGFs are produced by growth hormone-stimulated hepatocytes. In addition to endocrine actions, IGFs have important paracrine and autocrine functions and are locally produced by many tissues, including the prostate. More than 99% of circulating IGFs are bound to carrier proteins; to date, six insulin-like growth factor binding proteins (IGFBP-1 to IGFBP-6) have been identified. More than 90% of IGFs are bound to IGFBP-3 and another protein, acid labile subunit (ALS), to form a 150 kDa ternary complex. Immunoassays are available to measure free IGFs and total serum IGFs. Bound IGFs are storage forms with no biological activity. Certain proteases can cleave IGFBPs, thus releasing bioactive IGFs.

IGFs act by binding to IGF receptors. The type 2 IGF receptor is identical to the mannose-6-phosphate receptor and serves to clear IGF-2 from the circulation. The type 1 IGF receptor (IGF-1R) is homologous to the insulin receptor and has tyrosine kinase activity. IGF binding to this receptor initiates a signal transduction cascade, leading to cellular proliferation (mitogenesis) and cellular protection from apoptosis; this activity prompted scientists to hypothesize that the IGF axis plays a role in the initiation or progression of carcinogenesis.

In culture, normal prostate cell growth depends on presence of IGF-1 and IGF-2 (40). It has been shown that mRNA expression in BPH stroma is ten times higher than in normal tissue (41) and increased levels of IGF-1R are associated with BPH. In PCA, IGFBP-2 is elevated, while IGFBP-3 is decreased.

TGF-α (37,41–43) is 30% similar to EGF, which has a mitogenic effect on epithelial cells. Androgen deprivation causes regression of the prostate, and a decrease in EGF levels that can be reversed by testosterone administration. EGF stimulates growth of benign epithelium that also synthesizes and secretes EGF. In LnCaP-cells, EGF levels were described to be 100 times higher than TGF-α. Others have stated that EGF and EGF-receptor levels were the highest in prostate cancer tissue, supporting the role for EGF in prostate cancer (44).

Nine different genes (37) code for a group of related polypeptides known as the fibroblast growth factor (FGF) family (45). FGF-7 or keratinocyte growth factor (KGF) is the predominant form expressed in stroma (46) and a mitogen for epithelial cells that express the KGF-receptor (47). Therefore, KGF is considered important for mediating interaction of stroma and epithelium (48).

TGF-β (43,49) is a dimer of two gene products with 70% homology and occurs in three types. Androgen depletion increases both TGF-β1 and TGF-β1-receptor, while androgen supply restores the levels. In normal epithelium, TGF-β may inhibit proliferation. BPH or PCA diminishes control of proliferation maintained by TGF-β (50,51). Also, TGF-β upregulates production of the autocrine growth factor for prostatic tissue, bFGF. TGF-β1 and -2 are found in the prostate; however, TGF-β2 was shown to be elevated in BPH, in contrast to TGF-β1 (52).

Angiogenesis in the prostate. Angiogenesis is essential in development, wound repair, and reproduction (53). Dysregulation is common in malignant growth (54). As the prostate cells require a supply of nutrients, control of the capillary network is tightly regulated (53–55). Tissue hypoxia is a signal for vascular formation and supporting blood vessels are vital for every increase in benign or malignant tissue mass (56).

Vascular endothelial growth factor (VEGF) is a potent mitogen with angiogenic properties (57,58) produced in normal and malignant prostate cells in response to hypoxia (59), which forms new vessels. Androgen ablation impairs the capacity of PCA cells to synthesize VEGF (60,61), though angiogenesis is also affected by other factors such as platelet-derived growth factor (PDGF) and IGF-1, TGF-β, and interleukin-1α.

Blood flow regulation of the prostate. Endothelin 1 (ET-1) is the most powerful vasoconstrictor known today (62). Three types (ET-1 to ET-3) (63) have been identified as secretory products, found at their highest concentrations in human seminal plasma (64), where they generate contraction of prostatic smooth muscle. Two receptors (ET-A and ET-B) exist. Prostate stromal cells predominantly express ET-A-receptor, whereas ET-B-receptor is found in epithelium (65). However, ET-B is expressed in BPH stroma, signaling prostatic contraction (66). ET-1 has proliferative effects, synergistic with growth factors (67).

Nervous control of the contractile function of the prostate. Symptomatic benign prostatic enlargement is not solely an increase in amount of tissue, but is also—as evidenced by therapeutic effect of alpha-1-adrenergic antagonists to smooth muscle receptors—a function by some degree of contractile activity of smooth muscle (68).

Emission of prostatic secretion is due to smooth muscle contraction (69,70) by alpha-1-receptor signaling in adrenergic nerves (71). The major site of action is likely the stroma containing more than 95% of all receptors (68).

Secretory Products of the Prostate and Adjacent Gland

Ejaculate is composed of two different components—spermatozoa and seminal plasma. Spermatozoa account for less than 1% of ejaculate volume. The major contribution originates from the seminal vesicles ($\approx$1.5–2 mL), the prostate ($\approx$0.5 mL), Cowper's gland, and glands of Littre ($\approx$0.1–0.2 mL).

Human seminal plasma contains unusually high concentrations of zinc, potassium, citric acid, fructose, phosphorylcholine, spermine, free amino acids, prostaglandins, diamine oxidase, beta-glucuronidase, lactic dehydrogenase (LDH), and α-amylase (72–75). Enzymes constitute major components of prostatic secretions that may play key roles in enabling sperm to be motile and permit fertilization. Major prostatic secretory proteins are prostate-specific antigen (PSA), prostatic acid phosphatase (PAP), and prostate-specific protein 94 (PSP94 or beta-MSP).

Citric acid. Citric acid is secreted at 500- to 1,000-fold higher concentrations than in blood. In prostate epithelial cells, citrate is synthesized from aspartic acid (Asp) and glucose at concentration up to 30,000 nmoles per gram of tissue, and is secreted as one of the major anions in human seminal plasma. Up to 30 mmol/L of citrate binds divalent metal ions and approximately balances divalent metal ion levels (i.e., mainly calcium, 7 mmol/L; magnesium, 4 mmol/L; and zinc 2 mmol/L).

Fructose. Androgen-regulated biosynthesis of fructose by the seminal vesicles may contribute energy source for spermatozoa.

Spermine and spermidine. Prostate epithelium is the major contributor of up to 3.5 mg/mL of spermine. Polyamines like spermine and spermidine can also form covalent amide bonds to link them to protein carboxylic groups, which may be of regulatory significance. Spermine is synthesized from ornithine to putrescine, spermidine, and spermine (76). Diamine oxidase oxidizes polyamines to reactive aldehyde compounds with toxic properties for bacteria and sperm.

Phosphorylcholine. Found in prostatic secretions (22), this is a specific substrate for PAP, which causes rapid generation of free choline in the ejaculate.

Prostaglandins. Seminal vesicles are the richest sources of prostaglandins (22,77), which are found at levels of 100–300 µg/mL in seminal plasma. All are 20-carbon hydroxyl fatty acids with a cyclopentane ring and two side chains. All prostaglandins are potent pharmacological agents involved in a variety of functions in the male, including erection, ejaculation, sperm motility, and transport (78).

Zinc. The prostate has the highest levels of zinc of any organ (50 mg/100 g of dry weight) (79) and contributes high seminal plasma levels of zinc (2 mmol/L). Zinc levels are elevated or normal in benign hypertrophic tissue; markedly decreased zinc levels are associated with prostatic adenocarcinoma (22). Radioautography localized zinc-65 in epithelial cells (80). Many physiologic roles have been postulated for zinc and more recently, it has been shown that zinc ions may contribute powerful allosteric, reversible inhibition of hK2 and PSA activity.

Prostatic Secretory Proteins

Prostatic acid phosphatase (PAP). Human PAP is a dimeric glycoprotein with a molecular mass of 102 kDa. The protein can be dissociated into two 50-kDa subunits. Seminal plasma contains 0.3 to 1 g/L of PAP (22) and the enzymatic activity is more than 200-fold higher in prostate compared to any other tissue. Phosphorylcholine may be the natural substrate for PAP; PAP hydrolyzes protein tyrosine phosphate esters, although it is unknown whether PAP regulates tyrosyl protein kinase systems.

Gene products of the human kallikrein gene locus on chromosome 19q13.4. The genes for PSA, human glandular kallikrein 2 (hK2), and tissue kallikrein (hK1), together with 12 more recently discovered genes (81), span about 300 kilobases on the long arm of chromosome 19 (81–83). Each gene contains five exons and four introns. The two proteins, PSA and hK2, are most closely related with 79% identity in amino acid sequence (84). HK1 has 62% identity to PSA in amino acid sequence. Each gene product contains a signal peptide, short propeptide, and mature protein. Differences are noted with regard to pI values, molecular mass, immunological characteristics, and profiles of enzymatic activity. Recombinant protein expression provided critical prerequisites for detailed understanding of structure-function relationships of these gene products. Much less is presently known on biological roles of the more recently discovered gene products, though at least two of these, prostase/KLK-L1/hK4 and prostin/hK15, are expressed in prostatic tissue. This section will mainly focus on PSA and hK2.

Biochemistry of PSA. At levels up to 5 mg/mL in seminal fluid, PSA is one of the most abundant proteins (85,86). PSA is processed in steps from 261-amino acid prepro-PSA, through a 244-amino-acid zymogen (pro-PSA), to a 237-amino acid single-chain active serine protease (87). Release of the short propeptide at Arg_{-1} converts inactive pro-PSA to active enzyme, which can be accomplished in vitro by active hK2 at physiological ratios to pro-PSA (88–90) by trypsin (90) and prostin (91). However, it is still unknown whether these proteases regulate conversion of inactive proPSA to active 237-amino acid single-chain enzyme in vivo.

Heterogeneity of a single oligosaccharide covalently linked at Asp_{45} to the 26 kDa polypeptide confers multiple isoelectric points (6.8 to 7.5). The PSA molecule has a mass of about 28.4 kDa, established by mass spectrometry (92).

PSA has chymotrypsin-like serine protease activity (93–95). It hydrolyzes peptide bonds, mainly C-terminal, of certain tyrosine (Tyr) and glutamine (Gln) residues, but this activity is distinctly dissimilar to that of chymotrypsin (96). Contrary to earlier reports of PSA demonstrating trypsin-like activity [hydrolyzing peptide bonds C-terminal of arginine (Arg) and lysine (Lys) residues], PSA is virtually devoid of this activity (96,97). Major targets for PSA in vivo are the major gel-proteins, seminogelin I and seminogelin II (SgI & SgII), and fibronectin, in freshly ejaculated semen (94,98). Proteolytic fragmentation of fibronectin, SgI, and SgII by PSA liquefies semen (94,98–100) and releases progressively motile sperm.

In vitro studies have shown that increased levels of IGF-1 may result from inactivation of IGFBP3 due to proteolysis by PSA (101). However, several cleavages identified suggest that proteolysis of IGFBP3 might also result from trace contaminants (e.g., hK2 or trypsin) in PSA from seminal fluid. Other enzymatic actions of PSA in vitro include inactivation of parathyroid hormone-related protein (PTHrP) (102) expressed by neuroendocrine cells in prostatic tissue. Stimulation of mitogenic activity of osteoblasts, possibly through activation of TGF-β, proteolytic modification of cell-adhesion receptors (103), and anti-angiogenic activity (104) has also been attributed to the action of PSA. The in vivo significance of these actions is unknown, but suggest possible function for PSA in regulation of prostatic growth.

Human glandular kallikrein 2 (hK2). HK2-mRNA is expressed in prostatic epithelium at 10–50% of the levels of PSA-mRNA (105,106), though hK2-protein levels in seminal plasma are only about 1% of PSA-levels (107). The 237-amino acid hK2-polypeptide (84) with a single carbohydrate unit has a mass of 28.5 kDa by mass spectroscopy (108). PSA and hK2 have extensive similarity in 3-D structure and androgen-regulated tissue expression, but distinct differences in endoproteolytic substrate specificity.

Biochemistry of hK2. Similar to PSA, hK2-mRNA codes for a 261-amino-acid prepro-hK2 that is converted in steps to an active 237-amino-acid protease. Conversion of inactive pro-hK2 to active hK2 may be an autocatalytic process (109,110). HK2 has trypsin-like specificity, catalyzing cleavages C-terminal of certain single and double Arg-residues (108,109), distinct from the chymotrypsin-like PSA-activity. The in vivo significance of reported hK2-actions (88–90) is not known, although hK2 may be a likely physiological PSA-activator, considering that pro-PSA conversion occurs at physiological ratios of the two co-localizing proteins. HK2 can split SgI, SgII, and fibronectin—the primary PSA-targets—with a cleavage pattern distinctly different from that generated by PSA (111,112), and is of unclear physiological significance in vivo. Other reports suggest potentials for hK2 to regulate the urokinase plasminogen activator (uPA) system (90,113,114), which correlates with cancer invasion and metastatic potential. HK2 activates the single-chain uPA to active two-chain uPA, and hk2 inactivates PAI-1, the primary inhibitor of uPA, and forms complexes with protein C inhibitor (PCI is also known as PAI-3) (112). Thus hK2 may enhance PCA progression by activating uPA, and by inactivating PAI-1. Moreover, hK2 exhibits low kininogenase activity (115).

Prostase. Mainly expressed in prostate epithelial cells, prostase shares 47% amino acid sequence identity with PSA (81). Recent protein function data suggest that it can convert pro-PSA to active PSA (91).

Prostasin. A 40kDa serine protease, prostasin is expressed in normal prostate epithelial cells at mean levels of about 150 ng/mg of tissue and secreted to semen at concentrations up to 10 μg/mL (116). Extraprostatic expression has been found at much lower concentrations in kidneys and lungs. Its function is unclear. It has been suggested that prostasin suppresses PCA invasion in vitro because prostasin and prostasin mRNA are lacking in invasive prostate cancer (117).

Prostate-specific protein-94, β-microseminoprotein, or β-inhibin. Prostate-specific protein-94 (PSP-94 or β-MSP) is a major 94-amino-acid non-glycosylated protein of 16-kDa protein found in prostatic secretions. Clinical utility is limited due to a low and inconsistent expression in benign and malignant prostatic tissue (118). Further, transcripts of messenger RNA for this protein have also been identified in nongenital tissues (119), and high protein-levels have been detected primarily in mucous-producing glands in the pulmonary tract and in gastric mucosa (120).

Zn-α-2-glycoprotein. This 41-kDa glycoprotein is produced by a variety of normal epithelia (breast, liver, salivary glands). It induces lipolysis associated with cachexia in tumor animal models (121). Zn-α-2-glycoprotein is detected intensely by monoclonal antibodies in prostate epithelium but not in stroma or other parts of the prostate or the seminal vesicles.

Leucine aminopeptidase. Produced and secreted by prostate epithelial cells. leucine aminopeptidase is found in tissue extracts of cancer. However, tissue extracts of cancer contain less leucine aminopeptidase than extracts of benign tissue (122).

Immunoglobulins, C3 complement, and transferring. Immunoglobulins are found in prostate fluid and in seminal fluid at concentrations of 7–22 mg/100 mL (IgG) and 0–6-mg/100 mL (IgA) (123,124). Prostatic fluid contains the C3 component of complement (1.82 mg/100 mL). Increased levels of up to 10-fold (up to 16.9 mg/100 mL) are reported in fluid collected from patients with prostatic adenocarcinoma (125). Likewise, transferrin levels increase from normal prostatic fluid levels of 5.3 mg/100 mL to 42.4 mg/100 mL in prostatic carcinoma (125).

DISORDERS OF THE PROSTATE

The bulk of prostatic disorders are made up of three conditions: *benign prostatic hyperplasia* (BPH), *prostatitis,* and *adenocarcinoma of the prostate* (PCA), and these disorders can co-exist. This is true in particular for PCA and BPH. It is of utmost importance that a malignant process is ruled out before treatment of a non-malignant disorder is initiated

BPH

Background. The importance of BPH is stressed by its high prevalence in the same age group as men diagnosed with PCA (126). The symptoms of BPH consist of irritative and obstructive voiding disturbances of various degrees (127). It is not true that simple enlargement of the prostate causes BPH to manifest clinically. Only weak correlation exists between the degree of enlargement, the degree of subvesical bladder outlet obstruction (BOO), and subjective complaints of the patient (128,129). Patients with a relatively small prostatic volume can suffer massive obstructive and/or irritative symptoms, and patients with an extremely enlarged prostate may present only minor or no voiding difficulties at all (130).

Patients present with lower urinary tract symptoms (LUTS), consisting of one, several, or all of the following: weak urinary stream, intermittency, urgency, frequency, incomplete emptying of the bladder, straining, and nocturia. Further work-up clarifies whether the patient suffers from obstruction due to BPH or whether there are other underlying causes for patient complaints; e.g., urethral strictures, neurological disorders, neurological sequelae (neurogenic bladder in Parkinson's disease, multiple sclerosis), or diabetes.

Epidemiology, etiology and pathogenesis of BPH. Commonly, at the beginning of the fourth decade of life, hyperplastic growth of the glandular parts of the prostate is initiated in the periurethral parts of the prostate and the transition zone. Only about 8% of men at this age, but more than half of men between age 51 to 60, and more than 90% of men 70 years or older, have histological evidence of BPH (131,132). Clinical diagnosis of BPH (69% of 61–70 year-old men) corresponds to the estimated prevalence of pathologic BPH. This suggests that the proportion of men affected with *clinically* evident BPH is comparable to that with *pathologically* verified BPH, though there is poor correlation between symptoms, size and histology on an individual basis (133).

No risk factors other than age and inherited genetic components have been associated with the development of BPH (133,134). Androgens do not cause BPH; however, development of BPH requires androgen supply from early development to puberty and aging. Patients do not develop BPH if they have been castrated (8), or if they suffer from 5α-reductase deficiency (7) or other diseases that impair androgen supply, synthesis, or action. Nuclear androgen receptor expression levels remain high in the prostate throughout the entire life (135), unlike other androgen-dependent organs (e.g., penis) (136). Androgen receptor levels may be higher in hyperplastic than in normal tissue, and age-related increased estrogen levels may further increase expression levels of the androgen receptor. It is likely that androgens play a permissive, indirect role in prostatic growth via growth factors (137). Apart from androgen effects, interactions between epithelium and stroma are likely responsible for increased epithelial cell growth in BPH (137). Dysregulation of normal interactions of stroma-produced growth factors is likely to influence the balance between new cell formation and programmed cell death, which increases cellular volume.

Pathophysiology. As the prostate increases, it decreases the diameter of the prostatic urethra, thus elevating urethral resistance. The detrusor muscle compensates by increasing pressure to maintain outflow, which disturbs the normal storage function of the bladder. Prostate size does not correlate with the degree of outflow obstruction or symptoms. An important factor is the anatomical site of the enlargement and its relation to the urethra (3).

Smooth muscle comprises a significant amount of prostatic stroma in the normal and hyperplastic gland (138). Experimental stimulation leads to an increase, blockage of these muscles to a decrease, in prostatic urethral resistance (137). The most abundant receptor mediating muscular tone is the α-1-adreno-receptor (139), and receptor-blockage is a mainstay of conservative medical management of BPH (140).

Increased resistance results in detrusor instability or decreased detrusor compliance, presenting as frequency and urgency. Changes in detrusor contractility cause hesitancy, intermittency, increased residual urine volume, or acute urinary retention. Bladder decomposition may occur. Renal impairment due to obstruction can be observed in 10–15% of patients (137).

Treatment options for BPH can be divided into conservative and surgical management. Their necessity can be estimated by validated questionnaires such as the International Prostatic Symptom Score (IPSS) to help assess BPH and aid in decision-making for medical (5-α-reductase inhibitor, alpha-1-blocker) or surgical treatment. The mainstay of surgical treatment is transurethral resection in smaller prostates or open surgery.

Prostatitis

Background. The importance of prostatitis is due to its high incidence in men who are likely to harbor PCA. Prostatitis is rare in males under 30 (141) but is common in older males (142). Up to 50% of all men develop at least one episode of prostatitis in their lifetime. Prostatitis may be classified into four distinct types: acute bacterial prostatitis, chronic bacterial prostatitis, nonbacterial prostatitis (two subcategories), and asymptomatic inflammatory prostatitis (143) (see Table 1). The efficacy of antimicrobial therapy is limited due to poor antimicrobial penetration in the prostate. Therefore, long duration of treatment is required but failure rates are high at 30–40% (144).

Pathophysiology of prostatitis. Prostatic secretion maintains a slightly acidic pH of 6.6 to 7.6. Increasing age and prostatitis increase the pH range to 7 to 9, impairing its defense against pathogens. Bacterial invasion into the prostate may be due to ascending urethral infection or direct invasion of rectal bacteria. Lymphatic and hematogenous spread may occur. However, intraprostatic urinary reflux (145) may be the primary cause of most bacterial and nonbacterial prostatitis cases. Prostatic invasion of pathogens causes hyperperfusion, swelling, pain, and functional disturbances. The more acute the inflammatory process, the more likely is the progression of subclinical to clinical symptoms.

Acute bacterial prostatitis (NIH category I). Acute bacterial prostatitis is the least common type of prostatitis (146). It is accompanied by urinary tract infection with positive cultures from prostatic secretions. Blood cultures may show the same bacteria as urine culture due to hematogenous spread. It presents with sudden onset of fever, chills, low back, and perineal pain. Patients complain of obstructive and irritative voiding, generalized malaise, arthralgias, and myalgias. *Escherichia coli* is the most prevalent pathogen. Other microorganisms (*Proteus* and *Klebsiella*) may also be present. Antimicrobial therapy for 4–6 weeks is the mainstay of treatment.

Chronic bacterial prostatitis (CBP; NIH category II). CBP results from inadequate treatment of acute bacterial prostatitis due to antimicrobial resistance, relapse, or short-course therapy. Most common are recurrent urinary tract infections with obstructive and irritative urinary symptoms. Identification of bacteria from the prostate is key to the diagnosis of CBP.

Table 1 Classification of prostatitis

NIH classification	Definition
Category I	
Acute bacterial prostatitis	Acute infection of the prostate gland
Category II	
Chronic bacterial prostatitis	Recurrent infection of the prostate
Category IIIA	
Inflammatory CPPS	White cells in semen/EPS/voided bladder urine-3 (VB3 or postprostastic massage)
Category IIIB	
Non-inflammatory CPPS	No white cells in semen/EPS/VB3
Category IV	
Asymptomatic inflammatory prostatitis	Abnormal semen analysis
	Elevated PSA values
	Histological evidence of inflammation in prostatic biopsy

CPPS, chronic pelvic pain syndrome; EPS, expressed prostatic secretion.

Chronic prostatitis requires at least 10 to 12 weeks of antimicrobial therapy.

Nonbacterial prostatitis (NBP; NIH category IIIA/B). NBP is the most common type of prostatitis. There are two subforms, prostatitis with and without signs of infection. It occurs eight times more frequently than bacterial prostatitis and presents with the same signs and symptoms as bacterial prostatitis; however, prostatic fluid cultures are negative for bacteria. Inflammation is evident upon prostatic fluid analysis. Implicated pathogens include *Chlamydia trachomatis*, *Ureaplasma urealyticum*, and *Trichomonas vaginalis*. Treatment duration is approximately two to four weeks.

Asymptomatic inflammatory prostatitis (NIH category IV). In this condition, the patient is asymptomatic but has white blood cells in semen, or granulocytes and lymphocytes on histological evaluation of a biopsy specimen. PSA may be moderately elevated. This type of prostatitis is usually detected in the work-up for infertility or PCA screening.

Prostatic Intraepithelial Neoplasia (PIN)

A potentially premalignant state of proliferation in the prostate (147), PIN is present in up to 16% of men who undergo prostate biopsies (148–150). PIN alters cellular architecture, most commonly in the peripheral zone where the duct and gland architecture is preserved, and progressively disrupts the basal cell layer with increasing grades of PIN (147). Invasion of the stroma is lacking. Other changes also become apparent; these include loss of neuroendocrine and secretory differentiation, nuclear and nucleolar abnormalities, neovascularity, increased proliferative potential, genetic instability with variation of DNA content, and an increasing degree of nuclear aberration. PIN has a fragmented basal cell layer, whereas PCA lacks a basal cell layer. Basal cell-specific immunostaining for cytokeratin is present in PIN but absent in PCA areas (151). Severity of PIN is graded from lowest (Grade I) to highest grade (Grade III). PIN II–III should be summarized as high-grade PIN. High-grade PIN is associated with PCA and predates appearance of PCA by more than five years (147). High-grade PIN was found with PCA in 30–50% of biopsied men in various series (152). High-grade PIN, patient age, and PSA levels were highly significant predictors of PCA. Systematic rebiopsies should be performed after diagnosis of PIN to detect PCA (153).

Adenocarcinoma of the Prostate

Background. Adenocarcinoma of the prostate (PCA) is the most common noncutaneous malignancy in men and is one of the leading causes of cancer-related deaths in the United States and other western countries. In the U.S. alone, it is estimated that more than 198,000 new cases of PCA were diagnosed and 31,500 men died of the disease in 2001 (154,155).

Natural history of PCA. PCA represents a unique disease entity in several respects. Despite a 30–40% incidence of microscopic PCA in men above the age of 50 (156–158), only 9–11% of men develop clinically manifest disease, and only 2.6–4.3% die of the disease (159). In other words, the majority of histologically evident microscopic cancers do not impact the lifespan of the individual and may not need to be detected. This PCA category with indolent course, slow progression, low malignant potential, and no spread beyond the prostate capsule is unlikely to cause clinical disease or death. These clinically insignificant cancers correspond to those detected only on autopsy (160,161), and are typically found in patients in their eighth or ninth decade of life. Distinct from this group are cancers that develop in younger patients (e.g., in their 5th to 7th decade) with aggressive growth pattern and metastatic potential. If untreated, they will ultimately be the cause of death (162). In these patients, early diagnosis of PCA is vital, hence efforts should be made to identify the men who will benefit from curative treatment. The impact on health and life generated by an early stage PCA is difficult to quantify due to slow growth and long doubling time (average two to four years).

Prostate cancer is a cancer of elderly males. With increasing age, the likelihood of developing prostate cancer increases from 1 in 10,000 in men under age 39, to 1 in 103 in the range of 40 to 59 years, to 1 in 8 between the ages 60 to 79. Any treatment option must be considered in context with regard to age, adjusted life expectancy, and comorbidity according to Table 2, which shows that a white man who reaches age 65 can be

Table 2 Life tables for white and black U.S. males*

Age	Estimated life expectancy	
	White	Black
45	77.1	72.5
50	77.7	73.8
55	78.5	75.3
60	79.6	77.0
65	81.0	79.2
70	82.7	81.5
75	84.9	84.3
80	87.4	87.3

*National Vital Statistics Report, Vol 47, No 28; Dec 13, 1999.

expected to live 16 years longer, and a 55-year-old African-American has 20.3 years more to live.

Several studies examined conservative management of PCA. Of 536 unselected patients diagnosed with PCA who did not undergo curative treatment, 62% of all patients who lived longer than 10 years died from the disease. Moreover, the mortality rate persisted up to 25 years after PCA diagnosis. The median survival for well-differentiated, low-stage tumors was estimated to be 15 years. About 75% of men diagnosed with PCA before age 65 died of the disease when noncurative treatment was applied (163). A 15-year follow-up study (162) revealed the impact of tumor differentiation (Gleason Grade) with respect to survival of PCA patients treated conservatively. Survival was 91% when the Gleason score was 2–4, but decreased to 72% for patients with Gleason score 5–7 and to 49% for Gleason 8–10. Favorable Gleason scores of 2–4 were found in only 10% of patients, whereas 90% of the patients had Gleason scores of 5–7 and 8–10 (162). However, an earlier Swedish study analyzing the long-term survival of men with prostate cancer who were treated with expectant management, where average patient age was 72 years and a large proportion of men had very favorable pathology [i.e., 33% T1a-PCA and 66% well-differentiated, low-grade tumor burden (164)], found different results: only 13% of men diagnosed with PCA developed metastases, and only 11% died of PCA. This study population may be comparable to the Gleason score 2–4 from the study cited above in which only 10% of cancer cases had favorable pathology. It is therefore difficult to compare these results with those from patients who undergo definitive treatment in the U.S., and certainly it may be misleading to extrapolate survival rates of elderly men with low-grade cancer to men younger than 70 with Gleason scores of 6 or higher. It can be concluded that low-grade PCA in men over age 70 may be a slowly progressing tumor that might be managed conservatively. However, PCA in men aged 50–69 is progressing rapidly enough to be a major cause of death. Early detection and curative treatment strategies may be necessary to increase survival of these men with PCA.

Factors influencing PCA genesis. PCA incidence and mortality rates show striking differences in different populations. The lowest rates of PCA occur in Asian countries, where the rate of PCA is only 4% of those observed in U.S. (165). Factors other than genetic are likely to be important for tumorigenesis, as Asian populations migrating to the U.S. assume increased risks of developing PCA (166). Dietary factors are suggested as contributing to the reported incidence and mortality differences as they may contribute promotive [high fat, linoleic acid (167,168)], or preventive [vitamin E (169), vitamin D (170), selenium (171)] effects on PCA development.

In a defined population, ethnic origin is a risk factor for PCA development. In the U.S., PCA risk in African-American males is higher than in Caucasians, Hispanics, Asians, and men of North American origin (172–174). This includes earlier age of diagnosis, higher age-specific incidence and mortality, and more advanced stage at diagnosis. The incidence rate was 234.2 and death rate was 53.1 per 100,000 African-Americans, compared to an incidence of 144.6 and death rate of 22.4 per 100,000 in Caucasians (154). It is controversial whether differences in access to heath care for African-Americans compared to Caucasians contribute to these differences. Androgen exposure is essential for normal prostatic development, but also for the development of BPH and PCA. In men castrated for ritual reasons or males with 5-α-reductase type 2 deficiency, the prostate does not develop normal epithelium and PCA does not develop. Family risk of developing PCA is associated with the number of affected relatives (175). First-degree relatives affected at age 50 increases the relative risk seven-fold compared to brother or father diagnosed with PC at age 70 (176). Possible loci for putative PCA genes have been reported; strongest supported loci are on chromosome 1p (177) and on the X-chromosome (178).

Histological classification of prostate cancer. Ninety-five to 98% of all PCAs are adenocarcinomas that emerge from the epithelium of the acini and terminal ducts (179). Other, uncommon types of PCA include small cell carcinoma (180); mucinous adenocarcinoma (181); neuroendocrine differentiated carcinoma (182); prostatic ductal adenocarcinoma (emerging from the large ducts) (183); various types of sarcoma (184,185); primary and secondary lymphoma (186); and squamous cell carcinoma (187). These cancers tend to be more aggressive with worse prognosis than adenocarcinoma. This may in part be due to lack of PSA production, which results in detection of these tumors in a more advanced stage.

Diagnosis of PCA. Clinical symptoms relating to PCA typically do not manifest until the disease has spread beyond the prostate capsule, or metastasized to lymph nodes or bones, when curative treatment is no longer an option. Symptoms associated with advanced PCA include bone pain, obstructive and/or irritative voiding patterns, or lymphatic congestion in the lower extremities. Other symptoms are anemia and weight loss, both signs of extensive metastatic spread of cancer (188).

The possibility of diagnosing and successfully curing men with PCA is limited to the time frame when PCA is still organ-confined, a time in which PCA does not present any clinical signs. Fortunately, PCA is in its initial stages a slowly progressing tumor and might remain organ-confined for years (189).

DETECTION OF PCA

Digital rectal examination (DRE). While still a mainstay of prostatic evaluation, digital rectal examination (DRE) has important limitations for early diagnosis of PCA. In addition to estimating prostate size, DRE can identify PCA-suspected nodes in the peripheral zone. However, in patients with only small palpable PCA lesions, there are high rates of extracapsular extension of the cancer, reducing significantly the likelihood of cure. The limited efficiency of DRE screening for PCA is illustrated by reported pathology characteristics of PCA detected by DRE: more than two-thirds of patients had pathologically extraprostatic disease on radical prostatectomy specimens (190,191). Therefore, DRE does not serve as a sensitive tool for early PCA detection. Another limitation of DRE is the lack of specificity for PCA. Only 39% (1900/4939) of men with suspicious DRE are diagnosed with PCA after prostate biopsy (192). Other conditions causing prostatic indurations similar to PCA are chronic inflammatory processes or urogenital tuberculosis involving the prostate.

It is important to note that PCAs that are too small to be palpated may still be tumor lesions with clinically aggressive potential, and therefore would need to be detected and treated. Table 3 shows several studies evaluating the significance of nonpalpable (T1c) prostate cancer.

Transrectal ultrasonography (TRUS). Transrectal ultrasonography is the most common technique for prostate imaging. The typical presentation of PCA is that of a hypoechoic area (193) in the peripheral zone in about 60% of cases. The sensitivity of PCA detection using TRUS alone is poor. Additionally, PCA is understaged by TRUS, as it is with DRE.

TRUS-guided biopsy of the prostate: a gold standard for PCA detection. The introduction of TRUS-guided biopsy of six regions of the prostate revolutionized PCA detection. This procedure can be performed on an outpatient basis with little preparation (antimicrobial therapy) and low degree of discomfort and morbidity. Modifications of the original technique (194) to sample six parasagittal biopsies have been developed to improve PCA detection; e.g., by using a technique to direct six biopsies in a more lateral distribution, and to sample more from the anterior part of the peripheral zone, where PCA typically develops (195). Further modifications include an eight-core biopsy approach that has been reported to enhance PCA detection rates by 20% (196).

Repeated six-site biopsies are recommended in men with persistently elevated PSA due to the high likelihood of detecting PCA in men with initial negative biopsy. It has been reported that prostate cancer detection rates at first, second, and third rounds of biopsies were 34%, 19%, and 8%, respectively (197).

Table 3 Probability of prostate cancer on biopsy with negative DRE

	PSA <4.0 ng/mL	PSA >4.0 ng/mL
Cooner et al.	9	25
Hammerer et al.	4	12
Ellis et al.	6	24
Catalona et al.	—	32

Reprinted with permission from Polascik TJ, Oesterling JE, Partin AW. Prostate-specific antigen: a decade of discovery—what we have learned and where we are going. J Urol 1999;162(2):293–306.

PCA detection efficacy by biopsy is affected by prostate volume, as increased glandular volume increases the number of biopsies necessary to diagnose PCA, which is important due to high prevalence of BPH in these men (198). Sextant biopsy is still the most common biopsy procedure. Recent data suggest an increased number of biopsies—10 to 12 cores—but six cores might be sufficient for normally sized, small prostates.

Clinical Staging of Adenocarcinoma of the Prostate

Table 4 shows the 1992 TNM-Staging classification of PCA.

Grading of Adenocarcinoma of the Prostate

Introduced in 1974 (199), the Gleason Grading System of PCA is the most widely accepted grading system. The glandular tumor architecture at low magnification forms the basis of the Gleason grading system. Cytological features do not contribute to this grading system. The Gleason system describes the two most common patterns of dedifferentiation in one cancer with grades from 1 to 5. Grade 1 represents the most differentiated pattern, while the pattern continuously dedifferentiates from grades 2 to 4, while the Gleason grade 5 is anaplastic. The most common pattern of dedifferentiation is assigned the primary grade; the second most common pattern defines the secondary grade. Both primary and secondary Gleason grades contribute to PCA prognosis; that is why they are combined to a Gleason sum (e.g., Gleason grade $3 + 4 = 7$), synonymous for Gleason score. Therefore, Gleason sums range from 2 (Gleason grade $1 + 1 = 2$) to 10 for completely anaplastic cancers (Gleason grade $5 + 5 = 10$). It is most important to identify and distinguish Gleason grade 4 from grade 3 cancers, as the prognosis of the former is significantly worse (200). Therefore, predominance of Gleason grade 4 alters the prognosis unfavorably compared to a PCA with predominating grade 3.

The other common but less precise grading system is the World Health Organization (WHO) grades ranging from I to III, corresponding to well, moderately, or poorly differentiated PCA. WHO Grade I cancers correspond to Gleason sums 2 to 4, and WHO grade III cancers correspond to Gleason grades 8–10 cancers. However, the most common range of Gleason sum 5 to 7 does not correspond to WHO grade II cancer. This is because the prognosis of Gleason sum 5 cancers is significantly better than that of Gleason sum 7 cancers. Therefore, WHO grade II cancers do not reflect the significant differences in biological characteristics of Gleason sum 5 compared to Gleason sum 7 cancers.

Clinical-Pathological Features of Transition Zone Prostate Cancers

About 15–25% of all PCAs (2) and about 25% of nonpalpable PCAs (201) arise in the transition zone. They have a more favorable prognosis than peripheral zone cancers due to the significantly lower rate of capsular penetration, seminal vesicle invasion, and more favorable Gleason grades (202). Transition zones PCAs are difficult to diagnose, but PSA elevations in

Table 4 1992 American Joint Committee on Cancer TNM clinical staging of prostate cancer

Definition	Clinical stage
T — Tumor	
No evidence of primary tumor	T0
Tumor nonpalpable and nonvisible	**T1**
Incidental finding on TURP, <5% of resected tissue	T1a
Incidental finding on TURP, ≥5% of resected tissue	T1b
Tumor diagnosed by biopsy (PSA elevated in blood)	T1c
Tumor confined to the prostate	**T2**
Tumor involves half of one lobe or less	T2a
Tumor involves one lobe	T2b
Tumor involves both lobes	T2c
Extracapsular extension	**T3**
Unilateral extension	T3a
Bilateral extension	T3b
Seminal vesicle invasion	T3c
Tumor is fixed or invades adjacent structures other than seminal vesicles	**T4**
Bladder neck, external sphincter, rectum	T4a
Levator and/or pelvic wall	T4b
N — Regional lymph nodes	
Nodes of the true pelvis, essentially below the bifurcation of the common iliac artery (pelvic, hypogastric, obturator, iliac internal and external, periprostatic, and sacral).	
Laterality does not affect N classification.	
Regional nodes cannot be assessed	NX
No regional lymph node metastases	N0
Metastasis in regional lymph nodes	N1–N3*
M — Distant metastasis	
Distant metastasis cannot be assessed	MX
No distant metastasis	M0
Distant metastasis	M1a–M1c**

*N1 = one node ≤2 cm; N2 = one node 2–5 cm or multiple nodes <5 cm; N3 = node >5 cm.
**M1a = nonregional nodes; M1b = bone; M1c = other locations.

blood are frequently much more prominent in transition zone cancers compared to peripheral zone cancers. Transition zone cancers have a tendency to harbor large amounts of Gleason grade 2 cancers even at larger volume, even though Gleason grade 4/5 areas are found as well.

DESCRIPTION OF INDIVIDUAL TUMOR MARKERS

PSA in Serum

The potential of PSA in blood as a marker for prostate cancer was reported in the early 1980s (203–205). PSA is now known to outperform any other marker for prostatic malignancies (206).

PSA and antiproteases. Formation of stable, covalently-linked PSA complexes occurs slowly in vitro, by exposure of the active functional enzyme to many major extracellular antiproteases present in different body fluids, such as alpha-1-antichymotrypsin (ACT) (96,207,208); alpha-2-macroglobulin (AMG) (96,207,209); alpha-1-proteinase inhibitor (API) (208,210); protein C inhibitor (PCI) (209,211); and pregnancy zone protein (PZP) (96). Several of these inhibitors occur in blood at concentrations of 0.5–30 µmol/L, corresponding to 1,000-fold molar excess to PSA in blood.

PSA and antiproteases in seminal fluid. There are fundamental differences in the occurrence of PSA in blood compared to seminal fluid: the majority of PSA in seminal fluid, about 60–70% of PSA, manifests enzymatic activity and occurs at levels from 5–100 µmol/L (94,96). This corresponds to a more than 10-fold molar excess to antiprotease-levels contributed by the accessory sex glands, whereas less than 5% of PSA is complexed to antiproteases in seminal fluid (211). About 30–40% of PSA in seminal plasma is catalytically inactive. The majority of inactive PSA in seminal fluid occurs as internally cleaved, two- or multi-chain forms of the protein (96,212), resulting from cleavages C-terminal of Lys145 and Lys182 (96,212).

PSA and antiproteases in blood. PSA occurs normally at very low levels in blood, at concentrations that correspond to less than one-millionth of the levels found in seminal fluid. Unlike in seminal fluid, PSA does not manifest functional activity, i.e., it is essentially unreactive. The majority (typically 55–95%) of PSA in blood occurs in vivo in stable, covalently linked 1:1 molar ratio complexes with ACT (207,208). A minority, 5–45% of PSA in blood, is found in free noncomplexed forms. Free noncomplexed PSA forms are essentially unreactive with the large, normally greater than 10,000-fold excess of antiproteases such as ACT and AMG in blood (213). This contrasts with the reactions occurring when active PSA isolated from seminal fluid is added to blood in vitro, where PSA forms complexes in minutes, mainly with AMG but also with ACT (96,207,209). Serum levels of PSA-AMG-complexes are difficult to assess, mainly due to the fact that AMG conformation engulfs PSA, blocking access of PSA-antibodies, but also due to the very low (virtually nondetectable) levels of PSA-AMG found in vivo in freshly collected and carefully processed blood (213).

The different PSA forms are subject to different metabolic elimination pathways and therefore different elimination kinetics. A recent study elucidating the levels of different PSA forms before and after surgical manipulation of the prostate during radical prostatectomy showed that PSA-AMG levels were below the detection limits of the PSA-AMG assay (i.e., below 1.0–2.0 ng/mL) before, during, and after surgery. However, while free PSA levels increased 10-fold, neither PSA-ACT or AMG-PSA increased significantly, which suggests that free PSA released into blood by prostatic manipulation during surgery (and possibly by other conditions like inflammatory processes) does not manifest enzymatic action and forms no significant amounts of complexes with the vast excess of antiproteases in blood in vivo (213). However, PSA-AMG complexes have been reported to be readily detected by more sensitive assays, but this may be due to formation of PSA-AMG complexes in vitro due to nonoptimized, pre-analytical handling of sera stored frozen for a long time before testing (209). In addition, low concentrations of PSA-API complexes (contributing 1–2% of PSA immunodetected in blood) are found in blood (210,214).

Elimination kinetics of PSA occurring in blood have been studied in men exposed to curative radical prostatectomy for clinically localized PCA. The first reports focused on total PSA kinetics alone; the suggested half-life was 2.2 ± 0.8 days (215) to 3.2 ± 0.1 days (216). Following the design of specific assays for free PSA, PSA-ACT complexes, and total PSA, it was reported that free PSA elimination after radical prostatectomy could be explained by a bi-exponential, "two compartment" model. A primary, very rapid re-equilibration of intercellular and intravascular compartments (half-life <1 hour), and a second glomerular-filtration-dependent elimination rate of the 28.4-kDa free PSA with a half-life of 12–18 hours (213).

Other studies reported similar data on elimination rates of free PSA (217). Carefully processed serum samples collected immediately after prostatectomy and up to 14 days thereafter uncover the very slow, capacity-limited zero-order kinetic elimination rates of PSA-ACT in blood that corresponded to elimination rates of <0.8 ng/mL per day (218). While the smaller-sized free PSA molecule is subject to renal clearance, the >700-kDa PSA-AMG complexes (but not the ≈90-kDa PSA-ACT complex) are thought to be rapidly cleared from blood in vivo by an efficient hepatic AMG/low density lipoprotein receptor-related protein (LRP)-receptor pathway, giving half-life rates of <10 minutes for these complexes (219,220). The slow elimination kinetics of PSA-ACT complexes in human blood in vivo contribute significantly to the unique power of PSA testing in blood to detect and monitor malignant prostatic disease.

Isoforms of Free PSA

There is significant heterogeneity of free PSA in blood, consisting of molecular alterations of uncomplexed PSA molecules existing in several variants. Data on metabolism or synthesis are scarce at present; however, studies on clinical utility for the differentiation of benign and malignant prostatic disease are emerging (221–223).

Inactive pro-PSA (224). Recalling that pro-PSA is converted to PSA by cleavage of a seven-amino-acid sequence, it has been found that variations in the number of amino acids removed (3 or 5 amino acids) result in truncated forms of PSA: (-2)pPSA and (-4)pPSA. This may possibly correspond to more cancer-specific forms, such as the single-chain forms of PSA isolated from LNCaP-cells that are inactive due to lack of release of the short activation peptide in pro-PSA C-terminal of Arg_{-1} (221,225). Other free PSA forms are internally cleaved, nicked, or multi-chain PSA forms. These are generated by cleavages in the polypeptide chain at Lys145-Lys146 and Lys182-Ser183 positions (221,226).

Analytical considerations on immunoassays for PSA measurements in blood. The occurrence of several distinctly different PSA forms in the blood circulation has several important implications for the outcome of different designs of immunoassays used to measure total PSA levels in serum, plasma, or whole blood (227). Assays for detection of total PSA (i.e., the sum of free, noncomplexed PSA forms and the immunodetectable PSA complexes that essentially correspond to PSA-ACT) can be divided in two groups based on their relative ability to detect these major PSA forms. Equimolar PSA assays detect the free PSA forms and ACT-PSA by equally strong signal intensity and are largely unbiased by relative proportions of free PSA vs. ACT-PSA in serum. Other assay designs demonstrate a "skewed response" where free PSA levels are overestimated and PSA-ACT levels under-estimated. In these assays, free PSA forms are able to bind larger amounts of tracer antibody than PSA-ACT (207,227–229). Thus, when the proportion of free PSA (fPSA) increases, a higher amount of total PSA (tPSA) is measured and this in turn changes the percentage of the fPSA ratio to a lower level, falsely suggesting prostate cancer. Hence, the use of uniformly designed standard assay calibrators, and assay designs that provide essentially equimolar signal intensity detection of tPSA and fPSA is of great importance for generating results that are uniformly in agreement across different laboratories and that are independent of the assay manufacturer (230).

Measurements of PSA complexes. The first data reported on specific PSA-ACT complex measurements in blood demonstrated significant diagnostic enhancements by specific measurements of PSA-ACT complexes compared to conventional total PSA testing (208,231). However, they also indicated that these assays suffered from analytical problems due to nonspecific (i.e., false positive) background signals contributed by granulocyte-derived proteases such as cathepsin G, which also form complexes with ACT and attach to the solid phase surfaces of microtiter wells (227). Recently however, the design of an indirect immunodetection method of complexed PSA (cPSA) in serum was reported by Allard et al., where the capture antibody does not recognize free PSA due to the addition of a free-PSA-specific blocking antibody and therefore only captures complexed PSA in the sample (232). This assay has been granted regulatory approval by FDA in the U.S., and cPSA levels measured by this assay have been reported to correspond to the increment of free PSA subtracted from total PSA using assays that also have been granted regulatory approval by the FDA in the U.S. (233).

There exist also several analytical concerns regarding the specific measurements of free, non-complexed PSA forms in blood. According to recent reports, there are problems with lack of uniformity of manufactured free PSA assays that become amplified when free PSA levels are combined with total PSA levels to obtain free-to-total PSA ratios (230), as well as when total PSA assays do not detect free and complexed PSA forms with equimolar signal intensity as discussed above. High analytical precision is important for free PSA measurements, particularly at low levels of free PSA, to reduce the overlap in percent free-to-total PSA between men with PCA vs. those without cancer. Further, intra-individual day-to-day variation has been suggested to be higher for free PSA compared to PSA-ACT due to shorter half-life of in blood for free PSA compared to slow elimination of PSA-ACT complexes (218).

In vitro stability of PSA. A major concern in the analytical setting of PSA is that inappropriate sample handling might affect total PSA, free PSA, complexed PSA, or percentage fPSA. Woodrum et al. demonstrated a loss of 1% of fPSA per hour clotting time when serum was stored at 4 °C, and more importantly, about 0.9% decrease of fPSA per month when stored at –20 °C. Long-term storage (e.g., several months to years) should be undertaken at –70 °C as this condition did not show a significant loss in either analyte for a time period of two years. Piironen et al. demonstrated a significant decrease of fPSA in freshly collected samples stored at 4 °C after 23 hours in serum, after 86 hours in heparin-plasma, and after 71 hours in EDTA-plasma. However, there was no decrease of PSA-ACT levels during up to seven days storage of freshly collected samples (234–236).

Another aspect is the handling after the sample has been frozen and needs to be thawed for analysis. Leinonen et al. measured free PSA, total PSA, complexed PSA (cPSA), and percentage fPSA in sera that were stored at –20 °C for two years, subsequently thawed, and then stored at 4, 22, and 37 °C for a period of up to 11 days. They noted an 11% decrease in total PSA, which was mainly attributable to a 27% loss of cPSA, while a simultaneous increase in fPSA (63%) and a concomitant increase in percentage fPSA was noted (82%). The authors concluded that archival samples should be thawed only to pipette the amount needed (237). The decrease of cPSA in this study is likely explained by dissociation of the PSA-ACT complex, which has been shown to occur at high levels of pH.

Other data were based on analysis of serum and plasma samples stored at –20 °C for almost two decades. Samples were thawed, measured immediately, and also measured after exposure to room temperature for different periods of time. Contrary to what was found by Leinonen et al., this study found a very rapid and significant loss of fPSA but not cPSA levels in serum. In plasma however, thawed samples exposed for room temperature up to 24 hours did not have a significant change in neither fPSA nor cPSA concentrations. This suggests that plasma samples might have significant stability advantages as compared to serum in terms of long-term storage.

Human Glandular Kallikrein 2 and Antiproteases

Analogous to PSA, hK2 has been reported to form complexes with a large number of different extracellular antiproteases in serum and seminal fluid. Differences in amounts of complexed vs. free antigen and in types of antiproteases reacting with PSA and hK2 are noteworthy and are mainly due to different substrate specificity of the structurally similar proteases (97,112).

HK2 and antiproteases in seminal plasma and prostatic tissue. HK2mRNA is expressed in prostatic tissue at concentrations of about 20–50% of PSAmRNA (105,106,238). In seminal plasma, hK2 protein is found at concentrations of only 1% of PSA (107,239). HK2 in seminal plasma is enzymatically inactive and PCI is the major complexing ligand for hK2 (107,240). In vitro complex formation occurs with a panel of other antiproteases in addition to PCI, including AMG, antithrombin III (ATIII), α2-antiplasmin (α2-AP), ACT, C1-inactivator, and PAI-1 (108,113,114,240–242). When hK2 is complexed with PCI, PAI-1, or AMG, inhibition occurs more rapidly than with other antiproteases (114,240–242). In prostate cancer cells, about 10% of hK2 has been shown to enter complex formation with the intracellular serine protease inhibitor-6 (PI-6), which is possibly associated with tumor necrosis (243).

hK2 and antiproteases in blood. Compared to free and complexed PSA forms, concentrations of free and complexed hK2 correspond to only 1–2% of total PSA-levels. Based on gel-filtration data, the major proportion (80–95%) of detectable hK2 in serum is suggested to occur as free, noncomplexed 30-kDa forms. These may, in part, consist of catalytically inactive pro-hK2 forms (244). Only a minor proportion of hK2 (5–20%) has a 90-kDa size corresponding to that predicted for hK2 linked in complex with antiproteases, e.g., ACT or PCI (239–241,245,246).

Studies elucidating the elimination rates and kinetics of hK2 from blood are very limited. Based on similarities in clearance rates and size of free PSA and hK2, and the fact that the major proportion of hK2 in blood is likely to occur in free non-complexed forms (239,245,246), it has been suggested that glomerular filtration in the kidneys is the major elimination pathway of hK2 from blood.

Immunodetection of hK2 in serum—immunological cross-reactivity problems with PSA. There are extensive similarities, close to 80% identity, in primary structure between hK2 and PSA (84). However, as it has been suggested that there are significant differences in expression of these two proteins in benign vs. malignant prostate tissue (247,248), considerable efforts have been spent on exploring the potential of hK2 as an additional marker for prostate cancer. The similarity of hK2 and PSA complicates the immunodetection of hK2 in serum due to immunological cross-reactivity with PSA. Cross-reactivity and extensive characterization of the epitope structure of recombinant hK2 and hK2 has been studied using monoclonal anti-PSA antibodies (249,250), and has permitted development of sensitive and specific immunoassays for measurements of hK2 and PSA (239,244–246, 251–253).

Nonprostatic sources of PSA and hK2. Subsequent to the original reports that PSA, and more recently hK2, were expressed in an absolutely prostate-tissue specific pattern, more recently reported and carefully performed studies have elegantly shown that PSA and hK2 are expressed in both males and females, in several tissues other than the prostate, and are present in many biological fluids apart from blood and seminal plasma. It is however noteworthy that the contribution of PSA/hK2 to serum concentrations from these sources are likely to be insignificant under physiological conditions and may play no clinically significant role with respect to a pretreatment condition of prostate cancer. In the context of this chapter, only a short overview will be given for both proteins.

Tissues that produce PSA are the female periurethral glands (Skene's glands) (254), healthy breast tissue, and breast tumor extracts (255). Endometrial tissue produces PSA (256) as do some ovarian tumors (257), and PSA is present in amniotic fluid (258). Low levels of circulating PSA are detectable in female sera and in some cerebrospinal fluids (259). Various breast secretions contain PSA, including nipple aspirate fluid, milk of lactating women, and breast cyst fluid (258).

HK2 has been detected in normal and malignant breast tissue extracts (260) and in breast milk, amniotic fluid, breast cyst fluid (257), serum, urine, and saliva (240). In the latter, association is likely due to expression of hK2 in salivary glands.

Prostatic Acid Phosphatase (PAP, ACPP, ACP3)

Acid phosphatases (orthophosphoric monoester phosphohydrolases) are a group of enzymes capable of hydrolyzing esters of orthophosphoric acid in an acid medium. Enzymatic hydrolysis results in the splitting of O-P bands with the release of phosphoric acid (261). Four true isoenzymes (that is, forms with differences originating at the structural level of the gene) have been identified: erythrocytic, lysosomal, prostatic, and macrophagic acid phosphatases (262). More recently, a fifth acid phosphatase gene, termed testicular acid phosphatase (ACPT), has been cloned and found to be highly expressed in testes (263).

For prostate cancer, acid phosphatase (ACP) and its prostatic isoenzyme (PAP, ACPP, ACP3) have attracted considerable interest, since it was shown more than 60 years ago that serum levels are elevated in a proportion of patients with the disease, especially those with advanced stage and bone metastasis. The marker was used as an aid for diagnosis, staging, and monitoring.

Analytical considerations. Serum acid phosphatase originates from many tissues; only a minor fraction is contributed from the prostate. The majority is tartrate-resistant and probably originates in osteoclasts. For PCA applications, it is desirable to measure the prostatic form, which is strongly inhibited by tartrate ions. Although more sensitive immunological assays for PAP have been developed, their use does not offer any advantages. Major problems of ACP and PAP analysis include cross-reactivity/interference by various tissue forms of this enzyme, diurnal fluctuations, enzyme instability, and transient elevations due to prostatic massage, prostatic needle biopsy, cystoscopy, and prostatic infarctions. ACP elevations in serum may be associated with numerous malignant and nonmalignant diseases.

Most experts now agree that PAP analysis has no role in the diagnosis and monitoring of PCA and that PSA is clearly the superior marker. However, PAP analysis may contribute somewhat in specific clinical scenarios. A high pre-operative serum PAP value in a patient with clinically localized disease signifies that the patient has pathologic stage C or D disease and thus will not be a good candidate for surgical cure. PAP may be used in very rare patients whose tumors do not produce PSA, to monitor disease progression. Although PAP measurements alone have no value for disease screening or diagnosis, its incorporation into a neural network panel together with age, total PSA, free PSA, and creatine kinase appears to improve the specificity of the test, which is claimed to dramatically reduce the number of unnecessary biopsies (264). Recently, Han et al. reported that pre-operative PAP has independent predictive value for tumor recurrence following radical prostatectomy and may be used in multivariate models, along with other parameters, to identify those patients who are more likely to relapse (265). Dattoli et al. have further demonstrated that elevated pre-operative PAP, in patients who undergo radiation treatment for high-risk localized carcinoma, was the strongest predictor of long-term failure. For this application, PAP was stronger than Gleason score and pre-operative PSA (266).

Prostate-Specific Membrane Antigen (PSMA)

PSMA was discovered as a protein recognized by the murine monoclonal antibody 7E11, derived from mice immunized with purified fractions of cell membranes isolated from human prostate cancer LNCaP cells (267). By immunohistochemistry, it has been shown that PSMA is strongly expressed by the epithelial cells of the prostate and more intensely so in malignant tissues, compared to normal or hyperplastic prostates. Nonprostatic tissues also express lower amounts of PSMA, including the epithelia of small bowel and the proximal tubules of kidney (268).

The gene encoding PSMA consists of 19 exons, spanning approximately 60 kilobases (kb) of genomic DNA. The coding sequence of PSMA is 2.65 kb in length and encodes a 750-amino-acid type II transmembrane glycoprotein with a

100–120 kDa molecular mass. PSMA is composed of three structural domains: A 19-amino-acid N-terminal intracellular domain, a 24-amino-acid transmembrane domain, and a 707-amino-acid extracellular domain (269,270). The gene resides on the short arm of chromosome 11 (11p11 - 11p12). The gene is downregulated by androgens and is upregulated by various growth factors, including basic fibroplast growth factor (bFGF), TGF-α, and EGF.

The function of PSMA is not yet fully elucidated. PSMA has two enzymatic activities; one is folate hydrolase and the other is a carboxypeptidase. PSMA is capable of hydrolyzing gamma-linked terminal glutamates from folate in a sequential fashion. In the brain, PSMA releases glutamate from N-acetylaspartylglutamate. Thus, the formal name of PSMA is glutamate carboxypeptidase (EC 3.4. 17.21). Despite the fact that PSMA is highly expressed in prostatic cells, its function in this organ is currently unknown.

Clinical Applications of PSMA

Radioimmunoscintigraphy of PSMA. After prostate cancer treatment, extraprostatic spread of the tumor can occur in the prostatic fossa (local recurrence) or to regional and/or distinct lymphatics and/or in bone. Elevated levels of PSMA in serum is a very sensitive indicator of treatment failure but it does not indicate the sites of failure. Knowing the sites of failure is important for making further treatment decisions. Currently, patient exploration is undertaken with computed tomography (CT) and magnetic resonance imaging (MRI), or with guided needle biopsy. CT and MRI are dependent on the size of lymph node metastases and are not specific for the presence of prostate cancer cells; biopsy is invasive, operator-dependent, and prone to sampling errors.

The anti-PSMA murine monoclonal antibody 7E11 was linked to indium-111 to produce a radiodiagnostic marker suitable for in vivo detection of prostate cancer recurrence and metastasis (Prostascint®; Cytogen Corp., Princeton, NJ). The test was FDA-approved in 1997.

Multiple studies have evaluated the sensitivity and specificity of this procedure and compared it to CT, MRI, and biopsy data. In general, Prostascint was more sensitive (75%) and accurate (81%) in detecting local or regional lymph node spread than CT (36% sensitivity), or CT, MRI, and ultrasound combined (48% accuracy) (270). Prostascint can be combined with available algorithms and nomograms, as well as with single photon emission computed tomography (SPECT) imaging to further improve its predictive power. Some favorable features of this test include the membrane-bound nature of the antigen, its expression in dedifferentiated and metastatic cells, and its relative insensitivity to hormonal treatments or androgen resistance. Also, very few adverse effects have been reported with infusion of the antibody. The antibody currently used for this application binds to a cytoplasmic epitope of the antigen (a theoretical disadvantage). The recent availability of many monoclonal antibodies that bind to the extracellular domain may further improve the efficiency of this test.

Serum PSMA analysis. PSMA protein can now be detected by either Western blotting or a competitive enzyme-linked immunosorbent assay (ELISA) assay. There is very little information as to how PSMA molecules may be shed into the general circulation. Moreover, there is currently no convincing report that demonstrates any use of serum PSMA for diagnosis or monitoring of prostate cancer. Many researchers could not reproduce the original descriptions of circulating PSMA (268), which argues against any use of PSMA as a circulating marker of prostate cancer.

RT-PCR for detection of PSMA mRNA. Further details of reverse transcriptase-polymerase chain reaction (RT-PCR) are described in Chapter 9. Briefly, many authors compared the sensitivity of PSMA RT-PCR and PSA RT-PCR for detecting circulating prostate cancer cells for the purpose of "molecular staging." The data are quite variable with reported sensitivities between 39–91% for PSMA and 25–88% for PSA (270). Pooled sensitivities are around 65% and their combination may result in some improvement. The usefulness of this test has not as yet been accepted in clinical practice.

Therapeutic uses of PSMA. Several therapeutic approaches that target PSMA have been proposed for prostate cancer. These include immunotherapy with use of an artificial T-cell receptor (271) and pulsing of dendritic cells with PSMA peptides (272). Others have used the enzymatic activity of PSMA to liberate methotrexate from the precursor methotrexate triglutamate (273). Therapeutic antibodies loaded with toxins and targeting PSMA-positive prostate cells would be another approach currently under investigation (274).

An unexpected discovery is the expression of PSMA in the neovasculature of tumor cells (but not in the pre-existing vasculature of normal cells). This expression is found in many cancer types, not just prostate cancer, making PSMA a promising new target for antiangiogenic therapy.

Androgen Receptor and Carcinoma of the Prostate

The prostate is an androgen-regulated organ. The development and maintenance of the normal prostate gland requires a functional androgen-signaling axis comprising the following: biosynthesis of androgens in the testes, the transport of androgens to target tissues, conversion of testosterone (T) to its more active metabolite DHT, binding of T and DHT to the nuclear transcription factor androgen receptor (AR), and the transactivation of androgen-regulated genes (275–278). Prostate cancer is also intimately connected to this androgen axis and the components of the axis are now principal targets for hormonal therapies. For example, androgen ablation by surgery (orchiectomy) or administration of LHRH agonists or antagonists, bring about beneficial but transient effects. Similarly, AR antagonists are also used to block the action of androgens, either alone or in combination with LHRH agonists. In this section, we will briefly review the usefulness of studying AR alterations for prostate cancer predisposition, diagnosis, prognosis, or prediction of response to therapy.

Androgen receptor structure and function has been discussed previously in this chapter. Our knowledge that

- prostate growth and maintenance is dependent on the androgen axis,
- prostate cancer development and progression is connected to the androgen axis,
- prostate cancer therapy targeting the androgen axis is highly (but transiently) effective,
- prostate cancer cells ultimately grow and kill the patient despite androgen removal, and
- anti-androgens may ultimately stimulate prostate cancer cells (as clinically revealed by the anti-androgen withdrawal syndrome)

has stimulated research into the better understanding of AR function, AR polymorphisms, AR mutations, and AR amplification. Ultimately, this new information may lead to the development of testing as well as to new therapies for prostate cancer.

Androgen receptor polymorphisms. Most interest has focused on two polymorphic repeats $(CAG)_n$ and $(GGN)_n$ in exon 1 of the AR gene encoding for a polyglutamine and a polyglycine repeat. The CAG trinucleotide repeats have been implicated in the pathogenesis of Kennedy's disease (spinal bulbar muscular atrophy) (279) as well as an increased risk for prostate cancer (280–282). In Kennedy's disease, the expansion of the CAG repeats to >50 results in reduced transactivation activity of the AR and clinical symptoms of hypogonadism (279).

In the normal population, the number of CAG repeats range from 11 to 31 with an average of 21 ± 2. Higher prostate cancer risk is associated with shorter CAG alleles and the racial distribution of these alleles is supportive of this hypothesis. For example, African-Americans have about twice the incidence of prostate cancer than white men in the United States, and their CAG repeats average 18, in comparison to 21 for white men. Asians, who have the lowest risk, average 22 CAG repeats. It seems that shorter repeats are associated with increased transcriptionally active AR function (280). Others have reported that shorter CAG repeats may be associated with more aggressive forms and earlier onset of prostate cancers (282). The connection of CAG repeat length and risk or aggressiveness of prostate cancer has not been confirmed in all studies. Currently, the clinical benefit of genotyping individuals for CAG repeat length has not been demonstrated, despite the fact that such testing is technically simple (283).

Androgen receptor gene mutations. A database of all known AR gene mutations has been published (284) and is available at http://www.mcgill.ca/androgendb. Many germline mutations of AR cause Complete Androgen Insensitivity Syndrome (CAIS) which is outside the scope of this review. However, it is interesting to note that mutations found in PCA cluster mainly in two specific regions of the AR gene and cause gain of function rather than loss of function as in CAIS (285). Recently, Buchanan et al. analyzed the reported mutations of AR in experimental and clinical prostate cancer and concluded that these mutations are found in critical regions of the AR responsible for ligand binding, DNA binding, and transactivation domain (286). These mutations usually result in AR with altered androgen signaling and decreased specificity of ligand binding, leading to inappropriate receptor activation by estrogens, progestins, adrenal androgens, glucocorticoids, and/or androgen receptor antagonists, and even by nonsteroidal growth factors.

Despite the earlier reports of relatively rare somatic AR mutations in prostate cancer, it is now known that up to 40–50% of tumors may actually harbor such mutations (283,286), providing a reasonable explanation for the androgen independence of advanced prostate cancer (promiscuous activation of mutant AR by non-cognate steroids) and of the anti-androgen withdrawal syndrome (mutant AR activation by anti-androgens). Despite the fact that there is currently no practical clinical value to identifying such AR mutations in all prostate cancer patients, these investigations may shed further light into the role of mutant ARs in the establishment of androgen insensitivity. Such knowledge may lead to more effective treatments.

Androgen receptor amplification. AR amplification represents another potential mechanism by which tumor cells can adapt to low amounts of circulating androgens. AR amplification (5–60 copies of AR genes) was seen in about 25–30% of primary tumors after androgen deprivation or prostate cancer metastasis (287,288). It seems that AR amplification is not seen in tumors before androgen ablation. Again, although the phenomenon may help in the better understanding of androgen insensitivity, there is no clinical usefulness of determining AR amplification in all patients.

Insulin-Like Growth Factors and their Binding Proteins

Recently, measurement of circulating IGFs and some of their binding proteins revealed differences between nonaffected individuals and cancer patients. In particular, a number of prospective studies, using stored blood collected up to 14 years before the onset of the disease, have shown associations between IGF-1 levels and prostate cancer (289), premenopausal breast cancer (290), and colon cancer. The associations between prostate cancer and circulating IGFBP-3 levels was inconsistent, with some studies reporting an inverse relationship (289) and some reporting a direct relationship (291). Surprisingly, patients with acromegaly, who have chronically elevated levels of IGF-1, do not have an increased risk for prostate cancer but are more prone to benign prostatic hyperplasia (292,293). Acromegalics, though, do have a higher risk for colon and breast cancer.

Serum IGF-1 as a prostate cancer marker. A few studies have shown a small difference between mean concentration of serum IGF-1 of controls vs. prostate cancer patients (increased by about 7–8% in cancer) (289,291,294). Although statistically significant, this change is too small and the overlap between groups is quite substantial; this will predictably lead to low diagnostic specificity and sensitivity. Similar comments apply to breast and colon cancer.

Serum IGF-1 is age-dependent, and reference ranges should be adjusted accordingly. A few studies have addressed the issue of combining this measurement with serum PSA in screening programs. Despite the fact that a few authors reported some improvements over PSA alone, in the total PSA ranges of <3 µg/L (295) or 2.5–15 µg/L (296), most reports did not find such usefulness and they do not recommend IGF-1 analysis (292,297). PSA is clearly the superior marker. Furthermore, Yu et al. found no prognostic value of either IGF-1 or IGFBP-3 in prostate cancer (298) and Kurek et al. no differences after LHRH and anti-androgen treatment (299).

Until more convincing data are published, we currently do not recommend measurement of either IGF-1 or IGFBP-3 for screening, diagnosis, prognosis or risk assessment of patients with prostate cancer. The therapeutic and possibly preventive measures for cancer, targeting the IGF-axis, merit further investigation (290).

TUMOR MARKERS IN PROSTATIC DISEASES

Prostate-Specific Antigen in Benign Prostatic Hyperplasia

Patients with BPH and clinically localized PCA are commonly found to have elevated concentrations of PSA in serum that overlap significantly (216,300). BPH and PCA are commonly found simultaneously in the same prostate (301) and in a very significant proportion of men with histologically proven BPH (28%); PSA levels in serum have been found to be higher than 4.0 ng/mL. As it will be discussed in more detail below, PCA—in particular in men in their 8th and 9th decade—may often be clinically insignificant. However, the existence of PCA in a patient with BPH symptoms influences the treatment options for that patient, e.g., from a surgical approach such as transurethral resection (TURP) of the enlarged tissue to a medical treatment such as androgen ablation.

An important aspect is the impact of androgen treatment in men with BPH. Finasteride, a 5-α-reductase type 2 inhibitor, is a commonly used drug that reduces prostate tissue mass by blocking the conversion of T to DHT, which reduces serum PSA levels by 40–50% after treating for six months or more (302,303). It has been proposed that for patients on finasteride, multiplication of total PSA by a factor of two may simulate a presumably untreated state. Though the mean ratio of free to total PSA may remain unaffected from finasteride treatment, individual percentages have been reported to range from –81% to +20% of pretreatment levels (304). Alpha-blockers, the other common drug class for treatment of BPH, do not seem to have any impact on the total levels of PSA in serum (305).

Attempts to improve the value of PSA in the differential diagnosis of prostate cancer include the increase in PSA over time [PSA-velocity (306)], serum concentration of PSA relative to total (307), or transition zone prostate size (PSA-density, PSA-transition zone density, respectively; see ref. 308).

Age-specific PSA ranges (309) are discussed in the prostate cancer section.

Prostate-Specific Antigen and Prostatitis

All types of prostatitis are responsible for elevated serum PSA concentrations (310). Acute bacterial prostatitis can increase serum PSA considerably (by more than 10-fold). Other types of prostatitis with a less indolent or subclinical course may elevate PSA to a lesser extent but still in the range of total PSA-levels corresponding to those relevant for early detection of prostate cancer (311).

Prostate-Specific Antigen in Prostatic Intraepithelial Neoplasia

High-grade PIN may increase PSA concentration as compared to benign tissue only. However, coexisting benign tissue may contribute to increased serum levels and therefore mask the PSA elevation. The percentages of free PSA in men with benign disease and high-grade PIN have been shown to be similar and significantly higher than in prostate cancer patients (312).

Prostate-Specific Antigen and Adenocarcinoma of the Prostate

Prostate-specific antigen as a serum marker for prostatic tissue had higher impact on prostate cancer than any other tumor marker. Since its discovery in seminal plasma, its introduction into clinical use and finally its widespread application, PSA has revolutionized every aspect of prostate cancer: early detection, management, and follow-up (206). This is reflected by a continuous increase in the incidence of localized disease, while diagnosis of locally extensive or metastatic disease has steadily declined (313). In fact, there are concerns that PSA testing may cause detection and treatment of clinically insignificant tumors. Recently, a decrease in prostate cancer incidence in the U.S. has been observed in the SEER-data base, and today the incidence is only minimally higher than in the era before PSA was available (314). This may be evidence for the effectiveness of PSA screening. An effective screening method should increase the detection of a certain disease; however, the incidence should then decrease over time, if significant disease is detected by that screening method.

As a result of widespread PSA testing, the vast majority of newly diagnosed prostate cancers are detected only due to elevated PSA level in serum (315,316). These cancers have far more favorable pathology compared to those detected by digital rectal examination or transrectal ultrasonography. Thus, PSA contributes improved early detection of prostate cancer by the decrease in proportion of metastatic and locally advanced stage disease at the time of diagnosis. Still, there is clearly room for further improvement as only about 60% of T1c-prostate cancers are organ-confined (317,318). Moreover, PSA is the most sensitive marker for prostate cancer treatment, showing excellent correlation to therapeutic efficacy in response to curative and palliative treatment.

In this chapter, we will describe clinically relevant molecular forms of PSA for early detection, staging, curative treatment, and monitoring of prostate cancer as well as the impact of hormonal, anti-androgen, and chemotherapy of primary advanced or recurrent metastatic disease.

Total PSA in the Early Detection of Prostate Cancer

The diagnosis of prostate cancer is established by microscopic histopathological evaluation of tissue sections collected at biopsy. The likelihood of prostate cancer increases with increasing serum PSA concentrations, but also by the presence of a palpable lesion. When the results of total PSA testing in serum are added to DRE, the detection rate can increase by a factor of three to five (319). From retrospective studies, it is estimated that elevated PSA concentrations due to prostate cancer occur at a mean of 6.2 years before a palpable lesion can be identified (320), and that elevated PSA levels detects about 80% of all prostate cancers in a screening population (319). However, recently generated data, so far only reported in preliminary by Bjork et al. suggest that statistically significant changes of levels and proportions of different PSA forms and hK2 in men diagnosed with PCA were found in blood plasma collected up to 20 years before these men were diagnosed with PCA.

A biopsy is required to prove or rule out prostate cancer. The decision as to whether or not to perform a biopsy was traditionally based on DRE results. Pathological outcome and prognosis of cancers detected with DRE are unfavorable due to high incidence of extraprostatic extension of DRE-positive cancer. A common concern for the use of PSA in the early detection of prostate cancer is that clinically insignificant cancers may be diagnosed and subsequently treated. Recent definitions for clinically insignificant cancers take into account tumor volume and differentiation grade (321). More than 90% of insignificant cancers detected on autopsy have low volume (e.g., less than 0.5 cc) and low grade (Gleason grade of 1–2; i.e., Gleason sum of 4 or less) (322). Comparing these results with the pathologic features of screening-detected prostate cancers, fewer than 10% of these cancers meet the criteria of insignificance (323,324).

PSA is far from a perfect tumor marker. The three most common disorders of the prostate—prostate cancer, benign prostatic hyperplasia, and prostatitis—can all increase serum PSA concentrations. Other factors [physical activity, ejaculation (325), cystoscopy, prostate biopsy (326)] can increase the levels of PSA in serum as well. In addition, 5-α-reductase inhibitors, such as finasteride, used for treatment of symptomatic bladder outlet obstruction, decrease PSA levels in serum by approximately 50%, while the ratio of free to total PSA remains unchanged (303).

Both prostate cancer and benign prostatic hyperplasia increase serum PSA concentration. It has been suggested that each gram of benign tissue increases total levels of PSA in serum by approximately 0.3 ng/mL according to the polyclonal Yang assay, which overestimated PSA levels compared to presently accepted PSA measurements. Prostate cancer, on the other hand, was suggested to increase serum PSA about 10-fold as much as that contributed by benign tissue (215).

PSA in the early detection of prostate cancer: the rationale of PSA ranges. Total PSA levels in serum were commonly assigned to three different arbitrarily selected ranges, 0–4.0 ng/mL, 4.0–10.0 ng/mL, and >10.0 ng/mL (327). These ranges were useful to counsel a patient on his risk of prostate cancer and the necessity of a biopsy. Still, it is relevant that a cancer-suspicious finding revealed by carefully performed DRE may warrant biopsy, irrespective of the total PSA level in blood.

Total PSA <4.0 ng/mL. Total PSA levels in serum <4.0 ng/mL have been considered to be associated with a low risk for prostate cancer. Earlier recommendations suggested a restrictive strategy for prostate cancer detection in terms of performing a prostate biopsy in case of an unremarkable DRE. Today, however, analyses of prostate cancer incidence in the range below 4.0 ng/mL and nonsuspicious finding on DRE have shown that up to 22% of men with a total PSA in the range 2.6–4.0 ng/mL harbor significant disease. Moreover, the cancers removed, while still being clinically significant, were organ-confined in 81% of cases (328). Results from the multinational and multi-institutional European Randomized Screening Trial for Prostate Cancer (ERSPC), a study of patients with similar characteristics, demonstrated a detection rate of 19% of prostate cancers when total PSA was 2.0–3.9 ng/mL (329). Here, 84% of all cancers were confined to the prostate, as compared to 62% organ-confined disease when total PSA was 4.0–10.0 ng/mL. Data reported from another study within the ERSPC project, communicated by Lodding et al. found an increased detection of prostate cancer by 30% from the biopsy of men with total PSA levels of 3.0 to 4.0 ng/mL and that the majority of these cancers were considered clinically significant after radical prostatectomy (330).

Based on these data and similar findings reported by several other researchers, arguments are mounting in favor of trends to decrease cut-offs below 4.0 ng/mL. Presently, there are claims to use cut-offs ≥2.5 ng/mL for younger men in whom total PSA levels of 3 to 4.0 ng/mL may impose a more serious reason of concern than in men over the age of 70 years.

Total PSA levels ranging from 4.0 to 10.0 ng/mL. PSA levels ranging from 4.0 to 10.0 ng/mL have traditionally formed the basis for recommending additional clinical work-up, e.g., systematic sextant biopsies. It is commonly referred to as the diagnostic gray zone, because elevated total PSA levels caused by BPH and PCA largely overlap. Screening studies of men 50 years and older have shown that there are up to 10–12 % of men with total PSA levels of 4.0 ng/mL or higher (329). Biopsy-based results showed positive predictive values ranging from 12% to 32% (319,331–333) when there was a nonsuspicious DRE. There are concerns mainly for the costs but also for the morbidity of biopsy at total PSA levels of 4.0 to 10.0 ng/mL, since there would be no evidence of malignancy in three of four of the biopsied men.

Total PSA above 10.0 ng/mL. Patients with total PSA levels above 10.0 ng/mL on initial evaluation and nonsuspicious

DRE have a likelihood of more than 40–50% of harboring prostate cancer (323). It is therefore accepted that biopsy should be undertaken for all men in this range. It is noteworthy, however, that the likelihood of a pathologically organ-confined cancer may be as low as 25%.

Free PSA in the Early Detection of Prostate Cancer

It has been shown that the concentration of free (noncomplexed) PSA in blood does not contribute (on its own) any enhanced disease-specific information for the early detection of prostate cancer in comparison to the information provided by the complexed or total PSA levels. Therefore, free PSA measurements are used to generate the ratio of free to total PSA (%fPSA). The majority of PSA is found in stable complex with antiproteases, most notably alpha-1-antichymotrypsin. However, 5–45% of PSA occurs as free, uncomplexed forms in the circulation (207). A higher ratio of free to total PSA occurs in patients without evidence of cancer than in those with prostate cancer (231). Numerous studies have found that %fPSA significantly enhances the efficacy of early detection of prostate cancer, in particular within the diagnostic gray zone area of total PSA levels (4.0–10.0 ng/mL). These studies demonstrated that using %fPSA cut-offs between 14% and 28%, between 19% and 64% of unnecessary biopsies could have been avoided while maintaining a sensitivity of prostate cancer detection of 71–100% (231,334,335).

A large, prospective multi-center trial was able to confirm the retrospective studies. In these studies, a cut-off value for %fPSA of 25% detected 95% of cancers and reduced the biopsy rate by 20% in the total PSA range of 4.0–10.0 ng/mL (336). Measurements of %fPSA have been granted FDA approval in the U.S. for clinical use in the diagnostic gray zone range of 4.0–10.0 ng/mL levels of total PSA. However, these measurements may also be useful to enhance the diagnostic specificity at PSA levels <4.0 ng/mL, to improve the positive predictive value for an estimated 20% of men with total PSA in the 2.6–4.0 ng/mL range who may harbor significant prostate cancer. Evaluation of %fPSA in the total PSA range of 2.6–4.0 ng/mL demonstrated that a cut-off for %fPSA of 27% was able to detect 90% of cancers. An estimated 18% of unnecessary biopsies could be spared in the patients, thus encouraging the use of %fPSA in this lower total PSA range as well (328). Table 5 presents an overview of important studies. It is relevant to stress that it is possible that race might influence %fPSA, though there are also several other factors that impact on the outcome of these studies such as pre-analytical sample handling and instability of free PSA levels in serum (234–236). In terms of racial differences, one study analyzed %fPSA in 222 African-American and 298 Caucasian men with a total PSA of 2.5–9.9 ng/mL. It was reported that African-American men with prostate cancer on biopsy had higher %fPSA ratios than Caucasians (337).

Percent-free PSA has been found useful in identifying patients who develop highly aggressive cancer. Measurement of free and total PSA performed up to 10 years before diagnosis of prostate cancer with extraprostatic extension, lymph node, or bone metastases demonstrated statistically significant different %fPSA (p = 0.008) compared with patients who had prostate cancer and more favorable pathology (338). By contrast, total PSA levels failed to demonstrate any significant discrimination between the two groups (338).

Despite these encouraging results using %fPSA in the early detection of prostate cancer, problems with standardization and equimolarity of PSA assays must be kept in mind when %fPSA is used in clinical situations (230).

Prostatic manipulation causes about a 10-fold increase in free PSA levels; %fPSA increased from a pre-operative mean of 11.9% to 52.5% (213). Similar observations have been reported for DRE and prostate biopsy, although the magnitude of free PSA elevation is significantly smaller in less invasive manipulations (339). Moreover, cPSA levels are much less affected by DRE, cystoscopy, or prostate biopsy compared to free PSA (339). Therefore, measurements of free and total PSA levels and calculations of %fPSA are uncertain and should be avoided during the first 48 to 72 hours after any prostatic manipulation has been performed, such as DRE, cystoscopy, prostate biopsy, or other forms of urethral manipulation. More rapid elimination rates of fPSA compared to PSA-ACT (213) suggests that intra-individual, day-to-day variation of fPSA may be significantly higher than that of PSA-ACT. However, there is only indirect support from findings of higher intra-individual variation of tPSA levels in men with BPH (who have high %fPSA) compared to men with PCA (with lower %fPSA) (340). Analysis of PSA subfractions after radical prostatectomy demonstrated that virtually all PSA increases during surgery are due to release of free PSA (213).

Moreover, benign prostate gland volume influences %fPSA in prostate cancer patients (341). Only for normally small-sized prostates is there a statistically significant difference in the %fPSA ratio when patients with benign conditions are compared with prostate cancer patients (341) (Figure 5). A similar result was found when prostates <35cc vs. those ≥35cc were compared: A cut-off of 14% f%PSA for small prostates and 25% fPSA for larger prostates detected prostate cancer with 95% sensitivity (342). Therefore, differences in %fPSA of men with cancer from those with no cancer diminish with increasing total prostate volume; at large volumes there may be no significant differences in %fPSA concentrations in men with PCA compared to those without cancer.

In general, it is difficult to make generally valid recommendations on the reference value for %fPSA, as it is affected by multiple factors. Commonly recommended cut-offs range from 14% to 25% (231,335,336). The differences are mainly due to lack of uniformity in assay performance, lack of commonly accepted standardization, and lack of sufficiently validated preanalytical sample handling. It can be concluded that %fPSA improves specificity while maintaining a high sensitivity for prostate cancer in men with a total PSA of 2.6–10.0 ng/mL. There is less diagnostic impact of %fPSA measurements when DRE is suspicious, or if total PSA exceeds 10.0 ng/mL.

Table 5 Overview on the literature for the ratio of free to total PSA for the discrimination of benign vs. malignant prostatic disease

Authors	Year	Patients Benign/Cancer	DRE	tPSA range (ng/ml)	Cutoff %	Sensitivity %	Specificity
Christenson et al.	1993	not applicable	—	4–20 ng/ml	18%	71	95
Catalona et al.	1995	63/50	—	4–10 ng/ml	20%	90	38
		26/48	neg		23%	90	31
Prestigiacomo et al.	1996	20/28	—	4–10 ng/ml	23%	95	64
					14%	95	56
Catalona et al.*	1998	379/394	neg	4–10 ng/ml	25%	95	20
					22%	90	29
Catalona et al.	1997	73/259	neg	2.6–4 ng/ml	27%	90	18

*Multi-institutional.

Complexed PSA in the Early Detection of Prostate Cancer

As described previously, PSA is able to form stable, covalent 1:1 molar ratio complexes with alpha-1-antichymotrypsin. PSA is also able to form stable complexes with other serine protease inhibitors such as protein C inhibitor (PSA-PCI) and alpha-1-protease inhibitor (API-PSA) (208,211). In vivo, there may be no detectable levels of either PSA-PCI or PSA-AMG complexes in blood (211,231) and therefore the sum of ACT-PSA and API-PSA complexes represents the majority of PSA complexes. PSA-API represents a very small proportion of these complexes, i.e., no more than 1–2% of PSA in serum stored frozen for several years prior to analysis (214). PSA-ACT is the major form of PSA in serum and it is most strongly influenced by prostate cancer (208,231), but analytical difficulties with specific measurements of PSA-ACT complexes in blood has limited the implementation of these assays in clinical practice. However, recent progress has resulted from the design of a commercially available assay to measure complexed PSA (cPSA). Published reports from several research groups indicate that the measurement of cPSA enhances diagnostic performance relative to total PSA, although the level of enhancement differs among published reports. This may be due to differences in the patient populations tested.

The reported data show that measurements of cPSA in total PSA range from 2.5–4.0 ng/mL (233), 2.6–20.0 ng/mL (343), 0.37–117.0 ng/mL (344), and 4.1–10.0 ng/mL (345) demonstrated enhanced specificity for cPSA compared to total PSA at high sensitivity, whereas also small improvements in specificity could translate into reduction in unnecessary biopsies, cost savings, and reduced morbidity associated with the biopsy procedure.

Filella et al. evaluated the usefulness of cPSA in a study of 196 men with BPH and 55 patients with biopsy-confirmed PCA. For all samples tested, the specificity of cPSA was greater than total PSA at sensitivity range of 80–90%, though they did not find that the diagnostic utility of cPSA was greater than the %fPSA ratio within this range of sensitivity (346).

A study by Stamey et al. (347) differs with this conclusion; they included 90 patients who underwent two negative biopsies and 80 patients with prostate cancer who had at least 5 mm of prostate cancer on biopsy. These authors concluded that the diagnostic performance of cPSA provides marginal improvement relative to total PSA, where ROC analysis indicated that AUCs for total PSA, cPSA, free/total PSA, and complexed/total PSA ratios were 0.52, 0.57, 0.81, and 0.83, respectively. A prospective study of serum from more than 3,000 men with biopsy-confirmed benign prostatic hyperplasia and prostate cancer at total PSA levels of 2.0–20.0 and 2.0–10.0 ng/mL has been reported by Miller et al. For all samples, AUCs for tPSA, cPSA, and %fPSA were 0.52, 0.54, and 0.58, respectively (348).

Further, it has been reported that cPSA levels calculated from subtraction of levels of fPSA from tPSA (233) at tPSA levels of 2.5–4.0 ng/mL were comparable to measured cPSA, and also suggested improved cancer detection rates at this low and narrow PSA range by cPSA in comparison to %fPSA. Taken together, all reports to date have shown that cPSA enhances diagnostic performance over tPSA in the detection of PCA.

Subfractions of Free PSA in the Early Detection of Prostate Cancer

Subfractions of free PSA are unreactive with the large excess of anti-protease inhibitors in blood. Several types of PSA modifications have been distinguished:

- Internally cleaved, nicked, or multi-chain PSA forms cleaved at Lys_{145}-Lys_{146} and/or Lys_{182}-Ser_{183}-positions (this latter is known as BPSA; see below).
- Variable sizes of latent, single-chain proPSA-forms exist. Conversion of latent pro-PSA (to active single-chain 237-amino-acid PSA) occurs by release of the activation peptide C-terminal of Arg_{-1}.
- Intact PSA, an unreactive single chain isoform of free PSA isolated from LNCaP cells. Up to 50% of PSA from LNCaP cells consists of a single-chain 237-amino-acid mature form

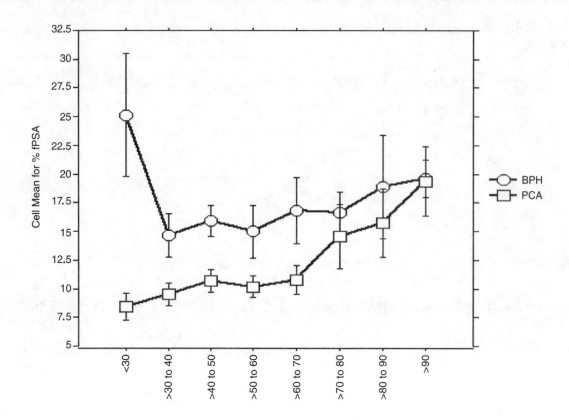

Figure 5 Impact of prostatic volume on %fPSA in volume groups (horizontal axis) for prostate cancer (PCA) and BPH. Reprinted with permission from Haese A, Graefen M, Noldus J, Hammerer P. Huland E, Huland H. Prostatic volume and ratio of free-to-total prostate specific antigen in patients with prostatic cancer or benign prostatic hyperplasia. J Urol 1997;158(6):2188–2192.

that under certain conditions does not manifest any enzymatic action (225).

BPSA. The principal feature of BPSA is an internal peptide cleavage at Lys_{182}-Ser_{183}; hence it is a multi-chain peptide of free PSA that may also contain internal peptide cleavage at Lys_{145}-Lys_{146}. BPSA was described in seminal plasma and nodular tissue samples of the transition zone of benign prostatic hyperplasia (226). A comparison of tissue from enlarged prostates due to BPH, normal prostates, and prostate cancer showed that BPSA is exclusively expressed in the transition zone. The expression of BPSA in normal prostates and in prostate cancer tissue was much less intense. The development of an immunoassay for the detection of BPSA in serum revealed a significant concentration of BPSA in serum of men with benign prostatic hyperplasia, whereas it was undetectable in normal control males. An estimated 15–50% of free PSA in serum was suggested to be BPSA (222). While it seems likely that BPSA reflects at least to some extent benign prostatic hyperplasia, and may have potential to monitor BPH under surgical or medical treatment, its role in the early diagnosis of prostate cancer remains to be clarified.

(-2)pPSA. This substance was found as a variant of free PSA that is expressed in large amounts in prostate cancer tissue (349). It is a single-chain polypeptide of 239 amino acids characterized by incomplete removal of the seven amino acids normally removed to activate pro-PSA. It was first described in prostate cancer tissue. When serum of prostate cancer (total PSA 6.0–24.0 ng/mL) was analyzed for (-2)pPSA, it could be shown that 25–95% of free PSA consisted of (-2)pPSA. Serum levels of men with no evidence of disease demonstrated an average of five-fold lower (-2)pPSA-concentrations. It is detectable at tPSA concentrations typical for the diagnostic gray zone. It is premature to speculate on the impact of (-2)pPSA on early detection of prostate cancer.

Intact PSA. Identification of monoclonal antibodies with capacity to discriminate single-chain free PSA forms (i.e., the sum of latent and mature PSA formats) from multi-chain PSA forms internally cleaved at Lys_{145}-Lys_{146} (221) has formed a basis for designing an assay to discriminate multi-chain forms of fPSA, nicked PSA or "PSA-N," from intact single-chain fPSA, "PSA-I" (221). Plasma samples with tPSA levels of >3.0 ng/mL from a subset of a screening study population in Sweden were used to report that proportions of intact-to-nicked fPSA were significantly higher in men with PCA than in those without (350). A second study analyzed 383 men (141 with no evidence of disease and 242 patients with biopsy-proven PCA) and demonstrated that measurements of intact PSA enhanced discrimination of patients with negative systematic prostate biopsy from those with biopsy-proven prostate cancer (223).

In summary, measurements of free PSA subfractions present encouraging results, though further evaluation is necessary, in addition to refinements in detection techniques and additional characterization of the exact nature of free PSA subfractions to asses their potential in the early detection of PCA.

Adenocarcinoma of the Prostate

Total PSA Derivatives in the Detection of Prostate Cancer

PSA derivatives are permutations of total PSA used to improve sensitivity and specificity of prostate cancer detection. To date, the reported permutations are PSA density, PSA velocity, and age-specific reference ranges.

PSA-Density (PSA-D). The concept of PSA-density was first described by Benson et al. (307). The rationale of PSA-density is the observation of a positive relationship between PSA levels in serum and volume of the prostate gland.

PSA-D is the result of a ratio of tPSA level in serum divided by prostatic volume. It was developed to normalize PSA levels with regard to the volume of the prostate, assuming that a certain volume of prostate cancer would increase PSA to a greater extent than benign prostatic hyperplasia, as reported by Stamey (215). However, several aspects limit the usefulness of PSA-D. First, measurements of prostate gland volume by TRUS are examiner-dependent; gland volumes measured by different examiners vary considerably. Secondly, the ratio of stroma to epithelium varies considerably between individuals. This influences PSA density as only the epithelium produces PSA and the stroma cannot be estimated from transrectal ultrasound (300,301). Therefore, results of PSA-D are discordant. A reported cut-off of 0.15 for PSA-D was found to enhance prostate cancer detection when PSA was <10.0 ng/mL (351). However, other studies have found that about 50% of all prostate cancers would be missed at this cut-off (352). Others could not find any difference in PSA-D for men with positive vs. negative biopsy (353). Therefore, the role of PSA-D in the early detection of prostate cancer has not been found useful.

A modification of PSA-D, transition zone density (PSA-TZD), is the normalization of PSA to the transition zone volume (308). It focuses on the assumption that histologically, hyperplasia occurs almost exclusively in the transition zone. In an initial study with a cut-off of 0.35 ng/mL/cc, PSA-TZD gave the highest positive predictive value (74%) for detection of prostate cancer (354). However, PSA-TZD suffers from methodological problems of volume measurement and epithelial-to-stroma ratio in the same way as PSA-D. As other centers have failed to reproduce the advantage of PSA-TZD, it cannot presently be considered to be a routine tool for prostate cancer detection.

PSA velocity in the early detection of prostate cancer. PSA velocity describes changes in PSA concentration over time. It was introduced to improve the ability of a single total PSA measurement for prostate cancer detection (306). PSA velocity uses the formula $1/2\%(PSA2-PSA1/time1$ in years $+ PSA3-PSA2/time2$ in years). PSA1 is the first PSA measurement, PSA2 the second, and PSA3 the third serum PSA measurement. These three measurements should be obtained in a two-year period or at least 12 to 18 months apart. Clinically, a PSA velocity of ≥ 0.75 ng/mL/year has been described to suggest the presence of prostate cancer with 72% sensitivity and 95% specificity. These significant differences of PSA velocity in BPH compared to prostate cancer were detectable up to nine years before prostate cancer had been diagnosed (306).

The clinical utility of the PSA velocity concept is limited by the fact that PSA is not cancer-specific, and that there is significant intra-individual day-to-day-variation of PSA concentration in blood. A study showed that when an increase in tPSA was less than 20–46%, it was more likely attributed to biological and assay variation than to prostate cancer development (340). Moreover, short episodes of PSA elevation (e.g., inflammatory processes) may interfere with the normal natural elevation of PSA over time (310,311). Finally, PSA results are different when measured on different PSA assays and add some degree of imprecision to PSA velocity determinations (230). Despite these limitations, a PSA velocity greater than 0.75 ng/mL/year may still be of some guidance in assessing the need for a prostate biopsy in patients with a total PSA below 10.0 ng/mL and unremarkable DRE.

Age-specific PSA ranges in the early detection of prostate cancer. The arbitrary upper limit of 4 ng/mL in PSA concentration does not compensate for increasing prostate volume with age, hence the introduction and development of the principle of age-specific PSA ranges (309) to improve sensitivity of prostate cancer detection in patients of younger age (e.g., age 50) with a PSA that might be much less of a concern for a patient at age 70.

Several studies examined age-specific PSA ranges. In the evaluation of almost 4,600 men, age-specific PSA ranges detected 74 additional cancers in men aged 60 years or younger. Pathologic work-up was favorable (Gleason score below 7, organ-confined or capsular penetration, no lymph node metastases or seminal vesicle invasion) in 80% of cancers. In younger men the detection of prostate cancer increased by 18% but decreased by 22% in older men (355). Comparison of age-specific PSA-ranges to normal PSA cut-offs of 4.0 ng/mL in a screening population showed that cancer detection increased by 8% when using age-specific ranges in men below age 59 (when DRE was unremarkable). Moreover, in men older than 60, 21% of biopsies could have been spared while missing only 4% of organ-confined cancers. It was concluded that age-specific PSA ranges improve sensitivity in the younger population (356). Other studies, however, concluded that the standard PSA cut-off of 4.0 ng/mL was optimal for all age groups (319) and in addition, the most cost-effective tool (357).

Race-corrected age-specific PSA ranges take reports into account that describe higher PSA in African-American as compared to Caucasian or Asian men, even when controlled for age, Gleason grade, or clinical stage. This has been associated with the detection of cancers with larger tumor volume at the time of diagnosis in African-American compared to Caucasian men (1.3–2.5 times larger) (309,358,359).

Human Glandular Kallikrein in the Early Detection of Prostate Cancer

Human glandular kallikrein and PSA (which is also called human kallikrein 3) share 80% identity in protein sequence (84). Both hK2 and PSA are expressed under androgen control (106). Despite similarities in organ specificity, hK2 has been suggested to be more intensely staining in high Gleason grade cancers (4–5) and lymph node metastases compared to low Gleason grade cancers, and still weaker in benign prostatic hyperplasia (247,248).

HK2 levels in blood correspond to about 1% of those of PSA. Serum concentrations of hK2, free hK2, and ACT-hK2 have been shown to be elevated in patients with prostate cancer (241,244,360–362). However, diagnostic enhancements contributed by hK2-measurements, in addition to testing for total and free PSA, may be moderate (363). The covariance of hK2 and tPSA concentrations is usually less than 60%, which suggest that hK2 might provide additional, independent information to that contributed by measurements of PSA (276, 283, 290, 364). Two scenarios for early diagnosis of prostate cancer exist:

- Increase of specificity in the total PSA-range between 4.0–10.0 ng/mL, where only 25% of men harbor prostate cancer and biopsy should be recommended. The specificity for cancer of the ratio of free-to-total PSA is about 31%. Hence, unnecessary biopsies are performed in about 70% of patients, a procedure that is costly and has some morbidity (365).
- Increase in sensitivity. Likewise, of interest is the patient group with PSA levels below 4.0 ng/mL. In this PSA range, up to 25% of men harbor clinically significant prostate cancer (366), which a cut-off at ≥4.0 ng/mL of total PSA in serum would fail to detect.

Saedi et al. (244) described increased concentrations of pro-hK2 in sera of patients with prostate cancer compared to sera of BPH patients, female sera, and healthy controls. Several other studies reported total hK2 concentrations using different research assays. In 937 archival serum samples of men with histologically confirmed prostate cancer or negative biopsy and a total PSA of 2.0–10.0 ng/mL, hK2, tPSA, and fPSA were measured (360). The ratio of total hK2/free PSA gave additional specificity in prostate cancer detection: In the PSA range of 4.0–10.0 ng/mL the risk of cancer was 23%; in the PSA range 2.0–4.0 ng/mL, 13%. Results were classified into three risk groups using %fPSA (cut-off 25%), resulting in a likelihood of cancer between 10% and 43%. A further subclassification using hK2/free PSA was devised. As a result, crude risk groups defined by %fPSA could be refined, yielding positive predictive values for cancer between 9 and 62%. Upon use of %fPSA and hK2/fPSA, 40% of cancers could have been detected, requiring a biopsy in only 16.5% of men in the PSA range of 2.0–4.0 ng/mL (360). Magklara et al. (367) analyzed hK2, total, and free PSA and merged hK2 and free PSA into the same algorithm, hK2/fPSA. On ROC-analysis, hK2/fPSA (AUC=0.69) was a stronger predictor of cancer than %fPSA (AUC=0.64). Moreover, at 95% specificity, hK2/fPSA identified 30% and 25% of cancers when PSA was 2.5–10.0 ng/mL and 2.5–4.0 ng/mL, respectively. They found hK2 valuable in identifying a subset of patients with low PSA but with high likelihood of cancer. Kwiatkowski et al. (368) calculated a median hK2/fPSA of 0.139 in prostate cancer patients versus 0.075 in BPH-patients. At a sensitivity of almost 95%, the specificity of hK2/fPSA was 60.4% compared to 27.6% for %fPSA.

Becker et al. (369) evaluated hK2-concentrations in a population-based screening study of 604 men with a total PSA of >3.0 ng/mL to evaluate the discriminative power of hK2 in prostate cancer detection. They merged hK2, total, and free PSA values into an algorithm (hK2xtPSA/fPSA). ROC-analysis revealed that the AUC for hK2xtPSA/fPSA was greater than that for total PSA and %fPSA. The respective ROC-curves are shown in Figure 6. Moreover, at a specificity of 90%, sensitivity was 55%, compared to 41% for %fPSA.

A cross-sectional study of 324 men (362) referred for prostate biopsy revealed significantly higher hK2 and hK2/fPSA levels in men with cancer compared to patients with a negative biopsy. The authors found a five- to eight-fold increased risk of prostate cancer with elevated hK2 and ratio of hK2/fPSA, hence improving selection criteria for patients referred for prostate biopsy. Studies performed so far show a moderate clinical potential for hK2 measurements that might add to the value of total and free PSA testing in the early detection of prostate cancer. Commercially available reagents for hK2 measurements are lacing, and the optimal utility of hK2 remains to be clarified. The low hK2 serum levels (about 1% of those of PSA) in normal healthy men makes it important to use hK2 assays with very low functional detection limits (<10 pg/mL) to detect hK2 levels in healthy men (246) and to use assay protocols that do not contribute significant cross-reaction from PSA (<0.01 %) (246).

STAGING OF PCA

Correct staging in men with prostate cancer is crucial not only for selecting appropriate therapy in clinically localized PCA but also for comparing outcomes of different treatment approaches. While surgical procedures offer the possibility of evaluating histological specimens (e.g., stage and grade of tumor), other therapies such as radiation do not offer such a possibility. Therefore,

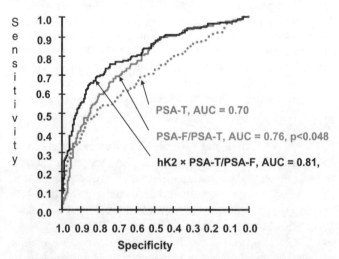

Figure 6 hK2, tPSA, and fPSA in combination for early detection of prostate cancer. Reprinted with permission from Becker C, Piironen T, Pettersson K, Hugosson J, Lilja H. Clinical value of human glandular kallikrein 2 and free and total prostate-specific antigen in serum from a population of men with prostate-specific antigen levels 3.0 ng/mL or greater. Urology 2000;55:694–699.

investigators need to rely to a much larger extent on accurate clinical staging of the disease. The TNM classification (see Table 4) describes local, lymphatic, and distant extension of PCA. However, severe limitations of TRUS and DRE significantly compromise the precision with which patients harboring PCA can be staged. Cancers confined to the prostate have far better prognosis than those showing extraprostatic extension (370,371). However, since extraprostatic extension may be detectable on microscopic evaluation only, it is logical that clinical assessment fails to detect this crucial step in cancer spread.

Total PSA in the Staging of Prostate Cancer

PSA and local staging. PSA has outperformed DRE-based prediction of stage, which showed unsuspected extraprostatic spread in up to 63% of cancer cases (372). Generally, PSA levels correlate with tumor volume and advancing clinical and pathological stage (216,300). When PSA ranges and staging results are analyzed, it can be shown that total PSA levels <4.0 ng/mL and >10.0 ng/mL correlate reasonably well with findings of organ-confined or extraprostatic cancer, respectively. At PSA levels <4.0 ng/mL, the likelihood of organ-confined cancer has been shown to be 81–84% when DRE was negative (328,329). The rates of organ-confined disease dropped to 53–67% at total PSA levels of 4.0–10.0 ng/mL (366), and to 31–55.9% when PSA was 10.0–20.0 ng/mL (330,373). Total PSA levels do not provide valuable staging information in the most frequently encountered PSA range of 4.0–10.0 ng/mL; they are not specific enough to permit predicting pathological stage in the most frequently encountered PSA range of 4.0–10.0 ng/mL. Therefore multi-parameter staging tools (nomograms and predictive algorithms) were developed to improve the accuracy of staging. These are described in a subsequent section.

PSA and distant metastasis. PSA has been shown to be a good predictor of a positive bone scan in patients with prostate cancer. Namely, if PSA is <20.0 ng/mL, the negative predictive value is 99.7% (374). This has resulted in a significant decrease in the number of bone scans performed in patients with PSA levels <20.0 ng/mL (374).

Ratio of Free Total PSA (%fPSA) for Staging of PCA

In contrast to its wide acceptance for the *detection* of PCA, studies that analyzed %fPSA in the staging of PCA have produced conflicting results. While some studies reported %fPSA to provide useful staging information, others failed to demonstrate such findings. Lerner et al. found statistically significant differences only in substages of prostate cancer (365), which is supported by data from Noldus et al. (375), where no difference was found in organ-confined compared to non-organ-confined cancers. However, a significantly lower %fPSA separated prostate cancers that invaded seminal vesicles from those who did not (375). Patient selection, study design, different immunoassays, and %fPSA cut-off values could influence the conclusions of each study. Therefore, to date, no established use of %fPSA exists for staging of PCA. Table 6 summarizes several studies on the use of %fPSA for PCA staging.

ACT-PSA Complex for Staging of Prostate Cancer

Only a limited number of studies evaluated ACT-PSA as a staging parameter for PCA. Most recently, PSA, PSA-density, ACT-PSA, and ACT-PSA density have been assessed in 62 patients with clinically localized PCA before radical prostatectomy. ROC-analysis showed that both ACT-PSA and ACT-PSA density had a larger, but not significantly larger, AUC compared to PSA and PSA-D. However, at a sensitivity of 100% for detecting organ-confined PCA, specificity was 37% and 42% for ACT-PSA and ACT-PSAD, compared to 19% and 24% for PSA and PSA-D (376). This is in accord with an earlier study of 652 patients, which concluded that ACT-PSA might replace PSA as a staging tool for prostate cancer (377). However, due to the limited amount of available data, no conclusions as to the utility of ACT-PSA for staging of prostate cancer can be made.

PSA in the Staging of Prostate Cancer: Algorithms and Nomograms

The weakness of PSA as a staging mechanism has resulted in the construction of nomograms that combine a number of clinically available variables to contribute independent prognostic significance (e.g., clinical stage, PSA, Gleason sum, or Gleason grade of prostatic biopsies) to provide more accurate preoperative estimation of pathological stage. PSA is an important contributing factor in predictive nomograms for lymphatic spread, pathological stage, or outcome of clinically localized PCA. A widely accepted tool for predicting pathologic stage is the Partin-Nomogram, which takes into account PSA, clinical stage, and the Gleason sum of the biopsy obtained. The Partin-Nomogram has been recently updated and validated. The most recent version is shown in Tables 7–10 (318). Another algorithm was developed and validated by Graefen et al., based on a CART-Analysis (CART=Classification And Regression Tree). This model performed a side-specific prediction of a pathologically organ-confined prostate cancer based on serum PSA and presence of Gleason grade 4/5 in the prostatic biopsies (378) (Figure 7).

Human Glandular Kallikrein 2 in the Staging of PCA

Human glandular kallikrein 2 has been studied in the early detection of PCA and proven to have potential in conjunction with PSA and %fPSA. More recently, studies evaluated the use of hK2 as a staging parameter for clinically localized prostate cancer. Detection of hK2, total, and free PSA in 68 sera from men scheduled for radical retropubic prostatectomy revealed that hK2 and a derived algorithm that combined hK2 with total PSA and free PSA (hK2xtPSA/fPSA) significantly improved the prediction of organ-confined (oc) vs. non-organ-confined (noc) prostate cancer, in a total PSA range up to 66.0 ng/mL (379) (Fig-

Table 6 %fPSA and staging of prostate cancer

Authors	Number of patients	pT2a/b	≥pT3a	Metastatic	Mean age	%fPSA useful
Graefen et al.	53	28	25	0	62.2	No[a]
Henricks et al.	70	46	24	0	NA	No[b]
Bangma et al.	123	81	19	23	NA	No[c]
Lerner et al.*	178*	100	78	0	63	No[d]
Pannek et al.	301	169	121	11	58.8	No[e]
Elgamal et al.**	69	37 T1c	32 ≥T2	0	69	Yes[f]
Pannek et al.	263	134	119	10	58.9	Yes[e]

NA, not applicable.
*Of the 290 initial patients, only 178 had RRP and were evaluated.
**Of the 117 initial patients, only 69 had RRP and were evaluated.
[a] DPC, Diagnostic Product Corporation
[b] Dianon
[c] DELFIA
[d] Research assay
[e] Hybritech
[f] Centrocor
p, pathologic stage; RRP, radical prostatectomy.
Reprinted with permission from Polascik TJ, Oesterling JE, Partin AW. Prostate-specific antigen: a decade of discovery—what we have learned and where we are going. J Urol 1999;162(2):293–306.

ure 8). Pre-treatment samples with total PSA levels <10.0 ng/mL were collected from another set of 161 patients diagnosed with PCA by the same group. Reported results were consistent with the original observations; measurements of hK2 alone, or used in combination with free and total PSA to generate a diagnostic algorithm, was significantly better in the prediction of pathological stage 2a/b-PCA than PSA (380) (Figure 9).

Recker et al. confirmed the improvement in staging accuracy. They found hK2 to be the only serum analyte that significantly discriminated pT2a/b-prostate cancers from ≥pT3a-PCA. Moreover, hK2 separated aggressive Grade 3 from less aggressive G1 and G2 PCAs (381).

These results encourage further studies to improve prostate cancer staging. As with the use of hK2 for detection of prostate cancer, potential uncertainties (lack of standardization, research assays, different word missing) must be kept in mind when hK2 is analyzed. Therefore, results from different centers and the performance of different assays, ideally as a multi-center trial, must be awaited to clarify the role of hK2 as a potential staging tool for PCA.

PSA and Radical Prostatectomy

Prostate-specific antigen has been proven to be the most powerful tool to identify those men in whom aggressive local therapy offers the best disease control (323). Radical retropubic prostatectomy is considered to be the standard of curative treatment and is widely recommended by urologists for intent-to-cure therapy in men diagnosed with early stage PCA (382,383), unless comorbidity or age suggests different treatment options. PSA is important in the context of a radical prostatectomy in several respects. First, PSA reliably identifies those men in whom radical prostatectomy may permit excellent cure rates (318,323,378). As outlined, PSA contributes alone or in combination with other parameters to predict the likelihood of success for patients who have to decide on treatment options. Pre-operative serum PSA levels are highly suggestive of cure vs. failure before radical prostatectomy (371). Figure 10 shows PSA-free survival after radical prostatectomy stratified by preoperative serum PSA-concentration.

PSA after Radical Prostatectomy

BPH (300), prostatitis (311), DRE, cystoscopy, biopsy (326), and PCA may influence serum PSA levels. After radical prostatectomy, PSA displays a truly unique feature: once the prostate is removed, contributing factors mentioned above are eliminated, and if PSA is detectable, it may be solely contributed from remaining PCA cells (384).

According to the first reports, total PSA levels drop to undetectable with a half-life of 2.2 to 3.3 days (215,216), though more recently generated data indicate that free and complexed PSA are eliminated by most dissimilar rates and elimination kinetics (213,218). The very slow clearance of complexed PSA from the circulation on the one hand, and the high sensitivity of current PSA immunoassays on the other hand, led to recommendations that total PSA measurements in blood after surgery should not be performed earlier than three months post-operatively (385). If taken too early, uncertainty remains whether or not detectable PSA is residual pre-operative PSA or PSA produced from prostate cancer cells left behind.

Failure to obtain undetectable PSA levels may be evidence for persisting PCA, though other explanations have been suggested, e.g., production of PSA by paraurethral glands. An undetectable PSA after radical prostatectomy is synonymous with a disease-free condition. This is the rationale for serial post-operative PSA testing (384).

In case of recurrent disease, PSA can be detected up to five years earlier than any clinical symptom and as such, is by far the most sensitive marker for PCA recurrence (371,384).

Recurrence of PCA typically occurs first as a PSA recurrence, which means, that PSA levels are rising from an undetectable level, to levels accessible to conventional or ultrasensitive PSA assays (386–388). In the absence of clinical signs of recurrence, this is called biochemical recurrence—any significant increase above the functional detectable limit, which is often about 0.1 ng/mL, on at least two subsequent post-operative samples (386). DRE or imaging studies do not provide any additional information in cases of biochemical failure (local recurrence or distant metastatic disease). Very sensitive PSA assays with detection limits up to 0.001 ng/mL PSA provide additional lead time of almost two years and may therefore be valuable for monitoring prostate cancer after radical prostatectomy (387,388).

A common definition of cure is disease-free state for a period of at least five years. This finding is not true for prostate cancer. Long-term follow-up studies from patients after radical prostatectomy indicate that 20–30% of cancers recur within the first five years after surgery. However, biochemical and clinical failure may occur even more than ten years after radical prostatectomy in 25–50% of cases (371,389,390). Others observed that patients with unfavorable pathological stages (seminal vesicle invasion, Gleason scores 8–10) or pre-treatment total PSA levels >10.0 ng/mL had high initial failure rates (within the first two years). By contrast, recurrence in patients with organ-confined cancers was observed also after five years. Very sensitive PSA assays will detect these failures long before they become clinically apparent.

PSA velocity after radical prostatectomy and PSA-progression. Follow-up of 304 deferred treatment patients who developed recurrent disease showed that the interval from biochemical PSA progression to development of clinically manifest metastatic disease was eight years (median). The mean time from metastatic disease to death was less than five years. When PSA recurrence occurs after radical prostatectomy, the rate at which PSA levels increase over time, i.e., postoperative PSA velocity, gives important information as to whether there is local or distant metastatic recurrent disease. Total PSA velocities of less than 0.75 ng/mL/year were shown to indicate local recurrent disease. PSA velocity exceeded this cut-off in more than 50% of patients with distant metastasis (391). Expectant management of PSA recurrent disease after radical prostatectomy may therefore have a prolonged survival and be an option in men with a life expectancy of less than 10 years at the time when recurrence is diagnosed and PSA velocity does not suggest rapidly progressing disease.

PSA AND HORMONAL THERAPY

Hormonal or androgen withdrawal therapy refers to treatment, in which the endogenous androgen biosynthesis is shut down to eliminate stimulative effects of androgen to hormone-sensitive PCA. No other treatment equals or outperforms the efficacy of androgen withdrawal therapy on advanced or recurrent PCA. However, despite undisputed efficacy in palliation (392), andro-

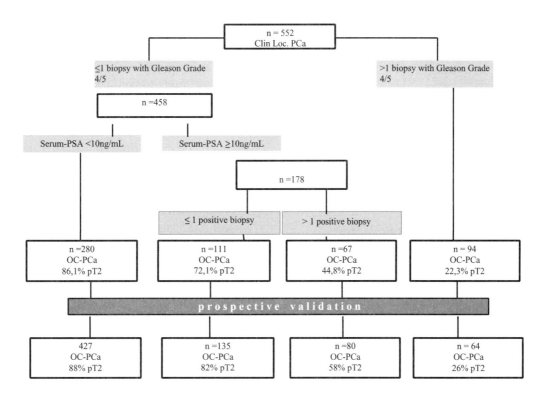

Figure 7 CART-analysis for prediction of a pathologically organ-confined prostate cancer. Reprinted with permission from Graefen M, Haese A, Pichlmeier U, Hammerer P, Noldus J, Butz K, Erbersdobler A, Henke RP, Michl U, Fernandez S, and Huland H. A validated strategy for side-specific prediction of organ-confined prostate cancer: a tool to select for nerve-sparing radical prostatectomy. J Urol 2001;165(3):857–863.

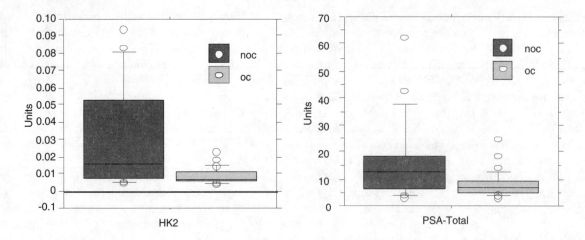

Figure 8 Human glandular kallikrein 2 (p = 0.0043) and PSA (p = 0.011) in the differentiation of organ- and non-organ-confined prostate cancer. Reprinted with permission from Haese A, Becker C, Noldus J, Grafen M, Huland E, Huland H, Lilja H. Human glandular kallikrein 2: a potential serum marker for predicting the organ confined vs. non-organ-confined growth of prostate cancer. J Urol 2000;163(5):1491–1497.

gen withdrawal is never a curative treatment due to inherent survival of PCA cells that do not rely on androgens to grow (393).

Pharmacologically, androgen withdrawal can be achieved at two different levels in the hypothalamic-pituitary-gonadal axis. Several drugs commonly referred to as LHRH-agonists achieve castrate levels of testosterone by overriding the pulsatile secretion of LHRH of the hypothalamus, which is responsible for appropriate LH and FSH secretion of the pituitary gland. Administration of these drugs elicits an initial *flare phenomenon* with aggravated symptoms due to initial rise of LH and testosterone resulting from supernormal stimulation of the pituitary and the Leydig cells. This may endure for two to three weeks before there is a decrease of testosterone to castration levels. Co-administration of anti-androgens should be performed, since this—while not preventing the flare-up phenomenon—will prevent androgen induced clinical exacerbation due to blockage of the excessive androgen (392).

Anti-androgens can be classified into nonsteroidal and steroidal anti-androgens. These agents shut down the effect of androgens by competing with the endogenous androgen for binding to the androgen receptor on the target cell (e.g., the PCA cell), thus preventing androgenic action. While nonsteroidal anti-androgens (flutamide, bicalutamide) do not alter serum testosterone levels, steroidal anti-androgens (cyproterone acetate, megrestol), have progestational activity, and inhibit testosterone production in addition to blocking the androgen receptor. The 5-α-reductase inhibitor finasteride prevents intracellular conversion of T to DHT as already described. Finally, LHRH-*antagonists* block the effect of LHRH on the pituitary gland. This group is relatively new and currently under comparison with LHRH-agonists and anti-androgens.

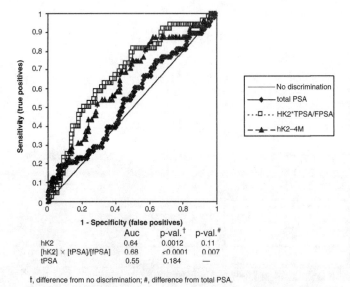

Figure 9 ROC-analysis of 161 patients with clinically localized prostate cancer for the prediction of pT2a/b vs. ≥pT3a-prostate cancer. From Haese A, Grafen M, Steuber T, Becker C, Pettersson K, Piironen T, Noldus, J, Huland H, Lilja, H. Human glandular kallikrein 2 levels in serum for discrimination of pathologically organ-confined from locally advanced prostate cancer in total PSA levels below 10 ng/mL. Prostate 2001;49(2):101–109. © 2001. Reprinted by permission of Wiley-Liss, Inc., a subsidiary of John Wiley & Sons, Inc.

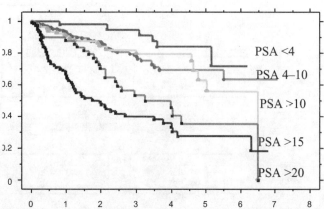

Figure 10 Biochemical (PSA) relapse-free survival in 789 patients after radical retropubic prostatectomy, stratified by pre-operative PSA concentration. Horizontal axis shows postoperative time in years.

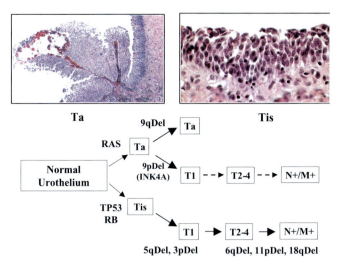

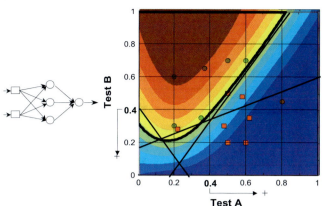

Figure 3 Genetic model of bladder cancer progression. Two different pathways have been proposed to characterize early tumorigenic events occurring in the urothelium, which may be associated in the production of papillary versus flat tumor lesions. These events are followed by secondary abnormalities that appear to be involved in tumor progression.
[See page 91.]

Figure 9 An MLP with two inputs, three hidden neurons, and a single output neuron. The three hidden neurons individually and independently implement three linear classifiers shown as three straight white lines. The output neuron superimposes the output from the three hidden neurons to form a nonlinear classifier shown as the black curve line.
[See page 138.]

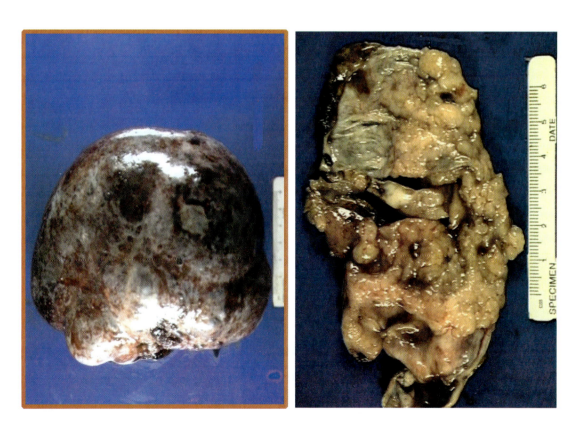

Figure 1 Gross appearance of an ovarian serous carcinoma, the most common type of ovarian cancer. The tumor is large (13 cm) and cystic, and it replaces the normal ovarian tissue which is not visible (right). On sectioning, the tumor appears to be papillary with numerous excrescences projecting into the cyst (left).
[See page 240.]

Plate 1

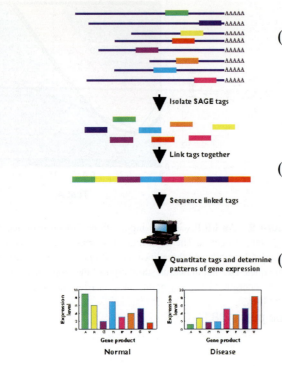

(1) A short sequence tag (10–14bp) contains sufficient information to uniquely identify a transcript provided that that the tag is obtained from a unique position within each transcript;

(2) Sequence tags can be linked together to from long serial molecules that can be cloned and sequenced;

(3) Quantitation of the number of times a particular tag is observed provides the expression level of the corresponding transcript.

Figure 2 The principles of serial analysis of gene expression (SAGE). The SAGE method is based on the isolation of unique sequence tags from individual transcripts and concatenation of tags serially into long DNA molecules. Rapid sequencing of concatemer clones reveals individual tags and allows quantitation and identification of cellular transcripts. Please visit http://www.sagenet.org/ for details of SAGE. [See page 248.]

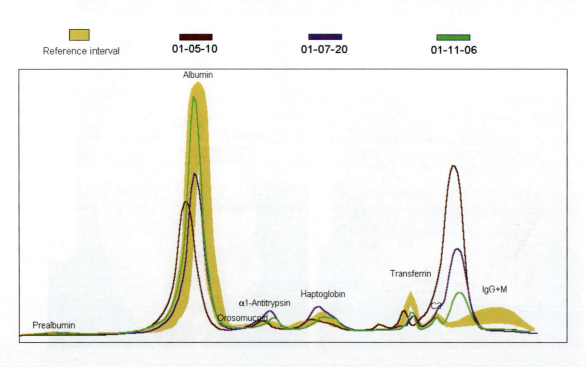

Figure 2 Graphical presentation of absorbance curves for samples from a patient with an IgE myeloma obtained before (brown curve), and 10 (blue curve) and 25 weeks (green curve) after, initiation of treatment with melphalan and prednisone. The yellow shaded area represents the normal reference interval for protein concentrations. The figure was obtained courtesy of Associate Professor Joyce Carlson, Department of Clinical Chemistry, Malmö University Hospital, Malmö, Sweden.
[See page 309.]

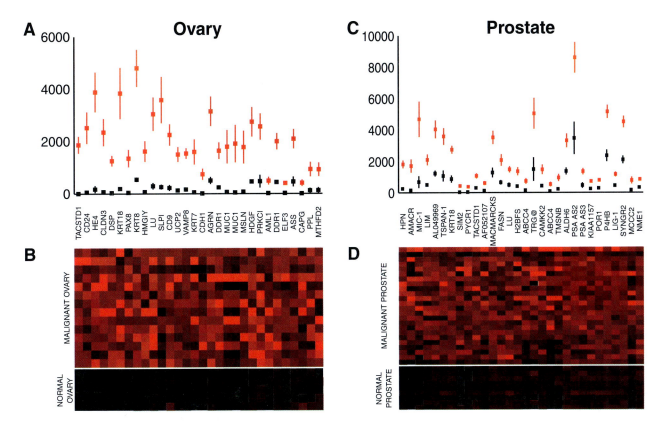

Figure 1 Expression of selected genes in normal and malignant tissue samples from ovary (A and B) and prostate (C and D). Thirty genes from each tissue type were selected for high differential expression in malignant compared to normal counterpart tissue. Ranking is based on a combined score that favors genes with large tumor (T) vs. normal (N) quotients, large T vs. N differences, and small p values in an unpaired t test (2). In A and C, the mean and 95% confidence interval for hybridization intensities (ordinate) is shown in a series of 30 genes in malignant (red) and normal (black) samples. In B and D, the expression level of each gene (column) in each normal and malignant sample (row) corresponds to the brightness of each square; high expression levels are shown as relatively bright red squares.
[See page 402.]

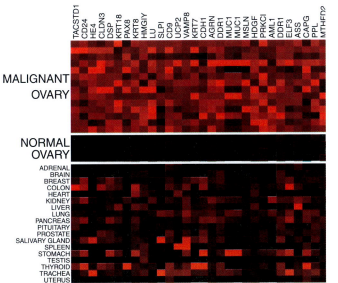

Figure 2 Gene expression in normal and malignant ovarian tissues compared to normal extra-ovarian tissues. Genes (in columns) were ranked for differential expression in malignant (upper rows) and normal (middle rows) ovarian tissues as in Figure 1. Expression levels in a panel of normal tissues (bottom rows) are shown for comparison.
[See page 403.]

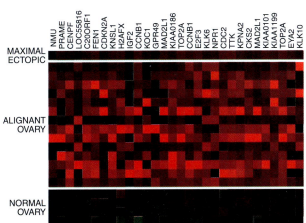

Figure 3 Gene expression in normal and malignant ovarian tissues compared to maximal expression in a panel of normal extra-ovarian tissues. Genes (in columns) were ranked for differential expression in malignant ovarian tissues (middle rows) compared to normal ovarian tissues (bottom rows). Genes whose maximal expression in a panel of normal extra-ovarian tissues was high were penalized in the ranking scheme, resulting in generally low "maximal ectopic" expression (upper row).
[See page 403.]

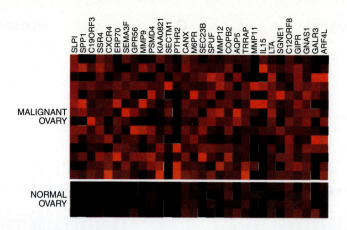

Figure 4 Gene expression in malignant (upper rows) and normal (lower rows) ovarian tissues. Only genes with annotations suggesting extracellularity of their encoded proteins were ranked. Genes were ranked for differential expression as in Figure 1.

[See page 404.]

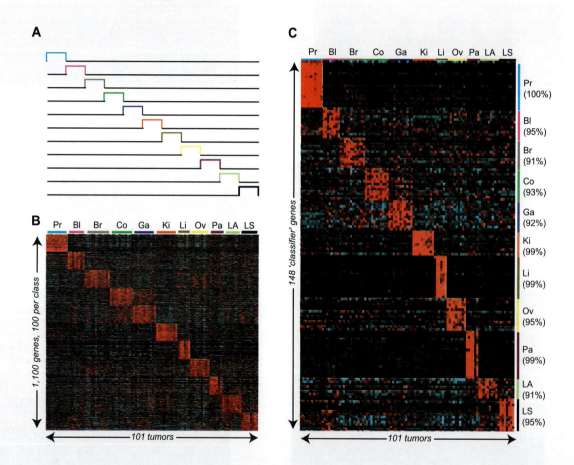

Figure 5 Selection of tumor-specific genes for cancer class prediction. (A) Schematic diagram depicting the idealized expression profile of tumor-specific genes that the method selects as classifiers. The shape of each profile represents genes that are highly expressed in each cancer type relative to all other tumors classes in the training set of tumors. (B) 100 genes per tumor class (1,100 total) with the most significant scores in a Wilcoxon rank sum test for equality were selected as likely candidates for tumor classifiers. Pr—prostate; Bl—bladder; Br—breast; Co—colorectal; Ga—gastroesophageal; Ki—kidney; Li—liver; Ov—ovary; Pa—pancreas; LA—lung adenocarcinomas; LS—lung squamous cell carcinoma. (C) The final refined set of gene classifiers was generated after ranking genes in (B) by SVM/LOOCV accuracy. For clarity, only 8 of 76 predictor genes for lung adenocarcinomas are depicted here. Levels of gene expression (depicted in each row) across all samples (columns) were median-centered and normalized by "Cluster" and output in "Treeview" (45). Red—increased gene expression; blue—decreased expression; black—median level of gene expression. The color intensity is proportional to the hybridization intensity of a gene from its median level across all samples. Reprinted with permission from AACR.

[See page 406.]

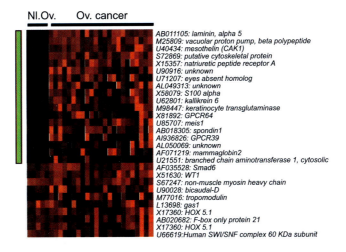

Figure 6 Tumor- and tissue-specific genes as class predictors of ovarian tumors. Shown are the expression levels of 28 highly predictive classifier genes (rows) in five normal (Nl. Ov., left columns) and 24 malignant (Ov. cancer, right columns) samples of ovarian tissue. The green bar indicates 18 of the genes that were significantly ($p < 0.01$ and fold change >3) upregulated in tumors as compared to normal tissues (tumor specificity); expression levels of the other 10 genes were similar in normal and malignant tissue samples (tissue, but not tumor, specificity). The order of genes was first determined using an unpaired, one-tailed t-test to measure the significance of differential expression in normal and tumor tissues, and secondarily by the difference in mean levels of expression. Reprinted with permission from AACR.
[See page 407.]

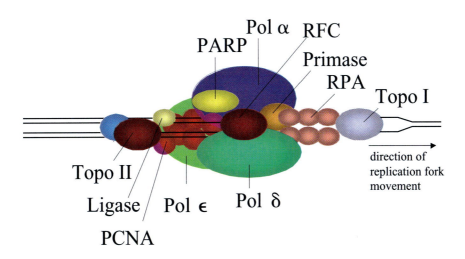

Figure 1 The proposed model for the mammalian DNA synthesome. The mammalian DNA synthesome is composed of DNA polymerases (pol) α, δ, and ε; proliferating cell nuclear antigen (PCNA); primase (primase); replication factor C (RF-C); poly(ADP)ribose polymerase (PARP); replication protein A (RP-A); DNA ligase; and the topoisomerases I and II (Topo I and II).
[See page 413.]

Plate 7

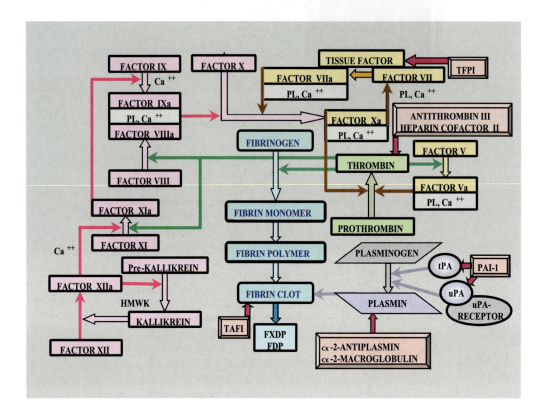

Figure 1 Blood coagulation cascade, fibrin formation, and fibrinolysis. Blood coagulation factors are primarily synthesized by the liver and released into the bloodstream. Usually, coagulation factors are synthesized as proteolytically inactive pro-enzymes, others serve as substrates or co-factors that can be transformed from an activate precursor state to the active form by various stimuli. All of the blood coagulation factors, except the cell membrane-associated tissue factor, are plasma proteins. Blood coagulation is initiated by tissue injury or factors affecting hemostasis.

Two different blood coagulation pathways are shown: the intrinsic pathway, known as *Contact Factor Pathway* (pink), and the extrinsic pathway, also named *Tissue Factor Pathway* (brown). The two pathways are interactive and meet at Factor IX and X, from where they initiate thrombin (green) and fibrin (cyan) formation. As a counterpart to fibrin clot formation, the fibrinolytic system (blue) is activated in a series of enzymatic reactions. It then generates the broad-spectrum serine protease plasmin from the proteolytically inactive plasma protein plasminogen by action of the plasminogen activators tPA (tissue-type plasminogen activator) or uPA (urokinase-type plasminogen activator). Plasmin destroys intravascular fibrin clots and, in addition to other proteins, fibrin contained within the extracellular matrix. Inhibitors are shown in red.

Under physiological conditions, such as wound healing, a critical balance between fibrin formation and fibrin degradation is maintained. In solid malignant tumors, excess production of uPA, and surprisingly of its inhibitor PAI-1, is associated with tumor cell invasion, metastasis, and early death of the cancer patient. (Scheme is based on the information provided by Kolde, H.J, Hemostasis, Pentapharm Ltd., 2001).

[See page 446.]

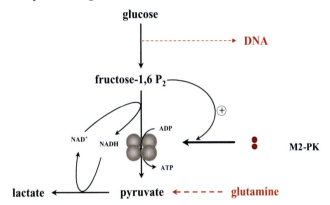

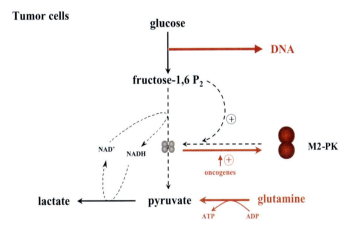

Figure 1 Metabolic scheme for the regulatory role of pyruvate kinase type M2. [See page 471.]

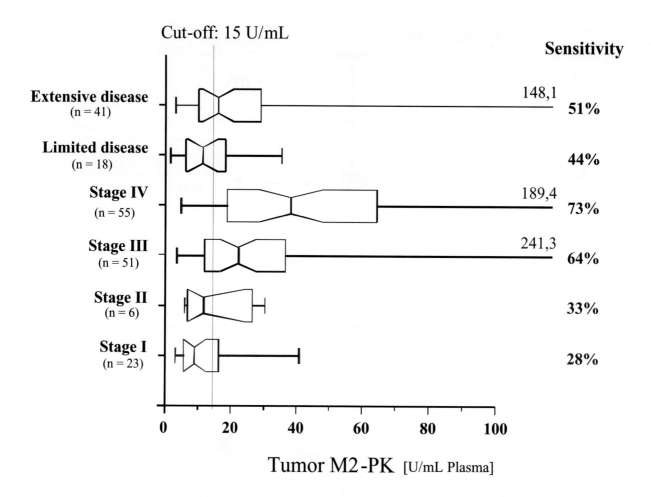

Figure 2 Correlation between Tumor M2-PK plasma concentrations and staging in lung cancer. The whiskers indicate the 25th and 75th percentiles. The center of the notches indicates the median. Lack of overlap indicates significant differences between the groups. Limited disease is compared with extensive disease for small-cell lung cancers. Stages I–IV are presented for all non-small-cell carcinomas. The sensitivity was calculated using the manufacturer's cut-off.
[See page 473.]

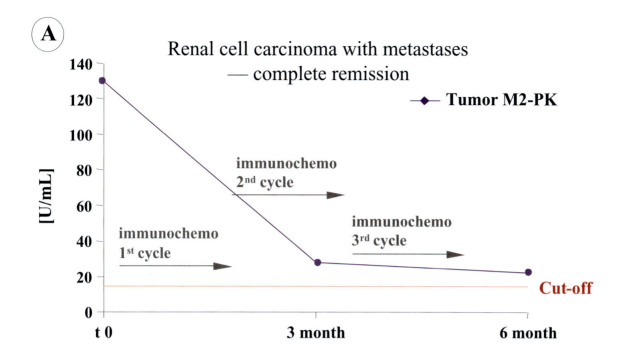

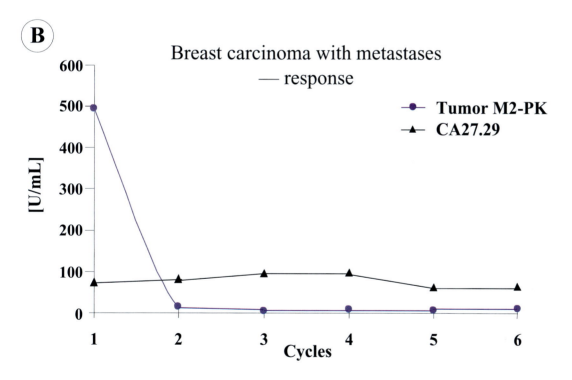

Figure 3 (A) Metastasized renal cell carcinoma: follow up with Tumor M2-PK. Tumor M2-PK levels in a patient with metastatic renal cell cancer (Robson IV) under immunochemotherapy, with complete remission after eight months. Radiological monitoring correlated well with Tumor M2-PK levels. (B) Longitudinal levels of Tumor M2-PK and CA27.29 levels in relation to response. Patient with partial response: elevated baseline level with prompt normalization after the start of chemotherapy.
[See page 474.]

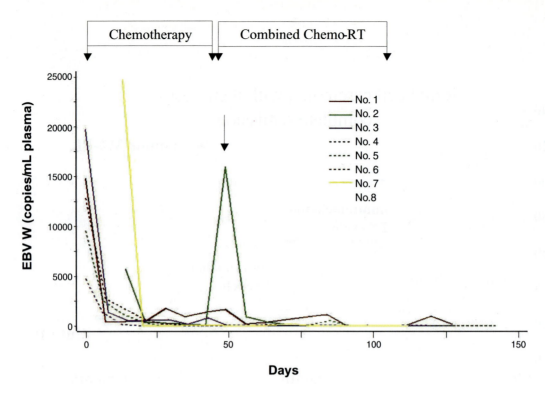

Figure 3 Monitoring response to chemotherapy with serial EBV DNA estimation. Note the rapid decrease in EBV DNA following the initiation of chemotherapy. In the one patient in whom there was a spike of EBV DNA (arrow), radiotherapy was delayed because of toxicity to chemotherapy (10).
[See page 492.]

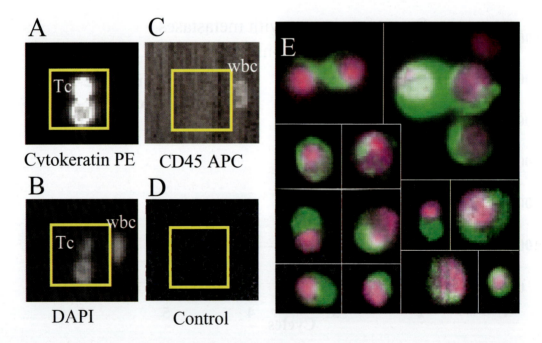

Figure 1 Identification of circulating tumor cells (CTC) by CellSpotter™.
The software identified a location in the Cellspotter™ chamber as potentially containing a CTC. The Cytokeratin-PE, DAPI, CD45-APC, and Control [DiOC16(3)] staining of this location is shown in Panels A, B, C, and D respectively, and the suspect area is indicated by the yellow box. A cluster of two tumor cells (Tc) and one white blood cell (wbc) can be discerned. Panel E shows twelve composites of the cytokeratin staining (green) and the nuclear staining (purple) of tumor cells identified in peripheral blood of breast cancer patients.
[See page 496.]

Table 7 Partin-Nomogram for clinical stage T1c prostate cancer (Tumor non-palpable, PSA elevated)

PSA (ng/mL)	Pathologic stage	Highest Gleason score in biopsy				
		2–4	5–6	3+4=7	4+3=7	8–10
0–2.5	OC	95 (89–99)	90 (88–93)	79 (74–85)	71 (62–79)	66 (54–76)
	EC	5 (1–11)	9 (7–12)	17 (13–23)	25 (28–24)	28 (20–38)
	SV	—	0 (0–1)	2 (1–5)	2 (1–5)	4 (1–10)
	LN	—	—	1 (0–2)	1 (0–4)	1 (0–4)
2.6–4.0	OC	92 (82–98)	84 (81–86)	68 (62–74)	58 (48–67)	52 (41–63)
	EC	8 (2–18)	15 (13–18)	27 (22–33)	37 (29–46)	40 (31–50)
	SV	—	1 (0–1)	4 (2–7)	4 (1–7)	6 (3–12)
	LN	—	—	1 (0–2)	1 (0–3)	1 (0–4)
4.1–6.0	OC	90 (78–98)	80 (78–83)	63 (58–68)	52 (43–60)	46 (36–56)
	EC	10 (2–22)	19 (16–21)	32 (27–36)	42 (35–50)	45 (36–54)
	SV	—	1 (0–1)	3 (2–5)	3 (1–6)	5 (3–9)
	LN	—	0 (0–1)	2 (1–3)	3 (1–5)	3 (1–6)
6.1–10.0	OC	87 (73–97)	75 (72–77)	54 (49–59)	43 (35–51)	37 (28–46)
	EC	13 (3–27)	23 (21–25)	36 (32–40)	47 (40–54)	48 (39–57)
	SV	—	2 (2–3)	8 (6–11)	8 (4–12)	13 (8–19)
	LN	—	0 (0–1)	2 (1–3)	2 (1–4)	3 (1–5)
>10.0	OC	80 (61–95)	62 (58–64)	37 (32–42)	27 (21–34)	22 (16–30)
	EC	20 (5–39)	33 (30–36)	43 (38–48)	51 (44–59)	50 (42–59)
	SV	—	4 (3–5)	12 (9–17)	11 (6–17)	17 (10–25)
	LN	—	2 (1–3)	8 (5–11)	10 (5–17)	11 (5–18)

Reprinted from Urology, 58, Partin AW, Mangold LA, Lamm DM, Walsh PC, Epstein JI, Pearson J. Contemporary update of prostate cancer-staging nomograms (Partin Tables) for the new millennium, 843–848. © 2001, with permission from Elsevier Science.

The Effect of Androgen Ablation on PSA

Androgen-sensitive cancers. Serum PSA is the most useful marker for monitoring response to androgen withdrawal and provides prognostic information of metastatic PCA. Initially, PSA drops to normal or subnormal (a mean 80% decrease) and occasionally to undetectable levels (<0.1 ng/mL) in more than 70% of men. This might take up to six months (394). During this time, androgen blockage (due to anti-androgen administration) and LHRH-induced shutdown of androgen pro-

Table 8 Partin–Nomogram for PCa with clinical stage T2a (tumor palpable on <50 of one side of the prostate)

PSA (ng/mL)	Pathologic stage	Highest Gleason score in biopsy				
		2–4	5–6	3+4=7	4+3=7	8–10
0–2.5	OC	91 (79–98)	81 (77–85)	64 (56–71)	53 (43–63)	47 (35–59)
	EC	9 (2–21)	17 (13–21)	29 (23–36)	40 (30–49)	42 (32–53)
	SV	—	1 (0–2)	5 (1–9)	4 (1–9)	7 (2–16)
	LN	—	0 (0–1)	2 (0–5)	3 (0–8)	3 (0–9)
2.6–4.0	OC	85 (69–96)	71 (66–75)	50 (43–57)	39 (30–48)	33 (24–44)
	EC	15 (4–31)	27 (23–31)	41 (35–48)	52 (43–61)	53 (44–63)
	SV	—	2 (1–3)	7 (3–12)	6 (2–12)	10 (4–18)
	LN	—	0 (0–1)	2 (0–4)	2 (0–6)	3 (0–8)
4.1–6.0	OC	81 (63–95)	66 (62–70)	44 (39–50)	33 (25–41)	28 (20–37)
	EC	19 (5–37)	32 (28–36)	46 (40–52)	56 (48–64)	58 (49–66)
	SV	—	1 (1–2)	5 (3–8)	5 (2–8)	8 (4–13)
	LN	—	0 (0–2)	4 (2–7)	6 (3–11)	6 (2–12)
6.1–10.0	OC	76 (56–94)	58 (54–61)	35 (30–40)	25 (19–32)	21 (15–28)
	EC	24 (6–44)	37 (34–41)	49 (43–54)	58 (51–66)	57 (48–65)
	SV	—	4 (3–5)	13 (9–18)	11 (6–17)	17 (11–26)
	LN	—	1 (0–2)	3 (2–6)	5 (2–8)	5 (2–10)
>10.0	OC	65 (43–89)	42 (38–46)	20 (17–24)	14 (10–18)	11 (7–15)
	EC	35 (11–57)	47 (43–52)	49 (43–55)	55 (46–64)	52 (41–62)
	SV	—	6 (4–8)	16 (11–22)	13 (7–20)	19 (12–29)
	LN	—	4 (3–7)	14 (9–21)	18 (10–27)	17 (9–29)

Reprinted from Urology, 58, Partin AW, Mangold LA, Lamm DM, Walsh PC, Epstein JI, Pearson J. Contemporary update of prostate cancer-staging nomograms (Partin Tables) for the new millennium, 843–848. © 2001, with permission from Elsevier Science.

duction causes apoptosis of PCA cells, and PSA is cleared from the circulation. Information relating to the time for serum PSA to reach treatment-baseline, or "PSA nadir," provides significant information with regard to the durability of the response. PSA nadir levels <4.0 ng/mL have longer median survival (40 months) compared to a PSA-nadir >4.0 ng/mL, when median survival may be only 18 months (395). Patients with PSA that does not drop to normal or subnormal levels may present a temporary decline above the normal range and a subsequent PSA rise, which is the first sign of androgen insensitivity. The vast majority of men, however, do not present any clinical complaints for 6–12 months despite a rising PSA (396).

The androgen-insensitive cancer. About 80% of all men with metastatic disease exhibit clinical and biochemical response upon androgen withdrawal. However, all cancers will become androgen-insensitive after a variable time span, which averages 24 to 36 months, while cancer control might be as short as six months or last more than a decade. Pre-treatment PSA-levels and histological cancer grade are important factors for determining the length of androgen control over the cancer. PSA is essential for detection of anti-androgen independent state, as the first sign is a continuously rising PSA. Androgen insensitivity develops as an adaptation of PCA cells to a continuously androgen-depleted environment. Mechanisms that permit progression to androgen insensitivity include a clonal selection of existing androgen-insensitive cells (397,398), upregulation of adaptive mechanisms that are depressed when androgens are present that may abort apoptosis of prostate cancer cells (399,400), mutations of the androgen receptor (401), or ligand-independent androgen receptor activation.

A noteworthy phenomenon occurs after long term anti-androgen treatment, called anti-androgen-withdrawal syndrome. While PSA values after initial successful treatment with anti-androgens and LHRH-agonists may rise and indicate androgen insensitivity, discontinuation of the anti-androgen may result in an up to 50% decrease of PSA in about 20–30% of patients. Median duration of anti-androgen withdrawal response was five months, while some patients experienced symptomatic improvement and disease regression for more than 10 months (392).

PSA AND RADIATION THERAPY
The Role of PSA in the Preradiation Setting

Comparable to the situation before surgical management, pre-radiation PSA correlates more accurately than clinical stage or Gleason grade with outcome after radiation therapy. The impact of pretreatment PSA on outcome is reflected in several series, reporting 69–90% biochemical disease-free rates three to five years after radiation therapy when pre-treatment PSA was <4.0 ng/mL. This rate consistently declined to 43–81% when PSA was 4.0–10.0 ng/mL, 27–59% in PSA ranges 10.0–20.0 ng/mL and 6–27% in ranges >20.0 ng/mL (364,402–406).

In these series, multivariate analysis of patients treated at seven institutions incorporated 1,765 patients with clinically localized PCA (stages T1b-T2). Most notably, PSA was the only parameter required to generate subgroup 1 with a PSA <9.2 ng/mL and subgroup 2 (PSA 9.2–19.7 ng/mL). Subgroups 3 and 4 required PSA and Gleason score (PSA >19.7 and Gleason score 2–6) and PSA >19.7 and Gleason score 7–10.

Table 9 Partin-Nomogram for PCa with clinical stage T2b (tumor palpable on >50 of one side of the prostate)

PSA (ng/mL)	Pathologic stage	Highest Gleason score in biopsy				
		2–4	5–6	3+4=7	4+3=7	8–10
0–2.5	OC	88 (73–97)	75 (69–81)	54 (46–63)	43 (33–54)	37 (26–49)
	EC	12 (3–27)	22 (17–28)	35 (28–43)	45 (35–56)	46 (35–58)
	SV	—	2 (0–3)	6 (2–12)	5 (1–11)	9 (2–20)
	LN	—	1 (0–2)	4 (0–10)	6 (0–14)	6 (0–16)
2.6–4.0	OC	80 (61–95)	63 (57–59)	41 (33–48)	30 (22–39)	25 (17–34)
	EC	20 (5–39)	34 (28–40)	47 (40–55)	57 (47–67)	57 (46–68)
	SV	—	2 (1–4)	9 (4–15)	7 (3–14)	12 (5–22)
	LN	—	1 (0–2)	3 (0–8)	4 (0–12)	5 (0–14)
4.1–6.0	OC	75 (55–93)	57 (52–63)	35 (29–40)	25 (18–35)	21 (14–29)
	EC	25 (7–45)	39 (33–44)	51 (44–57)	60 (50–68)	59 (49–69)
	SV	—	2 (1–3)	7 (4–11)	5 (3–9)	9 (4–16)
	LN	—	2 (1–3)	7 (4–13)	10 (5–18)	10 (4–20)
6.1–10.0	OC	69 (47–91)	49 (43–54)	26 (22–31)	19 (14–25)	15 (10–21)
	EC	31 (9–53)	44 (39–49)	52 (46–58)	60 (52–68)	57 (48–67)
	SV	—	5 (3–8)	16 (10–22)	13 (7–20)	19 (11–29)
	LN	—	2 (1–3)	6 (4–10)	8 (5–14)	8 (4–16)
>10.0	OC	57 (35–86)	33 (28–38)	214 (11–17)	9 (6–13)	7 (4–10)
	EC	43 (14–65)	52 (46–56)	47 (40–53)	50 (40–60)	46 (36–59)
	SV	—	8 (5–11)	17 (12–24)	13 (8–21)	19 (12–29)
	LN	—	8 (5–12)	22 (15–30)	27 (16–39)	27 (14–40)

Reprinted from Urology, 58, Partin AW, Mangold LA, Lamm DM, Walsh PC, Epstein JI, Pearson J. Contemporary update of prostate cancer-staging nomograms (Partin Tables) for the new millennium, 843–848. © 2001, with permission from Elsevier Science.

Table 10 Partin-Nomogram for PCa with clinical stage T2c (tumor palpable on both sides of the prostate)

PSA (ng/mL)	Pathologic stage	Highest Gleason score in biopsy				
		2–4	5–6	3+4=7	4+3=7	8–10
0–2.5	OC	86 (71–97)	73 (63–81)	51 (38–63)	39 (26–54)	34 (21–48)
	EC	14 (3–29)	24 (17–33)	36 (26–48)	45 (32–59)	47 (33–61)
	SV	—	1 (0–2)	5 (1–13)	5 (1–12)	8 (2–19)
	LN	—	1 (0–4)	6 (0–18)	9 (0–26)	10 (0–27)
2.6–4.0	OC	78 (58–94)	61 (50–70)	38 (27–50)	27 (18–40)	23 (14–34)
	EC	22 (6–42)	36 (27–45)	48 (37–59)	57 (44–70)	57 (44–70)
	SV	—	2 (1–5)	8 (2–17)	6 (2–16)	10 (3–22)
	LN	—	1 (0–4)	5 (0–15)	7 (0–21)	8 (0–22)
4.1–6.0	OC	73 (52–93)	55 (44–64)	31 (23–41)	21 (14–31)	18 (11–28)
	EC	27 (7–48)	40 (32–50)	50 (40–60)	57 (43–68)	57 (43–70)
	SV	—	2 (1–4)	6 (2–11)	4 (1–10)	7 (2–15)
	LN	—	3 (1–7)	12 (5–23)	16 (6–32)	16 (6–33)
6.1–10.0	OC	67 (45–91)	46 (36–56)	24 (17–32)	16 (10–24)	13 (8–20)
	EC	33 (9–55)	46 (37–55)	52 (42–61)	58 (46–69)	56 (43–69)
	SV	—	5 (2–9)	13 (6–23)	11 (4–21)	16 (6–29)
	LN	—	3 (1–6)	10 (5–18)	13 (6–25)	13 (5–26)
>10.0	OC	54 (32–85)	30 (21–38)	11 (7–17)	7 (4–12)	6 (3–10)
	EC	46 (15–68)	51 (42–60)	42 (30–55)	43 (29–59)	41 (27–57)
	SV	—	6 (2–12)	13 (6–24)	10 (3–20)	15 (5–28)
	LN	—	13 (6–22)	33 (18–49)	38 (20–58)	38 (20–59)

Reprinted from Urology, 58, Partin AW, Mangold LA, Lamm DM, Walsh PC, Epstein JI, Pearson J. Contemporary update of prostate cancer-staging nomograms (Partin Tables) for the new millennium, 843–848. © 2001, with permission from Elsevier Science.

When PSA was categorized into levels <10.0 ng/mL, 10.0–20.0 ng/mL, 20.0–30.0 ng/mL, and ≥30.0 ng/mL, it was shown that Gleason grade added only marginally to the predictive power of PSA alone (407).

Effects of Radiation Therapy on Serum PSA

The course of serum PSA after radiation therapy clearly differs from that observed after surgical removal of the prostate: the prostate remains *in situ*. Moreover, radioablative destruction of prostatic cells may take several months to exert full effect, since a double-strand break in DNA permits cellular survival until the next mitosis and cellular function may be intact. Therefore, serum PSA levels typically decline slowly over a period of up to 24 months to low but detectable concentrations. Transient increases in PSA (e.g., by ≥0.2 or ≥0.1 ng/mL) followed by decreases, termed bouncing PSA levels, occur frequently in men treated with radiation therapy and may be related to pretreatment PSA and radiation dose.

PSA to Estimate the Response of Radiation Therapy: PSA Nadir

PSA nadir precedes clinical failure by four to five PSA-doubling times, or three to four years. Therefore it has been accepted as a surrogate endpoint. After completion of radiation and attainment of nadir level, the only source of PSA is the remaining benign prostatic epithelium (if therapy is curative). The time at which nadir levels are reached, and the absolute PSA values that represent the nadir, are important factors in estimating the outcome of therapy. Nadir levels should be reached in 22–33 months and range from 0.4 to 0.5 ng/mL when external beam radiation therapy is curative. Nadir may be lower when external beam therapy is combined with interstitial therapy (e.g., <0.2 ng/mL). In case of local failure, PSA nadir is likely to be higher (2.0–3.0 ng/mL) and nadir occurs earlier (17–20 months). The chances of remaining free of recurrence are increased if the nadir is lower. If the nadir is <0.5 ng/mL, the likelihood of being disease-free after five years has been reported to be 75–90%, but may be less than 20% if the nadir 81.0 ng/mL.

Definition of Biochemical Failure

Interpretation of post-radiation PSA is certainly more difficult than in radical prostatectomy due to heterogeneity among patients in rate of PSA decline, duration of PSA nadir, and rate of PSA elevation. Since the prostate is not removed and is likely to produce some PSA, there are no clear-cut stringent definitions. On the other hand, the radiation technique *per se* may have an impact on nadir PSA. Two-thirds of patients may obtain a serum PSA of <0.2 ng/mL when a combination of external beam and brachytherapy is used (408), which is rarely achieved by external beam radiation alone. This implicates various definitions of cure vs. failure. Some investigators define failure as two or more rising PSA levels (409). Others applied a combination of threshold levels; e.g., two elevations of total PSA >1.0 ng/mL and above nadir PSA (364), ≥1.5 ng/mL and rising on two subsequent measurements (410), or >2.0 ng/mL and more than 1.0 ng/mL above the nadir PSA (411). According to the ASTRO (American Society of Therapeutic Radiation Oncologists) consensus conference, three consecutive PSA increases in PSA 3–4 months apart in the first two years after radiation therapy, and six months apart after two years after nadir, are reasonable to define biochemical failure. The time point at which biochemical failure occurred is backdated halfway between the last nadir value and the first of the three rising PSA values (412).

SCREENING FOR PROSTATE CANCER

Despite international efforts, early detection and treatment of PCA and screening strategies are controversial issues. While some claim the recent trend of decrease in mortality observed for PCA is due to extensive use of PSA (413), others state that to date, no controlled randomized trial has shown the efficiency of PSA to reduce mortality of PCA. However, prospective randomized trials initiated by the National Cancer Institute (414), the prostate, lung, colorectal, and ovarian (PLCO) screening trial and the European Randomized Study of Screening for Prostate Cancer (415) (ESPRC), have enrolled more than 50,000 and 80,000 men (in the group of men exposed to active screening), respectively, to investigate whether PSA screening will reduce mortality of PCA. Due to its natural history, more than a decade will be needed before an answer can be anticipated. When screening is performed, selection of screening tools is one issue, but the interval at which patients should be screened is as important.

The American Cancer Society and the American Urological Association (416) recommend an annual screening visit for early detection of PCA beginning at age 50. To reduce costs and prevent loss in quality of life for screened men however, others suggested an increase in screening intervals after adjusting for age or serum PSA.

Analysis of longitudinal screening studies shows that the initial screening PSA level is an important factor for developing cancer (417). For serum PSA <2.5 ng/mL at entry, the risk of cancer was shown to be about 1% within four years, but the risk increased to 12.7% and 38.4% in men with PSAs of 2.6–4.0 and 4.0–10.0 ng/mL, respectively. Results of the Baltimore Longitudinal Study of Aging showed a risk of only 4% for a man with initial PSA <2.0 ng/mL to progress to PSA of 4.1 to 5.0 ng/mL within four years (418). Therefore it can be suggested that patients with a low PSA (e.g., <2.0 ng/mL), might not be at risk when screening intervals are increased to a biannual schedule. Men with PSA levels >2.0 ng/mL should maintain annual screening (418). Other preliminary results of longitudinal follow-up suggest that the end of screening can be age- and PSA-adjusted; e.g., a 65-year-old man with a PSA level <1.0 ng/mL might stop screening with minimal risk of developing a cancer that will be the cause of death.

The age at which screening begins should take into account commonly accepted risk factors such as age, race, and family history. Earlier onset of screening has been shown to increase the likelihood of being diagnosed with an organ-confined cancer in any PSA range. See Table 11 (419).

Earlier onset of screening should also be performed in men with a positive family history due to increased risks for men with a first-degree relative affected with cancer. Hereditary cancers may account for 9% of all cancers, but have been suggested to make up to 40% of cancers diagnosed in men 55 years or younger (420,421). Therefore, it has been suggested that screening should start at age 40 for affected family members.

While the results of prospective randomized trails using PSA-based screening for prostate cancer are awaited, there is already strong evidence that PSA is beneficial for improving the early detection of prostate cancer while being a relatively inexpensive tool and having an acceptable sensitivity. As outlined previously, the initial increase in prostate cancer incidence followed by a decrease matches the assumed course of an effective screening tool. Adjustments in screening with respect to race, age, and family history might improve the screening modalities with respect to selecting those men (age, PSA, family history, ethnic background) in whom screening might be most useful.

REFERENCES

1. McNeal JE. The zonal anatomy of the prostate. Prostate 1981;2(1):35–49.
2. McNeal JE, Redwine EA, Freiha FS, Stamey TA. Zonal distribution of prostatic adenocarcinoma. Correlation with histologic pattern and direction of spread. Am J Surg Pathol 1988;12(12): 897–906.
3. McNeal JE. Origin and evolution of benign prostatic enlargement. Invest Urol 1978;15(4):340–345.
4. McNeal JE. Normal and pathologic anatomy of prostate. Urology 1981;17(Suppl 3):11–16.
5. Kastendieck H. Ultrastrukturpathologie der menschlichen prostatadruese: cyto-und histomorphogenese von atrophie, hyperplasie und karzinom. Veroeff Pathol 1977;106.
6. McPhaul M J, Marcelli M, Zoppi S, Griffin JE, Wilson JD. Genetic basis of endocrine disease. 4. The spectrum of mutations in the androgen receptor gene that causes androgen resistance. J Clin Endocrinol Metab 1993;76(1):17–23.
7. Imperato-McGinley J, Peterson RE, Gautier T, Sturla E. Male pseudohermaphroditism secondary to 5 alpha-reductase deficiency—a model for the role of androgens in both the development of the male phenotype and the evolution of a male gender identity. J Steroid Biochem 1979;11(1B):637–645.
8. Huggins C, Stevens RA. The effect of androgens on benign hypertrophy in man. J Urol 1940;43:705–714.
9. Huggins C, Hodges CV. The effect of castration, of estrogen and androgen injection on serum phosphatases in metastatic carcinoma of the prostate. Cancer Res 1941;1:293.

Table 11 Likelihood of harboring pathologically organ-confined prostate cancer as a function of total PSA and age at diagnosis

tPSA (ng/mL)	Age 40–50	Age 51–60	Age 61–70
2.5–4	89 (87–90)	83 (82–84)	78 (77–79)
4.1–6	87 (85–88)	81 (80–82)	74 (73–75)
6.1–8	84 (83–85)	78 (77–79)	71 (70–72)
8.1–10	83 (82–83)	75 (74–75)	67 (66–68)
>10	73 (65–80)	57 (52–62)	49 (45–53)

Reprinted with permission from Carter HB, Epstein JI, Partin AW. Influence of age and prostate-specific antigen on the chance of curable prostate cancer among men with nonpalpable disease. Urology 1999;53(1):126–130.

10. Yen SSC. Reproductive endocrinology: physiology, pathophsiology, and clinical management. In: Yen SSC, Jaffee RB, eds. Philadelphia: WB Saunders, 1986:33–74.
11. Carmel PW, Arani S, Ferrin M. Pituitary stalk portal collection in rhesus monkeys: Evidence of pulsatile release of gonadotropin-releasing hormone (GnRH). Endocrinology 1976;99:243–247.
12. Gitler MS, Barraclough CA. Locus coeruleus (LC) stimulation augments LHRH release induced by medial preoptic stimulation. Evidence that the major LC stimulatory component enters contralaterally into the hypothalamus. Brain Res 1987;422(1):1–10.
13. Bardin CW. Reproductive endocrinology: physiology, pathophsiology, and clinical management. In: Yen SSC, Jaffee RB, eds. Philadelphia: WB Saunders, 1986:177–199.
14. Walsh PC, Swerdloff RS, Odell WD. Feedback control of FSH in the male: role of oestrogen. Acta Endocrinol (Copenh) 1973; 74(3):449–460.
15. Walsh PC, Swerdloff RS, Odell WD. Feedback regulation of gonadotropin secretion in men. J Urol 1973;110(1):84–89.
16. Dorrington JH, Armstrong DT. Follicle-stimulating hormone stimulates estradiol-17beta synthesis in cultured Sertoli cells. Proc Natl Acad Sci USA 1975;72(7):2677–2681.
17. Winters SJ. Inhibin is released together with testosterone by the human testis. J Clin Endocrinol Metab 1990;70(2):548–550.
18. Carter JN, Tyson JE, Tolis G, Van Vliet S, Faiman C, Friesen HG. Prolactin-screening tumors and hypogonadism in 22 men. N Engl J Med 1978;299(16):847–852.
19. Simpson ER, Waterman MR. Steroid hormone biosynthesis in the adrenal cortex and its regulation by adrenocorticotropin. In: DeGroot LJ, ed. Endocrinology. Philadelphia: WB Saunders, 1989;2:1543–1556.
20. Trachtenberg J, Pont A. Ketoconazole therapy for advanced prostate cancer. Lancet 1984;2(8400):433–435.
21. Small EJ, Baron AD, Fippin L, Apodaca D. Ketoconazole retains activity in advanced prostate cancer patients with progression despite flutamide withdrawal. J Urol 1997;157(4):1204–1207.
22. Coffey DS. The molecular biology, endocrinology, and physiology of the prostate and seminal vesicles. In: Walsh PC, Retik AB, Stamey TA, Vaughan ED, eds. Campbell's urology. Philadelphia: WB Saunders,1992;1:221–266.
23. Vermeulen A. The physiologic state of testosterone in plasma. In: James VHT, Serio M, Martini L, eds. The endocrine function of the human testis. New York: Academic Press,1973;1:157–170.
24. Geller J. Effect of finasteride, a 5-alpha-reductase inhibitor on prostate tissue androgens and prostate-specific antigen. J Clin Endocrinol Metab 1990;71(6):1552–1555.
25. Gormley GJ, Stoner E, Bruskewitz RC, Imperato-McGinley J, Walsh PC, McConnell J D, Andriole GL, Geller J, Bracken BR, Tenover JS, et al. The effect of finasteride in men with benign prostatic hyperplasia. The Finasteride Study Group. N Engl J Med 1992;327(17):1185–1191.
26. DeKlerk DP, Heston WDW, Coffey DS. Studies on the role of macromolecular synthesis in the growth of the prostate. Benign prostatic hyperplasia. In: Grayhack JT, Wilson JD, Scherbenske MJ, eds. Proceedings of a workshop sponsored by the kidney disease and urology program of the NIAMDD. Washington, DC: US Government Printing Office,1976.
27. Carson-Jurica MA, Schrader WT, O'Malley BW. Steroid receptor family: structure and functions. Endocr Rev 1990;11(2): 201–220.
28. MacLean HE, Warne GL, Zajac JD. Localization of functional domains in the androgen receptor. J Steroid Biochem Mol Biol 1997;62(4):233–242.
29. Grover PK, Odell WD. Correlation of in vivo and in vitro activities of some naturally occurring androgens using a radioreceptor assay for 5-alpha-dihydrotestosterone with rat prostate cytosol receptor protein. J Steroid Biochem 1975;6(10):1373–1379.
30. Gleave ME, Sato N, Sadar M, Yago V, Bruchovsky N, Sullivan L. Butyrate analogue, isobutyramide, inhibits tumor growth and time to androgen-independent progression in the human prostate LNCaP tumor model. J Cell Biochem 1998;69(3):271–281.
31. Sadar MD, Gleave ME. Ligand-independent activation of the androgen receptor by the differentiation agent butyrate in human prostate cancer cells. Cancer Res 2000;60(20):5825–5831.
32. Walls R, Thibault A, Liu L, Wood C, Kozlowski JM, Figg WD, Sampson ML, Elin RJ, Samid D. The differentiating agent phenylacetate increases prostate-specific antigen production by prostate cancer cells. Prostate 1996;29(3):177–182.
33. Gkonos PJ, Ashby MH, Andrade AA. Vasoactive intestinal peptide stimulates prostate-specific antigen secretion by LNCaP prostate cancer cells. Regul Pept 1996;65(2):153–157.
34. Zhao XY, Ly LH, Peehl DM, Feldman D. 1alpha,25-dihydroxyvitamin D3 actions in LNCaP human prostate cancer cells are androgen-dependent. Endocrinology 1997; 138(8):3290–3298.
35. Fong CJ, Sutkowski DM, Braun EJ, Bauer KD, Sherwood ER, Lee C, Kozlowski JM. Effect of retinoic acid on the proliferation and secretory activity of androgen-responsive prostatic carcinoma cells. J Urol 1993;149(5):1190–1194.
36. Hobisch A, Eder IE, Putz, T, Horninger W, Bartsch G, Klocker H, Culig Z. Interleukin-6 regulates prostate-specific protein expression in prostate carcinoma cells by activation of the androgen receptor. Cancer Res 1998;58(20):4640–4645.
37. Culig Z, Hobisch A, Cronauer MV, Radmayr C, Trapman J, Hittmair A, Bartsch G, Klocker H. Androgen receptor activation in prostatic tumor cell lines by insulin-like growth factor-I, keratinocyte growth factor, and epidermal growth factor. Cancer Res 1994;54(20):5474–5478.
38. Gleave M, Hsieh JT, Gao CA, von Eschenbach AC, Chung LW. Acceleration of human prostate cancer growth in vivo by factors produced by prostate and bone fibroblasts. Cancer Res 1991; 51(14):3753–3761.
39. Tennant MK, Thrasher JB, Twomey PA, Birnbaum RS, Plymate SR. Insulin-like growth factor-binding protein-2 and -3 expression in benign human prostate epithelium, prostate intraepithelial neoplasia, annd adenocarcinoma of the prostate. J Clin Endocrinol Metab 1996;81:411–420.
40. Boudon C, Rodier G, Lechevallier E, Mottet N, Barenton B, Sultan C. Secretion of insulin-like growth factors and their binding proteins by human normal and hyperplastic prostatic cells in primary culture. J Clin Endocrinol Metab 1996;81:612–617.
41. Byrne RL, Leung H, Neal DE. Peptide growth factors in the prostate as mediators of stromal-epithelial interaction. Br J Urol 1996;77:627–663.
42. Sherwood ER, Lee C. Epidermal growth factor-related peptides in the epidermal growth factor receptor in normal and malignant prostate. World J Urol 1995;13:290–296.
43. Sikes RA, Kao C, Chung LWK. Autocrine and paracrine mediators for prostate growth in cancer progression. In: McGuire EJ, ed. Advances in urology. Chicago: Mosby Year Books, Inc., 1995; 8:21–60.
44. Wilding G, Valvaerius E, Knabbe C, Gelman EP. The role of transforming growth factor alpha in human prostate cancer cell growth. Prostate 1989;15:1–12.
45. Bikfalvi A, Klein S, Pintucci G, Rifkin DB. Biological roles of fibroblast growth factor-2. Endocr Rev 1997;18:26–40.

46. Ittmann M, Mansukhani A. Expression of fibroblast growth factors (FGFs) and FGF receptors in human prostate. J Urol 1997;157:353–356.
47. Nemeth JH, Zelner DJ, Land S, Lee C. Keratinocyte growth factor in ventral prostate: Androgen-independent expression. J Endocrinol 1998;156:115–125.
48. Yan G, Fukabori Y, Nikolaropoulos S, Wang F, McKeehan WL. Heparin-binding keratinocyte growth factor is a candidate stromal to epithelial cell andromedin. Mol Endocrinol 1992;6: 2123–2128.
49. Steiner MS. Role of peptide growth factors in the prostate: a review. Urology 1993;42(1):99–110.
50. Kyprianou N, Isaacs JT. Identification of a cellular receptor for transforming growth factor-beta in rat ventral prostate and its negative regulation by androgens. Endocrinology 1988;123(4): 2124–2131.
51. Steiner MS, Barrack ER. Transforming growth factor-beta 1 overproduction in prostate cancer: effects on growth in vivo and in vitro. Mol Endocrinol 1992;6(1):15–25.
52. Morikawa M, Harada N, Soma G, Yoshida T. Transforming growth factor-beta 1 modulates the effect of 1 alpha, 25-dihydroxyvitamin D3 on leukemic cells. In Vitro Cell Dev Biol 1990; 26(7):682–690.
53. Folkman J, Shing Y. Angiogenesis. J Biol Chem 1992;267(16): 10931–10934.
54. Campbell SC. Advances in angiogenesis research: relevance to urological oncology. J Urol 1997;158(5):1663–1674.
55. Montironi R, Diamanti L, Thompson D, Bartels HG, Bartels PH. Analysis of the capillary architecture in the precursors of prostate cancer: recent findings and new concepts. Eur Urol 1996; 30(2):191–200.
56. Folkman J, Klagsbrun M. Angiogenic factors. Science 1987; 235(4787):442–447.
57. Minchenko A, Bauer T, Salceda S, Caro J. Hypoxic stimulation of vascular endothelial growth factor expression in vitro and in vivo. Lab Invest 1994;71(3):374–379.
58. Ferrara N, Davis-Smyth T. The biology of vascular endothelial growth factor. Endocr Rev 1997;18(1):4–25.
59. Jackson MW, Bentel JM, Tilley WD. Vascular endothelial growth factor (VEGF) expression in prostate cancer and benign prostatic hyperplasia. J Urol 1997;157(6):2323–2328.
60. Joseph IB, Isaacs JT. Potentiation of the antiangiogenic ability of linomide by androgen ablation involves down-regulation of vascular endothelial growth factor in human androgen-responsive prostatic cancers. Cancer Res 1997;57(6):1054–1057.
61. Joseph IB, Nelson JB, Denmeade SR, Isaacs JT. Androgens regulate vascular endothelial growth factor content in normal and malignant prostatic tissue. Clin Cancer Res 1997;3(12 Pt 1): 2507–2511.
62. Yanagisawa M, Kurihara H, Kimura S, Tomobe Y, Kobayashi M, Mitsui Y, Yazaki Y, Goto K, Masaki T. A novel potent vasoconstrictor peptide produced by vascular endothelial cells. Nature 1988; 332(6163):411–415.
63. Levin ER. Endothelins as cardiovascular peptides. Am J Nephrol 1996;16(3):246–51.
64. Casey ML, Byrd W, MacDonald PC. Massive amounts of immunoreactive endothelin in human seminal fluid. J Clin Endocrinol Metab 1992;74(1):223–225.
65. Kobayashi S, Tang R, Wang B, Opgenorth T, Stein E, Shapiro E, Lepor H. Localization of endothelin receptors in the human prostate. J Urol 1994;151(3):763–766.
66. Webb ML, Chao CC, Rizzo M, Shapiro RA, Neubauer M, Liu EC, Aversa CR, Brittain RJ, Treiger B. Cloning and expression of an endothelin receptor subtype B from human prostate that mediates contraction. Mol Pharmacol 1995;47(4): 730–737.
67. Farnsworth WE. Prostate stroma: physiology. Prostate 1999; 38(1):60–72.
68. Kenny B, Ballard S, Blagg J, Fox D. Pharmacological options in the treatment of benign prostatic hyperplasia. J Med Chem 1997; 40(9):1293–1315.
69. Jacobs SC, Story MT. Exocrine secretion of epidermal growth factor by the rat prostate: effect of adrenergic agents, cholinergic agents, and vasoactive intestinal peptide. Prostate 1988;13(1): 79–87.
70. Wang JM, McKenna KE, Lee C. Determination of prostatic secretion in rats: effect of neurotransmitters and testosterone. Prostate 1991;18(4):289–301.
71. McVary KT, McKenna KE, Lee C. Prostate innervation. Prostate Suppl 1998;8:2–13.
72. Tauber PF, Zaneveld LJ, Propping D, Schumacher GF. Components of human split ejaculates. I. Spermatozoa, fructose, immunoglobulins, albumin, lactoferrin, transferrin, and other plasma proteins. J Reprod Fertil 1975;43(2):249–267.
73. Tauber PF, Zaneveld LJ, Propping D, Schumacher GF. Components of human split ejaculates. II. Enzymes and proteinase inhibitors. J Reprod Fertil 1976;46(1):165–171.
74. Mann T, Mann CL. Male reproductive function and semen. New York: Springer-Verlag,1981;269–336.
75. Aumuller G, Seitz J, Lilja H, Abrahamsson PA, von der Kammer H, Scheit KH. Species and organ specificity of secretory proteins derived from human prostate and seminal vesicles. Prostate 1990; 17(1):31–40.
76. Williams-Ashman HG, Pegg AE, Lockwood DH. Mechanisms and regulation of polyamine and putrescine biosynthesis in male genital glands and other tissues of mammals. Adv Enzyme Regul 1969;7:291–323.
77. Pourian MR, Kvist U, Bjorndahl L, Oliw EH. Rapid and slow hydroxylators of seminal E prostaglandins among men in barren unions. Andrologia 1995;27(2):71–79.
78. Fuchs AR, Chantharaski U. Prostaglandins and male fertility. In: Hafez ESE, ed. St. Louis, MO: Mosby, 1976.
79. Bedwal RS, Bahuguna A. Zinc, copper, and selenium in reproduction. Experientia 1994;50(7):626–640.
80. Chandler JA, Sinowatz F, Timms BG, Pierrepoint CG. The subcellular distribution of zinc in dog prostate studied by X-ray microanalysis. Cell Tissue Res 1977;185(1):89–103.
81. Diamandis EP, Yousef GM, Luo LY, Magklara A, Obiezu CV. The new human kallikrein gene family: implications in carcinogenesis. Trends Endocrinol Metab 2000;11(2):54–60.
82. Riegman PH, Vlietstra RJ, Klaassen P, van der Korput JA, Geurts van Kessel A, Romijn JC, Trapman J. The prostate-specific antigen gene and the human glandular kallikrein-1 gene are tandemly located on chromosome 19. FEBS Lett 1989; 247(1):123–126.
83. Riegman PH, Vlietstra RJ, van der Korput JA, Romijn JC, Trapman J. Characterization of the prostate-specific antigen gene: a novel human kallikrein-like gene. Biochem Biophys Res Commun 1989;159(1):95–102.
84. Schedlich LJ, Bennetts BH, Morris BJ. Primary structure of a human glandular kallikrein gene. DNA 1987;6(5):429–437.
85. Lilja H, Abrahamsson PA. Three predominant proteins secreted by the human prostate gland. Prostate 1988;12(1):29–38.
86. Wang TJ, Rittenhouse HG, Wolfert RL, Lynne CM, Brackett NL. PSA concentrations in seminal plasma. Clin Chem 1998;44(4): 895–896.

87. Lundwall A, Lilja H. Molecular cloning of human prostate-specific antigen cDNA. FEBS Lett 1987;214(2):317–322.
88. Kumar A, Mikolajczyk SD, Goel AS, Millar LS, Saedi MS. Expression of pro form of prostate-specific antigen by mammalian cells and its conversion to mature, active form by human kallikrein 2. Cancer Res 1997;57(15):3111–3114.
89. Lovgren J, Rajakoski K, Karp M, Lundwall A, Lilja H. Activation of the zymogen form of prostate-specific antigen by human glandular kallikrein 2. Biochem Biophys Res Commun 1997;238(2):549–555.
90. Takayama TK, Fujikawa K, Davie EW. Characterization of the precursor of prostate-specific antigen. Activation by trypsin and by human glandular kallikrein. J Biol Chem 1997;272(34):21582–21588.
91. Takayama TK, Carter CA, Deng T. Activation of prostate-specific antigen precursor (pro-PSA) by prostin, a novel human prostatic serine protease identified by degenerate PCR. Biochemistry 2001;40(6):1679–1687.
92. Belanger A, van Halbeek H, Graves HC, Grandbois K, Stamey TA, Huang L, Poppe I, Labrie F. Molecular mass and carbohydrate structure of prostate-specific antigen: studies for establishment of an international PSA standard. Prostate 1995;27(4):187–197.
93. Wang MC, Valenzuela LA, Murphy GP, Chu TM. Purification of a human prostate-specific antigen. Invest Urol 1979;17(2):159–163.
94. Lilja H. A kallikrein-like serine protease in prostatic fluid cleaves the predominant seminal vesicle protein. J Clin Invest 1985;76(5):1899–1903.
95. Lilja H, Abrahamsson PA, Lundwall A. Semenogelin, the predominant protein in human semen. Primary structure and identification of closely related proteins in the male accessory sex glands and on the spermatozoa. J Biol Chem 1989;264(3):1894–1900.
96. Christensson A, Laurell CB, Lilja H. Enzymatic activity of prostate-specific antigen and its reactions with extracellular serine proteinase inhibitors. Eur J Biochem 1990;194(3):755–763.
97. Malm J, Hellman J, Hogg P, Lilja H. Enzymatic action of prostate-specific antigen (PSA or hK3): substrate specificity and regulation by Zn(2+), a tight-binding inhibitor. Prostate 2000;45(2):132–139.
98. Lilja H, Oldbring J, Rannevik G, Laurell CB. Seminal vesicle-secreted proteins and their reactions during gelation and liquefaction of human semen. J Clin Invest 1987;80(2):281–285.
99. McGee RS, Herr JC. Human seminal vesicle-specific antigen is a substrate for prostate-specific antigen (or P30). Biol Reprod 1988;39(2):499–510.
100. Lee C, Keefer M, Zhao ZW, Kroes R, Berg L, Liu XX, Sensibar J. Demonstration of the role of prostate-specific antigen in semen liquefaction by two-dimensional electrophoresis. J Androl 1989;10(6):432–438.
101. Cohen P, Graves HC, Peehl DM, Kamarei M, Giudice LC, Rosenfeld RG. Prostate-specific antigen (PSA) is an insulin-like growth factor binding protein-3 protease found in seminal plasma. J Clin Endocrinol Metab 1992;75(4):1046–1053.
102. Iwamura M, di Sant'Agnese PA, Wu G, Benning CM, Cockett AT, Deftos LJ, Abrahamsson PA. Immunohistochemical localization of parathyroid hormone-related protein in human prostate cancer. Cancer Res 1993;53(8):1724–1726.
103. Killian CS, Corral DA, Kawinski E, Constantine RI. Mitogenic response of osteoblast cells to prostate-specific antigen suggests an activation of latent TGF-beta and a proteolytic modulation of cell adhesion receptors. Biochem Biophys Res Commun 1993;192(2):940–947.
104. Fortier AH, Nelson BJ, Grella DK, Holaday JW. Anti-angiogenic activity of prostate-specific antigen. J Natl Cancer Inst 1999;91(19):1635–1640.
105. Chapdelaine P, Paradis G, Tremblay RR, Dube JY. High level of expression in the prostate of a human glandular kallikrein mRNA related to prostate-specific antigen. FEBS Lett 1988;236(1):205–208.
106. Young CY, Andrews PE, Montgomery BT, Tindall DJ. Tissue-specific and hormonal regulation of human prostate-specific glandular kallikrein. Biochemistry 1992;31(3):818–824.
107. Deperthes D, Chapdelaine P, Tremblay RR, Brunet C, Berton J, Hebert J, Lazure C, Dube JY. Isolation of prostatic kallikrein hK2, also known as hGK-1, in human seminal plasma. Biochim Biophys Acta 1995;1245(3):311–316.
108. Mikolajczyk SD, Millar LS, Kumar A, Saedi MS. Human glandular kallikrein, hK2, shows arginine-restricted specificity and forms complexes with plasma protease inhibitors. Prostate 1998;34(1):44–50.
109. Lovgren J, Tian S, Lundwall A, Karp M, Lilja H. Production and activation of recombinant hK2 with propeptide mutations resulting in high expression levels. Eur J Biochem 1999;266(3):1050–1055.
110. Denmeade SR, Lovgren J, Khan SR, Lilja H, Isaacs JT. Activation of latent protease function of pro-hK2, but not pro-PSA, involves autoprocessing. Prostate 2001;48(2):122–126.
111. Deperthes D, Frenette G, Brillard-Bourdet M, Bourgeois L, Gauthier F, Tremblay RR, Dube JY. Potential involvement of kallikrein hK2 in the hydrolysis of the human seminal vesicle proteins after ejaculation. J Androl 1996;17(6):659–665.
112. Lovgren J, Airas K, Lilja H. Enzymatic action of human glandular kallikrein 2 (hK2). Substrate specificity and regulation by Zn2+ and extracellular protease inhibitors. Eur J Biochem 1999;262(3):781–789.
113. Frenette G, Tremblay RR, Lazure C, Dube JY. Prostatic kallikrein hK2, but not prostate-specific antigen (hK3), activates single-chain urokinase-type plasminogen activator. Int J Cancer 1997;71(5):897–899.
114. Mikolajczyk SD, Millar LS, Kumar A, Saedi MS. Prostatic human kallikrein 2 inactivates and complexes with plasminogen activator inhibitor-1. Int J Cancer 1999;81(3):438–442.
115. Charlesworth MC, Young CY, Miller VM, Tindall DJ. Kininogenase activity of prostate-derived human glandular kallikrein (hK2) purified from seminal fluid. J Androl 1999;20(2):220–229.
116. Yu JX, Chao L, Chao J. Prostasin is a novel human serine proteinase from seminal fluid. Purification, tissue distribution, and localization in prostate gland. J Biol Chem 1994;269(29):18843–18848.
117. Chen, LM, Hodge GB, Guarda LA, Welch JL, Greenberg NM, Chai KX. Down-regulation of prostasin serine protease: a potential invasion suppressor in prostate cancer. Prostate 2001;48(2):93–103.
118. Gagnon S, Tetu B, Dube JY, Tremblay RR. Expression of Zn-alpha 2-glycoprotein and PSP-94 in prostatic adenocarcinoma. An immunohistochemical study of 88 cases. Am J Pathol 1990;136(5):1147–1152.
119. Ulvsback M, Lindstrom C, Weiber H, Abrahamsson PA, Lilja H, Lundwall A. Molecular cloning of a small prostate protein, known as beta-microsemenoprotein, PSP94 or beta-inhibin, and

demonstration of transcripts in non-genital tissues. Biochem Biophys Res Commun 1989;164(3):1310–1315.
120. Weiber H, Andersson C, Murne A, Rannevik G, Lindstrom C, Lilja H, Fernlund P. Beta microseminoprotein is not a prostate-specific protein. Its identification in mucous glands and secretions. Am J Pathol 1990;137(3):593–603.
121. Hirai K, Hussey HJ, Barber MD, Price SA, Tisdale MJ. Biological evaluation of a lipid-mobilizing factor isolated from the urine of cancer patients. Cancer Res 1998;58(11):2359–2365.
122. Rackley RR, Yang B, Pretlow TG, Abdul-Karim FW, Lewis TJ, McNamara N, Delmoro CM, Bradley Jr EL, Kursh E, Resnick MI, et al. Differences in the leucine aminopeptidase activity in extracts from human prostatic carcinoma and benign prostatic hyperplasia. Cancer 1991;68(3):587–593.
123. Friberg J, Telly-Friberg I. Antibodies in human seminal fluid. In: Hafez ESE, ed. Human semen and fertility. St. Louis, MO: Mosby, 1976.
124. Gahankari DR, Golhar KB. An evaluation of serum and tissue-bound immunoglobulins in prostatic diseases. J Postgrad Med 1993;39(2):63–67.
125. Grayhack JT, Lee C. Evaluation of prostatic fluid in prostatic pathology. Prog Clin Biol Res 1981;75A:231–246.
126. Guess HA. Benign prostatic hyperplasia and prostate cancer. Epidemiol Rev 2001;23(1):152–158.
127. Okajima E, Ozono S, Ota M, Tanaka M, Tani M, Hirao Y. A study on international prostate symptom score in the assessment of therapeutic effects and severity of symptoms due to benign prostatic hyperplasia. Nippon Hinyokika Gakkai Zasshi 1995;86(9):1466–1474.
128. Andersen JT. Benign prostatic hyperplasia: symptoms and objective interpretation. Eur Urol 1991;20(Suppl 1):36–40.
129. Abrams P. Benign prostatic hyperplasia. Poorly correlated with symptoms. BMJ 1993;307(6897):201.
130. Atan A, Horn T, Hansen F, Jakobsen H, Hald T. Benign prostatic hyperplasia. Does a correlation exist between prostatic morphology and irritative symptoms? Scand J Urol Nephrol 1996;30(4):303–306.
131. Berry SJ, Coffey DS, Walsh PC, Ewing LL. The development of human benign prostatic hyperplasia with age. J Urol 1984;132(3):474–479.
132. Guess HA. Epidemiology and natural history of benign prostatic hyperplasia. Urol Clin North Am 1995;22(2):247–261.
133. Guess HA, Arrighi HM, Metter EJ, Fozard JL. Cumulative prevalence of prostatism matches the autopsy prevalence of benign prostatic hyperplasia. Prostate 1990;17(3):241–246.
134. Sidney S, Quesenberry Jr C, Sadler MC, Lydick EG, Guess HA, Cattolica EV. Risk factors for surgically treated benign prostatic hyperplasia in a prepaid health care plan. Urology 1991;38(1):13–19.
135. Barrack ER. The nuclear matrix of the prostate contains acceptor sites for androgen receptors. Endocrinology 1983;113(1):430–432.
136. Roehrborn CG, Lange JL, George FW, Wilson JD. Changes in amount and intracellular distribution of androgen receptor in human foreskin as a function of age. J Clin Invest 1987;79(1):44–47.
137. McDonnell JD. Epidemiology, etiology, pathopysiology, and diagnosis of benign prostatic hyperplasia. In: Walsh PC, Retik AB, Stamey TA, Vaughan ED, eds. Campbell's urology. Philadelphia: WB Saunders, 1998;2:1429–1449.
138. Shapiro E, Becich MJ, Hartanto V, Lepor H. The relative proportion of stromal and epithelial hyperplasia is related to the development of symptomatic benign prostate hyperplasia. J Urol 1992;147(5):1293–1297.
139. Kobayashi S, Tang R, Shapiro E, Lepor H. Characterization and localization of prostatic alpha 1 adrenoceptors using radioligand receptor binding on slide-mounted tissue section. J Urol 1993;150(6):2002–2006.
140. Atan A, Basar MM, Yildiz M, Akalin Z. The effect of age in the usage of alpha receptor blocker treatment in prostate patients. Arch Ital Urol Androl 1997;69(5):299–301.
141. Boneff A. Incidence of asymptomatic chronic prostatitis. Acta Urol Belg 1968;36(4):437–440.
142. Lipsky BA. Urinary tract infections in men. Epidemiology, pathophysiology, diagnosis, and treatment. Ann Intern Med 1989;110(2):138–150.
143. Krieger JN, Nyberg Jr L, Nickel JC. NIH consensus definition and classification of prostatitis. JAMA 1999;282(3):236–237.
144. Weidner W. Prostatitis—diagnostic criteria, classification of patients and recommendations for therapeutic trials. Infection 1992;20(Suppl 3):S227–31; discussion S35.
145. Sutor DJ, Wooley SE. The crystalline composition of prostatic calculi. Br J Urol 1974;46(5):533–535.
146. Meares Jr EM. Acute and chronic prostatitis: diagnosis and treatment. Infect Dis Clin North Am 1987;1(4):855–873.
147. Epstein JI. Pathology of prostatic intraepithelial neoplasia and adenocarcinoma of the prostate: prognostic influences of stage, tumor volume, grade, and margins of resection. Semin Oncol 1994;21(5):527–541.
148. Bostwick DG, Qian J, Frankel K. The incidence of high-grade prostatic intraepithelial neoplasia in needle biopsies. J Urol 1995;154(5):1791–1794.
149. Gaudin PB, Sesterhenn IA, Wojno KJ, Mostofi FK, Epstein JI. Incidence and clinical significance of high-grade prostatic intraepithelial neoplasia in TURP specimens. Urology 1997;49(4):558–563.
150. Wills ML, Hamper UM, Partin AW, Epstein JI. Incidence of high-grade prostatic intraepithelial neoplasia in sextant needle biopsy specimens. Urology 1997;49(3):367–373.
151. Wojno KJ, Epstein JI. The utility of basal cell-specific anti-cytokeratin antibody (34 beta E12) in the diagnosis of prostate cancer. A review of 228 cases. Am J Surg Pathol 1995;19(3):251–260.
152. Weinstein MH, Epstein JI. Significance of high-grade prostatic intraepithelial neoplasia on needle biopsy. Hum Pathol 1993;24(6):624–629.
153. Epstein JI. Pathology of adenocarcinoma of the prostate. In: Walsh PC, Retik AB, Stamey TA, Vaughan ED, eds. Campbell's urology. Philadelphia: WB Saunders 1998;3:2497–2498.
154. Howe HL, Wingo PA, Thun MJ, Ries LA, Rosenberg HM, Feigal EG, Edwards BK. Annual report to the nation on the status of cancer (1973 through 1998), featuring cancers with recent increasing trends. J Natl Cancer Inst 2001;93(11):824–842.
155. CDC. Prostate cancer: The public health perspective. [Online: www.cdc.gov/cancer/prostate/index.htm]. Department of Health and Human Services. Centers for Disease Control and Prevention. Accessed August 2001.
156. Franks LM, Durth MB. Latency and progression in tumors: the natural history of prostate cancer. Lancet 1956;17:1037–1039.
157. Guileyardo JM, Johnson WD, Welsh RA, Akazaki K, Correa P. Prevalence of latent prostate carcinoma in two US populations. J Natl Cancer Inst 1980;65(2):311–316.
158. Yatani R, Shiraishi T, Nakakuki K, Kusano I, Takanari H, Hayashi T, Stemmermann GN. Trends in frequency of latent prostate car-

cinoma in Japan from 1965–1979 to 1982–1986. J Natl Cancer Inst 1988;80(9):683–687.
159. Seidman H, Mushinski MH, Gelb SK, Silverberg E. Probabilities of eventually developing or dying of cancer—United States, 1985. CA Cancer J Clin 1985;35(1):36–56.
160. Boccon-Gibod L. Significant vs. insignificant prostate cancer—can we identify the tigers from the pussy cats? J Urol 1996; 156(3):1069–1070.
161. Walsh PC. The definition and pre-operative prediction of clinically insignificant prostate cancer. J Urol 1996;156(1):300–301.
162. Albertsen PC, Hanley JA, Gleason DF, Barry MJ. Competing risk analysis of men aged 55 to 74 years at diagnosis managed conservatively for clinically localized prostate cancer. JAMA 1998;280(11):975–980.
163. Aus G. Prostate cancer. Mortality and morbidity after non-curative treatment with aspects on diagnosis and treatment. Scand J Urol Nephrol Suppl 1994;167:1–41.
164. Johansson JE, Holmberg L, Johansson S, Bergstrom R Adami HO. Fifteen-year survival in prostate cancer. A prospective, population-based study in Sweden. JAMA 1997;277(6):467–471.
165. Whittemore AS. Colorectal cancer incidence among Chinese in North America and the People's Republic of China: variation with sex, age, and anatomical site. Int J Epidemiol 1989;18(3):563–568.
166. Parkin DM, Muir CS. Cancer incidence in five continents. Comparability and quality of data. IARC Sci Publ 1992;120:45–173.
167. Rose DP, Boyar AP, Wynder EL. International comparisons of mortality rates for cancer of the breast, ovary, prostate, and colon, and per capita food consumption. Cancer 1986;58(11):2363–2371.
168. Wang Y, Corr JG, Thaler HT, Tao Y, Fair WR, Heston WD. Decreased growth of established human prostate LNCaP tumors in nude mice fed a low-fat diet. J Natl Cancer Inst 1995; 87(19):1456–1462.
169. The effect of vitamin E and beta carotene on the incidence of lung cancer and other cancers in male smokers. The Alpha-Tocopherol, Beta Carotene Cancer Prevention Study Group. N Engl J Med 1994;330(15):1029–1035.
170. Zhao XY, Feldman D. The role of vitamin D in prostate cancer. Steroids 2001;66(3–5):293–300.
171. Clark LC, Combs Jr GF, Turnbull BW, Slate EH, Chalker DK, Chow J, Davis LS, Glover RA, Graham GF, Gross EG, Krongrad A, Lesher Jr JL, Park HK, Sanders Jr BB, Smith CL, Taylor JR. Effects of selenium supplementation for cancer prevention in patients with carcinoma of the skin. A randomized controlled trial. Nutritional Prevention of Cancer Study Group. JAMA 1996;276(24):1957–1963.
172. Smith DS, Bullock AD, Catalona WJ, Herschman JD. Racial differences in a prostate cancer screening study. J Urol 1996;156(4):1366–1369.
173. Gilliland FD, Key CR. Prostate cancer in American Indians, New Mexico, 1969 to 1994. J Urol 1998;159(3):893–897;discussion 897–898.
174. Cook LS, Goldoft M, Schwartz SM, Weiss NS. Incidence of adenocarcinoma of the prostate in Asian immigrants to the United States and their descendants. J Urol 1999;161(1):152–155.
175. Whittemore AS, Wu AH, Kolonel LN, John EM, Gallagher RP, Howe GR, West DW, Teh CZ, Stamey T. Family history and prostate cancer risk in black, white, and Asian men in the United States and Canada. Am J Epidemiol 1995;141(8):732–740.
176. Carter BS, Bova GS, Beaty TH, Steinberg GD, Childs B, Isaacs WB, Walsh PC. Hereditary prostate cancer: epidemiologic and clinical features. J Urol 1993;150(3):797–802.
177. Smith JR, Freije D, Carpten JD, Gronberg H, Xu J, Isaacs SD, Brownstein MJ, Bova GS, Guo H, Bujnovszky P, Nusskern DR, Damber JE, Bergh A, Emanuelsson M, Kallioniemi OP, Walker-Daniels J, Bailey-Wilson JE, Beaty TH, Meyers DA, Walsh PC, Collins FS, Trent JM, Isaacs WB. Major susceptibility locus for prostate cancer on chromosome 1 suggested by a genome-wide search. Science 1996;274(5291):1371–1374.
178. Monroe KR, Yu MC, Kolonel LN, Coetzee GA, Wilkens LR, Ross RK, Henderson BE. Evidence of an X-linked or recessive genetic component to prostate cancer risk. Nat Med 1995;1(8):827–829.
179. Peterson RO. The prostate. In: Biello LA, ed.Urologic pathology. Philadelphia: Lippincott,1986;613–646.
180. Tetu B, Ro JY, Ayala AG, Johnson DE, Logothetis CJ, Ordonez NG. Small-cell carcinoma of the prostate. Part I. A clinicopathologic study of 20 cases. Cancer 1987;59(10):1803–1809.
181. Epstein JI, Lieberman PH. Mucinous adenocarcinoma of the prostate gland. Am J Surg Pathol 1985;9(4):299–308.
182. Abrahamsson PA. Neuroendocrine differentiation and hormone-refractory prostate cancer. Prostate Suppl 1996;6:3–8.
183. Christensen WN, Steinberg G, Walsh PC, Epstein JI. Prostatic duct adenocarcinoma. Findings at radical prostatectomy. Cancer 1991;67(8):2118–21124.
184. Narayana AS, Loening S, Weimar GW, Culp DA. Sarcoma of the bladder and prostate. J Urol 1978;119(1):72–76.
185. Lauwers GY, Schevchuk M, Armenakas N, Reuter VE. Carcinosarcoma of the prostate. Am J Surg Pathol 1993;17(4):342–349.
186. Bostwick DG, Mann RB. Malignant lymphomas involving the prostate. A study of 13 cases. Cancer 1985;56(12):2932–2938.
187. Little NA, Wiener JS, Walther PJ, Paulson DF, Anderson EE. Squamous cell carcinoma of the prostate: 2 cases of a rare malignancy and review of the literature. J Urol 1993;149(1):137–139.
188. Kim ED, Grayhack JT. Clinical symptoms and signs of prostate cancer. In: Vogelzang NJ, Scardino PT, Shipley WU, Coffey DS, eds. Comprehensive textbook of genitourinary oncology 1. Baltimore, MD: Williams and Wilkins, 1996.
189. Schmid HP, McNeal JE, Stamey TA. Observations on the doubling time of prostate cancer. The use of serial prostate-specific antigen in patients with untreated disease as a measure of increasing cancer volume. Cancer 1993;71(6):2031–2040.
190. Chodak GW, Schoenberg HW. Early detection of prostate cancer by routine screening. JAMA 1984;252(23):3261–3264.
191. Thompson IM, Ernst JJ, Gangai MP, Spence CR. Adeno-carcinoma of the prostate: results of routine urological screening. J Urol 1984;132(4):690–692.
192. Brawer MK. The diagnosis of prostatic carcinoma. Cancer 1993;71(3 Suppl):899–905.
193. Lee F, Gray JM, McLeary RD, Lee Jr F, McHugh TA, Solomon MH, Kumasaka GH, Straub WH, Borlaza GS, Murphy GP. Prostatic evaluation by transrectal sonography: criteria for diagnosis of early carcinoma. Radiology 1986;158(1):91–95.
194. Hodge KK, McNeal JE, Terris MK, Stamey TA. Random systematic vs. directed ultrasound guided transrectal core biopsies of the prostate. J Urol 1989;142(1):71–74; discussion 74–75.
195. Terris MK, Wallen EM, Stamey TA. Comparison of mid-lobe vs. lateral systematic sextant biopsies in the detection of prostate cancer. Urol Int 1997;59(4):239–242.

196. Presti Jr JC, Chang JJ, Bhargava V, Shinohara K. The optimal systematic prostate biopsy scheme should include 8 rather than 6 biopsies: results of a prospective clinical trial. J Urol 2000; 163(1):163–166; discussion 166–167.
197. Keetch DW, Catalona WJ, Smith DS. Serial prostatic biopsies in men with persistently elevated serum prostate-specific antigen values. J Urol 1994;151(6):1571–1574.
198. Karakiewicz PI, Bazinet M, Aprikian AG, Trudel C, Aronson S, Nachabe M, Peloquint F, Dessureault J, Goyal MS, Begin LR, Elhilali MM. Outcome of sextant biopsy according to gland volume. Urology 1997;49(1):55–59.
199. Gleason DF, Mellinger GT. Prediction of prognosis for prostatic adenocarcinoma by combined histological grading and clinical staging. J Urol 1974;111(1):58–64.
200. McNeal JE, Villers AA, Redwine EA, Freiha FS, Stamey TA. Histologic differentiation, cancer volume, and pelvic lymph node metastasis in adenocarcinoma of the prostate. Cancer 1990; 66(6):1225–1233.
201. Stamey TA, Sozen TS, Yemoto CM, McNeal JE. Classification of localized untreated prostate cancer based on 791 men treated only with radical prostatectomy: common ground for therapeutic trials and TNM subgroups. J Urol 1998;159(6): 2009–2012.
202. Noguchi M, Stamey TA, Neal JE, Yemoto CE. An analysis of 148 consecutive transition zone cancers: clinical and histological characteristics. J Urol 2000;163(6):1751–1755.
203. Papsidero LD, Wang MC, Valenzuela LA, Murphy GP, Chu TM. A prostate antigen in sera of prostatic cancer patients. Cancer Res 1980;40(7):2428–2432.
204. Kuriyama M, Wang MC, Lee CI, Papsidero LD, Killian CS, Inaji H, Slack NH, Nishiura T, Murphy GP, Chu TM. Use of human prostate-specific antigen in monitoring prostate cancer. Cancer Res 1981;41(10):3874–3876.
205. Wang MC, Papsidero LD, Kuriyama M, Valenzuela LA, Murphy GP, Chu TM. Prostate antigen: a new potential marker for prostatic cancer. Prostate 1981;2(1):89–96.
206. Polascik TJ, Oesterling JE, Partin AW. Prostate-specific antigen: a decade of discovery—what we have learned and where we are going? J Urol 1999;162(2):293–306.
207. Lilja H, Christensson A, Dahlen U, Matikainen MT, Nilsson O, Pettersson K, Lovgren T. Prostate-specific antigen in serum occurs predominantly in complex with alpha 1-antichymotrypsin. Clin Chem 1991;37(9):1618–1625.
208. Stenman UH, Leinonen J, Alfthan H, Rannikko S, Tuhkanen K, Alfthan O. A complex between prostate-specific antigen and alpha 1-antichymotrypsin is the major form of prostate-specific antigen in serum of patients with prostatic cancer: assay of the complex improves clinical sensitivity for cancer. Cancer Res 1991;51(1):222–226.
209. Zhang WM, Finne P, Leinonen J, Vesalainen S, Nordling S, Rannikko S, Stenman UH. Characterization and immunological determination of the complex between prostate-specific antigen and alpha2-macroglobulin. Clin Chem 1998;44(12):2471–2479.
210. Zhang WM, Finne P, Leinonen J, Vesalainen S, Nordling S, Stenman UH. Measurement of the complex between prostate-specific antigen and alpha1-protease inhibitor in serum. Clin Chem 1999;45(6 Pt 1):814–821.
211. Christensson A, Lilja H. Complex formation between protein C inhibitor and prostate-specific antigen in vitro and in human semen. Eur J Biochem 1994;220(1):45–53.
212. Leinonen J, Zhang WM, Stenman UH. Complex formation between PSA isoenzymes and protease inhibitors. J Urol 1996;155(3):1099–1103.
213. Lilja H, Haese A, Bjork T, Friedrich MG, Piironen T, Pettersson K, Huland E, Huland H. Significance and metabolism of complexed and noncomplexed prostate-specific antigen forms, and human glandular kallikrein 2 in clinically localized prostate cancer before and after radical prostatectomy. J Urol 1999;162(6): 2029–2034; discussion 2034–2035.
214. Finne P, Auvinen A, Stenman UH. Prostate cancer screening. Lancet 2001;357(9263):1201;discussion 01–2.
215. Stamey TA, Yang N, Hay AR, McNeal JE, Freiha FS, Redwine E. Prostate-specific antigen as a serum marker for adenocarcinoma of the prostate. N Engl J Med 1987;317(15):909–916.
216. Oesterling JE, Chan DW, Epstein JI, Kimball Jr AW, Bruzek DJ, Rock RC, Brendler CB, Walsh PC. Prostate-specific antigen in the pre-operative and post-operative evaluation of localized prostatic cancer treated with radical prostatectomy. J Urol 1988;139(4):766–772.
217. Partin AW, Piantadosi S, Subong EN, Kelly CA, Hortopan S, Chan DW, Wolfert RL, Rittenhouse HG, Carter HB. Clearance rate of serum-free and total PSA following radical retropubic prostatectomy. Prostate Suppl 1996;7:35–39.
218. Bjork T, Ljungberg B, Piironen T, Abrahamsson PA, Pettersson K, Cockett AT, Lilja H. Rapid exponential elimination of free prostate-specific antigen contrasts the slow, capacity-limited elimination of PSA complexed to alpha 1-antichymotrypsin from serum. Urology 1998;51(1):57–62.
219. Pizzo SV, Mast AE, Feldman SR, Salvesen G. In vivo catabolism of alpha 1-antichymotrypsin is mediated by the Serpin receptor which binds alpha 1-proteinase inhibitor, antithrombin III, and heparin cofactor II. Biochim Biophys Acta 1988;967(2): 158–162.
220. Birkenmeier G, Struck F, Gebhardt R. Clearance mechanism of prostate-specific antigen and its complexes with alpha2-macroglobulin and alpha1-antichymotrypsin. J Urol 1999;162(3 Pt 1):897–901.
221. Nurmikko P, Vaisanen V, Piironen T, Lindgren S, Lilja H. Production and characterization of novel anti-prostate-specific antigen (PSA) monoclonal antibodies that do not detect internally cleaved Lys145-Lys146 inactive PSA. Clin Chem 2000;46 (10):1610–1618.
222. Mikolajczyk SD, Rittenhouse HG. BPSA and pPSA are complementary forms of PSA that are found, respectively, in the serum of men with benign and malignant prostate disease. J Clin Lig Assay (submitted 2001).
223. Nurmikko P, Steuber T, Haese A, Pettersson K, Hammerer P, Huland H, Lilja H. Discrimination of prostate cancer from benign disease by selective measurements in serum of subfractions of free PSA that are not internally cleaved at Lys145–Lys146. J. Ligand Assays 2001;in press.
224. Mikolajczyk SD, Graucr LS, Millar LS, Hill TM, Kumar A, Rittenhouse HG, Wolfert RL, Saedi MS. A precursor form of PSA (pPSA) is a component of the free PSA in prostate cancer serum. Urology 1997;50(5):710–714.
225. Vaisänen V, Lovgren J, Hellman J, Piironen T, Lilja H, Pettersson K. Characterization and processing of prostate-specific antigen (hK3) and human glandular kallikrein 2 (hK2) secreted by LNCaP cells. Prostate Cancer and Prostatic Diseases 1999;(2):91–97.
226. Mikolajczyk SD, Millar LS, Wang TJ, Rittenhouse HG, Wolfert RL, Marks LS, Song W, Wheeler HG, Slawin KM. "BPSA," a

specific molecular form of free prostate-specific antigen is found predominantly in the transition zone of patients with nodular benign prostatic hyperplasia. Urology 2000;55:41–45.
227. Pettersson K, Piironen T, Seppala M, Liukkonen L, Christensson A, Matikainen MT, Suonpaa M, Lovgren T, Lilja H. Free and complexed prostate-specific antigen (PSA): in vitro stability, epitope map, and development of immunofluorometric assays for specific and sensitive detection of free PSA and PSA-alpha 1-antichymotrypsin complex. Clin Chem 1995;41(10):1480–1488.
228. Piironen T, Villoutreix BO, Becker C, Hollingsworth K, Vihinen M, Bridon D, Qiu X, Rapp J, Dowell B, Lovgren T, Pettersson K, Lilja H. Determination and analysis of antigenic epitopes of prostate-specific antigen (PSA) and human glandular kallikrein 2 (hK2) using synthetic peptides and computer modeling. Protein Sci 1998;7(2):259–269.
229. Stenman UH, Paus E, Allard WJ, Andersson I, Andres C, Barnett TR, Becker C, Belenky A, Bellanger L, Pellegrino CM, Bormer OP, Davis G, Dowell B, Grauer LS, Jette DC, Karlsson B, Kreutz FT, van der Kwast TM, Lauren L, Leinimaa M, Leinonen J, Lilja H, Linton HJ, Nap M, Hilgers J, et al. Summary report of the TD-3 workshop: characterization of 83 antibodies against prostate-specific antigen. Tumor Biol 1999;20(Suppl 1):1–12.
230. Semjonow A, De Angelis G, Schmidt HP. Variability of immunoassays for PSA. In: Brawer MK, ed. Prostate-specific antigen 1. New York: Dekker, 2001.
231. Christensson A, Bjork T, Nilsson O, Dahlen U, Matikainen MT, Cockett AT, Abrahamsson PA, Lilja H. Serum prostate-specific antigen complexed to alpha 1-antichymotrypsin as an indicator of prostate cancer. J Urol 1993;150(1):100–105.
232. Allard WJ, Cheli CD, Morris DL, Goldblatt J, Pierre Y, Kish L, Chen Y, Dai J, Vessella RL, Chan DW, Schwartz MK, Zhou Z, Yeung KK. Multi-center evaluation of the performance and clinical utility in longitudinal monitoring of the Bayer Immuno 1 complexed PSA assay. Int J Biol Markers 1999;14(2):73–83.
233. Okihara K, Fritsche H, Ayala A, Johnston DA, Allard WJ, Babaian RJ. Can complexed prostate-specific antigen enhance prostate cancer detection in men with total prostate-specific antigen between 2.4 and 4 ng/mL? J Urol 2001;165:1930–1936.
234. Piironen T, Pettersson K, Suonpaa M, Stenman UH, Oesterling JE, Lovgren T, Lilja H. In vitro stability of free prostate-specific antigen (PSA) and prostate-specific antigen (PSA) complexed to alpha 1-antichymotrypsin in blood samples. Urology 1996;48(6A Suppl):81–87.
235. Woodrum D, French C, Shamel LB. Stability of free prostate-specific antigen in serum samples under a variety of sample collection and sample storage conditions. Urology 1996;48(6A):33–39.
236. Woodrum D, York L. Two-year stability of free and total PSA in frozen serum samples. Urology 1998;52(2):247–251.
237. Leinonen J, Stenman UH. Reduced stability of prostate-specific antigen after long-term storage of serum at −20 degrees C. Tumor Biol 2000;21(1):46–53.
238. Ylikoski A, Karp M, Pettersson K, Lilja H, Lövgren T. Simultaneous quantification of human glandular kallikrein 2 and prostate-specific antigen mRNAs in peripheral blood from prostate cancer patients. J Mol Diag 2001;(3):111–122.
239. Piironen T, Lovgren J, Karp M, Eerola R, Lundwall A, Dowell B, Lovgren T, Lilja H, Pettersson K. Immunofluorometric assay for sensitive and specific measurement of human prostatic glandular kallikrein (hK2) in serum. Clin Chem 1996;42(7):1034–1041.
240. Lovgren J, Valtonen-Andre C, Marsal K, Lilja H, Lundwall A. Measurement of prostate-specific antigen and human glandular kallikrein 2 in different body fluids. J Androl 1999;20(3):348–355.
241. Grauer LS, Finlay JA, Mikolajczyk SD, Pusateri KD, Wolfert RL. Detection of human glandular kallikrein, hK2, as its precursor form and in complex with protease inhibitors in prostate carcinoma serum. J Androl 1998;19(4):407–411.
242. Heeb MJ, Espana F. Alpha2-macroglobulin and C1-inactivator are plasma inhibitors of human glandular kallikrein. Blood Cells Mol Dis 1998;24(4):412–419.
243. Mikolajczyk SD, Millar LS, Marker KM, Rittenhouse HG, Wolfert RL, Marks LS, Charlesworth MC, Tindall DJ. Identification of a novel complex between human kallikrein 2 and protease inhibitor-6 in prostate cancer tissue. Cancer Res 1999;59(16):3927–3930.
244. Saedi MS, Hill TM, Kuus-Reichel K, Kumar A, Payne J, Mikolajczyk SD, Wolfert RL, Rittenhouse HG. The precursor form of the human kallikrein 2, a kallikrein homologous to prostate-specific antigen, is present in human sera and is increased in prostate cancer and benign prostatic hyperplasia. Clin Chem 1998;44(10):2115–2119.
245. Black MH, Magklara A, Obiezu CV, Melegos DN, Diamandis EP. Development of an ultrasensitive immunoassay for human glandular kallikrein with no cross-reactivity from prostate-specific antigen. Clin Chem 1999;45(6 Pt 1):790–799.
246. Becker C, Piironen T, Kiviniemi J, Lilja H, Pettersson K. Sensitive and specific immunodetection of human glandular kallikrein 2 in serum. Clin Chem 2000;46(2):198–206.
247. Darson MF, Pacelli A, Roche P, Rittenhouse HG, Wolfert RL, Young CY, Klee GG, Tindall DJ, Bostwick DG. Human glandular kallikrein 2 (hK2) expression in prostatic intraepithelial neoplasia and adenocarcinoma: a novel prostate cancer marker. Urology 1997;49(6):857–862.
248. Darson MF, Pacelli A, Roche P, Rittenhouse HG, Wolfert RL, Saeid MS, Young CY, Klee GG, Tindall DJ, Bostwick DG. Human glandular kallikrein 2 expression in prostate adenocarcinoma and lymph node metastases. Urology 1999;53(5):939–944.
249. Lovgren J, Piironen T, Overmo C, Dowell B, Karp M, Pettersson K, Lilja H, Lundwall A. Production of recombinant PSA and HK2 and analysis of their immunologic cross-reactivity. Biochem Biophys Res Commun 1995;213(3):888–895.
250. Eerola R, Piironen T, Pettersson K, Lovgren J, Vehniainen M, Lilja H, Dowell B, Lovgren T, Karp M. Immunoreactivity of recombinant human glandular kallikrein using monoclonal antibodies raised against prostate-specific antigen. Prostate 1997;31(2):84–90.
251. Finlay JA, Evans CL, Day JR, Payne JK, Mikolajczyk SD, Millar LS, Kuus-Reichel K, Wolfert RL, Rittenhouse HG. Development of monoclonal antibodies specific for human glandular kallikrein (hK2): development of a dual antibody immunoassay for hK2 with negligible prostate-specific antigen cross-reactivity. Urology 1998;51(5):804–809.
252. Klee GG, Goodmanson MK, Jacobsen SJ, Young CY, Finlay JA, Rittenhouse HG, Wolfert RL, Tindall DJ. Highly sensitive automated chemiluminometric assay for measuring free human glandular kallikrein-2. Clin Chem 1999;45(6 Pt 1): 800–806.
253. Finlay JA, Day JR, Evans CL, Carlson R, Kuus-Reichel K, Millar LS, Mikolajczyk SD, Goodmanson M, Klee GG, Rittenhouse HG. Development of a dual monoclonal antibody immunoassay for total human kallikrein 2. Clin Chem 2001;47(7):1218–1224.
254. Tepper SL, Jagirdar J, Heath D, Geller SA. Homology between the female paraurethral (Skene's) glands and the prostate.

Immunohistochemical demonstration. Arch Pathol Lab Med 1984;108(5):423–425.
255. Black MH, Diamandis EP. The diagnostic and prognostic utility of prostate-specific antigen for diseases of the breast. Breast Cancer Res Treat 2000;59(1):1–14.
256. Clements J, Mukhtar A. Glandular kallikreins and prostate-specific antigen are expressed in the human endometrium. J Clin Endocrinol Metab 1994;78(6):1536–1539.
257. Yu H, Diamandis EP, Levesque M, Asa SL, Monne M, Croce CM. Expression of the prostate-specific antigen gene by a primary ovarian carcinoma. Cancer Res 1995;55(8):1603–1606.
258. Magklara A, Scorilas A, Lopez-Otin C, Vizoso F, Ruibal A, Diamandis EP. Human glandular kallikrein in breast milk, amniotic fluid, and breast cyst fluid. Clin Chem 1999;45(10):1774–1780.
259. Melegos DN, Freedman MS, Diamandis EP. Prostate-specific antigen in cerebrospinal fluid. Clin Chem 1997;43(5):855.
260. Black MH, Magklara A, Obiezu C, Levesque MA, Sutherland DJ, Tindall DJ, Young CY, Sauter ER, Diamandis EP. Expression of a prostate-associated protein, human glandular kallikrein (hK2), in breast tumors and in normal breast secretions. Br J Cancer 2000;82(2):361–367.
261. Romas NA, Kwan DJ. Prostatic acid phosphatase. Biomolecular features and assays for serum determination. Urol Clin North Am 1993;20(4):581–588.
262. Moss DW, Raymond FD, Wile DB. Clinical and biological aspects of acid phosphatase. Crit Rev Clin Lab Sci 1995;32(4):431–467.
263. Yousef GM, Diamandis M, Jung K, Diamandis EP. Molecular cloning of a novel human acid phosphatase gene (ACPT) that is highly expressed in the testis. Genomics 2001;74(3):385–395.
264. Babaian RJ, Fritsche H, Ayala A, Bhadkamkar V, Johnston DA, Naccarato W, Zhang Z. Performance of a neural network in detecting prostate cancer in the prostate-specific antigen reflex range of 2.5 to 4.0 ng/mL. Urology 2000;56(6):1000–1006.
265. Han M, Piantadosi S, Zahurak ML, Sokoll LJ, Chan DW, Epstein JI, Walsh PC, Partin AW. Serum acid phosphatase level and biochemical recurrence following radical prostatectomy for men with clinically localized prostate cancer. Urology 2001;57(4):707–711.
266. Dattoli M, Wallner K, True L, Sorace R, Koval J, Cash J, Acosta R, Biswas M, Binder M, Sullivan B, Lastarria E, Kirwan N, Stein D. Prognostic role of serum prostatic acid phosphatase for 103Pd-based radiation for prostatic carcinoma. Int J Radiat Oncol Biol Phys 1999;45(4):853–856.
267. Horoszewicz JS, Kawinski E, Murphy GP. Monoclonal antibodies to a new antigenic marker in epithelial prostatic cells and serum of prostatic cancer patients. Anticancer Res 1987;7(5B):927–935.
268. Chang SS, Gaudin PB, Reuter VE, Heston WD. Prostate-specific membrane antigen: present and future applications. Urology 2000;55(5):622–629.
269. Gong MC, Chang SS, Sadelain M, Bander NH, Heston WD. Prostate-specific membrane antigen (PSMA)-specific monoclonal antibodies in the treatment of prostate and other cancers. Cancer Metastasis Rev 1999;18(4):483–490.
270. Elgamal AA, Holmes EH, Su SL, Tino WT, Simmons SJ, Peterson M, Greene TG, Boynton AL, Murphy GP. Prostate-specific membrane antigen (PSMA): current benefits and future value. Semin Surg Oncol 2000;18(1):10–16.
271. Gong MC, Latouche JB, Krause A, Heston WD, Bander NH, Sadelain M. Cancer patient T cells genetically targeted to prostate-specific membrane antigen specifically lyse prostate cancer cells and release cytokines in response to prostate-specific membrane antigen. Neoplasia 1999;1(2):123–127.
272. Tjoa BA, Simmons SJ, Bowes VA, Ragde H, Rogers M, Elgamal A, Kenny GM, Cobb OE, Ireton RC, Troychak MJ, Salgaller ML, Boynton AL, Murphy GP. Evaluation of phase I/II clinical trials in prostate cancer with dendritic cells and PSMA peptides. Prostate 1998;36(1):39–44.
273. Heston WD. Characterization and glutamyl preferring carboxypeptidase function of prostate-specific membrane antigen: a novel folate hydrolase. Urology 1997;49(3A Suppl):104–112.
274. Liu H, Rajasekaran AK, Moy P, Xia Y, Kim S, Navarro V, Rahmati R, Bander NH. Constitutive and antibody-induced internalization of prostate-specific membrane antigen. Cancer Res 1998;58(18):4055–4060.
275. Cude KJ, Dixon SC, Guo Y, Lisella J, Figg WD. The androgen receptor: genetic considerations in the development and treatment of prostate cancer. J Mol Med 1999;77(5):419–426.
276. Jenster G. The role of the androgen receptor in the development and progression of prostate cancer. Semin Oncol 1999;26(4):407–421.
277. Culig Z, Hobisch A, Bartsch G, Klocker H. Androgen receptor—an update of mechanisms of action in prostate cancer. Urol Res 2000;28(4):211–219.
278. Elo JP, Visakorpi T. Molecular genetics of prostate cancer. Ann Med 2001;33(2):130–141.
279. Mhatre AN, Trifiro MA, Kaufman M, Kazemi-Esfarjani P, Figlewicz D, Rouleau G, Pinsky L. Reduced transcriptional regulatory competence of the androgen receptor in X-linked spinal and bulbar muscular atrophy. Nat Genet 1993;5(2):184–188.
280. Chamberlain, NL, Driver ED, Miesfeld RL. The length and location of CAG trinucleotide repeats in the androgen receptor N-terminal domain affect transactivation function. Nucleic Acids Res 1994;22(15):3181–3186.
281. Schoenberg MP, Hakimi JM, Wang S, Bova GS, Epstein JI, Fischbeck KH, Isaacs WB, Walsh PC, Barrack ER. Microsatellite mutation (CAG24–>18) in the androgen receptor gene in human prostate cancer. Biochem Biophys Res Commun 1994;198(1):74–80.
282. Hardy DO, Scher HI, Bogenreider T, Sabbatini P, Zhang ZF, Nanus DM, Catterall JF. Androgen receptor CAG repeat lengths in prostate cancer: correlation with age of onset. J Clin Endocrinol Metab 1996;81(12):4400–4405.
283. Bharaj BS, Vassilikos EJ, Diamandis EP. Rapid and accurate determination of (CAG)n repeats in the androgen receptor gene using polymerase chain reaction and automated fragment analysis. Clin Biochem 1999;32(5):327–332.
284. Gottlieb B, Beitel LK, Trifiro MA. Variable expressivity and mutation databases: the androgen receptor gene mutations database. Hum Mutat 2001;17(5):382–388.
285. Tilley WD, Buchanan G, Hickey TE, Bentel JM. Mutations in the androgen receptor gene are associated with progression of human prostate cancer to androgen independence. Clin Cancer Res 1996;2(2):277–285.
286. Buchanan G, Greenberg NM, Scher HI, Harris JM, Marshall VR, Tilley WD. Collocation of androgen receptor gene mutations in prostate cancer. Clin Cancer Res 2001;7(5):1273–1281.
287. Visakorpi T, Hyytinen E, Koivisto P, Tanner M, Keinanen R, Palmberg C, Palotie A, Tammela T, Isola J, Kallioniemi OP. In vivo amplification of the androgen receptor gene and progression of human prostate cancer. Nat Genet 1995;9(4):401–406.

288. Koivisto P, Kononen J, Palmberg C, Tammela T, Hyytinen E, Isola J, Trapman J, Cleutjens K, Noordzij A, Visakorpi T, Kallioniemi OP. Androgen receptor gene amplification: a possible molecular mechanism for androgen deprivation therapy failure in prostate cancer. Cancer Res 1997;57(2):314–319.
289. Chan JM, Stampfer MJ, Giovannucci E, Gann PH, Ma J, Wilkinson P, Hennekens CH, Pollak M. Plasma insulin-like growth factor-I and prostate cancer risk: a prospective study. Science 1998;279(5350):563–566.
290. Hankinson SE, Willett WC, Colditz GA, Hunter DJ, Michaud DS, Deroo B, Rosner B, Speizer FE, Pollak M. Circulating concentrations of insulin-like growth factor-I and risk of breast cancer. Lancet 1998;351(9113):1393–1396.
291. Stattin P, Bylund A, Rinaldi S, Biessy C, Dechaud H, Stenman UH, Egevad L, Riboli E, Hallmans G, Kaaks R. Plasma insulin-like growth factor-I, insulin-like growth factor-binding proteins, and prostate cancer risk: a prospective study. J Natl Cancer Inst 2000;92(23):1910–1917.
292. Finne P, Auvinen A, Koistinen H, Zhang WM, Maattanen L, Rannikko S, Tammela T, Seppala M, Hakama M, Stenman UH. Insulin-like growth factor I is not a useful marker of prostate cancer in men with elevated levels of prostate-specific antigen. J Clin Endocrinol Metab 2000;85(8):2744–2747.
293. Grimberg A, Cohen P. Role of insulin-like growth factors and their binding proteins in growth control and carcinogenesis. J Cell Physiol 2000;183(1):1–9.
294. Giovannucci E. Insulin-like growth factor-I and binding protein-3 and risk of cancer. Horm Res 1999;51(Suppl 3):34–41.
295. Wolk A, Andersson SO, Mantzoros CS, Trichopoulos D, Adami HO. Can measurements of IGF-1 and IGFBP-3 improve the sensitivity of prostate-cancer screening? Lancet 2000;356(9245):1902–1903.
296. Djavan B, Bursa B, Seitz C, Soeregi G, Remzi M, Basharkhah A, Wolfram R, Marberger M. Insulin-like growth factor 1 (IGF-1), IGF-1 density, and IGF-1/PSA ratio for prostate cancer detection. Urology 1999;54(4):603–606.
297. Harman SM, Metter EJ, Blackman MR, Landis PK, Carter HB. Serum levels of insulin-like growth factor I (IGF-I), IGF-II, IGF-binding protein-3, and prostate-specific antigen as predictors of clinical prostate cancer. J Clin Endocrinol Metab 2000;85(11):4258–4265.
298. Yu H, Nicar MR, Shi R, Berkel HJ, Nam R, Trachtenberg J, Diamandis EP. Levels of insulin-like growth factor I (IGF-I) and IGF binding proteins 2 and 3 in serial post-operative serum samples and risk of prostate cancer recurrence. Urology 2001;57(3):471–475.
299. Kurek R, Tunn UW, Eckart O, Aumuller G, Wong J, Renneberg H. The significance of serum levels of insulin-like growth factor-1 in patients with prostate cancer. BJU Int 2000;85(1):125–129.
300. Partin AW, Carter HB, Chan DW, Epstein JI, Oesterling JE, Rock RC, Weber JP, Walsh PC. Prostate-specific antigen in the staging of localized prostate cancer: influence of tumor differentiation, tumor volume, and benign hyperplasia. J Urol 1990;143(4):747–752.
301. Stamey TA, Kabalin JN, McNeal JE, Johnstone IM, Freiha F, Redwine EA, Yang N. Prostate-specific antigen in the diagnosis and treatment of adenocarcinoma of the prostate. II. Radical prostatectomy treated patients. J Urol 1989;141(5):1076–1083.
302. Guess HA, Heyse JF, Gormley GJ, Stoner E, Oesterling JE. Effect of finasteride on serum PSA concentration in men with benign prostatic hyperplasia. Results from the North American phase III clinical trial. Urol Clin North Am 1993;20(4):627–636.
303. Pannek J, Marks LS, Pearson JD, Rittenhouse HG, Chan DW, Shery ED, Gormley GJ, Subong EN, Kelley CA, Stoner E, Partin AW. Influence of finasteride on free and total serum prostate-specific antigen levels in men with benign prostatic hyperplasia. J Urol 1998;159(2):449–453.
304. Gormley GJ, Ng J, Cook T, Stoner E, Guess H, Walsh P. Effect of finasteride on prostate-specific antigen density. Urology 1994;43(1):53–58;discussion 58–59.
305. Roehrborn CG, Oesterling JE, Olson PJ, Padley RJ. Serial prostate-specific antigen measurements in men with clinically benign prostatic hyperplasia during a 12-month placebo-controlled study with terazosin. HYCAT Investigator Group. Hytrin Community Assessment Trial. Urology 1997;50(4):556–561.
306. Carter HB, Pearson JD. PSA velocity for the diagnosis of early prostate cancer. A new concept. Urol Clin North Am 1993;20(4):665–670.
307. Benson, MC, Whang IS, Olsson CA, McMahon DJ, Cooner WH. The use of prostate-specific antigen density to enhance the predictive value of intermediate levels of serum prostate-specific antigen. J Urol 1992;147(3 Pt 2):817–821.
308. Djavan B, Zlotta AR, Byttebier G, Shariat S, Omar M, Schulman CC, Marberger M. Prostate-specific antigen density of the transition zone for early detection of prostate cancer. J Urol 1998;160(2):411–418;discussion 418–419.
309. Oesterling JE. Age-specific reference ranges for serum PSA. N Engl J Med 1996; 335(5):345–346.
310. Nadler RB, Humphrey PA, Smith DS, Catalona WJ, Ratliff TL. Effect of inflammation and benign prostatic hyperplasia on elevated serum prostate-specific antigen levels. J Urol 1995;154(2 Pt 1):407–413.
311. Hoekx L, Jeuris W, Van Marck E, Wyndaele JJ. Elevated serum prostate-specific antigen (PSA) related to asymptomatic prostatic inflammation. Acta Urol Belg 1998;66(3):1–2.
312. Ramos CG, Carvahal GF, Mager DE, Haberer B, Catalona WJ. The effect of high-grade prostatic intraepithelial neoplasia on serum total and percentage of free prostate-specific antigen levels. J Urol 1999;162(5):1587–1590.
313. Mettlin CJ, Murphy GP, Ho R, Menck HR. The National Cancer Data Base report on longitudinal observations on prostate cancer. Cancer 1996;77(10):2162–2166.
314. Wingo PA, Landis S, Ries LA. An adjustment to the 1997 estimate for new prostate cancer cases. Cancer 1997;80(9):1810–1813.
315. Plawker MW, Fleisher JM, Vapnek EM, Macchia RJ. Current trends in prostate cancer diagnosis and staging among United States urologists. J Urol 1997;158(5):1853–1858.
316. Ito K, Kubota Y, Suzuki K, Shimizu N, Fukabori Y, Kurokawa K, Imai K, Yamanaka H. Correlation of prostate-specific antigen before prostate cancer detection and clinicopathologic features: evaluation of mass screening populations. Urology 2000;55(5):705–709.
317. Partin AW, Kattan MW, Subong EN, Walsh PC, Wojno KJ, Oesterling JE, Scardino PT, Pearson JD. Combination of prostate-specific antigen, clinical stage, and Gleason score to predict pathological stage of localized prostate cancer. A multi-institutional update. JAMA 1997;277(18):1445–1451.
318. Partin AW, Mangold LA, Lamm DM, Walsh PC, Epstein JI, Pearson J. Contemporary update of prostate cancer-staging nomograms (Partin Tables) for the new millenium. Urology 2001;58(6):843–848.
319. Catalona WJ, Richie JP, Ahmann FR, Hudson MA, Scardino PT, Flanigan RC, deKernion JB, Ratliff TL, Kavoussi LR, Dalkin BL,

et al. Comparison of digital rectal examination and serum prostate-specific antigen in the early detection of prostate cancer: results of a multi-center clinical trial of 6,630 men. J Urol 1994;151(5):1283–1290.
320. Gann PH, Hennekens CH, Stampfer MJ. A prospective evaluation of plasma prostate-specific antigen for detection of prostatic cancer. JAMA 1995;273(4):289–294.
321. Epstein JI, Chan DW, Sokoll LJ, Walsh PC, Cox JL, Rittenhouse H, Wolfert R, Carter HB. Nonpalpable stage T1c prostate cancer: prediction of insignificant disease using free/total prostate-specific antigen levels and needle biopsy findings. J Urol 1998;160(6 Pt 2):2407–2411.
322. Belville WD. Are T1c tumors different from incidental tumors found at autopsy? The risk and reality of overdetection. Semin Urol Oncol 1995;13(3):181–186.
323. Catalona WJ, Smith DS, Ratliff TL, Basler JW. Detection of organ-confined prostate cancer is increased through prostate-specific antigen-based screening. JAMA 1993;270(8):948–954.
324. Mettlin C, Murphy GP, Lee F, Littrup PJ, Chesley A, Babaian R, Badalament R, Kane RA, Mostofi FK. Characteristics of prostate cancer detected in the American Cancer Society-National Prostate Cancer Detection Project. J Urol 1994;152(5 Pt 2): 1737–1740.
325. Herschman JD, Smith DS, Catalona WJ. Effect of ejaculation on serum total and free prostate-specific antigen concentrations. Urology 1997;50(2):239–243.
326. Oesterling JE, Rice DC, Glenski WJ, Bergstralh EJ. Effect of cystoscopy, prostate biopsy, and transurethral resection of prostate on serum prostate-specific antigen concentration. Urology 1993;42(3):276–282.
327. Catalona WJ, Smith DS, Ratliff TL, Dodds KM, Coplen DE, Yuan JJ, Petros JA, Andriole GL. Measurement of prostate-specific antigen in serum as a screening test for prostate cancer. N Engl J Med 1991;324(17):1156–1161.
328. Catalona WJ, Smith DS, Ornstein DK. Prostate cancer detection in men with serum PSA concentrations of 2.6 to 4.0 ng/mL and benign prostate examination. Enhancement of specificity with free PSA measurements. JAMA 1997;277(18):1452–1455.
329. Schroder FH, van der Cruijsen-Koeter I, de Koning HJ, Vis AN, Hoedemaeker RF, Kranse R. Prostate cancer detection at low prostate-specific antigen. J Urol 2000; 163(3):806–812.
330. Lodding P, Aus G, Bergdahl S, Frosing R, Lilja H, Pihl CG, Hugosson J. Characteristics of screening detected prostate cancer in men 50 to 66 years old with 3 to 4 ng/mL. Prostate-specific antigen. J Urol 1998;159(3):899–903.
331. Cooner WH, Mosley BR, Rutherford Jr CL, Beard JH, Pond HS, Terry WJ, Igel TC, Kidd DD. Prostate cancer detection in a clinical urological practice by ultrasonography, digital rectal examination, and prostate-specific antigen. J Urol 1990;143(6): 1146–1152; discussion 1152–1154.
332. Ellis WJ, Chetner MP, Preston SD, Brawer MK. Diagnosis of prostatic carcinoma: the yield of serum prostate-specific antigen, digital rectal examination, and transrectal ultrasonography. J Urol 1994;152(5 Pt 1):1520–1525.
333. Hammerer P, Huland H. Systematic sextant biopsies in 651 patients referred for prostate evaluation. J Urol 1994;151(1): 99–102.
334. Luderer AA, Chen YT, Soriano TF, Kramp WJ, Carlson G, Cuny C, Sharp T, Smith W, Petteway J, Brawer MK, et al. Measurement of the proportion of free to total prostate-specific antigen improves diagnostic performance of prostate-specific antigen in the diagnostic gray zone of total prostate-specific antigen. Urology 1995;46(2):187–194.
335. Prestigiacomo AF, Lilja H, Pettersson K, Wolfert RL, Stamey TA. A comparison of the free fraction of serum prostate-specific antigen in men with benign and cancerous prostates: the best case scenario. J Urol 1996;156(2 Pt 1):350–354.
336. Catalona WJ, Partin AW, Slawin KM, Brawer MK, Flanigan RC, Patel A, Richie JP, deKernion JB, Walsh PC, Scardino PT, Lange PH, Subong EN, Parson RE, Gasior GH, Loveland KG, Southwick PC. Use of the percentage of free prostate-specific antigen to enhance differentiation of prostate cancer from benign prostatic disease: a prospective multicenter clinical trial. JAMA 1998;279(19):1542–1547.
337. Fowler Jr JE, Sanders J, Bigler SA, Rigdon J, Kilambi NK, Land SA. Percent free prostate-specific antigen and cancer detection in black and white men with total prostate-specific antigen 2.5 to 9.9 ng/mL. J Urol 2000;163(5):1467–1470.
338. Carter HB, Partin AW, Luderer AA, Metter EJ, Landis P, Chan DW, Fozard JL, Pearson JD. Percentage of free prostate-specific antigen in sera predicts aggressiveness of prostate cancer a decade before diagnosis. Urology 1997;49(3):379–384.
339. Lynn NN, Collins GN, O´Reilly PH. Prostatic manipulation has minimal effect on complexed prostate-specific antigen levels. BJU Int 2000;86:65–67.
340. Nixon RG, Wener MH, Smith KMB. Biological variation of prostate-specific antigen levels in serum: an evaluation of day-to-day physiological fluctuations in a well-defined cohort of 24 patients. J Urol 1997;157:2183–2190.
341. Haese A, Graefen M, Noldus J, Hammerer P, Huland E, Huland H. Prostatic volume and ratio of free-to-total prostate-specific antigen in patients with prostatic cancer or benign prostatic hyperplasia. J Urol 1997;158(6):2188–2192.
342. Partin AW, Catalona WJ, Southwick PC, Subong EN, Gasior GH, Chan DW. Analysis of percent free prostate-specific antigen (PSA) for prostate cancer detection: influence of total PSA, prostate volume, and age. Urology 1996;48:55–61.
343. Mitchell IDC, Croal BL, Dickie A, Cohen NP, Ross IA. pros-pective study to evaluate the role of complexed prostate-specific antigen and free/total prostate-specific antigen ratio for the diagnosis of prostate cancer. J Urol 2001;165: 1549–1553.
344. Brawer MK, Cheli CD, Neaman IE, Goldblatt J, Smith C, Schwartz MK, Bruzek DJ, Morris DL, Sokoll LJ, Chan DW, Yeung KK, Partin AW, Allard WJ. Complexed prostate-specific antigen provides significant enhancement of specificity compared with total prostate-specific antigen for detecting prostate cancer. J Urol 2000;163:1476–1480.
345. Okegawa T, Noda H, Nutahara K, Higashihara E. Comparison of two investigative assays for the complexed prostate-specific antigen in total prostate-specific antigen between 4.1 and 10ng/mL. Urology 2000;55:700–704.
346. Filella X, Alcover J, Molina R, Corral JM, Carretero P, Ballesta AM. Measurement of complexed PSA in the differential diagnosis between prostate cancer and benign prostate hyperplasia. Prostate 2000;42(3):181–185.
347. Stamey TA, Yemoto CE. Examination of the 3 molecular forms of serum prostate-specific antigen for distinguishing negative from positive biopsy: relationship to transition zone volume. J Urol 2000;163(1):119–126.
348. Miller MC, O'Dowd GJ, Partin AW, Veltri RW. Contemporary use of complexed PSA and calculated percent free PSA for early detection of prostate cancer: impact of changing disease demographics. Urology 2001;57(6):1105–1111.
349. Mikolajczyk SD, Millar LS, Wang TJ, Rittenhouse HG, Marks LS, Song W, Wheeler TM, Slawin KM. A precursor form of

349. prostate-specific antigen is more highly elevated in prostate cancer compared with benign transition zone prostate tissue. Cancer Res 2000;60:756–759.
350. Nurmikko P, Pettersson K, Piironen T, Hugosson J, Lilja H. Discrimination of prostate cancer from benign disease by plasma measurement of intact, free prostate-specific antigen lacking an internal cleavage site at Lys145-Lys146. Clin Chem 2001; 47(8): 1415–1423.
351. Seaman E, Whang IS, Olsson CA, Katz AE, Cooner WH, Benson M. PSA-density (PSAD). Role in patient evaluation and management. Urol Clin North Am 1993;20:635.
352. Catalona WJ, Richie JP, de Kernion JB, Ahmann FR, Ratliff TL, Dalkin BL, Kavoussi LR, Mac Farlane MT, Southwick PC. Comparison of prostate-specific antigen concentration vs. prostate-specific antigen density in the early detection of prostate cancer: receiver operator characteristic curves. J Urol 1994;152: 2031.
353. Brawer MK, Aramburu EAG, Chen GL, Preston SD, Ellis WJ. The inability of prostate-specific antigen index to enhance the predictive value of prostate-specific antigen in the diagnosis of prostatic carcinoma. J Urol 1993;150:369.
354. Djavan B, Marberger M, Zlotta AR, Schulman CC. PSA, f/tPSA, PSAD, PSA-TZ and PSA-velocity for prostate cancer prediction: a multivariate analysis. J Urol 1998;159:898(A).
355. Partin AW, Criley SR, Subong EN, Zincke H, Walsh PC, Oesterling JE. Standard vs. age-specific prostate-specific antigen reference ranges among men with clinically localized prostate cancer: a pathological analysis. J Urol 1996;155:1336.
356. Reissigl A, Pointner J, Horninger W, Ennemoser O, Strasser H, Klocker H, Bartsch G. Comparison of different prostate-specific antigen cutpoints for early detection of prostate cancer: results of a large screening study. Urology 1995;46:662.
357. Littrup PJ, Kane RA, Mettlin C, Murphy GP, Lee F, Toi A, Badalament R, Babaian R, and Investigators of the American Cancer Society National Prostate Cancer Detection Project. Cost-effective prostate cancer detection. Reduction of low-yield biopsies. Cancer 1994;74:3146.
358. Oesterling JE, Kumamoto Y, Tsukamoto T, Girman CJ, Guess H, Masumori N, Jacobsen SJ, Lieber MM. Serum prostate-specific antigen in a community-based population of healthy Japanese men: lower values than for similarly aged white men. Br J Urol 1995;75:347.
359. Morgan TO, Jacobsen SJ, McCarthy WF, Jacobson DJ, McLeod DG, Moul JW. Age-specific reference ranges for prostate-specific antigen in black men. N Engl J Med 1996;335:304.
360. Partin AW, Catalona WJ, Finlay JA, Darte C, Tindall DJ, Young CY, Klee GG, Chan DW, Rittenhouse HG, Wolfert RL, Woodrum DL. Use of human glandular kallikrein 2 for the detection of prostate cancer: preliminary analysis. Urology 1999;54(5): 839–845.
361. Becker C, Piironen T, Pettersson K, Bjork T, Wojno KJ, Oesterling JE, Lilja H. Discrimination of men with prostate cancer from those with benign disease by measurements of human glandular kallikrein 2 (HK2) in serum. J Urol 2000;163(1):311–316.
362. Nam RK, Diamandis EP, Toi A, Trachtenberg J, Magklara A, Scorilas A, Papnastasiou PA, Jewett MA, Narod SA. Serum human glandular kallikrein-2 protease levels predict the presence of prostate cancer among men with elevated prostate-specific antigen. J Clin Oncol 2000;18(5):1036–1042.
363. Klee GG, Young CY, Tindall DJ. Human glandular kallikrein protein. In: Brawer MK, ed. Prostate-specific antigen 1. New York: Dekker, 2001:283–296.
364. Hanks GE, Perez CA, Kozar M, Asbell SO, Pilepich MV, Pajak TF. PSA confirmation of cure at 10 years of T1B, T2, N0, M0 prostate cancer patients treated in RTOG protocol 7706 with external beam irradiation. Int J Radiat Oncol Biol Phys 1994;30(2):289–292.
365. Lerner SE, Jacobsen SJ, Lilja H, Bergstralh EJ, Ransom J, Klee GG, Piironen T, Blute ML, Lieber MM, Zincke H, Pettersson K, Peterson D, Oesterling JE. Free, complexed, and total serum prostate-specific antigen concentrations and their proportions in predicting stage, grade, and deoxyribonucleic acid ploidy in patients with adenocarcinoma of the prostate. Urology 1996;48(2):240–248.
366. Narayan P, Gajendran V, Taylor SP, Tewari A, Presti Jr JC, Leidich R, Lo R, Palmer K, Shinohara K, Spaulding JT. The role of transrectal ultrasound-guided biopsy-based staging, pre-operative serum prostate-specific antigen, and biopsy Gleason score in prediction of final pathologic diagnosis in prostate cancer. Urology 1995;46(2):205–212.
367. Magklara A, Scorilas A, Catalona WJ, Diamandis EP. The combination of human glandular kallikrein and free prostate-specific antigen (PSA) enhances discrimination between prostate cancer and benign prostatic hyperplasia in patients with moderately increased total PSA. Clin Chem 1999;45(11):1960–1966.
368. Kwiatkowski MK, Recker F, Piironen T, Pettersson K, Otto T, Wernli M, Tscholl R. In prostatism patients the ratio of human glandular kallikrein to free PSA improves the discrimination between prostate cancer and benign hyperplasia within the diagnostic "gray zone" of total PSA 4 to 10 ng/mL. Urology 1998; 52(3):360–365.
369. Becker C, Piironen T, Pettersson K, Hugosson J, Lilja H. Clinical value of human glandular kallikrein 2 and free and total prostate-specific antigen in serum from a population of men with prostate-specific antigen levels 3.0 ng/mL or greater. Urology 2000; 55(5):694–699.
370. Epstein JI, Pizov G, Walsh PC. Correlation of pathologic findings with progression after radical retropubic prostatectomy. Cancer 1993;71(11):3582–3593.
371. Pound CR, Partin AW, Epstein JI, Walsh PC. Prostate-specific antigen after anatomic radical retropubic prostatectomy. Patterns of recurrence and cancer control. Urol Clin North Am 1997;24(2):395–406.
372. McNeal JE, Villers AA, Redwine EA, Freiha FS, Stamey TA. Capsular penetration in prostate cancer. Significance for natural history and treatment. Am J Surg Pathol 1990; 14(3): 240–247.
373. Partin AW, Yoo J, Carter HB, Pearson JD, Chan DW, Epstein JI, Walsh PC. The use of prostate-specific antigen, clinical stage, and Gleason score to predict pathological stage in men with localized prostate cancer. J Urol 1993;150(1):110–114.
374. Chybowski FM, Keller JJ, Bergstralh EJ, Oesterling JE. Predicting radionuclide bone scan findings in patients with newly diagnosed, untreated prostate cancer: prostate-specific antigen is superior to all other clinical parameters. J Urol 1991; 145(2):313–318.
375. Noldus J, Graefen M, Huland E, Busch C, Hammerer P, Huland H. The value of the ratio of free-to-total prostate-specific antigen for staging purposes in previously untreated prostate cancer. J Urol 1998;159(6):2004–2007;discussion 2007–2008.
376. Hara I, Miyake H, Hara S, Yamanaka N, Ono Y, Eto H, Takechi Y, Arakawa S, Kamidono S. Value of the serum prostate-specific antigen-alpha 1-antichymotrypsin complex and its density as a predictor for the extent of prostate cancer. BJU Int 2001;88(1): 53–57.

377. Kuriyama M, Ueno K, Uno H, Kawada Y, Akimoto S, Noda M, Nasu Y, Tsushima T, Ohmori H, Sakai H, Saito Y, Meguro N, Usami M, Kotake T, Suzuki Y, Arai Y, Shimazaki J. Clinical evaluation of serum prostate-specific antigen-alpha1-antichymotrypsin complex values in diagnosis of prostate cancer: a cooperative study. Int J Urol 1998;5(1):48–54.
378. Graefen M, Haese A, Pichlmeier U, Hammerer PG, Noldus J, Butz K, Erbersdobler A, Henke RP, Michl U, Fernandez S, Huland H. A validated strategy for side-specific prediction of organ confined prostate cancer: a tool to select for nerve sparing radical prostatectomy. J Urol 2001;165(3):857–863.
379. Haese A, Becker C, Noldus J, Graefen M, Huland E, Huland H, Lilja H. Human glandular kallikrein 2: a potential serum marker for predicting the organ confined vs. non-organ-confined growth of prostate cancer. J Urol 2000;163(5):1491–1497.
380. Haese A, Graefen M, Steuber T, Becker C, Pettersson K, Piironen T, Noldus J, Huland H, Lilja H. Human glandular kallikrein 2 levels in serum for discrimination of pathologically organ-confined from locally advanced prostate cancer in total PSA levels below 10 ng/mL. Prostate 2001;49(2):101–109.
381. Recker F, Kwiatkowski MK, Piironen T, Pettersson K, Huber A, Lummen G, Tscholl R. Human glandular kallikrein as a tool to improve discrimination of poorly differentiated and non-organ-confined prostate cancer compared with prostate-specific antigen. Urology 2000;55(4):481–485.
382. Lu-Yao GL, McLerran D, Wasson J, Wennberg JE. An assessment of radical prostatectomy. Time trends, geographic variation, and outcomes. The Prostate Patient Outcomes Research Team. JAMA 1993;269(20):2633–2636.
383. Gee WF, Holtgrewe HL, Blute ML, Miles BJ, Naslund MJ, Nellans RE, O'Leary MP, Thomas R, Painter MR, Mcycr JJ, Rohner TJ, Cooper TP, Blizzard R, Fenninger RB, Emmons L. 1997 American Urological Association Gallup survey: changes in diagnosis and management of prostate cancer and benign prostatic hyperplasia, and other practice trends from 1994 to 1997. J Urol 1998;160(5):1804–1807.
384. Pound CR, Partin AW, Eisenberger MA, Chan DW, Pearson JD, Walsh PC. Natural history of progression after PSA elevation following radical prostatectomy. JAMA 1999;281(17): 1591–1597.
385. Oh J, Colberg JW, Ornstein DK, Johnson ET, Chan D, Virgo KS, Johnson FE. Current follow-up strategies after radical prostatectomy: a survey of American Urological Association urologists. J Urol 1999;161(2):520–523.
386. Lange PH, Ercole CJ, Lightner DJ, Fraley EE, Vessella R. The value of serum prostate-specific antigen determinations before and after radical prostatectomy. J Urol 1989;141(4):873–879.
387. Stamey TA, Graves HC, Wehner N, Ferrari M, Freiha FS. Early detection of residual prostate cancer after radical prostatectomy by an ultrasensitive assay for prostate-specific antigen. J Urol 1993;149(4):787–792.
388. Haese A, Huland E, Graefen M, Hammerer P, Noldus J, Huland H. Ultrasensitive detection of prostate-specific antigen in the followup of 422 patients after radical prostatectomy. J Urol 1999;161(4):1206–1211.
389. Zincke H, Oesterling JE, Blute ML, Bergstralh EJ, Myers RP, Barrett DM. Long-term (15 years) results after radical prostatectomy for clinically localized (stage T2c or lower) prostate cancer. J Urol 1994;152(5 Pt 2):1850–1857.
390. Kattan MW, Wheeler TM, Scardino PT. Post-operative nomogram for disease recurrence after radical prostatectomy for prostate cancer. J Clin Oncol 1999;17(5):1499–1507.
391. Partin AW, Pearson JD, Landis PK, Carter HB, Pound CR, Clemens JQ, Epstein JI, Walsh PC. Evaluation of serum prostate-specific antigen velocity after radical prostatectomy to distinguish local recurrence from distant metastases. Urology 1994; 43(5):649–659.
392. Bruchowsky N. Androgens and anti-androgens. In: Holland JF, Frei E, Bast RC, et al, eds. Cancer medicine. Philadelphia: Lea & Fibiger, 1993:884–896.
393. Isaacs JT, Coffey DS. Adaptation vs. selection as the mechanism responsible for the relapse of prostatic cancer to androgen ablation therapy as studied in the Dunning R-3327-H adenocarcinoma. Cancer Res 1981;41(12 Pt 1):5070–5075.
394. Gleave ME, Goldenberg SL, Jones EC, Bruchovsky N, Sullivan LD. Biochemical and pathological effects of 8 months of neoadjuvant androgen withdrawal therapy before radical prostatectomy in patients with clinically confined prostate cancer. J Urol 1996; 155(1):213–219.
395. Miller JI, Ahmann FR, Drach GW, Emerson SS, Bottaccini MR. The clinical usefulness of serum prostate-specific antigen after hormonal therapy of metastatic prostate cancer. J Urol 1992;147 (3 Pt 2):956–961.
396. Bruchovsky N, Goldenberg SL, Akakura K, Rennie PS. Luteinizing hormone-releasing hormone agonists in prostate cancer. Elimination of flare reaction by pretreatment with cyproterone acetate and low-dose diethylstilbestrol. Cancer 1993; 72(5):1685–1691.
397. Isaacs JT, Wake N, Coffey DS, Sandberg AA. Genetic instability coupled to clonal selection as a mechanism for tumor progression in the Dunning R-3327 rat prostatic adenocarcinoma system. Cancer Res 1982;42(6):2353–2371.
398. Isaacs JT. The timing of androgen ablation therapy and/or chemotherapy in the treatment of prostatic cancer. Prostate 1984; 5(1):1–17.
399. Hsieh JT, Wu HC, Gleave ME, von Eschenbach AC, Chung LW. Autocrine regulation of prostate-specific antigen gene expression in a human prostatic cancer (LNCaP) subline. Cancer Res 1993; 53(12):2852–2857.
400. Nickerson T, Miyake H, Gleave ME, Pollak M. Castration-induced apoptosis of androgen-dependent shionogi carcinoma is associated with increased expression of genes encoding insulin-like growth factor-binding proteins. Cancer Res 1999;59(14): 3392 3395.
401. Taplin ME, Bubley GJ, Shuster TD, Frantz ME, Spooner AE, Ogata GK, Keer HN, Balk SP. Mutation of the androgen-receptor gene in metastatic androgen-independent prostate cancer. N Engl J Med 1995;332(21):1393–1398.
402. Zietman AL, Coen JJ, Shipley WU, Willett CG, Efird JT. Radical radiation therapy in the management of prostatic adenocarcinoma: the initial prostate-specific antigen value as a predictor of treatment outcome. J Urol 1994;151(3):640–645.
403. Kuban DA, el-Mahdi AM, Schellhammer PF. Prostate-specific antigen for pretreatment prediction and posttreatment evaluation of outcome after definitive irradiation for prostate cancer. Int J Radiat Oncol Biol Phys 1995;32(2):307–316.
404. Lee WR, Hanks GE, Schultheiss TE, Corn BW, Hunt MA. Localized prostate cancer treated by external-beam radiotherapy alone: serum prostate-specific antigen-driven outcome analysis. J Clin Oncol 1995;13(2):464–469.
405. Preston DM, Bauer JJ, Connelly RR, Sawyer T, Halligan J, Leifer ES, McLeod DG, Moul JW. Prostate-specific antigen to predict outcome of external beam radiation for prostate cancer: Walter

Reed Army Medical Center experience, 1988–1995. Urology 1999;53(1):131–138.
406. Crook J, Malone S, Perry G, Bahadur Y, Robertson S, Abdolell M. Postradiotherapy prostate biopsies: what do they really mean? Results for 498 patients. Int J Radiat Oncol Biol Phys 2000;48(2):355–367.
407. Shipley WU, Thames HD, Sandler HM, Hanks GE, Zietman AL, Perez CA, Kuban D A, Hancock SL, Smith CD. Radiation therapy for clinically localized prostate cancer: a multi-institutional pooled analysis. JAMA 1999;281(17):1598–1604.
408. Critz FA, Williams WH, Holladay CT, Levinson AK, Benton JB, Holladay DA, Schnell Jr FJ, Maxa LS, Shrake PD. Post-treatment PSA 70.2 ng/mL defines disease freedom after radiotherapy for prostate cancer using modern techniques. Urology 1999;54(6): 968–971.
409. Zagars GK, Pollack A, Kavadi VS, von Eschenbach AC. Prostate-specific antigen and radiation therapy for clinically localized prostate cancer. Int J Radiat Oncol Biol Phys 1995;32(2): 293–306.
410. Lee WR, Hanlon AL, Hanks GE. Prostate-specific antigen nadir following external beam radiation therapy for clinically localized prostate cancer: the relationship between nadir level and disease-free survival. J Urol 1996;156(2 Pt 1):450–453.
411. Crook JM, Bahadur YA, Bociek RG, Perry GA, Robertson SJ, Esche BA. Radiotherapy for localized prostate carcinoma. The correlation of pre-treatment prostate-specific antigen and nadir prostate-specific antigen with outcome as assessed by systematic biopsy and serum prostate-specific antigen. Cancer 1997;79(2): 328–336.
412. American Society for Therapeutic Radiology and Oncology Consensus Panel. Consensus statement: guidelines for PSA following radiation therapy. Int J Radiat Oncol Biol Phys 1997;37(5):1035–1041.
413. Merrill RM, Stephenson RA. Trends in mortality rates in patients with prostate cancer during the era of prostate-specific antigen screening. J Urol 2000;163(2):503–510.
414. Vanchieri C. Prostate cancer screening trials: fending off critics to recruit men. J Natl Cancer Inst 1998;90(1):10–12.
415. Schroder FH, Kranse R, Rietbergen J, Hoedemaeke R, Kirkels W. The European Randomized Study of Screening for Prostate Cancer (ERSPC): an update. Members of the ERSPC, Section Rotterdam. Eur Urol 1999;35(5–6):539–543.
416. Smith RA, Mettlin CJ, Davis KJ, Eyre H. American Cancer Society guidelines for the early detection of cancer. CA Cancer J Clin 2000;50(1):34–49.
417. Smith DS, Catalona WJ, Herschman JD. Longitudinal screening for prostate cancer with prostate-specific antigen. JAMA 1996;276(16):1309–1315.
418. Carter HB, Epstein JI, Chan DW, Fozard JL, Pearson JD. Recommended prostate-specific antigen testing intervals for the detection of curable prostate cancer. JAMA 1997;277(18): 1456–1460.
419. Carter HB, Epstein JI, Partin AW. Influence of age and prostate-specific antigen on the chance of curable prostate cancer among men with nonpalpable disease. Urology 1999;53(1):126–130.
420. Gronberg H, Isaacs SD, Smith JR, Carpten JD, Bova GS, Freije D, Xu J, Meyers DA, Collins FS, Trent JM, Walsh PC, Isaacs WB. Characteristics of prostate cancer in families potentially linked to the hereditary prostate cancer 1 (HPC1) locus. JAMA 1997; 278(15):1251–1255.
421. Walsh PC Partin AW. Family history facilitates the early diagnosis of prostate carcinoma. Cancer 1997;80(9):1871–1874.

Chapter **18**

Ovarian Cancer

Ie-Ming Shih, Lori J. Sokoll, and Daniel W. Chan

Ovarian cancer is the most lethal gynecologic malignancy (1,2). Although new chemotherapeutic agents have significantly improved the five-year survival rate, the overall mortality of ovarian cancer has remained unchanged (3). This is mainly because of a lack of success in diagnosing ovarian cancer at an early stage (nearly all patients with advanced stage of ovarian carcinoma die of the disease). On the other hand, 90% of those with the disease confined to the ovary survive.

Despite considerable efforts directed at early detection, no cost-effective screening tests have been developed (4). Although pelvic and, more recently, vaginal sonography have been used to screen high-risk patients, both techniques lack sufficient sensitivity and specificity as screening tools for the general population. Thus, the search for tumor markers capable of early detection of ovarian carcinoma is of profound importance and represents one of the most urgent subjects in the study of ovarian cancer.

Since the vast majority of ovarian cancers are of the epithelial type (carcinoma) and most studies on ovarian cancer markers focus on serological markers, this review will primarily focus on the secretory tumor markers in serum (or plasma) associated with ovarian carcinomas. First, the classification, epidemiology, tumorigenesis, and clinical management of ovarian cancer will be briefly reviewed to provide the essential background of ovarian cancer. Next, the current and potential tumor markers used in the diagnosis and follow-up in ovarian cancer patients will be summarized. Finally, new technologies that could lead to advances in identifying new markers for ovarian cancer will also be discussed.

OVERVIEW OF OVARIAN CANCER
Morphological Classification

Although ovarian cancer is often viewed as a single disease, it is considerably more complex and represents a family of related but distinct tumors including surface epithelial tumors, sex-cord stromal tumors, germ cell tumors, and metastatic tumors (5). Within each category, there are several histological subtypes. Among them, surface epithelial tumors (carcinomas) are the most common (Figure 1) and are divided, according to the Federation of Gynecology and Obstetrics (FIGO) and the World Health Organization (WHO) classifications, into five histologic types:

- serous,
- mucinous,
- endometrioid,
- clear cell, and
- transitional (6).

The different types of ovarian cancers are not only histologically distinct but may exhibit different clinical behavior, tumorigenesis, and probably gene expression pattern (7). Based on prevalence and mortality, the serous carcinoma is the most important, representing nearly 40% of all primary ovarian carcinomas with an overall five-year survival rate of approximately 30%. Unless otherwise specified, serous carcinoma is what is generally thought of as "ovarian cancer." Accordingly, in this review we will confine our discussions largely to serous carcinoma.

Epidemiology

Ovarian cancer represents 25% of gynecologic cancers but accounts for 50% of the deaths from all gynecologic tumors. Approximately 23,000 women are diagnosed with ovarian cancer each year in the United States and 14,000 women die of this disease annually (8,9).

Epidemiologic and molecular-genetic studies have identified several risk and protective factors associated with the development of ovarian cancer (10). The most significant risk factor is a family history of the disease, and genetic alterations in BRCA1 and BRCA2 tumor suppressor genes that occur in the majority of hereditary ovarian cancer. This hereditary form of ovarian cancer represents only 5% to 10% of all ovarian cancer patients, and the vast majority of ovarian cancers are sporadic (9). For women in the United States, the overall lifetime risk of developing ovarian cancer is 1.4% to 1.8%, whereas the risk increases to 9.4% for women with a family history (10). Additional risk factors include nulliparity and refractory infertility. Protective factors include multiparity, oral contraceptives, tubal ligation, and hysterectomy.

Pathogenesis

The development of improved strategies for the early detection of ovarian carcinoma depends on a better understanding of its pathogenesis—the morphological and molecular events in the development of ovarian cancer. Despite recent studies aimed at

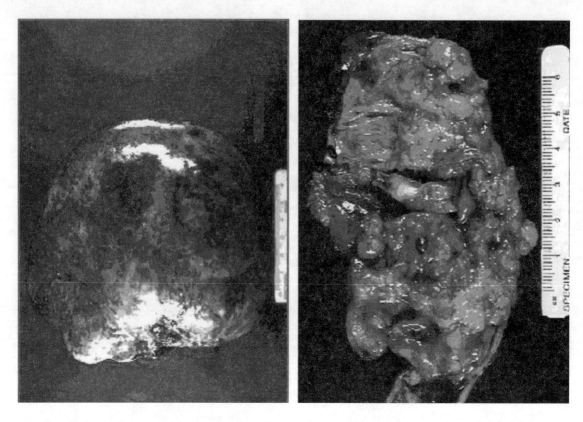

Figure 1 Gross appearance of an ovarian serous carcinoma, the most common type of ovarian cancer. The tumor is large (13 cm) and cystic, and it replaces the normal ovarian tissue which is not visible (right). On sectioning, the tumor appears to be papillary with numerous excrescences projecting into the cyst (left). **Color representation of figure appears on Color Plate 1.**

elucidating the molecular mechanisms of ovarian cancer, its pathogenesis is poorly understood (11). Several potential tumor suppressor genes have been identified: NOEY2, PTEN, and OVCA-1 and -2. Except for BRCA-1 and BRAC-2 in familial cases, little evidence has been reported suggesting that these genes are important in the pathogenesis of serous carcinomas (12–15). At present the most widely held view is that serous carcinoma arises directly from the transformation of the ovarian surface epithelium or its inclusion cysts through a "de novo" process (16,17). However, based on extensive studies of clinical, histopathological, and molecular genetic features of a large series of ovarian serous tumors, ovarian serous carcinoma may develop along different pathways (18,19).

In this new model, ovarian serous carcinomas are stratified into two morphological categories: conventional serous carcinomas and invasive micropapillary serous carcinoma (MPSC) that develop along distinctive pathways. In the first pathway, the conventional type of serous carcinoma develops by direct transformation from ovarian surface epithelium or inclusion cysts to a high-grade neoplasm without recognizable intermediate stages (the "de novo" pathway). These tumors demonstrate wild-type K-ras, frequent p53 mutations, and a high level of allelic imbalance even in early tumor development (20). The second is the "stepwise" pathway. The serous tumors develop from serous borderline tumor to a noninvasive micropapillary serous carcinoma, then to low-grade serous carcinoma (invasive micropapillary serous carcinoma). In contrast to conventional serous carcinoma, this process, which appears to develop in an indolent fashion, has clear-cut precursor lesions. These tumors exhibit frequent K-ras mutations, rare p53 mutations, and then gradually acquire more genetic abnormalities during tumor progression. For example, loss of 5q is associated with malignant transformation and loss of 1p with the acquisition of invasive phenotypes. Clinically, conventional serous carcinomas represent approximately 65% of all serous carcinoma and present as high-grade, high-stage aggressive neoplasms, whereas micropapillary serous carcinomas represents 35% of serous neoplasms and generally pursue a protracted indolent course.

Clinical Management

Most ovarian cancer patients do not present with specific clinical symptoms until their cancer has reached advanced stages (FIGO stage III or IV) (21). The strategies used to treat ovarian cancer are constantly evolving. Generally, surgical management represents the first-line treatment in all ovarian cancer patients (22,9). Following tumor resection or debulking surgery, the extent of disease involvement is determined (clinical staging) and combination chemotherapy using cisplatinum-based regimens is administrated to patients who have advanced-stage disease (9,23). These patients are followed by physical examination and imaging techniques, which are insensitive for detecting recurrence until tumors are quite advanced. In the past, second-look exploratory laparotomy was performed to evaluate the response to therapy; however, recently the benefit of this procedure has come into question because of its high morbidity and low sensitivity in detecting residual or recurrent carcinoma (9). Using a multi-modality approach to treatment, including aggressive cytoreductive surgery and combination chemotherapy, the five-year survival rates are 93% in stage I, 70% in stage II, 37% in stage III, and only 25% in stage IV (10).

OVARIAN CANCER BIOMARKERS

There are several current and potential biomarkers for ovarian cancer. The clinical applications of these biomarkers are summarized in Table 1.

CA125

Background and biochemistry. CA125 is currently the best tumor marker available for the management of a patient with ovarian cancer. Bast and colleagues identified the CA125 antigen in 1981 with the development of the OC 125 murine monoclonal antibody from cell line OVCA 433, which was derived from a patient with ovarian serous carcinoma (25). Historically, the CA125 antigen has been described as a mucin-like glycoprotein with a molecular mass ranging from 200 to 2000 kDa, although its function and role in ovarian cancer have yet to be elucidated. Recently, CA125 has been cloned with a partial cDNA sequence for the peptide core of the molecule identified (24). This new mucin molecule has been designated CA125/MUC16 (gene MUC16) and consists of a 156-amino-acid tandem repeat region in the N-terminus and a possible transmembrane region and tyrosine phosphorylation site in the C-terminus. Cloning the CA125 antigen will allow epitopes to monoclonal antibodies to CA125 to be identified. Workshops by the International Society of Oncodevelopmental Biology and Medicine (ISOBM) have characterized the two major antigenic domains of the CA125 antigen, classified as either OC 125-like or M 11-like (26,27).

The CA125 cell-surface antigen is expressed by epithelial ovarian tumors as well as other pathological and normal tissues of mullerian duct origin (28). Secretion of CA125 is linked to the signal transduction pathway of tyrosine kinase epithelial growth factor receptor (29). Elevation in serum concentrations in malignant disease is a result of vascular invasion, tissue destruction, and inflammation (30). In addition to secretion into blood, CA125 has been found in breast milk, ascites, cyst fluid, cervical secretions, uterine secretions, and amniotic fluid (26). The half-life of CA125 has been reported to range from 5 to 10 days (30). CA125 is released from the abdominal cavity during surgery and its synthesis may be modified by the taxol chemotherapeutic agent, although the effects of other medications have not been reproducible (31,32).

Analysis. The first immunoassay for CA125, commercialized in 1983 by Centocor (now Fujirebio Diagnostics), was a radioimmunometric assay with multiple CA125 determinants, allowing the OC 125 antibody to be used for both capture and detection (33,28). Due to a lack of purified CA125 for use in standardization, assay results were expressed as U(units)/mL. A second-generation assay was subsequently developed, incorporating the M11 antibody, which has a distinct non-overlapping epitope compared to OC 125. In this assay, termed CA125II, the M11 antibody functions as the capture antibody and the OC 125 antibody the labeled, detector antibody. As a result of the two distinct antibodies, the CA125II assay exhibited improved inter-assay precision, linearity, and diminished high-dose hook effect compared to the CA125 assay while displaying similar clinical characteristics (33). Assays for CA125 have since been adapted to automated platforms and characteristics of assays currently approved by the FDA are shown in Table 2. Despite the fact that the majority of manufacturers use a similar cut-off, concentrations of CA125 may vary among manufacturers due to assay methods and reagent specificities. Thus, values from different methods are not interchangeable and patients who are serially monitored should be re-baselined if there is a change in methodology (34). Laboratory reports should also indicate the specific assay used.

It is recommended that analysis be performed shortly after the prompt centrifugation of the specimen and separation of serum from the clot, and that specimens be stored at either 4 °C

Table 1 The clinical applications of current serum biomarkers for ovarian cancer

Serum Marker	Screening	Differential Diagnosis	Tumor Monitoring	Prognosis Prediction
CA125	No	?	Yes	?
CEA	No	No	Yes	No
TATI	No	No	Yes	?
Kallikreins 6, 10, 11	?	Yes	Yes	Yes
TPA	No	No	Yes	No
CASA	No	No	Yes	Yes
Fibrinolytic markers	No	?	?	Yes
IL-6	No	No	?	Yes
Prostasin	?	Yes	?	?
Urinary β-core hCG	No	No	?	Yes

TPA: Tissue polypeptide antigen; TATI: Tumor-associated trypsin inhibitor; CEA: Carcinoembryonic antigen; IL: interleukin; hCG: human chorionic gonadotropin; ?: the assay for the particular marker has not been performed or the results are not definitive.

Table 2 Characteristics of commercially available CA125 assays

Manufacturer/ Instrument	Name	Antibodies (C: Capture; D: Dectector)	Detection	Dynamic Range	Between-Run Precision	Comparative Method	Cut-off	Approved Indication*
Abbott AxSYM	CA125	C: Sheep polyclonal microparticles D: OC125 alkaline phosphatase	Fluorescence (MEIA)	2 U/mL– 600 U/mL	1.9%–4%	Y = 1.10 (Abbott RIA) – 7.36 U/mL, r = 0.969	35 U/mL	M
Bayer Immuno 1	CA125II	C: M11 immuno-magnetic particles D: OC125 alkaline phosphatase	Absorbance	.4 U/mL– 500U/mL	2.2%–3.6%	Y = 0.975 (Fujirebio) + 2.8 U/mL, Yr = 0.983	35 U/mL	R
Bayer ACS:180	OV	C: O125 para-magnetic particles D: M11 acridinium ester	Chemi-luminescence	1.7 U/mL– 1000 U/mL	4.5%–5.8%		35 U/mL	Q
DPC Immulite	OM-MA	C: M11 bead D: Rabbit polyclonal alkaline phosphatase	Chemi-luminescence	1 U/mL– 500 U/mL	4.6%–6.7%	Y = 0.77 (Fujirebio) – 3.7 U/mL, r = 0.974	21 U/mL	M, R
Fujirebio Diagnostics RIA	CA125II	C: M11 bead D: ^{125}I OC125	Radioactivity	0.4 U/mL– 500 U/mL	7.5%–9.8%		35 U/mL	R
Ortho Vitros	CA125II	C: M11 well via biotin-streptavidin D: OC125 horseradish peroxidase	Chemi-luminescence	1.2 U/mL– 1000 U/mL	4.0%–5.8%	Y = 0.97 (Elecsys) – 3.16 U/mL, r = 0.991	35 U/mL	M
Roche Elecsys 1010/2010	CA125II	C: M11 microparticles via biotin-streptavidin D: OC125 ruthenium	Electrochemi-luminescence	0.6 U/mL– 5000 U/mL	2.5%–4.2%	Y = 0.96 (Fujirebio) + 5.82 U/mL, r = 0.98	35 U/mL	M, R
Tosoh AIA-PACK	CA125	C: Mab B27.1 magnetic beads D: Mab B43.13 alkaline phosphatase	Fluorescence	2 U/mL– 1000 U/mL	3.2%–3.7%	y = 1.16 (Fujirebio) – 4.14 U/mL, r = 0.94	35 U/mL	M

*M: Serial measurement of CA125 to aid in the monitoring response to therapy; Q: Quantitative determination of CA125 in human serum; R: Aid in the detection of residual ovarian carcinoma in patients who have undergone first-line therapy and would be considered for second-look procedures

(1–5 days) or –20 °C (2 weeks–3 months) in the short term or –70 °C in the long term to ensure stability (32). Plasma is an acceptable specimen type for some assays. Similar to other immunoassays, assay interferences may be observed from the presence of heterophilic antibodies particularly as a result of therapeutic or diagnostic use of monoclonal antibodies.

Cut-off. A cut-off of 35 U/mL for the CA125 and CA125II assays was determined from the distribution of values in healthy individuals. Values tend to decline with menopause and aging. It has been recently reported that CA125II concentrations vary 20–50% by race in postmenopausal women, with concentrations in African and Asian women lower than in Caucasian women (35). Menstrual cycle variations can also be found with increases during the follicular phase. Elevations in values can be found in 1–2% of normals, 5% of those with benign diseases, and 28% of those with non-gynecologic cancers. CA125 is also used as a tumor marker for endometrial cancer. Elevations can occur in benign conditions, including pregnancy, endometriosis, ovarian cysts, pelvic inflammatory disease, peritonitis, cirrhosis, hepatitis, and pericarditis, and in other cancers such as fallopian tube, cervix, endometrium, pancreas, lung, breast, and colon (28,32,33).

Early detection. In women with epithelial ovarian cancer, 80% have CA125 levels >35 U/mL with elevations of 50% in clinically detected stage I disease, 90% in stage II, and >90% in stages III and IV (28). Concentrations correlate with tumor burden and stage. Due to the lack of sensitivity and specificity of the CA125 marker, it is not recommended for use in screening asymptomatic women. An NCI consensus development panel concluded that neither CA125 nor transvaginal ultrasonography effectively reduces mortality from ovarian cancer. The panel did recommend annual CA125 determinations, in addition to pelvic and ultrasound examinations, in women with a history of hereditary ovarian cancer who have an estimated lifetime risk of 40%.

To exploit the potential of CA125 in the early detection of cancer, a number of approaches have been performed to improve its specificity. Very high specificity is needed to achieve an acceptable positive predictive value of 10% with a prevalence of disease of 40 per 100,000 in women over age 50. A sensitivity of 67% and a specificity of 99.7% are needed for a 10% positive predictive value, which would result in 10 laparotomies or laparoscopies for each case of ovarian cancer detected (36). Strategies have included combining CA125 with ultrasound or employing a two-stage strategy in which ultrasonography is performed only if CA125 concentrations are elevated. In a study of 4,000 women, specificity of CA125 plus ultrasound was 99.9% compared to 98.3% for CA125 alone. The NIH-sponsored Prostate, Lung, Colon, and Ovary Cancer Screening Trial (32), a randomized prospective study initiated in 1993, will utilize both modalities with CA125 measurements at entry and annually for five years with transvaginal ultrasound at entry and annually for 3 years with 13 years of follow-up (36).

Other strategies that have been proposed to improve the specificity of CA125 for screening include the use of longitudinal measurements and the use of multiple markers. Skates et al. (37) developed a computer-generated algorithm for the risk of ovarian cancer using CA125II values measured over time. This was based on the observation in ovarian and other cancers that women with malignant disease have rising levels of the marker, while women without malignant disease do not. Data from a screening study in Stockholm were analyzed by examining the slopes and intercepts of the longitudinal CA125II measurements plotted as a function of time of patients with ovarian cancer compared to healthy subjects and patients with benign diseases or non-gynecologic malignancies. This yielded a specificity of 99.9%, a sensitivity of 83% and a positive predictive value of 16%. With respect to the use of additional markers, a large number of serum, plasma, and urine markers including oncofetal antigens, mucin-like proteins, enzymes, co-enzymes, enzyme inhibitors, receptors, cytokines, peptide hormones, proteins, phospholipids, and sialyated lipids (36) have been studied individually. However, the only marker to show a potential increase in sensitivity compared to CA125 was lysophosphatidic acid (LPA). Combining markers with CA125 that also show elevations in patients with ovarian cancer can increase specificity; however, sensitivity is often significantly compromised.

An alternative approach is to use markers complementary to CA125 to potentially increase sensitivity. Two markers studied in this capacity have been OVX1, a modified Lewis determinant expressed on a high molecular weight mucin found to be elevated in 47% of ovarian cancer patients who do not have elevations in CA125 and M-CSF, a cytokine dimer of 70 kDA that binds to the CSF-1 receptor encoded by the c-fms proto-oncogene (36,33). Combining data from two retrospective studies in which these three markers were measured showed CA125 elevation 69% in 89 patients with Stage I ovarian cancer compared to elevation of any of the 3 markers in 84% of patients. However, the sensitivity gained came at the expense of specificity, with 99% for CA125 alone compared to 89% for the multiple markers.

Discrimination of pelvic masses. Despite the controversy over the use of CA125 in the early detection of ovarian cancer, CA125 is more accepted as an adjunct in distinguishing benign from malignant disease in women, particularly in post-menopausal women presenting with ovarian masses (38, 3). In pre-menopausal women, benign conditions resulting in elevated CA125 levels may be a confounding factor. Sensitivities of 71–78% and specificities of 75–94% have been reported in different studies. Elevated concentrations of CA125 >95 U/mL in post-menopausal women can discriminate malignant from benign pelvic masses with a positive predictive value of 95% (33).

The multiple markers approach has been applied to the pre-operative discrimination of malignant and benign pelvic masses using a number of analytical techniques (39,40). Using an artificial neural network, a panel of the serum markers CA125II, CA 72-4, CA 15-3, and lipid-associated sialic acid (LASA) demonstrated improved specificity compared to CA125 alone (87.5% vs. 68.4%) with similar sensitivities (79.0% vs. 82.4%). Specificity was also improved in women less than 50 years of age (82.3% vs. 62%) (41).

Post-operative use. Initial studies on CA125 indicated that it was useful post-operatively in predicting the likelihood that a tumor would be found during a second-look operation. Thus CA125 assays were approved for this indication by the FDA (28,41). Elevations of CA125 over 35 U/mL after debulking surgery and chemotherapy indicated that residual disease was likely (>95% accuracy) and that further surgery was unlikely to be beneficial. However, due to a sensitivity of only 50%, if a value was less than the 35 U/mL cut-off, a second-look surgery was recommended. Currently, second-look laparotomy is controversial and suggested only for patients enrolled in clinical trials or in situations when surgical findings would alter clinical management. Monitoring with CA125 testing in women with elevated pre-operative CA125 concentrations, along with a routine history and physical, and recto-vaginal pelvic examination, has been advocated instead of surgery for asymptomatic women after primary therapy (38). Elevated, rising, or doubling CA125 concentrations predict relapse. However, negative values do not exclude disease presence. With the combination of parameters described, disease progression can be detected in 90% of patients with recurrence. Although monitoring intervals are undefined, current practice suggests following patients every three to four months for two years and then less frequently. Elevations in CA125 can precede clinical or radiological evidence or recurrence with a median time of two to six months, although there is no evidence that initiating salvage chemotherapy prior to clinical recurrence improves survival (42).

Prognosis. Use of CA125 levels, both pre-operatively and post-operatively, may be of prognostic significance, although results have varied. In patients who have a pre-operative CA125 concentration >65 U/mL, the five-year survival rates were significantly lower and conferred a 6.37-fold risk of death compared to patients who had values less than 65 U/mL (30,28). After primary surgery and chemotherapy, declines in CA125 concentrations during chemotherapy have generally been observed to be independent prognostic factors, and in some studies the most important indicator. Declines to normal concentrations are associated with negative second-look operations with improvements in survival and normalization of CA125 levels after one, two, or three courses of chemotherapy. Persistent elevations indicate a poor prognosis. In addition to the measured level, the half-life of the CA125 marker indicates prognosis. A half-life of less than 20 days, compared to an ideal regression rate of 7.6 days, was associated with significantly improved survival (28 months vs. 19 months) (33,44,44).

Monitoring treatment. CA125 concentrations may also play a role in monitoring response to chemotherapy. Declining CA125 concentrations appear to correlate with treatment response even when disease is not detectable by either palpation or imaging, and in a meta-analysis, serial CA125 concentrations in 89% of 531 patients correlated with clinical outcome of disease. Knowledge of treatment response, particularly in patients without detectable clinical disease, is important, as it would aid in the decision to continue a potentially toxic therapeutic regimen. Knowledge of treatment failure would spare patients a continuation of therapies that may be toxic or expensive and allow for salvage therapy or new treatments as part of a clinical trial. A number of approaches to assess treatment response have been developed and tested, including a computer algorithm incorporating serial CA125 concentrations at specific time intervals with benchmarks of a 50% decline after two elevated samples confirmed with a fourth sample, or a 75% decline over three consecutive samples. Further study is needed before these approaches are accepted into clinical practice (41,43,30). In addition to monitoring initial chemotherapeutic regiments, CA125 measurements may be useful in monitoring salvage therapy, because a doubling of values is associated with disease progression and treatment failure in more than 90% of cases. Disease progression may also occur without an increase in CA125, and therefore the presence of tumor should also be assessed by physical examination and imaging (32).

Other Markers

Other than CA125, several potential tumor-associated markers have been reported in serum or plasma of ovarian cancer patients. Although these experimental markers could represent promising new biomarkers for ovarian cancer screening, diagnosis, and monitoring, it is uncertain whether they will become viable clinical tools: sensitivity and specificity need to be addressed in a larger group of patients with stage I disease to validate their clinical usefulness.

Kallikrein family. The human kallikrein gene family is a subfamily of serine proteases and can be involved in the progression and metastasis of human cancers (45–47) (see also Chapter 46for more details). Expression of several members of the kallikrein family, including kallikreins 4, 5, 7, 8, 9, 10, and 11, have been reported in ovarian cancer. Kallikrein 4 is highly expressed in several neoplasms including prostate, breast, endometrial, and ovarian carcinomas. However, the protein has not as yet been measured in serum (48). In ovarian carcinoma, kallikrein 4 is expressed in the majority of serous carcinomas but rarely in normal ovarian surface epithelium (49,50). Kallikrein 4 expression is associated with more aggressive forms of ovarian cancer (higher clinical stage and tumor grade) and at univariate survival analysis revealed that patients with ovarian tumors positive for kallikrein 4 expression had an increased risk for relapse and death (50). Similarly, kallikrein 5 has been suggested to be a useful independent prognostic indicator in patients with stage I and II diseases (51). Assessment of kallikrein 5 expression could help oncologists determine those who are at higher risk of relapse. In contrast, using reverse transcription-PCR and direct sequencing, Magklara et al. have recently reported that kallikrein 8 (neuropsin/ovasin) is a novel favorable prognostic marker in ovarian cancer (52). Patients with higher kallikrein 8 expression in their tumors have lower-grade disease, lower residual tumor, longer survival, and low recurrence rate. In a multivariate analysis, higher kallikrein 8 expression was significantly associated with longer disease-free survival. Because kallikreins 4, 5, and 8 encode for predicted secreted proteins, their detection in serum or plasma may have potential clinical application in ovarian cancer patients. Similarly, human kallikrein 7 and 9 transcripts were shown to have prognostic significance in ovarian cancer (53,54). Among all kallikreins, human kallikrein 6 (hK6), human kallikrein 10 (hK10), and human kallikrein 11 (hK11) are the only ones that have been detected in serum to date, and they are all potential serological markers of the disease (55–57). Kallikrein 10, also known as normal epithelial cell-specific 1 protein, is a secreted serine protease produced by breast and other epithelial cells and carcinomas, including ovarian carcinoma (58). The development of a highly sensitive and specific immunoassay for kallikrein 10 has shown it to be a potential new serological marker for ovarian cancer diagnosis and monitoring (57). Serum kallikrein 10 is significantly elevated in 56% of the ovarian cancer patients and 15% of gastrointestinal cancer patients but not in healthy individuals or in patients who have other types of cancer. Cytosolic kallikrein 10 concentration in tumors correlates with an unfavorable prognosis (59). There is no correlation between kallikrein 10 and CA125 levels in ovarian cancer patients. In short, multiple kallikreins are potential ovarian cancer markers with hK6 and hK10 being the most promising.

Prostasin. Using cDNA microarray technology on RNA pooled from ovarian cancer and the human ovarian surface epithelial cell line, Mok et al. have identified an overexpressed gene that produces a secretory product, prostasin (60). Prostasin was originally isolated from human seminal fluid and is present at the highest level in the prostate gland (61). Using immunohistochemistry, prostasin is also expressed at much lower levels in a variety of human tissues including kidney, liver, pancreas, salivary gland, lung, and bronchus. Prostasin was detected more strongly in ovarian carcinoma than in normal ovarian tissue. The mean level of serum prostasin was 13.7 λg/mL in patients with ovarian cancer and 7.5 λg/mL in control subjects. In a series of patients with non-mucinous ovarian carcinoma, the combination of prostasin and CA125 gave a sensitivity of 92% and a specificity of 94% for detecting ovarian cancer. Although the above finding is promising, prostasin should be investigated further as a screening or tumor marker, alone and in combination with CA125.

Tissue polypeptide antigen (TPA). TPA is a single chain polypeptide with a molecular weight of 22–23 kD and probably consists of proteolytic fragments of the cytokeratins (62). Production of TPA may be associated with rapid cell turnover, and elevated TPA levels in serum have been reported in patients suffering from infectious diseases and cancers (63). In ovarian cancers of serous and mucinous type, TPA is reported to be strongly correlated with the FIGO stage. Thirty-three to 50% of the patients with stage I–II and 88–96% of patients with stage III–IV presented with elevated serum TPA. Serial TPA measurements correlated with the clinical course of ovarian cancer in 42–79% of the matched event. These findings suggest that TPA may be a potential marker for following ovarian cancer in patients.

Lysophosphatidic acid (LPA). An ovarian cancer-activating factor, comprised of various species of lysophosphatidic acid (LPA), was purified from the ascites of ovarian cancer patients and may play a biological role in ovarian cancer cell growth (64,65). In a preliminary study in a small number of patients, plasma LPA concentrations were elevated in 90% of women with stage I disease and 100% of women with advanced and recurrent disease compared to healthy controls, although 80% of women with other gynecologic cancers also had elevated levels. CA125 concentrations appeared to complement LPA levels thus the possibility exists to use these markers in combination. Further study of LPA is required, although current methods of measuring LPA involving lipid extraction followed by gas chromatography may limit its utility.

Tumor-associated trypsin inhibitor (TATI). TATI is a 60 kD protein and was first isolated from the urine of patients with ovarian cancer (66). The amino acid sequence and biochemical properties of TATI are identical to those of pancreatic secretory trypsin inhibitor (67). Elevated serum and urinary concentrations of TATI are frequently observed after in post-operative patients, in severe inflammatory diseases, and in various types of cancer, especially gynecological and pancreatic cancer (63). Frequent elevated TATI concentrations can be observed in ovarian cancers, especially the mucinous types. Generally, the elevated serum levels of TATI appear to correlate with higher stages of disease. In one report, the sensitivity is only 8% in patients with stage I–II and 62% of patients with stage III–IV (68). Several reports suggest that TATI is not a good marker for monitoring disease during therapy, as TATI had a lower sensitivity for residual tumor than CA125, and less than 50% of the matched clinical events are observed to correlate serum levels of TATI. Please also see Chapter 42.

Carcinoembryonic antigen (CEA). CEA is an oncofetal antigen (63). Elevated serum concentrations of CEA are frequently found in a variety of benign diseases and cancers, including ovarian carcinoma. The frequency of elevated concentration in ovarian carcinoma varies with the histological type and disease stage, generally being higher in patients with metastatic disease. The sensitivity of CEA as a marker to detect ovarian cancer is approximately 25%, and the positive predictive value of an elevated CEA concentration is only 14% (63). Although CEA is not a marker for early diagnosis due to its low sensitivity, CEA can be useful in determining treatment response in ovarian cancer patients whose changing levels of CEA are observed. More details on CEA can be found in other chapters of this book (e.g., Chapters 19, 21, and 31).

Cancer-associated serum antigen (CASA). CASA was initially defined by a monoclonal antibody that bound to an epitope on the polymorphic epithelial mucin (69). Elevated serum CASA concentration can be observed in individuals with late pregnancy, higher age, in smokers, and in patients with cancers. CASA is expressed in all histological types of ovarian cancer and seems to have a sensitivity of 46–73% in patients with ovarian cancer (63). Only a few studies have indicated that CASA is a potential useful marker in monitoring ovarian cancer. Ward et al. reported that inclusion of CASA in a diagnostic tumor panel might improve the detection of residual disease by increasing the sensitivity from 33% to 62% and the negative predictive value from 66% to 78% (70,71). Using CASA as a marker, some investigators have demonstrated that CASA can detect more cases with small volume disease than CA125, and that 50% of patients with microscopic disease are detected by

CASA alone (63). The prognostic value of post-operative serum CASA level is reported in one study showing that it is superior to CA125 and other parameters including residual disease, histological type, tumor grade, and the cisplatin-based chemotherapy (72).

Fibrinolytic markers. Fibrinolytic markers such as tissue-type plasminogen activator (tPA), urokinase-type plasminogen activator (uPA), plasminogen activator inhibitor-1 and -2 (PAI-1 and -2), and uPA receptor have been studied in ovarian cancer (73–77). In ovarian cancer, expression of uPA, PAI-1, and PAI-2 is significantly higher in the tumor tissue than in the control tissue, whereas tPA expression is significantly lower in the tumor tissue than in control tissue. The diagnostic and prognostic values of PAI-1 and PAI-2 have been recently reported in ovarian cancer (76). In this pilot study, PAI-1 appears to be an independent poor prognostic factor (74) as plasma levels of PAI-1 are significantly higher in patients with ovarian cancer, and their levels correlate with the diseases at higher clinical stages. Whether PAI-1 can be used clinically for the screening and/or monitoring ovarian cancer awaits further studies, including the correlation with clinical treatment events and comparison with CA125. In contrast, expression of PAI-2 in tumors has been shown to be a favorable prognostic factor in ovarian cancer patients (76).

Interleukin-6 (IL-6). IL-6 is a multifunctional cytokine displaying diverse biological functions that can be produced by a wide variety of normal and neoplastic cells types (78). High levels of IL-6 have been detected in the serum and ascites of ovarian cancer patients (78). IL-6 may be a useful serum marker for ovarian cancer, because it correlates with tumor burden, clinical disease status, and survival time of patients. Based on a multivariate analysis, investigators have found serum levels of IL-6 to be of prognostic value, but less sensitive than CA125 (79,80).

Human chorionic gonadotropin (hCG). hCG is a glycoprotein hormone composed of α and β subunits. This hormone is normally produced by trophoblast, and clinically it has been used as the surrogate serum or urine marker for pregnancy and gestational trophoblastic disease (81). Ectopic β-hCG production has been known in a variety of human cancers, and it has been more frequently detected in urine than in serum in those patients. Recent studies have demonstrated that the immunoreactivity of total β-hCG in serum and urine (urinary β-core fragment) represent a strong independent prognostic factor in ovarian carcinoma, and its prognostic value is similar to that of grade and stage (82,83). When serum β-hCG is normal, the five-year survival rate can be as high as 80%, but it is only 22% when β-hCG is elevated (82). In patients with stage III or IV and minimal residual disease, the five-year survival is 75% if β-hCG is not detectable compared with 0% if β-hCG is elevated. Similarly, β-core fragment can be detected in urine in 84% of ovarian cancer patients (83). The incidence of positive urinary β-core fragment correlates with disease progression (a higher proportion of patients is seen in advanced clinical stages). Although the availability of this marker before surgery could facilitate selection of treatment modalities, the clinical application of β-hCG for screening and diagnosis is limited.

Since several different types of tumors can produce β-hCG and only a small proportion of ovarian tumors express β-hCG, detection of serum β-hCG or urinary β-core fragment will not provide a specific or sensitive tool for screening or diagnosis in ovarian cancer.

Extracellular domain of C-erbB-2 or HER-2/NEU (P105). The c-erbB-2 oncogene expresses a transmembrane protein, p185, with intrinsic tyrosine kinase activity. Amplification of c-erbB-2 has been found in several human cancers, including ovarian carcinoma. The c-erbB-2 protein is expressed on the surface epithelium of normal ovaries; increased expression of c-erbB-2 has been shown in ovarian inclusion cysts and some ovarian carcinomas (84). After proteolytic activity, an extracellular domain (105 kD) of p185 is released from the surface of human cancer cells that overexpress p185. Accordingly, elevated serum levels of p105 have been identified in patients with various cancers known to overexpress c-erbB-2.

In ovarian cancer, 9% to 38% of patients have elevated p105 levels (85–87). In one report, measurement of c-erbB-2 alone or in combination with CA125 is not useful in differentiating benign from malignant ovarian tumors (87). However, elevated p105 in serum or immunohistochemically c-erbB-2 positive tumors are correlated with an aggressive tumor type, advanced clinical stages, and poor clinical outcome in patients (88). Thus, screening for an increased p105 levels could make it possible to identify a subset of high-risk patients (86). Furthermore, the test could be potentially useful for detecting recurrent disease. Further studies with a large series of cases should be undertaken to extend the preliminary finding and test whether analysis of p105 concentrations in serum is a valuable diagnostic tool for ovarian cancer patients.

AKT2 gene product. The AKT2 gene is one of the human homologues of v-akt, the transduced oncogene of the AKT8 virus, which experimentally induces lymphomas in mice. AKT2, which codes for a serine-threonine protein kinase, is activated by growth factors and other oncogenes such as v-Ha-ras and v-src through phosphatidylinositol 3-kinase in human ovarian cancer cells (89,90). Studies have shown that the AKT2 gene is amplified and overexpressed in approximately 12–36 % of ovarian carcinomas (91–93). In contrast, AKT2 alteration was not detected in 24 benign or borderline tumors.

Ovarian cancer patients with AKT2 alterations appear to have a poor prognosis. Amplification of AKT2 is more frequently found in histologically high-grade tumors or tumors at advanced stages (III or IV), suggesting that AKT2 gene overexpression, like c-erbB-2, may be associated with tumor aggressiveness (92).

PERSPECTIVES FOR IDENTIFYING NEW BIOMARKERS

Although the markers described above have shown some clinical potential in monitoring or predicting disease progression, they do not appear to be the candidate markers suitable for early detection in ovarian cancer patients. As the greatest potential for reducing mortality of ovarian cancer lies in the detection of asymptomatic, early stage disease, the exploration of new markers for such purpose using novel strategies and technologies holds the greatest promise to combat the disease (94–97). These emerging techniques include serial analysis for gene expression (SAGE), serological analysis of recombinant cDNA expression libraries (SEREX), nucleotide microarray, digital PCR-based assays, and proteomics using SELDI. It is expected that advances in the field of new cancer marker identification will be accelerated by these newly developed technologies and facilitated by the completion of the first phase of the Human Genome Project (96). Since nucleotide microarray and proteomics are described in separate chapters, in the following section, we will illustrate SAGE, SEREX, and digital PCR analysis, focusing on how they can be applied as a tool in identifying the new markers in ovarian cancer. Please refer to Chapters 33 and 34 for additional information on discovering new cancer markers.

Serial Analysis for Gene Expression (SAGE)

SAGE provides unprecedented quantities of genome-wide data on gene-expression patterns. The availability of this data does not depend on the prior availability of transcript information (98).

The SAGE method is based on the isolation of unique sequence tags from individual transcripts and concatenation of tags serially into long DNA molecules (Figure 2). Rapid sequencing of concatemer clones reveals individual tags and allows quantitation and identification of cellular transcripts (99). In the past few years, SAGE has been used to provide a comprehensive analysis of a variety of different tissue samples, each usually consisting of millions of cells. It is expected that SAGE can provide a novel avenue for the identification of new tumor-associated markers. This approach has recently been extended to permit analysis of gene expression in substantially fewer cells (microSAGE), thereby allowing analysis of heterogeneous tissue or microanatomical structures (95).

This new technique is especially important to identify markers in small early tumors. By comparing SAGE data from human tumors to their tissue of origin, many genes have been identified to be dramatically up-regulated in tumors. Morin et al. recently performed SAGE on several normal and tumor ovarian specimens (7,100). In their studies, a total of 385,000 tags have been sequenced, yielding over 56,000 genes expressed in nine individual libraries derived from ovarian tissues (100). These libraries included short-term culture of human ovarian surface epithelium, SV40-immortalized ovarian surface epithelial cells, SV-40 immortalized benign adenoma, conventional serous carcinomas, ovarian cancer cell lines, and a pool of ovarian cancer cell lines. Using the expression profiles generated by SAGE and stringent selection criteria, Morin et al. identified a number of preferentially expressed genes in carcinoma or normal ovarian epithelium (7,100). Some of the genes identified are already known to be overexpressed in ovarian cancer, but several represent novel candidates. Many of the genes up-regulated in ovarian cancer belong to surface or secreted proteins such as claudin-3 and -4, mucin-1, HE4, Epi-CAM (GA 733-2), and mesothelin representing the potential markers for ovarian carcinoma. A statistical analysis further shows that many genes are up-regulated in a coordinated manner in ovarian cancer, suggesting the presence of a few dominant molecular pathways, whose abnormal regulation is responsible for the overexpression of many genes (7). Several of the genes selected based on SAGE have been validated using immunohistochemistry and real-time PCR on ovarian specimens. These SAGE results have been deposited in the public domain (http://www.ncbi.nlm.nih.gov/SAGE) (96) and, unlike oligonucleotide or cDNA microarrays, the data can be directly compared with future ovarian carcinoma libraries generated by other investigators.

Although SAGE has great potential for identifying novel tumor markers in ovarian cancer, the validation of the candidate markers in management and analysis of the huge amounts of data have profound influence on the interpretation of the results. New computational analysis tools, like those designed for cDNA or oligonucleotide microarrays, may be required for optimal experimental design and meaningful data analysis.

Serological Analysis of Recombinant cDNA Expression Libraries (SEREX)

"De novo" molecular changes that occur during tumor development, including mutated, or aberrantly expressed/post-translational modified gene products, are often antigenic. The generation of circulating autologous antibodies against tumor antigens can be regarded as the systemic amplification by the host immune system of a signal that indicates the presence of the tumor. SEREX is a technique originally described by Sahin et al. to identify tumor antigens bound by autologous antibodies in cancer patients (101,102). The technique immunoscreens tumor cDNA expression libraries with sera that contain autologous antibodies from cancer patients, and then clones and characterizes the tumor antigens bound by antibodies. Furthermore, tumor antigens identified by SEREX are candidates for the development of cancer vaccine (103). More importantly, several studies have evaluated the diagnostic potential and prognostic relevance of autologous antibodies as serum markers, particularly for detection of small, early-stage lesions (104). The frequency of antibody responses to SEREX-defined antigens ranges from 14–27% in colon cancer and from 5–25% in renal cancer.

Recently, autologous tumor-specific antibody has been found in the serum of patients with ovarian cancer, but not of controls (105,106). Using this SEREX, Naora et al. found that 33% of ovarian cancer patients generated anti-HOXB7 antibody and the HOXB7, a homeobox gene, is expressed at high levels in primary ovarian carcinomas with different histological types and clinical stages but at very low level in ovarian surface epithelium (105). In another study using SEREX, Cao et al. screened cDNA library from a breast carcinoma cell line using antibodies isolated from cancer patients and found that RBP1L1, a retinoblastoma-binding protein-related gene, is

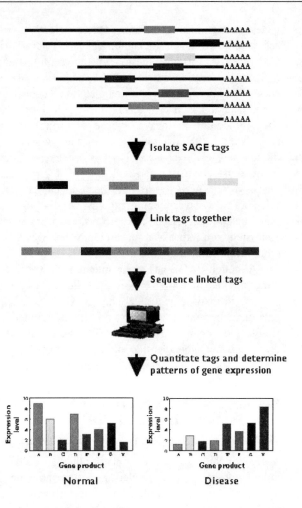

Figure 2 The principles of serial analysis of gene expression (SAGE). The SAGE method is based on the isolation of unique sequence tags from individual transcripts and concatenation of tags serially into long DNA molecules. Rapid sequencing of concatemer clones reveals individual tags and allows quantitation and identification of cellular transcripts. Please visit http://www.sagenet.org/ for details of SAGE. **Color representation of figure appears on Color Plate 2.**

overexpressed in the majority of carcinomas including ovarian cancer, but not in normal tissues except testis (106). Future studies will be undertaken to validate the observations in larger case/control studies to assess the potential of autologous antibodies reacting to HOXB7 and RBP1L1 or the HOXB7 and RBP1L1 themselves as diagnostic markers in ovarian cancer patients. For more information, please see Chapter 10.

Digital PCR-Based Analysis on Plasma DNA

Besides protein markers (as mentioned above), tumor-released DNA represents another unique marker in plasma or serum in cancer patients. It has been well known that tumors can release a significant amount of free DNA into the systemic circulation due to necrosis and/or apoptosis of cancer cells (107,108). Elevated amounts of circulating DNA can be detected in many patients with a variety of cancers (109–113). Tumor-released DNA is characterized by molecular genetic abnormalities, including microsatellite alterations (including loss of heterozygosity and microsatellite instability), and mutations in a variety of oncogenes and tumor-suppressor genes. Therefore, cancer patients theoretically can be diagnosed based on the presence of these molecular genetic alterations in their plasma or serum. Among these alterations, allelic imbalance (loss of heterozygosity) representing losses or gains of a defined chromosomal region is the most common molecular signature in human cancers (113). In normal tissue, the ratio of paternal allele to maternal allele of a specific chromosomal region is 1:1, and thus there is allelic balance in this region. In contrast, if the ratio is not 1:1, this indicates an imbalance in a certain chromosomal region between paternal and maternal alleles.

Using microsatellite markers, investigators have demonstrated allelic imbalance in the plasma or serum obtained from patients with lung cancer, breast cancer, head and neck squamous carcinoma, renal cell carcinoma, ovarian carcinoma, and melanoma (108). Moreover, allelic imbalance can be detected very early in tumor development (111). Although the results from these excellent studies appear encouraging, there are at least two main problems associated with the traditional assessment of allelic imbalance in serum. First, plasma or serum DNA is a mixture of neoplastic and non-neoplastic DNA. The DNA released from the non-neoplastic cells can mask allelic imbalance because it is difficult to quantify the allelic ratio using microsatellite markers. Second, such DNA is often degraded to a varying extent, producing artifactual enrichment of smaller alleles when microsatellite markers are used for analysis (114).

To overcome the obstacles associated with the molecular genetic analysis of allelic imbalance, a recently developed PCR-based approach called Digital Single Nucleotide Polymorphism (SNP) analysis was used in which the paternal or maternal alleles within a tumor sample were individually counted (115–118), thus allowing a quantitative measure of such imbalance in the presence of normal DNA. With digital SNP analysis, allelic imbalance in at least one of the eight SNP markers assayed can be found in 60% and 90% of stage I and III patients' plasma, respectively (119). In contrast, 50 patients without neoplastic disease do not contain allelic imbalance in their plasma DNA. The pattern of allelic imbalance in the plasma DNA is generally identical to the corresponding tumor (119). This finding suggests that it is possible to detect allelic imbalance in plasma DNA in a significant fraction of patients with potentially curable ovarian cancers. Future studies will aim at identifying the specific chromosomal regions with the allelic imbalance pattern specific to ovarian carcinoma to improve the specificity as a screening tool for ovarian carcinoma.

SUMMARY

Development of tumor markers that can be clinically applied to screening, differential diagnosis, monitoring, and prognostic prediction of ovarian cancer is crucial to improving the clinical outcomes in patients who have this devastating disease. Ideally, these tumor markers should provide a high sensitivity and specificity to such purposes. Unfortunately, these criteria are rarely met for the current ovarian cancer makers. CA125 is the only marker that has been applied in the clinical setting for the follow-up of patients with ovarian cancer; however, the low sensitivity and specificity limit its use as a screening tool for early detection and differential diagnosis. Recent advances in biotechnology and the completion of human genome project have great impact in accelerating the discovery of novel tumor markers associated with ovarian cancer. These emerging markers are expected to hold great promise in improving early diagnosis and monitoring in patients with ovarian cancer.

REFERENCES

1. Banks E, Beral V, Reeves G. The epidemiology of epithelial ovarian cancer: a review. Int J Gynecol Cancer 1997;7:425–438.
2. Parkin DM, Muir CS, Whelan SF. Cancer incidence in five continents. Lyon, France: IARC Scientific, 1992.
3. Ozols RF, Rubin SC, Thomas GB, Robboy SJ. Epithelial ovarian cancer. In: Hoskins WJ, Perez CA, Young RC, (eds.). Principles and practice of gynecologic oncology. 3rd ed. Philadelphia: Lippincott, Williams, and Wilkins, 2000:981–1057.
4. Paley PJ. Ovarian cancer screening: are we making any progress? Curr Opin Oncol 2001;13:399–402.
5. Young RH, Clement PB, Scully RE. The ovary. In: Sternberg SS, (ed.). Diagnostic surgical pathology. 3rd ed. Philadelphia: Lippincott, Williams, & Wilkins, 1999:2307–2394.
6. Scully RE. World health organization international histological classification of tumors. 2nd ed. New York, NY: Springer, 1999.
7. Hough CD, Cho KR, Zonderman AB, Schwartz DR, Morin PJ. Coordinately up-regulated genes in ovarian cancer. Cancer Res 2001;61:3869–3876.
8. Greenlee RT, Hill-Harmon MB, Murray T, Thun M. Cancer statistics, 2001. CA Cancer J Clin 2001;51:15–36.
9. Memarzadeh S, Berek JS. Advances in the management of epithelial ovarian cancer. J Reprod Med 2001;46:621–9; discussion 29–30.
10. Holschneider CH, Berek JS. Ovarian cancer: epidemiology, biology, and prognostic factors. Semin Surg Oncol 2000;19:3–10.
11. Berek JS, Martinez-Maza O. Molecular and biologic factors in the pathogenesis of ovarian cancer. J Reprod Med 1994;39:241–248.
12. Yu Y, Xu F, Peng H, Fang X, Zhao S, Li Y, et al. NOEY2 (ARHI), an imprinted putative tumor suppressor gene in ovarian and breast carcinomas. Proc Natl Acad Sci U S A 1999;96:214–219.
13. Obata K, Morland SJ, Watson RH, Hitchcock A, Chenevix-Trench G, Thomas EJ, et al. Frequent PTEN/MMAC mutations in endometrioid but not serous or mucinous epithelial ovarian tumors. Cancer Res 1998;58:2095–2097.
14. Schultz DC, Vanderveer L, Berman DB, Hamilton TC, Wong AJ, Godwin AK. Identification of two candidate tumor suppressor genes on chromosome 17p13.3. Cancer Res 1996;56:1997–2002.
15. Phillips NJ, Zeigler MR, Deaven LL. A cDNA from the ovarian cancer critical region of deletion on chromosome 17p13.3. Cancer Lett 1996;102:85–90.
16. Bell DA, Scully RE. Early de novo ovarian carcinoma. A study of fourteen cases. Cancer 1994;73:1859–1864.
17. Auersperg N, Edelson MI, Mok SC, Johnson SW, Hamilton TC. The biology of ovarian cancer. Semin Oncol 1998;25:281–304.
18. Seidman JD, Kurman RJ. Subclassification of serous borderline tumors of the ovary into benign and malignant types. A clinicopathologic study of 65 advanced stage cases. Am J Surg Pathol 1996;20:1331–1345.
19. Katabuchi H, Tashiro H, Cho KR, Kurman RJ, Hedrick Ellenson L. Micropapillary serous carcinoma of the ovary: an immunohistochemical and mutational analysis of p53. Int J Gynecol Pathol 1998;17:54–60.
20. Singer G, Kurman RJ, Chang H-W, Cho S, Shih I-M. Diverse tumorigenic pathways in ovarian serous carcinoma. Am J Pathol 2002;160:1223–1228.
21. Eltabbakh GH, Yadev PR, Morgan A. Clinical picture of women with early stage ovarian cancer. Gynecol Oncol 1999;75:476–479.
22. Stratton JF, Tidy JA, Paterson ME. The surgical management of ovarian cancer. Cancer Treat Rev 2001;27:111–118.
23. Christian J, Thomas H. Ovarian cancer chemotherapy. Cancer Treat Rev 2001;27:99–109.
24. Bast RC, Jr., Feeney M, Lazarus H, Nadler LM, Colvin RB, Knapp RC. Reactivity of a monoclonal antibody with human ovarian carcinoma. J Clin Invest 1981;68:1331–1337.
25. Yin BW, Lloyd KO. Molecular cloning of the CA125 ovarian cancer antigen: identification as a new mucin, MUC16. J Biol Chem 2001;276:27371–27375.
26. Nustad K, Bast RC, Jr., Brien TJ, Nilsson O, Seguin P, Suresh MR, et al. Specificity and affinity of 26 monoclonal antibodies against the CA125 antigen: first report from the ISOBM TD-1

workshop. International Society for Oncodevelopmental Biology and Medicine. Tumor Biol 1996;17:196–219.
27. Nap M, Vitali A, Nustad K, Bast RC, Jr., O'Brien TJ, Nilsson O, et al. Immunohistochemical characterization of 22 monoclonal antibodies against the CA125 antigen: 2nd report from the ISOBM TD-1 Workshop. Tumor Biol 1996;17:325–331.
28. Jacobs I, Bast RC, Jr. The CA125 tumor-associated antigen: a review of the literature. Hum Reprod 1989;4:1–12.
29. O'Brien TJ, Tanimoto H, Konishi I, Gee M. More than 15 years of CA125: what is known about the antigen, its structure, and its function. Int J Biol Markers 1998;13:188–195.
30. Meyer T, Rustin GJ. Role of tumor markers in monitoring epithelial ovarian cancer. Br J Cancer 2000;82:1535–1538.
31. Bidart JM, Thuillier F, Augereau C, Chalas J, Daver A, Jacob N, et al. Kinetics of serum tumor marker concentrations and usefulness in clinical monitoring. Clin Chem 1999;45:1695–1707.
32. Practice. Sol. Guidelines for the analytical performance and clinical utility of tumor markers. Washington, DC: The National Academy of Clinical Biochemistry, 1998.
33. Bast RC, Jr., Xu FJ, Yu YH, Barnhill S, Zhang Z, Mills GB. CA125: the past and the future. Int J Biol Markers 1998; 13:179–187.
34. Davelaar EM, van Kamp GJ, Verstraeten RA, Kenemans P. Comparison of seven immunoassays for the quantification of CA125 antigen in serum. Clin Chem 1998;44:1417–1422.
35. Pauler DK, Menon U, McIntosh M, Symecko HL, Skates SJ, Jacobs IJ. Factors influencing serum CA125II levels in healthy postmenopausal women. Cancer Epidemiol Biomarkers Prev 2001;10:489–493.
36. Bast RC, Urban N, Shrindhar V. Early detection of ovarian cancer: promise and reality. Cancer Treat Res 2002;107:61–97.
37. Skates SJ, Xu FJ, Yu YH, Sjovall K, Einhorn N, Chang Y, et al. Toward an optimal algorithm for ovarian cancer screening with longitudinal tumor markers. Cancer 1995;76:2004–2010.
38. Cancer O. NIH consensus conference. Ovarian cancer. Screening, treatment, and follow–up. NIH Consensus Development Panel on Ovarian Cancer. JAMA 1995;273:491–497.
39. Woolas RP, Conaway MR, Xu F, Jacobs IJ, Yu Y, Daly L, et al. Combinations of multiple serum markers are superior to individual assays for discriminating malignant from benign pelvic masses. Gynecol Oncol 1995;59:111–116.
40. Zhang Z, Barnhill SD, Zhang H, Xu F, Yu Y, Jacobs I, et al. Combination of multiple serum markers using an artificial neural network to improve specificity in discriminating malignant from benign pelvic masses. Gynecol Oncol 1999;73:56–61.
41. Fritsche HA, Bast RC. CA125 in ovarian cancer: advances and controversy. Clin Chem 1998;44:1379–1380.
42. Partridge EE, Barnes MN. Epithelial ovarian cancer: prevention, diagnosis, and treatment. CA Cancer J Clin 1999;49:297–320.
43. Duffy MJ. Clinical uses of tumor markers: a critical review. Crit Rev Clin Lab Sci 2001;38:225–262.
44. Verheijen RH, von Mensdorff-Pouilly S, van Kamp GJ, Kenemans P. CA125: fundamental and clinical aspects. Semin Cancer Biol 1999;9:117–124.
45. Diamandis EP, Yousef GM, Luo LY, Magklara A, Obiezu CV. The human kallikrein gene family implications in carcinogenesis. Trends Endocrinol Metab 2000;11:54–60.
46. Yousef GM, Diamandis EP. The new human tissue kallikrein gene family: structure, function and association to disease. Endocr Rev 2001;22:184–204.
47. Clements J, Hooper J, Dong Y, Harvey T. The expanded human kallikrein (KLK) gene family: genomic organization, tissue-specific expression, and potential functions. Biol Chem 2001; 382:5–14.
48. Obiezu CV, Soosaipillai A, Jung K, Stephan C, Scorilas A, Howarth DHC, et al. Detection of human kallikrein 4 (hK4) in normal and cancerous prostatic tissues by immunofluorometry and immunohistochemistry (submitted).
49. Dong Y, Kaushal A, Bui L, Chu S, Fuller PJ, Nicklin J, et al. Human kallikrein 4 (klk4) is highly expressed in serous ovarian carcinomas. Clin Cancer Res 2001;7:2363–2371.
50. Obiezu CV, Scorilas A, Katsaros D, Massobrio M, Yousef GM, Fracchioli S, et al. Higher human kallikrein gene 4 (klk4) expression indicates poor prognosis of ovarian cancer patients. Clin Cancer Res 2001;7:2380–2386.
51. Kim H, Scorilas A, Katsaros D, Yousef GM, Massobrio M, Fracchioli S, et al. Human kallikrein gene 5 (KLK5) expression is an indicator of poor prognosis in ovarian cancer. Br J Cancer 2001;84:643–650.
52. Magklara A, Scorilas A, Katsaros D, Massobrio M, Yousef GM, Fracchioli S, et al. The human KLK8 (neuropsin/ovasin) gene: identification of two novel splice variants and its prognostic value in ovarian cancer. Clin Cancer Res 2001;7:806–811.
53. Tanimoto H, Underwood LJ, Shigemasa K, Yan Yan MS, Clarke J, Parmley, O'Brien TJ. The stratum corneum chymotryptic enzyme that mediates shedding and desquamation of skin cells is highly overexpressed in ovarian tumor cells. Cancer 1999; 86:2074–2082.
54. Yousef GM, Kyriakopoulou LG, Scorilas A, Fracchioli S, Ghiringhello B, Zarghooni M, et al. Quantitative expression of the human kallikrein gene 9 (KLK9) in ovarian cancer: a new independent and favorable prognostic marker. Cancer Res 2001; 61:7811–7818.
55. Diamandis EP, Yousef GM, Soosaipillai AR, Bunting P. Human kallikrein 6 (zyme/protease M/neurosin): a new serum biomarker of ovarian carcinoma. Clin Biochem 2000;33:579–583.
56. Diamandis EP, Okui A, Mitsui S, Luo L-Y, Soosaipillai A, Grass L, et al. Human kallikrein 11: A new biomarker of prostate and ovarian carcinoma. Cancer Res (in press).
57. Luo L, Bunting P, Scorilas A, Diamandis EP. Human kallikrein 10: a novel tumor marker for ovarian carcinoma? Clin Chim Acta 2001;306:111–118.
58. Liu XL, Wazer DE, Watanabe K, Band V. Identification of a novel serine protease-like gene, the expression of which is down-regulated during breast cancer progression. Cancer Res 1996; 56:3371–3379.
59. Luo LY, Katsaros D, Scorilas A, Fracchioli S, Piccinno R, Rigault De La Longrais IA, et al. Prognostic value of human kallikrein 10 expression in epithelial ovarian carcinoma. Clin Cancer Res 2001;7:2372–2379.
60. Mok SC, Chao J, Skates S, Wong K, Yiu GK, Muto MG, et al. Prostasin, a potential serum marker for ovarian cancer: identification through microarray technology. J Natl Cancer Inst 2001; 93:1458–1464.
61. Yu JX, Chao L, Chao J. Prostasin is a novel human serine proteinase from seminal fluid. Purification, tissue distribution, and localization in prostate gland. J Biol Chem 1994;269: 18843–18848.
62. Sundstrom BE, Stigbrand TI. Cytokeratins and tissue polypeptide antigen. Int J Biol Markers 1994;9:102–108.

63. Tuxen MK, Soletormos G, Dombernowsky P. Tumor markers in the management of patients with ovarian cancer. Cancer Treat Rev 1995;21:215–245.
64. Xu Y, Shen Z, Wiper DW, Wu M, Morton RE, Elson P, et al. Lysophosphatidic acid as a potential biomarker for ovarian and other gynecologic cancers. JAMA 1998;280:719–723.
65. Pustilnik TB, Estrella V, Wiener JR, Mao M, Eder A, Watt MA, et al. Lysophosphatidic acid induces urokinase secretion by ovarian cancer cells. Clin Cancer Res 1999;5:3704–3710.
66. Stenman UH, Huhtala ML, Koistinen R, Seppala M. Immunochemical demonstration of an ovarian cancer-associated urinary peptide. Int J Cancer 1982;30:53–57.
67. Huhtala ML, Pesonen K, Kalkkinen N, Stenman UH. Purification and characterization of a tumor-associated trypsin inhibitor from the urine of a patient with ovarian cancer. J Biol Chem 1982;257:13713–13716.
68. Gadducci A, Ferdeghini M, Rispoli G, Prontera C, Bianchi R, Fioretti P. Comparison of tumor-associated trypsin inhibitor (TATI) with CA125 as a marker for diagnosis and monitoring of epithelial ovarian cancer. Scand J Clin Lab Invest Suppl 1991;207:19–24.
69. Zotter S, Hageman PC, Lossnitzer A, Moo WJ, Hilgers J. Tissue and tumor distribution of human polymorphic epithelial mucin. Cancer Rev 1988;11:55–101.
70. Ward BG, McGuckin MA. Are CASA and CA125 concentrations in peripheral blood sourced from peritoneal fluid in women with pelvic masses? Cancer 1994;73:1699–1703.
71. Ward BG, McGuckin MA, Ramm L, Forbes KL. Expression of tumor markers CA125, CASA, and OSA in minimal/mild endometriosis. Aust N Z J Obstet Gynaecol 1991;31:273–275.
72. Ward BG, McGuckin MA, Ramm LE, Coglan M, Sanderson B, Tripcony L, et al. The management of ovarian carcinoma is improved by the use of cancer-associated serum antigen and CA125 assays. Cancer 1993;71:430–438.
73. Ho CH, Yuan CC, Liu SM. Diagnostic and prognostic values of plasma levels of fibrinolytic markers in ovarian cancer. Gynecol Oncol 1999;75:397–400.
74. Chambers SK, Ivins CM, Carcangiu ML. Plasminogen activator inhibitor-1 is an independent poor prognostic factor for survival in advanced stage epithelial ovarian cancer patients. Int J Cancer 1998;79:449–454.
75. Gleeson NC, Hill BJ, Moscinski LC, Mark JE, Roberts WS, Hoffman MS, et al. Urokinase plasminogen activator in ovarian cancer. Eur J Gynaecol Oncol 1996;17:110–113.
76. Chambers SK, Ivins CM, Carcangiu ML. Expression of plasminogen activator inhibitor-2 in epithelial ovarian cancer: a favorable prognostic factor related to the actions of CSF-1. Int J Cancer 1997;74:571–575.
77. Chambers SK, Gertz RE, Jr., Ivins CM, Kacinski BM. The significance of urokinase-type plasminogen activator, its inhibitors, and its receptor in ascites of patients with epithelial ovarian cancer. Cancer 1995;75:1627–1633.
78. Gastl G, Plante M. Bioactive interleukin-6 levels in serum and ascites as a prognostic factor in patients with epithelial ovarian cancer. In: Bartlett JMS (ed.). Methods in molecular medicine—ovarian cancer. Totowa: Humana Press Inc., 2000:121–123.
79. Foti E, Ferrandina G, Martucci R, Romanini ME, Benedetti Panici P, Testa U, et al. IL-6, M-CSF, and IAP cytokines in ovarian cancer: simultaneous assessment of serum levels. Oncology 1999;57:211–215.
80. Scambia G, Testa U, Benedetti Panici P, Foti E, Martucci R, Gadducci A, et al. Prognostic significance of interleukin 6 serum levels in patients with ovarian cancer. Br J Cancer 1995;71:354–356.
81. Cole LA. hCG, its free subunits, and its metabolites. Roles in pregnancy and trophoblastic disease. J Reprod Med 1998;43:3–10.
82. Vartiainen J, Lehtovirta P, Finne P, Stenman UH, Alfthan H. Preoperative serum concentration of hCG-beta as a prognostic factor in ovarian cancer. Int J Cancer 2001;95:313–316.
83. Nishimura R, Koizumi T, Das H, Takemori M, Hasegawa K. Enzyme immunoassay of urinary ?-core fragment of human chorionic gonadotropin as a tumor marker for ovarian cancer. In: Bartlett JMS (ed.). Methods in molecular medicine—ovarian cancer. Totowa: Humana Press, Inc., 2000:135–141.
84. Katso RM, Manek S, O'Byrne K, Playford MP, Le Meuth V, Ganesan TS. Molecular approaches to diagnosis and management of ovarian cancer. Cancer Metastasis Rev 1997;16:81–107.
85. Meden H, Fattahi-Meibodi A, Marx D. ELISA-based quantification of p105 (c-erbB-2, HER-2/neu) in serum of ovarian carcinoma. In: Bartlett JMS (ed.). Methods in molecular medicine—ovarian cancer. Totowa: Humana Press, Inc., 2000:125–133.
86. Meden H, Kuhn W. Overexpression of the oncogene c-erbB-2 (HER-2/neu) in ovarian cancer: a new prognostic factor. Eur J Obstet Gynecol Reprod Biol 1997;71:173–179.
87. Cheung TH, Wong YF, Chung TK, Maimonis P, Chang AM. Clinical use of serum c-erbB-2 in patients with ovarian masses. Gynecol Obstet Invest 1999;48:133–137.
88. Hellstrom I, Goodman G, Pullman J, Yang Y, Hellstrom KE. Overexpression of HER-2 in ovarian carcinomas. Cancer Res 2001;61:2420–2423.
89. Liu AX, Testa JR, Hamilton TC, Jove R, Nicosia SV, Cheng JQ. AKT2, a member of the protein kinase B family, is activated by growth factors, v-Ha-ras, and v-src through phosphatidylinositol 3-kinase in human ovarian epithelial cancer cells. Cancer Res 1998;58:2973–2977.
90. Shayesteh L, Lu Y, Kuo WL, Baldocchi R, Godfrey T, Collins C, et al. PIK3CA is implicated as an oncogene in ovarian cancer. Nat Genet 1999;21:99–102.
91. Cheng JQ, Godwin AK, Bellacosa A, Taguchi T, Franke TF, Hamilton TC, et al. AKT2, a putative oncogene encoding a member of a subfamily of protein-serine/threonine kinases, is amplified in human ovarian carcinomas. Proc Natl Acad Sci U S A 1992;89:9267–9271.
92. Bellacosa A, de Feo D, Godwin AK, Bell DW, Cheng JQ, Altomare DA, et al. Molecular alterations of the AKT2 oncogene in ovarian and breast carcinomas. Int J Cancer 1995;64:280–285.
93. Yuan ZQ, Sun M, Feldman RI, Wang G, Ma X, Jiang C, et al. Frequent activation of AKT2 and induction of apoptosis by inhibition of phosphoinositide-3-OH kinase/AKT pathway in human ovarian cancer. Oncogene 2000;19:2324–2330.
94. Bichsel VE, Liotta LA, Petricoin EF. Cancer proteomics: from biomarker discovery to signal pathway profiling. Cancer J 2001;7:69–78.
95. Velculescu VE, Vogelstein B, Kinzler KW. Analyzing uncharted transcriptomes with SAGE. Trends Genet 2000;16:423–425.
96. Schaefer C, Grouse L, Buetow K, Strausberg RL. A new cancer genome anatomy project web resource for the community. Cancer J 2001;7:52–60.

97. Vlahou A, Schellhammer PF, Mendrinos S, Patel K, Kondylis FI, Gong L, et al. Development of a novel proteomic approach for the detection of transitional cell carcinoma of the bladder in urine. Am J Pathol 2001;158:1491–1502.
98. Velculescu VE, Zhang L, Vogelstein B, Kinzler KW. Serial analysis of gene expression. Science 1995;270:484–487.
99. Velculescu VE, Madden SL, Zhang L, Lash AE, Yu J, Rago C, et al. Analysis of human transcriptomes. Nat Genet 1999;23:387–388.
100. Hough CD, Sherman-Baust CA, Pizer ES, Montz FJ, Im DD, Rosenshein NB, et al. Large-scale serial analysis of gene expression reveals genes differentially expressed in ovarian cancer. Cancer Res 2000;60:6281–6287.
101. Sahin U, Tureci O, Pfreundschuh M. Serological identification of human tumor antigens. Curr Opin Immunol 1997;9:709–716.
102. Sahin U, Tureci O, Schmitt H, Cochlovius B, Johannes T, Schmits R, et al. Human neoplasms elicit multiple specific immune responses in the autologous host. Proc Natl Acad Sci U S A 1995;92:11810–11813.
103. Chen Y-T. Cancer vaccine: identification of human tumor antigens by SEREX. Cancer J 2001;6(suppl):s208–s217.
104. Soussi T. p53 Antibodies in the sera of patients with various types of cancer: a review. Cancer Res 2000;60:1777–1788.
105. Naora H, Yang YQ, Montz FJ, Seidman JD, Kurman RJ, Roden RB. A serologically identified tumor antigen encoded by a homeobox gene promotes growth of ovarian epithelial cells. Proc Natl Acad Sci U S A 2001;98:4060–4065.
106. Cao J, Gao T, Stanbridge EJ, Irie R. RBP1L1, a retinoblastoma-binding protein-related gene encoding an antigenic epitope abundantly expressed in human carcinomas and normal testis. J Natl Cancer Inst 2001;93:1159–1165.
107. Leon SA, Shapiro B, Sklaroff DM, Yaros MJ. Free DNA in the serum of cancer patients and the effect of therapy. Cancer Res 1977;37:646–650.
108. Anker P, Mulcahy H, Chen XQ, Stroun M. Detection of circulating tumor DNA in the blood (plasma/serum) of cancer patients. Cancer Metastasis Rev 1999;18:65–73.
109. Hickey KP, Boyle KP, Jepps HM, Andrew AC, Buxton EJ, Burns PA. Molecular detection of tumor DNA in serum and peritoneal fluid from ovarian cancer patients. Br J Cancer 1999;80:1803–1808.
110. Sozzi G, Conte D, Mariani L, Lo Vullo S, Roz L, Lombardo C, et al. Analysis of circulating tumor DNA in plasma at diagnosis and during follow-up of lung cancer patients. Cancer Res 2001;61:4675–4678.
111. Sozzi G, Musso K, Ratcliffe C, Goldstraw P, Pierotti MA, Pastorino U. Detection of microsatellite alterations in plasma DNA of non-small cell lung cancer patients: a prospect for early diagnosis. Clin Cancer Res 1999;5:2689–2692.
112. Taback B, Fujiwara Y, Wang HJ, Foshag LJ, Morton DL, Hoon DS. Prognostic significance of circulating microsatellite markers in the plasma of melanoma patients. Cancer Res 2001;61 5723–5726.
113. Lengauer C, Kinzler KW, Vogelstein B. Genetic instabilities in human cancers. Nature 1998;396:643–649.
114. Liu J, Zabarovska VI, Braga E, Alimov A, Klien G, Zabarovsky ER. Loss of heterozygosity in tumor cells requires re-evaluation: the data are biased by the size-dependent differential sensitivity of allele detection. FEBS Lett 1999;462:121–128.
115. Zhou W, Galizia G, Goodman SN, Romans KE, Kinzler KW, Vogelstein B, et al. Counting alleles reveals a connection between chromosome 18q loss and vascular invasion. Nat Biotechnol 2001;19:78–81.
116. Shih IM, Zhou W, Goodman SN, Lengauer C, Kinzler KW, Vogelstein B. Evidence that genetic instability occurs at an early stage of colorectal tumorigenesis. Cancer Res 2001;61:818–822.
117. Shih IM, Wang TL, Traverso G, Romans K, Hamilton SR, Ben-Sasson S, et al. Top-down morphogenesis of colorectal tumors. Proc Natl Acad Sci U S A 2001;98:2640–2645.
118. Shih IM, Yan H, Speyrer D, Shmookler BM, Sugarbaker PH, Ronnett BM. Molecular genetic analysis of appendiceal mucinous adenomas in identical twins, including one with pseudomyxoma peritonei. Am J Surg Pathol 2001;25:1095–1099.
119. Chang H-W, Cho S, Singer G, Sokoll LJ, Chan DW, Shih I-M. Tumor-release plasma DNA as a marker for ovarian cancer patients. Unpublished.

Chapter **19**

Tumor Markers for Colorectal Cancer

Morton K. Schwartz

Colorectal cancer affects about 5% of all Americans and represents 15% of all cancers. In 2001, it was projected that there would be about 135,400 cases of colorectal cancer and 56,700 deaths due to this disease (1). If detected early, the cancer is highly curable: the estimated five-year survival rate is 91% in persons with localized disease. On the other hand, the estimated five-year survival rate is 60% in individuals with regional spread, and only 6% in those with distant metastases. The availability of colonoscopy and fecal occult blood testing have reduced the mortality rate from this disease and enabled the detection of earlier-stage disease. The five-year survival rate for colon cancer increased from 41% in the 1950s to 54% in the 1980s; for rectal cancer, the rate rose from 41 to 52% (2).

There are numerous risk factors for colorectal cancer. These include genetic factors that lead to familial adenomatous polyposis syndrome, familial colorectal cancer, and other genetically related diseases. The gene for familial adenomatous polyposis has been identified, cloned, and sequenced, and it is located close to a marker at 5q21-22. In the progression from normal colon mucosa to frank adenocarcinoma, there are changes in the 5q chromosome and in the 15-*ras* oncogene (Figure 1). Other genes have been described at 5q21. Expression of C-*myc* is increased in mucinous and high-grade tumors, as is expression of *ras* in node-positive tumors. Other oncogenes have been enumerated and prognosis is inversely related to loss of *p53* and NM23-11s (3). Fecal occult blood testing is widely used in colorectal cancer screening despite the fact that there is a large incidence of false positives as well as false negatives. In a survey of six large studies including more than 150,000 individuals, the positive predictive value of fecal occult blood ranged from 4.7% to 17.7% (2). In another review of studies including 13,472 persons, the detection rate range was 5–18% in adenomas and 22–33% in cancer. DNA in exfoliated cells (k-*ras* and *p53* marker) has also had a large number of false negatives (4)(Table 1).

Numerous circulating antigens in body fluids have been described in colorectal cancer; the major emphasis of this chapter is to describe them and their utility in the management of the patient with cancer of the colon or rectum (Table 1).

CEA

Carcinoembryonic antigen (CEA) has been in use for more than two decades. It is well known that CEA is not specific for colorectal carcinoma and is elevated in many other cancers, including breast, lung, liver, and pancreas. Small amounts are found in normal tissue and benign tumors.

In the earliest studies, CEA was observed in fetal intestine, liver, and pancreas during the first six months of pregnancy and in cancerous liver, colon, or pancreas (5,6). Because it is a cell surface protein, it is shed into the circulation and found in serum. In a collaborative study of 35,000 serum samples from patients and controls, 98.7% of 1425 normal nonsmokers had serum levels less than 5 µg/L. In 857 smokers, elevations were seen in 33%. In 576 patients without clinical evidence of disease who had barium enemas, there were 23 cancers, 18 that expressed CEA values >2.5 µg/L (7).

Elevations are related to the extent of tumor burden and only a very small percentage of patients with early stage disease display serum elevations (Table 2). CEA levels are elevated in

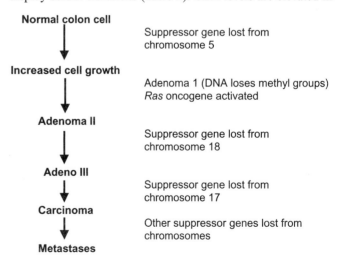

Figure 1 Evolution of colon cancer (1). Changes usually occur in order shown, but this order is not absolutely necessary.

Table 1 Tumor markers in gastrointestinal cancer

Circulating markers	Role
CEA	Most sensitive in colorectal cancer
CA19-9	Most sensitive in pancreatic cancer
CA195	Equally sensitive to CA19-9 in pancreatic cancer
CA72-4	Most sensitive in gastric cancer
CA50	Equally sensitive to CA19-9
Glycosyltransferases	Nonspecific
Tissue markers	**Role**
Lactic dehydrogenase	Prognosis
Ornithine decarboxylase	Prognosis
Genetic markers	**Role**
C-myc	Mucinous and high-grade tumors
RAS	Node-positive tumors
Ha-ras	Independent grade, stage, Ki-ras
Cathepsin B gene	Inversely related to stage MDR 1 — low-grade tumor
p53	Inversely correlated to metastases
nn23-Hi	Inversely correlated to metastatic disease
Growth factor (TGF2 and EGFR)	Related to tumor growth

40% of individuals with early stage disease compared to 65% of patients with distant metastases. Elevations are observed in 4% of Dukes' Stage A patients, 25% of those with stage B, 45% of those with Dukes' C, and 65% of patients with disease metastatic to liver, bone, or lung (8). Despite these limitations, a National Cancer Institute consensus panel concluded that "CEA is the best presently available non-invasive procedure for post-operative surveillance of patients to detect disseminated recurrence of colon-rectal cancer" (9).

Declining concentrations of CEA are indicative of effective therapy and rising levels indicate disease activity, although the increased CEA level may precede clinical symptoms of recurrence by months (10–12). This is undoubtedly still so, but it must be understood that not all patients with metastatic colon cancer exhibit elevations of serum CEA. (Table 3). In two patients with equally progressive disease, a crescendo-like rise in serum CEA concentration may occur in one patient while little or no increase is observed for the other (10). This probably reflects the pathology of the tumor. Well-differentiated tumors produce CEA while those that are undifferentiated or poorly differentiated produce little, if any CEA. In patients with metastatic gastric cancer, CEA elevations were never observed over a period of one year in individuals with undifferentiated cancers, whereas there was a mean rise of more than twenty times the pretreatment level in patients with highly differentiated tumors (12). Interpretation of CEA data would be more understandable and useful if the differentiation of the tumors was routinely reported with the CEA values.

During therapeutic monitoring, it is important to understand the significance of changes in CEA values. There is no definition of a meaningful decrease or increase of CEA. In general, a 25–35% change has been termed significant. Four patterns of change of serum CEA values may be observed. Two patterns are expected: an uninterrupted rise in patients who do not respond to treatment, and a fall in those who do. The remaining two patterns are these: (1) in patients who are responding to treatment, there may be a surge in CEA for weeks post-treatment, followed by the conventional fall; (2) in others, there may be an immediate but sustained fall in serum CEA, and then the rise that indicates lack of response. It is apparent that if CEA is to be used in evaluating response to therapy, an understanding of marker kinetics is essential (13).

A great deal is now known about the chemistry and immunology of CEA. It is a cell surface glycosylated (80%), monomeric protein with a molecular weight of 180–200 kDa. There are five major non-overlapping epitopes (Gold 1–5). These are broadly correlated with the domain organization without sequence localization (13). CEA is produced by fetal gut and colonic mucosa (differentiated surface epithelial cells) (15). Its half-life in the circulation is 3–11 days. After successful surgical

Table 2 Relation of carcinoembryonic antigen levels to state of disease in patients with primary colorectal cancer (37)

Stage	Number of patients	Percentage of patients				
		≤5.0 µg/L	5.1–10 µg/L	10.1–20 µg/L	21–100 µg/L	<100 µg/L
Benign	47	100	—	—	—	—
Dukes' A	58	97	3	—	—	—
Dukes' B	51	75	10	15	—	—
Dukes' C	63	56	14	13	11	3
Recurrent or metastatic	186	30	11	11	26	19

Table 3 CEA in recurrent colon cancer (37,38)

Study year	Number of patients	Positive % (5.0 µg/L)
1. 1974	53	68
2. 1976	12	67
3. 1976	82	77
4. 1976	23	87
5. 1978	19	89
6. 1979	18	61
7. 1980	18	94
Total	225	76

Table 4 CEA in "second look" surgery (37,38)

Study year	Number of patients		Recurrence %	Resected for cure %
1. 1978	Retrospective	22	86	27
	Prospective	18	94	72
2. 1978	14		100	50
3. 1980	16		94	27
4. 1981	14		78	7
5. 1981	37		89	43
6. 1981	15		100	27
7. 1985	146		95	55
Total	282		90	36

intervention, the serum CEA falls with a half-life ($T_{1/2}$) of about five days (11).

In the gene family related to CEA, there are at least four closely related genes involved in CEA control, and they are clustered in the long arm of chromosome 19. The structure of the molecule includes a 34-amino-acid leader peptide, a 108-amino-acid NH2 terminal domain, three homologous repeating domains of 178 amino acids and a 26-amino-acid hydrophobic C-terminal domain (15). It is hoped that the understanding of the CEA gene family may lead to the design of more specific CEA assays. Until the time when more specific assays are available, we must understand that about 25–30% of individuals with colon cancer metastatic to the liver will not demonstrate elevations throughout the course of their disease.

CEA methods have improved in detectability to less than 1 µg/L and have a precision of 5–10%, depending on the CEA concentration in the specimen. Standardization of methodology is possible because there is an available World Health Organization (WHO) standard (IRP 73/601). However, different methods yield different values and variation in intra-laboratory precision is very high. In a quality assurance study with four materials submitted to 30 Italian laboratories over a period of 30 months, the coefficients of variation (CVs) about the consensus means varied from 30 to 40%. Fourteen different assay methods were used by the laboratories in the study. In another study conducted by the UK NEQAS, 124 laboratories participated. Two manual test methods and 11 automated methods were represented. The acceptable limits for CEA were established as ±20% for bias and 20% for variability of the bias. In 1996, 5% of the participants exceeded the bias limits (15% in 1995) and 6% the variability limits (20% in 1995). In January 1998, 215 New York State laboratories took part in a CEA proficiency test. Eight methods, six of which were automated, were used. In a specimen with a mean value for all the laboratories of 4.4 ±0.6 µg/L (CV=13%) the variation was between 5.7 ±0.6 µg/L (CV=9.3%) for one instrument to 4.1 ±0.3 µg/L (CV=7.1%) for a manual Immunoradiometric Assay (IRMA) method. If 5.0 µg/L is used as the normal/abnormal reference range, two of the eight participants would report values construed as abnormal by the ordering physician (16).

Second-look surgery based solely on a rising CEA level has been recommended by several investigators (Table 4). In more than 90% of these patients, residual tumor has been found, but was resectable in only 7–43% of the patients. The problem of using CEA in second-look surgery is the time that elapses between the observation of the rising CEA titers and the decision to proceed with surgery. In a prospective study when surgical intervention occurred in a relatively short period after a rising CEA level, resectable tumor was found in 13 of 17 (76%) patients. Although the role of second-look surgery is not established, the data seem to indicate that the procedure will have little effect on survival. It can be expected that a five-year disease-free survival rate of 25% can be achieved in patients from whom hepatic metastases are removed. In CEA-directed second-look surgery, 16 of 43 (37%) were alive without disease after five years and in clinically directed second-look surgery, 11 of 32 (34%) were alive without disease after five years (17–18).

CEA can be a prognostic indicator. Pre-operative CEA values greater than 10 µg/L suggest metastatic disease. When the post-operative CEA falls to <5 µg/L, only 18% of patients will experience recurrence compared to 63% of patients in whom the CEA remains above 10µg/L. The lead time between elevation of CEA and recurrence is up to eight months (19).

The most useful application of serum/plasma CEA is in monitoring patients during therapy. However, monitoring CEA in patients with breast or colon cancer who are receiving chemotherapy has been the subject of controversy. The question has been "What extent of increase or decrease is meaningful?" In general, a 25–35% change in CEA level has been termed significant. It has been suggested that a baseline of at least two sequential values must be established during the first two months of therapy. Deviations from this value are highly significant. Survival was significantly longer ($p=0.00001$) in individuals whose titer decreased below the established baseline (20). The confusion surrounding CEA in evaluating therapy may be that most clinicians are unaware of the facts, repeated here, that four patterns in CEA may be observed: (1) the expected two, an uninterrupted rise in the titer of patients who do not respond and (2) a fall in that of those who do; the third, in which patients who are responding produce a surge in CEA that may last for weeks, with the conventional fall; and the last, in which there is an immediate but sustained fall in serum CEA and then a rise that indicates lack of response.

If CEA is to be used in evaluating response to therapy, an understanding of the kinetics is essential. Reports suggest that the difference between local recurrence and metastatic disease to the liver is a difference in the slope of increasing CEA levels over ten days of 0.17 μg/L and 2.2 μg/L. Others have proposed that increases of CEA of greater than 12% per month suggest recurrence. There is a logarithmic relationship between serum CEA and growth of metastatic tumor.

An important consideration in assaying CEA is the possible presence in the specimen of human anti-mouse antibody. This has become more important as the number of patients treated with mouse monoclonal antibodies increases. In one study, 58 specimens from 30 patients who received indium-labeled anti-CEA demonstrated abnormal CEA values (>5.0 μg/L). Addition of 200 μg of polyclonal mouse IgG reduced the number of CEA positive results to 37, and all the elevated specimens had lower values. When reagents specifically designed to reduce interference by heterophilic antibody were used, 47 of the 58 specimens had normal values (22).

When first described, CEA fulfilled all the requirements of an ideal tumor marker. It was apparently elevated in almost all patients with colorectal cancer (35/36 patients above 2.5 μg/L) but was normal after successful therapy and in all sera from normal persons and those with benign diseases of the colon. These observations have not been borne out over time. The expert panel of the American Society of Clinical Oncology (ASCO) has concluded that CEA cannot be used for screening, but pre-operative CEA may assist in staging and surgical treatment planning. Data are insufficient to recommend prognostic use. An expert panel also concluded that CEA elevations detect recurrence earlier than other techniques. CEA monitoring should be done monthly during the first three years after initial therapy, and then every three months for two years at the start of treatment and then every two to three months thereafter (23). In addition to understanding these recommendations, clinicians must be taught that smokers may have higher CEA values than nonsmokers and that different assay methods may yield different numbers. Laboratory staff must be aware of linearity, hook effects, and interference in the assays (16,22).

CEA in Other Body Fluids and in Solid Tissue

CEA has been measured in body fluids other than serum. Urinary CEA has a molecular weight of 90 kDa, much lower than plasma CEA. Since it has a relatively high molecular weight, it is suggested that in cancer of the genito-urinary tract, the source of CEA is distal to the kidney. In fact, urinary CEA levels more closely paralleled the extent of disease than did plasma CEA in patients with bladder cancer, but not those with prostate or testicular cancer (24). In lung cancer, bronchial lavage CEA was compared to bronchial cytology. Cytology was positive in 44% of patients and CEA in 56%. A combination of the two brought the positive detection rate to 75%. This combination may improve the diagnostic accuracy of lung cytology.

In colonic lavage obtained by attaching a modified dental irrigation unit to a colonoscope, CEA was observed in the supernatant from the captured lavage fluid. This represented CEA from exfoliated epithelial cells. CEA from patients with adenomas greater than one centimeter in size and in normal controls were similar, but significantly higher values were observed in patients with larger adenomas and adenocarcinoma, with increasing concentrations related to the extent of the cancer. The variability from patient to patient made the assays insufficiently accurate for diagnosis of colon cancer in individual patients (25).

CEA has also been measured in cerebrospinal fluid (CSF). Increased concentrations were observed in CSF from patients with leptomeningeal metastases. The ratio between plasma and CSF CEA ranged from 5–1000%. Serial CSF values seemed to monitor response to therapy. The data suggested that CEA may be a useful marker for detecting leptomeningeal metastases, but not intraparenchymal or epidural metastases (26).

Monoclonal antibodies against other antigens derived from colorectal cancer cell lines have been developed into diagnostic tests. These include CA50, CA195, CA19-9, and CA72-4. None of these appears to offer an advantage over CEA in cancer of the colon.

CA19-9

CA19-9 is the marker most useful in adenocarcinoma of the pancreas. It is more sensitive (70–95%) and specific (72%) than CEA (40–60%, and 70%, respectively). Combined measurement of both markers does not significantly augment the sensitivity of the test. CA19-9 is not elevated in islet cell carcinoma of the pancreas. The value of CA19-9 is obscured by the fact that benign conditions such as acute or chronic pancreatitis or cholelithiasis may cause elevations.

CA19-9 may be useful in monitoring patients who are receiving treatment. Many markers have been studied in patients with pancreatic cancer, but none has the sensitivity or specificity of CA19-9. Of considerable interest is that CA19-9 is only found in the serum of individuals who secrete Lewis antigen. It is not found in serum of nonsecretors. CA19-9 is not useful in colorectal cancer (27).

CA72-4

CA72-4 is a glycoprotein with a molecular weight of 220 to 400 kDa. It is clearly different from CEA, CA19-9, or other glycoprotein tumor markers. Although elevated in serum of patients with many different gastrointestinal cancers and only rarely in benign gastrointestinal diseases, it is more sensitive and specific than any other marker in gastric cancer. In one study, it was clearly shown that CA72-4 is inferior to CA19-9 in pancreatic cancer (where only 22% of patients were detected compared to 82% with CA19-9) and to CEA in colorectal cancer (where the sensitivity was 32% versus 58% with CEA). In gastric cancer, it identified 59% of the patients compared to 52% with CA19-9 and 25% with CEA. When combined with

CA19-9, 70% of the gastric cancer patients were identified (28).

ENZYMES

In many cancers, glycolytic enzymes have been found useful in monitoring metastatic disease and response to therapy. Serum glucose phosphate isomerase was elevated in 102/144 (71%) of patients with colorectal cancer; 60% of 33 patients with Stage I (Dukes' Stage A) disease; 72% with Stage II–III (Dukes' Stages B–C) cancer; and 65% of those with Stage IV (distant metastases) disease (29). Lactic dehydrogenase (LDH) is elevated in cancerous colon or rectal tissue. In 1968, Langvad observed that in colorectal carcinoma the LDH4/LDH2 ratio was 1.67 compared to 0.72 in normal tissue. In 1975, Langvad and Janec reviewed this data and concluded that the ratio was 0.92 ± 0.13 in individuals who had had a recurrence and died and 0.66 ± 0.07 in patients who survived (30). These ratios have been confirmed and extended. In normal colonic mucosa, LDH5 was $4.0 \pm 5.7\%$ of total LDH. In adenocarcinomas, LDH5 was $16.4 \pm 2.5\%$ of total LDH and in benign polyps, $10.9 \pm 8.1\%$. An important observation: increased LDH5 was observed in normal mucosa adjacent to tumor: $9.3 \pm 2.7\%$ at 2 cm; $7.9 \pm 3.1\%$ at 3 cm; $6.4 \pm 2.5\%$ at 6 cm; $6.2 \pm 2.8\%$ at 8 cm, and $4.8 \pm 1.9\%$ at 10 cm. Normal mucosa had $4.0 \pm 5.7\%$. Investigators concluded that shifts in LDH isoenzyme patterns in normal mucosa could be an early indicator of cancer before morphologic changes are observed. γ-Glutamyl transpeptidase (γ-GTP) and CEA have been used to achieve a better prediction rate of the presence of hepatic metastases. γ-GTP indicates the presence of liver disease and CEA discriminates between hepatomegaly due to metastatic disease or benign hepatic disease. This confirmation can be made six to nine months before clinical confirmation (31).

The glycosyltransferases catalyze the sequential addition of specific proteins to glycoprotein acceptors. Several of these enzymes have been examined as markers in colorectal cancer. Sialyltransferase catalyzes the transfer of sialic acid and is found in tissue and serum of cancer patients. It has been extensively studied in colorectal cancer. Increases in sialyltransferase activity are found in colon tumor tissue (1105 ± 413 units in normal colon, 2309 ± 677 units in cancerous tissue) and elevations are observed in serum from patients with colon cancer. Elevations were also observed in patients with rheumatoid arthritis, but not in individuals with cirrhosis or in pregnant women. Levels of galactosyltransferase are higher in normal than in cancerous colon tissue. An isozymic form of this enzyme has been observed in serum of patients with cancer.

Tissue enzyme activity has been used to identify individuals at high risk for colon cancer. The enzyme that has been studied the most in this regard is ornithine decarboxylase (ODC) (36). This enzyme catalyzes the decarboxylation of ornithine to form putrescine, the first compound in the polyamine biosynthesis pathway. ODC is probably the key enzyme in this synthesis. The polyamines putrescine, spermine, and spermidine are compounds that play an important role in cellular proliferation and differentiation. ODC has been measured in mucosa of patients with familial polyposis and in unaffected family members. In normal mucosa from 16 persons who were from unaffected branches of the family or from spouses of polyposis patients, the mean value was 1.02 units and all values were below 2.5 units. Thirteen patients with adenomas were studied. The ODC activity in flat normal-appearing mucosa, distant from the polyps, was over 2.5 units in 11 of 13 biopsies. The mean value was 3.05 units. In nine adenomatous polyps in this group, the mean value was 5.75 units; each of the nine had a value over 2.5. Similarly, each of nine polyps with dysplasia had values over 2.5 units. The mean activity was 7.61 units. This suggests that the higher the proliferative state of the colonic mucosa, the higher the ODC activity. The increased activity is associated with the potential development of polyps and the progression of adenomatous polyps to a dysplastic state. With 2.5 units as the normal/abnormal cut-off, colon mucosa ODC has a specificity of 100% and a sensitivity of 85% in separating normal individuals from those with polyps. ODC may be useful in detecting the asymptomatic carrier of the polyposis genotype.

Urinary aryl sulfatase B (one of the three isoenzymes of this enzyme) has been proposed as a marker in colorectal cancer (34). It was found in 12% of patients with Dukes' A disease, 63% of those with Dukes' B cancer, and 87% of those with Dukes' C and distant metastasis. The urinary aryl sulfatase correlated with serum CEA and values reflected the course of the disease.

SUMMARY

In colorectal cancer, tumor markers cannot be used in screening or for initial diagnosis. They can be prognostic indicators and may play an important role in monitoring response to therapy and detecting exacerbation of disease. The role of markers will not be realized until the genetic pathways in the development of colon cancer are elucidated and these are exploited as cancer tests.

REFERENCES

1. Greenlee RT, Hill-Harmon MB, Murray T, Thum M. Cancer statistics, 2001. CA Cancer J Clin 2001;51:15–31.
2. Winawer SJ. A quarter century of colorectal cancer screening: progress and prospects. J Clin Oncol 2001;19:63–125.
3. Kinzler KW, Vogelstein B. Lesion for heredity colorectal cancer. Cell 1976;87:159–170.
4. Alquist DA, Shuber AP. Stool screening for colorectal cancer: evolution from occult blood to molecular markers. Clin Chim Acta 2002;315:157–168.
5. Gold P, Freedman SO. Demonstration of tumor-specific antigens in human colon carcinomata by immunological tolerance and absorption techniques. J Expl Med 1965;122:467–481.
6. Thompson P, Krupey J, Freedman S, Gold P. The radioimmunoassay of circulating carcinoembryonic antigen of the human digestive system. Proc Nat Acad Sci 1969;64:161–169.

7. Hansen HJ, Snyder JJ, Miller E, Vanderoorder E, Miller ON, Hines LR, Burns JS. Carcinoembryonic antigen (CEA) assay. A laboratory adjunct in the diagnosis and management of cancer. Hum Path 1974;5:139–147.
8. Goldenberg DM, Neville AM, Carter AL, Go VLW, Holyoke ED, Isselbacher KJ, Schein B, Schwartz MK. CEA (carcinoembryonic antigen). Its role as a marker in the management of cancer. J Cancer Res Clin Oncol 1981;101:229–249.
10. Ladenson JH, McDonald JM, Schwartz MK. Colorectal cancer and carcinoembryonic antigen (CEA). Clin Chem 1980;26: 1213–1230.
11. Bidart JM, Thuillier F, Augereau C, Challas J, Daver A, Jacob N, Labrorsse F, Voitot H. Kinetics of serum tumor marker concentrations and usefulness in clinical monitoring. Clin Chem 1999;45: 1695–1707.
12. Maehara Y, Sugimachi K, Akagi M, Kakegawa T, Shimaza H, Tomita, M. Serum carcinoembryonic antigen level increases correlate with progression in patients with differentiated gastric cancer following non-curative resection. Cancer Res 1990;50: 3952–3955.
13. Kiang DT, Greenberg IJ, Kennedy BJ. Tumor marker kinetics in the monitoring of breast cancer. Cancer 1990;65:193–199.
14. Solassol I, Gramier C, Pelegrin A. Carcinoembryonic antigen continuous epitopes determined by the SPOT method. Tumor Biol 2001;22:184–190.
15. Zinnermann W, Orlieb B, Friedrich R, Von Kleist S. Isolation and characterization of cDNA clones encoding the human carcinoembryonic antigen reveal a highly conserved repeating structure. Proc Natl Acad Sci USA 1987;84:2960–2964.
16. Schwartz MK. Tumor markers into the twenty first century—retrospect and prospect. Proceedings of the UK NEQAS Meeting 1998;321–328.
17. Minton JP, Hoehm JL, Gerber DM, Hesley JS, Connelly DP, Valwan F, Fletcher WS, Cruz AB Jr., Getchell FG, Orieo M, et al. Results of 400 patient carcinoembryonic antigen second-look colorectal cancer study. Cancer 1985;550:1284–1290.
18. Moertal CG, Fleming TR, MacDonald JS, Haller DG, Lauril JA, Tangon C. An evaluation of the carcinoembryonic antigen (CEA) test for monitoring patients with resected colon cancer. JAMA 1993;270:943–978.
19. Wanebo HJ, Rao B, Pinsky CM, Hoffman RG, Stearns M, Schwartz MK, Oettgen HF. Pre-operative carcinoembryonic antigen as a prognostic indicator in colorectal cancer. New Eng J Med 1978;299:448–451.
20. Quentimer A, Schlay P, Hohenberger P, et al. Assessment of serial carcinoembryonic antigen: Determination to monitor the therapeutic progress of metastatic liver disease treated by regional chemotherapy. J Surg Oncol 1989;40:112–118.
21. Staab HJ, Andener FA, Stumpf F, et al. Slope analysis of the post-operative CEA time course and its possible application as an aid in diagnosis of disease progression in gastrointestinal cancer. Am J Surg 1978;136:322–327.
22. Price T, Beatty BG, Beatty JO, McNally AJ. Human anti-murine antibody interference in measurement of carcinoembryonic antigen assessed with a double antibody enzyme immunoassay. Clin Chem 1991;37:51–57.
23. American Society of Clinical Oncology. 1997 Update of recommendations for use of tumor markers in breast and colorectal cancer. J Clin Oncol 1998;16:793–795.
24. Fleisher M, Grabstald H, Whitmore Jr WF, Pinsky CM, Oettgen H, Schwartz MK. The clinical utility of plasma and urinary carcinoembryonic antigen in patients with genitourinary disease. J Urol 1977;117:635–637.
25. Winawer SJ, Fleisher M, Green S, Bhargara D. Leidner SP, Boyle C, Sherlock P. Carcinoembryonic antigen in colonic lavage. Gastroenterology 1977;73:719–722.
26. Blair O, Goldenberg DM. A correlative study of bronchial cytology, bronchial washing, carcinoembryonic antigen and plasma carcinoembryonic antigen in the diagnosis of bronchogenic cancer. Acta Cytol 1974;18:510–514.
27. Schold SC, Wasserstrom WR, Fleisher M, Schwartz MK, Posner JB. Cerebrospinal fluid biochemical markers in central nervous system metastases. Ann Neurol 1980;8:517–603.
28. Steinberg W, Felfand R, Anderson KK, et al. Comparison of the sensitivity and specificity of the CA19-9 and carcinoembryonic antigen assay in detecting cancer of the pancreas. Gastroenterology 1986;90:343–350.
29. Byrne DJ Browning MCK, Cuschieri A. CA72-4. A new tumor marker for gastric cancer. Br J Surg 1992;77:1010–1013.
30. Schwartz MK. Enzyme tests in cancer. Clinics in Lab Med. 1982; 2:479–491.
31. Langvad E, Jemnec B. Prediction of local recurrence in colorectal carcinomas. An LDH isoenzymatic assay. Brit J Cancer 1975; 31:661–664.
32. Cooper EH, Turner R, Steele L, Neville AM, MacKay AM. The combination of serum enzymes and carcinoembryonic antigen in the early diagnosis of metastatic colorectal cancer. Brit J Cancer 1975;31:111–117.
33. Morgan LR, Samuels MS, Thomas W, Krementz A, Meeker W. Arylsulfatase B in colorectal cancer. Cancer 1975;36:2332–2345.
34. Bosmann HB, Hall TC. Enzyme activity in invasive tumors of human breast and colon. Proc Natl Acad Sci USA 1974;71: 1833–1837.
35. Lamont JJ, Isselbacher RJ. Altered galactosyltransferase activity in human colon cancer. J Natl Cancer Inst. 1975;34:53–56.
36. Koo HB, Sigurdson ER, Daly JM, Berenson M, Green S, DeCosse JJ. Ornithine decarboxylase activity in levels in rectal mucosa of patients with colonic cancer. J Surg Oncol 1988;38: 240–243.
37. Ladenson JH, McDonald JM, Schwartz MK. Colorectal cancer and carcinoembryonic antigen. Clin Chem 1980;26:1628–1629.
38. Werner M, Schwartz MK. Are the so-called tumor markers really clinical markers? Giornale Italian di Chimica Clinica 1989;14: 245–256.

Chapter 20

Molecular Diagnostics of Hereditary Nonpolyposis Colorectal Cancer (HNPCC)

Michele Zysman and Bharati Bapat

Colorectal cancer (CRC) is a major health problem and a leading cause of cancer death in North America. About 5% of the population develops colon cancer in their lifetime. The etiology of CRC is heterogeneous and is regulated by the interplay between genetics and environment in different patients.

In recent years, significant advances have been made in understanding the molecular genetics and pathology of colon cancer. About 20% of all colon cancers occur in familial aggregations and patients in this group carry varying degrees of genetic predisposition to CRC (1,2). Both epidemiologic and family studies provide evidence for increased genetic contribution: individuals with a family history of colon cancer and those with familial aggregation of colon cancer consistent with an autosomal dominant mode of inheritance carry an increased risk of developing CRC. Familial adenomatous polyposis (FAP), characterized by numerous (100 or more) colorectal adenomatous polyps, accounts for approximately 1% of all cases of CRC. FAP is caused by germline mutations of the *APC* tumor suppressor gene. FAP patients are at increased risk of several extracolonic manifestations, including adenomas of the small intestine and stomach, desmoids, and cancers of the duodenum, periampullary region, brain, liver and thyroid. A mild variant of FAP is referred to as AAPC (attenuated APC) or AFAP (attenuated FAP), while the FAP variant associated with extracolonic manifestations is historically referred to as the Gardner syndrome. Among other rare inherited CRC syndromes, Peutz-Jeghers syndrome, characterized by distinct polyps in the colon, stomach and small bowel, is caused by mutations of the *STK11* gene; juvenile polyposis coli, recognized by hamartomatous polyps, is caused by defects in tumor suppressor genes, *PTEN* or *SMAD4/DPC4*.

The more common CRC predisposition syndrome is hereditary nonpolyposis colorectal cancer (HNPCC), which accounts for approximately 5–8% of all colon cancers (3). HNPCC is characterized by a predominantly right-sided colorectal cancer with an early age of onset (median age of 45 years) and an increased incidence of extra-colonic tumors, including cancers of the endometrium, small bowel, stomach, renal pelvis/ureter, ovary, and brain, as well as skin lesions. Colonic adenomas in HNPCC may develop at the same frequency as in the general population, but once formed, these adenomas progress to cancer much more rapidly than their sporadic counterparts. Therefore, a diagnosis of HNPCC based exclusively on clinical criteria is sometimes difficult due to the absence of an obvious clinical phenotype as seen in FAP, and due to presentations of a constellation of extra-colonic cancers in the family.

To address these issues, the International Collaborative Group on HNPCC (ICG-HNPCC) established research criteria for HNPCC (Amsterdam criteria I) (Table 1) in 1990. These criteria provided important guidelines for identifying HNPCC families for the purposes of collaborative studies and gene discovery. However, the Amsterdam criteria were deemed too restrictive since they primarily focused on site-specific colon cancer families. In response to these concerns, the Amsterdam criteria were subsequently revised (Amsterdam criteria II) to include extra-colonic cancers of HNPCC (Table 1). Germline mutations of a group of genes known as the mismatch repair (MMR) genes account for approximately 70% of Amsterdam criteria families. Germline mutations of as many as six different MMR genes, including *MSH2*, *MLH1*, *MSH6* (also known as *GTBP*), *MLH3*, *PMS1* and *PMS2* have been implicated in HNPCC (4). Mutations of *MLH1* and *MSH2* are responsible for approximately 80% of MMR mutation positive HNPCC cases (5), while germline mutations in *MSH6*, *MLH3*, *PMS1* and *PMS2* are less common and account for about 10-15% of HNPCC cases (6).

Mismatch repair genes function to maintain fidelity of DNA during replication. Mismatched nucleotides can arise in DNA from physical damage, misincorporation of nucleotides during DNA replication, small insertion/deletions due to DNA polymerase slippage or during genetic recombination. Mismatch repair proteins recognize and repair base-base mismatches and insertion-deletion loops made by DNA polymerase during replication. Base-base mismatches typically affect nonrepetitive DNA and result in substitution mutations. Errors in the insertion-deletion loops lead to gains or losses in repetitive DNA such as short tandem repeats or microsatellites. HNPCC tumors arise due to a complete inactivation of MMR, which results in microsatellite instability (MSI). This charac-

Table 1 Amsterdam/Bethesda criteria

*Amsterdam Criteria I**
There should be at least 3 relatives with CRC meeting the following criteria:
- One should be a first-degree relative of the other 2
- At least 2 successive generations should be affected
- At least 1 affected individual should be diagnosed before age 50
- Familial adenomatous polyposis (FAP) should be excluded
- Tumors should be verified by pathological examination

*Amsterdam Criteria II (Revised ICG-HNPCC criteria)***
There should be at least 3 relatives with an HNPCC-associated cancer (CRC, cancer of the endometrium, small bowel, ureter, or renal pelvis) meeting the following criteria:
- One should be a first-degree relative of the other 2
- At least 2 successive generations should be affected
- At least 1 should be diagnosed before age 50
- Familial adenomatous polyposis should be excluded in the CRC case(s) if any
- Tumors should be verified by pathological examination

Bethesda Criteria–modified§
- Individuals meeting Amsterdam Criteria I
- Individuals with 2 HNPCC cancers (including synchronous/metachronous CRCs)
- Individuals with CRC and a first-degree relative with CRC and/or HNPCC extracolonic cancer and/or colorectal adenoma (cancer at less than 50 years of age and adenoma at less than 40 years of age)

*Ref. 24; **Ref. 25; §Ref. 7.

teristic tumor feature is also referred to as replication error (RER) or mutator phenotype. In MSI+ tumors, inactivation of a mismatch repair gene leads to increased accumulation of mutations in other important genes implicated in cancer, particularly those with short repetitive sequences in their coding regions (e.g., *TGF-β-RII*, *BAX*). Mismatch repair genes *MSH3* and *MSH6* also contain coding region repeats and are susceptible to the development of somatic frameshift mutations.

Colorectal tumorigenesis can proceed via different genetic pathways leading to the formation of distinct tumor subtypes (7). In the more common "suppressor pathway," CRC tumors are predominantly left-sided, exhibit chromosomal instability and harbor mutations of tumor suppressor genes (e.g., *APC* or *p53*) and oncogenes (e.g., *Ki-ras*). In contrast, a subset of CRC tumors develops through the mutator pathway when both alleles of a mismatch repair gene are inactivated. As a result, these tumors display the MSI phenotype, are diploid in nature, and more frequently occur in the right colon. These tumors display characteristic pathologic features that include increased signet cells, a solid cribiform growth pattern and a tendency to form lymphoid aggregates. Recognition of this mutator phenotype led to the development of the Bethesda criteria (Table 1), which facilitates selection of tumors for MSI analysis.

Over 90% of HNPCC tumors (8) and about 15% of sporadic colorectal cancers (9) exhibit the MSI phenotype. A complete inactivation of *MSH2* or *MLH1* genes in tumors results in loss of expression of these proteins, which can be examined by immunohistochemistry (IHC) (10). Thus, analysis of immunohistochemical expression of MMR proteins in CRC complements tumor MSI analysis. In addition to colorectal cancer, approximately 15–20% of sporadic endometrial and gastric cancers also display MSI. The majority of these tumors lack MLH1 protein expression but do not carry mutations in the *MLH1* coding sequence (11). This points towards a role for inactivation of mismatch repair genes by other methods, including an epigenetic mechanism such as methylation. Many gene promoters contain CpG islands. The cytosine residues of CpG dinucleotides can acquire a methyl group, leading to transcription inhibition and gene silencing. In the majority of sporadic MSI+ colorectal and endometrial tumors, hypermethylation of the promoter region of the *MLH1* gene has been shown to be the principle mechanism of MMR inactivation. However, methylation of *MSH2* has not been observed in colorectal tumors (12).

CLINICAL APPLICATIONS

HNPCC patients carry a germline mutant MMR gene allele and acquire a second mutation in the remaining allele later in life, which leads to the formation of MSI+ tumors. In order to identify MSI+ tumors, the International Collaborative Group on HNPCC (ICG-HNPCC) and the National Cancer Institute have adopted sensitive and specific markers to perform standardized microsatellite instability analyses (13). In this assay, DNA obtained from matched normal and tumor specimens is analyzed for alterations in allele sizes, using a recommended panel of microsatellite markers. These include *BAT-25* and *BAT-26*, which encode two mononucleotide repeats, and *D2S123*, *D5S346* and *D17S250*, which encode three dinucleotide repeats. Tumors with 40% or more loci showing microsatellite instability (two of the five markers) are considered MSI-high (MSI-H), tumors with less than 30% microsatellite instability (only one of the five markers unstable) are MSI-low (MSI-L); and tumors with no instability are referred to as microsatellite stable (MSS). CRCs with MSI-L phenotype resemble MSS tumors clinically and pathologically and do not seem to be related to HNPCC.

Individuals who fulfill the revised Amsterdam Criteria, individuals with multiple HNPCC-associated primary cancers, and/or individuals who develop cancer at a young age of onset (< 35 years) with or without a family history, should be considered candidates for a possible diagnosis of HNPCC (Figure 1). Tumors from these patients should be tested for MLH1 and MSH2 expression by immunohistochemical analysis and for MSI status. IHC analysis can also aid in the diagnosis of MSI-H versus MSI-L status of the tumors, since loss of hMLH1 or hMSH2 expression is strongly correlated with the MSI-H but not the MSI-L phenotype. In cases where family history meets the Amsterdam criteria but the tumor is found to be MSS, the patient should be considered for other hereditary colorectal cancer conditions including attenuated adenomatous polyposis coli (AAPC), a milder form of colon cancer predisposition with

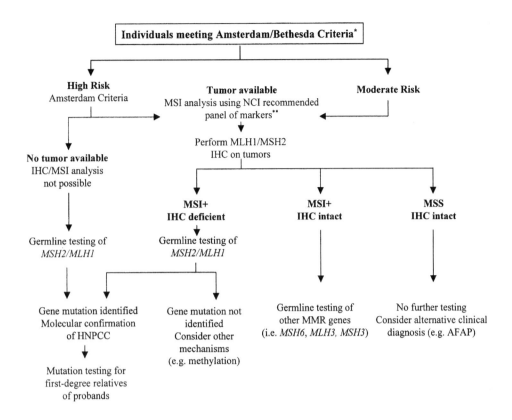

Figure 1 *Amsterdam Criteria I (Ref. 24), Amsterdam Criteria II (Ref. 25), Bethesda Criteria (Ref. 7). ** NCI recommended markers include BAT-25, BAT-26, D2S123, D5S346, and D17S250 (Ref. 13).

fewer adenomas, later onset, and lower cancer risk than is observed in familial adenomatous polyposis (FAP).

Once tumors are confirmed to be MSI+ and immunodeficient for either MSH2 or MLH1, germline molecular testing for the relevant gene should be undertaken. MMR gene mutations are quite diverse and include frameshift mutations, truncations, substitution mutations, and large deletions, and are distributed throughout the coding regions (14,15). The *MSH2* gene is encoded by 16 exons and *MLH1* is encoded by 19 exons. Sequencing of the entire coding region of the gene and of intron-exon boundaries is considered the gold standard for mutation analysis. Other mutation screening methods include single strand conformational polymorphism (SSCP) or denaturing gradient gel electrophoresis (DGGE), followed by DNA sequencing to confirm the nature of the mutation. Once a germline mutation is identified in an affected person, predictive genetic testing for the presence or absence of the same mutation can be offered to other first-degree members of his/her family.

It is important to emphasize that while a mutation-positive result in an affected person meeting Amsterdam/Bethesda criteria implicates a germline defect in a specific MMR gene, a negative result does not rule out the possibility of a mutation. In a study that investigated germline mutations of *MSH2* or *MLH1*, mutations were detected in only 70% of cases that fulfilled the Amsterdam criteria, even though 92% of the tumors displayed MSI (15). This suggests that mutations in other mismatch repair genes (e.g., *MSH6*) may also be responsible for the development of an MSI phenotype without identifiable mutations in *MLH1* or *MSH2*. As well, other mechanisms including loss of heterozygosity, large allelic deletions, unstable mutant proteins or methylation may account for the lack of MMR protein expression. Therefore, when there is a lack of MLH1 expression as determined from immunohistochemical analysis and when no mutations in MMR genes are identified, the tumor should be tested for methylation of the *MLH1* promoter. Finally, in some HNPCC families meeting the Amsterdam criteria, the underlying genetic defect may be in a gene unrelated to MMR (e.g., *TGF-β-RII*) (17).

FUTURE DIRECTIONS

Developing techniques with improved sensitivity and specificity for mutation detection will improve accurate and efficient identification of germline MMR defects underlying HNPCC. It is likely that mutation in one chromosomal allele may be obscured by the normal allele.

A recently described technique, conversion analysis, can overcome this problem. In this assay, the diploid genome is converted to a haploid state by fusion of the patient's lymphoblast cells to a novel recipient cell line, such as a rodent cell line. After a few passages in culture, the newly created hybrid cells contain only one copy of the gene in question. The monoallelic hybrids can then be screened for mutations using conventional techniques such as sequencing.

In a study of 22 patients with HNPCC, mismatch repair gene mutations were identified in 12 patients using conventional techniques. However, when conversion technology was used in conjunction with conventional methods, disease-causing alterations were identified in all 22 cases (18). Mutations exclusively identified by conversion technology were primarily expression-based mutations, including large deletions. Signals from such mutant alleles are often much weaker and therefore are masked by the signals from the normal allele when examined using manual or automated sequencing methods. Haploid conversion thus significantly increases the sensitivity of genetic tests for HNPCC.

In addition to better methods for diagnosing HNPCC, studies investigating the various treatment options available are essential to improving the outcomes for HNPCC patients. A study investigating the efficacy of 5-fluorouracil (5-FU)-based chemotherapy for patients with CRC found that the treatment was safe and provided an excellent prognosis for patients with tumors displaying MSI (19). In CRC, MSI+ status is associated with better prognosis. MSI+ colon tumors have been shown to have normal p53 without mutations or overexpression (20). Normal p53 is a marker indicating a good response to chemotherapy (21), further suggesting that patients with MSI+ CRCs would benefit from chemotherapy. However, other studies have reported conflicting results regarding the efficacy of chemotherapeutic agents in the treatment of CRC displaying MSI (22). Because CRCs with MSI have different molecular and pathologic profiles than MSS tumors, studies investigating the benefit of selective chemotherapeutic agents for the treatment of HNPCC-associated CRCs are still needed. Contrary to CRC, MSI+ status has been associated with a poor prognosis in a number of other cancers including sporadic endometrial cancer (23). Whether or not HNPCC-related endometrial cancer also exhibits this effect, as well as the effects of chemotherapy on other extra-colonic HNPCC-associated tumors, must also be assessed. Determining the effects of various chemotherapeutics including irinotecan or oxaliplatin on MSI+ CRCs must also be evaluated in conjunction with the effects on various other cancers in order to determine whether these treatments will improve survival of patients with HNPCC.

REFERENCES

1. Burt RW. Colon cancer screening. Gastroenterology 2000; 119:837–853.
2. Potter JD. Colorectal cancer: molecules and populations. J Natl Cancer Inst 1999;91:916–932.
3. Lynch HT, de la Chapelle A. Genetic susceptibility to non-polyposis colorectal cancer. J Med Genet 1999;36:801–818.
4. Samowitz WS, Curtin K, Lin HH, Robertson MA, Schaffer D, Nichols M, et al. The colon cancer burden of genetically defined hereditary nonpolyposis colon cancer. Gastroenterology 2001; 121:830–838.
5. Bocker T, Ruschoff J, Fishel R. Molecular diagnostics of cancer predisposition: hereditary non-polyposis colorectal carcinoma and mismatch repair defects. Biochim Biophys Acta 1999;1423:O1–O10.
6. Peltomaki P. Deficient DNA mismatch repair: a common etiologic factor for colon cancer. Hum Mol Genet 2001;10:735–740.
7. Rodriguez-Bigas MA, Boland CR, Hamilton SR, Henson DE, Jass JR, Khan PM, et al. A National Cancer Institute workshop on hereditary nonpolyposis colorectal cancer syndrome: meeting highlights and Bethesda guidelines. J Natl Cancer Inst 1997;89:1758–1762.
8. Aaltonen LA, Salovaara R, Kristo P, Canzian F, Hemminki A, Peltomaki P, et al. Incidence of hereditary nonpolyposis colorectal cancer and the feasibility of molecular screening for the disease. N Engl J Med 1998;338:1481–1487.
9. Lothe RA, Peltomaki P, Meling GI, Aaltonen LA, Nystrom-Lahti M, Pylkkanen L, et al. Rognum TO.Genomic instability in colorectal cancer: relationship to clinicopathological variables and family history. Cancer Res 1993;53:5849–5852.
10. Thibodeau SN, French AJ, Roche PC, Cunningham JM, Tester DJ, Lindor NM, et al. Altered expression of hMSH2 and hMLH1 in tumors with microsatellite instability and genetic alterations in mismatch repair genes. Cancer Res 1996;56:4836–4840.
11. Giardiello FM, Brensinger JD, Petersen GM. AGA technical review on hereditary colorectal cancer and genetic testing. Gastroenterology 2001;121:198–213.
12. Herman JG, Umar A, Polyak K, Graff JR, Ahuja N, Issa JP, et al. Incidence and functional consequences of hMLH1 promoter hypermethylation in colorectal carcinoma. Proc Natl Acad Sci USA 1998;95:6870–6875.
13. Boland CR, Thibodeau SN, Hamilton SR, Sidransky D, Eshleman JR, Burt RW, et al. A National Cancer Institute Workshop on Microsatellite Instability for cancer detection and familial predisposition: development of international criteria for the determination of microsatellite instability in colorectal cancer. Cancer Res 1998;58:5248–5257.
14. Peltomaki P, Vasen HF, and The International Collaborative Group on Hereditary Nonpolyposis Colorectal Cancer. Mutations predisposing to hereditary nonpolyposis colorectal cancer: database and results of a collaborative study. Gastroenterology 1997;113: 1146–1158.
15. Bapat BV, Madlensky L, Temple LK, Hiruki T, Redston M, Baron DL, et al. Family history characteristics, tumor microsatellite instability, and germline MSH2 and MLH1 mutations in hereditary colorectal cancer. Hum Genet 1999;104:167–176.
16. Liu B, Parsons R, Papadopoulos N, Nicolaides NC, Lynch HT, Watson P, et al. Analysis of mismatch repair genes in hereditary non-polyposis colorectal cancer patients. Nat Med 1996;2: 169–174.
17. Lu SL, Kawabata M, Imamura T, Akiyama Y, Nomizu T, Miyazono K, Yuasa Y. HNPCC associated with germline mutation in the TGF-beta type II receptor gene. Nat Genet 1998;19:17–18.
18. Yan H, Papadopoulos N, Marra G, Perrera C, Jiricny J, Boland CR, et al. Conversion of diploidy to haploidy. Nature 2000; 403:723–724.
19. Hemminki A, Mecklin JP, Jarvinen H, Aaltonen LA, Joensuu H. Microsatellite instability is a favorable prognostic indicator in patients with colorectal cancer receiving chemotherapy. Gastroenterology 2000;119:921–928.
20. Ionov Y, Peinado MA, Malkhosyan S, Shibata D, Perucho M. Ubiquitous somatic mutations in simple repeated sequences reveal a new mechanism for colonic carcinogenesis. Nature 1993;363:558–561.
21. Ahnen DJ, Feigl P, Quan G, Fenoglio-Preiser C, Lovato LC, Bunn PA Jr, et al. Ki-ras mutation and p53 overexpression predict the clinical behavior of colorectal cancer: a Southwest Oncology Group study. Cancer Res 1998;58:1149–1158.

22. Percesepe A, Benatti P, Roncucci L, Sassatelli R, Fante R, Ganazzi D, et al. Survival analysis in families affected by hereditary nonpolyposis colorectal cancer. Int J Cancer 1997;71:373–376.

23. Caduff RF, Johnston CM, Svoboda-Newman SM, Poy EL, Merajver SD, Frank TS. Clinical and pathological significance of microsatellite instability in sporadic endometrial carcinoma. Am J Pathol 1996;148:1671–1678.

24. Vasen HF, Mecklin JP, Khan PM, Lynch HT. The International Collaborative Group on Hereditary Non-Polyposis Colorectal Cancer (ICG-HNPCC). Dis Colon Rectum 1991;34:424–425.

25. Vasen HF, Watson P, Mecklin JP, Lynch HT. New clinical criteria for hereditary nonpolyposis colorectal cancer (HNPCC, Lynch syndrome) proposed by the International Collaborative group on HNPCC. Gastroenterology 1999;116:1453–1456.

Chapter 21

Serological Tumor Markers in Pancreatic Cancer

Matti Eskelinen and Ulf Haglund

Pancreatic cancer has a poor prognosis with a more than 99% mortality rate. The only curative treatment of pancreatic cancer is surgery with complete removal of the tumor. However, only 5–15% of tumors are detected early enough to allow radical resection (2). Early diagnosis may be the only means of improving treatment results. This chapter reviews the possibility of using serological tumor markers for earlier diagnosis of human pancreatic cancer. For a more detailed review and further references, the readers are directed to a recent review (3).

In the diagnosis of human pancreatic cancer, several serum tumor-associated antigens have been studied. Large numbers of markers have been tested separately in many studies, mostly by single-factor analyses, with varying cut-off levels and in varying patient populations. Therefore, evaluation of these studies is often difficult (3). According to many previous studies, it is obvious that the combined use of similar marker tests is unreasonable from both the clinical and the economic point of view.

CLINICAL APPLICATION OF TUMOR MARKERS FOR PANCREATIC CANCER

Glycoproteins

Carcinoembryonic antigen (CEA). CEA is a glycoprotein with a molecular weight of 180 kD. The major antigenic epitopes are localized on the protein portion of the molecule and at least six different epitopes are identified. CEA is normally present in the liver, pancreas, and gastrointestinal tract during fetal life, and in adolescence in small amounts in the colon and in endodermal tissue (3). Smoking can falsely elevate serum values of CEA, as can various benign diseases such as hepatic disease, extrahepatic cholestasis, and myocardial infarction (3). CEA is one of the most extensively studied tumor markers and can be regarded as a clinical reference for serum tumor markers for gastrointestinal cancers (3). CEA was for more than a decade the only serum tumor marker used clinically in the diagnosis of pancreatic cancer. The sensitivity (16–92%) and specificity (49–93%) of serum CEA (cut-off value 5μg/L) in the diagnosis of pancreatic cancer varies greatly (Table 1), and most studies have arrived at a level of sensitivity that is unacceptably low for clinical use (<50%).

Pancreatic oncofetal antigen (POA). POA is a glycoprotein developed by immunizing rabbits with extract of human fetal pancreas. The assay is very difficult to standardize. An elevated serum value of POA has been found in 15% to 35% of patients with gastrointestinal cancers and in 17% to 97% of patients with pancreatic cancer (Table 1). As such, the POA marker test hardly has a place in the workup aimed at early diagnosis of pancreatic cancer.

Cytokeratins

Tissue polypeptide antigen (TPA). TPA is a protein produced during the late S phase and G2 phase of cell division. Since the release of this antigen is a function of cell division, it differs from many other tumor marker tests, and possibly may be an indicator of the tumor proliferation rate rather than being a discriminator of the tumor burden. There are few data in the literature on the utility of the TPA assay in the diagnosis of pancreatic cancer, but its diagnostic value has been reported to be slightly inferior to that of CEA, CA50, CA19-9, and CA242 (Table 1) (3). When TPA was combined with the other markers, the specificity and efficiency improved clearly in all combinations, being highest in that of TPA and CA242 (specificity 95% and efficiency 87%) (3). These results indicate that the clinical utility of the TPA assay might be complementary.

Tissue polypeptide specific antigen (TPS.) TPS is the M3 specific epitope of TPA. It is produced during the late S and G2 phases and is released immediately after mitosis. Few data are available on the utility of serum TPS assay in the diagnosis of pancreatic cancer, and the sensitivity (50–98%) and specificity (22–73%) of serum TPS have varied considerably (Table 1). Pasanen et al. measured the serum values of TPS in a prospective series of 191 patients with pancreatic-biliary disease; 24 of them had pancreatic carcinoma and two patients had carcinoma of the papilla of Vater. The highest median serum TPS value was detected in patients with malignant liver disease, but high median values were also measured in patients with pancreatic cancer, bile duct cancer, or benign liver disease. The sensitivity of TPS was 50% with a specificity of 73%.

Table 1 Diagnostic sensitivity, specificity, and cut-off values for the most common used serological markers in human pancreatic adenocarcinoma (3)

Type of Marker	Sensitivity (range)	Specificity (range)	Cut-off value
Glycoproteins			
CEA	16–92 %	49–93 %	5.0 ng/mL
POA	17–97 %	65–100 %	NA*
Cytokeratins			
TPA	36–96 %	67–92 %	140–320 U/L
TPS	50–98 %	22–73 %	40–630 U/L
Enzymatic proteins			
Elastase-1	61–100 %	91–96 %	400 ng/dL
TATI	41–95 %	58–64 %	20–31 µg/L
Mucins			
DU-PAN-2	49–87 %	63–80 %	150–200 U/mL
SPAN-1	78–93 %	58–82 %	30 U/mL
Carbohydrate antigens			
CA19-9	69–93 %	46–98 %	37 U/mL
CA50	65–96 %	58–73 %	17 U/mL
CA242	57–83 %	79–90 %	20–30 U/mL
CA125	45–60 %	76–86 %	35 U/L
CA195	69–83 %	53–92 %	9 U/mL

*NA = cut-off value not available.

When TPS was combined with the other serum markers, the specificity and efficiency clearly improved.

Enzymatic Proteins

Tumor-associated trypsin inhibitor (TATI). TATI is a 6 kD peptide produced by several tumors and cell lines. It has been shown to be identical to pancreatic secretory trypsin inhibitor. In diagnosis of pancreatic cancer, sensitivity rates up to 85–95% have been recorded for TATI, but less favorable results have also been reported. A low specificity of TATI is a problem (3). When the serum values of TATI were measured in a prospective series of 154 patients, the sensitivity in diagnosing pancreatic cancer was 41.1% with a specificity of 63.5% and an efficiency of 61.0% (5).

Mucins

DU-PAN 2. DU-PAN is monoclonal antibody raised by immunization with a human pancreatic adenocarcinoma cell line recognizing an antigen on a mucin-like glycoprotein. The antigen has been detected in ductal epithelium in fetal pancreas as well as in normal adult pancreas and in normal biliary epithelium, but also in pancreatic adenocarcinomas. Elevated serum values of DU-PAN 2 tumor marker have been shown in 59% of patients with benign hepatobiliary disease, in 44–50% of patients with hepatoma, in 40–62% of patients with biliary cancer and in 19–28% of patients with gastric cancer. The diagnostic sensitivity of serum DU-PAN 2 marker in combination with a CA19-9 test in diagnosis of pancreatic cancer is reported to be 95%.

Recently it has been reported that the real epitope of DU-PAN-2 is LSTa (sialyllat-N-tetraose), the precursor of CA19-9. LSTa is found in sera of patients with the Lewis-negative phenotype; in this way the DU-PAN-2 test may have a complementary role in Lewis-negative and CA19-9-negative subjects suspected of having pancreatic cancer (3).

Span-1. Span-1 is a monoclonal antibody raised by immunization with a human pancreatic cancer cell line (SW 1990), reacting with a sialylated epitope with an CA19-9-like structure on a mucin. A sandwich radioimmunoassay has recently been developed and clinically tested for SPAN-1. The diagnostic sensitivity (78–93%) for the Span-1 tumor marker in serological diagnosis of pancreatic cancer has been shown to be higher than the diagnostic sensitivity (49–87%) for DU-PAN-2. The specificity levels used have varied considerably (Table 1) (3).

Carbohydrate Antigens

CA19-9. CA19-9 is defined by the mouse monoclonal antibody 1116 NS 19-9 (IgG1) (19-9-Ab), raised against a human colonic carcinoma cell line SW 1116. Its epitope is the sialylated Lewis A-antigen; in serum the CA19-9 antigen is associated with a mucin. CA19-9 was initially detected in meconium and colorectal cancer tissue, but has been found more widely distributed in normal fetal and adult pancreas, stomach, and biliary epithelium. Using an immunoradiometric assay, CA19-9 is found in most sera of healthy blood donors, but only 0.6% exceeds the recommended cut-off value of 37 U/mL. Smoking has not been shown to affect the serum concentrations. In benign gastrointestinal disease (excluding benign hepato-pancreatico-biliary diseases), the frequency of elevated serum CA19-9 levels is <15%. In acute and chronic pancreatitis, the frequency of elevated serum CA19-9 levels is in the range of 4–23%. In pancreatic cancer, CA 19-9 assay sensitivity varied between 69–93% and specificity between 46–98% (Table 1) (3). Those with Lewis-negative phenotype (about 10% of the general population) express CA19-9 antigen in only 40% of cases.

CA50. CA50 is defined by the monoclonal antibody C 50 developed against a colorectal cancer cell line, COLO 205. Increased concentrations of serum CA50 were originally observed in a high proportion of patients with gastrointestinal carcinomas. The frequency of elevated serum values of CA50 has varied between 13% and 91% in different malignant diseases (3).

Elevated serum CA 50 levels have been found in 65–96% of patients with pancreatic cancer (3). The cut-off value recommended by the manufacturer for CA50 (17 U/mL) is based on data from healthy blood donors. A sensitivity and specificity of 77% and 84%, respectively, have been reported using a higher (137 U/mL) cut-off level.

The interference of cholestasis and jaundice with the CA50 assays is unclear but it is likely nothing more than a correlation between serum bilirubin and CA50 levels (19,20).

CA242. CA242 is defined by a monoclonal antibody, C-242, which was obtained by immunizing mice with a human colorectal carcinoma cell line, COLO 205. An immunoassay for serum analysis of CA242 using the antibody against sialylated Lewis A as a catcher, and C 242 as a detector antibody, is available (6). Only 5% of normal healthy blood donors have a serum CA242 level above the recommended cut-off level of 20 U/mL. The reported overall sensitivity (57–83 %) (Table 2) is similar to that of CA19-9 or CA50. When comparing CEA, CA50, and CA242 by receiver operating characteristic (ROC) analysis, CA242 seems to have a higher sensitivity than CEA and CA50 at the high specificity levels (>0.90), but it is slightly less sensitive at low specificity levels (<0.60) (7). There is an interference of cholestasis and jaundice with the CA242 assays. Still CA242 seems to have better properties than CA19-9 for diagnosing pancreatic cancer.

CA195. CA195 is defined by a monoclonal antibody CC3C195 (IgM-type), which was obtained by immunizing mice with a membrane preparation from liver metastases of a human colonic cancer. Epitope analysis has shown that the monoclonal antibody binds to sialylated Lewis(a), as the monoclonal antibody C19-9, but also to the Lewis(a) glycolipid antigen itself. At the moment there are no studies available concerning the tissue distribution of CA195 in human pancreatic cancer. Only 1% of normal healthy individuals have a serum CA195 level above the recommended cut-off level of 20 U/mL in tests using an immunoradiometric assay (IRMA) for serum detection. The reported overall sensitivity (69–89.5%) and specificity (53–92%) levels of the CA195 assay for diagnosis of pancreatic cancer are quite similar to that of CA242 (Table 2).

CA125. CA125 is a high-molecular-weight glycoprotein of mucin type defined by a monoclonal antibody (IgG) raised against an ovarian cystadenocarcinoma cell line. CA125 is expressed in epithelial ovarian cancer tissue (>80%) and also in human pancreatic cancer (59%). The reported overall sensitivity (45–60%) and specificity (76–86%) levels in diagnosis of pancreatic cancer are comparable to many other serum tumor markers (Table 1). The clinical usefulness of CA125 in diagnosis of pancreatic cancer seems, however, to be limited, because patients with liver cirrhosis, hepatitis, pancreatitis, and jaundice related to other cancers also have elevated levels of CA125 (3).

FUTURE DIRECTIONS

CA494

The exact structure of the CA494 antigen is unknown, but it can be detected by a monoclonal antibody BW 494, which was initially isolated from BALB/c mice immunized with a human colon cancer cell line. Friess et al. found 90% sensitivity at a 94% specificity level in differentiating pancreatic cancer patients from patients with chronic pancreatitis (Table 2) (8). Although CA494 seems to be a promising marker for pancreatic cancer, further studies are needed to confirm the final clinical role of this marker.

CAM17.1

CAM17.1 was generated after immunization with colorectal cancer cells, and there is an enzyme-linked antibody sandwich assay (CAM 17.1/WGA) using this monoclonal antibody (Table 2). CAM17.1 is an IgM-type antibody with high specificity for intestinal mucus, particularly in the colon, small intestine, biliary tract, and pancreas. The epitope detected by the CAM17.1 antibody is a sialylated blood group antigen. Parker et al. (9) studied CAM17.1 as a serological marker in 79 patients with pancreatic cancer and 120 control patients and reported 78% sensitivity and 76% specificity. A study of patients with chronic pancreatitis, pancreatic cancer or other gastrointestinal cancer, and of healthy blood donors, revealed 67% sensitivity at 90% specificity level for serological CAM17.1/WGA assay in pancreatic cancer (10). The sensitivity of the CAM17.1 assay was similar to that of CA19-9, whereas the specificity of CAM17.1 assay was higher (90%). It is possible that the antigens studied are quite similar since the correlation between CA19-9 and CAM17.1 was high (correlation coefficient, r = 0.91) (10). Others (see 3) later confirmed these results.

K-ras Oncogene as a Serological Test

K-ras mutations were shown to be present in 95% of human carcinomas of the exocrine pancreas. Thereafter, point mutations of the K-ras oncogene have been shown to be the most common genetic change in pancreatic cancer (see Ref. 11 for a review) identified in 80–95% of pancreatic adenocarcinomas, but not in chronic pancreatitis. Recently Mulcahy et al. (12) (Table 2) collected plasma from 21 patients with pancreatic cancer and found a K-ras mutation in the plasma DNA in 17 of these (81%). In cases where both plasma and pancreatic tissue were available, DNA mutations were similar in both samples. Furthermore, K-ras mutations were found in the plasma of three patients with chronic pancreatitis at the time of testing.

Table 2 Diagnostic sensitivity, specificity, and cut-off values for the serological markers for human pancreatic adenocarcinoma (3)

Type of Marker	First Author (Ref. No)	Sensitivity (range)	Specificity (range)	Cut-off value
CA494	Friess et al. (8)	90 %	94 %	40 U/mL
CAM17.1	Parker et al. (9)	78 %	76 %	NA*
	Gansauge et al. (10)		67 %	90 % 37 U/mL
ras gene	Mulcahy et al. (12)	81 %	NA	±**
p53 gene	Laurent-Puig et al. (13)	21 %	96 %	±**

*NA = cut-off value not available; **± = serological marker absent or present.

All three were found to have clinically evident pancreatic cancer within a year later.

Tumor Suppressor Gene p53 as a Serological Test

The tumor suppressor gene p53 is located in the short arm of human chromosome 17 at the position 17p13.1. It is considered that mutations in the tumor suppressor gene p53 contribute to the development of up to 50% of all human cancers. Studies on gene p53 as a tumor marker of pancreatic cancer have not been very promising (3).

SUMMARY

Pancreatic cancer generally progresses without early symptoms and thus presents many discouraging unresolved problems in disease management. Theoretically, tumor markers would be ideal for early diagnosis of pancreatic cancer. However, the lack of specificity has been a major problem in their use; there are currently no markers sensitive and specific enough for early detection in clinical practice. However, using advances in molecular methods, attempts to develop new assays for serological diagnosis of pancreatic carcinoma are ongoing.

REFERENCES

1. Gudjonsson B. Cancer of the pancreas. 50 years of surgery. Cancer 1987;60:2284–2303.
2. Warshaw A, Fernandez del Castillo C. Pancreatic carcinoma. N Engl J Med 1992;326:455–465.
3. Eskelinen M and Haglund U. Developments in serologic detection of human pancreatic adenocarcinoma. Scand J Gastroenterol 1999;34:833–844.
4. Pasanen P, Eskelinen M, Partanen K, Pikkarainen P, Penttilä I, Alhava E. Diagnostic value of tissue polypeptide specific antigen in patients with pancreatic carcinoma. Tumor Biol 1994; 15:52–60.
5. Pasanen P, Eskelinen M, Pikkarainen P, Partanen K, Penttilä I, Alhava E. Tumor-associated trypsin inhibitor in the diagnosis of pancreatic carcinoma. J Cancer Res Clin Oncol 1994;120: 494–497.
6. Johansson C, Nilsson O, Lindholm L. Comparison of serological expression of different epitopes on the CA50-carrying antigen. Can Ag Int J Cancer 1991;48:757–763.
7. Pasanen P, Eskelinen M, Pikkarainen P, Partanen K, Alhava E, Penttilä I. ROC curve analysis of the tumor markers CEA, CA50 and CA242 in pancreatic cancer; results from a prospective study. Brit J Cancer 1993;67:852–855.
8. Friess H, Buchler M, Auerbach B, et al. CA 494—a new tumor marker for the diagnosis of pancreatic cancer. Int J Cancer 1993;53:759–763.
9. Parker N, Makin CA, Ching CK, et al. A new enzyme-linked lectin/mucin antibody sandwich assay (CAM 17.1/WGA) assessed in combination with CA 19-9 and peanut lectin binding assay for the diagnosis of pancreatic cancer. Cancer 1992; 70:1062–1068.
10. Gansauge F, Gansauge S, Parker N, et al. CAM 17.1– A new diagnostic marker in pancreatic cancer. Br J Cancer 1996;74: 1997–2002.
11. Eskelinen MJ and Haglund UH. Prognosis of human pancreatic adenocarcinoma: review of clinical and histopathological variables and possible uses of new molecular methods. Eur J Surg 1999;165:292–306.
12. Mulcahy HE, Lyautey J, Lederrey C, et al. A prospective study of K-ras mutations in the plasma of pancreatic cancer patients. Clin Cancer Res 1998;4:271–275.
13. Laurent-Puig P, Lubin R, Semhoun-Ducloux S, et al. Antibodies against p53 protein in serum of patients with benign or malignant biliary diseases. Gut 1995;36:455–458.

Chapter 22

Tumor Markers in Primary Malignancies of the Liver

Philip J. Johnson

This chapter focuses on primary tumors of the liver. Of these, hepatocellular carcinoma (HCC), also known as primary liver cell carcinoma (PLCC) or, less accurately, "hepatoma," is by far the most common and the one in which tumor markers play a major role in diagnosis and management. The clinical features of HCC, particularly those relevant to the application of tumor markers, are described first. The biology of alpha-fetoprotein (AFP) is then discussed in detail as it is the most important marker. Finally, other potential markers that have been investigated are then briefly described, together with a review of markers that may be used in other, less common, primary tumors of the liver.

HEPATOCELLULAR CARCINOMA

Hepatocellular carcinoma (HCC) is a common malignant tumor in many parts of the world and is a major public health problem. Tumor markers play an important role in the diagnosis and management of this disease.

Epidemiology and Etiology

Carriers of the hepatitis B virus (HBV), hepatitis C virus (HCV), or persons who have been exposed to the mycotoxin, aflatoxin, are at a very high risk of developing HCC. This accounts for the wide geographic variation in incidence, which ranges from less than 2/100,000 in Northern Europe and the USA to more than 100/100,000 in parts of sub-Saharan Africa and the Far East. Rates are higher for men than for women, and in 70–90% of cases, HCC is associated with hepatic cirrhosis. The histological features of the tumor are of little clinical significance except for the fibrolamellar variant of HCC that occurs in the young and carries a rather better prognosis than the "normal" type of HCC.

Presentation

The most common presentation is the triad of abdominal pain, weight loss, and hepatomegaly. Other presentations include decompensation of known hepatic cirrhosis, gastrointestinal bleeding, and tumor rupture. Increasingly, HCC is being detected at an asymptomatic stage following screening programs that use tumor markers.

Diagnosis

Initial investigations typically include imaging procedures, laboratory investigations (including tumor markers), and the histological confirmation of diagnosis. Ultrasound examination, which is usually the initial procedure, shows the tumor as hypoechoic when small, becoming progressively hyperechoic as it enlarges. Computerized tomography (CT) scanning is as sensitive as ultrasound and can also provide a detailed view of primary or secondary lesions outside the abdomen. These two imaging modalities are the primary parameters for assessing response to therapy and recurrence after surgical removal. Laboratory investigations include viral serology (HBV and HCV) and standard liver function tests as well as AFP estimation (discussed later in this chapter).

Natural History and Management

The only potentially curative treatment is surgical resection. Unfortunately, most cases fall within the "unresectable" category due to poor underlying liver function, extensive bilobar disease and/or invasion of the major vessels, extrahepatic spread, and coexistent serious medical conditions. In high-incidence areas the median survival from the time of diagnosis is, in the absence of resection, measured in weeks. In low-incidence areas, survival time is 6–12 months.

Alpha-fetoprotein (AFP)

AFP, one of the first serological tumor markers to be used in clinical practice, remains one of the most important. Western oncologists have the most experience with AFP in germ cell tumors (see Chapter 29); gastroenterologists use AFP as part of the screening strategy for HCC in patients with cirrhosis (discussed later in this chapter). In Asia, sub-Saharan Africa, and southern Europe, its role in the management of HCC is of primary importance.

Historical aspects. AFP was first identified as a distinct band, next to albumin (hence 'alpha'), by electrophoresis of human cord blood in 1956 (1), but the association with HCC was not made until 1963 when Abelev reported the detection of AFP in the plasma of mice with transplantable HCCs (2). The following year, Tatarinov reported finding AFP in the serum of patients with HCC (3) and these observations were confirmed by Stanislawski-Birenewajg et al. in chemically induced rat tumors and human subjects (4). Since then more sensitive assays have been developed, along with an increasing recognition of the spectrum of benign and malignant conditions that may result in elevated plasma levels; the structural and functional properties of this protein have also been deduced.

Structure and function. AFP is a glycoprotein comprised of 591 amino acids and 4% carbohydrate residues, giving a molecular mass of about 70 kD. The carbohydrate residue, purified from the ascitic fluid of a patient with HCC, was reported to consist of a single biantennary complex-type chain, N-linked to asparagine 232 of the protein backbone (Figure 1) (5,6). This basic structure has been confirmed by mass spectrometric analysis of AFP derived from the hepatoblastoma cell line Hep G2 (7,8), and by paper electrophoretic and chromatographic analysis of pooled human-cord serum AFP at term pregnancy (5). Human AFP exhibits microheterogeneity by isoelectric focusing (IEF) and lectin electrophoretic techniques (9,10,11). This microheterogeneity results from differing degrees of terminal sialylation and fucosylation of the sugar sidechain(s) (Figure 1) (12).

More sensitive analytical techniques, including fluorescence labeling, sequential exoglycosidase digestion, HPLC, and mass spectrometry, have revealed that up to eleven major types of sugar side chain ("glycans") can be detected. Of these, seven are N-linked and four are O-linked to the protein backbone (13). The structure of the N-linked glycans are, as suggested previously, of the biantennary complex-type with varying degrees of sialylation, fucosylation, and galactosylation. Of the O-linked glycans, three are of the mucin O-GalNAc type, with variable degrees of sialylation (Figure 1b). The finding of O-linked glycans was supported by the prediction of potential O-GalNAc glycosylation sites on the protein backbone by molecular modeling analysis of the AFP structure (13). These different "isoforms" of AFP may be disease-specific and therefore may form the basis of attempts to develop more specific assays for the detection of HCC.

Gene structure and localization. The *AFP* gene is a member of a supergene family that includes genes for serum albumin, vitamin D-binding protein, and alpha albumin; all are synthesized in the liver and secreted into serum. These genes are situated on the long arm of chromosome 4 (4q11-q13) and share a considerable degree of sequence homology (14).

Dynamics of AFP. Following removal of the tumor by either surgical resection or liver transplantation, AFP levels fall with a half-life of three to six days (15). Similar figures are found after cytotoxic chemotherapy on the rare occasion that it is effective. There is no "surge" of AFP into the blood following procedures that cause rapid tumor necrosis, presumably because the AFP is rapidly transferred out of cells and into the plasma rather than being stored in tumor cells.

Assay of AFP. Early studies applied immunodiffusion techniques and were essentially qualitative or semi-quantitative. A "positive" AFP test using these techniques represented a value of about 1–2 microgram/mL (i.e., 1000–2000ng/mL) or more. In a collaborative study involving several different countries and large numbers of patients, 60–75% of HCC cases were positive using a modified Ouchterlony technique (16). Not surprisingly, the higher figure was for those with a histological diagnosis and the lower figure for those with a "clinical" diagnosis. The occasional "false positive" results came from patients in the control group with cirrhosis, other primary tumors (stomach or pancreas), and testicular teratocarcinomas. Although it was stated that the results were not affected by race or by geographical factors, the high positivity rate probably reflected the fact that most patients came from high-HCC-incidence areas in Africa. Alpert et al., quantifying AFP levels using counter-immunoelectrophoresis, reported similar results, except that levels of positivity were significantly lower in Caucasian patients with HCC (17).

Reference range. In the early 1970s, several groups purified AFP from human serum and developed sensitive radioimmunoassays that could detect AFP in healthy adults, albeit at concentrations of less than 10 ng/mL (18–20). Masseyeff et al. reported a range of between 0.1 and 5.8 ng/mL (mean = 2.6 ± 1.6 ng/mL), as determined by radioimmunoassay, in normal subjects (19). However, routine assays are not very accurate at low levels and cut-off values for the upper limit of the reference range have since been variously set at 10 or 25 ng/mL. With this increased sensitivity, AFP could be detected in more than 80% of HCC cases but with an inevitable decrease in specificity. This loss of specificity involved patients with other malignant diseases, particularly of the GI tract (21–23), and others with benign chronic liver diseases (21,22,24,25).

Disease associations. In the case of HCC the *positivity rate* is around 80%, and the *range of values* from 1 to 10,000,000 ng/mL, with a median value of around 1000 ng/mL. Nonseminomatous germ cell tumors are the only other adult condition that has a similar positivity rate and a similar range of levels (26,27). For the patient with HCC, the positivity rate

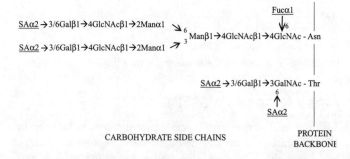

Figure 1 Structures of the main *N*- (upper) and *O*- (lower) linked glycans in human AFP. The charge heterogeneity depends on the number of sialic acid (SA) molecules at the sites underlined and, to a lesser extent, the fucose molecule, also underlined. The precise site of the attachment of the *O*-linked glycan(s) to threonine in the protein backbone is not known. The isoforms associated with HCC are predominantly the monosialylated species.

is not stage-dependent; if a tumor is "AFP-negative" at presentation, it remains so for the remainder of the clinical course. On the other hand, AFP levels do increase in patients with AFP-positive tumors with time; in the absence of treatment the doubling time is between five and 100 days.

AFP in benign diseases. Modest elevations of serum AFP concentration (10–500 ng/mL, and occasionally up to 1000 ng/mL) occur in adult patients with hepatitis (of any type) or liver cirrhosis. The frequency of elevation (>10 ng/mL) in chronic hepatitis and cirrhosis has been reported to be around 20% and 40%, respectively (21,22,24,25,28,29) and AFP elevations may be associated with the seroconversion from HBe antigenemia to HBe antibody positivity (30). These elevations appear to occur either when there is a high degree of inflammatory activity within the liver, or towards the end of an acute hepatitis when the liver function is recovering. These observations have often led to the suggestion that aberrant AFP secretion is related to cell proliferation or "hepatic regeneration." However, this certainly is not always the case since after hepatic resection, the classic initiator of liver cell regeneration, there is no increase in AFP levels (31). AFP levels between 10 ng/mL and 1,000 ng/mL therefore represent a "gray area," as benign conditions such as chronic hepatitis and cirrhosis and small HCCs may show values within this range (Figure 2). Since the clinician is often faced with the problem of determining if HCC has arisen in a patient with cirrhosis, the fact that AFP can be elevated in patients with chronic liver disease alone presents a major clinical problem.

Figures quoted for the frequency of AFP elevations should be taken with some caution. First, elevations close to the lower limits of the assay's limit of sensitivity can cause major changes in reported frequency. Second, there is often considerable fluctuation during the course of particular chronic liver diseases. For example there is probably a stage, during most cases of acute and chronic hepatitis, when AFP becomes transiently positive. Finally, serum AFP may be raised during the preclinical phase of HCC—before a tumor can be detected by imaging techniques. For this reason most series probably underestimate the true specificity of AFP for HCC (32).

AFP in other malignant diseases. The positivity rate is much lower in patients with malignant tumors other than HCC, as are the median and range. The major class of "other" malignant tumors that have been reported to secrete AFP is gastrointestinal (GI) tract tumors; these were first systematically studied by McIntire (23), who confirmed several earlier isolated reports (33,34). McIntire found raised levels in 15% of stomach cancer cases and 25% of cases of cancer of the biliary tract and pancreas. Levels were much lower than in patients with HCC—above 1000 ng/mL in over 40% of patients with HCC but in only 1% of patients with other GI tumors. These data have been confirmed over the years and are explained by the observation that the hepatic diverticulum, the pancreatic buds, and the stomach are all derived from the same endodermal lining of the foregut.

Diagnosis of HCC. Based on an evaluation of 239 cases of chronic hepatitis, 277 cases of cirrhosis, and 95 cases of HCC at varying clinical stages, Tekata demonstrated a sensitivity of 78.9% and a specificity of 78.1% when adopting a cut-off level of greater than 20 ng/mL for the diagnosis of HCC (35). At a cut-off level of 200 ng/mL, the specificity of the test rose to 99.6% at the expense of the sensitivity falling to 52.6%. Recognizing that modestly raised AFP levels occur in patients with chronic liver disease, a cut-off point of 400 or 500 ng/mL is now widely used in clinical practice.

Serum AFP levels may rise before the tumor can be detected by imaging techniques, so that the finding of a raised AFP without evidence of tumor is not necessarily a "false-positive" result. For accurate calculation of the specificity, AFP levels in cirrhotic patients followed for more than one year without evidence of HCC should be used, as is the case in the patients on which the data in Table 1 was based. An AFP level over 500 ng/mL in a patient known to have chronic liver disease is an indication for further detailed investigation. A hepatic mass by an imaging technique in the presence of chronic liver disease, accompanied by an AFP level of greater than 500 ng/mL, is virtually diagnostic of HCC.

A level below 500 ng/mL in a patient with chronic liver disease presents a diagnostic dilemma without clear management guidelines. Detailed investigation of all such patients will lead to some early and useful diagnoses of HCC, but it will be resource-intensive with numerous "false-positive" results. Most often when such raised levels are intensively investigated,

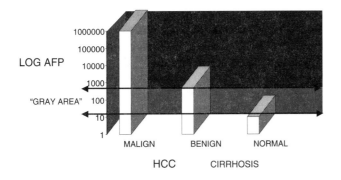

Figure 2 A diagrammatic representation of the range of AFP levels seen in normal subjects, patients with chronic liver disease, and those with hepatocellular carcinoma. The range between the upper limit of the reference range (10ng/mL) and 500 ng/mL is a "gray area." An AFP value falling in this range does not allow the clinician to make a confident diagnosis of HCC.

Table 1 Sensitivity and specificity of AFP for the diagnosis of HCC in patients with chronic liver disease using various cut-off points

Diagnostic criteria	Sensitivity (%)	Specificity (%)
AFP >615 ng/mL	56.4	96.4
AFP >530 ng/mL	56.4	94.5
AFP >445 ng/mL	56.4	94.5
AFP >100 ng/mL	72.6	70.9
AFP >20 ng/mL	87.1	30.9

The figures were calculated using patients with chronic liver disease who had been followed for >1 year to ensure that subclinical HCC was not present. Reference range: <20 ng/mL. Data courtesy of Dr. Terence CW Poon.

there is *no* associated hepatic inflammation; i.e., a markedly raised activity of serum AST. Otherwise a brief period of observation is in order. If levels continue to rise, this is suggestive of HCC. Conversely, if levels fall or fluctuate, then HCC is less likely. It should be noted that marked falls in AFP levels have also been observed in the terminal stage of HCC.

The option of careful follow-up in such patients is not without its problems. Lok et al. (36) reported that six patients with chronic liver disease had persistent or progressive increases in AFP levels and were confirmed to have HCC. However, in a further six patients in the same series, HCC was not identified despite elevations exceeding 200 ng/mL for more than six months. They concluded that monitoring time-trends of AFP levels alone is not an entirely satisfactory method for early diagnosis of HCC. However, steadily increasing levels of serum AFP above 1,000 ng/mL are usually an indication of AFP-producing tumors (37). These problems in the so-called gray area of AFP elevations have led to attempts to discover "tumor-specific" forms of AFP.

Factors influencing serum AFP levels. Gene expression is controlled mainly at the level of transcription. At presentation, levels can range from within the reference range up to 10,000,000 ng/mL (10 g/L) (Figure 2). About 40% of patients with HCC have AFP levels above 1,000 ng/mL (38). Well-differentiated small HCCs (<2 cm) seldom express detectable serum AFP (39), and the tumor cells do not show AFP by immunostaining. As small tumors have been increasingly detected by ultrasound screening since the 1970s, the number of AFP-negative tumors has increased and the sensitivity of the test for HCC has fallen.

Although small tumors tend to express lower levels of AFP, there is no clearly direct relationship between AFP levels and tumor size (29). Individual tumors appear to have different capacities to synthesize AFP, and it is difficult to accurately measure viable tumor cell mass and thereby investigate the correlation between viable tumor mass and AFP levels. Tumors that appear large on imaging procedures may in fact be necrotic and contain only a small number of viable cells. Male patients with HCCs tend to have slightly higher serum AFP concentrations than females (16,40) and serum AFP levels tend to be higher in younger patients (40,41).

Patients with HCC who are also seropositive for hepatitis B surface antigen (HBsAg) have a greater frequency of elevated AFP levels, but they also overlap to a greater extent with the AFP levels in HBsAg-positive patients with cirrhosis and/or chronic active hepatitis. The specificity of AFP for the detection of HCC in this serologically defined subgroup is thus decreased (42). Several studies have found a significantly higher AFP-positivity rate among HCC patients with underlying cirrhosis when compared to those without (43,44). The percentage of patients in Japan with HCC with serum AFP levels of <20 ng/mL at presentation increased from 3.6% to 29% during the nine-year period from 1978 to 1986, whereas the percentage with serum AFP > 10,000 ng/mL decreased from 53.5% to 6.4% over the same period (29). It seems likely that the larger number of HCCs with low AFP levels reflected more the introduction of sensitive imaging techniques such as ultrasound and computerized tomography.

Improving diagnostic specificity—disease-specific isoforms. The identification of "tumor-specific" glycoforms may improve the specificity of AFP for HCC. The most successful approach has been based on differences in binding affinity of AFP molecules from different sources to various lectins (35,44–50). AFP from patients with HCC binds to the lectin concanavalin A, whereas that from yolk-sac tumors does so to a lesser extent. Lentil lectin binds to AFP from HCC in preference to AFP from benign liver disease. By using other lectins such as *Lens culinarisa* and erythroagglutinating phytohemagglutinin, it is possible to differentiate, on the basis of different binding patterns, cord blood-type, HCC-type, GI tumor-type, and yolk sac-type AFPs (51). Commercially available assays based on this approach are now available and are useful in the early detection of HCC (52).

Isoelectric focusing (IEF) has also been used to directly identify isoforms of AFP (10,32,53). Three main bands are observed. The AFP+II band and AFP+III band are fairly specific for HCC and nonseminomatous germ cell tumors (NSGCT), respectively. A further band (+I) is found in patients with chronic liver disease without evidence of malignancy. In a study that followed a large cohort of patients with chronic liver disease, the band +II "hepatoma-specific AFP" was often detectable several months before ultrasound scanning could find the tumor (32). A qualitative assay of the tumor-specific band has led to an increase in positive predictive value from 41.5% with the conventional assay for total AFP to 73.1% with this specific isoform. The sensitivity and specificity are 86% and 77% respectively.

The structural basis of disease-specific isoforms. Studies by Yoshima et al. (5) and Yamashita et al. (6) described the basic structure of the asparagine (at position 232) N-linked sugar chain molecule of AFP. The charge heterogeneity of AFP and the molecular basis of the specific lectin binding are related to differences in terminal sialylation and fucosylation. It appears that the HCC-related AFP isoform has one terminal sialic acid, and its proximal N-acetyl glucosamine molecule is fucosylated (Figure 1) (6,12). We have recently confirmed these structures by direct sequencing of the AFP glycans from the serum of patients with HCC and NSGCT. However, it now appears that there are several other glycans, including some that are O-linked to the protein backbone. The "hepatoma-specific" bands seen on IEF do, in fact, represent a series of glycans, all of which are characterized by monosialation. Thus not only fucosylated monosialo biantennary complex-type N-glycans but also non-fucosylated monosialo biantennary complex-type N-glycans are the major carbohydrate structures of the HCC-specific AFP glycoforms (13).

Lectin binding and isoelectric focusing both appear to be of potent clinical value. However as they currently depend on some form of electrophoresis, they are unlikely to enter routine clinical practice until a simple, cheap, and robust assay of tumor-specific AFP becomes available. Since the biochemical differences between tumor- and non-tumor-related AFP are only minor, the development of such a routine assay is a technically difficult task.

Population screening and early diagnosis. Surgical resection or liver transplantation offers the only hope for long-term survival in people who have HCC. Both procedures are of very limited efficacy once symptoms develop; however, since we know the population in which most HCCs arise, screening asymptomatic subjects should, in theory, lead to more effective treatment. In an ideal world, prospective randomized studies would be undertaken before instituting a screening program, and only if such screening offered clear evidence of a decrease in disease-specific mortality would the program be introduced into clinical practice. At present no such data are available. Nonetheless, screening with AFP and ultrasound examination is in fact, widely practiced (54,55). Although at present it appears that ultrasound examination is the more useful of the two (particularly for small tumors) (56–58), two points should be noted. First, the AFP test is cheap and, if found to be positive simultaneously with the ultrasound (US) examination, it increases the specificity of the US result. Second, it is widely perceived that a positive AFP result in the absence of imaging evidence of a tumor indicates a "false positive" result. The possibility that the AFP is more sensitive than the imaging; i.e., there is a tumor present but not detectable by imaging methods, remains.

Staging and prognostic significance. In most clinical series of HCC patients, a raised serum AFP level is an adverse prognostic factor (59). This may reflect an intrinsically more aggressive tumor behavior or, in some cases, it may simply reflect the fact that patients with cirrhosis are more likely to be AFP-positive (60). One of the fundamental features of HCC that affects treatment decisions and prognosis is resectability, a decision that is based on both tumor-related factors (size and degree of vascular invasion) and the degree of underlying liver dysfunction. For this reason the conventional TNM staging system, which only considers tumor-related factors, has not been widely used in HCC. Although the TNM system does not take into account AFP, most other staging systems, built upon multivariate analysis of large cohorts of patients, have confirmed that a raised serum AFP level at the time of diagnosis predicts a poor prognosis compared to AFP-negative cases (61–63). The rate at which the AFP rises (expressed as doubling time) may also be of prognostic significance, presumably reflecting the rate of tumor growth (64).

Role of AFP in monitoring response to surgical and medical therapy. Serial estimation of serum AFP is useful for monitoring response to therapy. This practice was usually applied to surgical treatment, as non-surgical approaches have been, until recently, considered ineffective.

Surgery. Complete removal of an HCC by resection or liver transplantation rapidly decreases serum levels of AFP, with a half-life of 3.5–4 days. Poor survival rates are reported in patients showing longer AFP half-lives (64,65). The achievement of a "normal" level does not necessarily imply complete clearance of the disease. Patients often develop recurrent tumor after transplantation, despite the fact that their serum AFP level returned to the normal range in the immediate post-operative period (64,66,67). This presumably happens because micrometastases, the source of the recurrence, are too small to secrete sufficient AFP to raise the serum AFP level above the reference range. Even if resection appears complete, if the AFP did not achieve the normal range, residual nondetectable tumor is invariably present, presaging clinical tumor recurrence. Re-elevation of the AFP level in any situation is usually a strong indication of recurrence. Exceptions have, however, been described; a gradual rise in serum AFP levels was observed in seven patients without any evidence of post-operative recurrence (68). Conversely, patients with recurrent disease may occasionally show no AFP rise even when they were AFP-positive initially (69). Thus while factors influencing the absolute level of AFP in patients with HCC are still unclear, changes in serum AFP in the individual patient usually seem to mirror changes in tumor mass. These observations form the basis of the belief that changes in serum AFP may accurately reflect response to other, non-surgical forms of therapy.

Chemotherapy. Chemotherapy has been considered largely ineffective for HCC. However, some authors have found a broad correlation between AFP changes and tumor response. Patients classified as achieving a significant prolonged fall of AFP tended to survive longer than those with a transient fall, who in turn survived longer than those who had a continuously rising level (70–72). More effective combination systemic therapies are now becoming available and offer some important insights (73). In one such study, although only a modest number of partial remissions were achieved, a dramatic decrease in the AFP was seen in 75% of cases, and the normal range was attained in some of these (Figure 3). In about 20% of cases (most of those with "partial responses"), initially inoperable cases became operable. Histopathological examination of the resected specimen revealed either complete histological remission or only minimal residual disease. Such dramatic results were invariably associated with an AFP fall to within, or close to, the normal range. Conversely, when there was clearly progressive disease in those in whom AFP levels continued to rise, with a doubling time of 6.5 to 112 days (mean 41 days), the doubling times correlated positively with patient survival (64).

Radiotherapy. Radiotherapy for primary and secondary liver tumors results in a decrease in tumor markers more consistently than it does in changes in tumor size/volumes from CT images (74,75), and any reduction in tumor volume appears later than the fall in tumor marker levels. Experiences similar to that described for combination chemotherapy above have been reported in patients treated by selective internal radiation (SIR) therapy using yttrium-90 microspheres. Thus "partial responses," based on imaging criteria, may after tumor resection be shown to be complete pathological remissions (74–77). The discrepancy between the tumor marker levels and CT images may be due to fibrosis produced by the radiotherapy (74), and the size of tumor nodules on CT scans after treatment depends on a number of other factors, including the rate of the tumor cell death and reparative process (75). Tumor marker production may therefore cease completely following the death or damage of the tumor cells, while abnormalities persist on the CT images. It would be interesting to compare serum tumor markers such as AFP with an imaging modality such as positron emission tomography, which is capable of differentiating viable tumor from necrotic tissue.

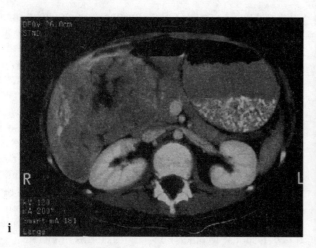 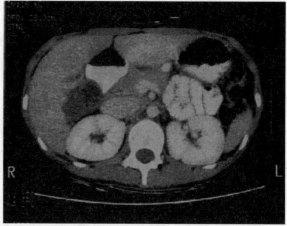

Figure 3a CT scans before (i) and after (ii) combined chemotherapy and radiotherapy. The tumor shrank initially in response to chemotherapy but then started to enlarge again. Subsequent treatment with internal radiotherapy (yttrium^{90}) resulted in further shrinkage although the overall response was still only "partial" by conventional radiological criteria.

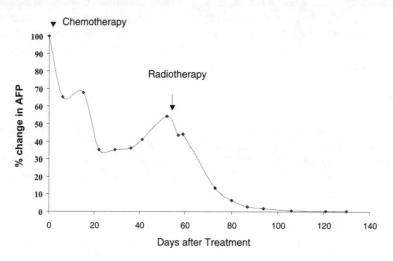

Figure 3b Note how the serum AFP level, over the same period, reflected the clinical changes but, whereas the radiological response was only partial, the AFP levels fell to within the reference range. This latter finding was in agreement with histopathological examination of the lesion after surgical resection where no viable tumor cells could be detected. Data courtesy of Dr. Thomas Leung.

Other Tumor Markers Used in HCC

Innumerable other markers have been studied in HCC, but to date none has found its way into routine clinical practice. The data on some of the potential markers are reviewed briefly here.

Serum ferritin. In early studies, estimation of serum ferritin had a poor specificity for HCC as raised levels were found as frequently in patients with uncomplicated cirrhosis (20 of 23, or 87%) as in patients with HCC (34 of 35, or 97%) (78). However in a later study, both its sensitivity and specificity were found to be superior to AFP as a diagnostic marker for HCC (79), and high ferritin levels were found to occur more frequently in low-AFP-producing HCCs. Serial determination of both markers has been suggested to increase the diagnostic sensitivity (80). Thus, the diagnostic rate for lesions of less than three centimeters in diameter was raised from 75% by measuring AFP alone, to 100% when both serum ferritin and AFP were measured. Ferritin may also be a useful marker for monitoring response to treatment, particularly in AFP-negative patients (81). Unlike AFP, there is usually an initial surge following effective treatment before levels fall with tumor regression.

γ-GTP isoenzyme. γ-GTP isoenzyme is a fetal isoenzyme. Activity is low in the adult liver but high in the fetal liver and in HCC tissue (82). Three isoforms of serum γ-GTP isoenzymes stand out as distinctive bands characteristic of HCC, among a total of 13 that appear during electrophoresis (29). One or more of the specific bands was detected in 109 of 200 patients with HCC but in only 1 of 57 patients with liver cirrhosis and 1 of 43 patients with chronic hepatitis. Although the HCC-specific γ-GTP occurs more frequently in patients with higher AFP levels, it was also found in 29 of 76 (38%) patients with AFP below 400 ng/mL and in 11 of 41 (27%) patients with AFP below 100 ng/mL. These HCC-specific isoenzymes may thus serve as a diagnostic marker that complements AFP. As with AFP, specificity is due to structural differences in the carbohydrate side chains that result from altered post-translational processing in the tumor cells. These structural differences give rise to distinct molecular weights, electrophoretic mobility, and lectin affinity.

Alkaline phosphatase (ALP). Variant ALP (VAALP) is less sensitive than AFP and γ-GTP but has a much higher specificity, as it is negative in patients with other types of cancer and in patients with benign hepatobiliary diseases (83). Since its prevalence is independent of the AFP level and the presence of γ-GTP, it may serve as a complementary marker to AFP or γ-GTP.

Des-γ-carboxy prothrombin (DCP). This marker is an abnormal prothrombin released into the blood when vitamin K-dependent carboxylase activity of the liver is inhibited, due to either the absence of vitamin K or the presence of a vitamin K antagonist. It is hardly detectable in normal subjects. Moderately raised levels were found in some patients with acute hepatitis, liver cirrhosis, and metastatic liver cancer (84). Sixty-nine of 76 patients (91%) with HCC showed high levels. At a cut-off value of 300 ng/mL, the test was positive in 67% of 76 patients with HCC and in one of 17 patients with metastatic liver cancer, but was negative in all 28 patients with chronic active hepatitis. Again, there was no correlation between AFP and DCP levels. Raised DCP levels were detected in 16 of 28 patients (57%) with HCC whose AFP levels were below 400 ng/mL (85). Furthermore, DCP is useful for monitoring response to treatment by surgery or chemotherapy. A recent study of 147 patients who underwent curative resection for HCC concluded that positivity of both DCP (>0.1 IU/mL) and AFP (>50 ng/mL) is one of the independent factors of poor prognosis for both overall survival and disease-free interval (86–90).

Alpha-1-antitrypsin (AAT). AAT is a 54 kD glycoprotein synthesized by the liver. It consists of a single polypeptide chain with four oligosaccharide side chains of two different types. The activity of AAT was found to be significantly higher in HCC than in benign liver diseases (91). There was no correlation between AAT and AFP levels, suggesting that AAT may be a useful marker to aid in the diagnosis of AFP-negative HCC. Serum AAT levels in Stage I HCC were significantly lower than those in Stage II or III (92). Patients with proven underlying cirrhosis had slightly higher levels than noncirrhotic patients. Among cases of AFP-negative HCC, AAT levels in HBsAg-positive patients were slightly higher than in HBsAg-negative patients. AAT levels increased with tumor size. HCC patients with well-encapsulated tumors and without tumor thrombus were found to have lower AAT levels than those with unencapsulated tumors or with capsular penetration, and also in those with vascular thrombi. Furthermore, tumor resectability was higher in patients with lower pre-operative AAT levels.

Aldolase A. High activity of aldolase A one of the key enzymes in the glycolytic pathway responsible for catalyzing the cleavage of fructose 1,6-diphosphate and fructose 1-phosphate, has been found in patients with HCC (93). Its serum level in benign liver disease such as cirrhosis and hepatitis was lower than in HCC. A positive aldolase A level was found in 11 of 17 patients (64.71%) with tumors ≤5 cm and in 23 of 29 patients (79.31%) with Stage I tumors (94), suggesting that the marker may be useful in early diagnosis. No parallel relationship between levels of aldolase A and AFP was found and the two markers appeared to be complementary. Aldolase A level returned to normal after complete resection of HCC and increased when there was recurrence.

5′-nucleotide phosphodiesterase V (5′-NPD). 5′-NPD is an enzyme that hydrolyzes a nucleotide to form a nucleoside and phosphoric acid. It was positive in 83.2% of 95 patients with HCC (95) and was detected in 8.3% of cases of cirrhosis and 13.3% of hepatitis (96). The positivity rate was 85.7% among AFP-positive HCC patients and 76.0% in AFP-negative cases. In a Japanese study, the diagnostic value of this enzyme for HCC was found to be relatively high, especially in patients with low or negative AFP levels (97). It was noted that jaundice caused a nonspecific false-positive reaction in the assay for this enzyme; it should not be used in patients with jaundice.

Tissue polypeptide antigen (TPA). TPA has been investigated for the detection of HCC in cirrhotic patients (98). The study involved two groups of cirrhotic patients, 35 with and 90 without HCC. There was a significant difference between the mean TPA levels in the two groups, and the best diagnostic accuracy for HCC with 48.6% sensitivity and 85.6% specificity was found at a cut-off value of 240 U/L. However, there is a significant correlation between TPA levels and liver enzymes so that great caution must be exercised when using TPA as a diagnostic aid: liver dysfunction may cause its elevation.

α-L-fucosidase. The serum α-L-fucosidase activity level in patients with HCC (575.76 ± 272.86 nmol/mL/h) was significantly higher than that in patients with cirrhosis (274.55 ± 138.97 nmol/mL/h) or other neoplasms (257.91 ± 128.12 nmol/mL/h; $p<0.001$) (99). With a sensitivity of 76% and a specificity of 90.9% at a cut-off value of 443 nmol/mL/h, α-L-fucosidase is considered a useful marker for detecting HCC when used in conjunction with AFP and ultrasound scan of the liver (100,101).

The Fibrolamellar Variant of Hepatocellular Carcinoma

This variant of HCC has a better prognosis than the common form of HCC and is composed of deeply eosinophilic cytoplasm and pyknotic nuclei interspersed with acellular collagen. The patients are young (mean age 26 years), the male:female ratio is 1:1, and the non-tumorous liver is usually not cirrhotic. The prognosis is rather better than for conventional HCC. Although resection rates are high, most patients will still die of their tumor with a median survival of around five years. Although AFP is not produced in excess, two other serum markers, the vitamin B_{12} binding protein (102,103) and neurotensin (104), may be useful. However, the rarity of this HCC variant makes detailed assessment of their value difficult.

Other Primary Liver Tumors: Cholangiocarcinoma

Cholangiocarcinomas account for about 10% of primary liver tumors and are of two types. *Intrahepatic cholangiocarcinomas* are derived from small bile duct cells and behave clinically in a manner similar to HCC. The second type, known as a "hilar" cholangiocarcinoma or "Klatskin" tumors, arises at or around the bifurcation of the common hepatic duct. The presentation is with pain, weight loss, and obstructive jaundice. A particularly difficult diagnostic problem is the development of cholangiocarcinoma in patients known to have sclerosing cholangitis. CA19-9 is the marker that has been used. In patients with intrahepatic cholangiocarcinomas, the sensitivity was 55% (at a cutoff of 100 U/mL) (105). Whether or not CA19-9 estimation has a role as determining if patients with sclerosing cholangitis have developed an associated cholangiocarcinoma remains contentious. Some workers find CA19-9 a valuable marker, with or without additional investigations such as positron emission tomography (PET) scanning (106), while others find it distinctly unreliable (107,108).

The Future—New Molecular Approaches

It is likely that novel approaches using proteome analysis will identify, in a systematic manner, many novel tumor markers for further investigation (109). In addition, the detection of cell free nucleic acids (110,111) and epigenetic abnormalities (such as p16 hypermethylation) in serum or plasma (112) offer an exciting new source of circulating molecular markers.

Acknowledgements

The author is indebted to the Kadoorie Charitable Foundations Limited and the Hong Kong Cancer Fund for their support of his work in the field of research.

REFERENCES

1. Bergstrand CG, Czar B. Demonstration of new protein fraction in serum from the human fetus. Scand J Clin Lab Invest 1956;8:174–176.
2. Abelev GI, Perova SD, Khramkova NI, et al. Production of embryonal α-globulin by transplantable mouse hepatomas. Transplant Bull 1963;1:174–180.
3. Tatarinov YS. Presence of embryo-specific α-globulin in the serum of patients with primary hepatocellular carcinoma. Vopi Med Khim 1964;10:90–91.
4. Stanislawski-Birenewajg M, Frayssinet C, Grabar P. Embryonic antigens in liver tumors in rats. Arch Immun Ther Exp 1966;14:730–735.
5. Yoshima H, Mizuochi T, Ishii M, et al. Structure of the asparagines-linked sugar chains of α-fetoprotein purified from human ascites fluid. Cancer Res 1980;40:4276–4281.
6. Yamashita K, Taketa K, Nishi S, et al. Sugar chains of human cord serum α-fetoprotein: characteristics of N-linked sugar chains of glycoproteins produced in human liver and hepatocellular carcinomas. Cancer Res 1993;53:2970–2975.
7. Tarelli E, Ashcroft AE, Calam DH, et al. Human alpha-fetoprotein. Molecular weight data from electrospray mass spectrometry (ESMS) analysis. Biol Mass Spect 1992;23:315–317.
8. Ferranti P, Pucci P, Marino G, et al. Human α-fetoprotein produced from Hep G2 cell line: structure and heterogeneity of the oligosaccharide moiety. J Mass Spect 1995;30:632–638.
9. Alpert E, Drysdale JW, Isselbacher KJ, et al. Human α-fetoprotein: isolation, characterization, and demonstration of microheterogeneity. J Biol Chem 1972;247:3792–3798.
10. Johnson PJ, Ho S, Cheng P, et al. Germ cell tumors express a specific alpha-fetoprotein variant detectable by isoelectric focusing. Cancer 1995;75:1663–1668.
11. Smith CJP, Kelleher PC. Alpha-fetoprotein molecular heterogeneity: physiologic correlations with normal growth, carcinogenesis, and tumor growth. Biochim Biophys Acta 1980;605:1–31.
12. Shimizu K, Katoh H, Yamashita F, et al. Comparison of carbohydrate structures for serum α-fetoprotein by sequential glycosidase digestion and lectin affinity electrophoresis. Clin Chim Acta 1996;254:23–40.
13. Johnson PJ, Poon TCW, Hjelm NM, et al. Glycan composition of serum alpha-fetoprotein in patients with hepatocellular carcinoma and non-seminomatous germ cell tumor. Br J Cancer 1999;81:1188–1195.
14. Belanger l, Roy S, Allard D. New albumin gene 3' adjacent to the alpha 1-fetoprotein locus. J Biol Chem 1994;269:5481–5484.
15. McIntire KR, Vogel CL, Primack A, et al. Effect of surgical and chemotherapeutic treatment on alpha-fetoprotein levels in patients with hepatocellular carcinoma. Cancer 1976;37:677–683.
16. O'Conor G, Tatarinov YS, Abelev GI, et al. A collaborative study for the evaluation of a serological test for primary cancer. Cancer 1970;25:1091–1098.
17. Alpert E, Hershberg R, Schur PH, et al. Alpha-fetoprotein in human hepatoma: improved detection in serum and quantitative studies using a new sensitive technique. Gastroenterology 1971;61:137–143.
18. Sell S. Diagnostic applications of alpha-fetoprotein: government regulations prevent full application of a clinically useful test. Hum Pathol 1981;12:959–963.
19. Masseyeff R, Bonet C, Drouet J, et al. Radioimmunoassay of α-fetoprotein: I. Technique and serum level in normal adult. Digestion 1974;10:17–28.
20. Ruoslahti E, Seppala M. Studies of carcino-fetal protein III. Development of a radioimmunoassay of alpha-fetoprotein. Demonstration of alpha-fetoprotein in serum of healthy human adults. Int J Cancer 1971;8:374–383.
21. Masopust J, Kithier K, Radl J, et al. Occurrence of fetoprotein in patients with neoplasms and nonneoplastic diseases. Intern J Cancer 1968;3:364–373.
22. Johnson PJ, Portmann B, Williams R. Alpha-fetoprotein concentration measured by radioimmunoassay in the diagnosing and excluding of hepatocellular carcinoma. Br Med J 1978;2:661–663.
23. McIntire R. Serum alpha-fetoprotein in patients with neoplasms of the gastrointestinal tract. Cancer Res 1975;35:991–996.
24. Bloomer JR, Waldmann TA, McIntire KR, Klatskin G. Relationship of alphafetoprotein to the severity and duration of illness in patients with viral hepatitis. Gastroenterology 1975;68:342–350.
25. Bloomer JR, Waldmann TA, McIntire KR. Klatskin G. Alpha-fetoprotein in nonneoplastic hepatic disorders. JAMA 1975;233:38–41.
26. Lange PH, Fralay EE. Serum AFP and HCG in the treatment of patient with testicular tumors. Urol Clin North Am 1977;4:393–406.
27. Javadpour N. The role of biologic tumor markers in testicular cancer. Cancer 1980;45:2166–2168.

28. Silver HK, Deneault J, Gold P, et al. The detection of alpha 1-fetoprotein in patients with viral hepatitis. Cancer Res 1974;34:244–247.
29. Sawabu N, Hattori N. Serological tumor markers in hepatocellular carcinoma. In: Okuda K, Ishak KG (eds.). Neoplasms of the liver. Tokyo: Springer-Verlag, 1987:227–238.
30. Liaw Y-F, Tai D-I, Chen T-J, et al. Alpha-fetoprotein changes in the course of chronic hepatitis: relation to bridging hepatic necrosis and hepatocellular carcinoma. Liver 1986;6:133–137.
31. Alpert E, Feller ER. Alpha-fetoprotein (AFP) in benign liver disease: evidence that normal liver regeneration does not induce AFP synthesis. Gastroenterology 1978;74:856–858.
32. Johnson PJ, Leung N, Cheng P, et al. "Hepatoma-specific" alphafetoprotein may permit preclinical diagnosis of malignant change in patients with chronic liver disease. Br J Cancer 1997;75:236–240.
33. Mehlman DJ, Bulkley BH, Wiernik PH. Serum alphafetoglobulin with gastric and prostatic carcinomas. N Engl J Med 1971;285:1060–1061.
34. Kozower M, Fawaz KA, Miller HM, et al. Positive alpha-fetoprotein in a case of gastric carcinoma. N Engl J Med 1971;285:1059–1060.
35. Taketa K. Alpha-fetoprotein. J Med Tech 1989;33:1380–1384.
36. Lok AS, Lai Cl. Alpha-fetoprotein monitoring in Chinese patients with chronic hepatitis B virus infection: role in the early detection of hepatocellular carcinoma. Hepatology 1989;9:110–115.
37. Sell S. Cancer markers of the 1990s. Clin Lab Med 1990;10: 1–37.
38. The Liver Study Group of Japan: Primary cancer in Japan. Sixth Report. Cancer 1987;60:1400–1411.
39. Kondo F, Wada K, Nagato Y, et al. Biopsy diagnosis of well-differentiated hepatocellular carcinoma based on new morphologic criteria. Hepatology 1989;9:751–755.
40. Mawas C, Buffe D, Burtin P. Influence of age on alphafetoprotein incidence. Lancet 1970;1:1292.
41. Namieno T, Kawata A, Sato N, et al. Age-related, different clinicopathologic features of hepatocellular carcinoma patients. Ann Surg 1995;221:308–314.
42. Lee HS, Chung YH, Kim CY. Specificity of serum α-fetoprotein in HBsAg+ and HbsAg-patients in the diagnosis of hepatocellular carcinoma. Hepatology 1991;14:68–72.
43. Melia WM, Wilkinson ML, Portmann BC. Hepatocellular carcinoma in the non-cirrhotic liver: a comparison with that complicating cirrhosis. Q J Med New Series LIII 1984;211:391–400.
44. Taketa K, Endo Y, Sekiya C, et al. A collaborative study for the elevation of lectin-reactive alpha-fetoproteins in early detection of hepatocellular carcinoma. Cancer Res 1993;53:5419–5423.
45. Aoyagi Y, Isemura M, Suzuki Y, et al. Fucosylated alphafetoprotein as a marker of early hepatocellular carcinoma. Lancet 1985;ii:1353–1354.
46. Aoyagi Y, Suzuki Y, Isemuna M, et al. Differential reactivity of alphafetoprotein with lectins and evaluation of its usefulness in the diagnosis of hepatocellular carcinoma. Gann 1984;75:809–815.
47. Buamah PK, Harris R, James DFW, et al. Lentil lectin-reactive alphafetoprotein in the differential diagnosis of benign and malignant liver disease. Clin Chem 1986;32:2083–2084.
48. Du MQ, Hutchinson WL, Johnson PJ, et al. Differential alphafetoprotein lectin binding in hepatocellular carcinoma. Cancer 1991;67:476–480.
49. Sato Y, Nakata K, Kato Y, et al. Early recognition of hepatocellular carcinoma based on altered profiles of alpha-fetoprotein. New Engl J Med 1993;328:1802–1806.
50. Taketa K, Izumi M, Ichikawa E. Distinct molecular species of human alpha-fetoprotein due to differential affinities to lectins. Ann NY Acad Sci 1983;417:61–68.
51. Taketa K. Alpha-fetoprotein in the 1990s. In: Sell S, ed. Serological Cancer Markers. Tolowa, NJ: The Humana Press, 1992:31–39.
52. Li D, Mallory T, Satomura S. AFP-L3: a new generation of tumor marker for hepatocellular carcinoma. Clin Chim Acta 2001;313:15–19.
53. Burditt LJ, Johnson MM, Johnson PJ, et al. Detection of hepatocellular carcinoma-specific alpha-fetoprotein by isoelectric focusing. Cancer 1994;74:25–29.
54. Colombo M. Screening for cancer in viral hepatitis. Clin Liver Dis 2001;5:109–122.
55. McMahon BJ, Bulkow L, Harpster A, Snowball M, Lanier A, Sacco F, Dunaway E, Williams J. Screening for hepatocellular carcinoma in Alaska natives infected with chronic hepatitis B: a 16-year population-based study. Hepatology 2000;32:842–846.
56. Okano H, Shiraki K, Inoue H, Ito T, Yamanaka T, Deguchi M, Sugimoto K, Sakai T, Ohmori S, Murata K, Takase K, Nakano T: Comparison of screening methods for hepatocellular carcinomas in patients with cirrhosis. Anticancer Res 2001;21:2979–2982.
57. Sherman M. Surveillance for hepatocellular carcinoma. Semin Oncol 2001;28:450–459.
58. Trevisani F, D'Intino PE, Morselli-Labate AM, Mazzella G, Accogli E, Caraceni P, Domenicali M, De Notariis S, Roda E, Bernardi M. Serum alpha-fetoprotein for diagnosis of hepatocellular carcinoma in patients with chronic liver disease: influence of HBsAg and anti-HCV status. J Hepatol 2001;34:603–605.
59. Nomura F, Ohnishi K, Tanabe Y. Clinical features and prognosis of hepatocellular carcinoma with reference to serum alpha-fetoprotein levels. Cancer 1989;64:1700–1707.
60. Johnson PJ, Melia WM, Palmer MK, Portmann B, Williams R. Relationship between serum alpha-fetoprotein cirrhosis and survival in hepatocellular carcinoma. Br J Cancer 1981;44:502–505.
61. Stuart KE, Anand AJ, Jenkins RL. Hepatocellular carcinoma in the United States. Prognostic features, treatment outcome, and survival. Cancer 1996;77:2217–2222.
62. Chevret S, Trinchet JC, Mathieu D, Rached AA, Beaugrand M, Chastang C. A new prognostic classification for predicting survival in patients with hepatocellular carcinoma. Groupe d'Etude et de Traitement du Carcinome Hepatocellulaire. J Hepatol 1999;31:133–141.
63. No authors listed. A new prognostic system for hepatocellular carcinoma: a retrospective study of 435 patients: the Cancer of the Liver Italian Program (CLIP) investigators. Hepatology 1998;28:751–755.
64. Johnson PJ, Williams R. Serum alpha-fetoprotein estimations and doubling time in hepatocellular carcinoma: influence of therapy and possible value in early detection. J Natl Cancer Inst 1980;64:1329–1332.
65. Sell S. Diagnostic applications of alpha-fetoprotein: government regulations prevent full application of a clinically useful test. Hum Path 1981;12:959–963.
66. Andorno E, Salizzoni M, Schieroni R, et al. Role of serum alpha-fetoprotein in pre- and post-orthotopic liver transplantation (OLT) for malignant disease. J Nucl Med All Sci 1989;33:132–134.
67. Urabe TS, Hayashi S, Terasaki M, et al. An assessment of therapeutic effect of hepatocellular carcinoma by the serial change of serum AFP value. Jpn J Gastroenterol 1990;87:100–108.

68. Curtin JP, Rubin SC, Hoskins WK, et al. Second-look laparotomy in endodermal sinus tumor: a report of two patients with normal levels of alpha-fetoprotein and residual tumor at re-exploration. Obst Gyne 1989;73:893–896.
69. Ezaki T, Yukaya H, Ogawa Y, Chang YC, Nagasue N. Elevation of alphafetoprotein level without evidence of recurrence after hepatectomy for hepatocellular carcinoma. Cancer 1988;61:1880–1883.
70. McIntire KR, Vogel CL, Primack A, et al. Effect of surgical and chemotherapeutic treatment on alpha-fetoprotein levels in patients with hepatocellular carcinoma. Cancer 1976;37:677–683.
71. Matsumoto Y, Suzuki T, Ono H, et al. Response of alpha-fetoprotein to chemotherapy in patients with hepatoma. Cancer 1974;34:1602–1606.
72. Johnson PJ, Williams R, Thomas H, et al. Induction of remission in hepatocellular carcinoma with doxorubicin. Lancet 1978;i:1006–1009.
73. Leung TWT, Patt YZ, Lau WY, et al. Complete pathological remission is possible with systemic combination chemotherapy for inoperable hepatocellular carcinoma. Clin Cancer Res 1999;5;1676–1681.
74. Barone RM, Byfield JE, Goldfarb PB, et al. Intra-arterial chemotherapy using an implantable infusion pump and liver irradiation for treatment of hepatic metastases. Cancer 1982;50:850–862.
75. Nauta RJ, Heres EK, Thoms DS, et al. Intra-operative single-dose radiotherapy. Observations on staging and interstitial treatment of unresectable liver metastases. Arch Surg 1987;122:1392–1395.
76. Lau WY, Leung WT, Ho S, Chan M, Leung NWY, Lin J, Metreweli C, Johnson PJ, Li AKC. Treatment of inoperable hepatocellular carcinoma with intrahepatic-arterial Yttrium-90 Microspheres—a phase I & II study. Br J Cancer 1994;70:994–999.
77. Lau WY, Ho S, Leung TWT, Chan M, Ho R, Johnson PJ, Li AKC. Selective internal radiation therapy for inoperable hepatocellular carcinoma with intra-arterial infusion of yttrium^{90} microspheres. Int J Rad Oncol Bio Phys 1998;40:583–592.
78. Melia WM, Bullock S, Johnson PJ, Williams R. Serum ferritin in hepatocellular carcinoma, comparison with alphafetoprotein. Cancer 1983;51:2112–2115.
79. Giannoulis E, Arvanitakis C, Nikopoulous A, et al. Diagnostic value of serum ferritin in primary hepatocellular carcinoma. Digestion 1984;30:236–241.
80. Nakano S, Kumada T, Sugiyama K, et al. Clinical significance of serum ferritin determination for hepatocellular carcinoma. Am J Gastroenterol 1984;79:623–627.
81. Tatsta M, Yamamura H, Iishi H, et al. Value of serum alpha-fetoprotein and ferritin in the diagnosis of hepatocellular carcinoma. Oncology 1986;43:306–310.
82. Fiala S, Fiala AE, Dixon B. γ-Glutamyl transpeptidase in transplantable chemically induced rat hepatomas and "spontaneous" mouse hepatomas. J Natl Cancer Inst 1972;48:1393–1401.
83. Szuki H, Iino S, Endo Y, et al. Tumor-specific alkaline phosphatase in hepatoma. Ann NY Acad Sci 1975;259:307–316.
84. Blanchard RA, Furie BC, Jorgensen M, et al. Acquired vitamin K-dependent carboxylation deficiency in liver disease. N Engl J Med 1981;305:242–245.
85. Liebmen HA, Furie BC, Tong MJ, et al. Des-γ-carboxy (abnormal) prothrombin as a serum marker for primary hepatocellular carcinoma. N Engl J Med 1984;310:1427–1431.
86. Shimada M, Takenaka K, Fujiwara Y, et al. Des-γ-carboxy prothrombin and α-fetoprotein status as a new prognostic indicator after hepatic resection for hepatocellular carcinoma. Cancer 1996;78:2094–2100.
87. Grazi GL, Mazziotti A, Legnani C, Jovine E, Miniero R, Gallucci A, Palareti G, Gozzetti G. The role of tumor markers in the diagnosis of hepatocellular carcinoma, with special reference to the des-gamma-carboxy prothrombin. Liver Transpl Surg 1995;1:249–255.
88. Sassa T, Kumada T, Nakano S, Uematsu T. Clinical utility of simultaneous measurement of serum high-sensitivity des-gamma-carboxy prothrombin and Lens culinaris agglutinin A-reactive alpha-fetoprotein in patients with small hepatocellular carcinoma. Eur J Gastroenterol Hepatol 1999;11:1387–1392.
89. Okuda H, Nakanishi T, Takatsu K, Saito A, Hayashi N, Takasaki K, Takenami K, Yamamoto M, Nakano M. Serum levels of des-gamma-carboxy prothrombin measured using the revised enzyme immunoassay kit with increased sensitivity in relation to clinicopathologic features of solitary hepatocellular carcinoma. Cancer 2000;88:544–549.
90. Mita Y, Aoyagi Y, Yanagi M, Suda T, Suzuki Y, Asakura H. The usefulness of determining des-gamma-carboxy prothrombin by sensitive enzyme immunoassay in the early diagnosis of patients with hepatocellular carcinoma. Cancer 1998;82:1643–1648.
91. Chio LF, Don CJ. Changes in serum alpha-antitrypsin, alpha acid glycoprotein and beta glycoprotein I in patients with malignant hepatocellular carcinoma. Cancer 1979;43:596–604.
92. Tu Z-X, Wu M-C. Clinical significance of serum alpha-1-antitrypsin determination in AFP-negative primary liver cancer. In: Tang Z-Y, Wu M-C, Xia S-S (eds.). Primary liver cancer. Beijing: China Acadcmic Publishcrs, 1989:262–268.
93. Asaka M, Nagasue K, Miyazaki, et al. Aldolase A isoenzyme levels in serum and tissue of patients with liver diseases. Gastroenterology 1983;84:155–160.
94. Zong M, Wu M-C. Clinical study of aldolase A in primary liver cancer. In: Tang Z-Y, Wu M-C, Xia S-S (eds.). Primary liver cancer. Beijing: China Academic Publishers,1989:269–276.
95. Lu HM, Chen Q. 5'-Nucleotide phosphodiesterase V and hepatocellular carcinoma. In: Tang Z-Y, Wu M-C, Xia S-S (eds.). Primary liver cancer. Beijing: China Academic Publishers, 1989:277–284.
96. Lu HM, Chcn Q, Szc PC, ct al. Thc significancc of 5'-nucleotide phosphodiesterase isoenzymes in the diagnosis of liver carcinoma. Int J Cancer 1980;26:21–35.
97. Fujiyama S, Tsude K, Sakai M, et al. 5'-Nucleotide phosphodiesterase isozyme-V in hepatocellular carcinoma and other liver diseases. Hepatogastroenterol 1990;37:469–473.
98. Leandro G, Zizzari S, Piccoli A, Manghisi OG. The serum tissue polypeptide antigen in the detection of hepatocellular carcinoma in cirrhotic patients. Hepatogastroenterol 1990;37:449–451.
99. Giardina MG, Matarazzo M, Varriale A, et al. Serum alpha-1-fucosidase. A useful marker for the diagnosis of hepatocellular carcinoma. Cancer 1992;70:1044–1048.
100. Hutchinson WL, Du M-Q, Johnson PJ, Williams R. Fucosyltransferases: Differential plasma and tissue alterations in hepatocellular carcinoma and chronic liver disease. Hepatology 91;13:683–688.
101. Hutchinson WL, Johnson PJ, Du M-Q, Williams R. Serum and tissue alpha–L–fucosidase activity in the preclinical and clinical stages of hepatocellular carcinoma. Clin Science 1991;81:177–182.

102. Kane SP, Murray–Lyon IM, Paradinas FJ, Johnson PJ, Williams R, Orr AH, Kohn J. Vitamin B12 binding protein as a tumor marker for hepatocellular carcinoma. Gut 1978;19:1105–1109.
103. Paradinas FJ, Melia WM, Wilkinson ML, Portmann B, Johnson PJ, Murray–Lyon IM, Williams R. High serum vitamin B12 binding capacity as a marker of the fibrolamellar variant of hepatocellular carcinoma. Br Med J (Clin Res Ed) 1982;285: 840–842.
104. Collier NA, Weinbren K, Bloom SR, Lee YC, Hodgson HJ, Blumgart LH. Neurotensin secretion by fibrolamellar carcinoma of the liver. Lancet 1984;1:538–540.
105. Patel AH, Harnois DM, Klee GG, LaRusso NF, Gores GJ. The utility of CA19–9 in the diagnoses of cholangiocarcinoma in patients without primary sclerosing cholangitis. Am J Gastroenterol 2000;95:204–207.
106. Nichols JC, Gores GJ, LaRusso NF, Wiesner RH, Nagorney DM, Ritts RE Jr. Diagnostic role of serum CA19–9 for cholangiocarcinoma in patients with primary sclerosing cholangitis. Mayo Clin Proc 1993;68:874–879.
107. Fisher A, Theise ND, Min A, Mor E, Emre S, Pearl A, Schwartz ME, Miller CM, Sheiner PA. CA19–9 does not predict cholaniocarcinoma in patients with primary sclerosing cholangitis undergoing liver transplantation. Liver Transpl Surg 1995;1: 94–98.
108. Torok N, Gores GJ, Bjornsson E, Kilander A, Olsson R. CA19–9 and CEA are unreliable markers for cholangiocarcinoma in patients with primary sclerosing cholangitis. Cholangiocarcinoma. Semin Gastrointest Dis 2001;12:125–132.
109. Poon TC, Johnson PJ. Proteome analysis and its impact on the discovery of serological tumor markers. Clin Chim Acta 2001;313:231–239.
110. Lo YMD, Chui R, Johnson PJ. Circulating nucleic acids in plasma or serum II. Ann NY Acad Sci 2001;945.
111. Jackson PE, Qian GS, Friesen MD, Zhu YR, Lu P, Wang JB, Wu Y, Kensler TW, Vogelstein B, Groopman JD. Specific p53 mutations detected in plasma and tumors of hepatocellular carcinoma patients by electrospray ionization mass spectrometry. Cancer Res 2001;61:33–35.
112. Wong IHN, Lo YMD, Zhang J, Liew CT, Ng MHL, Wong N, Lai PBS, Lau WY, Hjelm NM, Johnson PJ. Detection of aberrant p16 methylation in the plasma and serum of liver cancer patients. Cancer Res 1999;59:71–73.

Chapter 23

Bladder Cancer and Urine Tumor Marker Tests

Herbert A. Fritsche

Each year in the United States alone, nearly 54,000 new cases of bladder cancer are diagnosed and approximately 12,000 people die from this disease (1). The prevalence of bladder cancer in the United States is estimated at almost 600,000 cases. Almost twice as many cases of bladder cancer occur in men as compared to women.

Cigarette smoking is a leading cause of bladder cancer (2). Other risk factors include exposure to industrial carcinogens and chronic infection with *Schistosomiasis haematobium*. Bladder cancer can be detected early and treated effectively. Urine cancer markers can play important roles in the diagnosis and clinical management of this disease.

CLINICAL ASPECTS OF BLADDER CANCER

Table 1 lists some clinical features of bladder cancer. The most common cell type is transitional cell carcinoma (TCC) and the most frequent symptom is intermittent hematuria. Other symptoms are voiding problems, including irritation, increased frequency, urgency, or dysuria. In some cases, urine cytology is positive for tumor cells, but the diagnosis is usually established by cystoscopic evaluation and biopsy. Bladder cancer is staged pathologically and treated on the basis of the degree of tumor invasion into the bladder wall (3). Carcinoma *in situ* (Tis) and the superficial bladder cancers (stages Ta and T1) occur on the inner epithelial lining of the bladder and do not involve the muscle wall of the urinary bladder. Stage Ta tumors are confined to the mucosa, while stage T1 tumors superficially invade the lamina propria. Invasive tumors (stage T2) extend into the muscle and stage T3 tumors invade beyond the muscle into the perivesical fat layer. Metastatic tumors (stage T4) involve local nodes or distant organs.

The cellular morphology of superficial bladder tumors is graded on the degree of differentiation. The grading score consists of well-differentiated (grade 1), moderately differentiated (grade 2), and poorly differentiated (grade 3) tumors. Grading of cell morphology is important for establishing prognosis, as grade 3 tumors are the most aggressive and most likely to become invasive.

Noninvasive (superficial) bladder tumors are generally treated by transurethal resection of bladder (TURB) with or without intravesical treatments with Bacille Calmette-Guérin (BCG) immunotherapy or intravesical chemotherapy. Invasive tumors are usually treated by cystectomy, or with bladder-sparing therapies that consist of chemotherapy and radiation. Patients who have metastatic tumors require high-dose systemic chemotherapy with multiple anti-cancer agents (4).

Most bladder cancer patients (75%) are diagnosed with superficial tumors. Even though superficial tumors can be completely resected, about two-thirds of these patients will experience tumor recurrence within five years, and almost 90% will have a recurrence of their disease by 15 years. With intensive medical surveillance, the five-year survival rates for these patients ranges from 95% to 75% for Ta and T1 tumors, respectively. However, almost 25% of patients with these noninvasive tumors will eventually develop invasive disease. The five-year survival rate decreases with tumor invasiveness and the presence of metastasis. Patients with stage T2 tumors have a five-year survival rate of 60%, but only 35% of patients with stage T3 tumors and 10% of patients with stage T4 metastatic tumors will live for five years.

Thus, lifelong surveillance is required for bladder cancer patients who are initially diagnosed with noninvasive disease.

Table 1 Features of bladder cancer

• Cell Types:	Transitional, adenocarcinoma, squamous, and sarcoma
• Symptoms:	Hematuria (80–85%) and voiding problems (15–20%)
• Classes:	➢ Superficial (Stages Tis, Ta, T1) ➢ Invasive (Stages T2, T3, T4)
• Superficial Tumors:	➢ Treated locally by resection with intravesical treatment (Bacille Calmette-Guérin or chemotherapy) ➢ High risk of recurrence: 50–70% in 5 years ➢ Lifelong surveillance is required, which consists of periodic cystoscopy and cytology
• Invasive Tumors:	➢ Treated by cystectomy
• Metastatic Tumors:	➢ Treated with systemic chemotherapy

Current patient monitoring protocols generally consist of regularly scheduled cystoscopic evaluations, usually along with urine cytology, performed every three months during the first two years of follow-up, twice a year during years three and four, and annually thereafter, until disease recurrence is documented. When recurrent tumor is found, the surveillance protocol is repeated, starting again with year-one quarterly follow-up visits. The current surveillance protocols for detecting recurrent bladder cancer are costly and associated with some patient morbidity. This has led some urologists to consider using a less intensive monitoring protocol by reducing the frequency of patient follow-up visits, except for those patients who are at high risk for recurrence of their disease (5). However, the prognostic factors that have been proposed for defining high risk of recurrence, such as the tumor grade, number of lesions at diagnosis, and post-surgical recurrence detected at three months, are not generally accepted into routine clinical practice.

ROLE OF URINE TUMOR MARKERS IN DETECTING RECURRENT DISEASE

Various clinical applications have been proposed for bladder tumor markers. These include:

- serial testing for the earlier detection of recurrences,
- complementary testing to urine cytology to improve the detection rate,
- providing a less expensive and more objective alternative to the urine cytology test, and
- directing the cystoscopic evaluation in patient follow-up.

If cystoscopic evaluations are to be performed on the basis of a tumor marker test, the marker must have high sensitivity for the poorly differentiated (high-grade) noninvasive lesions. A false-negative test result will result in missing this high-risk lesion, which could become invasive and lead to a poor outcome for the patient. False-positive test results are not as critical as false-negative results because the most harm a false-positive tumor marker test result could do would be to initiate a cystoscopic exam, which would have been performed anyway under the current practice of regularly scheduled evaluations.

Until these highly sensitive and specific markers are identified, the objective of current bladder tumor markers is to complement cystoscopy and urine cytology in the early detection of tumor recurrence. Many new urine markers for bladder cancer have been reported and most of these appear to have value for this purpose.

BTA-STAT AND BTA-TRAK TESTS FOR COMPLEMENT FACTOR H AND RELATED PROTEINS

The BTA-Stat test (Polymedco; Cortlandt Manor, NY) detects complement factor H (CFH) or related proteins (CFH-rp) in urine (6). Factor H, a 155-kDa protein, has a central role in regulating the alternate pathway of complement activation to prevent complement-mediated damage to healthy cells. At least four other factor H-related proteins have been identified as products of a cluster of genes on chromosome 1 called the regulators of complement activation (RCA) locus, and although some of these proteins possess complement regulatory activity, others do not (7).

The production of CFH has been demonstrated for a variety of bladder cancer cell lines and has been suggested as a mechanism for the escape of tumor cells from immune surveillance. The BTA-Stat test provides semi-quantitative detection of CFH and the CFH-rp antigens using a double monoclonal antibody, immunochromatographic point-of-care device. The manufacturer reports no interference due to the presence of erythrocytes, leukocytes, hemoglobin, albumin, immunoglobulin G, uric acid, ascorbic acid, or a variety of anti-cancer drugs and antibiotics. False-positive test results are reported to occur in some patients after trauma, infection of the bladder or urinary tract, nephritis, or urinary calculi. The BTA-Stat test is reported to have high sensitivity for both superficial (Tis, Ta, T1) and invasive (T2–T4) tumors. The initial evaluation suggested that 50–60% of Tis and Ta tumors and 89% of T1 tumors could be detected by the BTA-Stat test (8). Clinical specificity was 72% for patients with non-cancerous genitourinary disease.

The BTA-Trak test is a quantitative enzyme immunoassay version of the BTA-Stat test. The manufacturer reports a sensitivity of 67% (Tis), 59% (Ta), 92% (T1), and 89% (T2–T4) for bladder cancer using a cut-off value of 14.0 U/mL. Specificities of 50–60% were observed in benign renal disease, urinary tract infections, and sexually transmitted diseases, and 80–90% for various other genitourinary diseases. Confirmatory reports have validated the high sensitivity of the BTA-Trak test in patients with recurrent disease (9,10). However, the test has not been generally accepted for patient surveillance, presumably due to its high false-positive rate (10,11).

Nuclear Matrix Protein 22

The nuclear matrix protein 22 (NMP22) test (Matritech; Newton, MA) is a double monoclonal antibody test for quantitative measurement of the nuclear mitotic apparatus (MUMA) protein. This component of the nuclear matrix that is overexpressed by bladder cancer is released into the urine. NMP22 is not stable in urine and the use of a protein preservative is recommended. Clinical trial data showed that the NMP22 test, when performed 6–40 days post-surgery, predicted the presence of recurrent disease at the first cystoscopic follow-up visit in 71% (24/34) of the patients (12). Of the subjects who had negative NMP22 test values, 86% (61/71) had no clinical evidence of disease at the first follow-up cystoscopy.

Subsequently, Miyanaga (13) compared the urine NMP22 test with voided urine cytology in subjects who had TCC of the bladder. In that study, NMP22 clearly performed better than voided urine cytology for detecting bladder cancer. However, they reported a 35% false-positive rate for NMP22. Rodriguez-Villanueva et al. (14) reported a similar experience with the NMP22 test. In a study of 205 patients, NMP22 values were determined on the day of or within 10 days before cystoscopic evaluation. There were 65 positive cystoscopies of recurrent bladder cancer confirmed by biopsy and the NMP22 test was abnormal in 45/65, or 63%. Most of the false-negatives (15/24) occurred in patients who had stage Ta tumors. Of the 181 negative cystoscopies, the NMP22 test was negative in 131 (specificity = 72%).

Confirmatory results were reported by Stampfer et al. in a multi-center study in which 171 patients had 274 cystoscopies (15). The sensitivity for all stages of disease was 68% (45/66) and the specificity was 80% (166/208). The sensitivity for non-invasive Ta, T1, and Tis disease stages was 61%, 100%, and 70%, respectively. The noninvasive tumors were subgrouped on the basis of risk for recurrence. "Low-risk" tumors were defined as stage Ta grades 1 and 2, and high-risk tumors were defined as stage Ta grade 3 and stage T1. For 39 low-risk tumors, 59% had abnormal NMP22 values, while 90% of the high-risk tumors had elevated NMP22 values. Urine cytology results were available for 26/39 low-risk subjects and 5/11 high-risk patients. Although the sensitivities for high-risk tumors were similar (60% for NMP22 and 80% for voided urine cytology), the sensitivity of NMP22 for low-risk tumors was almost twice that of voided urine cytology (54% vs. 23%). As was demonstrated in previous reports, NMP22 had greater sensitivity than voided urine cytology for detecting recurrent bladder cancer. While other reports have substantiated the high sensitivity of NMP22, the false-positive rate has limited its application to routine patient care (16).

Immunocyt

The Immunocyt test (Diagno-Cure Inc.; Sainte-Foy, Quebec, Canada) detects bladder cancer markers present on exfoliated cells using a cocktail of fluorescent antibodies (19A211, M344, and LDQ10). The monoclonal antibody 19A211 detects high molecular weight carcinoembryonic antigen, while M344 and LDQ10 detect a cancer-related mucin (17). One report has shown the test to have a sensitivity of 86% and specificity of 79% for detecting bladder cancer. The detection rate for Ta, T1, T2–T4, and Tis tumors was 86, 85, 83, and 100%, respectively. A limitation of the Immunocyt test is that it does require the presence of exfoliated cells. Immunocyt has been evaluated in several recent reports. In each case, the sensitivity was lower than previously reported, on the order of 50%. In addition, the test was subject to inter-observer variation and other technical limitations (18,19).

Cytokeratins (CK)

Cytokeratins are intermediate filament proteins that are characteristic of epithelial cells. Overexpression of certain cytokeratins occurs in transitional cell carcinoma of the bladder (20), and various urine CK assays have been developed. The tissue polypeptide antigen (TPA) test (Sangtec Medical; Sweden) was one of the first. It employs polyclonal antisera for detection of CK 8, 18, and 19. While the overall sensitivity is reported to be 80%, a false positive rate of 30–40% has limited its use in routine patient care (21). Subsequently, a tissue polypeptide specific (TPS) test (IDL Biotech; Sweden) was developed employing monoclonal antibodies for detecting CK 8 and 18 (22).

Another version, called the urinary bladder cancer (UBC) test, also detects CK 8 and 18. A preliminary report suggests a sensitivity of 65% and specificity of 92% for this test, but more confirmatory data is required (21,23).

Telomerase

Telomeres are regions located at the ends of human chromosomes. These regions are composed of many identical short repetitive sequences of TTAGGG. Their function is to stabilize and protect chromosomes (34,35). With each cell cycle, the ends of the telomeres shorten, until a critical length is reached after which cell division leads to breakdown of the telomere. Telomerase is a ribonucleoprotein enzyme that adds telomere repeats to maintain telomere length. Telomerase is inactivated in normal human epithelial tissue, but is reactivated in neoplasia (24). Telomerase has two major components, an RNA template and an enzymatic subunit. For more information, see Chapter 55.

The Telomeric Repeat Amplification Protocol (TRAP) assay (Geron; San Francisco, CA) measures enzymatic activity of telomerase. Telomeric repeats are synthesized *in vitro*, amplified by polymerase chain reaction (PCR), and the products are made visible by various methods (24). In a tissue study of bladder tumors, 86% (48/56) were shown to be telomerase-positive, but no activity was detected in non-neoplastic bladder tissue. The same study evaluated exfoliated cells in 109 urine samples from urological patients, 26 of which had bladder cancer. They reported 62% sensitivity and 96% specificity for telomerase activity in exfoliated urothelial cells (25). Advances in the measurement of telomerase include reverse transcriptase-PCR (RT-PCR) assays for the telomerase RNA (hTR) and messenger for telomerase reverse transcriptase (hTERT). These assays have demonstrated a sensitivity of 83% for hTR and 80% for hTERT (26,27). These results are encouraging for the use of telomerase as a marker for bladder cancer, but its measurement is limited to the presence of exfoliated cells.

BLCA-4

A bladder-cancer-specific nuclear matrix protein (BLCA-4) has been reported by Getzenberg et al (28). The proteins were identified on two-dimensional gels and sequenced, and antibodies were raised to synthetic peptides corresponding to those sequences. Preliminary immunoassay data suggest that the BLCA-4 protein is present in the urine of 53 of 54 bladder cancer patients (n = 4, for stage Tis; n = 25 for stages Ta-T1; n = 13, stages T2-T3; and n = 6, stage T4). All values for 51 healthy control subjects were below the upper limit of normal. However, 38 of 202 spinal cord-injured patients had elevated values. Superficial tumors were found in only 1 of these 38 cases (29). Since spinal cord injury patients are at high risk for developing bladder cancer, these subjects will require additional follow-up to assess the diagnostic role of BLCA-4. Clinical studies are under way to confirm the encouraging preliminary data on the utility of BLCA-4 in bladder cancer.

Survivin

The protein survivin is an inhibitor of apoptosis that is associated with the mitotic spindle. The expression of survivin is low in normal adult tissues but high in cancer tissues and transformed cell lines (31). Smith et al. have developed a polyclonal based, semi-quantitative immunoassay to assess the role of survivin as a urine marker for bladder cancer. The protein was detected in all of 46 new and recurrent cases of bladder cancer, but it was not detected in 17 healthy subjects. Survivin was present in 3 of 35 patients who had been previously treated for bladder cancer but who had negative cystoscopic evaluations (31). Additional studies are underway to establish the clinical value of this new marker.

Microsatellite Detection

Repetitive sequences of DNA containing from one to four base pairs each are contained throughout the genome and can undergo mutational changes. These mutations are associated with neoplasia, and can serve as genetic markers for cancer. The most common genetic change seen in bladder cancer is loss of heterogeneity (LOH) in chromosome 9. Sixty to 70 percent of bladder neoplasms show LOH in either the long or the short arm of chromosome 9, indicating that loss of suppressor genes may be the early initiating event in bladder carcinogenesis (32,33).

Using 20 microsatellite DNA markers, Mao et al. (34) detected 95% of patients with bladder cancer. Steiner et al. tested serial urine samples collected from 21 patients who had been treated for bladder cancer using two microsatellite markers. Recurrent lesions were detected in 10 of 11 patients who had recurrent disease. Both of the studies suggest that microsatellite analysis of exfoliated cells is potentially useful for the detection of bladder cancer.

Hyaluronic Acid (HA) and Hyaluronidase

Hyaluronic acid, the glycosaminoglycan ligand for CD44, has the ability to promote tumor cell adhesion, migration, and angiogenesis. Hyaluronidase degrades HA into angiogenically active fragments. Lokeshwar et al. (36) have demonstrated that the HA test had a sensitivity of 83% and specificity of 90% for detecting bladder cancer. Also, hyaluronidase was found to be from five to eight times elevated in the urine of patients with grade 2 and 3 tumors compared to the urine of normal individuals. Urinary hyaluronidase measurement has demonstrated a sensitivity of 100% and a specificity of 89% for detection of these high-grade bladder tumors in 139 patients (37). Both of these analytes deserve more study as urine markers for bladder cancer.

ROLE OF URINE MARKERS IN CANCER SCREENING

Almost all cases of bladder cancer are found during the work-up of patients who present with hematuria (38). But most cases of hematuria are not caused by bladder cancer. Urologic disease can be found in only 3–30% of various types of subjects who present with hematuria, and bladder cancer is detected in less than one-half of those patients (39–41).

The work-up of patients with hematuria is costly and usually requires cytology, cystoscopy, intravenous urography, or computed tomography (42). Thus, tumor markers could be useful for cancer screening in this high-risk group. Zippe et al. reported on the value of the urine NMP22 test in the evaluation of 330 patients with hematuria (43). The NMP22 test, when used with a cut-off value of 10.0 U/mL, detected all 18 cases of bladder cancer with only 45 false-positives (sensitivity = 100%, specificity = 85%). Thus in this study, 267 unnecessary cytoscopies could have been avoided if cytoscopy would have been directed by the NMP22 test.

In a clinical trial submitted to the Food and Drug Administration for pre-market approval (PMA), the NMP22 test was elevated in 69.6% of 56 bladder cancer patients that were detected in a high-risk group. The specificity was 67.7% (44). The NMP22 has been cleared by the FDA for use as a diagnostic aid for bladder cancer in individuals with risk factors or who have symptoms of bladder cancer. It is highly likely that urine markers may also have value for cancer detection in subjects who present with hematuria.

ROLE OF TISSUE MARKERS FOR PROGNOSIS

Considerable research effort continues to be directed to the identification of markers that would predict the aggressive nature of superficial bladder tumors. Such information could lead to more effective surveillance protocols and permit more aggressive treatments for those patients whose tumors will progress to invasive or metastatic disease (5). Stein et al. have performed an exhaustive review of a variety of biological markers reported to have prognostic value (45). More recently, p53 and other cell cycle control genes (46,47), as well as chorionic gonadotropin-beta gene transcripts, (48) have been reported to have prognostic value. However, at the present time, none of these markers has yet been proven for use in routine patient care.

SUMMARY

Many reports have established the value of urine tumor marker tests for the early detection of recurrent bladder tumors. These urine-based tests cannot replace cystoscopy and cytology in the management of bladder cancer patients. However, they can be used in a complementary manner to permit more effective utilization of clinical procedures, and thus reduce the cost of patient surveillance.

One major criticism of the urine-based tests, when they are used for assessing patients who present with hematuria or for patient surveillance, is the high false-positive rate. One report has evaluated the apparent false-positive rate for the BTA-Stat test. In 55 subjects who had a positive BTA-Stat test but a negative cystosocopy, additional work-up found nine cases of recurrence that cystoscopic evaluation missed. The remaining false-positives were attributed to urine infections, ongoing intravesical treatments, and unknown causes (49). Thus, better definition of the disease conditions that can produce a false-positive test value can lead to more effective use of the test for cancer detection.

Another criticism of the urine markers is the low sensitivity for detecting disease. However, in most studies, when these tests are used along with cytology and cytoscopy, there is a significant improvement in the detection rate for bladder cancer. It must also be recognized that voided urine cytology has limitations for detecting carcinoma *in situ* (Tis) and the low-grade bladder tumors (50). It appears that urine markers can assist in the early detection of recurrence in both of these patient groups. Finally, the stability of tumor marker analytes must be better defined to avoid apparent false-negative test values.

The overall effectiveness of urine markers for patient surveillance could also be improved by adjusting the intensity of the surveillance protocol on the basis of risk of recurrence (5). Patients with superficial lesions of low grade (Ta, grade 1, and 2) are of lower risk for recurrence than those with Ta grade 3 and T1 tumors, and these patients may need less intensive follow-up (15). The availability of many new markers for bladder cancer suggests the possibility of the combined use of markers either measured simultaneously or sequentially can further improve the cancer detection rate. The objective of such panel testing should be to improve both the sensitivity and the specificity for bladder cancer detection. Most certainly, prospective clinical trials are necessary to prove their clinical value before these tests can be implemented in routine patient care (51).

REFERENCES

1. Greenlee R, Hill-Harmon M, Murray T, Thun M. Cancer statistics 2001. CA Cancer J Clin 2001;51:15–36.
2. Vineis P, Esteve J, Hartge, et al. Effects of timing and type of tobacco in cigarette induced bladder cancer. Cancer Res 1998;48:3849–3852.
3. Lamm D, Torti F. Bladder cancer 1996. CA Cancer J Clin 1996;49:93–112.
4. Droller M. Bladder cancer—state of the art care. CA Cancer J Clin 1998;48:269–284.
5. Parmar M, Freedman L, Hargreave T, Tolley D. Prognostic factors for recurrence and follow-up policies in the treatment of superficial bladder cancer. Report from the British Medical Research Council Subgroups on Superficial Bladder Cancer. J Urol 1989;142:284–288.
6. Kinders R, Jones T, Root R, et al. Human bladder tumor antigen is a member of the RCA (regulators of complement activation) gene family. J Urol 1997;157:28.
7. Zipfel P, Skerka C: Complement factor H and related proteins: an expanding family of complement regulatory proteins. Immunol Today 1994;15:121–126.
8. Sarosdy M, Hudson M, Ellis W, et al. Improved detection of recurrent bladder cancer using the Bard BTA-Stat test. Urology 1997;50:349–353.
9. Thomas L, Leyh H, Murberger M, et al. Multi-center trial of the Quantitative BTA-Trak Assay in the detection of bladder cancer. Clin Chem 1999;45:472–477.
10. Mattioli S, Seregnis E, Caperna L. BTA Trak combined with urinary cytology is a reliable urinary indicator of recurrent transitional cell carcinoma of the bladder. Int J Biol Markers 2000;15:219–25.
11. Heicappall R, Weetig I, Schostak M, et al. Quantitative detection of human complement factor H-related protein in transitional cell carcinoma of the urinary bladder. Eur Urol 1999;35:81–87.
12. Soloway MS, Briggman J, Carpinito GA, et al. Use of a new tumor marker, urinary NMP22, in the detection of occult or rapidly recurring transitional cell carcinoma of the urinary tract following surgical treatment. J Urol 1996;156:363–367.
13. Miyanaga N, Akaza H, Ishikawa S, et al. Clinical evaluation of nuclear matrix protein 22 (NMP22) in urine as a novel marker for urothelial cancer. Eur Urol 1997;31:163–168.
14. Rodriguez-Villanueva J, Dinney C, Grossman H, Fritsche H. Evaluation of the NMP22 immunoassay in the detection of transitional cell carcinoma of the urinary tract. J Urol 1997;157:336.
15. Stampfer D, Carpinito G, Rodriguez-Villanueva J, et al. Evaluation of NMP22 in the detection of transitional cell carcinoma of the bladder. J Urol 1998;159:394–398.
16. Sharma S, Zippe L, Pondrangi L, et al. Exclusion criteria enhance the specificity and positive productive value of NMP22 and BTA Stat. J Urol 1999;162:53–157.
17. Mian C, Pycha A, Wiener H, et al. Immunocyt—a new tool for detecting transitional cell cancer of the urinary tract. J Urol 1999;161:1486–1489.
18. Bunting P, Fleshner N, Kapuesta L. Detection of bladder cancer via noninvasive methods: a direct comparison of NMP-22 and Immunocyt tests. J Urol 2000;163:592–597.
19. Vriesema J, Atsma F, Kiemeney L, et al. Diagnostic efficacy of the Immunocyt test to detect superficial bladder cancer recurrence. Urol 2001;58:367–371.
20. Southgate J, Harden P, Trejdosiewicz L. Cytokeratin expression patterns in normal and malignant urotheluim. Histol Histopath 1999;14:657–664.
21. Sanchez-Carbayo M, Herrero E, Mezias J, et al. Comparative sensitivity of urinary CYFRA 21-1, urinary bladder cancer antigen, tissue polypeptide antigen and NMP22 to detect bladder cancer. J Urol 1999;162:1951–1956.
22. Sanchez-Carbayo M, Urritia M, Silva J, et al. Urinary tissue polypeptide antigen for the diagnosis of bladder cancer. Urology 2000;55:526–532.
23. Miam C, Lodde M, Haitel A, et al. Comparison of the UBC-ELISA test and the NMP22 test for the detection of urothelial cell carcinoma of the bladder. Urology 2000;55:223–226.
24. Kim N, Piatyszek M, Prowse K, et al. Specific association of human telomerase activity with immortal cells and cancer. Science 1994;266:2011–2015.
25. Yoshida K, Sugino T, Tahara H, et al. Telomerase activity in bladder carcinoma and its implication for noninvasive diagnosis by detection of exfoliated cancer cells in urine. Cancer 1997;79:362–369.
26. Müller M, Krause H, Heicappell R, et al. Comparison of human telomerase RNA and telomerase activity in urine for diagnosis of bladder cancer. Clin Cancer Res 1998;4:1949–1954.
27. de Koh J, Ruers T, van Muijen G. Real-time quantification of human telomerase reverse transcriptase mRNA in tumors and healthy tissues. Clin Chem 2000;46:313–318.
28. Konety B, Nguyen T, Dhur R, et al. Detection of bladder cancer using a novel matrix protein, BLCA-4. Clin Cancer Res 2000;6:2618–2625.
29. Konety B, Nguyen T, Brenes G, et al. Clinical usefulness of the novel marker BLCA-4 for the detection of bladder cancer. J Urol 2000;164:634–639.

30. Ambrosini G, Adida D, Altieri D. A novel anti-apoptosis gene, survivin, expressed in cancer and lymphoma. Nature Med 1997;3: 917–921.
31. Smith S, Wheeler M, Plescia J, et al. Urine detection of survivin and diagnosis of bladder cancer. JAMA 2001;285:324–328.
32. Simoneau M, Aboulkassim TO, Rue HL, et al. Four tumor suppressor loci on chromosome 9q in the bladder cancer: evidence for two novel candidate regions at 9q22.3 and 9q31. Oncogene 1999;18:157–163.
33. Czerniak B, Chaturvedi V, Li L, et al. Superimposed histologic and genetic mapping of chromosome 9 in progression of human urinary bladder neoplasia: implications for a genetic model of multi-step urothelial carcinogenesis and early detection of urinary bladder cancer. Oncogene 1999;18:1185–1196.
34. Mao L, Schoenberg MP, Scicchitano M, Erozan YS, Merlo A, Schwab D, et al. Molecular detection of primary bladder cancer by microsatellite analysis. Science 1996;271:659–662.
35. Steiner G, Schoenberg MP, Linn JF, et al. Detection of bladder cancer recurrence by microsatellite analysis of urine. Nature Med 1997;3:621–624.
36. Lokeshwar V, Obek C, Pham H. Urinary hyaluronic acid and hyaluronidase hyaluronidase: markers for bladder cancer detection and evaluation of grade. J Urol 2000;163:348–356.
37. Pham H, Block N, Lokeshwar V: Tumor derived hyalouronidase. A diagnostic urine marker for high-grade bladder cancer. Cancer Res 1997;57:778–783.
38. Varkarakis M, Gaeta J, Moore R, et al. Superficial bladder tumor. Aspects of clinical progression. Urology 1990;32:838–845.
39. Grossfield G, Litwin M, Wolf S, et al. Evaluation of asymptomatic microscopic hematuria in adults. The American Urological Association Best Practice Policy—Part I: Definition detection, prevalence and etiology. Urology 2001;57:599–603.
40. Khadra M, Pickard R, Charlton M et al. A prospective analysis of 1930 patients with hematuria to evaluate current diagnostic practice. J Urol 2000;163:524–527.
41. Mariani J. Re: a prospective analysis of 1930 patients with hematuria to evaluate current diagnostic practice (Letter to the Editor). J Urol 2001;165:545–546.
42. Grossfield G, Litwin M, Wolf S, et al. Evaluation of asymptomatic microscopic hematuria in adults: The American Urological Association best preventive policy—Part II. Patient evaluation, cytology, voided markers, imaging, cytoscopy, nephrology evaluation, and follow-up. Urology 2001;57: 604–610.
43. Zippe C, Pandrangi L, Agarwal A. NMP22 is a sensitive, cost-effective test in patients at risk for bladder cancer. J Urol 1999; 161:62–65.
44. Matritech, Inc. PMA #940035. Submitted to the Food and Drug Administration, 1999.
45. Stein J, Grossfield C, Ginsberg D, et al. Prognostic markers in bladder cancer. A contemporary review of the literature. J Urol 1998;160:645–659.
46. Zlotta A, Schulman C. Biological markers in superficial bladder tumors and their prognostic significance. Urol Clinics N Amer 2000;27:179–189.
47. Grossman H, Libert M, Antelo M. p53 and RB expression predict progression in T1 bladder cancer. Clin Cancer Res 1998;4: 829–834.
48. Lazar V, Diez S, Laurent A. Expression of human chronic gonadotrophin B. Sub-unit genes in superficial and invasive bladder carcinomas. Cancer Res 1995;55:3735–3738.
49. Raitanen M, Kaasinen E, Lukkarinen O, et al. Analysis of false positive BTA-stat test results in patients followed up for bladder cancer. J Urol 2001;57:680–684.
50. Malik S, Murphy W. Monitoring patients for bladder neoplasms: what can be expected of urinary cytology consultations in clinical practice. Urology 1999;54:64–70.
51. Lokeshwar V, Soloway M. Current bladder tumor tests: does their projected utility fulfill clinical necessity? J Urol 2001;165: 1067–1077.

Chapter 24

Lung Cancer

Paul M. Schneider, Ralf Metzger, Jan Brabender, Sebastian Boehm,
Thomas Luebke, Kourosh Zarghooni, Klaus Prenzel, Sylke Schneider,
Peter H. Collet, and Arnulf H. Hoelscher

Lung cancer is the leading cause of cancer-related deaths in men and women in the western hemisphere. Survival from lung cancer depends mainly on cell type and stage of disease at presentation according to the international tumor-node-metastasis (TNM) classification system. The World Health Organization histologic classification of lung cancer describes two major entities dependent on cell-type: small-cell and non-small cell lung cancer (SCLC and NSCLC, respectively).

SCLC is a very aggressive disease with a poor clinical outcome and represents approximately 20% of lung cancer cases. Without treatment, median length of survival is one to three months. It is, however, responsive to both chemotherapy and radiotherapy. Combination chemotherapy has produced overall response rates on the order of 80%, with limited disease (LD) patients surviving a median of 14–16 months and extensive disease (ED) patients 8–11 months (1).

NSCLC is comprised of three major histological subtypes: squamous cell carcinoma (SCC), adenocarcinoma (AC), and large cell carcinoma (LC), which together represent approximately 75% of all lung cancer cases. Radical surgery with complete resection of the tumor offers the only chance for cure in patients with NSCLC and survival probabilities are mainly dependent on tumor stage (2). With acceptable morbidity and mortality rates, surgical resections remain the mainstay of therapy in stages I and II. In experienced centers, five-year survival rates are 70–75% for stage I, 40% for stage II, and 20% for selected patients with locally advanced stage III disease (3). Unfortunately, 70% of patients with NSCLC present with locally advanced (stage IIIA/B) or metastatic disease (stage IV), stages of progression that are not amenable to surgical therapy. Neoadjuvant treatment modalities are experimental therapies of choice for locally advanced NSCLC in stage IIIA/B but are currently not considered established standard therapies and should therefore be performed within controlled clinical trials. For the majority of patients with NSCLC, palliative treatment with different chemotherapy, radiation, or combined radiochemotherapy modalities, as well as best supportive care, are applied.

Tumor markers in lung cancer can serve as very valuable tools however, and apart from their inherent scientific interest, clinical application of such markers should significantly contribute to diagnosis or treatment. For reasons outlined above, the currently relevant markers are discussed separately for the two major forms of lung cancer, SCLC and NSCLC. In addition, the term "tumor marker" is broadly defined and includes not only substances measurable in the blood of patients (serum markers), but also abnormal parameters identified in lung tumors or their metastases, such as molecular markers, response prediction markers in neoadjuvant or adjuvant settings, and bone marrow or lymph node micrometastases.

SERUM MARKERS IN LUNG CANCER

In this section we discuss multiple serum markers for NSCLC and SCLC in terms of clinical application for diagnosis and treatment, assay sensitivities, and other issues. The most relevant information is briefly summarized in Table 1.

Serum Markers in NSCLC

Squamous cell carcinoma antigen (SCC-Ag). SCC-Ag is a glycoprotein secreted by NSCLC with a molecular weight (MW) of approximately 48 kDa. Normal serum levels are below 3.0 ng/mL in 95% of healthy controls. Elevated SCC levels occur in certain types of NSCLS, and also occur in association with liver or renal insufficiency. Smoking does not influence serum concentrations of SCC-Ag.

In squamous cell carcinoma, 35% of the patients have elevated SCC-Ag levels; among patients with non-squamous histology the frequency drops to 17%. Unlike carcinoembryonic antigen (CEA) or lactate dehydrogenase (LDH), SCC-Ag is not a marker for disease dissemination. The SCC-Ag serum level has a moderate diagnostic role in NSCLC. Both the pre-operative SCC-Ag level and its post-operative decrease have prognostic significance inferior to stage of disease (4,5).

Table 1 Serological tumor markers in lung cancer

Marker	Normal range	Sensitivity	Specificity	Prognostic value		Diagnostic value		Disease monitoring (recurrent disease)	
				SCLC	NSCLC	SCLC	NSCLC	SCLC	NSCLC
NSE[a]	10–25 ng/mL	0.55–0.9	0.85–0.97	++	+	++	−	++	
CYFRA 21-1[b]	2.1–3.6 ng/mL	0.19–0.68	0.89–0.96	++	++	+	++	+	++
CEA[c]	0–10 ng/mL	0.18–0.55	0.54	+	+	−	+	−	+
LDH[d]	120–240 U/L			+	−	+	−	+	−
ProGRP[e]	>100 pg/mL					+	−	+	−
TPA[f]	>100 U/L			+	+	+	+	+	+
SCC[g]	3.0 ng/mL			−	+	−	+	−	+

[a] False-positive conditions: metastatic neuroblastoma, brain tumor, prostatic carcinoma, hypernephroma, medullary thyroid carcinoma, malignant hematologic diseases, seminoma, apudoma, melanoma, pheochromocytoma, carcinoid tumor, bronchopneumonia, hepatic lesions, pulmonary fibrosis, hemolytic serum, long storage time, hemodialysis.

[b] False-positive conditions: hepatic metastasis, gynecological cancers [cervical carcinoma of the uterus (Se=37%), ovarian carcinoma (Se=36%)], bladder carcinoma, acute inflammatory diseases of the lung, trauma of cytokeratin-rich tissue, pancreatitis, gastrointestinal diseases, renal insufficiency, benign liver lesions, benign gynecological lesions, epidermoid.

[c] False-positive conditions: medullary thyroid cancer, gastrointestinal neoplasms, gynecological cancers, breast cancer, pheochromocytoma, hepatic lesions, nicotine abuse, pancreatitis, colitis ulcerosa, Morbus Crohn, inflammatory diseases of the lung, gastrointestinal ulcer, tuberculosis, autoimmune diseases, pulmonary emphysema, possibly renal insufficiency.

[d] False-positive conditions: myocarcial infarction, myocarditis, myopathy, congestion of liver, hepatitis, mononucleosis, toxic liver lesions, cholepathia, neoplasms, pulmonary infarction, pernicious anemia, hemolytic anemia.

[e] False-positive conditions: renal dysfunction, carcinoid syndrome.

[f] False-positive conditions: hepatitis, benign lung disease, liver cirrhosis, cholecystitis.

[g] False-positive conditions: liver and renal insufficiency, cervix carcinoma, larynx carcinoma, pharynx carcinoma.

Serum anti-p53 antibodies. Winter et al. have reported that p53-specific autoantibodies in the serum of NSCLC patients appeared to be dependent on the type of p53 mutation (6). Twenty-one percent of NSCLC patients contained autoantibodies against p53 and a positive titer for these autoantibodies was significantly correlated with positive immunohistochemical staining for p53. The serum p53 autoantibodies were not associated statistically with any clinical feature except for histological type. Serum p53 autoantibodies may be a clinical parameter for the presence of p53 mutations and p53 overexpression in NSCLC patients. The assay used had a sensitivity of 40% and a specificity of 92% (7) (see also Chapter 10).

While p53 antibodies are detected in the sera of patients with different kinds of cancer, including lung cancer, the presence of p53 antibodies in the serum of healthy subjects is extremely rare. In a recent study, serum antibodies were detectable in 35/109 patients (32.1%) with lung cancer. About 17/57 (29.8%) of NSCLC patients and 18/52 (34.6%) of those with SCLC were p53 autoantibody-positive. CEA, tissue polypeptide antigen(TPA), CYFRA 21-1, and neuron-specific enolase (NSE) sensitivity in lung cancer patients was 50.5%, 58.7%, 42.2%, and 35.8%, respectively. The lower sensitivity of serum p53 autoantibodies is connected with the higher specificity and diagnostic accuracy (100% and 69%, respectively). Therefore serum p53 autoantibody assessment is a simple and low-cost assay with a good specificity and diagnostic accuracy that can be used in lung cancer patients, at least in association with established tumor markers (8).

Cytokeratin 19 (CK 19) fragment and CYFRA 21-1. Cytokeratin 19 is a member of the intermediate filament group of proteins. It is found in the cytoplasm of epithelial tumor cells, including lung cancers. It has a molecular weight of 40 kDa and is an acid-type cytoplasmic protein. Upon cell death, it is released into the serum in the form of soluble fragments. CYFRA 21-1 is a CK 19 fragment that can be measured by enzyme-linked immunosorbent assay (ELISA). The CYFRA 21-1 half-life is reported to be 12 hours and a serum level up to 1.8 ng/mL is found in healthy volunteers regardless of age, gender, and smoking habits. Reasons for elevated serum CYFRA 21-1 levels are renal insufficiency, liver cirrhosis, trauma of cytokeratin-rich tissues, and benign pulmonary disease such as fibrosis, tuberculosis, and chronic obstructive pulmonary disease (COPD). These factors lead to reference values between 2.1 and 3.6 ng/mL with a 95% confidence interval (9).

CYFRA 21-1 is suggested to be a valuable marker in patients with NSCLC. CYFRA 21-1 levels do not differ between smoking and nonsmoking subjects and are significantly elevated in lung cancer cases, irrespective of cell type. CYFRA 21-1 is significantly elevated in squamous cell and adenocarcinoma varieties with the most prominent elevation in the squamous cell type. In lung cancer the specificity and sensitivity of CYFRA 21-1 are 92.3% and 52.2%, respectively. Sensitivity is 65.5% for all NSCLC, with 70.5% for squamous cell and 45.5% for adenocarcinoma varieties; the highest sensitivity rates were found in stage IIIA/IIIB (87.5%) and IV (75%) of squamous lung cancer. The CYFRA 21-1 level was significantly decreased after treatment in NSCLC patients.

The diagnostic value of CYFRA 21-1 in NSCLC has been established, with a sensitivity of 54% and a specificity of 96%

at a cut-off value of 3.3 ng/mL. In addition to their correlation with the presence of metastases (p = 0.017), CYFRA 21-1 (p = 0.017) and CA125 (p=0.03) were related to outcome. The presence of elevated levels of CYFRA 21-1 at any time during the disease course as selected by multivariate analysis was an additional predictor of poor survival (10).

CYFRA 21-1 was found to be the leading serum tumor marker in NSCLC due to its high specificity and sensitivity. CYFRA 21-1 has a diagnostic value in the detection of recurrent disease as well. Twenty-two out of 86 patients with NSCLC developed local recurrence or distant metastases following surgical resections. A CYFRA 21-1 increase preceded the detection of recurrence by two to 15 months in eight of 22 patients. CYFRA 21-1 therefore possesses a high specificity and sensitivity in the detection of recurrent disease in NSCLC patients.

The prognostic information given by a high CYFRA 21-1 level is independent of other well-known variables such as performance status and disease stage and is perennial throughout extended follow-up periods (11). CYFRA 21-1 can reliably diagnose squamous lung cancer (12).

Monoclonal antibodies 5E8, 5C7, and 1F10. The antibody 5E8 plus 5C7 plus 1F10 significantly surpassed SCC-Ag plus CEA in terms of sensitivity (p < 0.05) and proved to be the most accurate marker combination. Among single markers, 5E8 was most specific, 5C7 most sensitive, and 5C7 and 1F10 were each most accurate, but the differences from CEA alone were not significant. Sub-group analysis by histologic type and stage demonstrated similar findings, and marker combinations yielded little additional diagnostic benefit. 5E8, 5C7, and 1F10 performed marginally better than did CEA and SCC-Ag in patients with newly diagnosed NSCLC. Many limitations apply in defining a clinical niche for these tumor markers in NSCLC, although 5E8, 5C7, and 1F10 previously have demonstrated a modest prognostic value (13).

Nonspecific cross-reacting antigen 50/90 (NCA 50/90). NCA 50/90 belongs to the *CEA* gene family. Other members of this family are CEA, NCA 95, and pregnancy-specific beta-glycoprotein. Sensitivities of 70%, 39%, and 42% were found for lung cancer, colon cancer, and leukemia, respectively. The sensitivity for NSCLC was 85% compared to 50% for SCLC. These results suggest a clinical utility in the management of patients with NSCLC (14).

Progastrin-releasing peptide (ProGRP). Progastrin-releasing peptide is a stable 27-amino acid precursor peptide of the gastrin-releasing peptide, which was first isolated from porcine gastric cells and can be found in human gastrointestinal, broncho-alveolar, and neuronal cells. ProGRP is a specific tumor marker in patients with SCLC, and it has been reported that ProGRP levels are rarely elevated in patients with NSCLC (<3%) (15). However, if an NSCLC patient presents with a ProGRP level >100 pg/mL, the clinicopathologic features should be examined with regard to the small cell component, neuroendocrine differentiation, and renal dysfunction. (16).

Neuron-specific enolase (NSE). Neuron-specific enolase is a useful serum marker for the diagnosis and monitoring of SCLC. In addition to SCLC, elevated NSE levels are found in hemolysis and neuroendocrine disorders such as intestinal and pulmonary carcinoids, pheochromocytoma, pancreatic carcinoma, and melanoma. In NSCLC a high level of NSE prognosticates a poor outcome, probably by reflecting tumor heterogeneity and underestimated neuroendocrine differentiation (11).

Carcinoembryonic antigen (CEA). CEA is an oncofetal protein normally found in the embryonic and fetal gut and sometimes produced by malignant cells. It was first described by Gold and Freedman in 1965 in patients with adenocarcinoma of the colon. One of the most widely studied tumor markers in oncology, including lung cancer, CEA has a normal reference value of 5 ng/mL. Elevated CEA levels are found in NSCLC patients, including patients with adenocarcinoma, large cell carcinoma, and squamous cell carcinoma.

On the other hand, there are common conditions (other than cancer) in which CEA elevations are frequently registered. CEA elevations were observed in 13.6% of heavy smokers compared to1.8% of nonsmokers. Increased CEA levels are also frequently observed in patients with chronic obstructive pulmonary disease (COPD) and pulmonary infections, including tuberculosis. Other benign reasons for elevated CEA levels are hepatitis, liver cirrhosis, pancreatitis, ulcerative colitis, and Crohn's disease. However, the magnitude and frequency of elevations in CEA are considerably higher among those patients with malignant disease (5).

CEA levels have been shown to be lower in early-stage NSCLC patients as compared to patients with unresectable or metastatic disease. Also, CEA levels are significantly higher in patients with adenocarcinoma. There is a statistically significant relationship between CEA level and tumor size (12). Preoperative CEA levels seem to be of prognostic interest. In resectable Stage I NSCLC patients, for example, recurrences were observed in 12% of patients with levels ≤2.5 ng/mL, compared to 42% in patients with pre-operative CEA levels >2.5 ng/mL (p = 0.009).

CEA has an important role in determining metastatic disease, since elevated CEA levels were detected in unresectable NSCLC patients with distant metastases (12). In patients undergoing chemotherapy, responders were more likely to have decreases in CEA. Therefore CEA is a useful indicator of disease extent, a useful clinical therapeutic marker, and may potentially have prognostic value (17).

Tumor M2-PK. Significantly elevated tumor marker concentrations were found to correlate with advanced tumor stages. The best correlation with the tumor stage was observed for Tumor M2-PK and CYFRA 21-1. Generally higher sensitivity for NSCLC only was shown for Tumor M2-PK (65%), CEA (42%), and CYFRA 21-1 (58%). Therefore Tumor M2-PK and CYFRA 21-1 can be used to monitor disease for tumor progression or regression during chemotherapy (18).

CA125. CA125 serum levels are elevated in a variety of diseases such as liver cirrhosis, hepatitis, acute pancreatitis, and endometriosis. Increased levels of CA125 are found in 38% of patients with lung cancer. Compared with patients in whom normal CA125 levels are detected, patients with elevated CA125 values have a worse prognosis. CA125 levels have been shown to be lower in NSCLC patients with early-stage disease as compared to patients with nonresectable or metastatic disease. There is no statistically significant relationship between CA125 levels and histology, but a statistically significant relationship exists between CA125 level and tumor size. Responders to chemotherapy are more likely to have decreases in CA125. Therefore CA125 is a useful indicator of disease extent, resectability, and therapeutic success; and it may be a prognostic marker (5,17).

Tissue polypeptide antigen (TPA). Tissue polypeptide antigen (TPA) is a single-chain polypeptide that has been isolated from cell membranes and smooth endoplasmic reticulum of malignant cells. Benign reasons for increased TPA levels include hepatitis, liver cirrhosis, diabetes mellitus, and cholecystitis. NSCLC patients with elevated TPA levels, defined as at least 100 U/L, are associated with shortened survival. TPA occasionally precedes clinical recognition of recurrence or progression.

Serum Markers in SCLC

Neuron-specific enolase (NSE). In neurons and tumors with neuroendocrine differentiation (NE), high concentrations of NSE were identified and NSE classified as a neuroendocrine tumor marker (NE TM) and a marker for tumors with NE phenotype, especially SCLC. Although nonspecific for SCLC, the expression of NSE in serum seems rather persistent in this tumor type compared with NSCLC. Low or trace amounts of NSE have been proven in non-malignant "normal" tissues. NSE is a glycolytic neurospecific isoenzyme of enolase. It consists of two almost identical polypeptide chains, each with a molecular weight of 39 kDa. In 1965, enolase (2-phospho-D-glycerate hydrolase or phosphopyruvate hydratase) was isolated from beef brain by More and McGregor and described as a nerve-specific protein. Human enolases belong to an enolase gene family with different gene products: α, β, and γ isoenzymes with approximately 82% sequence homology. As have all eukaryotic enolases, the isoenzymes have a dimeric structure of three immunologically distinct subunits (α, β, γ) with five possible combinations: homodimeric αα, ββ, γγ, or heterodimeric αγ and αβ forms.

NSE is a soluble, metal-activated glycolytic metalloenzyme that provides components necessary for aerobic glycolysis. The β form is predominantly found in skeletal and cardiac muscles, and the α-enolase, called non-neuronal enolase (NNE), is widely distributed. The γ-enolase is primarily located in central and peripheral neuronal tissue, in tumors with neuroendocrine characteristics (e.g., SCLC, neuroblastomas, intestinal carcinoid). Furthermore, as NSE is also found in erythrocytes, plasma cells, and platelets, it may be released into serum if separation from red cells does not occur within 60 minutes of venipuncture.

The majority of the European studies are based on the S-NSE-RIA assay with a recommended upper reference limit of 12.5 µg/L. S-NSE-RIA (Pharmacia, Peapack, New Jersey, www.pnu.com) is a double-antibody radioimmunoassay (polyclonal antibodies, anti-rabbit IgG antibodies). NSE in the sample competes with a fixed amount of ^{125}I-labeled NSE for the binding sites of the specific antibodies. Bound and free NSE forms are separated by a second antibody. After centrifugation, the radioactivity in the pellet is inversely proportional to the quantity of NSE in the sample. The detection limit is <2.0 µg/L with a measuring range in mass concentration from 2.0–200 mg/L. No cross reactivity with NNE (αα-enolase) was detected until 13,000 µg/L NNE.

The S-NSE-DELFIA analysis (DELFIA) is a solid phase, two-site fluoroimmunometric assay based on the direct sandwich technique in which two monoclonal anti-mouse antibodies are directed against two separate antigenic determinants on the human NSE molecule. Sample NSE is bound by immobilized monoclonal antibodies and reacts subsequently with europium-labeled monoclonal antibodies against a different specific antigenic site. The cross reactivity with NNE is <0.001 %. The dynamic range covers three decades of NSE values from the detection limit of 1 µg/L to 1000 µg/L. The analytical sensitivity and reproducibility are superior for the DELFIA method compared to the S-NSE-RIA method. The DELFIA method is the easiest to perform with a turn-around time of a few hours, no isotopic waste, and a larger analytical range. The 95% confidence interval limits for healthy females and males are 2.9–9.6 and 3.4–11.7 µg/L, respectively.

The maximum diagnostic efficacy in SCLC for the two methods is 0.91 for both assays, and with identical diagnostic sensitivity, specificity, and discrimination power score. The two methods are for practical purposes interchangeable. The reproducibility and the precision are superior in the DELFIA assay compared to the RIA method.

In univariate studies S-NSE demonstrated significant prognostic value in SCLC not stratified for stage. For each 5 µg/L increment in S-NSE value, a reduction of 10% in median survival was observed, and pre-treatment S-NSE was found to be predictive for survival expectancy. Jorgensen and colleagues (18) attempted to derive a prognostic model for survival based on analysis of S-NSE in combination with other factors [stage, performance status (PS), age, sex, LDH, S-AP, and CEA] in 787 patients from nine centers in six countries. Multivariate regression analysis showed that elevated S-NSE was the most important adverse prognostic factor followed by PS and extensive disease stage. Another multivariate analysis confirmed the prognostic influence of S-NSE (19), and it was found to be superior to S-LDH. Based on S-NSE alone, a difference of 208 days was found in estimated median survival between patients with normal S-NSE and patients with S-NSE >75 µg/L. A more detailed prognostic stratification system was based on an algorithm including S-NSE, PS, and stage of the disease. The difference in estimated median survival between good and poor risk groups was 344 days. Thus, NSE is an independent prognostic factor of high significance in SCLC.

High pre-treatment S-NSE values are not incompatible with complete response (CR), and there seems to be no correlation to the type of response (19). In studies investigating the ability to discriminate between response types (18,20), the specificity of S-NSE was not sufficient to differentiate complete response (CR) from partial response (PR). There is general agreement that increasing S-NSE values during therapy are highly suggestive of progressive disease. S-NSE analysis however, cannot replace clinical evaluation during or after chemotherapy (18,20).

The cumulative data from more than 2,000 SCLC patients from about 20 countries show that increased S-NSE values were found in about 80% of all patients. The mean prevalence of increased NSE values at diagnosis was 0.68 in limited disease (LD) and 0.98 in extensive disease (ED). Results from studies in SCLC and NSCLC confirm that high S-NSE expressivity is a predominant characteristic in SCLC. The sensitivity of S-NSE in SCLC ranged from 55–99% compared to 5–21% for NSCLC. The tumor marker with the highest sensitivity in SCLC was S-NSE, followed by S-LDH. Although both S-NSE and S-LDH are correlated to the pre-treatment stage of disease, specific cut-off points could not be defined. S-NSE was positively correlated to the number of metastatic sites, but not to metastases in specific areas and was uninfluenced by brain metastases. In conclusion, S-NSE plays no role in staging and cannot be used as a surrogate for stage of disease.

In summary, S-NSE is not sensitive and specific enough to discriminate SCLC from NSCLC and it cannot replace histological evaluation. S-NSE could be a clinical guideline in cases (20%) where for various reasons it is not possible to establish a final diagnosis by biopsy. Decreasing values after primary treatment corresponding to the half-life period (one day for NSE) is the first sign of good prognosis and highly indicative for a treatment effect. Low pre-treatment S-NSE values, a significant decrease in S-NSE during initial treatment, and achievement of complete remission are important determinants of response duration. S-NSE was found to be unable to differentiate between partial and complete response to chemotherapy.

CYFRA 21-1 (Cytokeratin 19 fragment). Cytokeratin 19 (CK 19) is an acidic protein with a molecular weight of 40 kDa and is part of the cytoskeleton of epithelial cells (discussed in somewhat the same terms in a previous section). The distribution of the intermediate filament is exclusive to cells of simple and pseudostratified epithelium (such as the bronchial epithelium). Histopathological studies demonstrate that cytokeratin 19 is abundant in carcinomas of the lung. On the death of cells, it is released into the serum in the form of soluble fragments. CYFRA 21-1 is a CK 19 fragment found in serum that can be measured by a new immunoradiometric assay using two mouse monoclonal antibodies (mAbs), KS19-1 and BM 19-21. Since CYFRA 21-1 determines only fragments of cytokeratin 19, the test shows a higher specificity than the diagnostic assay for TPA, which identifies three antigens corresponding to cytokeratins 8, 18, and 19. CYFRA 21-1 has a half-life of 12 hours. Serum levels of CYFRA 21-1 have been determined in healthy individuals and those with benign lung disease (19). Of 711 healthy blood donors, 99.8 % had CYFRA 21-1 levels below 1.2 ng/mL; the 95% cut-off was 1.8 ng/mL without gender differences and influence of age and smoker status. In a group of 546 patients with benign lung disease (tuberculosis, acute inflammatory diseases of the lung, pulmonary fibrosis, COPD), 96 % had levels below 3.3 ng/mL (21). The sensitivity of CYFRA 21-1 in patients with SCLC ranges between 34% and 46%, respectively, 33% in limited disease, and up to 84%

in extensive disease of SCLC. Cell type heterogeneity may explain some differences between the published studies as to the sensitivity and specificity of CYFRA 21-1 in the various histologic subtypes of lung cancer. The magnitude of these differences is very small for NSCLC and rather large for SCLC. Elevated CYFRA 21-1 levels in SCLC could be either due to tumor heterogeneity with subpopulations of squamous cell differentiation or cytokeratin expression by the SCLC tumor cells.

CYFRA 21-1 is implicated as a parameter of tumor burden, tumor relapse after therapy, and also as an independent factor indicating a poor prognosis (22). But although serum concentrations of CYFRA 21-1 show significant correlation with tumor burden, there is no consistent relationship between production of this marker and tumor type. The majority of studies show that a higher CYFRA 21-1 level is correlated with advanced tumor stage. In addition, recent research correlates CYFRA 21-1 and tumor size and lymph node involvement. In lung cancer patients who have had tumor resection or chemotherapy, a rising serum CYFRA 21-1 level is an early indicator of tumor recurrence.

Anti-Hu antibodies. SCLC patients with paraneoplastic neurological manifestations (e.g., peripheral neuropathy, cerebellar degeneration) seem to have a more indolent course than those without. High-titer antineuronal antibodies (anti-Hu) are found in the serum and cerebrospinal fluid of patients with paraneoplastic encephalomyelitis/sensory neuronopathy from SCLC. In patients who received treatment, anti-Hu was associated with limited disease stage, complete response to treatment, and longer survival. Anti-Hu was found to be an independent predictive factor for complete response to therapy but not survival on multivariate analysis (23).

Carcinoembryonic antigen (CEA). CEA is a transmembrane glycoprotein with a MW of 180–200 kDa. It functions as a homotypic cell adhesion molecule and a heterotypic chemoattractant for neutrophils. CEA is one of the oncofetal antigens produced during embryonal and fetal development. CEA has a half-life of several weeks (24). Serum CEA is analyzed by means of a solid-phase immunoassay. CEA has a relatively high sensitivity for many advanced adenocarcinomas (primarily colon, but also breast, stomach, and lung cancer). Sensitivity of CEA measurement is greatest and serum CEA concentrations are highest in adenocarcinoma and large-cell carcinoma subtypes of NSCLC and SCLC. The applicability of CEA as a marker for SCLC is limited, for the proportion of patients with elevated levels at presentation has generally been reported as less than half. Although serum CEA assays have low sensitivity and specificity for diagnosing lung cancer, several reports have indicated that elevated pre-operative CEA levels are associated with more advanced disease and with very poor survival (9). No significant correlation with CEA concentrations could be shown between primary tumor size, TNM stage, number of organs involved, or sites of metastatic cancer. All in all, the exact mechanism of elevated serum CEA concentrations in lung cancers remains unclear.

Lactate dehydrogenase (LDH). LDH is an ubiquitous glycolytic enzyme, which catalyzes the reversible oxidation of lactate to pyruvate. It is widely distributed in many tissues, especially the myocardium, kidney, liver, muscle, and red blood cells. The enzyme LDH is present in SCLC tumor cells; however, its presence is traditionally understood to indicate liver involvement. Liver metastases are prevalent at diagnosis in 25% of patients with SCLC, and the negative influence of liver metastases has been emphasized previously. Several investigators found this simple biochemical test to be a good independent prognostic factor in SCLC. A retrospective review of 411 SCLC patients showed by means of Cox multivariate regression analysis that raised LDH and white blood cell counts were independent adverse prognostic factors, in addition to performance status, extent of disease, and age (23). The survival advantage for patients with normal LDH persisted even when adjustment was made for stage, performance status, and treatment protocol. In another study, a high proportion of patients with increased liver enzymes did not respond to therapy and high LDH levels carried low probability for complete response. Although LDH is correlated to pre-treatment stage of disease stage, specific cut-off points have not been defined. Serial measurements of LDH often mirror clinical response. During response, minor oscillations are usual and isolated abnormal values have been observed in few cases for LDH (18). Compared with LDH, however, the discriminative power of NSE is superior. Furthermore, Sagman et al. have reported that LDH levels are rarely normal in patients with bone marrow involvement. They recommended that patients with normal LDH levels need not be subjected to invasive bone marrow staging procedures (23).

Creatine kinase BB (CK-BB). Elevated levels of CK-BB (standard value: <10 ng/mL) can be found in the serum of SCLC patients. It is increased mainly in advanced stages, depending on tumor size (9). A strong correlation was found between the number of metastatic sites and the level of CK-BB (19% of all patients with a single metastasis and 100% with multiple metastases had elevated CK-BB). These authors observed a correlation with response to chemotherapy as well. No studies are available on its presence in sera from NSCLC and benign lung disease. The marker may be of prognostic value, but further studies must confirm its usefulness (24).

Chromogranin A (CgA). CgA is a 68-kDa protein found in secretory granules in normal tissues and in APUD (define) tumors. Concentrations of CGA are elevated in 65% of SCLC patients (standard value: <20 IU/L). In NSCLC sera and in sera from benign lung disease, CgA is found in 33% and 28%, respectively. Because positive sera are frequent in benign lung disease, CgA is less useful in discriminating between lung cancer and benign lung disease. CgA has particular relevance to the detection of treatment failure, for which it appears superior to other markers (24). The majority of patients who fail to respond to initial chemotherapy showed rising CgA levels during treatment and 78% of patients had increased levels at the time of recurrence (9).

Tissue polypeptide antigen (TPA). TPA is one of the oldest tumor markers (standard value: <60 IU/L). In controls, and in patients with benign lung disease, TPA-positive sera occur only with low frequency (9). TPA assays measure a mixture of cytokeratins 8, 18, and 19. Although serum concentrations of TPA show significant correlation with tumor burden, there is no consistent relationship between production of this marker and tumor type. In most cases, high TPA concentrations reflect advanced tumor stage and therefore suggest a bad prognosis. It is also useful for monitoring patients during chemotherapy (24).

Neural cell adhesion molecule (NCAM). NCAM is a 140–180 kDa sialoglycoprotein belonging to the immunoglobin superfamily (standard value: <20 IU/mL). It is implicated in mechanisms of adhesion, detachment, and aggregation processes that are thought to be involved in the metastatic behavior of cancer (24). High concentrations of NCAM were detected in sera of 21–51% of SCLC patients, while no serum from NSCLC patients or healthy controls were positive. Patients with elevated levels of this marker had significantly shorter survival times than patients with normal levels. Serial measurements of NCAM might be of value in monitoring response to therapy in those patients with SCLC whose pre-treatment levels are within pathological range (9).

Gastrin-releasing peptide (GRP). GRP is a growth-regulating peptide, characterized by its ability to release gastrointestinal hormones. The GRP peptide sequence is located at the N-terminal end of the GRP precursor molecule. The C-terminal end of the precursor is secreted in at least two major forms, which results in a stable product in plasma (24). Elevated serum concentrations of GRP are reported in 7–76% of SCLC cases (standard value: <50 pg/mL).

In another study, plasma GRP levels were elevated in 71% of patients with limited SCLC and in 80% of those with extensive disease (9). Both GRP and the C-terminal precursor fragment of GRP correlated with clinical stage during chemotherapy. Changes in GRP level showed excellent correlation with therapeutic response. Elevated levels of GRP have been found in the cerebrospinal fluid of 75% of SCLC patients suffering from meningeal carcinomatosis (9).

Atrial natriuretic peptide (ANP). ANP is present in several tissues, including SCLC. Increased plasma levels of ANP were observed in patients with inappropriate secretion of antidiuretic hormone (SIADH) due to SCLC (standard value: <33 ng/L). Some authors could demonstrate a relationship between ectopic production of ANP, serum sodium, and patient outcome in SCLC. Patients with extensive SCLC and hyponatremia had shorter survival times than patients with extensive stage SCLC and normal serum sodium values (24).

MOLECULAR MARKERS FOR LUNG CANCER

In this section, molecular alterations are discussed for the most relevant genetic abnormalities reported. A brief summary concerning the frequency and prognostic implication of these alterations is shown in Table 2.

Molecular Markers for NSCLC

p53. The tumor suppressor gene *p53* located at chromosome region 17p13.1 encodes a 53-kDa nuclear protein with a central

Table 2 Molecular markers in NSCLC

Genes	Abnormality	Frequency	Prognostic significance
p53	Overexpression Mutation Deletion	30%–70%	Controversial
c-erbB-2	Overexpression	30%	Controversial
K-ras	Mutation	30%–80%	Controversial
BCL-2	Overexpression	10%–35%	Controversial
p16	Mutation	70%	Unknown
Rb	Deletion Mutation	15%–30%	Controversial

role in the regulation of transcriptional events in the cell nucleus, particularly in response to DNA-damaging agents. It is the most frequently mutated gene in NSCLC. Mutations in the *p53* gene have been reported in 32–52% of NSCLC patients (25). The prevalent type of point mutation is a GC to TA transversion, causing missense mutations, and is believed to be related to benzo(a)pyrene-induced damage caused by tobacco smoking. The *p53* missense mutations usually lead to increased protein half-life, with higher p53 protein levels, that can be detected by immunohistochemistry. Although several studies observed that p53 alterations are a marker for poor prognosis, the lung cancer study group protocol 871 failed to show a prognostic impact in curatively resected NSCLC, but detected a weak negative survival correlation with positive p53 immunostaining ($p < 0.05$). Similarly, several other reports demonstrated that increased p53 immunostaining correlated with poor prognosis in resectable NSCLC. Other series, however, have shown no significant correlation between p53 expression and survival.

Clearly, further investigation will be necessary to clarify the conflicting information on the prognostic relevance of p53 expression and mutation in NSCLC. Because of the existence of directly conflicting data, the clinical usefulness must be considered limited at the present time (26).

c-erbB-2. The *c-erbB-2* gene (also known as *HER2/neu*) belongs to the family of transmembrane receptors that include the epidermal growth factor (EGFR or erbB-1) and encodes for transmembrane receptor-type tyrosine-protein kinases. The p185 protein is expressed at low levels in normal ciliated bronchial epithelium. Overexpression of HER2/neu, defined as a positive staining, was reported in 13–80% of adenocarcinomas, in 2–45% of squamous cell carcinomas, and in 0–20% of large cell carcinomas (25). Consequently, different results have been published concerning the impact of HER2/neu overexpression in NSCLC. Brabender et al. used real-time reverse transcriptase-polymerase chain reaction (RT-PCR), a method with high sensitivity and specificity for mRNA quantification of HER2/neu (27). In this study an individual expression value was calculated for each patient by calculating a tumor:normal expression ratio. Using this method, a high HER2/neu expression value was detected in 34.9% of NSCLC patients. Multivariate analysis revealed high HER2/neu expression as an independent prognostic factor for survival ($p = 0.041$) in NSCLC. Overexpression of EGFR in NSCLC has been reported in a variety of studies using immunohistochemical methods, with a frequency of overexpression between 32% and 47% in NSCLC. Most of the studies reported no correlation of EGFR overexpression to patient survival. High EGFR and HER2/neu protein co-overexpression was reported in 13% of patients by Tateishi and colleagues and 16.9% using HER2/neu mRNA in adenocarcinomas (27); these were associated with inferior five-year survival rates.

Ras. Members of the *ras* family (*H-ras, K-ras,* and *N-ras*) encode a membrane-associated 21-kDa guanine triphosphate (GTP) binding protein that is involved in signal transduction. These proteins are usually active only when GTP is bound and become inactive once GTP is hydrolyzed to GDP. However, dominant mutant oncogenes become continuously active through mutations in codon 12, 13, or 61. Continuously active ras protein causes unregulated interaction with effector proteins resulting in an uncontrolled signal cascade. Point mutations of *ras* genes are found in about 30% of NSCLC cases. The specific type of mutation varies between the histologic types. Mutations in the *K-ras* oncogene have been detected in about 30 to 80% of NSCLC cases, partly depending on methodology used. *K-ras* mutations seem associated with adenocarcinomas, and in particular, codon-12 mutation of *K-ras* seems to be associated with smoking-related adenocarcinomas. The existing data concerning the impact of *K-ras* mutations on survival are controversial (25*)*

Interestingly, presence of *K-ras* mutations in tumors could be used as a screening marker in bronchial washings in the future. Scott et al. have shown that in individuals with NSCLC adenocarcinoma containing *K-ras* codon-12 mutations, the identical mutations could be detected in 45% of sputum samples. Ahrendt et al. reported that 42% of NSCLC cases contain *K-ras* mutations and that the same mutation could be detected in 50% of bronchial lavage fluids (28).

BCL-2. The product of the *BCL-2* proto-oncogene expresses a protein that protects cells from apoptosis (see also Chapter 54). It is believed that this inhibition occurs by preventing the release of cytochrome C from the mitochondria as well as by inhibiting the apoptosis protease-activating factor-1 protein from initiating the proteinase caspase cascade that leads to DNA degradation in the apoptotic cell. Immunohistochemical studies have shown that BCL-2 protein is expressed at higher levels in 75–90% of SCLC compared with 10–35% of NSCLC, where the expression was higher in squamous cell carcinomas than in adenocarcinomas. Several reports demonstrated a survival benefit for patients with BCL-2-positive tumors, whereas the study from Anton et al. did not confirm this finding (29).

Retinoblastoma (*Rb*) gene. The first tumor suppressor gene discovered was the *Rb* gene, which predisposes to familial childhood retinoblastomas. This gene, located at chromosome region 13q14.11, encodes for a 105-kDa protein that is important in controlling the cell cycle during the G0/G1 phase.

The Rb protein is part of the p16/cyclin D1/CDK4/Rb pathway that is believed to be involved in most lung cancers. Nearly all tumors have abnormalities of one component of this pathway; abnormalities of the Rb protein are found in about 15–30% of NSCLCs. Xu et al. have shown that absence of Rb protein expression is associated with poor prognosis. These results however, were not confirmed by several other studies (26).

Cyclin E. Progression through the G1-S transition and S phase of the cell cycle is mediated by cyclin-dependent kinase 2 (cdk2), which interacts with several cyclins. Two of these, cyclin E and cyclin A2 (also known as cyclin A), are overexpressed in many cancers. Cyclin E2 and cyclin A1 are recently discovered cdk2-interacting cyclins that are found in malignant tumor cell lines and in acute myeloid leukemia, respectively. Muller-Tidow et al. (30) have analyzed expression and prognostic relevance of the cdk2-associated cyclins in non-small cell lung cancer (NSCLC) using fresh-frozen biopsies (n = 70) from completely resected tumors with stage I to IIIA NSCLC.

Gene expression was analyzed by quantitative real-time RT-PCR. Expression levels of cyclin E ($p = 0.04$) and cyclin A2 ($p = 0.004$) were significantly higher in the tumor samples than in normal controls. Cyclin A1, cyclin A2, and cyclin E2 expression levels did not have prognostic relevance for survival. The mean survival time associated with low and high levels of cyclin E was 69.4 and 47.2 months, respectively, which was statistically significant ($p = 0.03$). Differences in survival were particularly pronounced in stages I and II. Cyclin E was also closely associated with the development of distant metastasis ($p = 0.01$). Finally, immunohistochemistry analyses confirmed that cyclin E mRNA expression was closely associated with cyclin E protein expression.

Anton RC et al. (31) studied paraffin-embedded sections of NSCLC tissue immunostained with monoclonal antibody to cyclin D1 and cyclin E. Overall, 426 NSCLC patients positive for cyclin D1 and 360 NSCLC patients positive for cyclin E had adequate follow-up (median, 76 months) for survival analysis. Both cyclins independently showed significance in prognosis of SCC but not other cell types. For cyclin E, Stage I and II SCC with less than 50% immunopositivity had a worse prognosis ($p = 0.029$). Of 70 Stage I and II SCC cases immuno-stained for both monoclonal antibodies, 55% of patients with tumors that demonstrated both absence of cyclin D1 staining and cyclin E immunopositivity in less than 50% of cells were dead at five years compared to 35% of patients with tumors that demonstrated positive staining with cyclin D1 and cyclin E immunopositivity in more than 50% of cells.

Molecular Markers for SCLC

myc. The *myc* oncogenes—*c-myc* (cellular), *N-myc* (or *MYCN*, initially isolated from neuroblastoma cells), and *L-myc* (or *MYCL*, first isolated from SCLC cells)—encode for nuclear DNA-binding proteins, which are involved in transcriptional regulation. Their proto-oncogene product activates downstream genes that stimulate cell division after heterodimerization. Of the well-typified *myc* family of genes, *c-myc* is most frequently activated in non-small cell lung cancer (NSCLC) and small cell lung cancer (SCLC), whereas abnormalities of *N-myc* and *L-myc* usually occur only in SCLC. Generally, only one member of the *myc* family is activated in each individual tumor. Activation of *myc* genes results in protein overexpression through multiplied gene amplification (20 to 115 copies per cell).

Studies have shown that amplification of *c-myc* genes in the primary tumor correlates with adverse survival and that *myc* DNA amplification in tumor cell lines established from patients previously treated with chemotherapy were associated with significantly shortened survival. DNA amplification of the *myc* family occurs more commonly in specimens from chemotherapy-treated than from untreated patients. After progression from cytotoxic chemotherapy, between 28% and 36% of the cell lines demonstrated *myc* amplification, compared to frequencies from 8 to 11% of the untreated patient specimens. Additionally, amplification is seen more frequently in cell lines established from metastatic lesions than from primary tumors (32,33,34).

BCL-2. The *BCL-2* proto-oncogene product is—like p53—a key member of the normal apoptotic pathway because it protects cells from the normal apoptotic process. In most SCLC tumors (75–95%), BCL-2 protein immunohistochemical expression is present. BCL-2 expression has been discussed as a significant marker for survival of patients with SCLC, but recently it has been shown that it is not significantly correlated with the survival of SCLC patients (32).

p53. The most common genetic changes associated with SCLC involve mutations of the *p53* gene, a nuclear phosphoprotein that is important in cell cycle control. It is located on chromosome 17p13.1. Normally, when DNA damage has occurred, the cell arrests in the G1/S state because *p53* binds to DNA and leads to cell cycle arrest, blockage of DNA synthesis, and apoptosis. Loss of *p53* function allows survival of genetically damaged cells, leading to accumulation of multiple mutations and the evolution of a cancer cell (32,33).

Approximately 90% of SCLC tumors harbor mutated *p53*. The prevalent type of mutation is a GC:TA transversion and is related to exposure to benzopyrene from cigarette smoking. Overexpression of *p53* in SCLC is found in about 50% of all SCLC samples, and both its adverse prognostic impact and positive predictive potential for chemotherapy response is discussed controversially (35,36).

Retinoblastoma (*Rb*) gene. In more than 90% of SCLC tumors, abnormalities of Rb protein with either absent expression, deletion, or mutation of the pocket domain as well as hypophosphorylation are detectable. Since SCLC is Rb protein-negative in more than 90% of cases, and carcinoids of the lung are Rb protein-positive in approximately 92% of cases, immunohistochemical analysis for histological differential diagnosis of pulmonary neoplasms is advocated in critical cases. There is no correlation between Rb expression and the proliferation of lung cancer cells. Analysis of clinical data revealed no associations between Rb status and extent of disease, clinical response to chemotherapy, overall survival, or lymph node metastases (37,38).

METHYLATION MARKERS FOR LUNG CANCER

Alterations of DNA methylation patterns have been recognized as common changes in human cancers. These are thought to have important implications for abnormalities of gene expression, chromosome structure, and chromatin organization (39). Aberrant methylation of normally unmethylated CpG-rich areas, also known as CpG islands, which are located in or near the promoter region of many genes, has been associated with transcriptional inactivation of defined tumor suppressor genes (TSGs) in human cancer (40). Thus, aberrant methylation may serve as an alternative to the genetic loss of a TSG function by deletion or mutation (41).

Methylation Markers for NSCLC

Aberrant promoter methylation (referred to as methylation) has been described for several genes in various malignant diseases, including lung cancer (42). In NSCLC, methylation has been detected for

- the retinoic acid receptor β-2 (RARβ) in 40%,
- the tissue inhibitor of metalloproteinase 3 (TIMP3) in 26%,
- for p16^{INK4a} in 25%,
- for the O^6-methylguanine-DNA-methyltransferase (MGMT) in 21%,
- for the death-associated protein kinase (DAPK) in 19%,
- for E-cadherin (ECAD) in 18%,
- for p14^{ARF} in 8%, and
- for the glutathione S-transferase P1 (GSTP1) in 7% of primary tumor tissues.

It was not seen in the vast majority of the corresponding non-malignant tissues (42).

In this series, a total of 82% of the NSCLCs had at least one gene methylated, 22% two genes, 13% three genes, 8% four genes, and 2% of the NSCLCs had five methylated genes. This suggests that many NSCLCs hypermethylate a small percentage of genes, whereas a subset of tumors displays the "CpG island-methylator-phenotype (CIMP+)."

Subsequently, associations between aberrant DNA methylation and clinicopathological variables have been observed. Kim et al. (43) detected a significant association between hypermethylation of the DAPK promoter with advanced pathologic stage (p = 0.003), an increased tumor size (p = 0.009), and lymph node involvement (p = 0.04) in NSCLC. Of particular clinical interest is the association of aberrant methylation with prognosis for patients with NSCLC. For stage I NSCLC, Tang et al. (44) observed a significantly inferior five-year survival (p = 0.007) for patients harboring DAPK promoter methylation compared to patients lacking this epigenetic alteration, and Brabender et al. (45) reported a significantly worse survival (p = 0.041) for patients with high adenomatous polyposis coli (APC)-methylation status compared to patients with low APC-methylation status in curatively resected NSCLC. Moreover, methylation of p16^{INK}, MGMT, GSTPI, and DAPK has been described in serum DNA of NSCLC patients (46) and p16^{INK} methylation has been observed in precursor lesions of lung carcinomas (47), which suggests these epigenetic alterations as powerful candidate biomarkers for early diagnosis, estimation of prognosis, and surveillance of recurrence for NSCLC patients in the near future. The most current relevant data on gene methylation patterns in NSCLC are summarized in Table 3.

Methylation Markers for SCLC

In contrast to NSCLC, the role of CpG island methylation in SCLC has been studied less extensively. Virmani et al. (48) reported aberrant methylation of the retinoic acid receptor-beta (RARβ) P2 promoter in 72% (63/87) of SCLCs investigated, and methylation of the APC promoter 1A in 26% (13/50) SCLC cell lines tested (48). A high frequency of methylation of the tumor suppressor gene *RASSF1A* in SCLC has been reported independently from several groups. Agathanggelou et al. (49) reported *RASSF1A* methylation in 72%, Burbee et al. (50) in 100%, and Dammann et al. (51) in 79% of investigated SCLCs. Furthermore, aberrant methylation of the APC promoter 1A (21), the RARβ promoter P2 (52), and the RASSF1A promoter (49,50) was associated with loss of its gene expression in SCLC, suggesting a fundamental role of this epigenetic alteration in the pathogenesis of this malignant disease. The implication of this epigenetic alteration for diagnosis and treatment of SCLC has yet to be determined.

MICROMETASTASES IN LUNG CANCER
Lymph Node Micrometastases in NSCLC

In patients with lung cancer who do not have evidence of systemic tumor spread, the single most important prognostic factor is the presence or absence of regional lymph node metastases. On routine histopathological examination, tumor spread to the lymph nodes is likely to be underestimated. In fact, it has been calculated that a pathologist has only a 1% chance of identifying a small (three cell diameters) metastatic focus of cancer (1). Several studies have shown that the detection of disseminated tumor cells in lymph nodes by immunohistochemistry is an independent predictor of early relapse and would result in up-staging of many patients with NSCLC.

Chen et al. (53) used a polyclonal anti-cytokeratin antibody to examine regional lymph nodes from 60 patients with pN0 NSCLC. They demonstrated a much higher frequency of metastatic regional lymph nodes than stated by routine histopathology (Table 4). The median survival of patients with micrometastases (65.9 months) was shorter than that of patients without occult metastases (81.2 months). Passlick et al. (54) used the anti-epithelial monoclonal antibody Ber-EP-4 to study regional lymph nodes from 72 patients with node-negative

Table 3 Methylation markers in NSCLC

Gene	Stages	n	Association	p-value	Reference
DAPK	I–IV	185	Tumor stage	0.003	22
			Tumor size	0.009	
			Lymph node +	0.04	
DAPK	I	135	Five-year survival	0.007	12
APC	I–IIIA	91	Median survival	0.041	45
APC	I–IIIB	99	Median survival	0.015	24

Table 4 Micrometastases in lymph nodes detected by immunohistochemistry

Antibody	Stages	Frequency	Tissue prep	Staining	Marker	Reference
Polyclonal cytokeratin	I–III	38/60 (63%)	Paraffin	LSAB	Yes	53
Ber-EP-4	I–II	11/72 (15%)	Frozen	APAAP	Yes	54
Ber-EP-4	I–II	16/67 (24%)	Frozen	APAAP	Yes	34
CAM 5.2	I	31/44 (71%)	Paraffin	LSAB	Yes	40
AE1/3	I	21/104 (20%)	Paraffin	LSAB	Yes	23
p53	I–IV	14/31 (45%)	Paraffin	LSAB	Yes	20
Ber-EP-4, AE1/3	I	3/80 (4%)	Paraffin	Peroxidase	No	16
MNF116	I	3/49 (6%)	Paraffin	LSAB	No	9

LSAB, Labeled Strepavidin-Biotin method; APAAP, Alkaline Phosphatase Anti-Alkaline Phosphatase method.

NSCLC. Micrometastases were found in 15.2% of patients. The presence of occult tumor deposits was significantly associated with a shorter disease-free survival. After a median follow-up of 26 months, five of ten patients (50%) with micrometastases had recurrences, compared to eight of 56 patients (14.2%) without nodal metastases (p = 0.005). Izbicki et al. (34) used the same methodological setting and found that 24% of the 67 node-free NSCLC patients had occult lymph node involvement. The mean relapse-free survival and cancer-related survival rates were 41.1 months and 44.6 months for patients without micrometastases, compared to 29.0 months and 36.5 months for the 16 patients with occult nodal metastases (p = 0.008).

In a retrospective study by Marayuma et al. (40) on 44 patients with stage I NSCLC, occult nodal metastases were detected in 31 patients (70.5%) using the primary monoclonal antibody CAM 5.2 for cytokeratin staining. Disease-free survival was significantly shorter in patients with micrometastases than in node-negative patients (p = 0.004). In a recent study, Wu et al. (23) investigated 103 pN0 patients with T1 lung adenocarcinomas using the monoclonal anticytokeratin antibody AE1/3. They found occult metastases in lymph nodes of 21 patients (20.4%). The five-year survival rate of patients with occult metastases was significantly lower (62%) compared to patients without micrometastases (86%) (p = 0.0041). Dobashi and coworkers (20) investigated 47 patients with primary lesions stained positive for the p53 protein by immunohistochemistry. The histological tumor-free lymph nodes of 14/31 patients (45%) showed a positive staining for p53. Patients with p53 positive-lymph nodes had a significantly shorter survival than patients with no occult lymph node metastases (p = 0.0001).

In two other studies (9,16) no significant difference in survival rates between patients with and without immunohistochemically detected lymph node micrometastases was observed. Goldstein et al. (16) used the monoclonal antibodies AE1/3 and Ber-EP-4 in 80 patients with stage I adenocarcinoma. They found occult metastases in only three patients (4%). Nicholson et al. (9) used MNF11, a broad-spectrum anti-keratin antibody, in 49 patients with T1-2, N0 disease and showed micrometastases in the lymph nodes of 3 patients (6%) who were free from recurrence during follow-up. These controversial data demonstrate that it is difficult to compare the results obtained in different institutions on different material (snap-frozen, paraffin) with different antibodies and detection methods (APAAP, LSAB). Nevertheless, the majority of studies including those for other cancers (55) have consistently shown the clinical importance of occult micrometastatic lymph node disease.

More recently assays based on RT-PCR were established to detect occult metastases in lymph nodes from NSCLC patients (Table 5). Salerno et al. (17) detected MUC1 mRNA in 33 of 88 lymph nodes (38%) from 23 patients, which were classified negative (pN0) by routine histological examination. In 11 mediastinal lymph nodes from patients with benign thoracic pathology, MUC1 mRNA was absent. Thirteen of the 15 positive nodes identified by routine histological evaluation had detectable expression of MUC1 mRNA (87%). Hashimoto et al. (56) studied the lymph nodes from 31 NSCLC patients with p53- and K-ras-mutated primary tumors. They employed nested PCR and immunohistochemistry using the monoclonal antibody CAM 5.2 to detect occult metastases. Immunohistochemistry revealed 22/31 patients (77%) with micrometastases compared to 9/31 (29%) found by nested PCR. The concordance of the two methods was 77%, since 13 of 34 (34%) genetically positive lymph nodes could not be detected by immunohistochemistry. Of the 22 patients with pN0-disease, 6 (27%) were genetically positive and four (67%) of them died due to tumor relapse, whereas 17 (77%) were positive by immunohistochemistry and four (24%) died of cancer. Despite the small number of patients, the authors stated that genetically detected micrometastases in lymph nodes is of superior prognostic significance for early stage NSCLC than immunohistochemical results.

Currently there are only a limited number of studies available, with small numbers of patients in the study groups, evaluating micrometastases in lymph nodes of NSCLC by RT-PCR. A standardized protocol is not available so far and further studies are needed to assess the sensitivity and specificity of particular mRNA transcripts for lymph node classification in NSCLC.

Bone Marrow Micrometastases in NSCLC

The prognosis of patients with resectable lung cancer is also determined by the absence or presence of micrometastatic dissemination of cancer at the initial time of diagnosis and treatment, because primary treatment failure is secondary to undetectable systemic spread of tumor. Several recent studies have examined the presence of occult metastases in the bone marrow of resectable NSCLC patients (Table 6). In 1993, Pantel and cowork-

Table 5 Micrometastases in lymph nodes detected genetically

Target	Stage	Method	Detection rate	Sensitivity	Specificity	Prognostic significance	Reference
MUC1	I–IIIa	RT-PCR	16/23 (70%)	87%	100%	n.a.	17
p53, K-ras	I–IIIa	Nested-PCR	9/31 (29%)	n.a.	n.a.	Yes	56

n.a., not analyzed.

ers (57) demonstrated micrometastases in the bone marrow of 22/88 (25%) patients with operable NSCLC using immunohistochemistry and CK2, an antibody directed to cytokeratin polypeptide 18 (CK18). The detection of occult metastases in the bone marrow was significantly associated with size and histological grade of the primary tumor. Of patients with bone marrow micrometastases at the time of surgical resection, 66.7% showed a tumor relapse within 13 months. In contrast, only 36.6% of patients without occult metastases in the bone marrow relapsed in the same period of time (p <0.05). The same authors reported three years later on occult metastases in the bone marrow of 83 (60%) of 139 NSCLC patients without distant metastases (58). Tumors recurred in 19 (35%) of 54 patients without micrometastases compared to 9 (75%) of 12 patients with occult metastases in the bone marrow. Additionally it was shown that patients with pN0 disease who carried more than one cell per 4 $\times 10^5$ bone marrow nuclear cells were significantly more likely to suffer from relapse.

Cote et al. (59) used two cytokeratin-specific monoclonal antibodies, AE1 and CAM 5.2, in combination to detect the presence of tumor cells in the bone marrow of 43 patients with NSCLC. There was a strong association with the stage of disease; 29% of patients with stage I and II and 46% of patients with stage III disease had occult metastases in the bone marrow. Patients without micrometastases had a longer recurrence-free interval than patients with occult metastases, 35.1 vs. 7.3 months (p = 0.0009). Overall survival was also longer in patients without micrometastases: six (23%) of 26 patients without occult metastases died during follow-up compared to seven (41%) of 17 patients who showed positive staining for micrometastases in the bone marrow.

Ohgami et al. (60) investigated 39 patients with stage I-III NSCLC who underwent curative resection, using immunohistochemistry and the monoclonal antibody CK2. In addition they also performed immunostaining of the p53 protein in the corresponding tumors. Occult metastases were detected in 15 (39%) of 39 patients. Overexpression of p53 in the primary tumor was associated with the presence of CK18-positive cells in the bone marrow. Patients with occult bone marrow metastases demonstrated a significantly earlier tumor recurrence than those with tumor-free bone marrow (p = 0.0083).

Poncelet and coworkers (11) demonstrated the presence of occult metastases in the bone marrow in 22 (22%) of 99 patients with NSCLC, using immunohistochemistry with the monoclonal antibodies AE1 and CAM 5.2; however, they did not find any correlations to pathological T- or N-status. In contrast to the majority of studies, the detection of micrometastases was no predictor of early recurrence or reduced survival. Similar results were obtained by Hsu et al. (33), who found occult bone marrow metastases in 21 (22%) of 96 patients using the monoclonal antibodies AE1/AE3, Ber-EP-4, and clone MNF116. Similar disease-free survival (50.2% vs. 53.9%) and cumulative survival (66.7% vs. 67.8%) was shown in bone marrow-positive and bone marrow-negative patients.

It is possible that certain technical factors may account for these discrepancies. The choice of antibodies and technical skills involved in performing the procedures and interpreting the results may result in considerable variation and there is a certain imminent risk of false positive identification of non-epithelial cells.

Nevertheless there is accumulating evidence that the presence of micrometastatic cells in the bone marrow has a clinically significant effect in patients with NSCLC. A standardized protocol must be established in order to make the results of the different studies comparable.

Free Tumor Cells in Blood in NSCLC

An increasing number of studies report on PCR-based techniques for the detection of circulating tumor cells in the blood of NSCLC patients. These techniques rely on the fact that specific mRNA transcripts are selectively expressed in cancer cells of interest, but not in non-transformed normal cells. The presence of such transcripts is taken as indirect evidence for the presence of intact tumor cells within the sample, since RNA is degraded rapidly once released from the cells.

Table 6 Micrometastases in bone marrow of NSCLC patients detected by immunohistochemistry

Antibody	n	Stage	Detection rate	Sensitivity	Specificity	Prognostic significance	Reference
CK2	88	I–IIIb	22/88 (22%)	98.3%	95.5%	Yes	93
CK2	139	I–IIIb	83/139 (60%)	97.2%	n.a.	Yes	96
AE1, CAM 5.2	43	I–III	17/43 (40%)	100%	n.a.	Yes	55
CK2	39	I–III	15/39 (39%)	100%	n.a.	Yes	60
AE1/AE3, Ber-EP4, MNF116	96	I–IV	21/96 (22%)	100%	n.a.	No	33
AE1, CAM 5.2,	99	I–IV	22/99 (22%)	n.a.	n.a.	No	11

n.a., not analyzed.

Peck et al. (61) used nested RT-PCR to amplify CK19 mRNA and found a detection rate of 40% in adenocarcinoma and 41% in squamous cell carcinoma patients. The false positive rate was 1.6%. Castaldo et al. (62) investigated ten NSCLC patients with distant metastases and 14 patients with no evidence of distant metastases. They employed the RT-PCR dot-blot procedure to amplify CEA mRNA, which was found in ten (80%) of the patients with distant metastases and in four (29%) of the patients free of metastases.

Kurusu and coworkers (63) also amplified CEA mRNA in the blood of 103 patients with NSCLC before and after surgical resection. Sixty-two (60%) of the perioperative blood samples were positive. Of these 62 samples, 27 (44%) remained positive even after surgical resection, whereas the remaining 35 (56%) samples became negative. The incidence of positive CEA mRNA was highly related to the stage of the disease.

De Luca and coworkers (3) developed a RT-PCR assay for detection of circulating EGFR-mRNA expressing cells in the blood of patients with colon, breast, and lung cancer. They demonstrated occult metastases in 17 of 30 (57%) patients with stage IV NSCLC. The false-positive rate in 38 healthy volunteers was 10.5%. In contrast to the above studies, false-positive results have been reported due to illegitimate transcription of CEA or due to co-amplification of pseudogene sequences of the *CK19* gene (64). For this reason, the specificity of RT-PCR assays applied to the detection of occult metastases in the blood is controversial.

Lacroix et al. (65) amplified pre-progastrin-releasing peptide (preproGPR) mRNA to detect occult cancer cells in the peripheral blood from 25/92 NSCLC patients (27%). No positive results were obtained in the blood of 67 non-cancer patients. The occurrence of cancer cell dissemination showed no correlation to the disease stage. This could be explained by a lower transcription rate of the *preproGPR* gene in NSCLC cells, which makes the diagnostic relevance of this assay in NSCLC questionable. A recently published study (43) showed that it is difficult if not impossible to compare the results of RT-PCR-based assays obtained in different laboratories.

Until now the prognostic significance of disseminated metastases in the blood of patients with NSCLC has not been addressed. A summary of current results is shown in Table 7. For future studies, quantitative real time RT-PCR assays should be attempted for definition of thresholds and elimination of too many false-positive results in qualitative RT-PCR assays.

Micrometastases in SCLC

Bone marrow micrometastases in SCLC. The bone marrow is one of the most common metastatic sites in SCLC. Using immunohistochemical techniques that have the sensitivity to detect one in 10^4 cells, a number of small trials detected micrometastases in the bone marrow of 13–54% of newly diagnosed limited disease (LD) and in 44–77% extensive disease (ED) SCLC.

In a series by Leonard (66) using a panel of antibodies directed against cellular antigens characteristic of SCLC, residual tumor cells in the bone marrow of SCLC patients at clinical remission did predict tumor recurrence. Metastatic deposits of tumor cells were found in 8/12 patients (67%). Six of these had tumor recurrence, whereas the four patients without occult bone marrow metastases remained tumor-free.

Pasini et al. (67) used a monoclonal antibody that recognizes the neural cell adhesion molecule (NCAM/CD56) to detect metastases in the bone marrow from 17 of 44 patients. Patients with negative bone marrow showed a significantly better survival than those with immunohistochemically positive bone marrow (12 vs. 7 months, $p = 0.007$). Three years later the same group (68) found metastases in the bone marrow in 23/60 patients (38%). In striking contrast, only eight (13%) patients showed a bone marrow involvement by conventional staining procedures. They used the monoclonal antibody MluC1 directed against the Le^Y antigen, which is expressed by the cell membrane of SCLC cells. The authors combined the results obtained by immunohistochemistry and conventional bone marrow staining and found that patients with fewer than ten cells detected conventionally and no immunohistochemically visible metastases had a significantly longer survival than patients with more than ten cells and positive staining by immunohistochemistry. The authors concluded that the detection of bone marrow involvement may be improved by the use of MluC1 as an immunohistochemical marker. Nevertheless, no data concerning specificity and sensitivity were presented.

Although the bone marrow is the most common metastatic site in SCLC, the role of micrometastases is not well defined in this disease. A standard protocol has not yet been defined and it is questionable as to which antibody will give the highest sensitivity and specificity. Pelosi et al. (69) compared four different immunostaining methods using two monoclonal anti-NCAM antibodies on bone marrow aspirates of 37 SCLC patients. They obtained the best results in terms of sensitivity and specificity with a combination of the alkaline phos-

Table 7 Micrometastases in blood of NSCLC patients detected genetically

Target	Method	Detection rate	Sensitivity	Specificity	Reference
CK19	RT-PCR	26/64 (41%)	n.a.	98.4%	61
CEA	RT-PCR, Dot Blot	12/24 (50%)	80%	86%	62
CEA	RT-PCR	62/103 (60%)	n.a.	100%	63
EGFR	RT-PCR, Southern Blot	17/30 (57%)	n.a.	89.5%	3
PreProGRP	RT-PCR	25/92 (27%)	n.a.	100%	65

n.a., not analyzed.

Table 8 Micrometastases in bone marrow of SCLC

Antibody	Stage	Detection rate	Technique	Prognostic significance	Reference
Multiple	LD	8/12 (67%)	PAP	Yes	66
NCC-LU243	LD/ED	17/44 (39%)	APAAP	Yes	67
MLuC1	LD/ED	23/60 (38%)	APAAP	Yes	68
NCC-LU243 NCC-LU246	LD/ED	24/37 (65%)	APAAP+ SABAP	Yes	69

LD, limited disease; ED, extensive disease; PAP, peroxidase anti-peroxidase; APPAP, alkaline phosphatase anti-alkaline phosphatase; SABAP, streptavidin-biotin alkaline phosphatase complex.

phatase/anti-alkaline phosphatase and streptavidin-biotin/alkaline phosphatase complex methods. Twenty-four (65%) patients showed a positive staining by immunohistochemistry. Twelve patients with limited disease and negative bone marrow survived a median of 16.5 months whereas ten patients with limited disease and positive bone marrow survived only 13 months (p = 0.017). Fifteen patients suffered from extensive disease and had a median survival of nine months.

The survival rate of patients with SCLC is limited, yet the detection of occult metastases in the bone marrow of SCLC patients could lead to a more accurate staging, identifying patients without bone marrow involvement who may even benefit from a primary surgical or combined modality approach including surgery.

Free tumor cells in blood in SCLC. As in NSCLC, the impact of free tumor cells in the peripheral blood of patients with SCLC has not been evaluated thoroughly. The literature contains a small number of studies on the detection of tumor cells in the blood by RT-PCR or the presence of genetic alterations in plasma DNA. Peck et al. (61) demonstrated that four (27%) of 15 SCLC patients had circulating cancer cells using RT-PCR of cytokeratin 19 mRNA. Because the diagnostic value of cytokeratin 19 mRNA as a marker for micrometastatic disease is equivocal (64), the impact of this result is questionable.

Bessho and coworkers (70) used RT-PCR to amplify neuromedin B receptor (NMB-R) mRNA, one of the bombesin-like receptors that is highly expressed in SCLC cell lines. Fourteen of 44 patients (32%) were positive for NMB-R, and patients with extended diseased (ED) showed a higher rate of NMB-R than limited disease (LD) patients (44% vs. 19%) although the difference was not statistically significant (p = 0.16). Survival of NMB-R positive patients was marginally significantly shorter than NMB-R negative patients; however, in LD patients there was no significant difference in survival.

In a study by Lacroix et al. (65), seven different marker transcripts were amplified. The preprogastrin-releasing peptide RT-PCR assay was found to be highly sensitive for detecting cancer cells in peripheral blood and sputum of SCLC and NSCLC patients. The blood of 13/26 SCLC patients (50%) tested positive for disseminated cancer. Patients with extensive disease were positive in 69% (9/13) compared to 31% (4/13) of patients suffering from limited disease. This difference did not reach statistical significance (p = 0.11).

Due to the limited prognosis of SCLC patients, it seems to be difficult to establish a reliable mRNA marker for detecting micrometastases in peripheral blood of SCLC that will correlate with survival. The number of patients included in the above-mentioned studies (Table 9) is too low to allow definitive conclusions about the diagnostic potential of RT-PCR-based mRNA marker assays in the treatment of SCLC. Further prospective studies are needed for this technique to be exploited as a tool to monitor therapy response and to predict early relapse and therapeutic modifications.

Response Prediction Markers for Multimodality Therapy in Lung Cancer

As noted earlier, lung cancer is generally divided into small cell lung cancer (SCLC) and non-small cell lung cancer (NSCLC). SCLC is distinctive because of its high response rate to combination chemotherapy. The curative treatment for NSCLC, which accounts for about 80% of all lung cancers, is surgery. However, half of NSCLC patients present with inoperable disease (stage IIIb or IV). These patients are candidates for chemotherapy and radiotherapy. An additional 25% of patients with NSCLC present with locally advanced disease stage IIIa. These patients are now preferentially treated by induction chemotherapy or with radiochemotherapy followed by surgery (1,53).

In contrast to SCLC, patients with NSCLC show only limited sensitivity to chemotherapy, with relative response rates of 20–40%. This is mainly due to inherent drug resistance. Nevertheless there is recent evidence that multimodality therapy can prolong survival, therefore identification of the subset of patients responsive to chemotherapy or radiotherapy is critical to offering the most appropriate therapy.

Response Prediction Markers in NSCLC

Serum tumor markers CEA and CA125. CEA and CA125 are valuable serum tumor markers that can be used to monitor response to therapy in patients with various solid tumors. In a study by Salgia and co-workers (32), the levels of CEA and CA125 from 216 patients with newly diagnosed NSCLC were correlated with stage, histopathology, and response to chemotherapy. CEA and CA125 levels were shown to be lower in patients with early-stage disease as compared to patients with unresectable or metastatic disease. CEA levels were significantly higher among patients with adenocarcinoma, while

Table 9 Micrometastases in peripheral blood of SCLC patients

Target	Stage	Method	Detection rate	Sensitivity	Specificity	Prognostic significance	Author
CK 19	LD	RT-PCR	4/15 (27%)	n.a.	98.4%	n.a.	61
NMB-R	LD/ED	RT-PCR	14/44 (32%)	n.a.	n.a.	n.a.	70
PreProGRP	LD/ED	RT-PCR	13/26 (50%)	n.a.	100%	n.a.	65

n.a., not analyzed.

there was no statistically significant relationship between histology and CA125. There was a statistically significant difference in the CEA and CA125 levels dependent on tumor size. Thirty-seven patients were analyzed for responses to chemotherapy and responders are more likely to have decreases in CEA or CA125.

p53, c-erbB-2, and neuroendocrine markers. Several studies have suggested that NSCLC patients whose tumors have neuroendocrine features may be more responsive to chemotherapy. In addition, increased expression of p53 and c-erbB-2 may confer relative chemotherapy resistance and shortened survival. The Cancer and Leukemia Group B (CALGB) performed a series of studies involving sequential chemotherapy followed by radiation for patients with unresectable stage III NSCLC (28). The objectives of the study were to analyze pathological specimens using immunohistochemistry for p53, c-erbB-2, and the neuroendocrine markers (NE markers) NSE, Leu-7, and CgA to determine if there is a correlation between marker expression and response to the given therapy and survival. In conclusion, the study did not demonstrate that expression of NE markers, p53, and c-erbB-2 was predictive of response to chemotherapy or combined chemotherapy/radiation, or of survival.

Topo IIα, topo IIβ, Ki-67, and MRP. In vitro studies showed a relation between low topoisomerase (topo) IIα expression and resistance to chemotherapy in selected and unselected lung cancer cell lines (46,71). Dingemanns et al. (72) analyzed samples of 38 patients with NSCLC by immunohistochemical staining for topo IIα, topo IIβ, Ki-67, and multi-drug resistance associated protein (MRP). Additional mutation analysis of the *topo IIα* gene was performed. The survival analysis showed that the patients with high topo IIα-expressing tumors had a significantly worse survival compared to patients with low topo IIα-expressing tumors. In conclusion, no relation was observed between expression of topo IIα, topo IIβ, Ki-67, or MRP and response rate. Furthermore, contrary to the experiments with cell lines, worse survival was seen in patients with high topo IIα-expressing tumors.

Response Prediction Markers in SCLC

NSE and LDH. Neuron-specific enolase (NSE) and lactate dehydrogenase (LDH) are serum tumor markers of SCLC. The purpose of the study from Lim et al. (13) was to compare pretreatment serum levels of NSE and LDH for the prediction of response to chemotherapy in SCLC. In addition the use of dipyrimadole-modulated Tc-99m sestamibi (dipyrimadole-Mibi) single photon emission computed tomography (SPECT) was evaluated for its capacity to predict response to chemotherapy in SCLC patients.

The study showed that the change of tumor-to-normal lung ratio (T:NL) after infusion of dipyrimadole was significantly higher in responders compared to nonresponders. Pre-treatment serum levels of NSE and LDH did not correlate with response to chemotherapy. Increase of T:NL after dipyrimadole infusion was a strong negative predictor of chemotherapeutic response

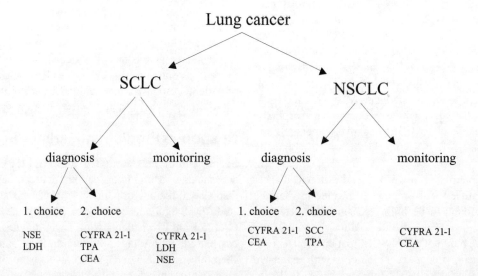

Figure 1 Flow sheet of currently recommended serum tumor markers in lung cancer for diagnosis and treatment at the University of Cologne, Germany.

in SCLC patients, whereas NSE and LDH levels could not predict response.

Topo IIα-, topo IIβ, MDR, p53, p21, BCL-2, Ki-67. Dingemanns et al. (73) evaluated the role of a number of markers for drug resistance, proliferation, and apoptosis in relation to response to chemotherapy and survival in patients with SCLC. Paraffin-embedded samples from primary tumors prior to chemotherapy were analyzed by immunohistochemistry for expression markers implicated in drug resistance: topo IIα, topo IIβ, MDR, p53, p21, BCL-2, and Ki-67. The following factors were found to be predictive for worse survival: high expression levels of topo IIα, Ki-67, and BCL-2. High topo IIβ expression was found to be predictive for lower overall and complete response rates. No relationship between apoptotic pathway markers or MRP and response to chemotherapy was observed.

SUMMARY

Despite tremendous efforts and progress over the past decades in tumor marker research, including the molecular biology of lung cancer, few applications are currently of clinical relevance. A flow chart of clinical useful markers in the daily routine for diagnosis and treatment of lung cancer patients is shown in Figure 1.

With mass application of modern molecular biology techniques, including chip technology, it is, however, expected that within a short period of time the field of clinical tumor marker application will dramatically change and improve.

REFERENCES

1. Guterson B, Ott R. Occult axillary lymph-node micrometastases in breast cancer. Lancet 1990;336:434–435.
2. Merlo A, Herman JG, Mao L, Lee DJ, Gabrielson E, Burger PC, Baylin SB, Sidransky D. 5′CpG island methylation is associated with transcriptional silencing of the tumor suppressor gene p16/CDKN2/MTS1 in human cancers. Nat Med 1995;1:686–692.
3. De Luca A, Pignata S, Casamassimi A, D´Ántonio A, Gridelli C, Rossi A, Cremona F, Pari V, De Matteis A, Normanno N. Detection of circulating tumor cells in carcinoma patients by a novel epidermal growth factor receptor reverse transcription-PCR assay. Clin Cancer Res 2000;6:1439–1444.
4. Vangsted, A. J. Serological tumor markers for small-cell lung cancer and their therapeutic implications. Apmis 1994;102:561–580.
5. Stieber P, Dienemann H, Hasholzner U, Fabricius PG, Schambeck C, Weinzierl M, Poley S, Samtleben W, Hofmann K, Meier W, et. al. Comparison of CYFRA 21-1, TPA, and TPS in lung cancer, urinary bladder cancer, and benign diseases. Int J Biol Markers 1994;9:82–88.
6. Wieskopf B, Demangeat C, Purohit A, Stenger R, Gries P, Kreisman H, Quoix E. Cyfra 21-1 as a biologic marker of non-small-cell lung cancer. Evaluation of sensitivity, specificity, and prognostic role. Chest 1995;108:163–169.
7. Ignacio I, Wistuba AF, Minna JD. Molecular genetics of small-cell lung carcinoma. Sem Oncol 2001;28(2,S4):3–13.
8. Cioffi M, Vietri MT, Gazzerro P, Magnetta R, D'Auria A, Durante A, Nola E, Puca GA, Molinari AM. Serum anti-p53 antibodies in lung cancer: comparison with established tumor markers. Lung Cancer 2001;33:163–169.
9. Nicholson AG, Graham, ANJ, Pezzella F, Agneta G, Goldstraw P, Pastorino U. Does the use of immunohistochemistry to identify micrometastases provide useful information in the staging of node-negative non-small-cell lung cancer? Lung Cancer 1997;18:231–240.
10. Brechot JM, Chevret S, Nataf J, Le Gall C, Fretault J, Chastang C. Diagnostic and prognostic value of Cyfra 21-1 compared with other tumor markers in patients with non-small-cell lung cancer: a prospective study of 116 patients. Eur J Cancer 1997;33:385–391.
11. Poncelet, AJ, Weynand B, Ferdin F, Robert AR, Noirhomme PH. Bone marrow micrometastasis might not be a short-term predictor of survival in early stages non-small-cell lung carcinoma. Eur J Cardio Thorac Surg 2001;20:481–488.
12. Tang X, Khuri FR, Lee JJ, Kemp BL, Liu D, Hong WK, Mao L. Hypermethylation of the death-associated protein (DAP) kinase promoter and aggressiveness in stage I non-small-cell lung cancer. J Natl Cancer Inst 2000;92:1511–1516.
13. Lim SC, Park KO, Kim YC, Na KJ, Song H, Bom HS. Comparison of Tc-99m sestamibi, serum neuron-specific enolase, and lactate dehydrogenase as predictors of response to chemotherapy in small-cell lung cancer. Cancer Biother Radiopharm 2000;14:381–386.
14. Allard WJ, Neaman IE, Elting JJ, Barnett TR, Yoshimura H, Fritsche HA, Yeung KK. Nonspecific cross-reacting antigen 50/90 is elevated in patients with breast, lung, and colon cancer. Cancer Res 1994;54:1227–1234.
15. Strauss GM. Prognostic markers in resectable non-small-cell lung cancer. Hematol Oncol Clin North Am 1997;11:409–434.
16. Goldstein NS, Mani A, Chmielewski G, Welsh R, Pursel S. Immunohistochemically detected micrometastases in peribronchial and mediastinal lymph nodes from patients with T1, N0, M0 pulmonary adenocarcinomas. Am J Surg Pathol 2000;24:274–279.
17. Salerno CT, Frizelle S, Niehans GA, Ho SB, Jakkula M, Kratzke RA, Maddaus MA. Detection of occult micrometastases in non-small-cell lung carcinoma by reverse transcriptase-polymerase chain reaction. Chest 1998;113:1526–1532.
18. Salgia R, Skarin AT. Molecular abnormalities in lung cancer. J Clin Oncol 1998;16(3):1207–1217.
19. Johnson BE, Russell E, Simmons AM. MYC family DNA amplification in 126 tumor cell lines from patients with small-cell lung cancer. J Cell Biochem Suppl 1996;24:210–217.
20. Dobashi K, Sugio K, Osaki T, Oka T, Yasumoto K. Micrometastatic p53-positive cells in the lymph nodes of non-small-cell lung cancer: prognostic significance. J Thorac Cardiovasc Surg 1997;114:339–346.
21. Virmani AK, Rathi A, Sathyanarayana UG, Padar A, Huang CX, Cunningham HT, Farinas AJ, Milchgrub S, Euhus DM, Gilcrease M, Herman J, Minna JD, Gazdar AF. Aberrant methylation if the adenomatous polyposis coli (APC) gene promoter 1A in breast and lung cancer. Clin Cancer Res 2001;7:1998–2204.
22. Kim DH, Nelson HH, Wiencke JK, Christiani DC, Wain JC, Mark EJ, Kelsey KT. Promoter methylation of DAP-kinase: association with advanced stage and non-small-cell lung cancer. Oncogene 2001;20:1765–1770.
23. Wu J, Ohta Y, Minato H, Tsunezuka Y, Oda M, Watanabe Y, Watanabe G. Nodal occult metastasis in patients with peripheral lung adenocarcinomas of 2.0 cm or less in diameter. Ann Thorac Surg 2001;71:1772–1778.
24. Usadel H, Brabender J, Danenberg KD, Jeronimo C, Harden S, Engles PV, Danenberg PV, Yang S, Sidransky D. Quantitative APC-promoter methylation analysis in tumor tissues, serum, and

plasma DNA of patients with lung cancer. Cancer Res 2002; 62(2):371–375.
25. Schneider J, Velcovsky HG, Morr H, Katz N, Neu K, Eigenbrodt E. Comparison of the tumor markers M2-PK, CEA, CYFRA 21-1, NSE, and SCC in the diagnosis of lung cancer. Anticancer Res 2000;20:5053–5058.
26. Zöchbauer-Müller S, Fong KM, Maitra A, Lam S, Geradts J, Ashfaq R, Virmani AK, Milchgrub S, Gazdar AF, Minna JD. 5′CpG island methylation of the FHIT gene is correlated with loss of gene expression in lung and breast cancer. Cancer Res 2001;61:3581–3585.
27. Brabender J, Danenberg KD, Metzger R, Schneider PM, Park J, Salonga D, Hölscher AH, Danenberg PV. Epidermal growth factor receptor and HER2-neu mRNA expression in non-small-cell lung cancer is correlated with survival. Clin Canc Res 2001;7:1850–1855.
28. Graziano SL, Tatum A, Herndon JE, Box J, Memoli V, Green MR, Kern JA. Use of neuroendocrine markers, p53, and HER2 to predict response to chemotherapy in patients with stage III non-small-cell lung cancer: a Cancer and Leukemia Group B study. Lung Cancer 2001;33:115–123.
29. Strauss GM, Skarin AT. Use of tumor markers in lung cancer. Hemat Oncol Clin North Am 1994;8:507–532.
30. Mountain CF. The international system for staging lung cancer. Semin Surg Oncol 2000;18(2):106–115.
31. Anton RC, Coffey DM, Gondo MM, Stephenson MA, Brown RW, Cagle PT. The expression of cyclins D1 and E in predicting short-term survival in squamous cell carcinoma of the lung. Mod Pathol 2000;13(11):1167–1172.
32. Salgia R, Harpole D, Herndon JE 2nd, Pisick E, Elias A, Skarin AT. Role of serum tumor markers CA 125 and CEA in non-small-cell lung cancer. Anticancer Res 2001;21:1241–1246.
33. Hsu C-P, Chen C-Y, Kwang P-C, Miao J, Hsia J-Y Shai S-E. Bone-marrow microinvolvement in non-small-cell lung cancer is not a reliable indicator of tumor recurrence and prognosis. Eur J Surg Oncol 2000;26:691–695.
34. Izbicki JR, Passlick B, Hosch SB, Kubuschock B, Schneider C, Busch C, Knoefel W, Thetter O, Pantel K. Mode of spread in the early phase of lymphatic metastases in non-small-cell lung cancer: significance of nodal micrometastasis. J Thorac Cardiovasc Surg 1996;112:623–630.
35. Esteller M, Sanchez-Cespedes M, Rosell R, Sidransky D, Baylin SB, Herman JG. Detection of aberrant promoter hypermethylation of tumor suppressor genes in serum DNA from non-small-cell lung cancer patients. Cancer Res 1999;59:67–70.
36. Qin J, Chen G, Wang X. The expression of p16 and Rb proteins in 106 cases of lung cancer. Zhonghua Jie He He Hu Xi Za Zhi 2000;23(10):588–590.
37. Schneider PM, Praeuer HW, Stoeltzing O, Boehm J, Manning J, Metzger R, Fink U, Wegerer S, Hoelscher AH, Roth JA. Multiple molecular marker testing (p53, c-Ki-ras, c-erbB-2) improves estimation of prognosis in potentially curative resected non-small-cell lung cancer. Br J Cancer 2000;83:473–479.
38. Pujol JL, Boher JM, Grenier J, Quantin X. Cyfra 21-1, neuron-specific enolase, and prognosis of non-small-cell lung cancer: prospective study in 621 patients. Lung Cancer 2001;31:221–231.
39. Antequere F, Boyes J, Bird A. High levels of de novo methylation and altered chromatin structure at CpG island cell lines. Cell 1990;62:503–514.
40. Maruyama R, Sugio K, Mitsudomi T, Saitoh G, Ishida T, Sugimachi K. Relationship between early recurrence and micrometastases in the lymph nodes of patients with stage I non-small-cell lung cancer. J Thorac Cardiovasc Surg 1997;114:535–543.
41. Baylin SB, Herman JG, Graff JR, Vertino PM, Issa JP. Alterations in DNA methylation: a fundamental aspect of neoplasia. Adv Cancer Res 1998;72:141–196.
42. Yip D, Harper PG. Predictive and prognostic factors in small-cell lung cancer: current status. Lung Cancer 2000;28:173–185.
43. Keilholz U, Wilhauck M, Rimoldi D, Brasseur F, Dummer W, Rass K, de Vries T, Blaheta J, Voit C, Lethe B, Burchill S. Reliability of reverse transcription-polymerase chain reaction (RT-PCR)-based assays for the detection of circulating tumor cells: a quality assurance initiative of the EORTC Melanoma Cooperative Group. Eur J Cancer 1998;34:750–753.
44. Takada M, Kusunoki Y, Masuda N, Matui K, Yana T, Ushijima S. Serum levels of progastrin-releasing peptide (31–98) as a tumor marker of small-cell lung cancer: comparative evaluation with neuron-specific enolase. Br J Cancer 1996;73:1227–1232.
45. Brabender J, Usadel H, Danenberg KD, Metzger R, Schneider PM, Lord RV, Wickramasinghe K, Lum CE, Park JM, Salonga D, Singer J, Sidransky D, Hölscher AH, Meltzer SJ, Danenberg PV. Adenomatous polyposis gene promoter hypermethylation in non-small-cell lung cancer is associated with survival. Oncogene 2001;20:3528–3532.
46. Eijdens EWHM, de Haas M, Timmermann AJ. Reduced topoisomerase II activity in multi-drug-resistant human non-small-cell lung cancer cell lines. Br J Cancer 1995;71:40–47.
47. Belinsky SA, Nikula KJ, Palmisano WA, Michels R, Saccomanno G, Gabrielson E, Baylin SB, Herman JG. Aberrant methylation of p16(INK4a) is an early event in lung cancer and a potential biomarker for early diagnosis. Proc Natl Acad Sci USA 1998;95:11891–11896.
48. Vassilakopoulous T, Troupis T, Sotiropoulou C, Zacharatos P, Katsaounou P, Parthenis D, Noussia O, Papiris S, Kittas C, Roussos C, Zatakynthinos S, Gorgoulis V. Diagnostic and prognostic significance of squamous cell carcinoma antigen in non-small-cell lung cancer. Lung Cancer 2001;32:137–144.
49. Agathanggelou A, Honorio S, Macartney DP, Martinez A, Dallol A, Rader J, Fullwood P, Chauhan A, Walker R, Shaw JA, Hosoe S, Lerma MI, Minna JD, Maher ER, Latif F. Methylation-associated inactivation of RASSF1A from region in 3p21.3 in lung, breast, and ovarian tumors. Oncogene 2001;20:1509–1518.
50. Burbee DG, Forgacs E, Zöchbauer-Müller S, Shivakumar L, Fong K, Gao B, Randle D, Virmani A, Bader S, Sekido Y, Latif F, Milchgrub S, Toyooka S, Gazdar AF, Lerman MI, Zabarovsky E, White M, Mina JD. Epigenetic inactivation of RASSF1A in lung and breast cancers and malignant phenotype suppression. J Natl Cancer Inst 2001;93:691–619.
51. Dammann R, Takahashi T, Pfeifer GP. The CpG island of the novel tumor suppressor gene RASSF1A is intensely methylated in primary small-cell lung carcinomas. Oncogene 2001;20:3563–3567.
52. Virmani AK, Rathi A, Zöchbauer-Müller S, Sacchi N, Fukuyama Y, Bryant D, Maitra A, Heba S, Fong KM, Thunissen F, Minna JD, Gazdar AF. Promoter methylation and silencing of the retinoic acid receptor-b gene in lung carcinomas. J Nat Cancer Inst 2000;92:1303–1307.
53. Chen ZL, Perez S, Holmes EC, Wang HJ, Coulson WF, Wen DR, and Cochran AJ. Frequency and distribution of occult micrometastases in lymph nodes of patients with non-small-cell lung cancer. J Natl Cancer Inst 1993;85:493–498.
54. Passlick B, Izbicki JR, Kubuschok B, Nathrath W, Thetter O, Pichelmeier U, Schweiberer L, Riethmüller G, Pantel K.

Immunohistochemical assessment of individual tumor cells in lymph nodes of patients with non-small-cell lung cancer. J Clin Oncol 1994;12:1827–1832.
55. Cote RJ, Hawes D, Chaiwun B, Beattie EJ. Detection of occult metastases in lung carcinomas: progress and implication for lung cancer staging. J Surg Oncol 1998;69:265–274.
56. Hashimoto T, Kobayshi Y, Ishikawa Y, Tsuchiya S, Okumura S, Nakagawa K, Tokuchi Y, Hayashi M, Nishida K, Hayashi S, Hayashi J, Tsuchiya E. Prognostic value of genetically diagnosed lymph node micrometatsasis in non-small-cell lung carcinoma cases. Cancer Res 2000;60:6472–6478.
57. Pantel K, Izbicki JR, Angstwurm M, Braun B, Passlick B, Karg O, Thetter O, Riethmüller G. Immunocytological detection of bone marrow micrometastasis in operable non-small-cell lung cancer. Cancer Res 1993;53:1027–1031.
58. Pantel K, Izbicki J, Passlick B, Angstwurm M, Häussinger K, Thetter O, Riethmüller G. Frequent prognostic significance of isolated tumor cells in bone marrow of patients with non-small-cell lung cancer without overt metastases. Lancet 1996;347:649–653.
59. Cote RJ, Beattie EJ, Chaiwun B, Shi S-RS, Harvey J, Chen S-C, Sherrod AE, Groshen S, Taylor TR. Detection of occult metastases in patients with operable lung carcinoma. Ann Surg 1995;222:415–425.
60. Ohgami A, Mitsudomi T, Sugio K, Tsuda T, Oyama T, Nishida K, Osaki T, Yasumoto K. Micrometastatic tumor cells in the bone marrow of patients with non-small-cell lung cancer. Ann. Thorac Surg 1997;64:363–367.
61. Peck K, Sher YP, Shih JY, Roffler SR, Wu CW, Yang PC. Detection and quantification of circulating cancer cells in the peripheral blood of lung cancer patients. Cancer Res 1998;58:2761–2765.
62. Castaldo G, Tomaiuolo R, Sanduzzi A, Bocchino ML, Ponticiello A, Barra E, Vitale D, Bariffi F, Sacchetti L, Salvatore F. Lung cancer metastatic cells detected in blood by reverse transcriptase-polymerase chain reaction and dot-blot analysis. J Clin Oncol 1997;15:3388–3393.
63. Kurusu Y, Yamashita J, Ogawa M. Detection of circulation tumor cells by reverse transcriptase-polymerase chain reaction in patients with resectable non-small-cell lung cancer. Surgery 1999;126:820–826.
64. Bostic PJ, Chatterjee S, Chi DD, Huynh KT, Giuliano AE, Cote R, Hoon DS. Limitations of specific reverse-transcriptase polymerase chain reaction markers in the detection of metastases in the lymph nodes and blood of breast cancer. J Clin Oncol 1998;16:2632–2640.
65. Lacroix J, Becker HD, Worner SM, Rittgen W, Drings P, v Knebel Doeberitz M. Sensitive detection of rare cancer cells in sputum and peripheral blood samples of patients with lung cancer by preProGRP-specific RT-PCR. Int J Cancer 2001;92:1–8.
66. Leonard RCF., Duncan LW, and Hay FG. Immunocytological detection of residual marrow disease at clinical remission predicts metastatic relapse in small-cell lung cancer. Cancer Res 1990;50:6545–6548.
67. Pasini F, Pelosi G, Mostacci R, Santo A, Masotti A, Spagnolli P, Recaldin E, and Cetto GL. Detection at diagnosis of tumor cells in bone marrow aspirates of patients with small-cell lung cancer (SCLC) and clinical correlations. Ann Oncol 1995;6:86–88.
68. Pasini F, Pelosi G, Verlato G., Guidi G, Pavanel F, Tummarello D, Masotti A, and Cetto L. Positive immunostainig with MluC1 of bone marrow aspirates predicts poor outcome in patients with small-cell lung cancer. Ann Oncol 1998;9:181–185.
69. Pelosi G, Pasini F, Pavanel F, Bresaol E, Schiavon I, and Iannucci A. Effects of different immunolabeling techniques on the detection of small-cell lung cancer cells in bone marrow. J Histochem Cytochem 1999;47:1075–1087.
70. Bessho A, Tabata M, Kiura K, Takata I, Nagata T, Fujimoto N, Kunisada K, Ueoka H, Harada M. Detection of occult tumor cells in peripheral blood from patients with small-cell lung cancer by reverse transcriptase-polymerase chain reaction. Anticancer Res 2000;20:1149–1154.
71. Giaccone G, Gazdar AF, Beck H, Zunino F, Capranico G. The multi-drug sensitivity phenotype of human lung cancer cells associated with topoisomerase II expression. Cancer Res 1992;52:1666–1674.
72. Dingemanns AM, van Ark-Otte J, Span S, Scagliotti GV, van der Valk P, Postmus PE, Giaccone G. Topoisomerase IIalpha and other drug resistance markers in advanced non-small-cell lung cancer. Lung Cancer 2001;32:117–128.
73. Dingemanns AM, Witlox MA, Stallaert RA, van der Valk P, Postmus PE, Giaccone G. Expression of DNA topoisomerase IIalpha and topoisomerase IIbeta genes predicts survival and response to chemotherapy in patients with small-cell lung cancer. Clin Cancer Res 1999;5:2048–2058.

Chapter 25

Monoclonal Gammopathies

Ingemar Turesson

Monoclonal gammopathies are disorders characterized by the existence of an immunoglobulin spike in serum and/or urine on protein electrophoresis. They all represent the proliferation of a clone arising from a single plasma cell precursor, and the cells produce a homogeneous (monoclonal) M-protein. Multiple myeloma is the prototype of a monoclonal plasma cell dyscrasia.

Waldenström was first to describe M-spikes in apparently healthy individuals; in 1961 he coined the term *benign monoclonal gammopathy* for this disorder, which is much more common than myeloma. When it became evident that a substantial proportion of these individuals later developed myeloma, the term *monoclonal gammopathy of undetermined significance* (MGUS) was introduced by Kyle and is now universally accepted. Other lymphoproliferative diseases included in this group are Waldenström's macro-globulinemia, AL-amyloidosis, and the heavy-chain diseases. A classification of monoclonal gammopathies is shown in Table 1.

EPIDEMIOLOGY

Multiple myeloma is generally a disease of the elderly, with few cases before 40 years. The median patient age is around 70 years and the incidence increases rapidly with age. It is somewhat more common in men, with a ratio of male/female of about 2:1. There is a wide geographical variation in reported incidence that could probably to a large extent be explained by different levels of case ascertainment. The total number of cases has increased in most western countries during the last decades due to an aging population. The annual age-adjusted incidence (adjusted to standard world population of 35–64 years) in the US from 1983–1987 was 4.7/100,000 in white men and 3.2/100,000 in white women. The incidence was higher in blacks (10.3 and 7.1, respectively) (1). Secular changes with increasing incidence over time have been reported in several studies. Such changes have not been observed in careful examination of well-defined populations from areas with a high level of case ascertainment. In Olmstead County in the US, the annual incidence per 100,000 population remained stable over the period 1945–1990 (5.4 and 2.8 for men and women, respectively, adjusted to the 1950 US population) (2). In Malmo, Sweden, the average annual incidence rate per 100,000 population during the period 1950–1979 was 4.9 for males and 3.7 for females (adjusted to the European age-standardized population) with a small trend for increase in men (3).These studies suggest that the increased incidence observed by others is mainly explained by higher levels of case ascertainment, especially among the elderly, and is perceived rather than real.

ETIOLOGY

The cause of multiple myeloma remains largely unknown. Associations have been reported with ionizing radiation and with a number of occupational exposures, including asbestos, benzene, pesticides, paints, and solvents, but the associations are weak and the results not consistent (1). Two studies of survivors of the atomic bomb explosion in Japan have given contradictory results (4). In several studies of agricultural workers, the relative risk has exceeded 1.0 but it has not been possible to identify any precise etiologic factors. Although reports exist of multiple myeloma in first-degree relatives, case control studies have given different results. The strongest factor associated with the risk of developing myeloma is the existence of a monoclonal gammopathy of undetermined significance (MGUS, see below).

BIOLOGY

Multiple myeloma is a malignant tumor of plasma cells, which produce and secrete immunoglobulin molecules. Since all cells derive from one ancestral cell, the secreted immunoglobulin product is homogeneous and can be identified in plasma and/or urine as an M-component or paraprotein. Multiple myeloma is thus a monoclonal malignant counterpart of normal antibody-producing plasma cell clones.

The bulk of tumor cells in multiple myeloma can be identified as plasma cells and proliferate in the bone marrow. Lymphocytes expressing the myeloma protein idiotype have been observed in the peripheral blood, and there is accumulating evidence that earlier stages in the B lymphocyte ontogeny are also involved (5).

In normal plasma cell development, activated mature B cells enter germinal centers in peripheral lymphoid tissues where they are stimulated to somatic mutation of their V genes and selected by antigen to survival or programmed cell death. The plasma blasts then undergo switch of the IgH isotype, migrate to the bone marrow and develop into long-lived plasma

Table 1 Classification of monoclonal gammopathies

I. Malignant monoclonal gammopathies.
   A. Multiple myeloma (IgG, IgA, IgD, IgE, and free light chain)
      1. Smoldering multiple myeloma
      2. Plasma cell leukemia
      3. Nonsecretory myeloma
      4. Osteosclerotic myeloma (POEMS syndrome)
      5. Plasmacytoma
         (a) Solitary plasmacytoma of bone
         (b) Extramedullary plasmacytoma
II. Waldenström's macroglobulinemia
III. Heavy-chain diseases (HCD)
   A. Gamma-HCD
   B. Alpha-HCD
   C. Mu-HCD
IV. Primary amyloidosis (AL)
V. Monoclonal gammopathies of undetermined significance (MGUS)
   A. Benign (IgG, IgA, IgD, IgM, and, rarely, free light chains)
   B. Biclonal gammopathies
   C. Idiopathic Bence Jones proteinuria.

From Kyle RA. Classification and diagnosis of monoclonal gammopathies. In: Rose NR, Friedman H, Fahey JL, eds. Manual of clinical laboratory immunology, 3rd ed. Washington, DC: American Society of Microbiology, 1998;152–167.

cells. Studies of Ig genes in multiple myeloma have demonstrated extensive somatic hypermutation and absence of intraclonal diversity (6). This supports the hypothesis that the cell of origin in multiple myeloma is a post-germinal B lymphocyte that has undergone antigenic selection and clonal expansion. The exact differentiation stage at which the malignant transformation occurs is unknown. The malignant plasma cells, like their normal counterparts, migrate to the bone marrow where they proliferate in close cooperation with accessory cells in the bone marrow microenvironment (7).

Karyotypic abnormalities are very common in multiple myeloma. They are often complex and accumulate during the development of the disease. With the more sensitive fluorescence in situ hybridization (FISH) technique, karyotype abnormalitites are detected in virtually all myeloma patients. Trisomies are the most common finding. Monosomy or deletions of chromosome 13 are of special interest since they occur in about 30% of all myeloma patients by conventional analysis and in 50–60% by FISH analysis and are unfavorable prognostic factors (7,8). The tumor suppressor retinoblastoma (*Rb*) gene is located on chromosome 13 but seems not to be involved since no effect on the expression of Rb protein has been observed in the monoallelic deletions in myeloma. Dysregulation of oncogenes by translocation to the IgH chain locus on chromosome 14 is a common event in other B lymphocyte tumors. The incidence of such translocations in myeloma is lower by conventional cytogenetic analysis but when examined with Southern blot, were observed in the vast majority of myeloma cell lines and fresh myeloma cell samples (7). Three common partner chromosomes and the involved oncogenes have been identified: 11q13 (*bcl1, cyclin D1*), 4p16.3 (*FGFR3* and *MMSET*), and 16q23 (*c-maf*). The translocations were typically into the switch region of the IgH chain gene and were found also in MGUS, indicating that they are early events in the evolution of the disease. Other common gene defects in myeloma are mutations of the *N-* and *K-ras* genes that have been reported in up to 49% of newly diagnosed myeloma cases. A model for the development of myeloma has been proposed where translocations into the IgH gene is an early event preceding clonal expansion, followed by genetic instability, deletions of chromosome 13, and *ras* mutations (7).

CLINICAL PRESENTATION AND ORGAN MANIFESTATIONS

Myeloma Bone Disease and Bone Marrow Microenvironment

Bone pain is the most common presenting feature in multiple myeloma and occurs in up to 90% of all patients. It is typically exacerbated by standing and relieved by resting. The most common localization is the back. Sudden exacerbation of back pain may be elicited by heavy lifting that causes a vertebral compression fracture. When lytic lesions engage the compact bone of the extremities, pathological fractures may also occur there. Headache is not a common symptom in spite of extensive lytic lesions, indicating that the cause of bone pain is probably microfractures elicited by strain on the skeleton by body weight and movement.

The myeloma bone disease is a result of close interaction between myeloma cells and osteoclasts, resulting in increased osteoclast recruitment and activity and increased bone resorption. The interaction involves both cell-to-cell adherence and the secretion of cytokines with osteoclast-activating effects such as tumor necrosis factor β (TNF-β), interleukin-1β (IL-1β), and interleukin 6 (IL-6) (9). Accumulating evidence supports the hypothesis that the interaction is reciprocal, resulting in bone marrow microenvironment stimulation of myeloma growth. Osteoclasts, osteoblasts, and stromal cells are induced to express and secrete myeloma growth-promoting cytokines. IL-6 may be the most important growth factor. It is produced in large amounts in multiple myeloma bone marrow by osteoclasts and stromal cells and its secretion is regulated by the IL1-β secreted by tumor cells. Thus a paracrine loop is established. (7,9).

In earlier stages of the disease, the myeloma cells are dependent on this interaction with the bone marrow stroma for proliferation. In advanced disease they may become IL-6-independent and extramedullary growth occurs. Infection of bone marrow dendritic cells in myeloma with herpes simplex virus 8 (HSV-8) has been reported and may be an alternative source of IL-6, since a homologue of human IL-6 has been identified in the HSV-8 genome (10). Myeloma cells interact also with endothelial cells and bone marrow microvessel density is significantly increased in myeloma bone marrow (11).

Anemia due to bone marrow suppression is common at diagnosis and is aggravated in the course of the disease. It causes weakness and can precipitate symptoms of coronary heart disease and congestive heart failure in the elderly population of myeloma patients. The anemia is usually normochromic and normocytic as in other types of malignancy. Bleeding due to thrombocytopenia is less common as a presenting feature.

Myeloma patients are prone to recurrent infections that may be the presenting symptom. The typical case is a bacterial infection of the upper respiratory tract (tonsillitis, sinusitis, bronchopneumonia). A defective humoral immune response reflected by low polyclonal serum immunoglobulin levels is the major factor explaining the increased occurrence of infections and predisposes the patients particularly to infections with encapsulated organisms such as *Streptococcus pneumoniae*. Later in the disease, neutropenia may develop both as a consequence of disease progression and from cytotoxic treatment, and it influences the infectious panorama. Less common presenting symptoms are caused by hypercalcemia, renal failure, spinal cord compression, hyperviscosity, and amyloidosis. In the course of the disease these complications occur with varying frequency.

Hypercalcemia has been reported to occur in 30% of myeloma patients some time during the disease. The primary event is bone degradation, but hypercalcemia may occur also in the absence of extensive bone lesions. The clinical picture is varied. Gastrointestinal symptoms include constipation, nausea, and vomiting. In persons with rapidly rising serum calcium levels, neurological symptoms may develop: drowsiness, lethargy, and coma. The hypercalcemic state causes polyuria and dehydration and can precipitate renal failure.

Impaired renal function occurs in about 50% of all myeloma patients some time in the course of the disease and is a very common finding at diagnosis (12). It is usually asymptomatic at this stage but acute or chronic renal failure may be a presenting symptom. Toxic effects of monoclonal light chains (Bence Jones protein) is the single most important factor causing tubular damage with atrophy and interstitial fibrosis. Free light chains are filtered at the glomerulus, reabsorbed, and catabolized by proximal tubules, and excess chains are secreted in the urine. Some patients may secrete large amounts of Bence Jones protein without renal damage; it is an unresolved question as to why some light chains are nephrotoxic and others not. In acute renal failure, tubules may be obstructed by large casts containing Bence Jones protein. Other less common forms of renal disease are glomerulonephritis with light chain depositions in the glomeruli, and nephrotic syndrome mostly associated with amyloidosis.

Spinal cord compression is an unusual but disastrous complication of myeloma. Careful examination has revealed that up to 12% of myeloma patients present with compressive symptoms (13). Radiating radicular back pain, weakness of lower extremities, and loss of sphincter control are signals that should lead to prompt diagnostic and therapeutic action to avoid permananent paraparesis.

Hyperviscosity develops in less than 10% of patients with myeloma as compared to 30–50% in Waldenström's macroglobulinemia, and is associated with very high levels of the M-protein. It is more common in IgA and IgG3 myeloma due to a greater tendency of these immunoglobins to form polymers. Hemorrhages from the skin and mucuous membranes, disturbance of vision, headache, and impairment of cerebral function are the most common symptoms.

In AL-amyloidosis, immunoglobulin light chains or fragments of them are deposited in the tissues of various organs in a characteristic, abnormal fibrillar form. This complication occurs in myeloma, but in most cases the underlying disease is a monoclonal gammopathy not fulfilling the diagnostic criteria of myeloma. The clinical picture, diagnosis, and treatment are described in a separate section.

Neuropathy is a rather uncommon complication in multiple myeloma and more often associated with Waldenström's macroglobulinemia or MGUS. In the POEMS syndrome, a progressive polyneuropathy is associated with a monoclonal gammopathy and osteosclerotic bone lesions, organomegaly, and endocrine disturbances (14).

Diagnosis

The diagnosis of multiple myeloma is based on the demonstration of a monoclonal immunoglobulin protein in plasma and/or urine, infiltration of plasma cells in the bone marrow, and typical lytic bone lesions on x-ray of the skeleton.

M-protein—a tumor marker of multiple myeloma. The M-component produced by the myeloma cells is unique among tumor markers since it is not produced or expressed by other cells at any stage of development, and it can be used for diagnosis as well as monitoring of disease during treatment. However, M-components are also seen in other monoclonal plasma cell proliferations, ranging from potentially benign conditions such as monoclonal gammopathy of undetermined significance (MGUS) to malignant tumors (solitary and extramedullary plasmocytomas, Waldenström's macroglobulinemia, heavy chain diseases, and primary amyloidosis) (see Table 1). Additional diagnostic procedures are thus required to differentiate among these conditions.

The M-protein is an immunoglobulin molecule with two identical heavy and two identical light polypeptide chains. Each chain has a constant (H) and a variable (V) part and a hinge (H) region connecting these. There are five heavy chains designated γ, α, μ, δ, and ε that determine the immungloblin class (G, A, M, D, and E respectively). IgG can be further divided into four subclasses and IgA into two. There are two types of light chains, κ and λ. Each immunoglobulin molecule consists of one type of heavy and one type of light chain, which are joined by a disulfide bridge.

In normal plasma cells there is a slight excess synthesis of light chains that are secreted as free light chains and can be detected in small amounts in serum. The variable parts of the heavy and light chain determine the antigen-binding site. Three regions, called hypervariable, are specifically responsible for forming the antigen-binding site, which is unique for all immunoglobulin molecules synthesized by one clone of plasma cells; this has been named the idiotype. This confers an identical electrical charge and is the basis for detection of M-protein with electrophoresis. The term isotype is used for the antigenic determinants on the constant part of the heavy chain and light chains and are present in all normal individuals.

The catabolic rate differs markedly between the different Ig classes, being considerably higher in IgA and IgG3 than in the other subclasses of IgG. The catabolism of IgG is concentration-dependent and more rapid in high serum levels of IgG. These differences may be relevant when M-protein concentrations are used to monitor changes in tumor cell burden. The characterization and metabolism of immunogloblins was recently reviewed (15).

The genes encoding the Ig chains are located on chromosome 14 (heavy chain), 2 (κ), and 22 (λ). The heavy chain gene contains variable (VH), diversity (DH), joining (JH), and constant (CH) gene segments; the light chain genes lack the joining segments but contain the other regions. In germline DNA these segments are not contiguous but separated. In the development of the B cell a sequential and ordered rearrangement of these genes occurs. In the heavy chain gene, D and J segments are first joined followed by V and C segments (Figure 1). Rearrangement of the heavy chain gene precedes that of light chain genes, and κ is rearranged before λ genes (16). After VDJH combination, the immunoglobulin chain class can switch from μ, δ to α and γ, occurring by deletion of segments in the switch region between JH and CH regions. VH and VL genes are divided into families. The rearrangement of the Ig gene segments results in the expression of immunoglobulin molecules on the membrane of virgin B lymphocytes. After contact with antigen, antibody diversity is generated by a process called somatic mutation that takes place in the germinal centers of peripheral lymphoid tissues. In this process cells are selected to survival or programmed cell death according to their affinity to the relevant antigen (17). Site mutations occur preferentially in a part of the heavy chain variable gene segments called the third complementary region (CDR III). The unique sequence of this region can be used for detecting monoclonality and residual cells in B cell maligancies by polymerase chain reaction (PCR)-based techniques (18).

Distribution of M-protein on Ig classes. In monoclonal gammopathy the distribution of M-proteins on Ig classes roughly reflects serum levels, and the number of plasma cells synthesizing them, in normal individuals. In a large series from the Mayo Clinic, 73% were IgG, 14% IgM, 11% IgA, and very few IgD or IgE. Sixty-two percent were of the κ type and 38% λ (19). There is some correlation between isotype and disease—IgM being very rare in myeloma but common in lymphoma, and λ being more common than κ in AL-amyloidosis. An excess synthesis of light chains is common in myeloma, and in about 20% of multiple myeloma cases the capacity to synthesize heavy chains is lost and only light chains are produced. Due to their lower molecular mass (22,000 Daltons), these undergo renal glomerular filtration, tubular reabsorption, and catabolism. When the capacity of the tubular cells is exceeded, light chains are secreted in the urine. Consequently examination of both serum and urine is required. In 2–3% of myeloma patients, no M-protein can be detected—this is termed non-secretory myeloma. In the majority of these cases, the monoclonal protein is located in the cytoplasm of the myeloma cells but not secreted. The distribution of M-protein on Ig classes in myeloma is shown in Table 2 (20).

High-resolution agarose gel electrophoresis is the best method to screen for M-components in serum. The M-protein is visible as a narrow band and the detection limit is about 1 g/L. Alternatively, capillary zone electrophoresis, which measures protein absorbance on-line and does not require protein staining, can be used (Figure 2). The immunoglobulin nature of the band and the heavy and light chain type is determined by immunofixation with antisera against heavy and light chains. In capillary zone electrophoresis this can also be obtained by immunosubtraction that might be less sensitive, however, in small bands (20,21). M-proteins in the urine are detected by the same methods. They usually consist of light chains only, but small amounts of complete Ig molecules may be filtrated in patients with glomerular disease.

The protein analysis should also include a quantification of the M-protein and the polyclonal immunoglobulin levels. Immune nephelometry and immune turbidimetry with antisera against the constant part of heavy and light Ig chains are satisfactory and reproducible methods and are widely used. Standardized antisera and other reagents and continuous quality control are mandatory. It is important that serum with high M-protein concentration is diluted so as to fall within the antigen-antibody assay range of the system. Densitometry of protein-stained agarose gel electrophoresis is an alternative method for quantification, but the results are not always in good accordance with immunological determinations. In IgG myeloma, an attempt should always be made to determine the concentration of the M-protein after subtraction of polyclonal IgG. This can be done by visual estimation of the polyclonal background in the agarose gel or by the use of densitometry (21). An analysis of a 24-hour specimen of urine should always

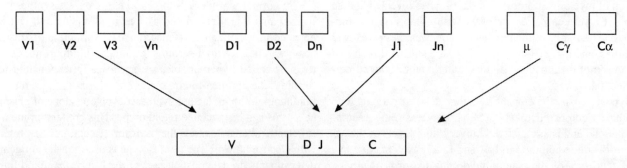

Figure 1 The immunoglobulin heavy chain gene is composed of four different segments. In the first DNA rearrangement, unique V, D, and J segments are joined, followed by joining to CH segments. The resulting gene is transcribed into messenger RNA and then translated into protein.

Table 2 Distribution (in percent) of monoclonal serum proteins in myeloma

Protein	St Bart's Hospital 1980–92 (n = 156)[a]	Mayo Clinic 1982–87 (n = 580)[b]
IgG	57	50
IgA	21	21
Light chain	18	17
IgD	1	2
Non secretory	2	9

[a] UK data: Malpas 1994.
[b] USA data: Kyle 1990.
From Malpas JS. Multiple myeloma: clinical presentation and diagnosis. In: Malpas JS, Bergsagel DE, Kyle R, Anderson K, eds. Myeloma: biology and management. Oxford: Oxford University Press, 1998;150–186.

be included to detect free light chains. Normal urine contains <10 mg/L of free light κ or λ chains. Quantitation of free light chains in serum, which may better reflect the synthetic rate, requires the use of antisera that detect determinants exposed only on free light chains. Such antisera have been raised but have not yet been widely tested (22). M-proteins with cryoglobulin qualities represent a special problem—in these cases the serum sample must be handled and analyzed at 37 °C.

The serum concentration of the M-protein is determined by the number of cells in the clone, the synthetic rate per cell, and the fractional catabolic rate. The synthetic rate differs markedly between different clones but remains relatively stable in each clone during the disease. The catabolic rate differs between Ig classes and among various subclasses in IgG. This makes it difficult to compare tumor cell burden in different myeloma patients from serum levels of the M-protein, but allows accurate estimations of changes in tumor cell burden in the individual patient. Determinations of M-protein levels in serum and/or urine are very helpful to monitor the effect of treatment, define response, and detect relapse. A decrease of the M-protein level in serum to <50% of the pretreatment level, and in urine to <0.2 g/24 hours, are generally accepted as criteria for a partial response (PR), while a complete response (CR) requires that no M-protein be detected with conventional methods and that the bone marrow contain less than 5% plasma cells. In responding patients, the M-protein level tends to stabilize in spite of further treatment, indicating that the disease has entered a stable plateau phase, which is often defined as <10% variation of M-protein level in three determinations at monthly intervals.

The achievement of a plateau phase is a favorable prognostic sign of greater significance than the degree of response. It can last for several years without cytotoxic treatment. Increasing M-protein levels signal relapse and need for reinitiation of therapy. In relapses, the doubling time of the M-protein level tends to be shorter, indicating a higher proliferative rate. In a few cases the protein synthetic rate of the M-protein may decrease in the terminal phase, which makes interpretation more difficult (23).

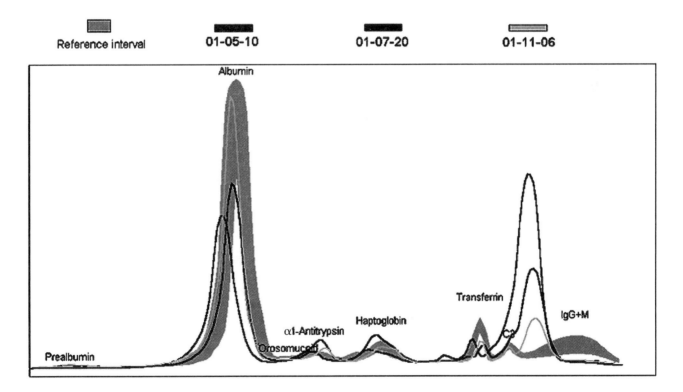

Figure 2 Graphical presentation of absorbance curves for samples from a patient with an IgE myeloma obtained before (brown curve), and 10 (blue curve) and 25 weeks (green curve) after, initiation of treatment with melphalan and prednisone. The yellow shaded area represents the normal reference interval for protein concentrations. The figure was obtained courtesy of Associate Professor Joyce Carlson, Department of Clinical Chemistry, Malmö University Hospital, Malmö, Sweden. **Color representation of figure appears on Color Plate 2.**

In myeloma patients who achieve a complete remission, there is a need to quantify M-protein levels below the detection limit with conventional methods. The use of anti-idiotypic antisera directed against the hypervariable part of the M-protein increases the sensitivity by 2–3 logs. The sensitivity could be further increased by the use of specific peptide mimotopes recognizing individual M-proteins and selected with phage display technology (24). An alternative is to trace residual myeloma cells in the bone marrow and/or blood. These techniques are more sensitive and avoid problems from changes in the protein synthetic rate but are open to sampling errors. Allele-specific PCR assay using probes directed to the CDR III region (25) is the most sensitive method and is estimated to detect one malignant B cell in 10^5–10^6 cells. Alternatively, flow cytometry has been used to identify myeloma cells with an aberrant phenotype, established at diagnosis (26).

Bone Marrow Biopsy. Multiple myeloma is a systemic disease and tumor cell infiltration is widespread in all hematopoetic bone marrow at presentation in most cases. May-Grunwald Giemsa-stained smears from aspiration biopsy from the sternum or the iliac crest are usually sufficient and the presence of at least 10% plasma cells is generally accepted as a diagnostic criterion.

The distribution of tumor cells in the bone marrow is not uniform and cases with fewer than 10% plasma cells do occur. Atypical morphology is common in myeloma and supports the diagnosis in these cases; morphologies include muclear/cytoplasmic asynchrony, nuclear abnormalities, and variations in size (27,28) (Figure 3). The growth pattern of the myeloma cells can be studied in a core biopsy. Both plasma cell morphology and growth pattern have been reported to add prognostic information (28,29). Monoclonality of the plasma cells can be demonstrated with antisera to heavy and light chains. This is helpful to confirm the diagnosis in non-secretory myelomas and solitary plasmocytomas that have no detectable M-protein.

Multiple myeloma is a slowly growing tumor. The labeling index (LI) can be determined by incubating tumor cells with DNA precursors such as tritiated thymidine or bromodeoxyuridine. Cells that are able to incorporate the DNA precursor are identified by autroradiography or staining with fluorescent antibodies to bromodeoxyuridine. The proportion of plasma cells in the S phase is only 1–3% in the majority of patients. LI is helpful to distinguish myeloma from MGUS, which is characterized by still lower LI (<1%) (30).

Karyotype analysis of myeloma cells is of limited diagnostic significance but adds important prognostic information. This subject has been dealt with in a previous section.

Radiography. Several imaging techniques have been used to study the bone lesions in myeloma. Conventional plain radiographs, scintigraphy with bone-seeking isotopes such as technicium-99, and computed tomography (CT) all show the bone reaction to the myeloma. Of these, scintigraphy has been repeatedly demonstrated to be less sensitive. This technique detects areas of new bone formation, while myeloma bone disease is characterized by bone resorption with impaired bone formation. CT is more sensitive than plain radiographs and may help to confirm the diagnosis in cases with bone pain and normal radiographs. It can also detect tumor extension into soft tissue (31).

In the majority of myeloma patients, conventional radiographs are sufficient and must still be considered the method of choice. The typical radiographic appearance is multiple punched-out lytic lesions without reactive sclerotic margins. They are most commonly seen in the skull but may engage also the ribs, vertebral column, pelvis, and bones of upper and lower extremities. The lesions erode the compact bone and can cause pathological fractures, observed in up to 50% of all cases. The most common localization is the vertebral column where compression fractures occur with high frequency. In some patients osteoporosis is the only manifestation and the diagnosis in these cases can be mistaken for senile osteoporosis if protein electrophoresis is not performed.

In a small percentage of myeloma patients the bone lesions are sclerotic. This is seen in the rare multisystemic syndrome POEMS, characterized by polyneuropathy, organomegaly, endocrinopathy, M-proteins, and skin changes (14).

Magnetic resonance imaging differs from the other techniques by visualizing the bone marrow directly and is considerably more sensitive in detecting bone marrow abnormalities. Small lytic foci that escape detection with the other techniques can thus be demonstrated. This may be helpful especially in those cases where plain radiographs show only osteoporosis. However plain radiographs show bony details better and MRI currently must be considered a complementary method where radiography is normal (32). MR imaging is also the method of choice to demonstrate spinal cord compression from tumor masses, a frequent complication of myeloma involving the spine that requires rapid therapeutic intervention.

Diagnostic Criteria. M-components are not unique for multiple myeloma and differentiation from other malignant plasma cell proliferations and MGUS is thus important. Diagnosis relies partially on arbitrary criteria and often requires observation of the patient for some time. Several lists of criteria have been published and although they differ only in details, there are no universally accepted minimal diagnostic

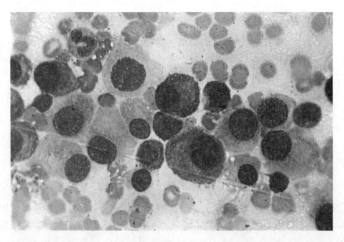

Figure 3 Bone marrow smear from a patient with multiple myeloma showing atypical plasma cells with size variation and asynchronous maturation of nucleus and cytoplasm with large nucleoli and loose chromatin structure.

criteria for myeloma. One representative example is presented in Table 3 (33). The term *smoldering myeloma* has been suggested for a group of patients with a stable disease that may not need treatment for several years. A number of staging systems have been developed with the intent of measuring tumor burden. The Durie/Salmon staging system uses hemoglobin concentration, calcium level, serum and urine M-protein levels, bone lesions, and serum creatinine level to define three stages (34). It has been widely used but better prognostic classifications have now been developed.

A consensus group was recently formed at the VIIIth International Myeloma Workshop with the aim of establishing uniform criteria for diagnosis and response to treatment and develop an international prognostic index.

MGUS

The demonstration of an M-protein spike in serum and/or urine on electrophoresis is a prerequisite for the diagnosis of a monoclonal plasma cell proliferation, except for the few cases of non-secretory myeloma (2–3 % of all myeloma cases). When electrophoresis is used for screening, the majority of patients with M-protein have no evidence of multiple myeloma, Waldenström's macroglobulinemia, AL-amyloidosis, or related conditions. For these cases, the term *monoclonal gammopathy of undetermined significance* (MGUS) has been introduced.

In a mass health control study in Sweden, M-protein was found in 64 of 6,995 subjects older than 25 years (0.9 %) (35). M-proteins were rare below the age of 50 and increased rapidly with age. Similar figures were then reported by other authors. In a study using high-resolution agarose gel electrophoresis and immunofixation, the prevalence of M-protein among individuals older than 90 years was 14% (36). In a Mayo Clinic series of 1,149 patients with an M-protein, 63% were classified as MGUS, 14% as myeloma, 4% as smoldering myeloma, and 10% as amyloidosis; the remaining were associated wih other lymphoproliferative diseases or solitary plasmocytoma (19).

Considering the prevalence of MGUS, it is evident that the differentiation from multiple myeloma is an important issue. In addition there is an inherent tendency for transformation of MGUS to myeloma, macroglobulinemia, or AL-amyloidosis with an actuarial rate of the development of these diseases of 16% at 10 years and 40% at 25 years (19). Methods to predict which cases will remain stable and which will progress are thus also important.

Patients with an M-protein spike who do not fulfill the diagnostic criteria for myeloma and have no evidence of other lymhpoproliferative disease are classified as MGUS, but it is evident that there is a grey zone where the arbitrary criteria cannot always distinguish malignant disease and that further differentiation is needed. Patients with myeloma tend to have higher levels of M-protein and β2-microglobulin in serum and lower levels of polyclonal immunoglobulins, but there is considerable overlap. Atypical plasma cell morphology is more common in myeloma. A plasma cell labeling index (PCLI) >1 speaks strongly for active myeloma, but approximtely 40% of myeloma patients have a normal PCLI. The presence of circulating plasma cells in the peripheral blood is also a good marker of active disease but careful examination has revealed circulating clonal cells also in MGUS and smoldering myeloma. An increased number of circulating plasma cells in smoldering myeloma does predict early transformation to active disease (37). Although lytic bone lesions would seem to be a clear-cut sign of myeloma, they may represent metastases of other malignant tumors in a patient with MGUS. Chromosomal abnormalities are common both in MGUS and myeloma (see above) but deletions of chromosome 13 and *ras* mutations seem to be related to evolution into myeloma. The cytokine IL-1β is expressed in the plasma cells in virtually all myeloma cases, 25% of MGUS cases, and not in normal individuals (38). This is an interesting observation since IL-1β is an osteoclast-activating factor, can increase expression of adherence molecules on plasma cells, and can induce paracrine IL-6 production, all important features in the development of myeloma.

In summary, there is no single clinical or biological factor that can clearly distinguish MGUS from myeloma or predict which cases will progress to myeloma. Consequently, careful follow-up with serial measurements of the M-protein and clinical evaluation is the only method useful for identifying those cases. The median duration from detection of an M-protein and development of active disease ranged from four to nine years in the Mayo Clinic series, and a stable level of the M-protein for several years did not exclude later transformation.

Prognostic Factors

The natural history of multiple myeloma is heterogeneous; survival times ranging from a few months to more than ten years. Prognostic classification is thus needed for providing correct information to the patient, for selecting treatment, and for stratification in clinical trials. A great number of biological and clinical characteristics have been reported to influence survival. These were recently reviewed by Rajkumar and Greipp (39) and can be grouped according to whether they reflect tumor burden or high proliferative activity as a sign of intrinsic malignancy. In recent years new prognostic factors have been identified that may be helpful in shedding light on the biology of the disease; these will be dealt with in more detail.

High proliferative activity is associated with a poor prognosis. A high PCLI predicts poor overall and progression-free

Table 3 Diagnostic criteria for multiple myeloma according to The Nordic Myeloma Study Group (NMSG)

A. M-protein IgG >30 g/L, IgA >20 g/L, IgD, or IgE irrespective of level *or* monoclonal light chains in urine >1g/24 hours.
B. M-protein in serum and/or urine in concentrations lower than mentioned above.
C. ≥10% plasma cells in bone marrow aspirate.
D. Lytic bone lesions at radiography.

The diagnosis of myeloma requires a combination of A + C or A + D or B + C + D. The criteria do not include nonsecretory myeloma.

survival and has been demonstrated to give independent prognostic information in multivariate analysis. Serum levels of thymidine kinase also reflect proliferative activity, and high levels indicate poorer prognosis. Plasmablastic morphology based on well-defined morphological criteria was a powerful prognostic factor in a large study from the ECOG. An increased number of circulating plasma cells is associated with poor prognosis.

Cytogenetic abnormalities in multiple myeloma are complex and related to stage, prognosis, and treatment. Deletions of chromosome 13 and abnormalities involving chromosome 11q appear to be particularly unfavorable (8,40). This variable is highly correlated to a high PCLI but in large samples retains independent information. The prognostic implication of translocations into the switch region of the Ig heavy chain gene on chromosome 14 are less clear.

A number of proteins, cytokines, and growth factors that can be measured in serum have been reported to give prognostic information. These include β2-microglobulin, C-reactive protein (CRP), interleukin-6 (IL-6), soluble IL-6-receptor (sIL-6R), hepatocyte growth factor (HGF), hyaluronan (HYA), and vascular endothelial growth factor (VEGF).

β2-microglobulin (β2-M). B2-microglobulin is the constant part of the human MHC (major histocompatibility complex) class I molecules located on the membrane of all nucleated cells. It is a small protein with a molecular mass of 11,800 Daltons. β2-M is shed from the surface into the extracellular space and is eliminated via glomerular filtration with a clearance similar to that of creatinine. The reference range of serum levels has been reported to 0.9–2.5 mg/L. The concentration is increased in renal failure and also in all lymphoproliferative diseases due to increased production. In myeloma there is a high correlation between serum level and tumor burden. A high β2-M serum level is a strong independent unfavorable prognostic factor in myeloma both after conventional chemotherapy and high-dose therapy (41,42).

Interelukin-6 and soluble interelukin-6 receptor. IL-6 is a polypeptide cytokine with multiple effects and plays a central role in the inflammatory response. The human IL-6 cDNA has been sequenced and predicts a protein with a molecular mass of 21 kDa. IL-6 exerts its effect by binding to a cell surface receptor. This consists of an 80-kDa binding molecule (IL-6Ralpha, CD 126) and a 130-kDa signal-transducing molecule (gp 130), which is also used by other cytokines. Binding of IL-6 to its receptor triggers homodimerization of gp 130, which then activates intracellular signaling systems and transcription factors. The IL-6 receptor also exists in a soluble form (sIL-6R) and the complex IL-6/sIL-6R is a more potent activator of gp 130 than IL-6 alone (43).

IL-6 is an essential survival factor for myeloma cells. It acts by preventing apoptosis induced by different stimuli. It is produced by bone marrow stromal cells, osteoblasts, and osteoclasts. The production is strongly enhanced in myeloma bone marrow as a consequence of adherence between myeloma and stromal cells and release of soluble factors such as IL-1β, TNF-α, and VEGF. The IL-6 receptor is expressed on a majority of myeloma cells and they also release the soluble form by prote-olytic degradation of the surface receptor and direct secretion. This results in a vicious cycle, with overproduction of the IL-6/sIL-6Ralpha complex in myeloma bone marrow. Myeloma growth is promoted and bone resorption is increased (43). In advanced cases of myeloma there has also been demonstrated an autocrine production of IL-6 by myeloma cells, making the clone less dependent on the bone marrow microenvironment.

Both IL-6 and sIL-6Ralpha can be measured in serum by immunoassays utilizing recombinant IL-6 and sIL-6Ralpha and monoclonal antibodies against these. Although the overproduction is a local paracrine event, sufficient amounts are released to be detectable in serum. Reported reference levels in healthy individuals vary but are in the range of 10–50 ng/mL for sIL-6R and below 3–10 pg/mL for IL-6. Several studies have reported increased serum levels in myeloma, and high levels were powerful prognostic factors associated with poor survival (44,45). Interestingly there was no significant correlation between serum levels of IL-6 and sIL-6Ralpha, and both were independent prognostic variables in multivariate analysis.

C-reactive protein. C-reactive protein (CRP) is an acute-phase reactant that is produced by hepatocytes on stimulation by IL-6 as part of the inflammatory response. Reported reference serum concentration in healthy individuals is below 5 mg/L. The serum level of CRP reflects the activity of IL-6 and can serve as a good surrogate for measurement of this cytokine. It is a strong prognostic factor associated with poor survival in myeloma (41). Substitution of CRP for IL-6 in a multivariate analysis of prognostic factors only marginally decreased the discriminant power of the model (45).

A number of prognostic systems combining factors with independent information have been proposed (39). Some factors (e.g., PCLI, cytogenetics, IL-6, sIL-6R) are not easily available in clinical practice, and prognostic systems based on simpler clinical and laboratory measures are currently used. In one study, the independent factors readily available (age, World Health Organization performance status, serum Ca, β2M, and CRP) gave excellent separation of prognostic groups (45).

Efforts are underway to establish an international prognostic index for myeloma using both simple and easily available parameters and those that require more advanced laboratory methods.

Treatment

Multiple myeloma is a fatal disease with a median survival of about 30 months, and no curative therapy exists. The goal of treatment is to achieve a response, improve quality of life, and prolong survival. Asymptomatic patients with stable disease do not benefit from early treatment, which should be deferred (46). Measurements of serum and urine M-proteins are the best methods for evaluating response. Criteria for partial remission (PR) and complete remission (CR) are described in a previous section. A typical feature of the response is the achievement of a plateau phase (stable response) that is usually defined by <10% variation in M-protein level in three determinations at monthly intervals. Continued cytotoxic therapy in this situation does not prolong survival and should not be given. The mechanism behind this plateau phenomenon, which may last for several years, is unclear but suggests establishment of a control mechanism. Eventually the disease relapses and although new responses can be achieved, they are of shorter duration. The disease enters a terminal phase characterized by progressive increase in regrowth rate and pancytopenia (47).

Cytotoxic therapy. Intermittent treatment with melphalan and prednisone (MP) was introduced in the 1960s and is still the recommended treatment for the majority of myeloma patients. The courses are given at 4–6 week intervals and induce a partial response in 50–60 % of patients, but complete remissions are rare and survival has not improved during the three decades that MP has been the standard therapy for myeloma.

Combination chemotherapy was introduced in the 1970s with the intention of improving the quality of response. The VAD regimen, which combines continuous intravenous (i.v.) infusion of vincristine and doxorubicin for four consecutive days with oral high doses of dexamethasone for three four-day periods per month, is the best known. Several other combinations of vincristine (V), BCNU (B), cyclophosphamide (C), melphalan (M), adriamycin (A), prednisone (P), and dexamethasone (D) have been described (VBMCP, VBAP/VMCP, VCAD, VAMP). Although higher response rates can be achieved by combination therapy as compared to MP, a careful meta-analysis of 6,633 patients from 27 studies demonstrated no survival benefit from combination therapy (48). High doses of corticosteroids are part of most combination regimens and may be the most important constituent of these. In fact, dexamethasone alone is an effective agent in myeloma and can induce remissions with almost the same frequency as VAD. It is therefore an attractive therapeutic option in patients with bone marrow toxicity from cytotoxic therapy (47).

Interferon-α (IFN) is active as a single agent in myeloma but the response rate is lower than with MP. A prolongation of remission duration from IFN given during the plateau phase was reported in several studies and confirmed in a meta-analysis of 4,012 patients from 24 trials (33,49). This overview also reported a modest improvement in survival of four months, which should be weighed against side effects that can be considerable.

In 1983 McElvain et al. reported high response rates using higher doses of melphalan. This treatment was complicated by pronounced bone marrow toxicity. Introduction of techniques for mobilization and harvest of hematopoetic stem cells have since then been introduced and allowed treatment with high doses of melphalan with autologous stem cell support and acceptable toxicity at least in younger patients (below 60–65 years). High response rates and improved survival were reported early by several groups, and high-dose treatment has been widely used although comparative studies have been lacking. A randomized study from the French Myeloma Group compared combination therapy (VMCP/VBAP) with high-dose melphalan (200 mg/m^2) and total body irradiation (TBI) in newly diagnosed patients younger than 60 years (50). Autologous stem cells from bone marrow were used as support. A significant prolongation of survival was observed (five-year survival rates of 28 and 52% respectively). The Nordic Myeloma Study Group compared the outcome of 274 patients below the age of 60 years treated with melphalan (200 mg/m^2) with an historical group of 274 patients conventionally treated in a population-based study with a very high inclusion rate (51). Survival was significantly improved in the high-dose group (risk ratio 1.62; p <0.001). In this study, autologous stem cells were mobilized and harvested from the peripheral blood, which is more convenient and allows more rapid bone marrow recovery. Intensification of treatment by tandem transplantation may improve results (52). No study, however, has demonstrated a plateau phase of the survival curve and the treatment is not curative. Since relapses may be caused by tumor cells contaminating the stem cell harvests, efforts have been made to improve results by in vitro purging, thus far without success.

Allogeneic stem cell transplantation has been performed in a limited number of patients. The largest published series is from the European Bone Marrow Transplantation Group (EBMT) (53). This procedure was complicated by a high treatment-related toxicity, and a mortality of 40% was observed. Although transplantation-related mortality has decreased over the years, it is still about 30%, and cure has not been unequivocally proven. A graft vs. myeloma effect has been demonstrated, and studies that evaluate conditioning regimens with reduced intensity and/or donor lymphocyte transfusions in relapse are ongoing.

Non-cytotoxic therapy. Thalidomide is an anti-angiogenic agent that was recently reported to produce responses in one-third of patients with refractory, advanced myeloma. In addition to inhibiting myeloma bone marrow angiogenesis, this drug has multiple effects on myeloma cell adhesion and myeloma-triggered production of IL-6 and TNF-α, growth factors for myeloma cells. It can also induce apoptosis directly in myeloma cells. A response rate of about 30% in refractory or relapsed cases has been confirmed in several studies (54).Thalidomide is not toxic to the bone marrow. Combination of thalidomide and cytotoxic agents and/or coroticosteroids are now tested in ongoing randomized trials.

A number of new drugs with anti-myeloma effects *in vitro* will be tested in clinical trials in the nearest future. They include immunomodulatory drugs (analogs of thalidomide), proteasome inhibitors that act by inhibition of the transcription factor NF-kB, and arsenic trioxide. Another future development is vaccination strategies using idiotype vaccine or DNA vaccines.

Bisphosphonates are drugs with potent inhibitory effects on osteoclast-mediated bone resorption. They are very effective in the treatment of myeloma-associated hypercalcemia when given as an i.v. infusion. The nitrogen-containing bisphosphonates (pamidronate, risedronate, ibandronate, and zoledronate) act by inhibition of the mevalonate pathway in osteoclasts and tumor cells and are more potent than etidronate and clodronate. In a randomized, placebo-controlled study, intermittent i.v. infusion of pamidronate, 90 mg over four-week intervals, was reported to delay and reduce skeletal complications in myeloma patients (55). Studies using oral bisphosphonate preparations have reported similar results but with smaller and not always significant differences that may be due to the low absorption of these drugs. By decreasing production of cytokines such as IL-6 by osteoclasts as well as by directly inducing apoptosis of myeloma cells, bisphosphonates may also have an anti-tumoral effect in myeloma. A survival benefit in a subgroup of patients has been reported (55).

Management of Complications

Erythropoetin was reported in a pilot study to improve anemia in 11/13 myeloma patients with a normal renal function. These results have then been confirmed in several randomized studies demonstrating a response rate of 50–60% (56).

In acute renal failure, plasmapheresis is an efficient method to remove circulating light immunoglobulin chains and decrease the load on the kidney, but the clinical benefit from this treatment in recovering renal function has been only modest. Plasmapheresis may also be a valuable tool in patients with hyperviscosity syndrome.

Spinal cord compression is an acute complication that requires prompt therapeutic intervention to avoid permanent paresis. Radiotherapy and dexamethasone are the recommended treatment with results not inferior to surgical laminectomy. In some cases surgery may be neccessary to stabilize the spine.

Bone pain is the dominating symptom in myeloma and effective pharmacological treatment of this is mandatory. Opioid analgesics are usually necessary and should be prescribed liberally. Slow-release oral preparations of morphine, transdermal administration of phentanyl, and continuous i.v. infusion of morphine with aid of a portable pump are options.

Radiotherapy

Myeloma cells are usually very sensitive to irradiation and local radiotherapy of painful bone lesions is effective in reducing pain. Radiotherapy with curative intent is the cardinal method for treatment of solitary skeletal plasmacytoma or extramedullary plasmacytoma. Total body irradiation has been used by many groups as part of the conditioning treatment before autologous or allogeneic stem cell support while others have avoided this procedure because of the increased toxicity.

WALDENSTÖM´S MACROGLOBULINEMIA

In 1944 Jan Waldenström published a paper describing two patients with oronasal bleeding, elevated sedimentation rate, lymphadenopathy, hyperviscosity, and lymphoid infiltration of the bone marrow. The hyperviscosity was caused by a high-molecular-weight globulin that was later identified as a monoclonal IgM. He postulated a new syndrome that was later named after him. Waldenström's macroglobulinemia (WM) is a malignant lymphoma, and in the revised European-American classification of lymphoid neoplasms it is included in the group of lymhpo-plasmacytic lymphoma. The characteristic features of the disease are, however, caused by the presence of the high-molecular-weight macroglobulin that determines most of the clinical manifestations. The M-protein in WM is not only a tumor marker but contributes considerably to the morbidity of the disease.

Epidemiology and Etiology

WM is a rare disease with an age-adjusted annual incidence of $0.34/10^5$ for men and $0.17/10^5$ for women (57). As in myeloma the incidence increases rapidly with age, but in contrast to myeloma the disease is more common in whites than in blacks. Incidence figures are, however, uncertain, since the distinction of macroglobulinemia from other lymphoproliferative diseases and MGUS is only arbitrary. The cause of macroglobulinemia remains largely unknown. No precise environmental factors have been identified.

Biology

Biologically, WM has many similarities to multiple myeloma (MM). Both are monoclonal B cell malignancies and the cells secrete a homogeneous M-protein. Accumulating data support the hypothesis that the cell of origin, as in myeloma, is a postgerminal center B cell which has undergone somatic mutation and antigen selection.

Some fundamental differences exist. In contrast to myeloma, the B cell clone in WM is characterized by intraclonal differentiation and maturation from small lymphocytes through intermediate stages to mature plasma cells (58). The monoclonal IgM is expressed on the cell membrane in the earlier maturation stages and secreted in the later stages. Several other B cell antigens are expressed (CD19, CD20, CD22, CD79a) but not CD5 (59). The tissue distribution is different and although bone marrow is always involved in WM, the clone is not dependent on the bone marrow microenvironment for proliferation but grows equally well in peripheral lymphoid organs. Circulating monoclonal B lymphocytes expressing the surface IgM can be demonstrated by flow cytometry and these cells can undergo spontaneous maturation in vitro to IgM-secreting plasma cells (60). Abnormal karyotypes have been observed regularly in WM but the number of patients examined are relatively few and none of the abnormalities is specific (reviewed in 61).

Clinical Presentation and Organ Manifestations

The presenting features of WM are heterogeneous. Some of them are caused by infiltration of the neoplastic cells into the bone marrow and peripheral lymphoid tissues and are shared with other types of disseminated lymphoma: fatigue, anorexia, weight loss, night sweats, and symptoms of bone marrow failure. Enlargement of the liver, spleen, and peripheral lymph nodes is common but not seen in all patients. Another set of manifestations is caused by biological effects of the M-protein. These are determined by physicochemical properties of the M-protein, protein-protein interactions involving the M-protein, and auto-antibody activity of the macroglobulin. Several reviews of the clinical manifestations of WM have ben published recently (59,62–64).

Hyperviscosity is the most common complication related to the M-protein. The clinical picture and complex pathogenetic mechanisms were recently reviewed (65). The pentameric IgM molecule has a tendency to form aggregates, bind water, and increase red cell aggregation, impairing blood flow. The plasma volume is expanded. Common symptoms are headache, vertigo, blurred vision, mucosal bleeding, and heart failure. There is a rough correlation between serum IgM level and symptoms, hyperviscosity being relatively rare with IgM concentrations below 50 g/L, but there is considerable interindividual variation. Ophthalmoscopy shows a characteristic picture with distended veins and retinal bleeding.

In cryoglobulinemia type I the M-protein precipitates at low temperatures due to physicochemical properties that are poorly understood. This results in impaired blood flow in small vessels, preferentially in areas with lower body temperature. Common symptoms are Raynaud's phenomenon; acrocyanosis and necrosis of fingers, toes, and nose tip; and leg ulcers.

Cryoglobulinemia type II is also characterized by precipitation at low temperature, but the nature of the precipitates and the clinical manifestations are different. In this syndrome the monoclonal IgM has antibody activity against immunoglobulin (rheumatoid factor activity), and the resulting immune complexes increase rapidly in size at low temperature. The consequence is an immune complex-mediated vasculitis of small vessels aggravated by exposure to cold. The most serious complication is a membranoproliferative glomerulonephritis that may develop to renal failure.

Auto-antibody activity of the monoclonal IgM causes two other common manifestations of WM: peripheral neuropathy and cold agglutinin syndrome. Clinical evidence of peripheral neuropathy was reported in 14% in a large consecutive series of patients with WM (62). The common form is a distal symmetric demyelinating neuropathy affecting both sensory and motor functions. In approximately half of the patients with neuropathy, antibody activity was demonstrated against a myelin-associated glycoprotein (MAG), but other auto-antibody activities against constituents of nerve tissue have been reported.

Cold agglutinin disease is caused by monoclonal IgM with antibody activity against red cell antigens, mainly with I/i specificity resulting in a mild chronic hemolytic anemia that can be aggravated by exposure to cold. It was reported in 4% of patients (62). Anemia in WM is more often caused by bone marrow infiltration and dilution due to the expanded plasma volume. Mucosal bleeding and purpura are common manifestations in WM. The symptoms are related to hyperviscosity but protein/protein interactions of the macroglobulin also play an important role. High levels of IgM coat platelets and impair both adhesion and aggregation. In addition, monoclonal IgM interacts with clotting factors, disturbing the coagulation cascade (63).

Less common manifestations of WM are caused by lymphoid infiltration of other organs. They include pulmonary nodules and pleural effusions, urticarial skin lesions, and rarely, lytic bone lesions. Monoclonal IgM may be deposited in the lamina propria of the small intestine and cause malabsorption. Light immunoglobulin chain amyloidosis is a rare complication of WM.

Diagnosis

The diagnosis of WM requires the demonstration of a monoclonal IgM in serum and bone marrow infiltration with lymphocytes, plasmacytoid cells, and mature plasma cells. The techniques for identification and quantitation of the M-protein have been discussed in an earlier section. If the monoclonal IgM has cryoglobulin properties, it is essential that blood is collected and separated at 37 °C. Free light chains (Bence Jones protein) in the urine are a common finding, but this seldom amounts to more than 1 g/24 hours. A core biopsy of bone marrow is necessary since aspiration biopsy often results in "dry tap." A lymph node biopsy can support the diagnosis when lymphadenopathy is present. There are no uniform diagnostic criteria for WM. The extent of bone marrow infiltration and the size of the M-protein have been used as criteria to distinguish WM from other lymphoproliferative diseases and MGUS, but the cutoff values reported show considerable variation. A serum IgM concentration of >30 g/L was used as a criterion in a large series from the Mayo Clinic. Patients with smaller IgM spikes may, however, require treatment due to extensive bone marrow infiltration of lymphoplasmacytic lymphoma and/or constitutional symptoms. They have a similar clinical course and survival and differ only with respect to the size of the M-protein and the absence of hyperviscosity (66) . Patients with small IgM spikes and no overt signs of lymphoma are classified as MGUS, but symptoms related to the biological effect of the macroglobulin such as polyneuropathy and cold agglutinin disease have also been described in this group. The inherent tendency for MGUS to transform into malignant lymphoproliferative disease was discussed in a previous section. In a long-term follow-up of 242 patients with MGUS of the IgM type, 17% developed a serious disease (WM, other lymphoma, amyloidosis, or chronic lymhpocytic leukemia) (66).

Treatment and Prognosis

The clinical course of WM is heterogeneous. The median survival reported is influenced by the diagnostic criteria used but has in most series been about five years. Both the rarity of the disease and the lack of uniform diagnostic criteria have hampered efforts to establish reliable prognostic models. In a large series of 144 patients with clinically overt macroglobulinemia, these independent prognostic factors were associated with poor survival: hemoglobin <90 g/L, age >70 years, weight loss, and cryoglobulinemia (67).

Asymptomatic patients with WM may follow a stable clinical course for several years and do not benefit from early treatment. When symptoms appear, two therapeutic strategies exist: cytotoxic treatment with the aim to reduce tumor cell burden, and plasmapheresis with the aim to rapidly reduce the M-protein level and symptoms caused by its biological effects. The choice and combination of these therapeutic options depend on the clinical situation. The treatment of WM was recently reviewed (68).

Plasmapheresis is a very effective means to rapidly reduce the circulating IgM and should always be used as initial therapy in patients with symptoms of hyperviscosity. In cryoglobulinemia it may be necessary to perform the procedure in a warm environment. Plasmapheresis may also be used as initial treatment in polyneuropathy. A symptomatic improvement can support the decision of later initiation of cytotoxic therapy. In patients with low tumor burden and no other manifestations of the disease, and particularly in patients who do not tolerate cytotoxic treatment, plasmapheresis at regular intervals can avoid or postpone the initiation of cytotoxic therapy for a long period. However in the majority of patients with WM, specific cytotoxic therapy directed against the tumor cells is indicated.

Chlorambucil has for a long time been the standard treatment of WM. A response is achieved in about 50% and no difference between intermittent or continuous treatment was observed (69). Maintenance therapy after achievement of response does not prolong survival. As in myeloma, there is no evidence that combinations of different alkylating agents, vinca alkaloids, or anthracyclines improve the outcome. The nucleoside analogs fludarabine and 2-chlorodeoxyadenosine (cladribin) are effective in various types of indolent lymhpomas and have shown promising results in WM (reviewed in 64,68). Response rates of up to 80% in first-line treatment and in one-third of previously treated patients have been reported, and the response is more rapid than with chlorambucil. The nucleoside analogs suppress monocytes as well as $CD4^+$ and $CD8^+$ lymphocytes, which increases the risk of opportunistic infections.

Randomized studies comparing the long-term outcome in patients treated with alkylating agents versus nucleoside analogs are not yet reported. The majority of the malignant cells in WM express the CD 20 antigen; the chimeric anti-CD20 monoclonal antibody rituximab has been used in a limited number of patients. About one third of previously treated patients do benefit from this therapy. High-dose therapy with autologous stem cell support may increase the rate of complete remissions, but the long-term outcome is not known and the number of patients treated is limited. None of the therapeutic options is curative.

AL-AMYLOIDOSIS

In AL-amyloidosis, fragments of light immunoglobulin chains or rarely, heavy chains, are deposited in various tissues in a pathognomic abnormal fibrillar form called amyloid. Immunoglobulins are only one of several proteins that can serve as precursor protein to amyloid. Serum amyloid protein A (SAA, an acute phase reactant), β2-microglobulin, transthyretin, and Aβ protein precursor (associated with Alzheimer's disease) are other precursor proteins. Amyloid substance also contains glucosaminoglycans and a minor nonfibrillar constituent, amyloid P component, derived from the plasma protein serum amyloid P component.

In this section only AL-amyloidosis will be discussed. Amyloidosis may complicate multiple myeloma or more seldom, Waldenström's macroglobulinemia, but in the majority of cases the tumor cell mass of the underlying monoclonal plasma cell dyscrasia is small and the manifestations of the disease are entirely dependent on the effects of the amyloid deposits.

Epidemiology

AL-amyloidosis is an uncommon disease with a reported annual incidence of 0.8 per 100,000/year. The median age is about 73 years (70).

Biology

The fundamental question in amyloidosis is why certain protein precursors are amyloidogenic. The primary structure of the protein is important but very little is known about the structure of amyloidogenic Ig chains. In contrast to myeloma where κ chains are more common, λ light chains predominate in AL-amyloidosis with overrepresentation of the λ_{VI} subclass (70). In the course of the disease amyloid deposits accumulate and their physical presence disrupts tissue organization and damages organ function.

Clinical Manifestations

The clinical manifestations of AL-amyloidosis are the clue to an early diagnosis. Several reviews have recently been published (70,71). The four most common syndromes are congestive heart failure, nephrotic syndrome, polyneuropathy, and hepatomegaly. The heart is involved in the majority of cases and restrictive cardiomyopathy is the presenting feature in about one third of all cases. Arrhythmias are common. Amyloid deposits in the kidneys cause nonselective proteinuria with nephrotic syndrome and eventually end-stage renal failure. Peripheral neuropathy occurs in about 20% of patients. Other less common manifestations are macroglossia, autonomic neuropathy with orthostatic hypotension, digestive tract involvement with motility disturbances, and malabsorption and carpal tunnel syndromes. Bleeding diathesis, which may be a serious complication, may be associated with deficiency of coagulation factor X but is more often explained by amyloid deposits in the vessels.

Diagnosis

The diagnosis of AL-amyloidosis requires the demonstration of amyloid in a tissue biopsy and either immunocytochemical identification of the amyloid as light immunoglobulin-derived or the finding of a monoclonal immunoglobulin in serum and/or urine. When amyloid is stained with Congo red and examined in polarized light, it gives a red-green birefringence which is pathognomic. Abdominal subcutaneous fat and bone marrow are the biopsy sites with the highest prevalence of positive staining (72). If these are negative but the clinical suspicion of amyloidosis remains, biopsy of the involved organ (e.g., kidney, heart, liver) may be necessary. Scintigraphy with radiolabeled serum amyloid P component has been used to determine the distribution of amyloid deposits and for quantitation during treatment (71).

Immunocytochemical demonstration of immunoglobulin light chain determinants in amyloid is subject to technical problems. The presence of an M-protein in serum and/or urine can be taken as a strong indirect evidence that the amyloidosis is of the AL type. A monoclonal light chain is found in serum and/or urine in 90% of patients with AL-amyloidosis (73). In the remaining cases, a monoclonal plasma cell infiltration in the bone marrow is almost always detectable by immunocytochemistry. The number of tumor cells is low in most cases with the exception of amyloidosis complicating myeloma.

Prognosis and Treatment

The only treatment presently available for amyloidosis is aimed at reducing the supply of protein fibril precursors. Response is defined both by the effect on the M-protein concentration and bone marrow plasma cell percentage, and by improvement of organ function. Standard treatment with melphalan and prednisone (MP) elicits responses in about 30% of patients, but the reported median survivals are short. In two randomized studies, MP was superior to colchicin, and the median survival ranged from 12.2 to 17 months (74,75). High-dose therapy (HCT), with autologous stem cell support, has been used in several phase II studies with higher response rates, but phase III trials comparing HCT with standard therapy have yet not been performed (reviewed in 76). An interesting new approach is the use of agents that can dissolve established amyloid deposits. The doxorubicin analogue 4'-iodo-4'-deoxydoxorubicin has been reported to have effects in a small series of patients (77).

Congestive heart failure is the most important adverse factor for survival and is a common cause of death. Heart transplantation in end-stage amyloid cardiomyopathy has been performed in selected cases, but indications for selecting patients who benefit from this procedure have not yet been established. Patients with end-stage renal failure are candidates for chronic dialysis and renal tranplantation, which both are effective in AL-amyloidosis.

REFERENCES

1. Herrinton LJ, Weiss NS, Olshan AF. Epidemiology of myeloma. In: Malpas JS, Bergsagel DE, Kyle R, Anderson K, eds. Myeloma: biology and management. Oxford: Oxford University Press, 1998;150–186.
2. Kyle RA, Beard CM, O'Fallon M, Kurland LT. Incidence of multiple myeloma in Olmstead County, Minnesota: 1978–1980, with a review of the trend since 1945. J Clin Oncol 1994;12: 1577–1583.
3. Turesson I, Zettervall O, Cuzick J, Waldenström GJ, Velez R. Comparison of trends in the incidence of multiple myeloma in Malmö, Sweden, and other countries. New Engl J Med 1984;310: 421–424.
4. Preston DL, Kusumi R, Tomonaga M, Izumi S, Ron E, Kuramoto A, et al. Cancer incidence in atomic bomb survivors, Part III: leukemia, lymphoma, and multiple myeloma, 1950–87. Radiation Research 1994;137:S68–S97.
5. Billadeau D, Quam L, Thomas W, Kay N, Greipp P, Kyle R, et al. Detection and quantitation of malignant cells in the peripheral blood of multiple myeloma patients. Blood 1992;80:1818–1824.
6. Vescio RA, Cao J, Hong CH, Lee JC, Wu CH, Der Danielian M, et al. Myeloma Ig heavy chain V region sequences reveal prior antigenic selection and marked somatic mutation but no intraclonal diversity. J Immunol 1995;155:2487–2497.
7. Hallek M, Bergsagel PL, Anderson KC. Multiple myeloma: increasing evidence for a multi-step transformation process. Blood 1998;91:3–21.
8. Tricot G, Barlogie B, Jagannath S, Bracy D, Mattox S, Vesole DH, et al. Poor prognosis in multiple myeloma is associated only with partial or complete deletions of chromosome 13 or abnormalities involving 11q and not with other karyotype abnormalities. Blood 1995;86:4250–4256.
9. Mundy G. Myeloma bone disease. In: Mundy G, ed. Bone remodeling and its disorders. London: Martin Dunitz Ltd., 1999; 147–161.
10. Rettig MB, Ma HJ, Vescio RA, Pold M, Schiller G, Belson D, et al. Kaposi's sarcoma-associated herpes virus infection of bone marrow dendritic cells from multiple myeloma patients. Science 1997;276:1851–1854.
11. Rajkumar SV, Leong T, Roche PC, Fonseca R, Dispenzieri A, Lacy MQ, et al. Prognostic value of bone marrow angiogenesis in multiple myeloma. Clin Cancer Res 2000;6:3111–3116.
12. Iggo N. Management of renal complications. In: Malpas JS, Bergsagel DE, Kyle R, Anderson K, eds. Myeloma: biology and management. Oxford: Oxford University Press, 1998;150–186.
13. Spiess JL, Adelstein DJ, Hines JD. Multiple myeloma presenting with spinal cord compression. Oncology 1988;45:88–92.
14. Takatsuki K, Sanada I. Plasma cell dyscrasia with polyneuropathy and endocrine disorder: clinical and laboratory features of 109 reported cases. Japanese Journal of Clinical Oncology 1983;13:543–555.
15. Joshua DJ. Immunoglobulins. In: Malpas JS, Bergsagel DE, Kyle R, Anderson K, eds. Myeloma: biology and management. Oxford: Oxford University Press, 1998;3–28.
16. Blackwell TK, Alt FW. Immunoglobulin genes. In: Hames BD, Glover MD, eds. Molecular Immunology. Oxford: IRL Press, 1989;1–60.
17. McLennan I. Immunology. The center of hypermutation. Nature 1991;354:352–353.
18. Billadeau D, Blackstadt M, Greipp P, Kyle RA, Oken MM, Kay N, Van-Ness B. Analysis of B-lymphoid malignancies using allele-specific polymerase chain reaction: a technique for sequental quantitation of residual disease. Blood 1991;78:3021–3029.
19. Kyle RA, Rajkumar SV. Monoclonal gammopathies of undetermined significance. In: Kyle RA, Gertz MA, eds. Monoclonal Gammopathies and related disorders. Hematology/Oncology Clinics of North America 1999;13:1181–1202.
20. Malpas JS. Clinical presentation and diagnosis. In: Malpas JS, Bergsagel DE, Kyle R, Anderson K, eds. Myeloma: biology and management. Oxford: Oxford University Press, 1998;150–186.
21. Carlson J. From paper electrophoresis to computer-supported interpretation of capillary electrophoresis—clinical plasma protein analysis in Malmö, Sweden. Clin Chem 2001;(in press).
22. Bradwell AR, Carr-Smith HD, Mead GP, Tang LX, Showell PJ, Drayson MT, Drew R. Highly sensitive, automated immunoassay for immunoglobulin free light chains in serum and urine. Clin Chem 2001;47:673–680.
23. Bladé J, Samson D, Reece D, Apperley J, Björkstrand B, Gahrton G, et al. Criteria for evaluating disease response and progression in patients with multiple myeloma treated with high dose therapy and hematopoetic stem cell transplantation. Br J Hematol 1998;102:115–123.
24. Szecsi PB, Riise E, Roslund LB, Engberg J, Turesson I, Buhl L, et al. Identification of patient-specific peptides for detection of M-proteins and myeloma cells. Brit J Hematol 1999;107: 357–364.

25. Rasmussen T, Poulsen TS, Honore L, Johnsen HE. Quantitation of minimal residual disease in multiple myeloma using an allele-specific real-time PCR assay. Exp Hematol 2000;28:1039–1045.
26. Almeida J, Orfao A, Ocqueteau M, Mateo G, Corral M, Caballero MD, et al. High-sensitive immunophenotyping and DNA ploidy studies for the investigation of minimal residual disease in multiple myeloma. Br J Hematol 2000;110:751–753.
27. Turesson I. Nucleolar size in benign and malignant plasma cell proliferation. Acta Med Scand 1975;197:7–14.
28. Greipp PR, Leong T, Bennett JM, Gaillard JP, Klein B, Stewart JA, et al. Plasmablastic morphology—an independent prognostic factor with clinical and laboratory correlates: Eastern Cooperative Oncology Group (ECOG) Myeloma Trial E9486 report by the ECOG Myeloma Laboratory Group. Blood 1998;91:2501–2507.
29. Bartl R, Frisch B, Wilmanns W. Bone and marrow findings in multiple myeloma and related disorders. In: Wiernik PH, Canellos GH, Durcher JP, Kyle RA, eds. Neoplastic diseases of the blood. New York: Churchill Livingstone, 1996.
30. Greipp PR, Witzig TE, Gonchoroff TJ, Habermann TM, Katzmann JA, O'Fallon WM, Kyle RA. Immunofluorescence labeling indices in myeloma and related monoclonal gammapathies. Mayo Clin Proc 1987;62:969–977.
31. Solomon A, Rahamani R, Seligsohn U, Ben-Artzi F. Multiple myeloma: early vertebral involvement assessed by computed tomography. Skeletal Radiology 1984;11:258–261.
32. Mouolopoulos LA, Varma DG, Dimopoulos MA, Leeds NE, Kim EE, Johnston DA, et al. Multiple myeloma: spinal MR imaging in patients with untreated newly diagnosed disease. Radiology 1992;185:833–840.
33. Hjorth M, Westin J, Dahl IM, Gimsing P, Hippe E, Holmberg E, et al. Interferon-alfa-2b added to to melphalan-prednisone for initial and maintenance therapy in multiple myeloma: a randomized controlled trial. Ann Intern Med 1996;124:212–222.
34. Durie BG, Salmon SE. A clinical staging system for multiple myeloma. Correlation of measured myeloma cell mass with presenting clinical features, response to treatment, and survival. Cancer 1975;36:842–854.
35. Axelsson U, Bachmann R, Hällén J. Frequency of pathological proteins (M-components) in 6,995 sera from an adult population. Acta Med Scand 1966;179:235–247.
36. Crawford J, Eye MK, Cohen HJ. Evaluation of monoclonal gammapathies in the "well" elderly. Am J Med 1987;82:39–45.
37. Witzig TE, Kyle RA, O'Fallon WA, Greipp PR. Circulating peripheral blood plasma cells as a predictor of disease course in patients with smoldering multiple myeloma. Br J Hematol 1994;87: 266–272.
38. Lacy MQ, Donovan KA, Heimbach JK, Ahmann GJ, Lust JA. Comparison of interleukin-1 beta expression by in situ hybridization in monoclonal gammopathy of undetermined significance and multiple myeloma. Blood 1999;93:300–305.
39. Rajkumar SV, Greipp PR. Prognostic factors in multiple myeloma. In: Kyle RA, Gertz MA, eds. Monoclonal gammopathies and related disorders. Hematology/Oncology Clinics of North America 1999;13:1295–1314.
40. Desikan R, Barlogie B, Sawyer J, Ayers D, Tricot G, Badros A, et al. Results of high-dose therapy for 1,000 patients with multiple myeloma: durable complete remissions and superior survival in the absence of chromosome abnormalities. Blood 2000;95: 1008–1010.
41. Bataille R, Boccadoro M, Klein B, Durie B, Pileri A. C-reactive protein and serum β2microglobulin produce a simple and powerful myeloma staging system. Blood 1992;80:733–737.
42. Facon T, Avet-Loiseau H, Guillerm G, Moreau P, Genevieve F, Zandecki M, et al. Chromosome 13 abnormalities identified by FISH analysis and serum beta2-micro-globulin produce a powerful myeloma staging system for patients receiving high-dose therapy. Blood 2001;97:1566–1571.
43. Barille S, Bataille R, Amiot M. The role of interleukin-6/interleukin-6 receptor-alpha complex in the pathogenesis of multiple myeloma. Eur Cytokine Netw 2000;11:546–551.
44. Greipp PR. Prognosis in myeloma. Mayo Clin Proc 1994;69: 895–902.
45. Turesson I, Abildgaard N, Ahlgren T, Dahl I-M, Holmberg E, Hjorth M, et al. Prognostic evaluation in multiple myeloma: an analysis of the impact of new prognostic factors. Brit J Hematol 1999;106:1005–1012.
46. Hjorth M, Hellquist L, Holmberg E, Magnusson B, Rödjer S, Westin J. Initial versus deferred melphalan-prednisone therapy for asymptomatic multiple myeloma stage I: a randomized study. Eur J Hematol 1993;50:95–102.
47. Bergsagel DE. Chemotherapy of myeloma. In: Malpas JS, Bergsagel DE, Kyle R, Anderson K, eds. Myeloma: biology and management. Oxford: Oxford University Press, 1998: 269–302.
48. Myeloma Trialists' Collaborative Group. Combination chemotherapy versus melphalan plus prednisone as treatment for multiple myeloma: An overview of 6,633 patients from 27 randomized trials. J Clin Oncol 1998;16:3832–3842.
49. Myeloma Trialists' Collaborative Group. Interferon as therapy for multiple myeloma: an individual patient data overview of 24 randomized trials and 4012 patients. Br J Hematol 2001;113: 1020–1034.
50. Attal M, Harousseau JI, Stoppa AM, Sotto JJ, Fuzibet JG, Rossi JF, et al. A prospective, randomized trial of autologous bone marrow transplantation and chemo-therapy in multiple myeloma. N Engl J Med 1996;335:91–97.
51. Lenhoff S, Hjorth M, Holmberg E, Turesson I, Westin J, Nielsen JL, et al. Impact on survival of high-dose therapy with autologous stem cell support in patients younger than 60 years with newly diagnosed multiple myeloma: a population-based study. Blood 2000;95:7–11.
52. Barlogie B. High-dose therapy and innovative approaches to treatment of multiple myeloma. Semin Hematol 2001;38:21–27.
53. Björkstrand B. European Group for Blood and Marrow Transplantation Registry studies in multiple myeloma. Semin Hematol 2001;38:219–225.
54. Barlogie B, Zangari M, Spencer T, Fassas A, Anaissie E, Badros A, et al. Thalidomide in the management of multiple myeloma. Semin Hematol 2001;38:250–259.
55. Berenson JR, Lichtenstein A, Porter L, Dimopoulos MA, Bordoni R, George S, et al. Efficacy of pamidronate in reducing skeletal events in patients with advanced multiple myeloma. N Engl J Med 1996;334:448–493.
56. Osterborg A. The role of recombinant human erythropoietin in the management of anemic cancer patients: focus on hematological malignancies. Med Oncol 2000;17 suppl 1:17–22.
57. Groves F, Travis LB, Devesa SS, Ries LA, Fraumeni JF. Waldenström's macroglobulinemia. Incidence patterns in the United States 1988–1994. Cancer 1998;82:1078–1081.
58. Aoki H, Takishita M, Kosaka M, Saito S. Frequent somatic mutations in D and/or JH segments of Ig gene in Waldenström's macroglobulinemia and chronic lymphocytic leukemia (CLL) with Richter's syndrome but not in common CLL. Blood 1995;85: 1913–1919.

59. Gertz MA, Fonseca R, Rajkumar SV. Waldenström's macroglobulinemia. The Oncologist 2000;5:63–67.
60. Levy Y, Fermand JP, Navarro S, Schmitt C, Vainschenker W, Seligmann M, Brouet JC. Interleukin 6 dependence of spontaneous in vitro differentiation of B cell from patients with IgM monoclonal gammopathies. Proc Natl Acad Sci USA 1990;87:3309–3313.
61. Dewald GW, Jenkins RB. Cytogenetic studies on patients with monoclonal gammopathies. In: Dutcher JP, Kyle RA, eds. Neoplastic diseases of the blood, 3rd ed. New York, NY: Churchill Livingstone, 1996;515.
62. Merlini G. Waldenström's macroglobulinemia—clinical manifestations and prognosis. 41st annual meeting of the American Society of Hematology Educational Book. 1999:358–369.
63. Kyle RA. Waldenström's macroglobulinemia. In: Malpas JS, Bergsagel DE, Kyle R, Anderson K, eds. Myeloma: biology and management. Oxford: Oxford University Press, 1998:639–662.
64. Dimopoulos MA, Galani E, Matsouka C. Waldenström's macroglobulinemia. In: Kyle RA, Gertz MA, eds. Monoclonal gammopathies and related disorders. Hematol Oncol Clin North Am, 1999;13:1351–1366.
65. Gertz MA, Kyle RA. Hyperviscosity syndrome. J Intensive Care Med 1995;10:128–141.
66. Kyle RA, Garton JP. The spectrum of IgM monoclonal gammopathy in 430 cases. Mayo Clin Proc 1987;62:719–731.
67. Gobbi PG, Bettini R, Montecucco C, Cavanna L, Morandi S, Pieresca C, et al. Study of prognosis in Waldenström's macroglobulinemia: a proposal for simple binary classification with clinical and investigational utility. Blood 1994;83:2929–2945.
68. Dimopoulos MA. Waldenström's macroglobulinemia—therapy. In: 41st annual meeting of the American Society of Hematology education program book. Washington, DC: American Society of Hematology, 1999;370–375.
69. Kyle RA, Greipp PR, Gertz MA, Witzig TE, Lust JA, Lacy MQ, Therneau TM. Waldenström's macroglobulinemia: a prospective study comparing daily versus intermittent oral chlorambucil. Br J Hematol 2000;108:737–742.
70. Gertz M, Lacy MQ, Dispenzieri A. Amyloidosis. In: Kyle RA, Gertz MA, eds. Monoclonal gammopathies and related disorders. Hematol Oncol Clin North Am, 1999;13:1211–1233.
71. Hawkins, PN, Pepys MB. Amyloidosis. In: Malpas JS, Bergsagel DE, Kyle R, Anderson K, eds. Myeloma: biology and management. Oxford: Oxford University Press, 1998;559–603.
72. Westermark P. The pathogenesis of amyloidosis: understanding general principles. Am J Pathol 1998;152:1125–1127.
73. Kyle RA, Gertz M. Primary systemic amyloidosis: clinical and laboratory features in 474 cases. Semin Hematol 1995;32:45–59.
74. Kyle RA, Gertz M, Greipp PR, Witzig TE, Lust JA, Lacy MQ, Therneau TM. A trial of three regimens for primary amyloidosis: colchicine alone, melphalan and prednisone, and melphalan, prednisone, and colchicin. N Engl J Med 1997;336:1202–1207.
75. Skinner M, Anderson J, Simms R, Falk R, Wang M, Libbey C, et al. Treatment of 100 patients with primary amyloidosis: a randomized trial of melphalan, prednisone, and colchicin versus colchicin only. Am J Med 1996;100:290–298.
76. Comenzo RL. High-dose therapy for the treatment of primary systemic amyloidosis. In: 41st annual meeting of the American Society of Hematology education program book. Washington, DC: American Society of Hematology, 1999;347–357.
77. Gianni L, Bellotti, Gianni AM, Merlini G. New drug therapy of amyloidoses: resorption of AL-type deposits with 4'-iodo-4'-deoxydoxorubicin. Blood 1995;86:855–861.

Chapter **26**

Leukemias and Lymphomas

Joseph A. DiGiuseppe and Michael J. Borowitz

"Solid" malignancies may be characterized by surrogate markers that are produced by tumor cells, which are identified and quantified in serum using biochemical techniques or immunoassay. By contrast, in leukemias and lymphomas, the neoplastic cells themselves may be identified and quantified in peripheral blood and/or bone marrow specimens. Thus, with the significant exception of lactate dehydrogenase, and to a lesser extent β-2-microglobulin, conventional serum tumor markers do not play a large role in the current clinical management of patients with leukemias or lymphomas.

Instead, much of the work in this area has focused on molecular genetic methods for identifying tumor-specific nucleic acid as an indicator of the presence of rare neoplastic cells. Other techniques are designed to directly identify rare residual neoplastic cells using immunologic techniques, most commonly multi-parameter flow cytometry. These techniques have no useful role in screening normal individuals, in large part because of the low incidence of hematopoietic malignancies. However, in several specific instances, detection of "minimal residual disease" (MRD) has prognostic value in patients with leukemias and lymphomas in remission. The goal of identifying MRD is to identify patients in whom tumor burden is comparatively low, in the hope that this might render subsequent therapy more effective. Moreover, the detection of MRD after initial therapy may enable more effective therapy to be administered specifically to high-risk patients, while sparing those with low-risk disease the attendant therapeutic toxicities.

In this chapter, we review some of the "conventional" serum markers that have been evaluated in leukemia/lymphoma. The remainder of the chapter, however, is devoted to a review of those specific types of leukemia and lymphoma in which the immunophenotypic or molecular detection of MRD has established prognostic significance.

"CONVENTIONAL" SERUM MARKERS IN LEUKEMIA AND LYMPHOMA

Lactate Dehydrogenase

The most widely used conventional serum marker in the clinical evaluation of patients with non-Hodgkin's lymphomas (NHLs) is lactate dehydrogenase (LDH), a cytoplasmic enzyme whose elevation in serum is associated with increased cellular turnover. NHLs are often divided clinically into low-grade (indolent) and intermediate- or high-grade (aggressive) lymphomas on the basis of their histopathologic features. Nonetheless, within each of these two broad categories, there is considerable clinical heterogeneity. Among patients with aggressive non-Hodgkin's lymphomas, a serum LDH level above the upper limit of normal is one of five independent predictors of death (1). Age, stage, number of extranodal sites involved, performance status, and LDH level comprise the International Prognostic Index (IPI), a widely used clinical model that stratifies patients with aggressive NHLs into low, low-intermediate, high-intermediate, and high-risk groups, and in turn permits administration of risk-adjusted therapy (1). Although originally evaluated in aggressive NHLs, the IPI, including LDH, appears to predict likelihood of response to therapy and survival among patients with all grades of NHL (2,3). Additionally, although this has not been rigorously studied, a rising LDH in a patient with a history of lymphoma in remission often triggers a more extensive search for evidence of recurrent disease.

β-2-Microglobulin

β-2-microglobulin is the light chain of class I major histocompatibility (MHC) antigens, and serum levels appear to correlate with systemic lymphoid and plasmacytic activation and proliferation. Though the literature in lymphoma is not as extensive as that in multiple myeloma (see chapter 25), elevated β-2-microglobulin levels predict lower complete response rates and shorter time to treatment failure (TTF) in patients with either indolent (4) or aggressive (5) NHLs. Serum β-2-microglobulin levels also correlate with disease progression and predict poor prognosis in patients with B-cell chronic lymphocytic leukemia (B-CLL) (6). Although the published experience of some institutions would support more widespread use of β-2-microglobulin, in contrast with LDH, many clinicians do not routinely incorporate β-2-microglobulin levels into their evaluation of patients with NHL.

CD23

CD23 is a B-cell surface membrane antigen characteristically expressed in B-CLL, and a soluble form of CD23 (sCD23) shed from these neoplastic cells may be measured in serum by immunoassay. Patients with sCD23 levels above the median at presentation have a worse rate of survival compared with those whose sCD23 is below median (7). Perhaps more importantly, among patients with clinically early-stage disease, whose subsequent rate of disease progression is difficult to predict, a doubling in the level of sCD23 is associated with a 15-fold increase in risk of disease progression, with elevation in sCD23 preceding disease progression by four years (7). When combined with β-2-microglobulin levels, sCD23 may provide yet more precise prognostic information in B-CLL (8). At this time, however, measurement of sCD23 has not become part of routine clinical practice.

Other Potential Markers

In addition to those described above, many other serum markers, including soluble forms of membrane proteins and cytokines, have been suggested to have prognostic utility in lymphomas and leukemias (Table 1). Although not yet used in routine clinical practice, roles for some of these other potential markers may become established as additional supporting data become available. Note that of the markers listed in Table 1, only assays for LDH, β-2-microglobulin, interleukin-6, and CA125 are currently available outside research laboratories.

IMMUNOPHENOTYPIC AND MOLECULAR MARKERS IN LEUKEMIA AND LYMPHOMA

In patients with acute leukemia, clinical remission is defined as reduction in the percentage of neoplastic cells (blasts) in the bone marrow to fewer than 5%. At diagnosis, however, the total burden of leukemic cells may number 10^{12} (25); thus a patient in clinical remission may still harbor more than 10^{10} leukemic cells. A similar principle is applicable in patients with NHLs, which may involve the bone marrow at levels below the detection limit of microscopic examination. Through the use of flow cytometric immunophenotyping (FCI) or polymerase chain reaction (PCR), it has become feasible to detect and quantify residual neoplastic cells in patients who are in clinical remission. Because patients with acute leukemia who fail to enter remission have a very poor prognosis, the detection of such "minimal residual disease" (MRD) following initial therapy might potentially identify those patients who are most likely to relapse, thus suggesting a new definition of remission (26). If used to monitor patients, detection of MRD could also potentially indicate imminence of relapse of patients in remission. The sensitivity and specificity of these measurements have not been nearly as well established as those of the usual solid tumor markers, and repeated monitoring of these markers in the management of patients with these diseases is of uncertain value. However, detection of either leukemic cells or their nucleic acid markers has been shown to provide prognostic information in many of these diseases. The remainder of this chapter will review this topic.

Acute Lymphoblastic Leukemia (ALL)

MRD detection has been extensively studied in children with acute lymphoblastic leukemia. In general, MRD has been evaluated using either PCR or FCI. PCR has been used in the majority of published studies to detect clone-specific antigen-receptor (i.e., immunoglobulin heavy chain [IGH] or T-cell receptor [TCR]) gene rearrangements. The great majority of cases will show one or more of these unique clonal markers. In those cases with balanced translocations, reverse transcriptase-PCR (RT-PCR) is used to detect fusion transcripts (27–30), though only a subset of patients with leukemia will have informative markers of this type. Although there are difficulties involved in PCR-based quantification, analyses have been done in a semi-quantitative fashion using limiting dilution, competitor templates, and more recently, real-time quantification (reviewed in 27, 28).

By contrast, FCI enables simultaneous detection and quantification of leukemic cells on the basis of aberrant combinations of surface membrane antigens (31) or in the case of the more common B-lineage ALL, deviation from predictable patterns of antigen expression seen in normal B-cell precursors (hematogones) (32). These tumor-specific phenotypes can be found in greater than 95% of cases of precursor B-cell ALL (32). Novel markers identified by DNA microarray analysis can further help to identify unique phenotypes (33). In comparative studies, both FCI and PCR yield similar results (34,35); thus, optimal screening might incorporate both methods, which would minimize the potential for loss of the genetic or immunophenotypic targets as a result of tumor progression (34,36).

Table 1 "Conventional" serum tumor markers in leukemia and lymphoma

Serum Marker	Associated Disease(s)	Assay Methodology	References
LDH	NHL	Enzymatic	1–3
β-2-microglobulin	B-CLL, NHL	Immunoassay	4–6
CD23	B-CLL	Immunoassay	7,8
Nm23-H1	NHL, AML	Immunoassay	9–12
Interleukin-6	B-CLL, NHL,	Immunoassay	13,15,16
Interleukin-10	B-CLL, HL, NHL	Immunoassay	13,14,17
CD44	B-CLL, NHL	Immunoassay	18,19
CA125	NHL	Immunoassay	20,21
Thymidine kinase	B-CLL	Enzymatic	22
BFGF	NHL	Immunoassay	23
VEGFR-2	B-CLL	Immunoassay	24

Abbreviations: NHL, non-Hodgkin's lymphoma; B-CLL, B-cell chronic lymphocytic leukemia; AML, acute myeloid leukemia; HL, Hodgkin's lymphoma; bFGF, basic fibroblast growth factor; VEGFR-2, vascular endothelial growth factor receptor-2.

Three large prospective series of patients with pediatric ALL established the prognostic significance of MRD detection at different times following therapy (37–39). Using FCI with a sensitivity of 10^{-4}, Coustan-Smith et al. studied a series of 158 children with precursor B- or T-cell ALL at remission induction and at several time points during and at the completion of continuation therapy (37). Detectable disease at remission induction was associated with the presence of Philadelphia chromosome-positivity and rearrangements involving the mixed lineage leukemia (*MLL*) gene, both of which are adverse prognostic factors (37). Moreover, MRD detectable at any time point was associated with a higher risk of relapse (37). Using a semi-quantitative PCR method for detection of clone-specific antigen receptor rearrangements, van Dongen et al. studied a series of 240 patients with precursor B- and T-cell ALL at remission induction and a number of times thereafter (38). On the basis of the levels of MRD detected at the end of induction and prior to consolidation ($<10^{-4}$, 10^{-3}, or $>10^{-2}$), patients could be stratified with respect to their three-year relapse rate into low- (2%), intermediate- (23%), and high- (75%) risk groups (38). At all times, low-level (i.e., 10^{-3} in this study) MRD conferred a lower risk of relapse compared with high-level (i.e., $>10^{-2}$) MRD; nonetheless, at later times after remission induction, even low-level disease was associated with a poor outcome (38). In a multi-center study employing a competitive PCR assay, Cave et al. quantified MRD at several times after remission induction in a series of 178 patients with precursor B- and T-cell ALL (39). Again, at all time points studied, detectable MRD was associated with an increased risk of relapse, and the amount of MRD was an important factor; patients with high-level MRD (defined as $>10^{-2}$) had the highest rate of relapse (39). A number of studies describing smaller cohorts of children with precursor B- and/or T-cell ALL have yielded similar conclusions (40–44).

Although there is no current consensus on the optimal times or frequency of monitoring children with ALL, early positivity appears to be a consistently poor prognostic factor. For example, in a recent study of 68 patients with precursor B- or T-cell ALL, no relapses were observed among 14 patients with fewer than 10^{-4} blasts at day 15, compared with 16 (30%) of 54 patients with 10^{-3} or more blasts at day 15 (45). In another study of 195 patients with ALL, those with detectable MRD at remission induction, but in whom MRD was undetectable at week 14 or week 32 of continuation therapy, fared significantly better than those in whom MRD was persistently detectable (46). Data regarding adult ALL are comparatively sparse, but MRD detection is likely to be informative in this setting as well (47).

Analysis of MRD may also be useful in patients with ALL who undergo bone marrow transplantation (BMT). In a series of 71 children who underwent allogeneic BMT for ALL, MRD was detected following transplantation in 88% of patients who relapsed compared with 22% of those who remained in continuous remission (48). Therapy for patients who relapse following allogeneic BMT often involves administration of donor leukocytes to elicit a graft vs. leukemia effect; targeting this form of treatment to the subset of MRD+ allogeneic BMT patients may not only be more effective prior to frank relapse, but may also spare many MRD-negative patients the toxicities associated with graft-versus-host disease (GVHD). Potentially more significant would be identification of patients prior to transplantation in whom standard allogeneic BMT is unlikely to be successful. In a retrospective study of 64 children with ALL who underwent allogeneic BMT, two-year event-free survival was 0%, 36%, and 73% in patients with high-level (10^{-2} to 10^{-3}), low-level (10^{-3} to 10^{-5}), or undetectable MRD, respectively (49). MRD analysis prior to allogeneic BMT, therefore, could potentially identify patients who may require additional therapy prior to transplantation (49).

In contrast to myeloid leukemias (see below), there are relatively scant data on the use of PCR to assess leukemia-specific fusion transcripts in patients with ALL. In one study of 36 patients with Philadelphia chromosome-positive ALL who underwent BMT, detection of the BCR/ABL fusion transcript by RT-PCR was associated with a much higher risk of relapse compared with a negative assay (50).

Acute Myeloid Leukemia

In acute myeloid leukemia (AML), antigen receptor genes are not typically rearranged, and thus, are not suitable targets for MRD detection. Detection of MRD in patients with AML has generally been accomplished through detection of aberrant combinations of antigen expression by FCI, or through RT-PCR-mediated amplification of disease-specific translocation transcripts. However, in contrast with ALL, in which >90% of cases (46) display aberrant immunophenotypic combinations detectable by FCI, only 70–75% of cases of AML manifest such immunophenotypic aberrations (51,52). An additional limitation to the flow cytometric detection of MRD in AML is the tremendous immunophenotypic plasticity seen in AML. For example, in a recent series of 136 patients with AML whose blasts were analyzed by FCI both at diagnosis and at first relapse, immunophenotypic changes, including complete loss or gain of distinct leukemic cell populations, were seen at relapse in 124 cases (91%); in this series, a panel of 16 different antibodies was required to ensure detection of relapse in all cases (53). This contrasts with the experience in ALL, in which immunophenotypic changes at relapse are comparatively infrequent and insubstantial (54). Molecular detection of MRD in AML is also complicated by the presence of the more common recurrent translocations in only 20–30% of cases (55). Even with an optimized multiplex RT-PCR assay, which detects 29 different translocations seen in acute leukemias, a fusion transcript was detected in only 45 of 102 cases (44%) of AML (56).

Notwithstanding these technical limitations, immunophenotypic and molecular detection of MRD in AML appears to have clinical value in certain settings. Using three-color FCI, two groups have independently shown the prognostic value of MRD in patients with AML (51,52,57). In a study of 56 patients with AML whose leukemias showed an abnormal immunophenotype, Venditti et al. found that the presence of $>3.5 \times 10^{-4}$ leukemic cells after consolidation (but not after remission induction) correlated with adverse cytogenetics, the multi-drug resistance (MDR) phenotype, and shorter relapse-free survival (RFS) and overall survival (OS), compared with patients with fewer leukemic cells (51). More recently, San Miguel et al. studied 126 patients with AML at first morphologic remission by FCI (52). In this series, patients could be stratified on the basis of MRD levels into different risk groups with respect to incidence of relapse and OS (52). In multivariate analysis, MRD levels were the most important predictor of RFS (52). These findings hold the promise for risk-adjusted post-induction therapy in AML patients, in the hopes of improving survival in this generally poor-prognosis disease.

Acute Promyelocytic Leukemia [AML with t(15;17)]

In virtually all cases, acute promyelocytic leukemia (APL) is associated with a translocation juxtaposing the *PML* and *RAR*α genes on chromosomes 15 and 17, respectively (58), and the fusion transcript produced in this distinct form of AML is a suitable target for MRD detection by RT-PCR. In general, detection of MRD by RT-PCR following consolidation therapy (but not immediately following induction) is associated with a significantly elevated risk of relapse (reviewed in 58). In a prospective study of 163 patients with APL using an RT-PCR assay with a sensitivity of 10^{-4}, Diverio et al. found that 20 of 21 (95%) patients who converted to MRD+ status during post-consolidation follow-up relapsed at a median of three months following molecular conversion, compared with 8 of 142 (6%) who were persistently MRD-negative (59). On the strength of these data, patients in this trial are now offered salvage therapy at molecular relapse (59). Patients with APL who relapse may be offered autologous bone marrow transplantation in second complete remission (CR). However, a prospective study of 15 such patients demonstrated that positivity for MRD by RT-PCR in second CR was invariably associated with relapse following transplantation, while six of the eight MRD-negative patients remained in CR (60). Thus, while monitoring patients with APL for the presence of molecularly detectable PML-RARα RNA clearly helps to identify those at risk of relapse, to date there are no satisfactory therapeutic options when such patients are identified.

Acute Myeloid Leukemias with Core Binding Factor Translocations

The most common balanced translocations in AML involve core binding factor, and the significance of detecting these leukemia-associated transcripts by RT-PCR is controversial. In AML with t(8;21), a translocation between *ETO* and *AML-1* (*CBF*α), most patients in sustained CR for up to 12.5 years following therapy [61]) still harbor AML1/ETO fusion transcripts detectable by RT-PCR (27). Indeed, clonogenic progenitor cells expressing the fusion transcript have also been isolated from the marrow of these patients (61), illustrating the viability and proliferative capacity of the cells constituting the MRD. Similarly, patients with AML with inv(16)(p13;q22) or t(16;16)(p13;q22) (rearrangements that juxtapose *CBF*β and *MYH11* genes), a form of AML that is pathogenetically related to t(8;21) AML (62), also show fusion transcripts detectable by RT-PCR in long-term remission (63,64). However, recent studies suggest that quantitative and repetitive molecular monitoring may provide some useful clinical information. In one recent study of 25 patients with t(8;21) AML, for example, relapses were limited to those patients with $>2 \times 10^3$ molecules of fusion transcript/μg of peripheral blood or bone marrow RNA (65). Likewise, serial monitoring for increases in the level of fusion transcript using real-time RT-PCR has the potential to identify patients with inv(16) AML in clinical remission who are about to relapse (66).

Chronic Myeloid Leukemia

Chronic myeloid leukemia is a disease characterized by proliferation of morphologically unremarkable granulocytes. Because routine methods cannot readily distinguish leukemic from non-leukemic granulocytes, and because it is relatively easy to induce a hematologic remission in CML, having a tumor-specific marker to monitor therapy in CML is of critical importance. Juxtaposition of the *bcr* and *abl* genes, the molecular correlate of the Philadelphia chromosome [t(9;22)(q34;q11)], produces a fusion transcript that is a suitable target for molecular detection of MRD in patients with CML (reviewed in 27, 67). Measurement of this transcript has taken on a crucial role as a surrogate marker to evaluate the success of therapy in CML, either by allogeneic bone marrow transplantation (67), after interferon (67,68), or more recently, following administration of the *bcr-abl* kinase-specific therapy, STI-571 (69). This assay has also been used to monitor patients with CML in remission, and predict those who are likely to relapse. However, in a series of 346 patients with CML after bone marrow transplantation, Radich and colleagues found that the timing of the assay was critical in interpreting its significance (70). Positivity for MRD at 6–12 months post-BMT was associated with a 26-fold elevated risk of relapse, while a positive result at three months was not predictive of relapse (70). Moreover, the great majority of CML patients with a positive result at 18 months or later following transplantation remained in complete remission in a more recent large study (71). Therefore, in patients with CML following transplantation, a single positive qualitative result in an individual patient may be of limited usefulness.

Quantitative, serial RT-PCR assays for BCR/ABL transcripts, however, appear to provide more refined prognostic information in CML patients. In a prospective study of 98 patients with CML following transplantation, Lin et al. found that only 1 of 69 patients (1%) with decreasing BCR/ABL levels or <50 BCR/ABL transcripts/μg of RNA subsequently relapsed, compared with 21 of 29 (72%) with increasing BCR/ABL levels or persistently >50 BCR/ABL transcripts/μg of RNA (72). Even among patients tested early after transplantation (3–5 months), when a positive qualitative assay is not associated with relapse (70), quantification of BCR/ABL transcripts provides significant prognostic information (73).

Non-Hodgkin's Lymphomas

MRD detection in the B-cell NHLs has most commonly been evaluated using PCR analysis with primers derived either from the *IGH* genes or from regions surrounding translocation breakpoints specific for the lymphoma being studied [e.g., t(14;18) in follicular lymphoma, juxtaposing *IGH* and *BCL-2* genes, and t(11;14) in mantle cell lymphoma, juxtaposing *CCND-1* and *IGH* genes] (reviewed in 74). Several groups have reported series of patients with follicular lymphoma, either following high-dose chemotherapy plus autologous stem cell transplantation (75–77) or conventional-dose chemotherapy alone (78). Detection of the t(14;18) translocation in blood and/or bone marrow autografts of patients transplanted for follicular lymphoma was associated with a higher risk of relapse, and achievement of PCR-negative status following therapy was associated with a reduced risk of relapse in these studies (75–78). However, the value of serial monitoring to predict patients likely to relapse following long-term remission of follicular lymphoma has not been conclusively demonstrated. In patients with mantle cell lymphoma, which is incurable even with high-dose chemotherapy plus autologous stem cell rescue, PCR-negative status is seldom achieved (77,79).

Finally, it is worth noting that therapy impacts the clinical significance of MRD detection. For example, when patients with B-cell chronic lymphocytic leukemia/small lymphocytic lymphoma (B-CLL) are treated with high-dose chemotherapy plus autologous stem cell rescue, persistence of detectable MRD is essentially universal (74). However, in a recent study of B-CLL patients treated with CAMPATH-1H (a humanized monoclonal antibody directed against the surface antigen, CD52) and/or fludarabine followed by autologous peripheral blood stem cell transplant (PBSCT) and studied by flow cytometry, 19 of 25 (76%) became MRD-negative (80). Thus, as was the case with novel therapies for CML, detection of MRD can be used as a surrogate marker to determine the effectiveness of new treatments in CLL.

SUMMARY

With the notable exception of LDH, conventional serum tumor markers do not play a major role in the current clinical management of patients with leukemia and lymphoma. However, a number of promising markers are currently being evaluated, and some of these may ultimately prove clinically useful. In the last decade, detection of tumor-specific cellular markers based on unique molecular sequences or immunologically defined abnormal phenotypes has been studied extensively in patients with ALL, AML, CML, and NHLs (Table 2). In most cases, the presence of a certain level of MRD in clinical remission imparts an elevated risk of subsequent relapse, and in pediatric ALL, as well as in APL, clinical trials are currently underway to ascertain whether the earlier intervention made possible by MRD detection improves outcome. In addition, in some circumstances, these tumor-specific markers have been used as surrogates to evaluate the effectiveness of novel therapies.

Table 2 "Cellular" tumor markers in leukemias and lymphomas

Marker	Type	Associated Disease(s)
Abnormal immunophenotype	Cell surface membrane antigens	ALL, AML, B-CLL
Clonotypic antigen receptor (IGH or TCR)	DNA	ALL, NHL
BCR/ABL	RNA	CML, ALL
PML/RARα	RNA	APL
AML1/ETO	RNA	t(8;21) AML
CBFB/MYH11	RNA	inv(16) AML
IGH/BCL-2	DNA	FL
CCND-1/IGH	DNA	MCL

See text for descriptions of individual markers. Abbreviations: ALL, acute lymphoblastic leukemia; AML, acute myeloid leukemia; NHL, non-Hodgkin's lymphoma; CML, chronic myeloid leukemia; APL, acute promyelocytic leukemia; FL, follicular lymphoma; MCL, mantle cell lymphoma.

REFERENCES

1. The International Non-Hodgkin's Lymphoma Prognostic Factors Project. A predictive model for aggressive non-Hodgkin's lymphoma. N Engl J Med 1993;329:987–994.
2. Hermans J, Krol AD, van Gronigen K, KluinNelemans JC, Kramer MH, Noordijk EM, et al. International prognostic index for aggressive non-Hodgkin's lymphoma is valid for all malignancy grades. Blood 1995;86:1460–1463.
3. Federico M, Vitolo U, Zinzani PL, Chisesi T, Clo V, Bellesi G, et al. Prognosis of follicular lymphoma: a predictive model based on a retrospective analysis of 987 cases. Blood 2000;95:783–789.
4. Litam P, Swan F, Cabanillas F, Tucker SL, McLaughlin P, Hagemeister FB, et al. Prognostic value of serum beta-2 microglobulin in low-grade lymphoma. Ann Int Med 1991;114:855–860.
5. Suki S, Swan F, Tucker S, Fritsche HA, Redman JR, Rodriguez MA, et al. Risk classification for large cell lymphoma using lactate dehydrogenase, beta-2 microglobulin, and thymidine kinase. Leukemia & Lymphoma 1995;18:87–92.
6. Keating MJ. Chronic lymphocytic leukemia. Semin Oncol 1999;26:107–114.
7. Sarfati M, Chevret S, Chastang C, Biron G, Stryckmans P, Delespesse G, et al. Prognostic importance of serum soluble CD23 level in chronic lymphocytic leukemia. Blood 1996;88:4259–4264.
8. Molica S, Levato D, Cascavilla N, Levato L, Musto P. Clinicoprognostic implications of simultaneous increased serum levels of soluble CD23 and beta2-microglobulin in B-cell chronic lymphocytic leukemia. Eur J Haematol 1999;62:117–122.
9. Niitsu N, Okabe-Kado J, Kasukabe T, Yamamoto-Yamaguchi Y, Umeda M, Honma Y. Prognostic implications of the differentiation inhibitory factor nm23-H1 protein in the plasma of aggressive non-Hodgkin's lymphoma. Blood 1999;94:3541–3550.
10. Niitsu N, Okabe-Kado J, Okamoto M, Takagi T, Yoshida T, Aoki S, et al. Serum nm23-H1 protein as a prognostic factor in aggressive non-Hodgkin lymphoma. Blood 2001;97:1202–1210.

11. Niitsu N, Okamato M, Okabe-Kado J, Takagi T, Yoshida T, Aoki S, et al. Serum nm23-H1 protein as a prognostic factor for indolent non-Hodgkin's lymphoma. Leukemia 2001;15: 832–839.
12. Niitsu N, Okabe-Kado J, Nakayama M, Wakimoto N, Sakashita A, Maseki N, et al. Plasma levels of the differentiation inhibitory factor nm23-H1 protein and their clinical implications in acute myeloid leukemia. Blood 2000;96:1080–1086.
13. Fayad L, Keating MJ, Reuben JM, O'Brien S, Lee BN, Lerner S, Kurzrock R. Interleukin-6 and interleukin-10 levels in chronic lymphocytic leukemia: correlation with phenotypic characteristics and outcome. Blood 2001;256–263.
14. Vassilakopoulos TP, Nadali G, Angelopoulou MK, Siakantaris MP, Dimopoulou MN, Kontopidou FN, et al. Serum interleukin-10 levels are an independent prognostic factor for patients with Hodgkin's lymphoma. Haematologica 2001;86:274–281.
15. Fayad L, Cabanillas F, Talpaz M, McLaughlin P, Kurzrock R. High serum interleukin-6 levels correlate with a shorter failure-free survival in indolent lymphoma. Leukemia & Lymphoma 1998;30:563–571.
16. Seymour JF, Talpaz M, Cabanillas F, Wetzler M, Kurzrock R. Serum interleukin-6 levels correlate with prognosis in diffuse large-cell lymphoma. J Clin Oncol 1995;13:575–582.
17. Blay JY, Burdin N, Rousset F, Lenoir G, Biron P, Philip T, et al. Serum interleukin-10 in non-Hodgkin's lymphoma: a prognostic factor. Blood 1993;82:2169–2174.
18. Molica S, Vitelli G, Levato D, Giannarelli D, Gandolfo GM. Elevated levels of soluble CD44 can identify a subgroup of patients with early B-cell chronic lymphocytic leukemia who are at high risk of disease progression. Cancer 2001;92:713–719.
19. Ristamaki R, Joensuu H, Lappalainen K, Teerenhovi L, Jalkanen S. Elevated serum CD44 level is associated with unfavorable outcome in non-Hodgkin's lymphoma. Blood 1997;90:4039–4045.
20. Lazzarino M, Orlandi E, Klersy C, Astori C, Brusamolino E, Corso A, et al. Serum CA 125 is of clinical value in the staging and follow-up of patients with non-Hodgkin's lymphoma: correlation with tumor parameters and disease activity. Cancer 1998;82:576–582.
21. Benboubker L, Valat C, Linassier C, Cartron G, Delain M, Bout M, et al. A new serologic index for low-grade non-Hodgkin's lymphoma based on initial CA 125 and LDH serum levels. Ann Oncol 2000;11:1485–1491.
22. Hallek M, Langenmayer I, Nerl C, Knauf W, Dietzfelbinger H, Adorf D, et al. Elevated serum thymidine kinase levels identify a subgroup at high risk of disease progression in early, non-smoldering chronic lymphocytic leukemia. Blood 1999;93:1732–1737.
23. Salven P, Teerenhovi L, Joensuu H. A high pretreatment serum basic fibroblast growth factor concentration is an independent predictor of poor prognosis in non-Hodgkin's lymphoma. Blood 1999;94:3334–3339.
24. Ferrajoli A, Manshouri T, Estrov Z, Keating MJ, O'Brien S, Lerner S, et al. High levels of vascular endothelial growth factor receptor-2 correlate with shortened survival in chronic lymphocytic leukemia. Clin Cancer Res 2001;7:795–799.
25. Radich JP. Clinical applicability of the evaluation of minimal residual disease in acute leukemia. Curr Opin Oncol 2000;12:36–40.
26. Pui CH, Campana D. New definition of remission in childhood acute lymphoblastic leukemia. Leukemia 2000;14:783–785.
27. Radich JP. The use of PCR technology for detecting minimal residual disease in patients with leukemia. Rev in Immunogenet 1999;1:265–278.
28. Deptala A, Mayer SP. Detection of minimal residual disease. Methods Cell Biol 2001;64:385–420.
29. van Dongen JJM, Macintyre EA, Gabert JA, Delabesse E, Rossi V, Saglio G, et al. Standardized RT-PCR analysis of fusion gene transcripts from chromosome aberrations in acute leukemia for detection of minimal residual disease. Report of BIOMED-1 concerted action: Investigation of minimal residual disease in acute leukemia. Leukemia 1999;13:1901–1928.
30. Hokland P, Pallisgaard N. Integration of molecular methods for detection of balanced translocations in the diagnosis and follow-up of patients with leukemia. Semin Hematol 2000;37:358–367.
31. Campana D, Coustan-Smith E. Detection of minimal residual disease in acute leukemia by flow cytometry. Cytometry 1999;38: 139–152.
32. Weir EG, Cowan K, LeBeau P, Borowitz MJ. A limited antibody panel can distinguish B-precursor acute lymphoblastic leukemia from normal B precursors with four color flow cytometry: implications for residual disease detection. Leukemia 1999;13:558–567.
33. Chen J-S, Coustan-Smith E, Suzuki T, Neale GA, Mihara K, Pui C-H, Campana D. Identification of novel markers for monitoring minimal residual disease in acute lymphoblastic leukemia. Blood 2001;97:2115–2120.
34. Neale GA, Coustan-Smith E, Pan Q, Chen X, Gruhn B, Stow P, et al. Tandem application of flow cytometry and polymerase chain reaction for comprehensive detection of minimal residual disease in childhood acute lymphoblastic leukemia. Leukemia 1999; 13:1221–1226.
35. Malec M, Bjorklund E, Soderhall S, Mazur J, Sjogren A-M, Pisa P, et al. Flow cytometry and allele-specific oligonucleotide PCR are equally effective in detection of minimal residual disease in ALL. Leukemia 2001;15:716–727.
36. Goulden N, Oakhill A, Steward C. Practical application of minimal residual disease assessment in childhood acute lymphoblastic leukemia. Br J Haematol 2001;112:275–281.
37. Coustan-Smith E, Behm FG, Sanchez J, Boyett JM, Hancock ML, Raimondi SC, et al. Immunological detection of minimal residual disease in children with acute lymphoblastic leukemia. Lancet 1998;351:550–554.
38. van Dongen JJ, Seriu T, Panzer-Grumayer ER, Biondi A, Pongers-Willemse MJ, Corral L, et al. Prognostic value of minimal residual disease in acute lymphoblastic leukemia in childhood. Lancet 1998;352:1731–1738.
39. Cave H, van der WerfftenBosch J, Suciu S, Guidal C, Waterkeyn C, Otten J, et al. Clinical significance of minimal residual disease in childhood acute lymphoblastic leukemia. N Engl J Med 1998;339:591–598.
40. Dibenedetto SP, Lo Nigro L, Mayer SP, Rovera G, Schiliro G. Detectable molecular residual disease at the beginning of maintenance therapy indicates poor outcome in children with T-cell acute lymphoblastic leukemia. Blood 1997;1226–1232.
41. Goulden NJ, Knechtli CJ, Garland RJ, Langlands K, Hancock JP, Potter MN, et al. Minimal residual disease analysis for the prediction of relapse in children with standard-risk acute lymphoblastic leukemia. Br J Haematol 1998;100:235–244.
42. Gruhn B, Hongeng S, Yi H, Hancock ML, Rubnitz JE, Neale GA, Kitchingman GR. Minimal residual disease after intensive induction therapy in childhood acute lymphoblastic leukemia predicts outcome. Leukemia 1998;12:675–681.
43. Evans PA, Short MA, Owen RG, Jack AS, Forsyth PD, Shiach CR, et al. Residual disease detection using fluorescent polymerase chain reaction at 20 weeks of therapy predicts clinical outcome in

childhood acute lymphoblastic leukemia. J Clin Oncol 1998;16:3616–3627.
44. Biondi A, Valsecchi MG, Seriu T, D'Aniello E, Willemse MJ, Fasching K, et al. Molecular detection of minimal residual disease is a strong predictive factor of relapse in childhood B-lineage acute lymphoblastic leukemia with medium risk features. A case control study of the International BFM study group. Leukemia 2000;14:1939–1943.
45. Panzer-Grumayer ER, Schneider M, Panzer S, Fasching K, Gadner H. Rapid molecular response during early induction chemotherapy predicts a good outcome in childhood acute lymphoblastic leukemia. Blood 2000;95:790–794.
46. Coustan-Smith E, Sancho J, Hancock ML, Boyett JM, Behm FG, Raimondi SC, et al. Clinical importance of minimal residual disease in childhood acute lymphoblastic leukemia. Blood 2000;96:2691–2696.
47. Brisco J, Hughes E, Neoh SH, Sykes PJ, Bradstock K, Enno A, et al. Relationship between minimal residual disease and outcome in adult acute lymphoblastic leukemia. Blood 1996;87:5251–5256.
48. Knechtli CJ, Goulden NJ, Hancock JP, Harris EL, Garland RJ, Jones CG, et al. Minimal residual disease status as a predictor of relapse after allogeneic bone marrow transplantation for children with acute lymphoblastic leukemia. Br J Haematol 1998;102: 860–871.
49. Knechtli CJC, Goulden NJ, Hancock JC, Grandage VLG, Harris EL, Garland RJ, et al. Minimal residual disease status before allogeneic bone marrow transplantation is an important determinant of successful outcome for children and adolescents with acute lymphoblastic leukemia. Blood 1998;92: 4072–4079.
50. Radich J, Gehly G, Lee A, Avery R, Bryant E, Edmands S, et al. Detection of bcr-abl transcripts in Philadelphia chromosome-positive acute lymphoblastic leukemia after marrow transplantation. Blood 1997;89:2602–2609.
51. Venditti A, Buccisano F, Del Poeta G, Maurillo L, Tamburini A, Cox C, et al. Level of minimal residual disease after consolidation therapy predicts outcome in acute myeloid leukemia. Blood 2000;96:3948–3952.
52. San Miguel JF, Vidriales MB, Lopez-Berges C, Diaz-Mediavilla J, Gutierrez N, Canizo C, et al. Early immunophenotypical evaluation of minimal residual disease in acute myeloid leukemia identifies different patient risk groups and may contribute to post-induction treatment stratification. Blood 2001;98: 1746–1751.
53. Baer MR, Stewart CC, Dodge RK, Leget G, Sule N, Mrozek K, et al. High frequency of immunophenotype changes in acute myeloid leukemia at relapse: implications for residual disease detection (Cancer and Leukemia Group B Study 8361). Blood 2001;97:3574–3580.
54. Czuczman MS, Dodge RK, Stewart CC, Frankel SR, Davey FR, Powell BL, et al. Value of immunophenotype in intensively treated adult acute lymphoblastic leukemia: Cancer and Leukemia Group B Study 8364. Blood 1999;93:3931–3939.
55. Sievers EL, Radich JP. Detection of minimal residual disease in acute leukemia. Curr Opin Hematol 2000;7:212–216.
56. Pallisgard N, Hokland P, Riishoj DC, Pedersen B, Jorgensen P. Multiplex reverse transcription-polymerase chain reaction for simultaneous screening of 29 translocations and chromosomal aberrations in acute leukemia. Blood 1998;92:574–588.
57. San Miguel JF, Martinez A, Macedo A, Vidriales MB, Lopez-Berges C, Gonzales M, et al. Immunophenotyping investigation of minimal residual disease is a useful approach for predicting relapse in acute myeloid leukemia. Blood 1997;2465–2470.
58. Lo Coco F, Diverio D, Falini B, Biondi A, Nervi C, Pelicci PG. Genetic diagnosis and molecular monitoring in the management of acute promyelocytic leukemia. Blood 1999;94:12–22.
59. Diverio D, Rossi V, Avvisati G, DeSantis S, Pistilli A, Pane F, et al. Early detection of relapse by prospective reverse transcriptase-polymerase chain reaction analysis of the PML/RARalpha fusion gene in patients with acute promyelocytic leukemia enrolled in the GIMEMA-AIEOP multi-center "AIDA" trial. Blood 1998;92: 784–789.
60. Meloni G, Diverio D, Vignetti M, Avvisati G, Capria S, Petti MC, et al. Autologous bone marrow transplantation for acute promyelocytic leukemia in second remission: prognostic relevance of pretransplant minimal residual disease assessment by reverse transcription-polymerase chain reaction of the PML/RAR alpha fusion gene. Blood 1997;90:1321–1325.
61. Miyamoto T, Nagafuji K, Akashi K, Harada M, Kyo T, Akashi T, et al. Persistence of multi-potent progenitors expressing AML1/ETO transcripts in long-term remission patients with t(8;21) AML. Blood 1996;87:4789–4796.
62. Liu PP, Hara A, Wijmenga C, Collins FS. Molecular pathogenesis of the chromosome 16 inversion in the M4Eo subtype of acute myeloid leukemia. Blood 1995;85:2289–2302.
63. Hebert J, Cayuela JM, Daniel MT, Berger R, Sigaux F. Detection of minimal residual disease in acute myelomonocytic leukemia with abnormal eosinophils by nested polymerase chain reaction with allele specific amplification. Blood 1994;84: 2291–2296.
64. Tobal K, Johnson PR, Saunders MJ, Harrison CJ, Liu Yin JA. Detection of CBFB/MYH11 transcripts in patients with inversion and other abnormalities of chromosome 16 at presentation and remission. Br J Haematol 1995;91:104–108.
65. Tobal K, Newton J, Macheta M, Chang J, Morgenstern G, Evans PA, et al. Molecular quantitation of minimal residual disease in acute myeloid leukemia with t(8;21) can identify patients in durable remission and predict clinical relapse. Blood 2000;95:815–819.
66. Krauter J, Hoellge W, Wattjes MP, Nagel S, Heidenreich O, Bunjes D, et al. Detection and quantification of CBFB/MYH11 fusion transcripts in patients with inv(16)-positive acute myeloblastic leukemia by real-time RT-PCR. Genes Chrom Cancer 2001;30:342–348.
67. Faderl S, Talpaz M, Kantarjian HM, Estrov Z. Should polymerase chain reaction analysis to detect minimal residual disease in patients with chronic myelogenous leukemia be used in clinical decision making? Blood 1999;93:2755–2759.
68. Hochhaus A, Reiter A, Saussele S, Reichert A, Emig M, Kaeda J, et al. Molecular heterogeneity in complete cytogenetic responders after interferon-alpha therapy for chronic myelogenous leukemia: low levels of minimal residual disease are associated with continuing remission. German CML Study Group and the UK MRC CML Study Group. Blood 2000;95:62–66.
69. Shah NP, Snyder DS, Nicoll JM, McMahon RJ, Hsu NC, Forman SJ, et al. PCR-negative molecular remissions in chronic-, accelerated-, and blast crisis-phase CML patients treated with STI571, an Abl-specific kinase inhibitor. Blood 2000;96:471a.
70. Radich JP, Gehly G, Gooley T, Bryant E, Clift RA, Collins S, et al. Polymerase chain reaction detection of the BCR-ABL fusion transcript after allogeneic marrow transplantation for chronic

myeloid leukemia: results and implications in 346 patients. Blood 1995;85:2632–2638.
71. Radich JP, Gooley T, Bryant E, Chauncey T, Clift R, Beppu L, et al. The significance of *bcr-abl* molecular detection in chronic myeloid leukemia patients "late," 18 months or more after transplantation. Blood 2001;98:1701–1707.
72. Lin F, van Rhee F, Goldman JM, Cross NC. Kinetics of increasing BCR-ABL transcript numbers in chronic myeloid leukemia patients who relapse after bone marrow transplantation. Blood 1996;87:4473–4478.
73. Olavarria E, Kanfer E, Szydlo R, Kaedo J, Rezvani K, Cwynarski K, et al. Early detection of *BCR-ABL* transcripts by quantitative reverse transcriptase-polymerase chain reaction predicts outcome after allogeneic stem cell transplantation for chronic myeloid leukemia. Blood 2001;97:1560–1565.
74. Corradini P, Ladetto M, Pileri A, Tarella C. Clinical relevance of minimal residual disease monitoring in non-Hodgkin's lymphomas: a critical reappraisal of molecular strategies. Leukemia 1999;13:1691–1695.
75. Gribben JG, Neuberg D, Freedman AS, Gimmi CD, Pesek KW, Barber M, et al. Detection by polymerase chain reaction of residual cells with the bcl-2 translocation is associated with increased risk of relapse after autologous bone marrow transplantation for B-cell lymphoma. Blood 1993;81:3449–3457.
76. Zwicky CS, Maddocks AB, Andersen N, Gribben JG. Eradication of polymerase chain reaction detectable immunoglobulin gene rearrangement in non-Hodgkin's lymphoma is associated with decreased relapse after autologous bone marrow transplantation. Blood 1996;88:3314–3322.
77. Corradini P, Astolfi M, Cherasco C, Ladetto M, Voena C, Caracciolo D, et al. Molecular monitoring of minimal residual disease in follicular and mantle cell non-Hodgkin's lymphomas treated with high-dose chemotherapy and peripheral blood progenitor cell autografting. Blood 1997;89:724–731.
78. Lopez-Guillermo A, Cabanillas F, McLaughlin P, Smith T, Hagemeister F, Rodriguez MA, et al. The clinical significance of molecular response in indolent follicular lymphomas. Blood 1998;91:2955–2960.
79. Andersen NS, Donovan JW, Borus JS, Poor CM, Neuberg D, Aster JC, et al. Failure of immunologic purging in mantle cell lymphoma assessed by polymerase chain reaction detection of minimal residual disease. Blood 1997;90:4212–4221
80. Rawstron A, Kennedy B, Evans PAS, Davies FE, Richards SJ, Haynes AP, et al. Quantitation of minimal residual disease levels in chronic lymphocytic leukemia using a sensitive flow cytometric assay improves the prediction of outcome and can be used to optimize therapy. Blood 2001;98:29–35.

Chapter **27**

Tumor Markers in Primary and Metastatic Brain Tumors

Susanne M. Arnold and Roy A. Patchell

Despite our growing understanding of tumor biology, the molecular mechanisms of central nervous system (CNS) tumors remain poorly understood. In part, this is because the brain is physiologically distinct from other organs by virtue of the blood-brain-barrier (BBB), autoregulation of blood flow, lack of lymphatic drainage, and lack of regenerative capacity after injury (1,2,3). Because of the BBB, serum tumor markers are much less likely to be clinically applicable in primary or metastatic brain tumors. In addition, tumor markers from the brain parenchyma are complex; multiple oncoproteins have been implicated in each step of tumorigenesis. Although our understanding of CNS tumor markers remains in its infancy, some progress has been made in the last decade and will be described in this chapter. We will focus on parenchymal tumor markers in astrocytomas and oligodendrogliomas, where the most data are available, and describe other markers that are unique to medulloblastomas and pineal tumors. Finally we will describe what is known about parenchymal and cerebrospinal fluid (CSF) markers in tumors metastatic to the brain.

PRIMARY TUMORS OF THE CENTRAL NERVOUS SYSTEM—GENERAL PRINCIPLES OF TREATMENT

The most common and well-studied primary tumors of the CNS are astrocytomas, which are classified into the following grades by the World Health Organization (WHO):

- pilocytic and other low-grade astrocytomas (grade I),
- fibrillary astrocytomas (grade II),
- anaplastic astrocytomas (grade III), and
- glioblastoma multiforme (GBM) (grade IV) (4).

Within this classification, high-grade astrocytomas are the most common type of primary brain tumor in adults and make up about half of all primary brain tumors. Aggressive surgical resection and post-operative radiation therapy are the principal treatments for high-grade astrocytomas (5,6). Post-operative radiation therapy, when given at doses of 6,000 to 7,000 cGy, produces a statistically significant increase in median survival time (6,7). The addition of chemotherapy to primary radiation also improves survival in the non-operative setting (8). Within the category of high-grade astrocytomas two distinct entities have emerged: primary GBMs (arising *de novo*) and secondary GBMs (developing through malignant progression from lower grade astrocytomas) (9). Even with the most aggressive treatment, however, the median survival of patients with GBMs is less than one year, with primary GBMs having shorter survival times than secondary GBMs.

The overall prognosis for patients with low-grade gliomas is significantly better than for those with high-grade astrocytomas. The median five-year survival time for low-grade infiltrating astrocytomas ranges from 21% to 55% following surgery and is 10–43% at ten years (7). There is little doubt that surgery has diagnostic and therapeutic value; however, the role of radiotherapy is less clear. Several retrospective studies have suggested that survival time increases when post-surgical radiotherapy is used (10), but the definitive dose remains controversial (11). Within the broad category of astrocytomas, significant prognostic variables include grade, age, duration of symptoms, performance status, contrast enhancement on computed tomography (CT), and corticosteroid dependence (12,13).

Other histologic subtypes of interest in the discussion of CNS tumor markers include oligodendrogliomas, medulloblastomas, and pineal region tumors of childhood. Oligodendrogliomas are slow-growing tumors that occur primarily in the cerebral hemispheres; they account for about 10% of primary brain tumors. Attempts at surgical removal of oligodendrogliomas are often incomplete; in tumors that cannot be totally resected, several retrospective reviews have suggested that survival time is enhanced by post-operative radiotherapy (14,15). Furthermore, oligodendrogliomas are one of the few brain tumors to demonstrate chemosensitivity. Procarbazine-CCNU-vincristine (PCV) has prolonged patient survival times in the adjuvant setting after incomplete resection prior to radiation (16,17) and improves overall survival times in recurrent tumors (18). When treated with chemotherapy and radiation, pure oligodendrogliomas have a median survival time of 5.3 years, while mixed oligoastrocytomas have a median survival time of 1.3 years (19).

Medulloblastomas are the most common brain tumors in children; they occur in the posterior fossa, and have a strong tendency to spread in the CSF. Using both CSF cytology and myelography, evidence of leptomeningeal spread is present in about 30% of patients at diagnosis (20). Surgery is the first treatment used, and there is a relationship between the extent of resection and subsequent length of survival (21). Unfortunately, all patients treated with surgery alone ultimately relapse regardless of the degree of initial resection. A dramatic increase in survival has been found with the addition of adjuvant radiation and chemotherapy (most pronounced in patients with advanced stage tumors) with a five-year survival rate of 55–59% (22).

Germ cell tumors of the pineal region include germinomas, embryonal cell carcinomas, teratomas, choriocarcinomas, and endodermal sinus tumors. Germinomas are the most common CNS germ cell tumor, and account for about 60% of the total. Radiation therapy is the mainstay of treatment, and the five-year survival rate for histologically confirmed germinomas is 60 to 90% (23).

Current Diagnostic and Monitoring Procedures

The best diagnostic tests for primary brain tumors are contrast-enhanced magnetic resonance imaging (MRI) and to a lesser extent, CT (24,25). Surgical or stereotactic needle biopsy is the mainstay of diagnosis for most brain tumors. Historically, pathologists have used immunohistochemical (IHC) tumor markers to determine the cell of origin for specific brain tumors. The most important of these is glial fibrillary acidic protein (GFAP). GFAP is a marker of fibrillary astrocytes whose expression is especially useful in the recognition of astrocytic neoplasms. However, it is also expressed in oligodendrogliomas, ependymomas, choroid plexus papillomas, and other primary CNS neoplasms (26). Its expression has not reliably been correlated with neoplastic progression (27), and its utility lies in the realm of a diagnostic marker rather than a prognostic one. Neurofilament proteins are composed of three subunits of different molecular weight, each encoded by a separate gene. The neurofilament proteins are useful markers of well-differentiated ganglion cell tumors, some medulloblastomas, neurocytomas, and pineocytomas, but have little prognostic value at this time (26). Synaptophysin is the major calcium-binding protein of the presynaptic vesicle membrane. Synaptophysin IHC (reviewed in Wilkstrand et al.) (26) is useful in identifying medulloblastomas, neurocytomas, pinoecytomas, and ganglion cell tumors (26). It is also found in peripheral neuroendocrine tumors such as pheochromocytomas, carcinoids, and small-cell lung cancer (28). The classic tumor markers are used diagnostically but have little role in predicting prognosis or in making therapeutic decisions.

In the majority of CNS tumors, no serum or CSF markers are commonly used to follow primary brain tumors. In contrast to the rest of neuro-oncology, serum and CSF tumor markers have a defined role in the diagnosis and management of specific intracranial germ cell tumors, predominantly a pediatric disease. Specifically, alpha-fetoprotein (AFP), human chorionic gonadotrophin (HCG), and placental alkaline phosphatase (PAP) are often elevated in the CSF of patients with nongerminomatous germ cell tumors (embryonal carcinomas, endodermal sinus tumors, choriocarcinomas, and immature teratomas) (Table 1). These markers are considered part of the required work-up of pediatric patients with intracranial germ cell tumors (usually located in the pineal region). While they remain an essential part of the diagnostic evaluation, they are also prognostic. Elevation of tumor markers in nongerminomatous germ cell tumors portends a poorer prognosis in several studies to date (29–31). In children with markedly elevated tumor markers, it has been suggested that craniospinal dissemination can be prevented in patients with a relative increase in AFP or HCG by early, aggressive surgical therapy (31).

The majority of tumor markers that are considered in the following sections are well-established immunohistochemical (IHC) markers in brain parenchyma, unless otherwise indicated. Currently, these markers have practical diagnostic application for neuropathologists, neurosurgeons, and neuro-oncologists and are gradually being incorporated into therapeutic decision-making.

Specific Markers for Primary Brain Tumors

Proliferating cell nuclear antigen and Ki-67/MIB-1. The most widely investigated molecular markers in primary tumors of the CNS include two markers of cell proliferation: prolifer-

Table 1 Cerebrospinal fluid levels of alpha-fetoprotein (AFP), human chorionic gonadotrophin (HCG), and placental alkaline phosphatase (PAP) in patients with intracranial nongerminomatous germ cell tumors

Tumor Marker	Intracranial Germ Cell Tumor					
	Germinoma	Immature Teratoma	Embryonal Carcinoma	Mature Teratoma	Choriocarcinoma	Endodermal sinus tumor
Alpha-fetoprotein	−	±	+	−	−	+++
Human chorionic gonadotrophin-β	±	−	++	−	+++	−
Placental Alkaline Phosphatase	++	−	−	−	−	−

−, negative; ± may or may not be elevated; +, slightly elevated; ++, modestly elevated; +++, markedly elevated.

ating cell nuclear antigen (PCNA) and Ki-67/MIB-1. PCNA is a nuclear protein present in G1, S, and G2 phases of the cell cycle, and functions as an auxiliary to DNA polymerase. The test uses immunocytochemical-coupling flow cytometry and light microscopy, which is cumbersome and fraught with high inter-observer variability. Multiple studies have investigated the utility of PCNA in predicting clinical outcome and prognosis, but no overall consensus has been reached (12,32). Ki-67 is a nuclear protein present in all but G0 of the cell cycle and has two available antibodies, Ki-67 and MIB-1 (MIB-1 may be used on paraffin-embedded specimens). Because of its convenience, Ki-67/MIB-1 is now the preferred method of assessing proliferative potential of brain tumors. The majority of studies available for analysis are retrospective and have conflicting results, primarily because of inconsistent methodologies and high inter-observer variability. Several studies have shown indeterminate prognostic value of Ki-67 by IHC in low-grade astrocytomas (33), a variety of astrocytomas and oligodendrogliomas (34–36), and in GBMs (37). Generally, Ki-67 labeling correlates with poorer survival in diffuse astrocytomas in adults (38–41), in oligodendrogliomas (42), and in anaplastic, non-pilocytic astrocytomas in children (43). While there is a massive amount of data regarding MIB-1's reliability in predicting disease response, no widely accepted use of MIB-1 as a specific tumor marker can be delineated.

Despite the lack of generalizability to all brain tumors, there are several circumstances where MIB-1 labeling has a prognostic or diagnostic role (44). MIB-1 expression in greater than 8% of tumor cells has been predictive of malignant transformation and shortened survival times in patients with grade II astrocytomas (45) and in gliomas in general (40). In oligodendrogliomas, a MIB-1 labeling index greater than 5% predicts a significantly shorter patient survival time in two different studies (46,47). Another area where proliferative indices may be helpful is in standardizing other IHC marker testing (i.e., sampling for mitosis; p53 expression by IHC). At least one author has suggested parallel Ki-67 immunostaining be used as a guide to the most proliferative areas of a tumor with which to quantitate other tumor markers (48). At this time, MIB-1 may be considered a prognostic guide but is not considered an adequate tumor marker for primary brain tumors, with the exception of grade II astrocytomas.

Chromosome 1p and 19q. Chromosomal loss has been noted in many brain tumors, but in the case of oligodendrogliomas, loss of chromosomes 1p and 19q specifically correlates with outcome. Loss of 1p and 19q is found in 50–70% of oliogodendrogliomas (25). Interestingly, loss of 1p correlates with increased sensitivity to chemotherapy (49), while concomitant loss of 19q was associated with longer recurrence-free survival after chemotherapy using loss of heterozygosity (LOH) assays in tumor DNA in a landmark study by Cairncross. These findings have been replicated using fluorescence in-situ hybridization techniques, showing a clear association of 1p and 19q loss with the prolonged overall survival in pure oligodendrogliomas by univariate and multivariate analysis, but not in astrocytomas or mixed oligoastrocytomas (50). In a recent study of anaplastic oligodendrogliomas (51), 1p and 19q abnormalities (as determined by LOH assay) allowed oligodendrogliomas to be stratified into four therapeutic and prognostic categories. Patients with a combined loss of 1p and 19q (without other mutations) had a significantly longer response to chemotherapy and a survival time of greater than 123 months. Those with 1p loss (with or without other chromosomal abnormalities) also responded well to chemotherapy, but with shorter responses and a median survival time of 71 months. Patients without 1p loss but with p53 mutations had a median survival time of 71 months, and did respond to chemotherapy, but relapsed more quickly than those in the previous group. Those without 1p loss and without p53 mutations were poorly responsive to chemotherapy and died rapidly. It has also been shown that radiation sensitivity may be predicted by the isolated loss of both 1p and 19q in oligodendrogliomas (52). Clearly, loss of chromosome 1p and 19q not only aids in the diagnosis of oliogodendroglioma, but correlates with improved length of survival; specific loss of 1p is predictive of chemosensitivity. These chromosomal abnormalities (loss of 1p and 19q) provide the strongest argument to date for the incorporation of tumor markers into therapeutic decision-making in neuro-oncology and future prospective trials.

O^6-methyl-guanine-DNA methyltransferase. The gene for DNA-repair enzyme O^6-methyl-guanine-DNA methyltransferase (MGMT) is located on chromosome 10. It removes mutagenic and cytotoxic adducts from the O^6 position of guanine, thus inhibiting the ability of alkylating agents such as 1,3-bis(2-chloroethyl)-1-nitrosurea to kill tumor cells. When the MGMT's promoter is methylated, gene activity is turned off. Several studies have demonstrated increased MGMT activity by *in vitro* assays and have shown increased activity of this DNA repair protein in astrocytomas (53). In novel work from Esteller and colleagues (54), glioma samples were analyzed via polymerase chain reaction (PCR) for the presence of methylation within the *MGMT* promoter. Methylation was associated with regression of tumor after alkylator therapy and prolonged overall and disease-free survival times. Remarkably, the presence of this MGMT tumor marker within the glioma was a stronger independent prognostic factor than other, more traditional factors such as age, stage, tumor grade, or performance status in the 47 patients evaluated (54). While not in common practice, *MGMT* methylation by PCR or *in vitro* assay has demonstrated a powerful ability to detect therapeutic response, based on biologic differences between tumors and to predict outcome. Tumor markers such as these will likely be commonplace in the future.

Epidermal growth factor receptor. The product of the v-$erbB_1$ oncogene on chromosome 7p, epidermal growth factor receptor (EGFR) is a transmembrane tyrosine kinase receptor involved in ligand binding and intracellular signaling cascades. It is present in 40–50% of astrocytomas and is associated with poor prognosis and decreased survival times (55,56). Both reverse transcriptase PCR (RT-PCR) and Southern blotting have been used reliably in the study of EGFR in brain tumors (55), but IHC has also been studied and can reliably predict activation of EGFR and overexpression of the most common mutant form in astrocytomas, EGFRvIII (deletion of exons 2–7) (57). In diffuse astrocytomas, IHC expression of EGFR is an independent predictor of decreased disease-free survival (39). Primary GBMs tend to show EGFR overexpression or amplification, compared with secondary GBMs (58), and EGFR expression and amplification is thought to be the main reason for the poor outcome in primary GBMs (59). While oligodendrogliomas are generally thought to arise from molecular events distinct from astrocytomas, they demonstrate EGFR overexpression in over 50% of tumors (60). EGFR is another very promising tumor marker in brain parenchyma because of its dominant overexpression in astrocytomas, its practical application in IHC, and multiple studies showing reliable correlation with length of survival.

The EGFR tumor marker has special significance due to a variety of biologic therapies based on EGFR overexpression, including both iodine-125 labeled (61) and non-labeled anti-EGFR monoclonal antibodies (62, 63) used in high-grade gliomas and recurrent astrocytomas, intratumoral anti-EGFR therapy (64), antisense EGFR therapies (65), and immunotoxin therapy (using EGFRvIII fused to *Pseudomonas* exotoxin) (66). While EGFR expression has shown conflicting results in some tumor tissues, it has prognostic value and likely will have significant therapeutic value in the future as EGFR-based therapies enter the mainstream and identification of appropriate patients becomes necessary.

p53 and Mouse Double Minute-2. The *p53* gene located on chromosome 17p plays a major role in cell cycle regulation, apoptosis, and response to DNA damage. Nuclear accumulation of p53 confers a more aggressive phenotype in many cancers (67) and is found in about 35% of all astrocytomas (68). Primary GBMs have been shown to lack *p53* mutations (through DNA sequencing), but have amplification of Mouse Double Minute-2 (MDM-2) and EGFR. They carry a very poor prognosis in general. Secondary GBMs have frequent *p53* mutations, rare EGFR gene amplification, and a superior prognosis to primary GBMs (69,70). In this setting, p53 is diagnostic and prognostic and clearly aids in predicting clinical outcome. It has significant potential as a reliable tumor marker in GBMs but has not been widely accepted yet.

While *p53* mutation in GBMs is prognostic and predictive of overall length of survival, the data regarding low-grade astrocytomas are less compelling. Using IHC expression of p53 in a group of diffuse astrocytomas, multivariate analysis revealed that p53-labeling index was an independent predictor of overall survival in one study (71), but had no association with survival time in several others (34,72). In oligodendroglioma, IHC expression of p53 in tumor cells was associated with a decreased length of survival in several studies (73,74). While *p53* mutations are frequently found in those low-grade astrocytomas that eventually progress to GBMs, the evidence for a causative effect is circumstantial. To date, p53 IHC is not used as a definitive tumor marker of low-grade astrocytomas.

Despite conflicting results between *p53* mutations and length of patient survival, the use of p53 as a tumor marker holds promise as a prognostic indicator when used on tumor tissue directly (based on some studies, showing correlation between tumor and overall survival time). Because of its frequent mutation in many cancers, it is nonspecific for the brain, but likely would be most informative in combination with other tumor markers in CNS tumors.

The *MDM-2* oncogene located on chromosome 12q binds to and inactivates p53 protein, playing a major role in the p53-dependent carcinogenesis cascades. It is amplified in primary GBMs that show no *p53* mutation (75) and correlates with a worse prognosis. While IHC studies of astrocytomas have revealed a significant correlation between p53 and MIB-1 expression on the one hand, and tumor grade on the other, MDM-2 has shown no clear relationship with other prognostic variables (76). Although it appears to correlate with outcome in some brain tumors, it is not widely accepted as a tumor marker at this time.

Matrix metalloproteinases and tissue inhibitors of metalloproteinases. Matrix metalloproteinases (MMPs) are a family of zinc-dependent endopeptidases that degrade many elements of the extracellular matrix (?) (ECM) allowing progression of tumor locally and distantly. They have been divided into four subgroups:

- matrilysin;
- collagenases, metalloelastase, and stromelysins;
- gelatinases; and
- transmembrane-containing metalloproteinases or MT-MMPs (77,78).

They are regulated by tissue inhibitors of metalloproteinases (TIMPs), which bind to and inhibit the active forms of MMPs, blocking endogenous enzymatic activity and thus degradation of the ECM. While the complex balance between MMPs and TIMPs is not fully understood in primary brain tumors, several authors have begun to elucidate interesting patterns. Kachra and colleagues (79) analyzed a variety of brain tumor specimens using IHC and Western blotting, concluding that several MMPs were overexpressed in high-grade tumors (MMP-9: anaplastic astrocytomas and anaplastic oligodendrogliomas; MMP-12: GBMs). TIMP-1 and TIMP-2 expression was significantly lower in higher-grade tumors (grade II and III astrocytomas and oligodendrogliomas) as compared to low-grade brain tumors, implying a lack of control over the invasive phenotype as one mechanism of tumor progression. This ratio of high MMP expression and low TIMP expression may be useful in determining which brain tumors are likely to need more aggressive therapy, although this has not been proven conclusively in clinical studies. While the use of TIMPs and MMPs is not routine, they have a good potential as tumor markers in the future.

Telomerase. Telomerase is a ribonucleoprotein that synthesizes telomeric DNA on the ends of chromosomes in order to protect central coding regions of chromosomes. Telomere-shortening is thought to be the basis for one avenue of cellular senescence and increased telomerase production is present in a variety of cancers (80). In grade II and anaplastic astrocytomas, telomerase activity correlated with early tumor progression and reduced survival. In general, increased aggressiveness accompanies increased telomerase activity in astrocytomas. High telomerase activity was also exhibited in oligodendrogliomas (81). While several studies have demonstrated increased telomerase activity in human brain tumor tissues (82), no clear-cut role for telomerase as a tumor marker has yet been demonstrated. For more information on telomerase, please see Chapter 55.

Neurotrophin receptor kinase C. Neurotrophins are a family of four trophic factors that have broad effects on developing, mature, and injured CNS cells. Each binds preferentially to neurotrophin receptor kinases to regulate cell proliferation, differentiation, and death. Neurotrophin receptor kinase C (TrkC) mRNA expression has been studied in medulloblastoma by fluorescence in-situ hybridization in several studies (83,84). Increased TrkC expression apparently activates multiple signaling pathways, including early expression of the oncogenes *c-jun* and *c-fos*, thus promoting apoptosis. In one study (84), high TrkC expression was found to be the strongest predictor of a favorable outcome when compared with established clinical prognostic factors and laboratory variables. It has been suggested that this putative tumor marker be used to help plan treatment for patients with medulloblastoma, although no prospective clinical studies have been reported to validate this claim.

While many other growth factors (platelet-derived growth factor, vascular endothelial growth factor), growth factor receptors, oncogenes (*bcl-2* and retinoblastoma gene), and cyclin-dependent kinases (cdk-2, 4, and 6) have been studied in brain tumors, none of these has been validated as a true tumor marker in the clinical practice of neuro-oncology.

BRAIN METASTASES: GENERAL PRINCIPLES OF THERAPY

Metastases to the brain are the most common type of intracranial tumor; 25% of adults and 10% of children with systemic cancer develop brain metastases during their lifetime (85,86). Because most patients present with multiple metastases, whole brain radiotherapy (WBRT) is the treatment of choice for most patients with brain metastases (79,80). The accepted dose of therapeutic WBRT is from 3600–5040 cGy(87–89). In the patient with a single brain metastasis, two prospective randomized trials support the use of surgical removal (90,91), while one trial did not find an advantage to surgery (92). Newer techniques such as gamma knife radiosurgery are being studied as possible alternatives to surgical resection. One randomized trial (93) has explored the benefit of post-operative radiation in this setting, and has shown decreased tumor recurrence and death from neurological causes, although no significant difference in survival was shown.

The growth of tumors within the brain requires many steps: detachment from the primary tumor site, response to chemotactic factors, invasion and degradation of the brain's particular ECM, angiogenesis, and successful growth within the brain (1,2,3,94). Whether these metastatic steps are unique to the brain or common to a universal metastatic process is unknown, although it is central to the development of directed therapies and prevention of brain metastasis. At the cellular level, numerous oncoproteins have been evaluated in brain metastasis (including p53, bcl-2, MMPs, e-cadherin, CD44, and nerve growth factor), but no standard of care exists for using serum, CSF, or brain tissue tumor markers as indicators of prognosis or treatment. While the use of tumor markers for monitoring brain metastases remains in its infancy, there are exciting investigations on the horizon in which tumor markers may play an integral role in cancer management.

Specific Tumor Markers for Metastatic Tumors to the Brain

p53. A highly significant proportion of brain metastases (>90%) overexpress p53 by IHC, as do the tumors from which they metastasize (95). It is likely that deregulation of the G1-S cell cycle checkpoint is necessary for metastasis, although this is probably not specific to brain metastases, given that *p53* is frequently mutated in metastatic tumors (67). The use of p53 as a tumor marker for brain metastasis may be impractical because it is so commonly mutated in brain metastasis and primary brain tumors and is therefore not brain-specific.

Cell adhesion molecules. The cell adhesion molecule CD44 exists in multiple splice forms and is thought to influence metastasis formation. It is considered a homing receptor and is found in primary brain tumors and metastasis (96). Techniques such as reverse transcriptase-polymerase chain reaction (RT-PCR) (97) and IHC (98) have shown variant forms of CD44 to be overexpressed in metastatic brain tumors. Further, primary brain tumors show only weak expression of CD44, and no CD44 expression is seen in tumors metastatic to the spine, leading to the conclusion that CD44 expression influenced the tumor cell's choice of end-organ metastasis. While CD44 has not been connected to clinical prognosis in brain metastasis, its role as a homing device to the brain makes it attractive as a tumor marker. If it can be predictive of which tumors will eventually spread to the brain, it could significantly influence therapeutic decision making.

E-cadherin (EC) is a calcium-dependent transmembrane glycoprotein that allows cell-cell adhesion and invasion-suppression in epithelial cells. Its expression is often lost during tumor progression (99,100). In one study using IHC, it was shown to be overexpressed in the vast majority of brain metastases. (95). The balance of cell adhesion in brain metastases appears to rely on increased expression of cell-cell adhesion molecules once the cells have spread to the brain. This may represent a reactivation of cell adhesion once tumor cells arrive at the targeted end organ. Cell adhesion molecule overexpression may be specific to the brain in the cases of CD44 and EC, but both await validation prior to being accepted as tumor markers.

MMPs and TIMPs. MMPs degrade many elements of the ECM, allowing tumor invasion into distant sites. Several studies have shown a correlation between increased MMP expression and increased metastatic potential (78,101). Native TIMPs inhibit *in vivo* metastasis in animal models (102). Several studies have demonstrated a striking pattern of MMP overexpression by IHC in brain metastases [specifically MMP-9 (95) and MMP-2 (103)], suggesting that MMP production is a common feature of brain metastasis. In addition, TIMPs appear to be downregulated in brain metastases that overexpress MMPs (95,104). This implies a disruption in the normal balance between MMPs and TIMPs in the ECM of the brain during metastasis. It is unknown whether these markers will be prognostic in a brain metastasis' response to therapy or predictive of which primary tumors will spread to the brain.

GT1B. Another group of cellular adhesion molecules, gangliosides, and plasma membrane proteins are involved in metastasis and are thought to be lineage-specific. GT1b is brain-specific and is overexpressed not only in brain metastasis, but in primary tumors that eventually spread to the brain (105). Although this report is preliminary, GT1b appears to target the brain as a site of metastasis, and may be necessary for tumors to metastasize to the brain.

SUMMARY

Currently, tumor markers play a role in the diagnosis and treatment of some primary CNS tumors (astrocytomas, GBMs, and oligodendrogliomas, in particular). The most significant advances in CNS tumor markers have allowed physicians to predict response to specific chemotherapy, as in the case of 1p and 19q loss in oligodendrogliomas and MGMT methylation in grade III and IV astrocytomas. As we discover more about the oncogenic pathways that are active in CNS tumors and metastases, we will likely find that some are unique to the brain, while others are common to a universal process of tumorigenesis. Those that are unique to the brain, or selectively altered in specific situations, will likely aid in the development of reliable CNS tumor markers in the future. Brain parenchyma and CSF appear to provide the most reliable tissues for future study because of the brain's unique microenvironment. Molecules that specifically localize to the brain are particularly attractive in predicting spread of tumors into the CNS. Characterizing CNS tumor markers will permit optimal use of new therapies including EGFR-based therapies, MMP, and angiogenesis inhibitors.

REFERENCES

1. Liotta LA, Stetler-Stevenson WG, Steeg PS. Cancer invasion and metastasis: positive and negative regulatory elements. Cancer Inv 1991;9:543–551.
2. Nicholson GL, Menter DG, Herrman J, Cavanaugh P, Jia L, et al. Tumor metastasis to brain: role of endothelial cells, neurotrophins, and paracrine growth factors. Crit Rev Oncog 1994;5:451–471.
3. DeClerck YA, Shimada H, Gonzales-Gomez I, Raffel C. Tumoral invasion in the central nervous system. J Neurooncol 1994;18:111–121.
4. Kleihues P, Burger PC, Scheithauer BW. The new WHO classification of brain tumors. Brain Pathol 1993;3:225–268.
5. Shapiro WR. Treatment of neuroectodermal brain tumors. Ann Neurol 1982;12:231–237.
6. Walker MD, Green SB, Byar DP, Alexander E Jr, Batzdorf U, et al. Randomized comparisons of radiotherapy and nitrosoureas for the treatment of malignant glioma after surgery. N Engl J Med 1980;303:1323–1329.
7. Levin VA. Management of gliomas, medulloblastomas, and CNS germ cell tumors. In: Cavalli F, Hansen HH, Kaye SB (eds.). Textbook of medical oncology. London: Martin Dunitz, 1997:309–323.
8. Prados MD, Larson DA, Lamborn K, McDermott MW, Sneed PK, et al. Radiation therapy and hydroxyurea followed by the combination of 6-thioguanine and BCNU for the treatment of primary malignant brain tumors. Int J Radiat Oncol Biol Phys 1998:40:57–63.
9. von Deimling A, von Ammon K, Schoenfeld D, Wiestler OD, Seizinger BR, et al. Subsets of glioblastoma multiforme defined by molecular genetic analysis. Brain Pathol 1993;3:19–26.
10. Berger MS, Leibel, SA, Bruner JM, et al. Primary central nervous system tumors of the supratentorial compartment. In: Levin VA (ed.). Cancer in the nervous system. New York: Churchill Livingstone,1995:57–68.
11. Karim AB, Maat B, Hatlevoll R, Menten J, Rutten EH, et al. A randomized trial on dose-response in radiation therapy of low-grade cerebral glioma: European Organization for Research and Treatment of Cancer (EORTC) Study 22844. Int J Radiat Oncol Biol Phys 1996;36:549–556.
12. Grzybicki DM, Moore SA. Implications of prognostic markers in brain tumors. Clin Lab Medicine 1999;19:833–847.
13. Lote K, Egeland T, Hager B, Stenwig B, Skullerud K, et al. Survival, prognostic factors, and therapeutic efficacy in low-grade gliomas: A retrospective study in 379 patients. J Clin Oncol 1997;15:3129–3140.
14. Roberts M, German WJ. A long-term study of patients with oligodendrogliomas. Follow-up of 50 cases, including Dr. Harvey Cushing's series. J Neurosurg 1966;24:697–700.
15. Chin HW, Hazel JJ, Kim TH, Webster JH. Oligodendrogliomas. I. A clinical study of cerebral oligodendrogliomas. Cancer 1980;45:1458–1466.
16. Cairncross G, Macdonald D, Ludwin S, Lee D, Cascino T, et al. Chemotherapy for anaplastic oligodendroglioma. National Cancer Institute of Canada Clinical Trials Group. J Clin Oncol 1994;12:2013–2021.
17. Macdonald DR, Gaspar LE, Cairncross JG. Successful chemotherapy for newly diagnosed aggressive oligodendroglioma. Ann Neurol 1990;27:573–574.
18. Cairncross JG, Macdonald DR. Successful chemotherapy for recurrent malignant oligodendroglioma. Ann Neurol 1988;23:360–364.
19. Winger MJ, Macdonald DR, Cairncross JG. Supratentorial anaplastic gliomas in adults: the prognostic importance of extent of resection and prior low-grade glioma. J Neurosurg 1989;71:487–493.
20. Deutsch M. The impact of myelography on the treatment results for medulloblastoma. Int J Radiat Oncol Biol Phys 1984;10:999–1003.
21. Park TS, Hoffman HJ, Hendrick EB, Humphreys RP, Becker LE. Medulloblastoma: clinical presentation and management. Experience at the hospital for sick children, Toronto, 1950–1980. J Neurosurg 1983;58:543–552.
22. Tait DM, Thornton-Jones H, Bloom HJG, Lemerle J, Morris-Jones P, et al. Adjuvant chemotherapy for medulloblastoma:

the first multi-center control trial of the International Society of Pediatric Oncologists (SIOP I). Eur J Cancer 1990;26: 464–469.
23. Sano K, Matsutani M. Pinealoma (Germinoma) treated by direct surgery and post-operative irradiation. A long-term follow-up. Childs Brain 1981;8:81–97.
24. Davis PC, Hudgins PA, Peterman SB, Hoffman JC. Diagnosis of cerebral metastases: double-dose-delayed CT vs. contrast enhanced MR imaging. AJNR 1991;12:293–300.
25. Sze G, Milano E, Johnson C, Heier, L. Detection of brain metastases: comparison of contrast-enhanced MR with unenhanced MR and enhanced CT. AJNR 1990;1:785–791.
26. Wilkstrand CJ, Fung K, Trojanowski JQ, Mclendon RE, Bigner DD. Antibodies and molecular immunology: Immunohistochemistry and antigens of diagnostic significance. In: Bigner DD, McLendon RE, Bruner (eds.). Russell and Rubinstein's pathology of tumors of the nervous system (6th ed). New York, NY: Oxford University Press,1998:251–304.
27. Duffy PE, Huang YY, Rapport MM, Graf L. Glial fibrillary acidic protein in giant cell tumors of brain and other gliomas. A possible relationship to malignancy, differentiation, and pleomorphism of glia. Acta Neuropathol 1980;52:51–57.
28. Wiedenmann B, Huttner WB. Synaptophysin and chromogranins/secretogranins—widespread constituents of distinct types of neuro-endocrine vesicles and new tools in tumor diagnosis. Virchows Arch B Cell Pathol Incl Mol-Pathol 1989; 58:95–121.
29. Schild SE, Haddock MG, Scheithauer BW, Marks LB, Norman MG, et al. Nongerminomatous germ cell tumors of the brain. Int J Radiat Oncol Biol Phys 1996;36:557–563.
30. Itoyama Y, Kochi M, Yamamoto H, Kuratsu J, Uemura S, et al. Clinical study of intracranial nongerminomatous germ cell tumors producing alpha-fetoprotein. Neurosurgery 1990;27: 454–460.
31. Nishizaki T, Kajiwara K, Adachi N, Tsuha M, Nakayama H, et al. Detection of craniospinal dissemination of intracranial germ cell tumors based on serum and cerebrospinal fluid levels of tumor markers. J Clin Neurosci 2001;8:27–30.
32. Lafuente JV, Alkiza K, Garibi JM, Alvarez A, Bilboa J, et al. Biologic parameters that correlate with the prognosis of human gliomas. Neuropathology 2000;20:176–183.
33. Nakamura M, Konishi N, Tsunoda S, Nakase H, Tsuzuki T, et al. Analysis of prognostic and survival factors related to treatment of low-grade astrocytomas in adults. Oncology 2000;58: 108–116.
34. Cunningham JM, Kimmel DW, Scheithauer BW, O'Fallon JR, Novotny PJ, et al. Analysis of proliferation markers and p53 expression in gliomas of astrocytic origin: relationships and prognostic value. J Neurosurg 1997;86:121–130.
35. Ehrmann J Jr, Rihakova P, Hlobilkova A, Kala M, Kolar Z. The expression of apoptosis-related proteins and the apoptotic rate in glial tumors of the brain. Neoplasma 2000;47:151–155.
36. Reis-Filho JS, Faoro LN, Carrilho C, Bleggi-Torres LF, Schmitt FC. Evaluation of cell proliferation, epidermal growth factor receptor, and bcl-2 immunoexpression as prognostic factors for patients with World Health Organization grade 2 oligodendroglioma. Cancer 2000;88:862–869.
37. Korshunov A, Golanov A, Sycheva R, Pronin I. Prognostic value of tumor-associated antigen immunoreactivity and apoptosis in cerebral glioblastomas: an analysis of 168 cases. J Clin Pathol 1999;52:574–580.
38. McKeever PE, Strawderman MS, Yamini B, Mikhail AA, Blaivas M. MIB-1 proliferation index predicts survival among patients with grade II astrocytoma. J Neuropathol Exp Neurol 1998; 57:931–936.
39. Korkolopoulou P, Christodoulou P, Kouzelis K, Hadjiyannakis M, Priftis A, et al. MDM2 and p53 expression in gliomas: a multivariate survival analysis including proliferation markers and epidermal growth factor receptor. Br J Cancer 1997;75: 1269–1278.
40. Di X, Nishizaki T, Harada K, Kajiwara K, Nakayama H, et al. Proliferative potentials of glioma cells and vascular components determined with monoclonal antibody MIB-1. J Exp Clin Cancer Res 1997;16:389–394.
41. Wakimoto H, Aoyagi M, Nakayama T, Nagashima G, Yamamoto S, et al. Prognostic significance of Ki-67 labeling indices obtained using MIB-1 monoclonal antibody in patients with supratentorial astrocytomas. Cancer 1996;77:373–380.
42. Kros JM, Hop WC, Godschalk JJ, Krishnadath KK. Prognostic value of the proliferation related antigen Ki-67 in oligodendrogliomas. Cancer 1996;78:1107–1113.
43. Ho DM, Wong TT, Hsu CY, Ting LT, Chiang H. MIB-1 labeling index in nonpilocytic astrocytoma of childhood: a study of 101 cases. Cancer 1998;82:2459–2466.
44. Heesters MA, Koudstaal J, Go KG, Molenaar, WM. Analysis of proliferation and apoptosis in brain gliomas: prognostic and clinical value. J Neurooncol 1999;44:255–266.
45. Schiffer D, Cavalla P, Chio A, Richiardi P, Giordana MT. Proliferative activity and prognosis of low-grade astrocytomas. J Neurooncol 1997;34:31–35.
46. Coons SW, Johnson PC, Pearl DK. The prognostic significance of Ki-67 labeling indices for oligodendrogliomas. Neurosurgery 1997;41:878–884.
47. Dehghani F, Schachenmayr W, Laun A, Korf HW. Prognostic implication of histopathological, immunohistochemical, and clinical features of oligodendrogliomas: a study of 89 cases. Acta-Neuropathol- (Berl) 1998;95:493–504.
48. Sallinen PK, Sallinen SL, Helen PT, Rantala IS, Rautiainen E, et al. Grading of diffusely infiltrating astrocytomas by quantitative histopathology, cell proliferation, and image cytometric DNA analysis. Comparison of 133 tumors in the context of the WHO 1979 and WHO 1993 grading schemes. Neuropathol Appl Neurobiol 2000;26:319–331.
49. Cairncross JG, Ueki K, Slatescu M, Lisle D, Finkelstein D, et al. Specific genetic predictors of chemotherapeutic response and survival in patients with anaplastic oliogodendrogliomas. J Natl Cancer Inst 1998; 90:1473–1479.
50. Smith J, Perry A, Borelli T, Lee Hi, O'Fallon J, et al. Alterations in chromosome arms 1p and 19q as predictors of survival in oligodendrogliomas, astrocytomas, and mixed oligoastrocytomas. J Clin Oncol 2000; 18:636–645.
51. Ino Y, Betensky RA, Zlatescu MC, Sasaki H, Macdonald DR, et al. Molecular subtypes of anaplastic oligodendroglioma: Implications for patient management at diagnosis. Clin Cancer Res 2001;7:839–845.
52. Bauman GS, Ino Y, Ueki K, Zlatescu M, Fisher BJ, et al. Allelic loss of chromosome 1p and radiotherapy plus chemotherapy in patients with oligodendrogliomas. Int J Radiat Oncol Biol Phys 2000;48:825–830.
53. Silber J, Bobola M, Ghatan S, Blank A, Kolstoe DD, et al. 0⁶-methyl-guanine-DNA methyltransferase activity in adult gliomas: relation to patient and tumor characteristics. Cancer Res 1998;58:1068–1073.
54. Esteller M, Garcia-Foncillas J, Andion E, Goodman SN, Hidalgo O, et al. Inactivation of the DNA-repair gene MGMT and the

clinical response of gliomas to alkylating agents. New Engl J Med 2000;343:1350–1354.
55. Worm K, Dabbagh P, Schwechheimer K. Reverse transcriptase polymerase chain reaction as a reliable method to detect epidermal growth factor receptor exon 2-7 gene deletion in human glioblastomas. Hum Pathol 1999;30:222–227.
56. Von Deimling A, Louis DN, Wiestler OD. Molecular pathways in the formation of gliomas. Glia 1995;15:328–338.
57. Feldkamp, MM, Lala P, Lau N, Roncari L, Guha A. Expression of activated epidermal growth factor receptors, ras-guanosine triphosphate, and mitogen-activated protein kinase in human glioblastoma multiforme specimens. Neurosurgery 1999;45:1442–1453.
58. Kleihues P, Ohgaki H. Phenotype vs. genotype in the evolution of astrocytic brain tumors. Toxicol Pathol 2000;28:164–170.
59. Von Deimling A. Molecular genetic classification of astrocytomas and oligodendroglial tumors. Brain Pathol 1997;7:1311–1313.
60. Reifenberger J, Reifenberger G, Ichimura K, Schmidt EE, Wechsler W, et al. Epidermal growth factor receptor expression in oligodendroglial tumors. Am J Path 1996;149:25–35.
61. Brady L-W. A new treatment for high-grade gliomas of the brain. Bull Mem Acad R Med Belg 1998;153:255–261.
62. Faillot T, Magdelenat H, Mady E, Stasiecki P, Fohanno D, et al. A phase I study of an anti-epidermal growth factor receptor monoclonal antibody for the treatment of malignant gliomas. Neurosurgery 1996;39:478–483.
63. Sampson JH, Crotty LE, Lee S, Archer G-E, Ashley DM, et al. Unarmed, tumor-specific monoclonal antibody effectively treats brain tumors. Proc Natl Acad Sci USA 2000;97:7503–7508.
64. Yang W, Barth RF, Adams DM, Soloway AH. Intratumoral delivery of boronated epidermal growth factor for neutron capture therapy of brain tumors. Cancer Res 1997;57:4333–4339.
65. Tian XX, Lam P, Chen J, Pang JCS, To SST, et al. Antisense EGFR RNA transfection in human malignant gliomas cells leads to inhibition of proliferation and in detection of differentiation. Neuropathol Applied Neurobiol 1998; 24:389–396.
66. Archer GE, Sampson JH, Lorimer IA, McLendon RE, Kuan CT, et al. Regional treatment of epidermal growth factor receptor vIII-expressing neoplastic meningitis with a single-chain immunotoxin, MR-1. Clin Cancer Res 1999;5:2646–2652.
67. Vogelstein B, Fearon ER, Hamilton S, Kern S, Preisinger A, et al. Genetic alterations during colorectal tumor development. N Engl J Med 1988;319:525–532.
68. Louis DN. The p53 gene and protein in human brain tumors. J Neuropathol Exp Neurol 1994;1:163–170.
69. Watanabe K, Tachibana O, Sato K, Yonekawa Y, Kleihues P, et al. Overexpression of the epidermal growth factor receptor and p53 mutation are mutually exclusive in the evolution of primary and secondary glioblastomas. Brain Pathol 1996;6:217–223.
70. Ng H, Lam P. The molecular genetics of central nervous system tumors. Pathology 1998;30:196–202.
71. Korkolopoulou P, Kouzelis K, Christodoulou P, Papanikolaou A, Thomas-Tsagli E. Expression of retinoblastoma gene product and p21 (WAF1/Cip 1) protein in gliomas: correlations with proliferation markers, p53 expression, and survival. Acta Neuropathol (Berl) 1998;95:617–624.
72. al Sarraj S, Bridges LR. P53 immunoreactivity in astrocytomas and its relationship to survival. Br J Neurosurg 1995;9:143–149.
73. Kros JM, Godschalk JJ, Krishnadath KK, van Eden CG. Expression of p53 in oligodendrogliomas. J Pathol 1993;171:285–290.
74. Pavelic J, Hlavka V, Poljak M, Gale N, Pavelic K. P53 immunoreactivity in oligodendrogliomas. J Neurooncol 1994;22:1–6.
75. Reifenberger G, Liu L, Ischimura K, Schmidt EE, Collins VP. Amplification and overexpression of the MDM2 gene in a subset of human malignant gliomas without p53 mutations. Cancer Res 1993;53:2736–2739.
76. Dietzmann K, von-Bossanyi P, Sallaba J, Kirches E, Synowitz HJ, et al. Immunohistochemically detectable p53 and mdm-2 oncoprotein expression in astrocytic gliomas and their correlation to cell proliferation. Gen Diagn Pathol 1996;141:339–344.
77. Powell WC, Matrisian LM. Complex role of matrix metalloproteinases in tumor progression. Curr Top Microbiol Immunol 1996;213:1–21.
78. Stetler-Stevenson WG, Liotta L, Kleiner DE. Extracellular matrix 6: Role of matrix metalloproteinases in tumor invasion and metastasis. FASEB 1993;J7:1434–1441.
79. Kachra Z, Beaulieu E, Delbecchi L, Mousseau N, Berthelet F, et al. Expression of matrix metalloproteinases and their inhibitors in human brain tumors. Clin Exp Metastasis 1999;17:555–566.
80. Hastie ND, Dempster M, Dunlop MG, Thompson AM, Green DK, et al. Telomere reduction in human colorectal carcinoma and with aging. Nature 1990;346:866–868.
81. Nakatani K, Yoshimi N, Mori H, Yoshimura S, Sakai H, et al. The significant role of telomerase activity in human brain tumors. Cancer 1997;80:471–476.
82. Hiraga S, Ohnishi T, Izumoto S, Miyahara E, Kanemura Y, et al. Telomerase activity and alterations in telomere length in human brain tumors. Cancer Res 1998;58:2117–2125.
83. Kim JY, Sutton ME, Lu DJ, Cho TA, Goumnerova LC, et al. Activation of neurotrophin-3 receptor TrkC induces apoptosis in medulloblastomas. Cancer Res 1999;59:711–719.
84. Grotzer MA, Janss AJ, Fung KM, Biegel JA, Sutton LB, et al. TrkC expression predicts good clinical outcome in primitive neuroectodermal brain tumors. J Clin Oncol 2000;18:1027–1035.
85. Posner JB. Clinical manifestations of brain metastases. In: Weiss L, Gilbert HA, Posner JB, eds. Brain Metastases. Boston: GK Hall, 1980:189–207.
86. Zimm S, Wampler GL, Stablein D, Hazra T, Young HF. Intracranial metastases in solid tumor patients: natural history and results of treatment. Cancer 1981;48:384–394.
87. Gelber RD, Larson M, Borgelt BB, Kramer S. Equivalence of radiation schedules for the palliative treatment of brain metastases in patients with favorable prognosis. Cancer 1981;48:1749–1753.
88. Gregor A, Cull A, Stephens RJ, Kirkpatrick JA, Yarnold JR, et al. Prophylactic cranial irradiation is indicated following complete response to induction therapy in small-cell lung cancer: results of a multi-center randomized trial. United Kingdom Coordinating Committee for Cancer Research (UKCCCR) and the European Organization for Research and Treatment of Cancer (EORTC). Eur J Cancer 1997;33:1752–1758.
89. Epstein BE, Scott CB, Sause WT, Rotman M, Sneed P, et al. Improved survival duration in patients with unresected solitary brain metastasis using accelerated hyperfractionated radiation therapy at total doses of 54.4 gray and greater. Results of the Radiation Therapy Oncology Group 85-28. Cancer 1993;7:1362–1367.
90. Patchell RA, Tibbs PA, Walsh JW, Dempsey R, Maruyama Y, et al. A randomized trial of surgery in the treatment of single metastases to the brain. N Engl J Med 1990;322:494–500.
91. Vecht CJ, Haaxma-Reiche H, Noordijk EM, Padberg G, Voormolen J, et al. Treatment of single brain metastasis: radio-

therapy alone or combined with neurosurgery. Ann Neurol 1993;33:583–590.
92. Mintz AH, Kestle J, Rathbone M, Gaspar L, Hugenholtz H, et al. A randomized trial to assess the efficacy of surgery in addition to radiotherapy in patients with single cerebral metastasis. Cancer 1996;78:1470–1476.
93. Patchell RA, Tibbs A, Regine WF, Dempsey R, Mohiuddin M, et al. Post-operative radiotherapy in the treatment of single metastases to the brain: a randomized trial. J Am Med Assoc 1998;280:1485–1489.
94. Folkman J. Tumor angiogenesis. Adv Cancer Res 1985;43: 175–185.
95. Arnold SM, Young AB, Munn RK, Patchell RA, Markesbery WR. Expression of p53, bcl-2, E-cadherin, matrix metalloproteinase-9, and tissue inhibitor of metalloproteinases-1 in paired primary tumors and brain metastasis. Clin Cancer Res 1999;5:4028–4033.
96. Weber G, Ashkar S. Molecular mechanisms of tumor dissemination in primary and metastatic brain cancers. Brain Res Bull 2000;53:421–424.
97. Resnick DK, Resnick NM, Welch WC, Cooper DL. Differential expressions of CD44 variants in tumors affecting the central nervous system. Mol Diag 1999;4:219–232.
98. Harabin-Slowinska M, Slowinska J, Koneki J, Mrowka R. Expression of adhesion molecule CD44 in metastatic brain tumors. Folia Neuropathol 1998;36:179–184.
99. Behrens J, Lowrick O, Klein-Hitpass L, Birchmeier W. The E-cadherin promoter: Final analysis of a G:C-rich region and an epithelial cell-specific palindromic regulatory element. Proc Natl Acad Sci USA 1991;88:11495–11499.
100. Mattijssen V, Peters HM, Schalkwijk L, Manni J, van't Hof-Grootenboer B, et al. E-cadherin expression in head and neck squamous cell carcinoma is associated with clinical outcome. Int J Cancer 1993;55:580–585.
101. Ennis BW, Matrisian LM. Matrix-degrading metalloproteinases. J Neurooncol 1994;18:105–109.
102. Stetler-Stevenson WG, Aznavoorian S, Liotta L. Tumor cell interactions with the extracellular matrix during invasion and metastasis. Ann Rev Cell Biol 1993;9:541–573.
103. Jaalinoja J, Herva R, Korpela M, Hoyhtyp M, Turpeenniemi-Hujanen R. MMP-2 immunoreactive protein is associated with poor grade and survival in brain neoplasms. J Neurooncol 2000;46:81–90.
104. Kachra Z, Beaulieu E, Delbecchi L, Mousseau N, Berthelet F, et al. Expression of matrix metalloproteinases and their inhibitors in human brain tumors. Clin Exp Metastasis 1999;17: 553–566.
105. Hamasaki H, Aoyagi M. Kasama T, Handa S, Hirakawa K, et al. GT1b in human metastatic brain tumors: GT1b as a brain metastasis-associated ganglioside. Biochimica et Biophysica Acta 1999;1437:93–99.

Chapter **28**

Neuroendocrine Tumors

Kjell Öberg and Mats Stridsberg

Neuroendocrine tumors derive from neuroendocrine cells (defined as highly specialized cells), which upon specific stimulation secrete hormones regulating various bodily functions. In this chapter we will discuss the following neuroendocrine tumors: carcinoids, endocrine pancreatic tumors, neuroblastomas, medullary thyroid carcinomas, and pheochromocytomas.

The so-called "diffuse" neuroendocrine cell system of the gastrointestinal (GI) tract is the largest endocrine organ of the body and was described by Feyrter in 1938 (1). Pearse noted the Amine Precursor Uptake and Decarboxylation (APUD) properties of neuroendocrine cells and introduced the concept that these cells were derived from the neural crest (2). Fujita emphasized the striking similarities between gut, neuroendocrine cells, neurons, and other endocrine cells (e.g. parathyroid, pituitary) and regarded neuroendocrine cells as paraneurons, which formed a separate division of the nervous system (3).

The hypothesis that gut neuroendocrine cells originate from the neural crest received some support from studies of hybrid insulin genes in transgenic mice (4), but a series of studies favors the idea that neuroendocrine cells originated from endodermal stem cells (5,6). Fifteen different neuroendocrine cell types of the GI tract have been identified, each of which has specific hormone products and regulatory function (7). Today we recognize more than 30 gut peptide hormone genes, which express more than 100 bioactive peptides. It has been suggested that gut hormones should be regarded as general intracellular messengers in the body and not only as regulators of the GI tract (8). This concept was based on the following observations:

- Hormone families can be assembled with structural homologies, e.g. the secretin, insulin, epidermal growth factor, gastrin, pancreatic polypeptide, tachykinin, and somatostatin families.
- Gut hormone genes are widely expressed, not only in neuroendocrine cells and neurons but also in unrelated tumor cells.
- The same hormone gene can have a cell-specific expression in different cell types.
- The hormone gene can give rise to multiple bioactive peptides.
- The hormone-producing cells utilize endocrine, paracrine, neurocrine, or autocrine regulatory mechanisms.

The processing and secretion of hormones and amines is exemplified in Figure 1, showing the EC-cell that constitutes the largest neuroendocrine cell population of the gut (9). The cytoplasm of the EC cells is occupied by a large number of secretory granules of varying electron density, size, and shape (100–400 nm in diameter) and is the storage site of secretory products (e.g., serotonin and tachykinin).

Serotonin (5-HT) is synthesized from the amino acid tryptophan by hydroxylation and decarboxylation. The rate-limiting step in the 5-HT synthesis is a conversion of tryptophan to 5-HTP by tryptophan 5-hydroxylase, which occurs in the cytoplasm of the EC cells. Serotonin is subsequently taken up into the secretory granules by an active transport mechanism, Vesicular MonoAmine Transporter (VMAT) (10). Upon specific stimulation, granules are translocated to the cell membrane and their content released by exocytosis. Secreted 5-HT may influence adjacent cells by paracrine actions or exert hormonal effects on distant cells via the circulation. Most of the secreted 5-HT is taken up by the platelets, while free 5-HT is rapidly degraded by monoamine oxidase (MAO) in the liver and lung. After dehydrogenation, the 5-HIAA metabolite is excreted in the urine in free or conjugated form (11,12). Peptide prohormones are synthesized in the rough endoplasmatic reticulum (RER) together with chromogranin A and other granular proteins. Chromogranins may serve as substrates for proteolytic enzymes and thereby modulate this process (see below). The products are then transported to the Golgi apparatus for packaging into prosecretory granules. Sorting of chromogranin A occurs via selective aggregations and the secretory granules are formed (13). CgA can be further hydrolized into smaller fragments, e.g. vasostatins, pancreastatin, chromostatin. Upon stimulation, the secretory products are released from the granules by exocytosis (Figure 1).

The processes described above generally work in most neuroendocrine cells but also in tumors derived from the same cell system. Secretory products from such tumors may serve as markers for diagnosis but also as surrogate markers during treatment and follow-up.

CHROMOGRANINS

The chromogranin/secretogranin family consists of chromogranin A (CgA), chromogranin B (CgB; sometimes called secretogranin I), secretogranin II (SgII; sometimes called chro-

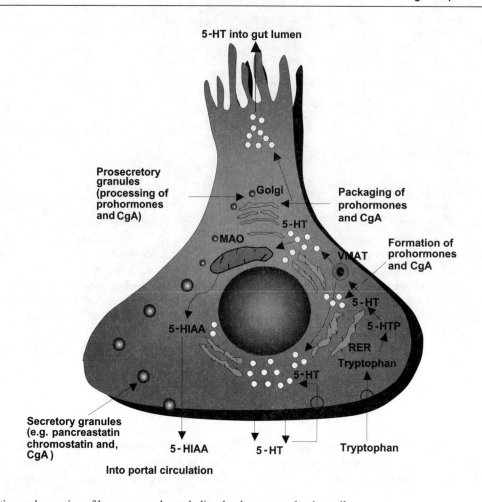

Figure 1 Production and secretion of hormones and metabolites by the neuroendocrine cell.

mogranin C), secretogranin III (often called 1B1075), secretogranin IV (often called HISL-19), and secretogranin V (often called 7B2) (14). CgA, originally called secretory protein I, was first isolated as a water-soluble protein present in chromaffin cells from bovine adrenal medulla (15–17). Later, CgB was also isolated from the adrenal medulla (18). SgII was isolated from the anterior pituitary (19,20).

Chromogranins are found in neuroendocrine cells throughout the body, thus forming the neuroendocrine system. Chromogranins are also located in the neuronal cells in the central and peripheral nervous system. Neuroendocrine cells are capable of synthesizing and releasing amines and hormones (neuropeptides, regulatory peptides). These are stored intracellularly in secretory granules and are released upon stimulation. Besides the hormones, the granules contain one or more members of the chromogranin/secretogranin family of proteins. Adrenal chromaffin granules contain about 40 different proteins and the chromogranins account for about 40% of the soluble proteins (18). In adrenal chromaffin cells, CgA and CgB are present in about equal amounts, while SgII is less abundant (21,22). However, secretory granules from other neuroendocrine tissues contain different relative amounts of chromogranins and secretogranins. For example, parathyroid cells and enterochromaffin cells in the stomach contain mostly CgA, and very little CgB (21,23). On the other hand, prostasomes, the secretory products from the prostate, contain mostly CgB (24).

The members of the chromogranin/secretogranin family have some common structural features, which are more or less unique to these proteins. They are synthesized with an N-terminally located signal peptide, which directs the chromogranins/secretogranins through Golgi apparatus to the regulated secretory pathway. They are hydrophilic and highly acidic with a high content glutamic acid, giving an isoelectric point of about 5 (16). They have multiple pairs of basic amino acids distributed along the molecules, but more abundantly in the C-terminal parts. These sites are potential cleavage sites for producing biologically active peptides. Heat-stable, they can resist high temperatures, even boiling, without denaturation (14,19), and they can bind calcium and other divalent cations, which can induce conformational changes (25,26). The proteins may be O-glycosylated, phosphorylated, and sulphated (19,27).

In addition, CgA and CgB have a similar structure in the N-terminal parts, where two cystein residues, at amino acid positions 17 and 38 for CgA and 16 and 37 for CgB, respectively, form an SS-bridge. This will probably give the N-terminal a more rigid "loop" formation in the three-dimensional structure than the rest of the molecule, which displays mostly a random coil structure. Furthermore, this N-terminal part is well conserved between different species, which indicates its biological importance. This structure is not seen in the secretogranins (14).

Chromogranins are processed post-translationally. CgA isolated from bovine adrenal medulla exhibits five phosphorylation sites and two O-glycosylation sites (27). Six of these post-translational modifications were located in regions with highly conserved amino acid sequences, indicating the importance for biological functions. This biological importance was shown for the antibacterial peptide chromacin (corresponding to human CgA176-225), which was biologically inactive without glycosylation (28). Post-translational modifications have also been identified in human CgA (29). Some of the modifications in the human CgA were found at corresponding positions compared to the bovine sequence. However, the human CgA was isolated from urine collected from a patient who had a carcinoid tumor, and it is thus possible that the post-translational processing may be somewhat different from that in a "normal" human CgA.

CgA can also be sulphated. It has been shown that CgA isolated from the bovine parathyroid gland is sulphated on tyrosine residues, while CgA isolated from bovine adrenals is sulphated mainly on oligosaccharide residues. CgB from bovine adrenals, on the other hand, was sulphated on tyrosine residues (30). This shows that different neuroendocrine cells are capable of processing the chromogranins differently. It is therefore possible that the post-translational differences may affect both the metabolism and the biological functions of the chromogranins.

Peptide hormones and neuropeptides are synthesized as pro-peptides and specifically processed to biologically active peptides within the secretory granules before release. The best-known example is the processing of proinsulin to active insulin and C-peptide. The cleavage is, to a large extent, mediated by the pro-hormone convertases PC1/3 and PC2, which are present almost exclusively in neuroendocrine tissue (31,32). These enzymes act preferentially on the C-terminal side of sites with two basic amino acids, usually Lys-Arg or Arg-Arg and sometimes also at single Arg residues. Chromogranins and secretogranins are stored with the hormones and neuropeptides within the secretory granules, and since they also have several pairs of basic amino acids a specific cleavage of chromogranins will probably occur. This pro-hormone convertase cleavage will generate specific chromogranin-related peptides that can have biological importance. Indeed, a recent study has shown that the endocrine cells within the pancreatic islets process the CgA molecule differently, giving rise to different fragments of CgA (33).

BIOLOGICAL EFFECTS OF CHROMOGRANINS AND CHROMOGRANIN-RELATED PEPTIDES

Intracellularly located chromogranins have been suggested to play a role in the formation, function, and regulation of secretory granules and their contents (34). As indicated above, chromogranins can also serve as precursors for generation of biologically active peptides. Several chromogranin-related peptides have been identified in biological tissues and fluids and some of these have also been shown to have biological function.

The biological functions of the chromogranin-related peptides are located in different parts of the molecules. The N-terminal part of CgA has vasodilatory functions. The central and the C-terminal parts of CgA have autocrine or paracrine inhibitory functions on hormonal release. The C-terminal part of CgB has antibacterial functions. The middle part of SgII (secretoneurin) influences migration of monocytes.

Unspecific degradation of Cg starts both at the C terminal and at the N terminal (35). It has also been shown that CgA is filtered in the kidneys, where it is taken up in the proximal tubuli cells and degraded in the lysosomal pathway (36). However, due to its size, the intact CgA molecule is not filtered in normal kidneys, but requires either a cleavage of the entire molecule or a kidney dysfunction affecting glomerular filtration, to be released to the urine (37,38). Like other small proteins and peptides, fragments of CgA can be both filtered in the glomeruli and metabolized in the proximal tubules.

Tumors of neuroendocrine origin usually present with increased plasma levels of CgA. The neuroendocrine tumors are derived from the neuroendocrine cells; typical neuroendocrine tumors include carcinoid tumors, pheochromocytomas, neuroblastomas, small cell lung cancers, hyperparathyroid adenomas, pituitary tumors, prostate cancers, and pancreatic islet tumors including the multiple endocrine neoplasia (MEN)1 and 2 syndromes. This also includes the different pancreatic islet cell syndromes, namely the insulinomas, the glucagonomas, the somatostatinomas, the Zollinger-Ellison syndrome, the Verner-Morrison syndrome, the pancreatic polypeptide-producing tumors, and the non-functioning neuroendocrine tumors.

The most useful assays for tumor detection have been those that measure the whole molecule. Assays measuring specifically defined parts of the molecule usually have lower sensitivity in detecting patients with neuroendocrine tumors (39).

Today, measurements of CgA are routine procedures in the management of neuroendocrine tumours. Most CgA methods are classical competitive assays that use one polyclonal antibody. However, some methods are non-competitive assays that use two antibodies, which bind to different parts of the CgA molecule. This approach may be less useful since it requires binding to a larger part of the CgA molecule. As chromogranins are often cleaved into smaller fragments, these methods may give false low values in some patients. The ideal assay would be one that measures both intact CgA and fragments of CgA. Commercial kits for determining CgA are available. Two of them are non-competitive radioimmunoassays, one with polyclonal antibodies and one with monoclonal antibodies. The third is a competitive radioimmunoassay.

In most neuroendocrine tumors, CgA is more abundant than CgB, and thus CgA is usually a better circulating tumor marker than CgB. However, in some tumor patients one can find increased circulating CgB even when CgA is normal. Therefore, both CgA and CgB should be analyzed to increase the sensitivity when chromogranins are used as tumor markers.

The most common non-tumor associated increase of CgA is decreased renal function (37). Other important non-tumor associated increases of CgA are type A gastritis and treatments with proton pump inhibitors (40). However, none of these parameters affects the measurements of CgB (41).

Concentrations of CgA, measured in the assays using purified chromogranin as standard, are mostly presented in ng/mL (µg/L). Usually, the circulating levels of CgA in humans are measured to about 50–100 µg/L. The measured concentration in a given sample is dependent on what epitopes the antibodies recognize and how they can bind to these epitopes. Different pairs of antibodies can give different measured concentrations, as described for development of non-competitive methods (42,43). One explanation of this behavior is that some antibody-binding epitopes on CgA may be masked by the three-dimensional folding of the molecule. This has been shown earlier when an antibody specific for pancreastatin did not bind to intact CgA, but showed a partial binding to partly processed CgA (38). When the standard preparations are more defined, i.e., when synthesized peptides are used, concentrations are usually given in pmol/L. Since plasma chromogranins are circulating both in the intact form and as fragments, the molar presentation may be a more accurate way to express concentrations of chromogranins.

CARCINOID TUMORS

The carcinoid tumors have been divided according to the presumed embryological origin of the precursor cells. They were thus divided into foregut (stomach, duodenum, pancreas); midgut (jejunum, ileum, appendix, and caecum); and hindgut: distal colon and rectum (44). This classification has been of value for the clinical management of carcinoid tumors and also the understanding of biological differences between various types of carcinoids.

A revised classification of all neuroendocrine tumors has been proposed. This classification takes into account tumor location, size, angioinvasion, hormone production, degree of neuroendocrine differentiation, histological grade, and proliferation index. Such classifications also take into account the clinical behavior of the tumor (benign, low grade, or high-grade malignancy). The new classification from WHO recognizes three main categories: well-differentiated endocrine tumors (classical midgut carcinoids), differentiated endocrine carcinoma (atypical carcinoid), and poorly differentiated carcinoma (45). The histopathological investigation of carcinoid tumors includes immunostaining for chromogranin A, synaptophysin, neuron-specific enolase (NSE), and serotonin. These are the standard immunostainings that should be performed in all patients. As an option, the proliferation marker Ki-67 (MIB-1) should be analyzed, as well as expression of various growth factor (IGF-1, PDGF, TGF-α, TGF-β) and somatostatin receptor subtypes. There exist at the moment five somatostatin receptor subtypes, SST1-5, which are mediating different intracellular signals (46). About 80–90% of carcinoid tumors express the type 2 receptor, which can be used as a target for diagnosis and treatment (47). There is a scintigraphic technique using the somatostatin analog octreotide bound to ^{111}Indium, which is an important method for staging of the disease (48). Tumors expressing somatostatin receptor type 2 can also be treated with somatostatin analogs (octreotide, lanreotide). Other therapeutic options for low proliferating carcinoid tumors are α-interferons, but therapeutic options for tumors with high proliferation capacity are cytotoxic agents such as streptozotocin, doxorubicin, 5-FU, cisplatinum, etoposide (49,50).

TUMOR MARKERS IN CARCINOIDS
Foregut Carcinoids

Foregut carcinoids display varied clinical symptoms and hormone products. These tumors can produce any of the characterized hormones in the body, most often in combinations, which give rise to mixed clinical presentations. A substantial proportion (13–50%) of patients is asymptomatic, and the tumors are detected on routine chest X-ray (51).

Carcinoid syndrome. Carcinoid syndrome, which includes flushing, diarrhea, cardiac, fibrosis, wheezing, and dyspnea, is rather rare (<10%). This syndrome is related to production of serotonin and tachykinins (neuropeptide-K, substance-P) (52,53). However, a small number of patients produce an atypical syndrome with prolonged flushing, headache, palpitation, and bronchoconstriction. In this syndrome, histamine is one of the main mediators besides 5-hydroxytryptamine (54).

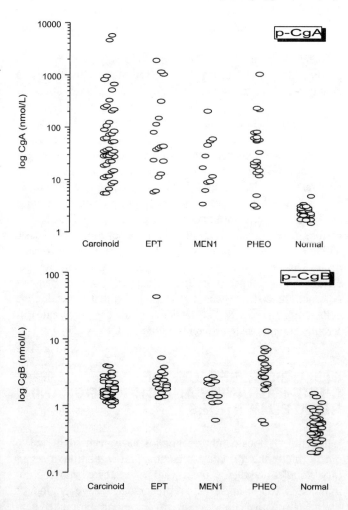

Figure 2 Plasma levels of chromogranin A and chromogranin B in patients with neuroendocrine tumors.

Lung carcinoids might also present with Cushing's syndrome, due to ectopic ACTH production (55) or acromegaly due to ectopic secretion of GHRH (56). Gastric and duodenal tumors are able to secrete gastrin, giving rise to the Zollinger-Ellison syndrome with recurrent ulcers, diarrhea, and gastric pain.

Recommended markers. The following markers are recommended: CgA, CgB, gastrin, somatostatin, ACTH, GHRH, GH, IGF-1, hCG-α/β subunits, urine-5-HIAA, urine histamine metabolites, and urine cortisol.

The most important general marker is chromogranin A. Other markers are usually analyzed when clinical symptoms indicate a particular syndrome.

Midgut Carcinoids

This type of carcinoid is also called "classical" carcinoid. Its more uniform clinical presentation usually involves malignant tumors (which present in more than 60% of the patients who have the carcinoid syndrome) as well as flushing, diarrhea, cardiac fibrosis, and dyspnea. These symptoms are related to secretion of serotonin, tachykinins, bradykinins, and kallikrein. Prostaglandin has also been implicated in the development of diarrhea (12,52,53).

Recommended markers. These include CgA, plasma neuropeptide-K (NPK), neurokinin-A (NKA) and substance P.

The serotonin metabolite 5-HIAA is the most important urinary marker in this group of patients. A combination of chromogranin A and U-5-HIAA gives a correct diagnosis in more than 95% of patients with malignant midgut carcinoid tumors.

Hindgut Carcinoids

Hindgut carcinoids present clinically as non-functional tumors (non-functional with respect to production of hormones). These patients present with abdominal pain, gastrointestinal bleeding, and an enlarged liver with metastases (12).

Recommended markers. These include plasma, CgA, pancreatic polypeptide (PP), peptide YY (PYY), and hCG-α and hCG-β subunits.

ENDOCRINE PANCREATIC TUMORS

These tumors include insulinomas, gastrinomas, vasoactive intestinal polypeptide (VIP)-omas, glucagonomas, somatostatinomas, and non-functioning pancreatic tumors (57). The tumors are named after the main secretory product but the majority of them are malignant and produce several different hormones at the same time or sequentially.

Insulinomas are the most common of the functioning tumors of the pancreas. In about 80% of cases, the tumors are benign and can be radically resected. In about 10–15% of cases, the tumors are malignant and produce insulin, pro-insulin, and sometimes also gastrin and glucagon (58). These tumors are subjected to treatment with cytotoxic drugs including streptozotocin, 5-FU, and doxorubicin (57).

Gastrin-producing tumors present with the so called "Zollinger-Ellison syndrome": recurrent ulcers, diarrhea, and abdominal cramping. These tumors can also be found in the duodenum and are mostly malignant. Lymph nodes and liver metastases are present in 75–80% of the patients at the time of diagnosis (59). The main secretory product is gastrin, stimulating acid secretion in the stomach, thus causing the clinical symptoms. Surgery combined with cytotoxic treatments is a standard procedure. One-third of these patients belong to families with multiple endocrine neoplasia type 1 (MEN-1), which also presents with hyperparathyroidism, pituitary tumors, and sometimes adrenocortical lesions.

VIP-secreting tumors give rise to the Verner-Morrison syndrome, which results from hypersecretion of VIP and sometimes also peptide histidine methionin (PHM) or calcitonin. The syndrome includes characteristic watery diarrhea (up to 15 litres/day), with dehydration, hypopotassemia, and sometimes episodes of cutaneous flushing (60). The treatment is similar to insulinomas and gastrinomas but also includes therapy with somatostatin analogs, which might ameliorate the diarrheas.

Glucagonomas account for about 4% of all endocrine pancreatic tumors. They present quite often with necrolytic migratory erythema and are generally first diagnosed by dermatologists. Other features of the syndrome include diabetes mellitus, weight loss, normochronic and normocytic anemia, glossitis, and deep vein thrombosis (61). The syndrome is caused by glucagon and the treatment is similar to that for VIP-secreting tumors.

Somatostatinomas are very rare endocrine pancreatic tumors that mostly secrete somatostatin and can be found both in the pancreas and duodenum (62). Duodenal somatostatinomas are frequently associated with von Recklinghausen disease. Syndrome of somatostatinomas is associated with gall bladder stones, diabetes mellitus, and diarrhea with steatorrhea. The treatment is similar to that for other endocrine pancreatic tumors. Another rare type of endocrine pancreatic tumors, the so called GRF-omas, secrete growth-hormone-releasing hormone (GHRH) and lead to acromegaly.

Non-functioning pancreatic tumors constitute about 30% of all endocrine pancreatic tumors (63). Their symptomatology varies with size. In the beginning they are generally asymptomatic and are discovered only by chance when diagnostic imaging procedures are performed for other reasons. In the more advanced stages, they present with metastases and symptoms such as epigastric pain, weight loss, and jaundice. Their clinical silence in the beginning may be due to a combination of various factors, including low or inactive peptide production, secretion of peptide inhibitors, and down-regulation of peripheral receptors. The tumors secrete a variety of markers such as chromogranin A, chromogranin B, hCG-α and hCG-β subunits, pancreatic polypeptide, and somatostatin.

Localization procedures for the various subtypes of endocrine pancreatic tumors include computerized tomography, magnetic resonance imaging, ultrasonography, somatostatin receptor scintigraphy, and positron emission tomography. Endoscopic ultrasound is capable of detecting small endocrine pancreatic tumors, particularly in the head of the pancreas. Today, somatostatin receptor scintigraphy is the most important imaging tool used in screening for endocrine pancreatic tumors (48).

Recommended Markers

These general markers for all subtypes of endocrine pancreatic tumors include CgA, CgB, pancreatic polypeptide, and hCG-α and hCG-β subunits.

Specific markers and additional tests. These include the following, grouped by type of tumor.

- Insulinomas: Plasma insulin, pro-insulin including 48-hour fasting with analysis of blood glucose, plasma insulin, and pro-insulin.
- Gastrinomas: Plasma gastrin, secretin infusion test with analysis of plasma gastrin.
- Others: Plasma VIP for VIP-omas, plasma glucagon for glucagonomas, plasma somatostatin for somatostatinomas, and plasma GHRH for GRF-omas. A meal stimulatory test with analyzing plasma pancreatic polypeptide and gastrin is particularly useful in early diagnosis of patients with multiple endocrine neoplasia type 1 and the suspicions of endocrine pancreatic tumors.

Pheochromocytoma

Pheochromocytoma tumors derive from the neural crest and are located in the adrenal medulla and sympathetic ganglia. Tumors that arise from extra-adrenal chromaffin cells are usually called extra adrenal pheochromocytomas or paragangliomas.

About 80–90% of pheochromocytomas are benign. The tumors are dangerous because of their capacity to produce and release catecholamines in large amounts, which can cause hypertensive crisis. Pheochromocytomas are rare; less than 1% of hypertensive patients have chromaffin tumors as the cause of increased blood pressure. However, these tumors are important since misdiagnosed or improperly treated tumors may be fatal. Correctly diagnosed and treated, pheochromocytoma is curable.

The clinical manifestations of pheochromocytoma are largely predictable from the physiological and pharmacological effects of catecholamines. Symptoms include sustained hypertension that is resistant to conventional treatment, and hypertensive crisis with malignant hypertension, hypertensive encephalopathy, or manifestations suggestive of aortic dissection or myocardial infarction. Also paroxysmal attacks suggestive of seizure disorders, anxiety attacks, and hyperventilation can occur. Severe hypertensive reactions during incidental surgery or in association with trauma can be fatal. The characteristic paroxysmal crisis of pheochromocytoma is the consequence of catecholamine release from the tumor, but the manifestations are variable. Hypertension is the most common feature and occurs in more than 90% of patients. It is usually sustained and may be without definite crisis, essentially resembling hypertension. Unstable blood pressure is usually present, and many patients with sustained hypertension also have distinct paroxysm. The hypertension is often severe and occasionally malignant with retinopathy and severe proteinuria. Headache, sometimes severe, can occur in more than 80% of patients. Excessive sweating and palpitations are also common (64,65).

Biosynthesis and storage of catecholamines in chromaffin cell tumors may be different than in normal adrenal medulla. However, chromaffin granules from pheochromocytomas are morphologically, physically, and functionally similar to chromaffin granules of the adrenal medulla. The increase in tissue turnover of catecholamines in vivo and in vitro in some tumors suggests an alteration in the regulation of catecholamine biosynthesis, possibly because of an impairment in feedback inhibition of tyrosine hydroxylase. Changes in the tumor blood flow, direct pressure, chemicals, and drugs may initiate catecholamine release.

Most pheochromocytomas contain more noradrenalin than adrenalin, unlike the normal adrenal medulla, which contains 85% adrenalin. However, in most cases it is impossible to predict the pattern of catecholamine secretion from the clinical features. Extra adrenal pheochromocytomas usually secrete only noradrenalin. Excretion of dopamine and metabolites such as HVA is not increased in patients with benign pheochromocytoma. Pheochromocytomas may synthesize neuropeptides, usually those normally found in the adrenal medulla.

Pheochromocytomas are occasionally inherited as autosomal dominant traits and may be parts of multiple endocrine neoplasia type 2 (MEN-2). The trait is autosomal dominant. MEN-2A is also known as Sipple's syndrome and consists of pheochromocytoma, medullary carcinoma of the thyroid, and hyperparathyroidism. The genetic basis for this syndrome involves germ-line mutations in the RET proto-oncogene, which encodes for a cell surface receptor tyrosine kinase involved in the regulation of cell growth and differentiation. The specific mutations affect the extra-cellular ligand-binding domain of the protein. Pheochromocytoma occurs in 40–50% of affected individuals in MEN-2A kindred and is responsible for a substantial portion of MEN-2A morbidity and mortality. Pheochromocytoma in MEN-2A originates from adrenomedullary hyperplasia and usually secretes adrenalin. Extra adrenal pheochromocytomas are rare.

Multiple endocrine neoplasia MEN-2B is also known as the mucosal neuroma syndrome. It includes medullary carcinoma of the thyroid, pheochromocytoma, and multiple mucosal neuromas, and is often in association with a marphanoid habitus. Although this syndrome is also caused by mutations in the RET proto-oncogene of chromosome 10, these mutations affect the tyrosine kinase catalytic site in the intra-cellular domain of the protein.

Von Hippel-Lindau disease is an autosomal dominant disorder consisting of retinal angioma, hemoangioblastoma of the central nervous system, renal carcinoma, renal and pancreatic cysts, and epidermal cyst-adenoma. Pheochromocytoma occurs in 10–20% of these patients. Variations of the disease cluster within the affected families and pheochromocytoma may be present in more than 90% of affected members, or it may be rare. Among patients with pheochromocytoma, about 20% may have von Hipple-Lindau disease. The gene responsible for this disorder is located on human chromosome 3 tand appears to function as a tumor suppressor gene.

Neurofibromatosis can occur in two variants. Pheochromocytoma is occasionally seen in the type-1 disease. The underlying mutations in this disorder are inactivating mutations in the neurofibromatosis-1 gene, a putative tumor suppressor gene located on chromosome 17.

The diagnosis of pheochromocytoma is usually established by demonstrating increased urinary excretion of catecholamines or catecholamine metabolites. Assays used to diagnose pheochromocytoma include VMA, HVA, metanephrines, and catecholamines. Usually one or two 24-hour urine collections are used for the diagnosis. Creatinine can be measured and the excretion of catecholamines can be expressed in relation to the creatinine excretion. Urinary catecholamines and their metabolites are fairly easy to measure with HPLC techniques. The main drawback is too many false positive results. This is probably a consequence of different stress factors that increase the activity of the sympathetic nervous system. Such factors can be expected to be more important in a stressful diagnostic situation. One possible way to overcome this ordinary daytime stress would be to base the diagnosis on urine collected during the night.

Plasma catecholamine determinations are of limited usefulness in the diagnosis. Some studies claim that analyses of plasma metanephrines can increase the diagnostic sensitivity, but these studies have not compared the use of chromogranins, and the results have not been confirmed by other research groups (66).

Plasma measurements of neuropeptide Y (NPY) and vasoactive intestinal polypeptide (VIP) have been reported to be elevated in patients with pheochromocytoma (67,68). Plasma levels of NSE also can be increased in patients with pheochromocytoma, at least in patients who have malignant tumors (65). However, the diagnostic sensitivity of these neuropeptides is usually low compared to measurement of urinary catecholamines or chromogranin A.

Several studies have pointed out the value of measuring CgA in patients with pheochromocytoma (41,69–72). The

Table 1 Overview of circulating markers for different neuroendocrine tumors

Tumor marker	Carcinoid tumors	Endocrine pancreatic tumors	Pheocromocytoma	Medullary thyroid cancer	Neuroblastoma
Plasma markers					
Chromogranin A (CgA)	X	X	X	X	X
Chromogranin B (CgB)	X	X	X	X	X
Neuron-specific enolase (NSE)	X	X	X	X	X
α-subunit of glycoprotein hormones	X	X	X	X	X
hCG-beta	X	X	X	X	X
Gastrin		X			
Glucagon		X			
Insulin		X			
Proinsulin		X			
Pancreatic polypeptide (PP)		X			
Somatostatin		X			
Substance P	X				
Neuropeptide K (NPK)	X				
Neuropeptide Y (NPY)			X		X
Vasoactive intestinal polypeptide (VIP)			X		X
Calcitonin				X	
Carcinoembryonic antigen (CEA)				X	
Metanephrins			X		X
Urinary markers					
5-Hydroxyindoloacetic acid (5-HIAA)	X				
Tele-methylimidazoleacetic acid (MelmII)		X			
Noradrenalin			X		X
Adrenalin			X		X
Homovallinic acid (HVA)			X		X
Vanillylmandelic acid (VMA)			X		X
Dopamine			X		X

reported diagnostic sensitivities are high, up to 90%, and highest for the studies where CgA was measured with competitive assays. Measurements of NSE and the alpa-subunit of glycoprotein hormones usually give less information than CgA measurements (67). It has also been shown that CgA is proportional to tumor size in and can be a used for screening familiar pheochromocytoma (69). Normal adrenal medulla expresses both CgA and CgB. Although one study has shown the high sensitivity of CgB, measurements of CgA was slightly more sensitive (71).

Recommended Markers

Urinary measurements of noradrenalin, adrenalin, VMA, HVA, and metanephrines, in combination with plasma measurements of CgA, will probably give the correct diagnosis in almost all cases. In follow-up and in screening of family members, CgA is the marker of first choice. Plasma measurements of catecholamines or metanephrines are probably of lesser value for diagnosis and monitoring of treatments.

MEDULLARY THYROID CARCINOMA

Medullary thyroid carcinoma accounts for about 10% of thyroid malignancies. It usually occurs after the age of 40 and is slightly more common in women. The carcinoma readily invades the intraglandular lymphatics and spreads to other parts of the gland and in the pericapsular and regional lymph nodes. It also regularly spreads via the blood to the lungs, bone, and liver.

This carcinoma arises from the C-cells of the thyroid and secretes characteristic hormones like calcitonin. The tumors occur in both sporadic and familial forms, the latter making up about 20% of the total. The disease is associated with MEN-2A and MEN-2B (73).

Measurement of calcitonin is the most important tumor marker, but elevations of carcinoembryonic antigen (CEA) are also often observed. Calcitonin is a 32-amino acid polypeptide, which is expressed in and secreted from thyroid C-cells. Normally, calcitonin can be released by acute hypercalcemia. Also some gastrointestinal hormones, i.e. gastrin, can stimulate calcitonin release.

Calcitonin is measured in serum by immunochemical methods. The circulating half-life is short, only a few minutes. The diagnostic sensitivity is about 75–90% for medullary thyroid carcinoma (71) and can be increased by stimulating calcitonin release with pentagastrin. Elevated levels of calcitonin are occasionally observed in patients who have other neuroendocrine tumors, e.g., small-cell lung cancer, carcinoid tumors, and pancreatic endocrine tumors. Calcitonin can also be increased in patients with breast, stomach, liver, and kidney tumors. Non-tumor associated increases in calcitonin can be observed in patients with decreased liver function. Elevated levels of CgA have been reported in about 25% of patients with medullary thyroid carcinoma, mostly those with more advanced disease (74).

Recommended Markers

Plasma measurement of calcitonin is the marker of first choice for medullary thyroid carcinoma. Samples taken before and after stimulation with pentagastrin can increase the diagnostic sensitivity. Serum CEA might be an additional adjunct.

Neuroblastoma

Neuroblastoma is a malignant tumor that appears in early childhood. It is characterized by rapid growth and widespread metastases.

Most patients present with metastases at diagnosis. The tumors are derived from the neural crest and are located in the adrenal medulla and sympathetic ganglia. Neuroblastoma is often associated with excessive production of catecholamines and catecholamine metabolites. The biology is poorly understood. The immature tumors appear to have a latent capacity to differentiate into more mature tissue, and this feature may account for some of the spontaneous remissions that have occurred. However, in younger patients, the tumor is more aggressive and less likely to undergo spontaneous regression.

The prognosis is poorest for those tumors of adrenal medullary origin. There have been considerable improvements in the prognosis of other pediatric solid tumors during the last 30 years, but neuroblastoma is still accompanied by a mortality rate of approximately 25–50%, despite multi-modality treatment with chemotherapy, radiotherapy, and surgery (75).

Biochemical markers are used to confirm the diagnosis, to monitor the effects of treatment, and to detect relapses. Markers used for the diagnosis of neuroblastoma include catecholamine metabolites such as vanillylmandelic acid (VMA), dopamine (DA), and homovallinic acid (HVA), assayed in 24-hour urine samples according to recommendations made by the European Neuroblastoma Study Group in 1995. The urinary concentrations of HVA and VMA are not proportional to the tumor burden but are elevated in approximately 90% of patients. However, urine sampling in small children may pose practical problems and sometimes demands an indwelling catheter.

Neuron-specific enolase (NSE) is a glycolytic enzyme, which is found in high concentrations in the serum of patients with advanced neuroblastoma, but elevated NSE levels have also been reported in Wilm's tumor, Ewing's sarcoma, and acute leukemias. Hence, there is a clinical need for simple, reproducible, and reliable biochemical factors, preferably serum markers for neuroblastoma. Measurements of neuropeptide Y and vasoactive intestinal polypeptide have been used, but these do not seem to offer any additional information about the tumors.

CgA has a high sensitivity for neuroblastoma, and the plasma levels are proportional to tumor size (76). Furthermore, CgA levels can be used to predict survival (76). Others, however with few patients, have found both higher and lower sensitivity (71,77). Although more experience with this marker may be needed, CgA seems the most promising for confirming neuroblastoma, since it offers both high sensitivity tund correlates to tumor burden and survival.

Recommended Markers

Because of the high sensitivity and the correlation to tumor burden and survival, CgA is most suitable marker. However, urinary measurements of VMA, HVA, and DA are standard procedures, although they seem to offer less information about tumor growth. NSE can be used if CgA or the urinary markers are not available.

REFERENCES

1. Feyrter F. Über diffuse endokrine epitheliale organe. Leipzig: Barth, 1938.
2. Pearse AG. Common cytochemical and ultrastuctural characteristics of cells producing polypeptide hormones (the APUD series) and their relevance to thyroid and ultimobranchial C cells and calcitonin. Proc R Soc Lond B Biol Sci 1968;170:71–80.
3. Fujita T. The gastro-enteric endocrine cell and its paraneuronic nature in chromaffin, enterochromaffin, and related cells. 1976; 14:191–208.
4. Alpert S, Hanahan D, Teitelman G. Hybrid insulin genes reveal a developmental lineage for pancreatic endocrine cells and imply a relationship with neurons. Cell 1988;53:295–308.
5. Andrew A, Kramer B, Rawdon BB. The origin of gut and pancreatic endocrine (APUD) cell—the last word? J Pathol 1998;186:117–118.
6. Wright N. The origin of gut and pancreatic neuroendocrine (APUD) cells. J Pathol 1999;189:439–440.
7. Rindi G, Villanacci V, Ubiali A. Biological and molecular aspects of gastroenteropancreatic neuroendocrine tumors. Digestion 2000;62:19–26.
8. Rehfeld JF. The new biology of gastrointestinal hormones. Physiol Rev 1998;78:1087–1108.
9. Portela-Gomes GM, Grimelius L, Bergström R. Enterochromaffin (Argentaffin) cells of the rat gastrointestinal tract: an ultrastructural study. Acta Pathol Microbiol Immunol Scand (A). 1984;92:83–89.
10. Erickson JD, Eiden LE, Schafer MK. Reserpine- and tetrabenazine-sensitive transport of (3)H-histamine by the neuronal isoform of the vesicular monoamine transporter. J Mol Neurosci 1995;6:277–287.
11. Feldman J, Moore J. Biogenic amines in carcinoid tumors. Biogenic Amines 1989;6:247–252.
12. Feldman JM. Carcinoid tumors. In: Massafferi EL et al. (eds.). Endocrine tumors. Boston: Blackwell Scientific Publications, 1993;700–722.
13. Huttner WB, Gerdes HH, Rosa P. The granin (chromogranin/secreto-granin) family. Trends Biochem Sci 1991; 16:27–30.
14. Winkler H, Fischer-Colbrie R. The chromogranins A and B; the first 25 years, and future perspectives. Neuroscience 1992;49:497–528.
15. Banks P, Helle K. The release of protein from the stimulated adrenal medulla. Biochem J 1965;97:40C–1C.
16. Smith AD, Winkler H. Purification and properties of an acidic protein from chromaffin granules of bovine adrenal medulla. Biochem J 1967;103:483–492.
17. Blaschko H, Comline RS, Schneider FH, Silver M, Smith AD. Secretion of a chromaffin granule protein, chromogranin, from the adrenal gland after splanchnic stimulation. Nature 1967;215:58–59.
18. Fischer-Colbrie R, Frischenschlager T. Immunological characterization of secretory proteins of chromaffin granules: Chromogranin A, chromogranin B, and enkephalin-containing peptides. J Neurochem 1985;44:1854–1861.
19. Rosa P, Hille A, Lee RHW, Zanini A, Decamilli P, Huttner WB. Secretogranins I and II, two tyrosin-sulphated secretory proteins common to a variety of cell- secreting peptides by the regulated pathway. J Cell Biol 1985;101:1999–2011.
20. Fischer Colbrie R, Hagn C, Kilpatrick L, Winkler H. Chromogranin C: a third component of the acidic proteins in chromaffin granules. J Neurochem 1986;47:318–321.
21. Hagn C, Schmid KW, Fischer Colbrie R, Winkler H. Chromogranin A, B, and C in human adrenal medulla and endocrine tissues. Lab Invest 1986;55:405–411.
22. Schober M, Fischer Colbrie R, Schmid KW, Bussolati G, O'Connor DT, Winkler H. Comparison of chromogranins A, B, and secretogranin II in human adrenal medulla and pheochromocytoma. Lab Invest 1987;57:385–391.
23. Buffa R, Mare P, Gini A, Salvadore M. Chromogranins A and B and secretogranin II in hormonally identified endocrine cells of the gut and the pancreas. Basic Appl Histochem 1988;32:471–484.
24. Stridsberg M, Fabiani R, Lukinius A, Ronquist G. Prostasomes are neuroendocrine-like vesicles in human semen. Prostate 1996;29:287–295.
25. Yoo SH. Identification of the calcium-dependent calmodulin-binding region of chromogranin A. Biochemistry 1992;31:6134–6140.
26. Yoo SH. pH-dependent binding of chromogranin B and secretory vesicle matrix proteins to the vesicle membrane. Biochim Biophys Acta Mol Cell Res 1993;1179:239–246.
27. Strub JM, Sorokine O, Van Dorsselaer A, Aunis D, Metz-Boutigue MH. Phosphorylation and O-glycosylation sites of bovine chromogranin a from adrenal medullary chromaffin granules and their relationship with biological activities. J Biol Chem 1997;272:11928–11936.
28. Strub JM, Goumon Y, Lugardon K, Capon C, Lopez M, Moniatte M, et al. Antibacterial activity of glycosylated and phosphorylated chromogranin A-derived peptide 173–194 from bovine adrenal medullary chromaffin granules. J Biol Chem 1996;271:28533–28540.
29. Gadroy P, Stridsberg M, Capon C, Michalski JC, Strub JM, Van Dorsselaer A, et al. Phosphorylation and O-glycosylation sites of human chromogranin A (CGA79–439) from urine of patients with carcinoid tumors. J Biol Chem 1998;273:34087–34097.
30. Gorr SU, Cohn DV. Secretion of sulfated and nonsulfated forms of parathyroid chromogranin A (secretory protein-I). J Biol Chem 1990;265:3012–3016.
31. Steiner DF, Smeekens SP, Ohagi S, Chan SJ. The new enzymology of precursor-processing endoproteases. J Biol Chem 1992;267:23435–23438.
32. Creemers JW, Jackson RS, Hutton JC. Molecular and cellular regulation of prohormone processing. Semin Cell Dev Biol 1998;9:3–10.
33. Portela-Gomes GM, Stridsberg M. Selective processing of chromogranin A in the different islet cells in human pancreas. J Histochem Cytochem 2001;49:483–490.
34. Deftos LJ. Chromogranin A: its role in endocrine function and as an endocrine and neuroendocrine tumor marker. Endocr Rev 1991;12:181–187.
35. Metz-Boutigue M-H, Garcia-Sablone P, Hogue-Angeletti R, Aunis D. Intracellular and extracellular processing of chromo-

granin A—determination of cleavage sites. Eur J Biochem 1993; 217:247–257.
36. Weiler R, Steiner H, Fischer Colbrie R, Schmid KW, Winkler H. Undegraded chromogranin A is present in serum and enters the endocytotic lysosomal pathway in kidney. Histochemistry 1991; 96:395–399.
37. Hsiao RJ, Mezger MS, O'Connor DT. Chromogranin A in uremia: Progressive retention of immunoreactive fragments. Kidney Int 1990;37:955–964.
38. Stridsberg M, Hellman U, Wilander E, Lundqvist G, Hellsing K, Öberg K. Fragments of chromogranin A are present in the urine of patients with carcinoid tumors: development of a specific radioimmunoassay for chromogranin A and its fragments. J Endocrinol 1993;139:329–337.
39. Stridsberg M, Öberg K, Li Q, Engström U, Lundqvist G. Measurements of chromogranin A, chromogranin B (secretogranin I), chromogranin C (secretogranin II), and pancreastatin in plasma and urine from patients with carcinoid tumors and endocrine pancreatic tumors. J Endocrinol 1995;144:49–59.
40. Sanduleanu S, Stridsberg M, Jonkers D, Hameeteman W, Biemond I, Lundqvist G et al. Serum gastrin and chromogranin A during meals. Aliment Pharmacol Ther 1999;13: 145–153.
41. Stridsberg M, Husebye ES. Chromogranin A and chromogranin B are sensitive circulating markers for pheochromocytoma. European J Endocrinol 1997;136:67–73.
42. Corti A, Gasparri A, Chen FX, Pelagi M, Brandazza A, Sidoli A, Siccardi AG. Characterization of circulating chromogranin A in human cancer patients. Br J Cancer 1996;73:924–932.
43. Degorce F, Goumon Y, Jacquemart L, Vidaud C, Bellanger L, Pons-Anicet D et al. A new human chromogranin A (CgA) immunoradiometric assay involving monoclonal antibodies raised against the unprocessed central domain (145–245). Br J Cancer 1999;79:65–71.
44. Williams ED, Sandler M. The classification of carcinoid tumors. Lancet 1963;1:238–239.
45. Solcia E, Klöppel G, Sobin LH. Histological typing of endocrine tumors. In: World Health Organization international histological classification of tumors, 2nd ed. Berlin: Springer, 2000.
46. Patel YC, Srikant CB. Subtype selectivity of peptide analogs for all five cloned human somatostatin receptors (hsstr 1–5). Endocrinology 1994;135:2814–2817.
47. Eriksson B, Öberg K. Summing up of 15 years of somatostatin analog therapy in neuroendocrine tumors: future outlook. Ann Oncol 1999;10:31–38.
48. Krenning EP, de Jong M, Kooij PM. Radiolabeled somatostatin analog(s) for peptide receptor scintigraphy and radionuclide therapy. Ann Oncol 1999;10:23–29.
49. Öberg K. The use of chemotherapy in the management of neuroendocrine tumors. Endocrinol Metab Clin North Am 1993;22: 941–952.
50. Öberg K. Interferon in the management of neuroendocrine GEP-tumors. Digestion 2000;62:92–97.
51. Mendonca C, Baptista C, Rames M, Yglesias de Oliveira JA. Typical and atypical lung carcinoids: clinical and morphological diagnosis. Microsc Res Tech 1997;38:468–472.
52. Oates J, Sjoerdsma A. A unique syndrome associated with secretion of 5-hyroxytryptophan by metastatic gastric carcinoids. Am J Med 1962;32:333–342.
53. Norheim I, Wilander E, Öberg K. Tachykinin production by carcinoid tumors in culture. Eur J Cancer Clin Oncol 1987;23: 689–695.
54. Pernow B, Waldenström J. Paroxysmal flushing and other symptoms caused by 5-hydroxytryptamine and histamine in patients with malignant tumors. Lancet 1954;II:951.
55. Dusmet ME, McKneally MF. Pulmonary and thymic carcinoid tumors. World J Surg 1996;20:189–195.
56. Ezzat S, Asa SL, Stefaneanu L, Whittom R, Smyth HS, Horvath E, Kovacs K, Frohman LA. Somatotroph hyperplasia without pituitary adenoma associated with a longstanding growth hormone-releasing hormone-producing bronchial carcinoid. J Clin Endocrinol Metab 1994;78:555–560.
57. Öberg K. Neuroendocrine gastrointestinal tumors: a condensed overview of diagnosis and treatment. Ann Oncol 1999;10: S3–S8.
58. Creutzfeldt W. Insulinomas: clinical presentation, diagnosis, and advances in management. In: Mignon M, Jensen RT (eds.). Endocrine tumors of the pancreas: recent advances in research and management. Basel: Karger,1995;148–165.
59. Mignon M, Jais PH, Cadiot G. Clinical features and advances in biological diagnostic criteria for Zollinger-Ellison syndrome. In: Mignon M, Jensen RT (eds.). Endocrine tumors of the pancreas: recent advances in research and management. Basel: Karger, 1995;223–239.
60. Long RG, Bryant MG, Mitchell SJ. Clinicopathological study of the pancreatic and ganglioneuroblastoma tumors secreting vasoactive intestinal polypeptide (vipomas). BMJ 1981;282: 1767–1771.
61. Guillausseau PJ, Guillausseau C, Villet R. Les glucagonomes. Aspects cliniques, biologiques, anatomopathologiques, et thérapeutiques: revue générale de 130 cas. Gastroenterol Clin Biol 1982;6:1029–1041.
62. Vinik AI, Strodel WE, Eckhauser FE. Somatostatinomas, PPOmas, neurotensinomas. Semin Oncol 1987;14:263–281.
63. Eriksson B, Öberg K. Ppomas, nonfunctioning endocrine pancreatic tumors: clinical presentation, diagnosis, and advances in management. In: Mignon M, Jensen RT (eds.). Endocrine tumors of the pancreas: recent advances in research and management. Basel: Karger, 1995;208–222.
64. Young WF, Jr. Pheochromocytoma. Trends Endocrinol Metab 1993;4:122–127.
65. Grahame PE, Smythe GA, Edwards GA, et al. Laboratory diagnosis of pheochromocytoma: which analytes should we measure? Ann Clin Biochem 1993;30:129–134.
66. Eisenhofer G, Lenders JW, Linehan WM, Walther MM, Goldstein DS, Keiser HR. Plasma normetanephrine and metanephrine for detecting pheochromocytoma in von Hippel-Lindau disease and multiple endocrine neoplasia type 2. N Engl J Med 1999;340: 1872–1879.
67. Grouzmann E, Gicquel C, Plouin Pf, Schlumberger M, Comoy E, Bohuon C. Neuropeptide Y and neuron-specific enolase levels in benign and malignant pheochromocytomas. Cancer 1996;66: 1833–1835.
68. Gröndal S, Eriksson B, Hamberger B, Theodorsson E. Plasma chromogranin A+B, neuropeptide Y, and catecholamines in pheochromocytoma patients. J Intern Med 1991;229:453–456.
69. Nobels FR, Kwekkeboom DJ, Coopmans W, Schoenmakers CH, Lindemans J, De Herder WW, et al. Chromogranin A as serum marker for neuroendocrine neoplasia: comparison with neuron-specific enolase and the alpha-subunit of glycoprotein hormones. J Clin Endocrinol Metab 1997;82:2622–2628.
70. Hsiao RJ, Neumann HPH, Parmer RJ, Barbosa JA, O'Connor DT. Chromogranin A in familial pheochromocytoma: diagnostic

screening value, prediction of tumor mass, and post-resection kinetics indicating two-compartment distribution. Am J Med 1990;88:607–613.
71. Boomsma F, Bhaggoe UM, `t Veld AJMI, Schalekamp MADH. Sensitivity and specificity of a new ELISA method for determination of chromogranin A in the diagnosis of pheochromocytoma and neuroblastoma. Clin Chim Acta 1995;239:57–63.
72. Baudin E, Gigliotti A, Ducreux M, Ropers J, Comoy E, Sabourin JC, et al. Neuron-specific enolase and chromogranin A as markers of neuroendocrine tumors. Br J Cancer 1998;78: 1102–1107.
73. DeLellis RA, Dayal Y, Tischler AS, et al. Multiple endocrine neoplasia (MEN) syndromes: cellular origins and interrelationships. Int Rev Exp Pathol 1986;28:163–215.
74. Guignat L, Bidart JM, Nocera M, Comoy E, Schlumberger M, Baudin E. Chromogranin A and the α-subunit of glycoprotein hormones in medullary thyroid carcinoma and pheochromocytoma. Br J Cancer 2001;84:808–812.
75. Brodeur GM and Castleberry RP. Neuroblastoma. In: Pizzo PA and Poplack DG (eds.). Principles and practice of pediatric oncology. Philadelphia: JB Lippincott, 1993:739–767.
76. Hsiao RJ, Seeger RC, Yu AL, O'Connor DT. Chromogranin A in children with neuroblastoma: serum concentration parallels disease stage and predicts survival. J Clin Invest 1990;85: 1555–1559.
77. Kimura N, Hoshi S, Takahashi M, Takeha S, Shizawa S, Nagura H. Plasma chromogranin a in prostatic carcinoma and neuroendocrine tumors. J Urol 1997;157:565–568.

Chapter 29

Markers for Testicular Cancer

Ulf-Håkan Stenman and Henrik Alfthan

Of the malignant tumors arising in the testis, about 95% are germ cell tumors, most of the rest being lymphomas, Leydig cell tumors, and mesotheliomas (Table 1). Germ cell tumors consist of two major types: seminomas and nonseminomatous germ cell cancers of the testis (NSGCT). Testicular cancers comprise only about 1% of all malignancies, but they are the most common tumors in men under 45 years of age. Thus, they may have a considerable impact on lost years of life, but thanks to efficient therapy, more than 90% of the cases are cured (1).

A minority of germ cell tumors originate from extragonadal sites mainly in the sacrococcygeal region, mediastinum, and pineal gland (2). These are treated and monitored according to the same principles used to manage testicular tumors. Germ cell tumors are rare in women, representing about 1% of ovarian cancers. (Ovarian dysgerminoma is the female counterpart of seminoma.)

Table 1 Histological classification of testicular neoplasms

Germ cell tumors
    Seminoma
        Classic (typical)
        Anaplastic
        Spermatocytic
    Embryonal carcinoma
    Teratoma
        Mature
        Immature
        Mature or immature, with malignant transformation
    Choriocarcinoma
    Yolk-sac tumor (endodermal-sinus tumor)
    Mixed germ-cell tumor (specify all individual cell types)
Sex-cord-stromal tumors
    Sertoli-cell tumor
    Leydig-cell tumor
    Granulosa-cell tumor
Both germ-cell and gonadal stromal elements
    Gonadoblastoma
Adnexal and paratesticular tumors
    Adenocarcinoma of rete testis
    Mesothelioma
Miscellaneous neoplasms
    Carcinoid
    Lymphoma
    Cysts

Tumor marker determinations in serum play a central role in the treatment of patients with testicular cancer. Applications include staging, evaluating response to therapy, and monitoring disease. Treatment of a relapse may even be initiated on the basis of increasing marker concentrations alone.

The most useful serum markers are alpha-fetoprotein (AFP) and human chorionic gonadotropin (hCG); most cases of NSGCT have elevated serum levels of either marker, while hCG and its free beta subunit (hCGβ) are useful in detecting seminomas. Lactate dehydrogenase (LDH) and placental alkaline phosphatase (PLAP) can be used to detect seminomas and nonseminomatous germ cell cancers. Several other markers, especially placental proteins, have been evaluated but provide limited additional clinical information.

HISTOLOGICAL TYPES OF TESTICULAR CANCER

Different histological classifications of germ cell tumors are used, which complicates comparisons of marker expression in various studies (3). The most widely used WHO-Mostofi classification subdivides testicular cancers into two main types—seminomas and nonseminomatous germ cell tumors (NSGCT)—that differ with respect to treatment and marker expression. The peak incidence of seminoma occurs in the fourth decade of life, and the peak incidence of NSGCT in the third.

Seminomas are subdivided into pure seminomas and the rare spermatocytic seminomas that occur in elderly men. NSGCTs usually contain a mixture of various histological types including seminomatous components, embryonal carcinomas, choriocarcinomas, yolk sac tumors (also called endodermal sinus tumors), and teratomas. Teratomas are further classified as mature or immature. Teratoma with malignant transformation denotes somatic cancers of various types that occasionally develop from a teratoma. Any component occurring in the primary tumor can be expressed in metastases, which sometimes contain components not detected in the primary tumor (3). Testicular tumors are described on the basis of the contents of various histologically defined tissue types, with fewer than 10% of testicular tumors containing a single type (Table 2).

Immunohistochemistry facilitates detection of minor tumor components, e.g., syncytiotrophoblasts with hCG anti-

Table 2 Frequency of various histological types of testicular cancer (3)

Pure forms		Mixed forms	
Pure seminoma	26.9%	ECa+YST+T+SCT	14.3%
Spermatocytic seminoma	2.4%	Seminoma + SCT	8.1%
Embryonal carcinoma	3.1%	ECa +YST+T+S+SCT	7.4%
Yolk sac tumor	2.4%	ECa +YST+Teratoma	4.7%
Teratoma	2.7%	YST+Teratoma	2.5%
Choriocarcinoma	0.1%	ECa +T (TCa)	1.4%
ITMGC	0.6%	Other combinations	24.0%

Abbreviations: ECa, embryonal carcinoma; ITMGC, intratubular malignant germ cells; SCT, syncytiotrophoblasts; S, seminoma; TCa, teratocarcinoma; T, teratoma; YST, yolk sac tumor.

bodies, that may be missed by histological examination. The frequency of different histological types and combinations of these are shown in Table 2 (4).

MARKER EXPRESSION IN VARIOUS TUMOR TYPES

AFP is detected by immunohistochemistry in nearly all yolk sac tumors and in 10–20% of embryonal carcinomas and teratomas. AFP expression may appear in metastases from the rare AFP-negative primary yolk sac tumors. PLAP is detected in virtually all seminomas and embryonal carcinomas and in half of the yolk sac tumors and choriocarcinomas, but only rarely in teratomas. Tissue expression of hCG is detected in virtually all syncytiotrophoblasts and in about 30% of seminomas but not in other tissue types. In seminomas, the expression occurs especially in syncytio-trophoblast components. There is some controversy as to whether these tumors should be considered pure seminomas (3) but most authors include them among seminomas because they are treated as such (5,6). Reports on hCG expression in teratoma are conflicting, and positive results have been ascribed to expression in neighboring trophoblastic cells.

BIOLOGY, BIOCHEMISTRY, AND ASSAY OF MARKERS

AFP

AFP is a single-chain, 69 kDa glycoprotein containing 590 amino acids. It displays 30% homology with albumin, which like AFP, functions as a carrier protein for low molecular weight substances like fatty acids and steroid hormones (7). AFP belongs to a multigene family that, in addition to albumin, consists of vitamin D-binding protein (also called group-specific component, GC) and α-albumin/afamin (AFM). These proteins are encoded by genes that are clustered on chromosome 4 tq11-13 (8). During fetal life, AFP is first produced by the yolk sac and later by the fetal liver, resulting in very high plasma concentrations (9). The AFP concentration in fetal plasma peaks at about 3g/L in the 12th–14th week of gestation and towards term decreases to around 10–200 mg/L (10). After birth, AFP levels decrease with a half-life of five days, reaching adult levels at 8–10 months of age (11,12).

It is important to recognize the high normal values in early childhood because AFP is a sensitive marker for testicular yolk sac tumors, which is the most common testicular neoplasm in children (13,14). AFP is also a reliable marker for mixed tumors containing yolk sac tumor components in adults, and is expressed by some embryonal cancers (Table 3). Elevated serum concentrations of AFP are also caused by hepatocellular carcinomas and occasionally by other gastrointestinal cancers. (Benign liver disease can cause moderately elevated AFP levels.) AFP derived from the liver and the yolk sac display differences in carbohydrate composition (15), and lectin-binding can be used to differentiate between elevated levels caused by testicular cancer and liver disease, respectively. However, this approach it is not widely used (16).

Assay. At present, most commercial methods for determining AFP are sandwich assays that use monoclonal antibodies or a combination of monoclonal and polyclonal antibodies. The results obtained by these assays are similar to those obtained by earlier radioimmunoassays (RIAs) based on the binding inhibition principle. Most manufacturers calibrate their assays against the WHO standard 72/225, in which one International Unit (IU) of AFP corresponds to 1.21 ng (17). Differences in glycosylation patterns between AFP from various sources do not affect immunoreactivity, and antibody selection is not critical for assay performance (18).

Reference values. In spite of variation in assay calibration, the upper reference limit used by most centers is 10–15 µg/L. Careful determination of reference values has shown that concentrations of AFP increase with age. With one particular method the reference range was 0.6–9.3 kIU/L in subjects under 40 years of age, and 1.4–12.6 kIU/L in those above this age (18). It is recommended that age-specific reference values be established for each assay.

Table 3 Immunohistochemical expression of various markers in tumor components of various histological types (4)

Histological type	Marker expression		
	AFP	hCG	PLAP
Seminomas	Neg.	30–50%	>95%
Yolk sac tumors	90–95%	Neg.	40%
Embryonal cell carcinoma	10%	Neg.	95%
Syncytiotrophoblasts	Neg.	90–95%	40–50%
Teratoma	20%	Neg%	<5%

HCG and hCGβ

HCG is a heterodimeric glycoprotein hormone consisting of an α-(hCGα) and a β-subunit (hCGβ). The α-subunit, which contains 92 amino acids, is common to hCG, luteinizing hormone (LH), follicle-stimulating hormone (FSH), and thyroid-stimulating hormone (TSH), while the β chains are unique and determine the biological activity. The β chains of hCG and LH share about 80% homology, and hCG and LH act through the same receptor. HCGβ contains 145 amino acids, including a 24-amino-acid C-terminal extension not present in LHβ. The molecular weight of hCG is about 37 kDa, that of hCGβ is 22 kDa, and that of hCGα 15 kDa (19). The subunits lack hCG activity but hCGβ has been shown to enhance the growth of tumor cells in culture by preventing apoptosis (20).

hCGα is encoded by a single gene on chromosome 12q21.1-23, while hCGβ is encoded by six nonallelic genes clustered on 19q13.3, together with the gene encoding LHβ. The genes are called *CGβ1* (or *β1*) to *CGβ9*. *β1* and *β2* are pseudogenes that are not expressed, and *β4* encodes LH while *β7* and *β9* are alleles to *β6* and *β3*, respectively. *β6* and *β7*, which are called type I genes, encode a protein with alanine at position 117 while the protein encoded by the type II genes *β3/9*, *β5*, and *β8* contains aspartic acid at this position (21).

hCG is produced at high concentrations by syncytiotrophoblasts of the placenta and by trophoblastic tumors. It is also secreted at low levels by the pituitary, producing plasma levels that are measurable by sensitive methods. The secretion of hCG is regulated by gonadotropin-releasing hormone (GnRH) and thus the levels parallel those of LH. Therefore the serum concentrations increase with age both in men and in women, especially after the menopause (22). In addition to the pituitary, the testis, breast, prostate, and skeletal muscle express the mRNA for both subunits but the levels are 1000-fold lower than those in the placenta (21).

Sensitive assays can detect hCGβ in serum, but the levels are lower than those of hCG and they are not age-dependent (23). In addition to tissues expressing both subunits, normal bladder, adrenal, colon, thyroid, and uterus have also been shown to express hCGβ mRNA at levels about 10,000-fold lower than those in the placenta. These and other normal tissues expressing this mRNA are potential sources of hCGβ in the plasma of men and nonpregnant women, but the relative contribution of the various tissues is not known (21). Expression of hCGβ in normal nontrophoblastic tissues is usually caused by type I gene expression, but type II genes are expressed in the normal testis. Placenta and malignant tumors express predominantly type II genes (21). Moderately elevated serum concentrations occur in 30–70% of various nontrophoblastic and nongonadal cancers (24,25).

hCG and hCGβ are excreted into urine at concentrations similar to those in plasma. They are partially degraded during excretion; a major part of the hCG immunoreactivity in urine consists of a fragment of hCGβ called the core fragment (26), abbreviated as hCGβcf. Because the protein concentrations in urine are highly dependent on urinary flow rate, urine measurements of hCG, hCGβ, and hCGβcf should not be used to monitor cancer patients.

Nomenclature. The nomenclature used for various hCG assays is confusing: the expressions "β-hCG" or "hCG-beta assay" mostly denote assays that measure both hCG and hCGβ, but they are sometimes used even if the assay measures only intact hCG. These expressions stem from the use of polyclonal antisera prepared by immunization with hCGβ to establish the first immunoassays that did not crossreact with LH (27). According to the nomenclature recommended by the International Federation of Clinical Chemistry (IFCC), hCG denotes the intact αβ heterodimer, hCGβ the free β-subunit, and hCGα the free α-subunit. Assays should be defined according to what they measure, i.e., hCG and hCGβ separately or hCG and hCGβ together (28).

Standards. The third international standards (3rd IS) are currently used for intact hCG (code 75/537), hCGβ (code 75/551), and hCGα (75/569). The hCG standard was calibrated against the second standard by bioassay, whereas the subunits were assigned values on the basis of their protein content, one µg corresponding to one IU. Thus the substance concentrations corresponding to one IU of hCGβ is 15-fold and that of hCGα 22-fold that of 1 IU of hCG. The relationship between the various units is shown in Table 4. Cross-reactivity of the various forms of hCG should be expressed on the basis of molar concentrations. New standards for various forms of hCG are being developed and these will be primarily calibrated on the basis of their substance concentrations, i.e., in mol/L (28).

Various forms of hCG and assay design. Several variants of hCG have been identified, especially in cancer patients, e.g., nicked and hyperglycosylated forms, and variants lacking the C-terminal extension of hCGβ. These forms are detected to various degrees by different assays (29) depending on the epitope specificity of the antibodies used. Several epitopes have been defined on hCG and its subunit. Two epitopes called β8 and β9 on the C-terminal portion of hCGβ are completely specific for hCG and hCGβ and are therefore widely used in commercial assays. However, these antibodies have a relatively low affinity that limits assay sensitivity (30), and they do not react with hCG lacking the C-terminal extension on hCGβ (29). Assays specific for intact hCG can be constructed by using a sandwich assay with a catcher antibody to hCGβ and a tracer antibody to hCGα. Alternatively, antibodies recognizing two epitopes present on intact hCG (called c1 and c2) but not on the subunits can be used. Such assays tend to underestimate nicked hCG, which, however, has not been found to be a problem in the diagnosis of testicular cancer (31). Antibodies with high affinity for hCG and hCGβ often show a slight cross-reactivity with LH (0.1–0.3%), and therefore they are not widely used in commercial assays. The cross-reactivity is not a diagnostic problem, and such antibodies are required for measurement of

Table 4 Comparison of various units for the third international standards for hCG and its subunits

Abbreviation	MW	µg/IU	pmol/IU
hCG	37000	0.11	3
hCGβ	22000	1.0	45
hCGα	15000	1.0	67

the low physiological concentrations of hCG in men and nonpregnant women (22). Assays recognizing both hCG and hCGβ with an eight-fold over-recognition of hCGβ have been recommended for monitoring testicular cancer. Such assays are not currently available (29). Therefore, optimal detection of testicular cancer requires separate assays for hCG and hCGβ.

Reference values. The introduction of monoclonal antibodies and sandwich assays has facilitated the measurement of the low plasma concentrations of hCG and hCGβ occurring in males and nonpregnant women. The concentrations of hCG in nonpregnant subjects are around 3–10% of the LH concentrations when expressed in IUs based on bioactivity (22). The upper reference limit (based on the 97.5th percentile) is 5–10 IU/L in postmenopausal women and 3 IU/L in menstruating women (Table 5). The reference limits for men under 50 years of age is 0.7 IU/L and for men over this age 2.1 IU/L. In spite of the lower reference limits in men and differences in assay calibration, 5 IU/L is most often used as a cut-off value for patients with testicular cancer. Although most men with testicular cancer are young, the hCG levels often correspond to those in older men because testicular malfunction is common and this may lead to a slight increase in hCG levels. Furthermore, the detection limit of many commercial assays does not allow reliable measurement of levels below 5 IU/L. It should be noted that chemotherapy causes gonadal suppression that increases hCG levels. Therefore, levels increasing from < 2 up to 5–8 IU/L during chemotherapy are often iatrogenic and do not necessarily indicate a relapse. This can be confirmed by short-term testosterone treatment, which suppresses pituitary secretion of hCG (32). A more simple check is to measure serum LH and FSH. Levels above 30–50 IU/L indicate that the hCG originates in the pituitary.

The upper reference limit for hCGβ is 2 pmol/L, which corresponds to 0.044 IU/L of the 3rd IS. The reference range is not dependent on age or gender, and elevated levels are not caused by benign diseases (23). hCGβ assays are especially important in patients with seminoma. Of all hCG-producing seminomas, 30–40% have elevated serum levels of both hCG and hCGβ, 25% of hCG only, and 35% of hCGβ alone. When expressed in comparable molar concentrations, the upper reference limit for hCG (5.3 IU/L) is 15.5 pmol/L while that of hCGβ is 2 pmol/L and that for hCG + hCGβ 18 pmol/L (23). Therefore a seminoma producing only hCGβ will be detected later by an assay measuring both hCG and hCGβ rather than by a specific hCGβ assay.

Lactate Dehydrogenase (LDH)

LDH is a 134 kDa enzyme expressed in many tissues. It is a tetrameric enzyme that may contain various combinations of three subunits; LDH-A, LDH-B, and LDH-C. LDH-A and LDH-C are encoded by genes (*ldh-a* and *ldh-c*) located on chromosome 11, while the gene for LHD-B (*ldh-b*) is located on chromosome 12 (33). LDH-C is only expressed in the testis and on sperm and is not detected in serum.

The five isoenzymes occurring in plasma consist of the five possible combinations of LDH-A and B. Thus, LDH-1 consists of four B subunits (B_4), LDH-2 of B_3A_1, LDH-3 of B_2A_2, LDH-4 of B_1A_3, and LDH-5 of A_4. The elevation of LDH-1 has been linked to the regular occurrence of multiple copies of an isochromosome of chromosome 12, i(12p), in most cases of testicular cancer (34).

The serum concentrations of LDH are mainly measured enzymatically, and the values are method-dependent. The degree of elevation is therefore expressed in relation to the upper reference limit. LDH-1 is the most specific isoenzyme for testicular cancer (35). It may be determined by zymography, by assays utilizing immunoprecipitation of the other isoenzymes and catalytic determination of residual catalytic activity. Although elevated levels are caused by a wide variety of diseases, LDH is a useful serum marker both for staging and monitoring seminoma and NSGCT (35).

Placental Alkaline Phosphatase (PLAP)

Expression of a tumor-associated isoenzyme of alkaline phosphatase was first described in a patient with lung cancer and named the Regan isoenzyme after the name of the patient. This isoenzyme corresponds to placental alkaline phosphatase (PLAP), which is one of four alkaline phosphatases. Three organ-specific isoenzymes—the intestinal, germ cell, and placental alkaline phosphatases—are 90–98% homologous and are encoded by genes on chromosome 2q34-37. The fourth isoenzyme—tissue-nonspecific ALP—is encoded by a gene on chromosome 1p36.1-p34 and shows about 70% homology with the other isoenzymes.

The alkaline phosphatases are dimers. The two subunits in PLAP contain 479 amino acids (36). PLAP can be determined by zymography, immunoassay (37), or enzymatic assay after immunocapture (38). Due to the high degree of homology, antibody selection is critical. PLAP may provide unique information not obtained by other markers (38,39), and it is especially useful in patients with seminoma, where elevated levels occur in 60–70% of cases (38,40). Elevated results are common in

Table 5 Reference values of hCG and hCGβ in serum of women and men. The values have been established with highly sensitive time-resolved immunofluorometric assays calibrated against the 3rd IS for hCG and hCGβ (23). Higher reference values are mostly obtained by less sensitive methods

	Upper reference limit (IU/L)			
	Women		Men	
	<50 yr	≥50 yr	<50 yr	≥50 yr
hCG	3.0	5.3	0.7	2.0
hCGβ	0.04	0.04	0.04	0.05
	Upper reference limit (pmol/L)			
	Women		Men	
	<50 yr	≥50 yr	<50 yr	≥50 yr
hCG	8.6	15.5	2.1	6.1
hCGβ	1.6	2.0	1.9	2.1

smokers (38). This, along with the paucity of commercial assays, limits the clinical use of PLAP.

Immunohistochemical staining of PLAP is useful for characterizing germ cell tumors, which greatly facilitates detection of intratubular testicular neoplasia, which is a precursor of testicular cancer (4).

Other Markers

Several other markers have been studied. For example, pregnancy-specific beta-1 glycoprotein, also called SP1, is a fairly sensitive marker but its expression is very similar to that of hCG, which is a superior marker (41). Thus these markers have not been found to add sufficient new information to be clinically useful. Neuron-specific enolase (NSE) is elevated in about 30–50% of patients with seminomas and less often in NSGCT patients (42,43). The use of NSE is limited in spite of these promising results.

CLINICAL USE OF MARKER DETERMINATIONS

Serum Markers at Presentation

The marker expression in serum is dependent on tumor load and type i.e., stage and histological type of the tumor. Seminoma patients have elevated serum levels of hCG in 10–30% of cases, of LDH in about 60%, and PLAP in 50–60%. At least one marker is elevated in 80–90% of seminoma cases (40,44,45). Patients with NSGCT have elevated serum hCG in 40–50% of cases, and of AFP in 50–60%. Either one is elevated in 80–90% of cases. LDH is elevated in about 40–60% (45). The hCG concentrations in seminoma patients are usually below 300 IU/L while levels above 1000 IU/L are associated mostly with NSGCT. Very high levels, above 10000 IU/L, mainly occur in patients with pure choriocarcinoma.

Tumor classification is based on histological examination of the primary tumor, but a tumor histologically classified as a seminoma is reclassified as NSGCT and treated accordingly, if serum AFP is elevated. This finding indicates that nonseminomatous components occurring in the primary tumor or metastasis have been missed.

Serum Markers and Staging

Determination of marker levels in serum can be used to predict the presence of lymph node metastasis after orchiectomy in patients with clinical stage I disease. Elevated levels that are not accounted for by the metabolic decay rate of marker produced by the primary tumor reliably indicate metastatic disease and higher stage. Normal marker levels do not exclude the presence of metastases (46). Marker levels are used for staging of testicular cancers in the last edition of the TNM classification. Stage I is subdivided into tumors with or without lymphatic or vascular invasion and cases with elevated serum concentrations of AFP, hCG, or LDH in the absence of clinical or radiographic evidence of metastatic disease. Stage II disease includes retroperitoneal nodal disease without distant metastases, with or without serum markers elevations. Stage III comprises patients with only distant metastases or elevated serum marker levels (1,47).

Markers as Prognostic Factors

Elevated serum concentrations of AFP, hCG, and LDH in serum are associated with adverse prognosis in testicular germ cell tumors (45,48,49). A high serum hCG concentration is the strongest prognostic factor, and the risk increases with increasing concentration (50). Various cut-off levels are used to indicate high risk, e.g., AFP values above 500–1000 IU/L and hCG values above 1000–10000 IU/L (51–53).

The prognostic impact of markers is dependent on histological type and stage. Moderately elevated serum hCG levels in patients with pure seminoma are not associated with an adverse outcome (54), and high serum hCG concentrations (>300 IU/L) mostly indicate NSGCT (55). In Stage I NSGCT, the prognostic value of markers is dependent on the presence of vascular invasion. Absence of vascular invasion in combination with an elevated AFP has actually been found to be associated with low risk and the opposite combination with high risk (56).

Chemotherapy often induces a surge, i.e., a transient increase in marker concentrations, during the first week of treatment (57). A surge of AFP, but not of hCG, is an independent prognostic factor for disease progression (58). Testicular tumors grow very rapidly and growth rate is reflected in the marker doubling time. Patients with metastatic disease and a doubling time under four days have a worse prognosis than those with longer doubling times (59).

Monitoring of Therapy

If the concentrations of AFP or hCG are elevated before therapy, the rate of marker decline reflects the response to therapy. Persistent marker elevation after chemotherapy indicates residual disease and the need for further therapy (60,61). The normal half-life of hCG is about 1.5 days and that of AFP 5 days (62,63). Marker half-lives exceeding 3.5 days for hCG and 7 days for AFP during chemotherapy are strong predictors of recurrence and adverse prognosis (64). Marker half-life is determined by regression analysis of the logarithm of the marker concentration versus time. The half-life can be calculated by the following formula:

$$T_{1/2} = \text{Log } 2 \times (T2 - T1)/[\log (\text{conc. 1} - \text{conc. 2})]$$

Conc. 1 denotes the concentration at the first time point (T1) and conc. 2 that at time point 2.

It is preferable to use marker concentrations from several time points and to calculate the half-life from the slope of the regression line for the logarithm of the marker concentration (y-axis) plotted against time (x-axis) using the following formula:

$$T_{1/2} = \log 2/\text{slope}$$

The half-life calculation should be performed during two cycles of chemotherapy using regression analysis of weekly determinations between days 7 and 56, i.e., after the initial marker surge. Estimation of marker decline is especially important in poor-risk patients, in whom treatment failure is common. In patients with abnormal marker decline, a change to more aggressive therapy has been found to improve outcome (64).

Surveillance

Tumor marker determinations and imaging with computed tomography (CT) reliably detect relapse of testicular tumors. The prognosis of Stage I NSGCT is generally good and if metastases are not detected by CT or by elevated marker levels after primary surgery, further therapy is given only if a relapse occurs. About one-fourth of the cases relapse—90% within the first year—while relapses after two years are rare. During the first year after primary treatment, surveillance with serum marker determinations is usually performed at four weeks and CT at three-month intervals. Monitoring is continued at less frequent intervals during the following five years (Table 6). Practically all relapses are detected by a combination of CT and tumor marker determinations; about 70% of patients have elevated tumor marker levels at relapse (56,65).

The optimal frequency of tumor marker monitoring has been calculated on the basis of the marker doubling time. If serum markers are measured frequently enough, an increase can be detected before the levels reach the concentrations associated with an adverse prognosis, i.e., serum AFP >500 IU/L and hCG >1000 IU/L. On this basis, weekly determinations have been recommended for surveillance of Stage I tumors (66). Less frequent monitoring with a combination of marker assay and imaging is used by most centers (Table 6).

False-Positive and -Negative Marker Results

Increasing serum levels of AFP, hCG, or both during follow-up indicate active disease. If false positive results can be ruled out, this finding is a sufficient reason to initiate treatment even in the absence of positive clinical and radiological findings. It is therefore important to identify false-positive and -negative results.

Patients with testicular cancer may have elevated AFP levels caused by other diseases. Elevated AFP levels occur in about 70% of patients with hepatoma and in 10–20% of those with other cancers of the upper gastrointestinal tract. These diseases rarely occur in patients with testicular cancer. The most common causes are liver damage induced by chemotherapy and hepatitis (67). Apparently false-negative AFP results may be associated with loss or shift of marker expression during chemotherapy (68). Therapy may also eliminate all malignant tissue despite the persistence of a teratoma requiring surgery (69). Moderately elevated values that do not increase suggest that the elevation is not due to cancer (70).

Elevated levels of hCG are extremely rarely caused by other tumors, but the physiological elevation caused by therapy-induced gonadal suppression must be kept in mind (32). Depending on the method used, the levels may increase to 5–12 IU/L (70), which corresponds to those in post-menopausal women (23). A truly false elevation of serum hCG is occasionally caused by heterophilic antibodies, which link the catcher antibody to the tracer antibody, causing a signal indistinguishable from a specific one. This problem has so far been reported to occur mainly in women (71) because of the widespread use of hCG assays for diagnosis of pregnancy, but there is no reason why it cannot occur in men. If suspected, such false-positive results can be checked by analysis of hCG in urine or by addition of mouse IgG or serum to block the heterophilic antibodies. Because various assays differ with respect to this interference, it is useful to control the result with another assay (29). Apparently false-negative hCG results can be obtained if a tumor produces only hCGβ but not hCG. While this is most likely to occur in seminoma (72), it has also been reported in NSGCT patients (73).

Elevated LDH values are caused by a multitude of diseases, e.g., myocardial infarction, lung and liver disease, and hemolysis. It is therefore important to rule out concomitant disease when evaluating the impact of an elevated LDH value. Hemolysis of the sample is an important cause of falsely elevated values.

Elevated levels of PLAP are common in smokers, with levels tenfold those found in nonsmokers being fairly common. The high degree of homology between placental and other alkaline phosphatase is a potential problem in immunological PLAP assays. This can be controlled by careful selection of antibodies (38). However, this problem has not been extensively studied due to lack of widely available methods.

Table 6 Follow-up schedule of patients with Stage I NST-GCT, recommended by Gels et al. (65)

Year	Schedule	
1	Every 4 weeks	PE, TM
	Every 3 months	PE, TM, CTa, CTc
2	Every 8 weeks	PE, TM
	Every 6 months	PE, TM, CTa, CTc
3	Every 3 months	PE, TM
	Every 12 months	PE, TM, CTa, CTc
4 and 5	Every 6 months	PE, TM
	Every 12 months	PE, TM, CTa, CTc

PE, physical examination; TM, tumor markers AFP and hCG; CTa, computed tomogram of the abdomen; CTc, computed tomogram of the chest.

REFERENCES

1. Bosl GJ, Motzer RJ. Testicular germ-cell cancer. N Engl J Med 1997;337:242–253.
2. Mead GM, Stenning SP, Parkinson MC, Horwich A, Fossa SD, Wilkinson PM, Kaye SB, Newlands ES, Cook PA. The Second Medical Research Council study of prognostic factors in non-seminomatous germ cell tumors. Medical Research Council Testicular Tumor Working Party. J Clin Oncol 1992;10:85–94.
3. Mostofi FK, Sesterhenn IA, Davis Jr CJ. Developments in histopathology of testicular germ cell tumors. Semin Urol 1988; 6:171–188.

4. Mostofi FK, Sesterhenn IA, Davis CJ, Jr. Immunopathology of germ cell tumors of the testis. Semin Diag Pathol 1987;4: 320–341.
5. Javadpour N. The role of biologic tumor markers in testicular cancer. Cancer 1980;45:1755–1761.
6. Lange PH, Nochomovitz LE, Rosai J, Fraley EE, Kennedy BJ, Bosl G, Brisbane J, Catalona WJ, Cochran JS, Comisarow RH, Cummings KB, deKernion JB, Einhorn LH, Hakala TR, Jewett M, Moore MR, Scardino PT, Streitz JM. Serum alpha-fetoprotein and human chorionic gonadotropin in patients with seminoma. J Urol 1980;124:472–478.
7. Morinaga T, Sakai M, Wegmann TG, Tamaoki T. Primary structures of human alpha-fetoprotein and its mRNA. Proc Natl Acad Sci USA 1983;80:4604–4608.
8. Nishio H, Dugaiczyk A. Complete structure of the human alpha-albumin gene, a new member of the serum albumin multigene family. Proc Natl Acad Sci USA 1996;93:7557–7561.
9. Abelev GI. Alpha-fetoprotein as a marker of embryo-specific differentiations in normal and tumor tissues. Transplant Rev 1974; 20:3–37.
10. Gitlin D, Boesman M. Serum alpha-fetoprotein, albumin, and gamma-G-globulin in the human conceptus. J Clin Invest 1966; 45:1826–1838.
11. Blohm ME, Vesterling-Horner D, Calaminus G, Gobel U. Alpha 1-fetoprotein (AFP) reference values in infants up to 2 years of age. Pediatr Hematol Oncol 1998;15:135–142.
12. Brewer JA, Tank ES. Yolk sac tumors and alpha-fetoprotein in first year of life. Urology 1993;42:79–80.
13. Huddart SN, Mann JR, Gornall P, Pearson D, Barrett A, Raafat F, Barnes JM, Wallendsus KR. The UK Children's Cancer Study Group: testicular malignant germ cell tumors 1979–1988. J Pediatr Surg 1990;25:406–410.
14. Carroll WL, Kempson RL, Govan DE, Freiha FS, Shochat SJ, Link MP. Conservative management of testicular endodermal sinus tumor in childhood. J Urol 1985;133:1011–1014.
15. Ruoslahti E, Adamson E. Alpha-fetoproteins produced by the yolk sac and the liver are glycosylated differently. Biochem Biophys Res Commun 1978;85:1622–1630.
16. de Takats PG, Jones SR, Penn R, Cullen MH. Alpha-foetoprotein heterogeneity: what is its value in managing patients with germ cell tumors? Clin Oncol 1996;8:323–326.
17. Mann K. Tumor markers in testicular cancer. Urologe A 1990;29: 77–86.
18. Christiansen M, Hogdall CK, Andersen JR, Norgaard-Pedersen B. Alpha-fetoprotein in plasma and serum of healthy adults: preanalytical, analytical, and biological sources of variation and construction of age-dependent reference intervals. Scand J Clin Lab Invest 2001;61:205–215.
19. Pierce JG, Parsons TF. Glycoprotein hormones: structure and function. Annu Rev Biochem 1981;50:465–495.
20. Butler SA, Ikram MS, Mathieu S, Iles RK. The increase in bladder carcinoma cell population induced by the free beta subunit of human chorionic gonadotropin is a result of an anti-apoptosis effect and not cell proliferation. Br J Cancer 2000;82:1553–1556.
21. Bellet D, Lazar V, Bieche I, Paradis V, Giovangrandi Y, Paterlini P, Lidereau R, Bedossa P, Bidart JM, Vidaud M. Malignant transformation of nontrophoblastic cells is associated with the expression of chorionic gonadotropin beta genes normally transcribed in trophoblastic cells. Cancer Res 1997;57:516–523.
22. Stenman UH, Alfthan H, Ranta T, Vartiainen E, Jalkanen J, Seppälä M. Serum levels of human chorionic gonadotropin in non-pregnant women and men are modulated by gonadotropin-releasing hormone and sex steroids. J Clin Endocrinol Metab 1987;64:730–736.
23. Alfthan H, Haglund C, Dabek J, Stenman U-H. Concentrations of human chorionic gonadotropin, its β-subunit and the core fragment of the β-subunit in serum and urine of men and non-pregnant women. Clin Chem 1992;38:1981–1987.
24. Alfthan H, Haglund C, Roberts P, Stenman U-H. Elevation of free β-subunit of human choriogonadotropin and core β fragment of human choriogonadotropin in the serum and urine of patients with malignant pancreatic and biliary disease. Cancer Res 1992;52: 4628–4633.
25. Marcillac I, Troalen F, Bidart JM, Ghillani P, Ribrag V, Escudier B, Malassagne B, Droz JP, Lhomme C, Rougier P, et al. Free human chorionic gonadotropin beta subunit in gonadal and nongonadal neoplasms. Cancer Res 1992;52:3901–3907.
26. Papapetrou PD, Nicopoulou SC. The origin of human chorionic gonadotropin β-subunit-core fragment excreted in the urine of patients with cancer. Acta Endocrinologica 1986;112:415–422.
27. Vaitukaitis JL. Human chorionic gonadotropin as a tumor marker. Ann Clin Lab Sci 1974;4:276–80.
28. Stenman U-H, Bidart JM, Birken S, Mann K, Nisula B, O'Connor J. Standardization of protein immunoprocedures. Choriogonadotropin (CG). Scand J Clin Lab Invest Suppl 1993; 216:42–78.
29. Cole LA, Shahabi S, Butler SA, Mitchell H, Newlands ES, Behrman HR, Verrill HL. Utility of commonly used commercial human chorionic gonadotropin immunoassays in the diagnosis and management of trophoblastic diseases. Clin Chem 2001;47: 308–315.
30. Berger P, Sturgeon C, Bidart J-M, Paus E, Gerth R, Niang M, Fougeat L, Bristow A, Birken S, Stenman U-H. An important step towards user-orientated standardization of pregnancy and tumor marker diagnosis: assignment of epitopes to the 3D structure of diagnostically and commercially relevant monoclonal antibodies (mAbs) directed against human chorionic gonadotropin (hCG) and derivatives. Tumor Biology (in press).
31. Hoermann R, Berger P, Spoettl G, Gillesberger F, Kardana A, Cole LA, Mann K. Immunological recognition and clinical significance of nicked human chorionic gonadotropin in testicular cancer. Clin Chem 1994;40:2306–2312.
32. Catalona WJ, Vaitukaitis JL, Fair WR. Falsely positive specific human chorionic gonadotropin assays in patients with testicular tumors: conversion to negative with testosterone administration. J Urol 1979;122:126–128.
33. Li SS, Luedemann M, Sharief FS, Takano T, Deaven LL. Mapping of human lactate dehydrogenase-A, -B, and -C genes and their related sequences: the gene for LDHC is located with that for LDHA on chromosome 11. Cytogenet Cell Genet 1988;48:16–18.
34. von Eyben FE, de Graaff WE, Marrink J, Blaabjerg O, Sleijfer DT, Koops HS, Oosterhuis JW, Petersen PH, van Echten-Arends J, de Jong B. Serum lactate dehydrogenase isoenzyme 1 activity in patients with testicular germ cell tumors correlates with the total number of copies of the short arm of chromosome 12 in the tumor. Mol Gen Genet 1992;235:140–146.
35. von Eyben FE. Biochemical markers in advanced testicular tumors: serum lactate dehydrogenase, urinary chorionic gonadotropin, and total urinary estrogens. Cancer 1978;41: 648–652.
36. Le Du MH, Stigbrand T, Taussig MJ, Menez A, Stura EA. Crystal structure of alkaline phosphatase from human placenta at 1.8 Å resolution. Implication for a substrate specificity. J Biol Chem 2001;276:9158–9165.
37. Fishman WH. Perspectives on alkaline phosphatase isoenzymes. Am J Med 1974;56:617–650.

38. De Broe ME, Pollet DE. Multi-center evaluation of human placental alkaline phosphatase as a possible tumor-associated antigen in serum. Clin Chem 1988;34:1995–1999.
39. Lange PH, Millan JL, Stigbrand T, Vessella RL, Ruoslahti E, Fishman WH. Placental alkaline phosphatase as a tumor marker for seminoma. Cancer Res 1982;42:3244–3247.
40. Weissbach L, Bussar-Maatz R, Mann K. The value of tumor markers in testicular seminomas. Results of a prospective multi-center study. Eur Urol 1997;32:16–22.
41. de Bruijn HW, Sleijfer DT, Schraffordt Koops H, Suurmeijer AJ, Marrink J, Ockhuizen T. Significance of human chorionic gonadotropin, alpha-fetoprotein, and pregnancy-specific beta-1-glycoprotein in the detection of tumor relapse and partial remission in 126 patients with nonseminomatous testicular germ cell tumors. Cancer 1985;55:829–835.
42. Kuzmits R, Schernthaner G, Krisch K. Serum neuron-specific enolase. A marker for responses to therapy in seminoma. Cancer 1987;60:1017–1021.
43. Fossa SD, Qvist H, Stenwig AE, Lien HH, Ous S, Giercksky KE. Is post-chemotherapy retroperitoneal surgery necessary in patients with nonseminomatous testicular cancer and minimal residual tumor masses? J Clin Oncol 1992;10:569–573.
44. Koshida K, Uchibayashi T, Yamamoto H, Hirano K. Significance of placental alkaline phosphatase (PLAP) in the monitoring of patients with seminoma. Br J Urol 1996;77:138–142.
45. von Eyben FE, Blaabjerg O, Hyltoft-Petersen P, Madsen EL, Amato R, Liu F, Fritsche H. Serum lactate dehydrogenase isoenzyme 1 and prediction of death in patients with metastatic testicular germ cell tumors. Clin Chem Lab Med 2001;39:38–44.
46. Bosl GJ, Lange PH, Fraley EE, Goldman A, Nochomovitz LE, Rosai J, Waldmann TA, Johnson K, Kennedy BJ. Human chorionic gonadotropin and alphafetoprotein in the staging of nonseminomatous testicular cancer. Cancer 1981;47:328–332.
47. Sobin L, Wittekind C. TNM classification of malignant tumors. International Union Against Cancer 1997;1–227.
48. Droz JP, Kramar A, Ghosn M, Piot G, Rey A, Theodore C, Wibault P, Court BH, Perrin JL, Travagli JP, et al. Prognostic factors in advanced nonseminomatous testicular cancer. A multivariate logistic regression analysis. Cancer 1988;62:564–568.
49. Mead GM, Stenning SP. The International Germ Cell Consensus Classification: a new prognostic factor-based staging classification for metastatic germ cell tumours. Clin Oncol (R Coll Radiol) 1997;9:207–209.
50. Vogelzang NJ. Prognostic factors in metastatic testicular cancer. Int J Androl 1987;10:225–237.
51. Aass N, Klepp O, Cavallin-Stahl E, Dahl O, Wicklund H, Unsgaard B, Baldetorp L, Ahlstrom S, Fossa SD. Prognostic factors in unselected patients with nonseminomatous metastatic testicular cancer: a multi-center experience. J Clin Oncol 1991;9:818–826.
52. Dearnaley DP, Horwich A, A'Hern R, Nicholls J, Jay G, Hendry WF, Peckham MJ. Combination chemotherapy with bleomycin, etoposide, and cisplatin (BEP) for metastatic testicular teratoma: long-term follow-up. Eur J Cancer 1991;27:684–691.
53. Mead GM, Stenning SP. Prognostic factors in metastatic non-seminomatous germ cell tumors: the Medical Research Council studies. Eur Urol 1993;23:196–200.
54. Weissbach L, Bussar-Maatz R, Lohrs U, Schubert GE, Mann K, Hartmann M, Dieckmann KP, Fassbinder J. Prognostic factors in seminomas with special respect to HCG: results of a prospective multi-center study. Seminoma Study Group. Eur Urol 1999;36:601–608.
55. Ruther U, Rothe B, Grunert K, Bader H, Sessler R, Nunnensiek C, Rassweiler J, Luthgens M, Eisenberger F, Jipp P. Role of human chorionic gonadotropin in patients with pure seminoma. Eur Urol 1994;26:129–133.
56. Klepp O, Dahl O, Flodgren P, Stierner U, Olsson AM, Oldbring J, Nilsson S, Daehlin L, Tornblom M, Smaland R, Starkhammar H, Abramsson L, Wist E, Raabe N, Edekling T, Cavallin-Stahl E. Risk-adapted treatment of clinical stage 1 non-seminoma testis cancer. Eur J Cancer 1997;33:1038–1044.
57. Vogelzang NJ, Lange PH, Goldman A, Vessela RH, Fraley EE, Kennedy BJ. Acute changes of alpha-fetoprotein and human chorionic gonadotropin during induction chemotherapy of germ cell tumors. Cancer Res 1982;42:4855–4861.
58. de Wit R, Collette L, Sylvester R, de Mulder PH, Sleijfer DT, ten Bokkel Huinink WW, Kaye SB, van Oosterom AT, Boven E, Stoter G. Serum alpha-fetoprotein surge after the initiation of chemotherapy for non-seminomatous testicular cancer has an adverse prognostic significance. Br J Cancer 1998;78:1350–1355.
59. Price P, Hogan SJ, Bliss JM, Horwich A. The growth rate of metastatic nonseminomatous germ cell testicular tumours measured by marker production doubling time—II. Prognostic significance in patients treated by chemotherapy. Eur J Cancer 1990;26:453–457.
60. Toner G. Serum tumor-marker half-life during chemotherapy allows early prediction of complete response and survival in non-seminomatous germ cell tumors. Cancer Res 1990;50:5904–5910.
61. Coogan CL, Foster RS, Rowland RG, Bihrle R, Smith JR ER, Einhorn LH, Roth BJ, Donohue JP. Post-chemotherapy retroperitoneal lymph node dissection is effective therapy in selected patients with elevated tumor markers after primary chemotherapy alone. Urology 1997;50:957–962.
62. Kohn J. The dynamics of serum alpha-fetoprotein in the course of testicular teratoma. Scand J Immunol (Suppl 8) 1978;8:103.
63. Lange PH, Vogelzang NJ, Goldman A, Kennedy BJ, Fraley EE. Marker half-life analysis as a prognostic tool in testicular cancer. J Urol 1982;128:708–711.
64. Mazumdar M, Bajorin DF, Bacik J, Higgins G, Motzer RJ, Bosl GJ. Predicting outcome to chemotherapy in patients with germ cell tumors: the value of the rate of decline of human chorionic gonadotrophin and alpha-fetoprotein during therapy. J Clin Oncol 2001;19:2534–2541.
65. Gels ME, Hoekstra HJ, Sleijfer DT, Marrink J, de Bruijn HW, Molenaar WM, Freling NJ, Droste JH, Schraffordt Koops H. Detection of recurrence in patients with clinical stage I nonseminomatous testicular germ cell tumors and consequences for further follow-up: a single-center 10-year experience. J Clin Oncol 1995;13:1188–1194.
66. Seckl MJ, Rustin GJ, Bagshawe KD. Frequency of serum tumor marker monitoring in patients with non-seminomatous germ cell tumors. Br J Cancer 1990;61:916–918.
67. Germa JR, Llanos M, Tabernero JM, Mora J. False elevations of alpha-fetoprotein associated with liver dysfunction in germ cell tumors. Cancer 1993;72:2491–2494.
68. Czaja JT, Ulbright TM. Evidence for the transformation of seminoma to yolk sac tumor, with histogenetic considerations. Am J Clin Pathol 1992;97:468–477.
69. Prow DM. Germ cell tumors: staging, prognosis, and outcome. Semin Urol Oncol 1998;16:82–93.
70. Morris MJ, Bosl GJ. Recognizing abnormal marker results that do not reflect disease in patients with germ cell tumors. J Urol 2000;163:796–801.

71. Cole LA, Rinne KM, Shahabi S, Omrani A. False-positive hCG assay results leading to unnecessary surgery and chemotherapy and needless occurrences of diabetes and coma. Clin Chem 1999;45:313–314.
72. Saller B, Clara R, Spottl G, Siddle K, Mann K. Testicular cancer secretes intact human choriogonadotropin (hCG) and its free beta-subunit: evidence that hCG (+hCG-beta) assays are the most reliable in diagnosis and follow-up. Clin Chem 1990;36:234–239.
73. Summers J, Raggatt P, Pratt J, Williams MV. Experience of discordant beta hCG results by different assays in the management of non-seminomatous germ cell tumours of the testis. Clin Oncol 1999;11:388–392.

Chapter **30**

Tumor Markers in Melanoma

Steven D. Trocha, Rishab K. Gupta, and Donald L. Morton

Between 1973 and 1995, the incidence of melanoma in the United States rose by more than 125%. Unfortunately, melanoma tends to strike in the prime of life (35% of cases occur in individuals between the ages of 35 and 54), with a median age of 56 years at diagnosis (1). Although early-stage disease is curable by surgery, the prognosis associated with metastasis to distant sites is poor—median survival is only four to six months. These statistics reflect melanoma's unpredictable pattern of recurrence and the lack of sensitive tools to monitor therapy and follow-up (2). In addition, melanoma is very resistant to radiation and chemotherapy (3). These factors underline the importance of early detection of disease and sensitive monitoring of the response to therapy.

Evaluating the usefulness of the tools for monitoring melanoma requires an understanding of the current American Joint Committee on Cancer (AJCC) staging system. This system stages melanoma by the Breslow thickness or Clark level of invasion of the primary tumor (T), metastasis to regional in-transit sites or lymph nodes (N), and metastasis beyond the regional lymph nodal basin (M) (4). The most significant prognostic tool in the melanoma staging system remains the tumor status of the regional lymph nodes. Other prognostic factors include Breslow thickness, anatomic site of the primary, patient age, and number of organs involved. However, these factors have many shortcomings. For instance, even in "thin" melanomas (<1 mm) that should be readily cured by surgery alone, there is a 10% failure rate that increases to 25–30% for patients with AJCC stage II disease.

It has been argued that the inadequacy of current prognostic tools, especially in patients with clinically node-negative melanoma, is due to initial understaging of disease, i.e., failure to identify occult regional metastasis. To improve the sensitivity and accuracy of lymph node evaluation, Morton et al. (5) developed a selective biopsy technique called sentinel lymphadenectomy. This minimally invasive technique begins with injection of a tracer (vital dye and/or radioisotope) in the periphery of a tumor. The tracer is followed along the lymphatics that drain the primary melanoma until they reach the first (sentinel) lymph node. Because this node is the most likely site of regional metastasis, it is excised and examined for tumor cells. The sentinel node specimen is much smaller than a conventional lymphadenectomy specimen and thus can be quickly and cost effectively examined with highly sensitive immunohistochemical and molecular techniques.

Tumor marker assays can be applied to a variety of sample types. These include the primary tumor, draining lymph node basins, metastatic sites, serum, and blood. The majority of markers in melanoma have focused on the primary tumor and/or serum samples with recent emphasis on whole blood using reverse transcriptase-polymerase chain reaction (RT-PCR) methods. This review identifies standard and potential tumor markers in melanoma (Table 1) and describes their diagnostic and prognostic roles.

MELANIN-RELATED METABOLITES

The rate of melanin synthesis in melanocytes governs skin pigmentation. In malignant disease the synthesis of melanin is elevated, as are the metabolites of this process. Melanin synthesis in the melanocyte is based on the conversion of tyrosine to dopa and dopaquinone by way of tyrosinase. Dopaquinone is converted to 5-S-cysteinyldopa (5SCD) and pheomelanin or 5-6-dihydroxyindole (5,6DHI), then to 5(6)-hydroxy-6(5)-methoxyindole-2-carboxylic acid (6H5MI2C), and ultimately to eumelanin (Figure 1). These natural precursors of melanin have been investigated as tumor markers (6,7).

5-S-Cysteinyldopa (5SCD)

5SCD is a very specific marker of melanin metabolism that can be detected in urine or serum (8). Urine 5SCD determinations have focused primarily on advanced melanomas because earlier studies have noted that fewer than 2% of stage I–III melanomas had high 5SCD urine excretion (>0.4 mg per 24 hr). In contrast, 60% of stage IV patients had high urinary levels (8). In support of these findings, a separate study of 50 patients found no elevated urine excretion in stage I–III disease. However, all 12 of the stage IV patients had significantly elevated values, especially those with liver metastasis (9).

In simultaneous collections of urine and serum, 5SCD levels were elevated earlier in serum and more accurately reflected melanoma recurrence or progression (8). Serum detection of 5SCD employs high-pressure liquid chromatography (HPLC). Other investigators have demonstrated that plasma 5SCD level increased from twofold to fourfold to 450-fold as disease progressed from stage I/II to III to IV (10). Another study confirmed that plasma 5SCD levels of 252 patients were significantly different for clinical stage I vs. III disease and for clini-

Table 1 Melanoma tumor marker categories

Melanin-related metabolites	Adhesion molecules	Immunoregulatory molecules
• 5-S-Cysteinyldopa	• CD44	• MART-1
• 6H5MI2C	• Alphavbeta3	• Tyrosinase
	• Beta 1 and 3	
	• MUC18	
	• ICAM-1	
Cytokines and receptors	**Cell growth factors**	**Apoptosis**
• IL-2/IL-2R	• AP-2	• Fas
• IL-6/IL-6R	• MITF	• Bcl-2
• IL-10	• nm-23	• TRAIL
	• c-myc	• FLIP
	• Ki-67	
	• Cell Cycle Regulators	
	• MIA	
Angiogenesis factors	**Extracellular matrix proteins**	**Others**
• VEGF	• MMP-2	• LDH
• bFGF	• MMP-9	• TA90-IC

cal stage II vs. III disease (11). However, these differences carried no prognostic significance.

The value of 5SCD in monitoring the response to immunochemotherapy was evaluated in a study of 11 patients (12). Decreasing serum 5SCD concentrations *during* therapy with IL-2, IFN-α, and dacarbazine correlated with significantly longer survival. Furthermore, changes in 5SCD levels following the initiation of therapy discriminated responders from nonresponders.

ADHESION MOLECULES

Adhesion molecules are cell-surface proteins that mediate the recognition and adhesion of cells to a substrate and to other cells. Although a tumor cell's ability to attach to the endothelium and migrate across cell-cell barriers is essential for metastasis, very few adhesion molecules have been evaluated as tumor markers. This is in large part due to the wide range of techniques required for their assessment.

Immunoglobulin Superfamily

CD44 (Pgp-1, HCAM). This membrane glycoprotein has a cellular receptor for hyaluronic acid. It is expressed on leukocytes and erythrocytes and allows lymphocytes to adhere to high endothelial venules. The expression of this glycoprotein on tumor cells could potentially influence leukocyte adhesion and enhance or compromise immune surveillance. Alternatively, adherence of tumor cells to endothelial venules could target these cells to transmigrate and invade the microvasculature or lymphatics.

CD44 exists as a standard form (CD44std) and as ten isoforms (v1-v10) that are the result of several alternative splicings of mRNA (13). In 292 patients with clinical stage I disease, CD44 IHC expression was significantly reduced. Reduction in CD44 expression independently predicted a shorter disease free-survival (DFS) and overall survival (OS) (14). In a separate study of 52 patients, serum levels of CD44 were significantly decreased (15). On other hand, Dietrich et al. (16).

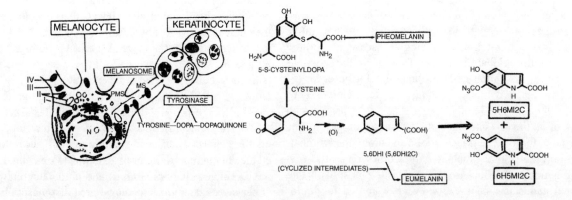

Figure 1 Melanin synthesis pathway within the melanocyte. Both eumelanin and pheomelanin pigments are synthesized from the common metabolic pathway (i.e., conversion of tyrosine to dopa and dopaquinone in the presence of tyrosinase). 5-6-Dihydroxyindole (5,6DHI), its carboxylic acid form (5,6DHI2C), and 5-*S*-cysteinyldopa are the major metabolites of eumelanin and pheomelanin synthesis. 5,6DHI2C is subsequently *O*-methylated to form 5(6)-hydroxy-6(5)-methoxyindole-2-carboxylic acid [5(6)H6(5)MI2C]. (Reprinted with permission from reference 6.)

suggested that high CD44 expression significantly reduced survival. Schaider et al. (17) reported that the circulating forms of CD44std, v5, v6, and v10 were not significantly elevated in melanoma patients, although a few patients did have higher levels of circulating CD44std.

The value of CD44 as a diagnostic or prognostic marker needs further investigation with special emphasis on standard vs. isoform measurements, because one isoform may compensate for the quantitative changes in another.

Melanoma cell adhesion molecule (MCAM). MCAM is an integral membrane glycoprotein with Ca(2+)-independent cell adhesion properties. This protein demonstrates heterophilic cell-to-cell interactions that result in dynamic actin-cytoskeleton rearrangements (18). Cytoskeleton rearrangements can facilitate cell detachment and migration, which are key functions in metastasis and invasion. MCAM has been mapped to chromosome 11 band q23.3 (19). Its expression depends on cAMP response element-binding protein (CREB), and immunohistochemistry (IHC) has demonstrated a limited number of tissues that express MCAM such as melanoma, gestational trophoblastic lesions, and endothelial cells (20). Others have demonstrated a diagnostic role for MCAM by noting that it is highly expressed in most melanoma cells but not in normal melanocytes (18,19,21). The loss of MCAM could significantly affect cell-cell contact and disrupt the actin-cytoskeleton (18). In fact, one group of investigators demonstrated that in vitro inhibition of MCAM led to the loss of melanoma cell-to-cell adhesion and a decreased tumorigenic phenotype. On the other hand, the in vivo expression of MCAM mRNA and protein levels was directly proportional to the development of metastatic deposits in mice (22). In humans MCAM expression has been shown to correlate with tumor thickness and confer metastatic potential in one study, while in a separate study that evaluated seven immunohistochemical markers, MUC18 did not retain prognostic significance (23,24). MCAM remains a promising marker in melanoma, but future studies must focus on multi-marker comparisons and clinical outcome correlation.

ICAM-1 (CD54). This adhesion molecule is found on the surface of antigen-presenting cells (APCs), T cells, and vascular endothelial cells, and its expression is a marker of poor outcome. ICAM-1 expression plays an important role in neutrophil adhesion and transendothelial migration, the significance of which is demonstrated in ischemia-reperfusion pathology and other promoters of inflammation. ICAM-1 may be membrane-associated (mICAM-1) and/or soluble (sICAM-1) (25). mICAM-1 has been detected by IHC in 69% of primary and 89% of metastatic lesions and is associated with a shorter DFS (26,27). sICAM-1 has been demonstrated in 52 primary melanomas, but in concentrations that were not significantly different from controls (15). In advanced metastatic disease, however, pretreatment elevation of sICAM-1 was significantly higher in bone/liver metastasis and was a prognostic indicator of survival (28,29).

Integrins

Integrins mediate a diverse array of functions. As cell surface proteins they mediate functions of antigen-presenting cells (APCs), act in leukocyte migration, and modulate adherence of cells to each other and their surrounding extracellular matrix (i.e., vitronectin or fibronectin). These transmembrane adhesion molecules form heterodimers composed of an alpha and a beta chain. The target ligands are most often fibronectin or vitronectin in the extracellular matrix.

Alphavbeta3. The in vitro ligation of alphavbeta3 (a vitronectin receptor) has demonstrated an increase in protein kinase C (PKC) activity with a subsequent increased expression of urokinase plasminogen activator receptor mRNA and plasmin. The result was increased cell invasiveness (30). Others have noted that ligation of this integrin upregulates the expression of matrix metalloproteinase-2 (MMP-2) and increases tumor invasiveness (31). Additional reports have attributed angiogenic properties to alphavbeta3, which may potentiate invasiveness (32,33).

IHC shows that alphavbeta3 expression is restricted to melanoma cells but differs among different types of melanomas (34). Thus, acral and superficial melanoma demonstrated only 50% staining whereas lymph nodes and cutaneous metastases stained 60% and 80%, respectively (35). This could be due to the fact that alphavbeta3 is first expressed when melanoma changes from a radial to vertical growth phase; its appearance thus may herald progression to an invasive phenotype. Several investigators have demonstrated a significant relationship between the expression of alphavbeta3 in nonacral lesions and tumor thickness, recurrence, and outcome (36). Their findings suggest that this integrin may have significant prognostic potential in thicker and metastatic melanomas.

Beta1 and beta3. Although antibodies do not distinguish between different alpha subunits of beta1 and beta3, different integrin complexes have distinctly different ligands and potentially different functional consequences. An IHC study of 111 intermediate-thickness melanomas reported expression of beta1 and beta3 in 52% and 64%, respectively. Beta3 expression was associated with a greater mortality (37). In another study, the expression of beta3 in 130 samples increased with tumor thickness, but the strong expression of beta3 by Spitz nevi limits the diagnostic potential of this subunit (38).

Beta1 expression in 38 metastatic melanomas demonstrated a relatively low positivity of 39%. Contrary to alphavbeta 3 data, increased expression of the beta1 subunit correlated with longer DFS and overall survival (OS) (39).

IMMUNOREGULATORY MOLECULES

Immunoregulatory molecules are antigens that elicit a number of diverse immune actions and reactions. Immune surveillance, recognition, and destruction are the primary modes by which tumor cells are removed from the circulation. This surveillance is based on antigen recognition, but in tumor cells these antigens are often mutated or dysregulated. The best studied of these antigens are the melanocyte differentiation antigens: melanoma antigen recognized by T cells (MART-1) and tyrosinase.

MART-1 / Melan-A

MART-1 is a protein of 118 amino acids, and its expression is limited to melanocytes of the skin and retina. The MART-1 gene encodes an HLA-A2 restricted peptide epitope recognized by CD8+ cytotoxic T-lymphocytes (CTLs) and a HLA-DR4 recognized by CD4+ T cells. There are two antibodies for IHC detection of this single epitope: M2-7C10/MART-1 and A103/Melan-A antibody (40,41). Both antibodies, which recognize the same antigen, have been reported to be more sensitive than HMB-45, although Melan-A has demonstrated cross-reactivity with steroid-producing tumors (41). Therefore, when discussing this protein, the specific antibody is referenced.

One report demonstrated IHC detection of MART-1 in 90% of primary melanomas. Progression of disease, increasing Breslow thickness, and reduction in DFS and OS were associated with a significant loss of MART-1 expression (42). Similar results were noted by De Vries et al. (43), who used IHC to compare expression of MART-1, gp100, S-100, and tyrosinase in 80 paraffin-embedded primary melanomas and in locoregional metastasis, lymph node, and visceral metastases. Staining was negatively correlated with Clark level, and nodal metastases demonstrated less staining than primary tumors from the same patients. S-100 was the most sensitive marker, and there was no significant difference among the remaining three markers. Because IHC staining for MART-1 was unable to distinguish between Spitz nevus, melanoma, and melanocytes, this marker has limited potential to differentiate benign disease from malignant melanoma (44).

Results of RT-PCR analysis of MART-1 expression in the peripheral blood are conflicting. A study of 10 patients found 100% detection in whole blood but *none* in the serum or plasma (45). RT-PCR analysis of specimens from 80 patients reported no correlation of tyrosinase or MART-1 with disease stage (46). However, another study found that the expression of MART-1 was much lower in patients with disseminated disease than in those with locoregional disease. A recent study comparing MART-1 and tyrosinase expression in 299 patients found a progressive increase with disease stage (42%, 65%, 82%, and 81% for stages I, II, III, and IV, respectively) but no clear distinction between each stage (47).

Tyrosinase

Tyrosinase is an important enzyme in melanin synthesis and represents a marker of melanocytic differentiation. T311 is an antityrosinase monoclonal antibody identified by strong IHC expression in 84% of paraffin-embedded metastatic melanoma specimens but only poorly reactive in desmoplastic or spindle cell types (48). In a multi-marker comparison of T311, S-100, HMB45, and A103 (anti-Melan-A), S-100 was the most sensitive and HMB45 the most specific marker (49). Although T311 did not demonstrate an advantage over A103, T311 was considered a reliable marker of melanocytes by IHC. IHC staining for T311 significantly decreased with the progression of melanoma from primary to visceral metastasis. This suggests that the loss of tyrosinase may be a marker of progression.

Approximately 0.1% of viable cells from a primary melanoma enter the circulation. The clinical significance of these circulating cells is currently under intense investigation, in part due to the rapid development of RT-PCR markers. The detection of tyrosinase mRNA as an indicator of circulating melanoma cells was first demonstrated by Smith et al. (50) in stage IV patients. Recently, Tsao et al. (51) performed a meta-analysis of studies that examined tyrosinase mRNA in melanoma. This marker was expressed in 28%, 19%, 30%, and 45% of patients with stage I, stage I/II, stage III, and stage IV melanoma, respectively. The lack of correlation with outcome and the relatively low positivity rates limit the usefulness of this marker.

TUMOR-ASSOCIATED GLYCOPROTEIN ANTIGEN (TA90)

This 90 kD glycoprotein tumor-associated antigen is immunogenic in the host. An endogenous humoral immune response against TA90 has been detected in melanoma patients. A monoclonal antibody-based ELISA was developed to detect TA90-specific immune complexes (TA90-IC) in cancer patients. This complex is found in the serum (63%) and urine (68%) of melanoma patients (52). TA90-IC has also been identified in patients with breast cancer, sarcoma, lung cancer, and colon cancer (53).

Kelley et al. (54) evaluated the efficacy of TA90-IC in detecting subclinical metastasis of early-stage melanoma and predicting survival. Of the 56 clinical stage I melanoma patients that were identified to have subclinical disease, 43 (77%) were positive for TA90-IC preoperatively. Subclinical disease was defined by positive nodes on post-operative pathology or subsequent development of recurrence. In distinction, only 14 of 58 pathological stage I patients were positive for TA90-IC. Thus, sensitivity and specificity for the detection of occult metastasis were 77% and 76%, respectively. Furthermore, 15 of 18 (83%) node-positive cases and 34 of 46 (74%) recurrences were accurately predicted. In subsequent studies of patients with stage II and III disease, TA90-IC status was an independent prognostic marker for both DFS and OS (55). TA90-IC was elevated postoperatively in 54 of 78 (69%) patients who developed recurrent disease. These patients had elevated TA90-IC levels at a median of 19 months *before* clinically detectable disease.

During the last 30 years we have actively pursued vaccine protocols for metastatic melanoma and have aggressively defined markers of therapeutic efficiency. In 125 patients who received adjuvant immunotherapy with a polyvalent vaccine after complete resection of AJCC stage IV melanoma, post-operative/pre-vaccine TA90-IC levels strongly correlated with survival (56). Median DFS was seven versus four months, and five-year OS was 49% versus 27% for patients with negative versus positive TA90-IC results. This is the first serum marker shown to be important in predicting the survival of melanoma patients receiving adjuvant immunotherapy after complete resection of distant metastases.

LACTATE DEHYDROGENASE (LDH)

Because LDH is found throughout the body, nearly every type of cancer as well as many other diseases can elevate serum LDH levels. Therefore, this marker cannot be used for screening or diagnosis, but it can be used to monitor the course of melanoma. Persistent or recurrent elevation of LDH after treatment usually indicates that the disease is still present or has recurred. In 121 stage II and 58 stage III patients, LDH indicated recurrence with a sensitivity/specificity of 72% and 97%, respectively (57). As an indicator of liver metastasis the sensitivity/specificity was 95 and 82% for stage II and 86 and 57% for stage III melanoma, respectively. In addition, the median survival of patients with an elevated LDH was 5.9 months.

More recently, LDH has been compared in multivariate analysis to several other tumor markers including S-100 and melanoma inhibitory activity (MIA), and consistently found to be the most predictive factor for a poor outcome (58). This and several other reports have led the AJCC to propose a subtype of distant metastatic disease based on an elevated LDH serum level (M3) (149).

CYTOKINES AND/OR RECEPTORS

The correlation between cytokines and cancer is complex. Cytokines are not only expressed by cancer cells but also have a suppressive effect on autocrine and paracrine systems. In addition, they induce other cytokines of the same family and their receptors. Although the focus on cytokines has been primarily therapeutic, interleukins 2, 6, and 10 have been investigated as tumor markers.

IL-2 has been used in the treatment of melanoma for many years. The mechanism of action is thought to be through stimulated CTLs. Soluble IL-2 receptor (sIL-2R) is found in high levels in patients with metastatic disease and has been shown to interfere with IL-2 therapy; as many as 80% are nonresponders (59,60). In patients undergoing IL-2 treatment, elevated sIL-2 receptor expression correlated with shorter median survival and was statistically associated with disease progression and tumor load (59,61).

IL-6 is elevated in stage IV disease. In patients undergoing cisplatin/IL-2/IFN-α therapy, IL-6 serum levels were significantly elevated pretreatment and during therapy in nonresponders, suggesting a potential mechanism for resistance to biochemotherapy (61). Thus, endogenous IL-6 may provide valuable information for monitoring the response to biotherapy in patients with metastatic malignant melanoma (61,62). The mechanism may be related to the intracellular expression of IL-6 and its receptor (IL-6R). One study of fine-needle aspirates from stage IV lymph nodes and visceral metastases reported a correlation between nonresponse to biochemotherapy and decreased intracellular IL-6 and IL-6R expression in the presence of elevated IL-6 serum levels (63). This suggests that resistance to biochemotherapy is the result of an intracellular defect in IL-6/IL-6R and not the elevated serum IL-6 levels.

Although IL-10 has both immunosuppressive and anti-inflammatory functions (64), the correlation between IL-10 and tumor growth and survival is unclear. Some investigators have noted that decreased serum levels of IL-10 are associated with tumor growth (65). On the other hand, serum IL-10 levels >10 pg/mL by ELISA were associated with a poorer survival in 41 patients (66). In an attempt to understand these conflicting results, one group evaluated the gene promoter for IL-10 in 165 melanoma patients and found that IL-10—1082 AA (the predominant genotype) was associated with low expression of IL-10 and advanced disease, whereas several other genotypes were significantly associated with overexpression of IL-10 and radial (not vertical) growth (67). Clearly, the role of IL-10 in prognosis needs further investigation and standardization.

APOPTOSIS INHIBITORS

Apoptosis is emerging as an important mechanism in cell proliferation and immune surveillance. The proteins associated with apoptosis are pro-apoptotic (induce cell death) or anti-apoptotic (allow unregulated growth or escape from immune destruction). Among the several proteins and their ligand-receptors that have been investigated in melanoma are Fas, TRAIL, and the Bcl family of proteins.

Fas (APO-1,CD95)

Fas is a member of the tumor necrosis factor-receptor (TNFR) superfamily of transmembrane receptors. The Fas receptor (Fas), Fas ligand (FasL), and their soluble forms (sFas and sFasL) are components of this family of pro-apoptotic effectors. Originally believed to be restricted to T cells and natural killer (NK) cells, it has now been identified in many other cell types including melanoma. FasL expression may target T cells, eliminate them from the circulation, and thereby downregulate the immune system (68).

Fas and FasL are expressed in normal skin, and benign and malignant lesions, but Fas expression is significantly higher in normal skin and FasL is higher in melanoma (69). FasL expression increases with thickness of the primary tumor, whereas Fas expression decreases.

An enzyme-linked immunosorbent assay (ELISA) was used to monitor sFas and sFasL before and after biochemotherapy in 45 patients. No significant changes were noted in responders, but pretreatment sFasL levels were elevated in nonresponders and remained elevated post-therapy. sFas levels of nonresponders were also elevated post-therapy. These findings suggest a role for sFasL in identifying patients that may be refractory to therapy and a role for sFas in monitoring responses during therapy (70).

IHC studies show that FasL expression is high in primary melanomas thicker than 0.75 mm and in lymph nodes, whereas it is low or absent in benign and melanoma in situ lesions (71). FasL expression, however, does not correlate with apoptotic events in melanoma lesions and may play more of a role in escape from immune surveillance (69).

These results appear to conflict with the anticipated results for FasL overexpression, which would include increased apoptotic cell death. One possible explanation might be the induction of significant T-cell death, which would provide an escape from immune surveillance. Alternatively, anti-apoptotic proteins might be upregulated. Fas and FasL have been demonstrated in numerous melanoma cell cultures; however, very few of these cell lines undergo apoptosis. These *inducible* apoptotic cell lines interestingly had decreased expression of the anti-apoptotic proteins Bcl-2 and BcL-xL as compared to eight other cell culture lines that were not inducible (72).

Bcl-2 Family

This large group of proteins can exhibit anti- or pro-apoptotic effects. Recent studies using RT-PCR have shown that Bcl-2 (an anti-apoptotic protein) is expressed in 87% of metastatic and 53% of primary lesions. Bcl-xL, an anti-apoptotic protein in the mitochondria of cells, was found in 84% of primary lesions and 100% of metastases, suggesting a strong association with metastatic progression of primary melanoma (73). Thus, Bcl-2 and Bcl-xL expression could reflect an increased malignant potential resulting from inhibition of apoptosis. Flow cytometric evaluation of 42 lymph node metastases showed that 15 patients were positive for Bcl-2; this marker was an independent indicator of prognosis and its expression correlated with shorter overall survival (74).

TNF-related apoptosis-inducing ligand (TRAIL)

TRAIL induces apoptosis through a caspase-dependent mechanism. TRAIL has two pro-apoptotic receptors (R1 and R2) and two inhibitory receptors called decoys (R3 and R4). Transfection in vitro with R3 or R4 increases the resistance to TRAIL-induced apoptosis (75). This relatively new apoptotic factor has been identified in 68% of melanoma cell lines (75). Curiously, TRAIL can lead to the activation of NF-kappaB through activation of TRAIL R1 or R2, the result of which is inactivation of caspase 8 and subsequently apoptosis (76). Low TRAIL R expression was noted in fresh isolates from eight patients, suggesting a method by which melanoma may evade the immune system's apoptotic stimuli (77). Most recently, FLIP (FLICE inhibitory protein) has been identified in melanoma. This protein is an intracellular inhibitor of caspase 8, which controls numerous intracellular apoptotic functions, including the effectors of Fas and TRAIL. IHC revealed an 83% rate of FLIP expression in melanoma and zero in benign lesions (78).

ANGIOGENESIS FACTORS

Vascularity is a requirement for tumor growth. Several studies have demonstrated that microvessel density increases with the thickness of a primary melanoma, and that increased density correlates with decreased DFS (79,80). Of the numerous factors that play a role in angiogenesis, very few have been evaluated as tumor markers. Vascular endothelial growth factor (VEGF) and basic fibroblast growth factor (bFGF) are the most commonly cited.

VEGF

VEGF is a multi-functional, homodimeric peptide cytokine. Serum ELISA revealed elevated VEGF in all patients with melanoma, with higher levels in advanced disease and following transition from horizontal to vertical growth (81,82). Elevated levels have also been correlated with progression of melanoma (82). IHC evaluation of primary melanomas, however, has revealed only 42% VEGF expression and, interestingly, no expression in benign lesions (83). Additionally, eleven of 19 primary lesions and 15 of 20 metastatic lesions demonstrated IHC staining for VEGF in a separate study (85).

bFGF

This heparin-binding polypeptide is expressed by many cell types but not melanocytes. In human skin reconstructs, bFGF has been noted to be a critical factor in transducing melanoma cells from an *in situ* phase to a vertical growth phase and thereby conferring tumorigenicity in vivo (84). Birck et al. (85) compared expression of bFGF and VEGF in paired primary and metastatic melanoma from the same patients and demonstrated bFGF IHC expression occurred earlier and in more samples than VEGF. However, IHC expression did not correlate with recurrence or DFS (86). By contrast, others have noted that elevated *serum* levels correlated with advanced disease and shorter DFS and OS (82).

EXTRACELLULAR MATRIX-DEGRADING ENZYMES

A tumor cell's ability to invade and metastasize requires invasion of the basement membrane, degradation of local connective tissue, and subsequent migration into the surrounding stroma, vessels, and lymphatics. The matrix is degraded by several proteinases, including members of the aspartate, serine, cysteine, and matrix metalloproteinases (MMPs). The two most common families of proteinases found in conjunction with melanoma are MMPs and serine proteinases (87).

Matrix Metalloproteinases

The 26 human MMPs thus far identified have been classified into four subgroups based on their extracellular matrix substrate (ECM): interstitial collagenases, gelatinases, stromelysins, and membrane-type (MT-MMP) (87). Most investigators have focused on gelatinase A (MMP-2) and gelatinase B (MMP-9), which act on type IV collagen in basement membranes. Tissue inhibitors of metalloproteinases (TIMP) act in concert with MMPs to keep a dynamic and balanced activity in ECM degradation (88,89). Although considered to be important in the late phase of invasion and metastasis, gelatinase B as detected by IHC is reportedly expressed more strongly in melanomas < 1.6 mm (90). In one IHC study, 64% of primary paraffin-embedded melanomas stained positive for

MMP-2, and overexpression of this marker (defined as >34% positive cells) correlated with a poorer five-year survival (91).

CELL GROWTH FACTORS

One of the initiating events in melanoma progression is dysregulated cell proliferation, which begins when the melanocyte precursor loses control over the cell cycle. Melanoma cell growth is mediated by transcription factors, tumor suppressor genes, and a variety of proteins.

AP-2

AP-2 is a 52-kD, DNA-binding transcription factor that has been shown to control gene expression in epidermal cell lineages (92). Three AP-2 human genes have been cloned: TFAP2A, TFAP2B, and TFAP2C (93). These genes encode AP2alpha, AP2beta, and AP2gamma, respectively. The gene products appear to have regulatory control over several other genes including cKIT, E-cadherin, MMP-2, MCAM, p21(WAF-1), and c-erbB-2 (94,95). In melanoma, the loss of AP-2 expression results in the subsequent loss of cKIT expression and upregulation of MCAM with a significant increase in invasiveness.

The prognostic value of IHC-detected expression of AP-2 was addressed in a study of 369 patients with clinical stage I melanoma (96). In this group of patients, loss of AP-2 expression was predictive of decreased DFS and OS. It was also associated with reduced p21 expression and with greater Breslow thickness and Clark level.

Microphthalmia Transcription Factor (MITF)

MITF is a melanocyte-specific basic helix-loop-helix nuclear protein critical for melanocyte viability, maturation, and regulation of melanin synthesis. In vitro, MITF has been shown to activate promoters of tyrosinase, tyrosinase-related protein-1(TRP-1), and TRP-2, which can potentiate tumorigenicity (97–99). MITF has demonstrated a significant pattern of positive staining in melanoma. In one study, all 76 melanoma specimens and none of the 60 nonmelanoma specimens were positive for MITF (99). Another study demonstrated 82% nuclear staining of intermediate-thickness cutaneous melanomas; loss of MITF expression correlated with decreased DFS and OS (100). In 266 melanoma patients, 88% had tumors that stained positive for MITF, a rate that equaled or surpassed the rate of staining for S-100 or HMB45 (101). However, the specificity was poor, especially using the D5 antibody against MITF for detection (102).

nm23

This metastasis suppressor gene has two variants, nm23-H1 and nm23-H2, that encode for nucleoside diphosphate kinases (NDPK) A and B, respectively (103). These oligomers can be soluble or membrane-bound. Originally, nm23 was detected in human melanoma cell lines that were transplanted into mice; increased nm23 mRNA expression correlated with decreased metastatic potential (104). In a study that involved nm23 evaluation by IHC of 157 clinical stage I specimens, strong immunoreactive positivity was found to correlate with an improved survival (105). A smaller series found nm23 expression to be lowest in the thickest melanomas and those with lymph node metastasis. However, nm23 expression was not correlated with organ metastasis or subsequent five-year survival (106).

c-myc

This nuclear oncoprotein forms a heterodimer with c-myc associated factor X (MAX) family of proteins and produces a functional DNA binding transcription factor that is required for the transition of a cell from G1 to S phase (92). C-myc is overexpressed in many tumors including colon and prostate cancers. A recent study reported c-myc expression in 96% of 48 melanoma specimens, and noted that this marker had a stronger prognostic correlation than other clinicopathological parameters, including nodal positivity (107). However, another study of 40 patients with tumors thicker than 1 mm demonstrated only a 47% rate of c-myc positivity and no correlation with survival (108). Overexpression was most significant in vertical growth patterns and in metastatic versus primary tumors (109,110). Acral lentigo melanoma had the greatest overall expression, and elevated c-myc expression predicted shorter DFS and OS (111).

Ki-67 (MIB-1 Antibody)

This nonhistone DNA-binding nuclear protein is found during late G1, S, G2, and M phases but not in the G0 phase. Therefore, it represents a powerful marker to differentiate between proliferating and nonproliferating cells (112). As a diagnostic marker, Ki-67 staining can distinguish Spitz nevus and other benign skin lesions from melanoma (113). Because Ki-67 expression increases during a cell's transition from radial to vertical growth (114), this marker also has prognostic significance. IHC staining with MIB-1 demonstrated a progressive increase in Ki-67 expression from benign tumors to primary melanomas to metastatic lesions. The MIB-1 score of primary melanomas correlated significantly with tumor thickness and Clark level of invasion (115). Another study of 55 fresh samples from primary melanomas <1.5 mm in thickness reported a significant correlation between Ki-67 positivity and tumor thickness, S phase fraction, and metastasis (116).

In 60 patients undergoing chemoimmunotherapy for metastatic melanoma, low Ki-67 expression was significantly associated with blood vessel density. Because of the importance of angiogenesis in tumor growth and invasiveness, it is not surprising that low Ki-67 expression prior to treatment was an independent prognostic factor for longer DFS and OS (117).

Cell-Cycle Regulators

The cyclins (A, B, D1, D2, D3, and E) bind and activate specific cyclin-dependent protein kinases (CDK1, 2, 4, and 6) to modulate the transition of cells from the G1 to S phase. This transition can be significantly decreased by CDK inhibitors, of which there are two groups. INK4 inhibitors act on CDK4, CDK6, and cyclin D through p16, p15, p18, and p19. KIP inhibitors act on CDK2 and CDK4 through p21/WAF1, p27, and p57 (118).

The most commonly evaluated CDKs are CDK1, 2, and 4. IHC studies show that expression of CDK2 increases progressively from benign to primary to metastatic lesions (119,120). Western blot has demonstrated a threefold to eightfold increase of the CDK2 protein in metastatic lesions (121). A similar relationship has not been demonstrated for either CDK 1 or CDK 4.

Both IHC and Western blot show increased expression of cyclin A in melanoma (119,121). The overexpression of cyclin A correlates with the Ki-67 index (proliferative index), tumor thickness, Clark level, and decreased survival (119,121). IHC shows that expression of cyclin B is higher in metastatic melanomas than in benign or primary lesions. This suggests a prognostic role for cyclin B in patients with advanced disease.

Cyclin D has several subtypes including D1, D2, and D3, each with different diagnostic and prognostic significance. Overall, Western blot analyses have revealed a significantly higher expression of cyclin D in metastatic melanoma specimens than in benign lesions (121). With attention to subtypes, however, there is a greater variability in expression. IHC studies show that D1 is expressed in 62% of primary and 29% of metastatic lesions with rare staining in benign disease (122). Cyclin D2 appears to be elevated in metastatic disease and not in primary melanomas (120). Cyclin D3, by contrast, demonstrates 96% and 97% heterogeneous staining in primary vs. metastatic melanoma and is rarely seen in benign lesions (122). Elevated expression of cyclin D3, defined as >5% of the sample, was greater in nodular (42%) than superficial (22%) melanoma but had a significant correlation with survival only in superficial melanomas.

KIP family. The best characterized member of this family is p21, a protein that can lead to tumor suppression (123). An IHC study noted no expression of p21 in 30% of primary and 40% of metastatic melanomas (124). In addition, p21 expression decreased with metastatic progression of primary melanoma. A study of 369 stage I melanoma patients demonstrated that decreased expression of p21 was inversely related to Breslow thickness, recurrence, TNM stage, and age but not to DFS or OS (125). Studies since then have noted expression of this inhibitory protein in 60% in situ, 29–61% primary, and 33–48% metastatic samples (126,127). These contradictory reports based on IHC suggest that the diagnostic and prognostic usefulness of p21 needs further investigation with Western blot and RT-PCR.

INK4 family. The best studied member of this family is the *CDKN2A* gene, which encodes two separate inhibitor proteins, p16INK4a and p14ARF. Loss or mutation of these tumor-suppressor proteins dysregulates cell proliferation. An IHC study showed that p16INK4a, which inhibits CDK 4 and 6, was expressed in 92% of *in situ* lesions, 50% of primary lesions, and 64% of metastatic melanomas (127). By contrast, p16INK4a expression was low or absent in 45% of primary lesions and 77% of metastatic lesions in 200 patients with vertical growth phase melanomas (128). The ten-year survival rate was 37% versus 77% for patients with p16INK4a-negative versus p16INK4a-positive melanomas, respectively, making this protein an independent predictor of survival.

Melanoma Inhibitory Activity (MIA)

MIA is an 11-kDa, soluble protein of 131 amino acids, with a gene locus at 19q13.32 (129). MIA is secreted by melanoma cells and chondrocytes. Addition of MIA to cell culture results in melanoma cells rounding up in a short time period, suggesting that this protein may be involved in metastasis and/or invasiveness of melanoma (130). ELISA studies have detected a stage-related increase in MIA expression in the serum of patients with melanoma (131,132). MIA levels have been noted to normalize after resection of disease, and several investigators have reported a correlation between decreased MIA levels and stabilization or regression of disease (131–134).

RT-PCR detection of MIA in peripheral blood has been disappointing. One study demonstrated only 27% positivity in stage I /II and 28% in stage III or IV using a RT-PCR-ELISA method. Of interest, MIA mRNA was detected in 85% of patients with stage IV disease, in 26% of patients undergoing chemotherapy, and in no stage IV patients without evidence of disease (134). Unfortunately, a recent report has noted that low levels of MIA mRNA could also be detected in other neoplastic and normal cells (135).

S-100 and S-100b

S-100 is a 21-kD, acidic, calcium-binding protein composed of isomeric alpha and beta subunits. This heterodimer is associated with glial cells and melanoma. It is believed to be involved in cell cycle progression and differentiation (136). S-100 was first reported by our group in the 1980s to be a marker for human melanoma (137–138). S-100 IHC staining has subsequently become the method of choice for diagnosing malignant melanoma on pathological section, although it is not very specific.

With the introduction of two assays to detect serum S-100 levels, several conflicting studies have emerged to define the prognostic significance of this protein. In the four largest studies, S-100 levels were elevated in 4–9% of patients with stage I, 8–19% of stage III, and 48–89% of stage IV disease (139–142). Therefore, serum levels correlate with stage of disease and have an 81% rate of correlation with clinical outcome. S-100 levels have also been correlated with the number of affected organs, presence of liver or bone metastasis, and response to chemotherapy or immunotherapy. For example, in a study of 64 stage IV patients, 78% of nonresponders demonstrated elevated S-100b levels at four weeks after initiation of therapy and 84% had elevations by the end of therapy (143). For responders, 95% demonstrated a stable or decreased S-100b expression at four weeks and 98% by the end of treatment. Rising levels of S-100b were specific and sensitive for tumor progression and detected disease 5–23 weeks before other clinical or radiographic methods. Of note was the significant decrease in S-100 among patients who had been rendered NED (no evidence of disease).

SENTINEL NODE AND TUMOR MARKERS

Lymph nodes remain the most significant prognostic marker in melanoma. Since the advent and acceptance of sentinel lymphadenectomy for staging of melanoma, it has become apparent that nodal metastasis ranges from single cells to micrometastatic or macrometastatic deposits. While in the past pathologists were forced to review all the lymph nodes resected with a specimen, we now are able to focus on one or two with the greatest likelihood of harboring disease.

Wang et al. (144) presented some of the earliest data on RT-PCR detection of tyrosinase in the lymph nodes of melanoma patients. In his study of 29 nodes, 11 were histologically positive whereas 19 were positive by RT-PCR. This set the stage for other studies that have noted a 21% (87/417) rate of positive findings by tyrosinase RT-PCR (145). In another study, 47 of 91 pathologically negative nodes were positive by RT-PCR for tyrosinase (146), and recurrence rates reached 61% when nodes were positive by both histologic and molecular techniques. Similarly, Blaheta et al. (147) demonstrated recurrence rates of 67% for histopathologically positive nodes, 25% for RT-PCR positive nodes, and 6% for nodes negative by both techniques.

SUMMARY

The use of S-100 and HMB45 as standard markers for identification and differentiation of melanoma from other benign and malignant lesions has been challenged by the introduction of FLIP, MIA, tyrosinase (T311), MART-1 (A103), MITF, cyclin D3, and MIB-1. The most promising of these new markers appears to be MITF, which recently has been compared to S-100, tyrosinase, MART-1, and HMB45 (101). In this multimarker IHC comparison, 266 melanoma specimens were evaluated as positive if 10% of cells were stained. S-100 and tyrosinase demonstrated 90% positivity, MITF 88%, MART-1 78%, and HMB45 66%. Unfortunately, MITF failed to identify most of the desmoplastic melanomas. Tyrosinase and MART-1 have had additional multi-marker IHC comparisons that have uniformly noted S-100 to be the most sensitive and HMB45 to be most specific, leaving T311 and A103 antibodies in the intermediate range (49,148). Thus, no single marker can identify all melanomas with high-enough diagnostic sensitivity and specificity; however, *in combination* these markers may be very powerful diagnostic tools.

A major limitation of the IHC technique is that the tumor specimen must be available. For this reason it is desirable to focus on a marker that can persist in serum and be detected with ease. With few exceptions, none of the markers for melanoma has withstood the test of time. The few exceptions are TA90-IC, S-100, and MIA. TA90-IC is immunogenic in the host and the latter two are not. TA90-IC is very sensitive in early-stage disease. This property makes it an important marker for melanoma because it can identify the subgroup of patients with stage I and II disease, who are at higher risk of developing recurrent disease and are therefore ideal candidates for adjuvant therapies. Clearly, it is in the thin and intermediate-thickness melanomas that we need to better define those patients with poor DFS and/or OS.

In metastatic melanoma, expression of ICAM-1, bFGF, and MMP-2 has been associated with changes in DFS and OS. Interestingly, the marker with the greatest range and utility for melanoma appears to be LDH, which has prognostic value in stage II, III, and IV disease. As previously noted, LDH is so strong a predictor of poor outcome in stage IV disease that the forthcoming revised AJCC staging for melanoma will use this tumor marker for the first time to denote a separate stage subtype, M3 (149).

The most significant prognostic marker in most cancers and melanoma remains the lymph node status. In this area tumor markers have begun to make revolutionary contributions. This is especially true of RT-PCR markers such as tyrosinase. As noted earlier, a significant number of pathologically negative nodes demonstrate RT-PCR positivity that has been shown to predict higher rates of recurrence than would have been predicted by standard pathologic examination with hematoxylin and eosin staining.

REFERENCES

1. Cancer Facts and Figures—1998 (SEER data), American Cancer Society (ACS), Atlanta, Georgia, 1998.
2. Weiss M, Loprinzi CL, Creagan ET, et al. Utility of follow-up tests for detecting recurrent disease in patients with malignant melanoma. CA Cancer J Clin 1996;46:225–244.
3. Balch CM. Cutaneous melanoma: prognosis and treatment results worldwide. Semin Surg Oncol 1992;8:400–414.
4. Fleming ID, Cooper JS, eds. AJCC Cancer Staging Manual, 5th ed. Philadelphia/New York: Lippincott-Raven, 1997:163–170.
5. Morton DL, Wen DR, Wong JH, Economou JS, Cagle LA, Storm FK, et al. Technical details of intraoperative lymphatic mapping for early stage melanoma. Arch Surg 1992;127:392–399.
6. Jimbow K, Lee SK, King MG, Hara H, Chen H, Dakour J, et al. Melanin pigments and melanosomal proteins as differentiation markers unique to normal and neoplastic melanocytes. J Invest Dermatol 1993;100(3 Suppl):259s–268s.
7. Karnell R, Kagedal B, Lindholm C, Nilsoon B, Arstrand K, Ringborg U. The value of cysteinyldopa in the follow-up of disseminated malignant melanoma. Melanoma Res 2000;10:363–369.
8. Agrup G, Agrup P, Andersson T, Hafstrom L, Hansson C, Jacobsson S, et al. Five years' experience of 5-S-cysteinyldopa in melanoma diagnosis. Acta Derm Venereol 1979;59:381–388.
9. Horikoshi T, Ito S, Wakamatsu K, Onodera H, Eguchi H. Evaluation of melanin-related metabolites as markers of melanoma progression. Cancer 1994;73:629–636.
10. Peterson LL, Woodward WR, Fletcher WS, Palmquist M, Tucker MA, Ilias A. Plasma 5-S-cysteinyldopa differentiates patients with primary and metastatic melanoma from patients with dysplastic nevus syndrome and normal subjects. J Am Acad Dermatol 1988;19:509–515.

11. Banfalvi T, Glide K, Boldizsar M, Kremmer T, Otto S. Serum levels of S-100 protein and 5-S-cysteinyldopa as markers of melanoma progression. Pathol Oncol Res 1999;5:218–222.
12. Wimmer I, Meyer JC, Seifert B, Dummer R, Flace A, Burg G. Prognostic value of serum 5-S-cysteinyldopa for monitoring human metastatic melanoma during immunochemotherapy. Cancer Res 1997;57:5073–5076.
13. Sy MS, Mori H, Liu D. CD44 as a marker in human cancers. Curr Opin in Oncol 1997;9:108–112.
14. Karjalainen JM, Tammi RH, Tammi MI, Eskelinen MJ, Agren UM, Parkkinen JJ, et al. Reduced level of CD44 and hyaluronan associated with unfavorable prognosis in clinical stage I cutaneous melanoma. Am J Pathol 2000;157:957–965.
15. Yasasever V, Tas F, Duranyildiz D, Camlica H, Kurul S, Dalay N. Serum levels of the soluble adhesion molecules in patients with malignant melanoma. Pathol Oncol Res 2000;6:42–45.
16. Dietrich A, Tanczos E, Vanscheidt W, Schopf E, Simon JC. High CD44 surface expression on primary tumors of malignant melanoma correlates with increased metastatic risk and reduced survival. Eur J Cancer 1997;33:926–930.
17. Schaider H, Rech-Weichselbraun I, Richitig E, Seidl H, Soyer HP, Smolle J, et al. Circulating adhesion molecules as prognostic factors for cutaneous melanoma. J Am Acad Dermatol 1997;36(2 Pt 1): 209–213.
18. Satyamoorthy K, Muyrers J, Meier F, Patel D, Herlyn M. Mel-Cam-specific genetic suppressor elements inhibit melanoma growth and invasion through loss of gap junctional cummunication. Oncogene 2001;20:4676–4684.
19. Kuske MD, Johnson JP. Assignment of the human melanoma cell adhesion molecule gene (MCAM) to chromosome 11 band q23.3 by radiation hybrid mapping. Cytogenetics Cell Genetics 1999; 87:258.
20. Jean D, Bar-Eli M. Regulation of tumor growth and metastasis of human melanoma by the CREB transcription factor family. Mol Cell Biochem 2000;212:19–28.
21. Shih IM, Elder DE, Speicher D, Johnson JP, Herlyn M. Isolation and functional characterization of the A32 melanoma-associated antigen. Cancer Res 1994;54:2514–2520.
22. Shih IM. The role of CD146 (Mel-CAM) in biology and pathology. J Pathol 1999;189:4–11.
23. Ostmeier H, Fuchs B, Otto F, Mawick R, Lippold A, Krieg V, et al. Prognostic immunohistochemical markers of primary human melanomas. Br J Dermatol 2001;145:203–209.
24. Luca MR, Bar-Eli M. Molecular changes in human melanoma metastasis. Histol Histopathol 1998;13:1225–1231.
25. Alexander CL, Edward M, MacKie RM. The role of human melanoma cell ICAM-1 expression on lymphokine activated killer cell-mediated lysis, and the effect of retinoic acid. Br J Cancer 1999;80:1494–1500.
26. Kageshita T, Yoshii A, Kimura T, Kuriya N, Ono T, Tsujisaki M, et al. Clinical relevance of ICAM-1 expression in primary lesions and serum of patients with malignant melanoma. Cancer Res 1993;53:4927–4932.
27. Ciotti P, Pesce GP, Cafiero F, Rainero ML, Sementa A, Nicolo G, et al. Intercellular adhesion molecule-1 (ICAM-1) and granulocyte-macrophage colony stimulating factor (GM-CSF) co-expression in cutaneous malignant melanoma lesions. Melanoma Res 1999; 9:253–260.
28. Vuoristo MS, Laine S, Huhtala H, Parvinen LM, Hahka-Kemppinen M, Korpela M, et al. Serum adhesion molecules and interleukin-2 receptor as markers of tumor load and prognosis in advanced cutaneous melanoma. Eur J Cancer 2001;37:1629–1634.
29. Boyano MD, Garcia-Vazquez MD, Lopez-Michelena T, Gardeasabal J, Bilbao J, Canavate ML, et al. Soluble interleukin-2 receptor, intercellular adhesion molecule-1, and interleukin-10 serum levels in patients with melanoma. Br J Cancer 2000; 83:847–852.
30. Khatib AM, Nip J, Fallavollita L, Lehmann M, Jensen G, Brodt P. Regulation of urokinase plasminogen activator/plasmin-mediated invasion of melanoma cells by the integrin vitronectin receptor alphavbeta3. Int J Cancer 2001;91:300–308.
31. Danen EH, Van Muijen GN, Ruiter DJ. Role of integrins as signal-transducing cell adhesion molecules I human cutaneous melanoma. Cancer Surv 1995;24:43–65.
32. Maeshima Y, Yerramalla UL, Dhanabal M, Holthaus KA, Barbashov S, Kharbanda S, et al. Extracellular matrix-derived peptide binds to alpha(v)beta(3) integrin and inhibits angiogenesis. J Biol Chem 2001;276:31959–31968.
33. Minamiguchi K, Kumagai H, Masuda T, Kawada M, Ishizuka M, Takeuchi T. Tiolutin, an inhibitor of HUVEC adhesion to vitronectin, reduces paxillin in HUVECs and suppresses tumor cell-induced angiogenesis. J Cancer 2001;93:307–316.
34. Johnson JP. Cell adhesion molecules in the development and progression of malignant melanoma. Cancer Metastasis Rev 1999; 18:345–357.
35. Natali PG, Hamby CV, Felding-Habermann B, Liang B, Nicotra MR, Di Filippo F, et al. Clinical significance of alphavbeta3 integrin and intercellular adhesion molecule-1 expression in cutaneous malignant melanoma lesions. Cancer Res 1997;57: 1554–1560.
36. Kageshita T, Hamby CV, Hirai S, Kimura T, Ono T, Ferrone S. Differential clinical significance of alphavbeta3 expression in primary lesions of acral lentiginous melanoma and of other melanoma histotypes. Int J Cancer 2000;89:153–159.
37. Hieken TJ, Ronan SG, Farolan M, Shilkaitis AL, Das Gupta TK. Molecular prognostic markers in intermediate-thickness cutaneous malignant melanoma. Cancer 1999;85:375–382.
38. Vihinen P, Hikkola J, Vlaykova T, Hahka-Kemppinen M, Talve L, Heino J, et al. Prognostic value of beta1 integrin expression in metastatic melanoma. Melanoma Res 2000;10:243–251.
39. Van Belle PA, Elenitsas R, Satyamoorthy K, Wolfe JT, Guerry 4th D, et al. Progression-related expression of beta3 integrin in melanomas and nevi. Hum Pathol 1999;30:562–567.
40. Fetsch PA, Marincola MD, Abati A. The new melanoma markers: MART-1 and Melan-A (The NIH experience). Letter. Am J Surg Pathol 1999;23:607–613.
41. Busam KJ, Jungbluth AA. Melan-A, a new melanocytic differentiation marker. Adv Anat Pathol 1999;6:12–18.
42. Berset M, Cerottini JP, Guggisberg D, Romero P, Burri F, Rimoldi D, et al. Expression of Melan-A/MART-1 antigen as a prognostic factor in primary cutaneous melanoma. Int J Cancer 2001;95: 73–77.
43. De Vries TJ, Smeets M, de Graaf R, Hou-Jensen K, Brocker EB, Renard N, et al. Expression of gp100, MART-1, tyrosinase, and S100 in paraffin-embedded primary melanomas and locoregional, lymph node, and visceral metastases: implications for diagnosis and immunotherapy. A study conducted by the EORTC Melanoma Cooperative Group. J Pathol 2001;193:13–20.
44. Bergman R, Azzam H, Sprecher E, Manov L, Munichor M, Friedman-Birnbaum R, et al. A comparative immunohistochemical study of MART-1 expression in Spitz nevi, ordinary

melanocytic nevi, and malignant melanoma. J Am Acad Dermatol 2000;42:496–500.
45. Hasselmann DO, Rappl G, Rossler M, Ugurel S, Tilgen W, Reinhold U. Detection of tumor-associated circulating mRNA in serum, plasma, and blood cells from patients with disseminated malignant melanoma. Oncol Rep 2001;8:115–118.
46. Kulik J, Nowecki ZI, Rutkowski P, Ruka W, Rochowska M, Skurzak H, et al. Detection of circulating melanoma cells in peripheral blood by a two-marker RT-PCR assay. Melanoma Res 2001;11:65–73.
47. Brownbridge GG, Gold J, Edward M, MacKie RM. Evaluation of the use of tyrosinase-specific and melanA/MART-1-specific reverse transcriptase-coupled-polymerase chain reaction to detect melanoma cells in peripheral blood samples from 299 patients with malignant melanoma. Br J Dermatol 2001;144:279–287.
48. Jungbluth AA, Iversen K, Coplan K, Kolb D, Stockert E, Chen YT, et al. T311—an anti-tyrosinase monoclonal antibody for the detection of melanocytic lesions in paraffin embedded tissues. Pathol Res Pract 2000;196:235–242.
49. Clarkson KS, Sturdgess IC, Molyneux AJ. The usefulness of tyrosinase in the immunohistochemical assessment of melanocytic lesions: a comparison of the novel T311 antibody (anti-tyrosinase) with S100, HMB45, and A103 (anti-Melan A). J Clin Pathol 2001;54:196–200.
50. Smith B, Selby P, Southgate J, Pittman K, Bradley C, Blair GE. Detection of melanoma cells in peripheral blood by means of reverse transcriptase and polymerase chain reaction. Lancet 1991;338:1227–1229.
51. Tsao H, Nadiminti U, Sober AJ, Bigby M. A meta-analysis of reverse transcriptase-polymerase chain reaction for tyrosinase mRNA as a marker for circulating tumor cells in cutaneous melanoma. Arch Dermatol 2001;137:325–330.
52. Gupta RK, Morton DL. Monoclonal antibody-based ELISA to detect glycoprotein tumor-associated antigen-specific immune complexes in cancer patients. J Clin Lab Anal 1992;6:329–336.
53. Euhus DM, Gupta RK, Morton DL. Characterization of a 90–100 kDa tumor-associated antigen in the sera of melanoma patients. Int J Cancer 1990;45:1065–1070.
54. Kelley MC, Jones RC, Gupta RK, Yee R, Stern S, Wanek L, et al. Tumor-associated antigen TA-90 immune complex assay predicts subclinical metastasis and survival for patients with early stage melanoma. Cancer 1998;83:1355–1361.
55. Kelley MC, Gupta RK, Hsueh EC, Yee R, Stern S, Morton DL. Tumor-associated antigen TA90 immune complex assay predicts recurrence and survival after surgical treatment of stage I–III melanoma. J Clin Oncol 2001;19:1176–1182.
56. Hsueh EC, Gupta RK, Qi K, Yee R, Leopoldo ZC, Morton DL. TA90 immune complex predicts survival following surgery and adjuvant vaccine immunotherapy for stage IV melanoma. Cancer J Sci Am 1997;3:364–370.
57. Finck SJ, Giuliano AE, Morton DL. LDH and melanoma. Cancer 1983;51:840–843.
58. Deichmann M, Benner A, Bock M, Jackel A, Uhl K, Waldmann V, et al. S100-beta, melanoma-inhibiting activity, and lactate dehydrogenase discriminate progressive from non-progressive American Joint Committee on Cancer stage IV melanoma. J Clin Oncol 1999;17:1891–1896.
59. Boyano MD, Garcia-Vazquez MD, Lopez-Michelena T, Gardeazabal J, Bilbao J, Canavate ML, et al. Soluble interleukin-2 receptor, intercellular adhesion molecule-1, and interleukin-10 serum levels in patients with melanoma. Br J Cancer 2000;83:847–852.
60. Gooding R, Riches P, Dadian G, Moore J, Gore M. Increased soluble interleukin-2 receptor concentration in plasma predicts a decreased cellular response to IL-2. Br J Cancer 1995;72:452–455.
61. Vuoristo MS, Laine S, Huhtala H, Parvinen LM, Hahka-Kemppinen M, Korpela M, et al. Serum adhesion molecules and interleukin-2 receptor as markers of tumor load and prognosis in advanced cutaneous melanoma. Eur J Cancer 2001;37:1629–1634.
62. Mouawad R, Benhammouda A, Rixie O, Antoine EC, Borel C, Weil M, et al. Endogenous interleukin 6 levels in patients with metastatic malignant melanoma: correlation with tumor burden. Clin Cancer Res 1996;2:1405–1409.
63. Mouawad R, Khayat D, Merle S, Antoine EC, Gil-Delgado M, Soubrane C. Is there any relationship between interleukin-6/interleukin-6 receptor modulation and endogenous interleukin-6 release in metastatic malignant melanoma patients treated by biochemotherapy? Melanoma Res 1999;9:181–188.
64. Walos S, Szary J, Szala S. Inhibition of tumor growth by interleukin 10 gene transfer in B16(F10) melanoma cells. Acta Biochimica Polonica 1999;46:967–970.
65. Nemunaitis J Fong T, Shabe P, Martineau D, Ando D. Comparison of serum interleukin-10 (IL-10) levels between normal volunteers and patients with advanced melanoma. Cancer Invest 2001;19:239–247.
66. Huang S, Ullrich SE, Bar-Eli M. Regulation of tumor growth and metastasis by interleukin-10: the melanoma experience. J Interferon Cytokine Res 1999;19:697–703.
67. Howell WM, Turner SJ, Bateman AC, Theaker JM. IL-10 promoter polymorphisms influence tumor development in cutaneous malignant melanoma. Genes Immunity 2001;2:25–31.
68. Hahne M, Rimoldi D, Schroter M, Romero P, Schreier M, French LE, et al. Melanoma cell expression of Fas (Apo-1/CD95) ligand: implications for tumor immune escape. Science 1996;274:1363–1366.
69. Sprecher E, Bergman R, Meilick A, Kerner H, Manov L, Reiter L, et al. Apoptosis, Fas, and Fas-ligand expression in melanocytic tumors. J Cutan Pathol 1999;26:72–77.
70. Mouawad R, Khayat D, Soubrane C. Plasma Fas ligand, an inducer of apoptosis, and plasma-soluble Fas, an inhibitor of apoptosis, in advanced melanoma. Melanoma Res 2000;10:461–467.
71. Maeda A, Aragane Y, Tezuka T. Expression of CD95 ligand in melanocytic lesions as a diagnostic marker. Br J Dermatol 1998;139:198–206.
72. Ugurel S, Seiter S, Rappl G, Stark A, Tilgen W, Reinhold U. Heterogeneous susceptibility to CD95-induced apoptosis in melanoma cells correlates with bcl-2 and bcl-x expression and is sensitive to modulation by interferon-gamma. Int J Cancer 1999;82:727–736.
73. Leiter U, Schmid RM, Kaskel P, Peter RU, Krahn G. Antiapoptotic bcl-2 and bcl-xL in advanced malignant melanoma. Arch Dermatol Res 2000;292:225–232.
74. Grover R, Wilson GD. Bcl-2 expression in malignant melanoma and its prognostic significance. Eur J Surg Oncol 1996;22:347–349.
75. Zhang XD, Franco AV, Nguyen T, Gray CP, Hersey P. Differential localization and regulation of death and decoy receptors for TNF-related apoptosis-inducing ligand (TRAIL) in human melanoma cells. J Immunol 2000;164:3961–3970.

76. Franco AV, Zhang XD, Van Berkel E, Sanders JE, Zhang XY, Thomas WD, et al. The role of NF-kappa B in TNF-related apoptosis-inducing ligand (TRAIL)-induced apoptosis of melanoma cells. J Immunol 2001;166:5337–5345.
77. Nguyen T, Zhang XD, Hersey P. Relative resistance of fresh isolates of melanoma to tumor necrosis factor-related apoptosis-inducing ligand (TRAIL)-induced apoptosis. Clin Cancer Res 2001;7(3 Suppl):966s–973s.
78. Bullani RR, Huard B, Viard-Leveugle I, Byers HR, Irmler M, Saurat JH, et al. Selective expression of FLIP in malignant melanocytic skin lesions. J Invest Dermatol 2001;117:360–364.
79. Viac J, Schmitt D, Claudy A. Circulating vascular endothelial growth factor (VEGF) is not a prognostic indicator in malignant melanoma. Cancer Lett 1998;125:35–38.
80. Vlaykova T, Laurila P, Muhonen T, Hahka-Kemppinen M, Jekunen A, Alitalo K, et al. Prognostic value of tumor vascularity in metastatic melanoma and association of blood vessel density with vascular endothelial growth factor expression. Melanoma Res 1999;9:59–68.
81. Erhard H, Rietveld FJ, van Altena MC, Brocker EB, Ruiter DJ, de Waal RM. Transition of horizontal to vertical growth phase melanoma is accomplished by induction of vascular endothelial growth factor expression and angiogenesis. Melanoma Res 1997; Suppl 2:S19–S26.
82. Ugurel S, Rappl G, Tilgen W, Reinhold U. Increased serum concentration of angiogenic factors in malignant melanoma patients correlates with tumor progression and survival. J Clin Oncol 2001;19:577–583.
83. Bayer-Garner IB, Hough AJ Jr, Smoller BR. Vascular endothelial growth factor expression in malignant melanoma: prognostic versus diagnostic usefulness. Mod Pathol 1999;12:770–774.
84. Meier F, Nesbit M, Hsu MY, Martin B, Van Belle P, Elder DE, et al. Human melanoma progression in skin reconstructs: biological significance of bFGF. Am J Pathol 2000;156:193–200.
85. Birck A, Kirkin AF, Zeuthen J, Hou-Jensen K. Expression of basic fibroblast growth factor and vascular endothelial growth factor in primary and metastatic melanoma from the same patients. Melanoma Res 1999; 9:375–381.
86. al-Alousi S, Barnhill R, Blessing K, Barksdale S. The prognostic significance of basic fibroblast growth factor in cutaneous malignant melanoma. J Cutan Pathol 1996;23:506–510.
87. Brinckerhoff CE, Rutter JL, Benbowe U. Interstitial collagenases as markers of tumor progression. Clin Cancer Res 2000;6: 4823–4830.
88. Henriet P, Blavier L, Declerck YA. Tissue inhibitors of metalloproteinases (TIMP) in invasion and proliferation. APMIS 1999; 107:111–119.
89. Hofmann UB, Westphal JR, Van Muijen GN, Ruiter DJ. Matrix metalloproteinases in human melanoma. J Invest Dermatol 2000; 115:337–344.
90. Van den Oord JJ, Paemen L, Opdenakker G, de Wolf-Peeters C. Expression of gelatinase B and the extracellular matrix metalloproteinase inducer EMMPRIN in benign and malignant pigment cell lesions of the skin. Am J Pathol 1997;151:665–670.
91. Vaisanen A, Kallioinen M, Taskinen PJ, Turpeenniemi-Hujanen T. Prognostic value of MMP-2 immunoreactive protein (72 kD type IV collagenase) in primary skin melanoma. J Pathol 1998; 186:51–58.
92. Karjalainen JM. Transcription factors and other dysregulated proteins in melanoma prognosis. Curr Oncol Rep 2001;3: 368–375.
93. Williamson JA, Bosher JM, Skinner A, et al. Chromosomal mapping of the human and mouse homologues of two new members of the AP-2 family of transcription factors. Genomics 1996;35: 262–264.
94. Jean D, Gershenwald JE, Huang S, Luca M, Hudson MJ, Tainsky MA, et al. Loss of AP-2 results in up-regulation of MCAM.MUC18 and an increase in tumor growth and metastasis of human melanoma cells. J Biol Chem 1998;273:16501–16508.
95. Bar-Eli M. Role of AP-2 in tumor growth and metastasis of human melanoma. Cancer Metastasis Rev 1999;18:377–385.
96. Karjalainen JM, Kellokoski JK, Eskelinen MJ, Alhava EM, Kosma V. Downregulation of transcription factor AP-2 predicts poor survival in stage I cutaneous malignant melanoma. J Clin Oncol 1998;16:3584–3591.
97. Fisher DE. Microphthalmia: a signal responsive transcriptional regulator in development. Pigment Cell Res 2000;13(Suppl 8):145–9.
98. Fang D, Setaluri V. Role of microphthalmia transcription factor in regulation of melanocyte differentiation marker TRP-1. Biochem Biophys Res Commun 1999;256:657–663.
99. King R, Weilbaecher KN, McGill G, Cooley E, Mihm M, Fisher DE. Microphthalmia transcription factor. A sensitive and specific melanocyte marker for melanoma diagnosis. Am J Pathol 1999;155:731–738.
100. Salti GI, Manougian T, Farolan M, Shilkaitis A, Majumdar D, Das Gupta TK. Microphthalmia transcription factor: a new prognostic marker in intermediate-thickness cutaneous malignant melanoma. Cancer Res 2000;60:5012–5016.
101. Miettinen M, Fernandez M, Franssila K, Gatalica Z, Lasota J, Sarlomo-Rikala M. Microphthalmia transcription factor in the immunohistochemical diagnosis of metastatic melanoma: comparison with four other melanoma markers. Am J Surg Pathol 2001;25:205–211.
102. Busam KJ, Iversen K, Coplan KC, Jungbluth AA. Analysis of microphthalmia transcription factor expression in normal tissue and tumors, and comparison of its expression with S-100 protein, gp100, and tyrosinase in desmoplastic malignant melanoma. Am J Surg Pathol 2001;25:197–204.
103. Hamby CV, Abbi R, Prasad N, Stauffer C, Thomson J, Mendola CE, et al. Expression of a catalytically inactive H118Y mutant of nm23-H2 suppresses the metastatic potential of line IV Cl 1 human melanoma cells. Int J Cancer 2000;88:547–553.
104. Meng L. Expression of the tumor metastatic suppressor gene in mouse melanoma model: inverse association to metastatic potential. J Tongji Med Univ 1998;18:28–32.
105. McDermott NC, Milburn C, Curran B, Kay EW, Barry Walsh C, Leader MB. Immunohistochemical expression of nm23 in primary invasive malignant melanoma is predictive of survival outcome. J Pathol 2000;190:157–162.
106. Dome B, Somlai B, Timar J. The loss of nm23 protein in malignant melanoma predicts lymphatic spread without affecting survival. Anticancer Res 2000;20:3971–3974.
107. Grover R, Ross DA, Wilson GD, Sanders R. Measurement of c-myc oncoprotein provides an independent prognostic marker for regional metastatic melanoma. Br J Plast Surg 1997; 50:478–482.
108. Ricaniadis N, Kataki A, Agnantis N, Androulakis G, Karakousis CP. Long-term prognostic significance of HSP-70, c-myc, and HLA-DR expression in patients with malignant melanoma. Eur J Surg Oncol 2001;27:88–93.
109. Schlagbauer-Wadl H, Griffioen M, van Elsas A, Schrier PI, Pustelnik T, Eichler HG, et al. Influence of increased c-myc expression on the growth characteristics of human melanoma. J Invest Dermatol 1999;112:332–336.

110. Ross DA, Wilson GD. Expression of c-myc oncoprotein represents a new prognostic marker in cutaneous melanoma. Br J Surg 1998;85:46–51.
111. Grover R, Chana J, Grobbelaar AO, Hudson DA, Forder M, Wilson GD, et al. Measurement of c-myc oncogene expression provides an accurate prognostic marker for acral lentiginous melanoma. Br J Plast Surg 1999;52:122–126.
112. Korabiowska M, Brinck U, Middel P, Brinkmann U, Berger H, Radzun HJ, et al. Proliferative activity in the progression of pigmented skin lesions, diagnostic and prognostic significance. Anticancer Res 2000;20:1781–1785.
113. Bergman R, Malkin L, Sabo E, Kerner H. MIB-1 monoclonal antibody to determine proliferative activity of Ki-67 antigen as an adjunct to the histopathologic differential diagnosis of Spitz nevi. J Am Acad Dermatol 2001;44:500–504.
114. Kaleem Z, Lind AC, Humphrey PA, Sueper RH, Swanson PE, Ritter JH, et al. Concurrent Ki-67 and p53 immunolabeling in cutaneous melanocytic neoplasms: an adjunct for recognition of the vertical growth phase in malignant melanoma. Mod Pathol 2000;13:217–222.
115. Sparrow LE, English DR, Taran JM, Heenan PJ. Prognostic significance of MIB-1 proliferative activity in thin melanomas and immunohistochemical analysis of MIB-1 proliferative activity in melanocytic tumors. Am J Dermatopathol 1998;20:12–16.
116. Moretti S, Spallanzani A, Chiarugi A, Fabiani M, Pinzi C. Correlation of Ki-67 expression in cutaneous primary melanoma with prognosis in a prospective study: different correlation according to thickness. J Am Acad Dermatol 2001;44:188–192.
117. Vlaykova T, Talve L, Hahka-Kemppinen M, Hernberg M, Muhonen T, Franssila K, et al. MIB-1 immunoreactivity correlates with blood vessel density and survival in disseminated malignant melanoma. Oncology 1999;57:242–252.
118. Palazzo JP. Cyclin-dependent kinase inhibitors—a novel class of prognostic indicators. Hum Pathol 2001;32:769–770.
119. Tran TA, Ross JS, Carlson JA, Mihm MC Jr. Mitotic cyclins and cyclin-dependent kinases in melanocytic lesions. Hum Pathol 1998;29:1085–1090.
120. Georgieva J, Sinha P, Schandendorf D. Expression of cyclins and cyclin-dependent kinases in human benign and malignant melanocytic lesions. J Clin Pathol 2001;54:229–235.
121. Tang L, Li G, Tron VA, Trotter MJ, Ho VC. Expression of cell cycle regulators in cutaneous malignant melanoma. Melanoma Res 1999;9:148–154.
122. Florenes VA, Faye RS, Maelandsmo GM, Nesland JM, Holm R. Levels of cyclin D1 and D3 in malignant melanoma: deregulated cyclin D3 expression is associated with poor clinical outcome in superficial melanoma. Clin Cancer Res 2000;6:3614–3620.
123. Jiang H, Lin J, Su ZZ, Herlyn M, Kerbel RS, Weissman BE, et al. The melanoma differentiation-associated gene mda-6, which encodes the cyclin-dependent kinase inhibitor p21, is differentially expressed during growth, differentiation and progression in human melanoma cells. Oncogene 1995;10:1855–1864.
124. Maelandsmo GM, Holm R. Fodstad O, Kerbel RS, Florenes VA. Cyclin kinase inhibitor p21WAF1/CIP1 in malignant melanoma: reduced expression in metastatic lesions. Am J Pathol 1996;149:1813–1822.
125. Karjalainen JM, Eskelinen MJ, Kellokoski JK, Reinikainen M, Alhava EM, Kosma VM. P21(WAF1/CIP1) expression in stage I cutaneous malignant melanoma: its relationship with p53, cell proliferation, and survival. Br J Cancer 1999;79:895–902.
126. Trotter MJ, Tang L, Tron VA. Overexpression of the cyclin-dependent kinase inhibitor p21 (WAF1/CIP1) in human cutaneous malignant melanoma. J Cutaneous Pathol 1997;24:265–71.
127. Sparrow LE, Eldon MJ, English DR, Heenan PJ. P16 and p21 WAF1 protein expression in melanocytic tumors by immunohistochemistry. Am J Dermatopathol 1998;20:255–261.
128. Strume O, Sviland L, Akslen LA. Loss of nuclear p16 protein expression correlates with increased tumor cell proliferation (Ki-67) and poor prognosis in patients with vertical growth phase melanoma. Clin Cancer Res 2000;6:1845–1853.
129. Koehler MR. Assignment of the human melanoma inhibitory activity gene (MIA) to 19q13.4 by fluorescene in situ hybridization (FISH). Genomics 1996;271:490–495.
130. Bosserhoff AK, Golob M, Buettner R, Landthaler M, Hein R. MIA. Biological functions and clinical relevance in malignant melanoma. Hautarzt 1998;49:762–769.
131. Bosserhoff AK, Lederer M, Kaufmann M, Hein R, Stolz W, Apfel R, et al. MIA, a novel serum marker for progression of malignant melanoma. Anticancer Res 1999;19:2691–2693.
132. Stahlecker J, Gauger A, Bosserhoff A, Buttner R, Ring J, Hein R. MIA as a reliable tumor marker in the serum of patients with malignant melanoma. Anticancer Res 2000;20:5041–5044.
133. Bosserhoff AK, Dreau D, Hein R, Landthaler M, Holder WD, Buettner R. Melanoma inhibitory activity (MIA), a serological marker of malignant melanoma. Recent Results Cancer Res 2001;158:158–168.
134. Muhlbauer M, Langenbach N, Stolz W, Hein R, Landthaler M, Buettner R, et al. Detection of melanoma cells in the blood of melanoma patients by melanoma-inhibitory activity (MIA) reverse transcription-PCR. Clin Cancer Res 1999;5:1099–1105.
135. De Vries TJ, Fourkour A, Punt CJ, Diepstra H, Ruiter DJ, van Juijen GN. Melanoma-inhibiting activity (MIA) mRNA is not exclusively transcribed in melanoma cells: low levels of MIA mRNA are present in various cell types and in peripheral blood. Br J Cancer 1999;81:1066–1070.
136. Jackel A, Deichman M, Waldmann V, et al. S-100B protein in serum, a tumor marker in malignant melanoma—current state of knowledge and clinical experiences. Hautarzt 1999;50:250–6.
137. Gaynor, R, Herschman HR, Irie, R, Jones P, Morton DL, Cochran A. S100 protein: a marker for human malignant melanomas? Lancet 1981;1:869–871.
138. Gaynor, R, Irie R, Morton DL, Herschman HR. S100 protein is present in cultured human malignant melanomas. Nature 1980;286:400–401.
139. Von Schoultz E, Hansson LO, Dijureen E, et al. Prognostic value of serum analysis of S-100B protein in malignant melanoma. Melanoma Res 1996;6:133–137.
140. Kaskel P, Berking C, Snader S, et al. S-100 protein in peripheral blood: a marker for melanoma metastasis: a prospective 2-center study of 570 patients with melanoma. J Am Acad Dermatol 1999;41:962–969.
141. Ghanem G, Loir B, Sales F, et al. Serum protein S-100 is a useful marker in metastatic melanoma. Melanoma Res 1997;7(Suppl 1):S55.
142. Berking C, Schlupen EM, Schrader A, et al. Tumor markers in peripheral blood of patients with malignant melanoma: multimarker RT-PCR versus a luminoimmunometric assay for S-100. Arch Dermatol Res 1999;291:479–484.
143. Hauschild A, Engel G, Brenner W, Glaser R, Monig H, Henze E, Christophers E. Predictive value of serum S100B for monitoring patients with metastatic melanoma during chemotherapy and/or immunotherapy. Br J Dermatol. 1999;140:1065–1071.

144. Wang X, Heller R, VanVoorhis N, Cruse CW, Glass F, Fenske N, Berman C, Leo-Messina J, Rappaport D, Wells K. Detection of submicroscopic lymph node metastases with polymerase chain reaction in patients with malignant melanoma. Ann of Surg 1994;220:768–774.
145. Blaheta HJ, Schittek B, Breuninger H, Maczey E, Kroeber S, Sotlar K, Ellwanger U, Thelen MH, Rassner G, Bultmann B, Garbe C. Lymph node micrometastases of cutaneous melanoma: increased sensitivity of molecular diagnosis in comparison to immunohistochemistry. Inter J of Cancer 1988;79: 318–323.
146. Shivers SC, Wang X, Li W, Joseph E, Messina J, Glass LF, et al. Molecular staging of malignant melanoma: correlation with clinical outcome. JAMA 1998;280:1410–1415.
147. Blaheta HJ, Ellwanger U, Schittek B, Sotlar K, MacZey E, Breuninger H, et al. Examination of regional lymph nodes by sentinel node biopsy and molecular analysis provides new staging facilities in primary cutaneous melanoma. J Invest Dermatol 2000;114;637–642.
148. De Vries TJ, Smeets M, de Graaf R, Hou-Jensen K, Brocker EB, Renard N, et al. Expression of gp100, MART-1, tyrosinase, and S100 in paraffin-embedded primary melanomas and locoregional, lymph node, and visceral metastases: implications for diagnosis and immunotherapy. A study conducted by the EORTC Melanoma Cooperative Group. J Pathol 2001;193:13–20.
149. Balch CM, Buzaid AC, Seng-Jaw S, Atkins MB, Cascinelli N, Coit DG, et al. Final version of the American Joint Committee on Cancer staging system for cutaneous melanoma. J Clin Oncol 2001;19:3635–3648.

Chapter **31**

Gastric Cancer

Sten Hammarström and Torgny Stigbrand

The gastrointestinal tract harbors more tumors than any other organ system in the body. Five tumor sites dominate, i.e., cancers of colorectal, gastric, pancreatic, esophageal, and hepatocellular origin. An interesting feature of this entire group of tumors is the large variability in morbidity and mortality, which probably reflects local environment, rather than racial or other genetic factors, as crucial for the etiology. Thus when people move from geographical high-risk regions to low-risk locations, the incidence of tumors also changes, reflecting the risk of that new region.

Gastric cancer is ranked as the fourth most common cause of cancer death in the European Union (1), and the long-term survival rate is low (7–15%) even in cases treated with radical surgery. Chemotherapy has not proven successful as a treatment strategy. In the Western world the incidence of this disease has decreased in recent decades, but in parts of Asia almost 100 deaths per 100,000 is observed in some populations. In the U.S., in contrast, a death rate of only 6 per 100,000 people has been reported. In Europe, incidence values between 7 and 46 have been reported.

Gastric carcinomas are rare before the age of 40, and the incidence increases with age. It occurs more commonly in men than in women (incidence sex ratio is 2.2 in Europe). Environmental factors including infection with *Helicobacter pylori,* high salt consumption, and lack of fresh fruit and vegetables in the diet are considered to be risk factors for stomach cancer. Gastric tumors generate early hematogenic metastases to the liver, lungs, brain, and skeleton. Microscopically, the tumors are adenocarcinomas with marked variability in histopathology.

Gastroscopy, biopsy, double contrast radiography, and chest x-ray or liver sonography usually establish the gastric cancer diagnosis.

Three tumor markers are frequently used to monitor gastric cancer: carcinoembryonic antigen (CEA), CA19-9, and CA72-4. The "European Group on Tumor Markers" has also considered these markers to hold promise for monitoring of gastric cancer but to require further evaluation (2).

CARCINOEMBRYONIC ANTIGEN (CEA)

CEA is one of the oldest tumor markers and probably the best characterized, at present. Gold and Freedman originally discovered CEA in colon carcinoma in 1965 (3). CEA was independently cloned and sequenced in 1987 by several research groups [for references see Hammarström 1999 (4)] and was, together with a number of related molecules, shown to form a separate subfamily—the CEA subfamily—within the immunoglobulin superfamily. The CEA subfamily can be divided into two subgroups: the CEA subgroup with seven expressed members, and the pregnancy-specific glycoprotein (PSG) subgroup with 11 expressed members. The entire family of genes is located within a region of 1.8 megabases (Mb) on chromosome 19q13.2 (for details see 4).

The structures of the molecules in the CEA subgroup are shown in Figure 1. The molecules are made up of a varying number of immunoglobulin domains. However, there is always only one N-terminal IgV-like domain followed by zero to six IgC2-like domains. The molecules are associated with the plasma membrane of the cell in either of two ways: through a membrane-spanning peptide or via a glycosyl phosphatidyl inositol moiety (GPI). The N-terminal IgV-like domain is unusual in that it lacks the intrachain disulfide bridge; instead there is an intrachain salt bridge. The CEA family of molecules has recently been renamed to indicate the cell adhesive properties of its members (5) and is now called CEACAMs (Figure 1). For historical reasons, the name CEA is used when referring to the protein, whereas the CEA gene is termed CEACAM5).

CEA is the largest molecule in the family. It consists of seven immunoglobulin domains and is linked to the cell membrane via a GPI linkage. A heavily glycosylated glycoprotein (molecular weight ≈ 180 kDa), CEA contains about 50% carbohydrate. The carbohydrate chains are of the complex multiantennary type linked to the peptide via N-acetyl glucosamine to asparagine.

Compared to most other members of the CEA subfamily, CEA shows a relatively limited expression in normal adult tissues. It is most abundantly expressed in columnar epithelial cells and goblet cells in the colon. It is also expressed in mucous neck cells and pyloric mucous cells in the stomach, in squamous epithelial cells of the tongue, esophagus and cervix, in secretory epithelia and duct cells of sweat glands, and in epithelial cells of the prostate (6–9). CEA expression commences during the early fetal period (week 9–14) and seems to persist throughout life (8). Thus contrary to earlier belief, CEA is not a so-called oncofetal antigen. In normal colon, CEA expression is related to the degree of differentiation of the epithelial cells. Thus fully differentiated epithelial cells at the

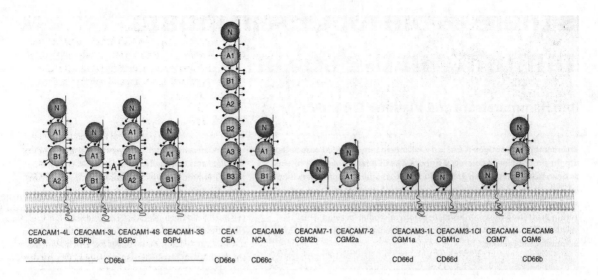

Figure 1 Models of the molecules in the carcinoembryonic antigen (CEA) subgroup. The immunoglobulin (Ig)V-like amino-terminal domains are dark and the IgC-like domains (A and B) are grey. The glycosylphosphatidylinositol (GPI) linkage to the cell membrane is shown as an arrowhead. Two forms of CEACAM1 cytoplasmic domains (long and short) that are derived by alternative mRNA splicing are shown. Glycosylation sites are shown as lollipops. Names are given in three different nomenclature systems. The upper line refers to the new nomenclature agreed upon in 1999 (reference 5). For historical reasons, CEA is used when referring to the protein, whereas the CEA gene is termed *CEACAM5*. The middle line gives the original names of these molecules: biliary glycoprotein (BGP); carcinoembryonic antigen (CEA); nonspecific cross-reacting antigen (NCA); CEA gene family members 1,2,3,4, and 6 (CGM1-CGM4, CGM6). The lower line gives the cluster of differentiation (CD) names of five of the molecules. Three molecules are not named in the CD system. (Hammarström and Baranov. Trends Microbiol 2001;9:119–125.) (Reproduced with permission from Elsevier, London).

free luminal surface express the highest levels of CEA, while immature epithelial cells at the bottom of the crypt express no or very little CEA (10,11). Similarly, well-differentiated colon carcinomas express high levels of CEA (4). Whether CEA expression is related to normal cellular differentiation in the stomach is unclear at present. It is however known that only some parts of the normal stomach i.e., gastroesophageal and gastroduodenal junctions and antrum, are CEA-positive, but not cardia or corpus (8). Well-differentiated gastric adenocarcinomas express CEA mRNA. Interestingly, however, this is also the case in the majority of poorly differentiated gastric tumors (12). It would also seem as if the mRNA level of CEA is upregulated in the tumor tissue as compared to the adjacent normal tissue in most patients with gastric adenocarcinoma (12,13). As a matter of fact, all four CEA family members that can be detected in epithelia, namely CEA, CEACAM1, CEACAM6, and CEACAM7, were found to be upregulated in gastric adenocarcinoma (12). CEACAM7 may be an interesting new candidate marker for gastric cancer. However no specific CEACAM7 immunoassay has so far been developed.

A number of commercial immunoassays for the analysis of CEA in the blood are available. They are with very few exceptions highly specific for CEA, and cut-off levels are typically around 5 ng/mL. Elevated levels of CEA are sometimes seen among smokers. The lung produces small amounts of CEA and smoking appears to re-route some of this CEA to the blood. In a recent prospective cohort study, we found three elevated serum CEA samples out of 248 randomly selected gender-, age-, and date-of-sampling-matched controls from the Northern Sweden Health and Disease Cohort. All three positive controls were smokers and had moderately elevated (7.2–8.0 ng/mL) CEA levels (14). Thus smoking habits of the patient should be investigated and/or the plasma levels of cotinine, the major metabolite of nicotine, should be determined. Benign liver and bowel diseases such as cirrhosis, chronic active hepatitis, viral hepatitis, obstructive jaundice, diverticulitis, inflammatory bowel disease, peptic ulcers, polyps, and pancreatitis may occasionally give rise to elevated serum CEA levels.

The positivity rate of serum CEA in gastric cancer is typically between 15 and 35 % (15–19). This is clearly lower than for colorectal cancer and limits the usefulness for diagnosis when used alone. However as seen below, when combined with CA19-9 and CA72-4, positivity rates increase significantly. CEA can also be detected in the gastric juice. However, there is no correlation between serum CEA and gastric juice CEA in patients with gastric cancer, and the latter measurement appears to lack diagnostic value (20,21).

In a study involving a total of 549 patients with gastric cancer who underwent gastrectomy, Ishigami et al. (17) analyzed CEA and CA19-9 serum levels preoperatively and determined the prognostic utility of increased marker values. It was found that surgical outcomes of patients who were CEA-positive and CA19-9-positive were poorer than those of patients with normal CEA and CA19-9. Using a higher cut-off (10 ng/mL) for CEA, the authors concluded that raised preoperative CEA levels were an important prognostic factor for patients with gastric cancer. In another similar study (18), it was demonstrated that a low three-year cumulative survival rate was significantly associated with elevated serum levels of CEA ($p < 0.001$). The measurement of CEA, CA19-9, and Sialyl Tn[1] was also shown to be of prognostic value for chemotherapy of gastric cancer (22). Using the criterion that all three markers should decrease by at least 50% compared to pretreatment levels and remain stable for at least one month, it was shown that the median survival time for responders was 17 months as compared to six months for nonresponders.

Chimeric monoclonal antibodies against CEA are also considered for immunotargeting (diagnostic/therapeutic) of CEA-positive (CEA+) gastric tumors. Thus in a nude mouse model, in which the animals were carrying CEA+ MNK-45 gastric cancer cells, it was demonstrated that a chimeric anti-CEA mAb will target the tumor with a high degree of specificity (23–25). Recently, CEA was considered as a target for gene therapy of gastric cancer (26). In this study, a novel bifunctional Moloney murine leukemia virus-based recombinant retroviral vector, which displayed a chimeric envelope protein containing a single-chain variable fragment antibody to CEA carrying the iNOS gene in the genome was constructed. The bifunctional vector induced apoptosis in the tumor cells, causing direct and efficient killing of CEA+ carcinoma cells.

Almost half of the patients with gastric cancer invading beyond the serosal surface will die of progression of peritoneal micrometastases. Detection of peritoneal micrometastases of gastric cancer is presently based on peritoneal wash cytology alone. It was, however, recently demonstrated (27) that the use of a combination of CEA reverse transcriptase-polymerase chain reaction (RT-PCR) and cytological assay (both on peritoneal washes) improves the detection of peritoneal recurrence.

CA19-9

The sialylated lactofucopentanose, or sialyl Lewis^a (SLe^a), is a well-known carbohydrate tumor marker determinant related to the Lewis blood group system. It is used to monitor several gastrointestinal malignancies such as pancreatic, gall bladder, gastric, and colorectal cancers. The original discovery was made by Koprowski et al. (28) in 1979, and the marker belongs to the established tumor markers for gastrointestinal cancer. The SLe^a epitope initially was defined by the monoclonal antibody "19-9," which was raised against a monosialoganglioside on colorectal carcinoma cells. The epitope is present both as a carbohydrate component of cell surface glycoproteins and as a membrane-associated glycolipid. It appears in the fetal epithelium of the stomach, small and large intestine, liver, and pancreas. In adults, the epitope is expressed in trace amounts in pancreas, liver, gallbladder, and lung. The epitope is expressed on mucosal cells.

In patients with malignant diseases, the epitope typically appears in blood present on high molecular weight glycoproteins (>1000 kDa). In a recent report from the International Society for Oncodevelopmental Biology and Medicine (ISOBM) a number of monoclonal antibodies against this epitope were compared with respect to specificity and affinity, and out of 20 selected anti-CA19-9 monoclonal antibodies, 19 reacted with the sialyl Lewis^a-epitope, but also with the structurally closely related SLe^x and the desialylated form, Le^a (29). Only a minor fraction of the antibodies tested were specific for SLe^a, which indicates that possibilities for improvements in the assays still exist. The different carbohydrate epitopes are presented in Table 1.

The galactosyltransferase [UDP-galactose:beta N-acetylglucosamine beta-1,3-galactosyltransferase (beta 3Gal-T5)] responsible for the synthesis of all type 1 Lewis antigens was recently cloned (30). This enzyme is involved in the synthesis of the sialyl Lewis epitope.

The biological half-life of CA19-9 has been reported to be seven hours in cell culture. The normal range has been determined to < 37 or < 60 U/mL, depending on the methods used. The circulating antigen was reported to be eliminated exclusively via the bile. Thus even slight cholestasis can sometimes cause considerable rises in CA19-9 levels. Values above 10,000 U/mL usually indicate metastatic disease.

The clinical significance of CA19-9 as a tumor marker is obvious for pancreatic cancer (see Chapter 21), but this antigen also serves as a valuable marker in combination with CEA for gastric cancer. Both CA19-9 and CEA have been reported separately to give a sensitivity of 18–30% (17), and when used in combination, the sensitivity is raised to 50–60 %. Serum levels of CEA and CA19-9 were positively correlated with depth of invasion and hepatic metastasis and negatively correlated with curability. A significant but weak correlation between CEA and CA19-9 marker values was also observed (r = 0.24) (17).

Interestingly, this tumor marker seems to be inappropriate for those individuals with mutations in the *FUT3* gene, which encodes an alpha-1,4-fucosyltransferase necessary for the synthesis of the epitope. Recent studies have revealed pronounced differences between heterozygous (Le/le) and homozygous

Table 1 Structures of oligosaccharides related to the Lewis blood group system and the CA19-9 epitope

Name	Structure
SLe^a (CA19-9)	Galβ1–3GlcNAc-R ↑2,3 ↑1,4 Neu 5Acα Fucα
SLe^x	Galβ1–3GlcNAc-R ↑2,3 ↑1,3 Neu 5Acα Fucα
Le^a	Galβ1–3GlcNAc-R ↑1,4 Fucα
Le^x	Galβ1–3GlcNAc-R ↑1,3 Fucα

---

[1] The Tn antigen is a core oligosaccharide (GalNAc-O-Ser) present in mucins. The GalNAc residue is normally substituted at the 3-position with Gal. In a number of human tumors, the core oligosaccharide is substituted with sialic acid, forming Sialyl Tn.

(Le/Le) individuals, which strongly suggests that immunoassays should be "allele-corrected" to improve the outcome of the assay. Individuals with the blood group Le a-/b- (7–10% of the normal population) are unable to synthesize CA19-9.

Several recent publications have indicated CA19-9 to be of value for detecting recurrent gastric cancer (15,16). In a series of 35 patients with recurrent gastric cancer who had undergone curative gastrectomy, serum CA19-9 was elevated in 57%, compared to 34% for CEA. (15). In another study (16) 35% of patients with gastric cancer had elevated preoperative CA19-9 values while patients with recurrent disease had elevated CA19-9 values in 56% of the cases. Values for CEA in the same investigation were 16% CEA+ preoperatively and 44% at disease recurrence (16). When the tumor marker CA 72-4 was added, the sensitivity for recurrent disease was increased to 87%. Using all three markers, Ychou et al. (31) obtained a sensitivity of 75% for gastric cancer. Marker specificity, evaluated in 58 disease-free patients, was 79% for CEA, 74% for CA19-9, and 97% for CA72-4 (16). When the prognostic values of CEA, CA19-9, and CA72-4 were compared, only CA72-4 was found to have a significant prognostic value (4.2-fold higher risk of death with high values of CA72-4 than with low levels) (18).

It should, however, be noted that both CEA and CA19-9 can be elevated in benign diseases like acute hepatitis, chronic active hepatitis, biliary disease, cystic fibrosis, pancreatitis, and rheumatic diseases. None of these markers has so far proven useful for screening or diagnosing early gastric cancer.

CA 72-4

The tumor marker CA72-4 initially was defined as an antigen recognized by two different monoclonal antibodies, i.e., CC49 and B72-3 (32). The CC49 antibody was generated against a highly purified mucin-like tumor-associated glycoprotein TAG72, with a molecular weight between 220 and 400 kDa. The other antibody, B72-3, was generated against a membrane-enriched fraction, derived from the cells of a human breast carcinoma metastasis. The protein appears in several fetal tissues, but rarely appears in adult human tissues. Immunohistochemically, the antigen is associated with adenocarcinomas in several organs including colon, ovaries, esophagus, breast, non-small cell lung cancer, and carcinomas of the stomach.

The upper normal range for this marker in serum is between 2.5 and 4 ng/mL and several assays are commercially available. The correlation coefficient between different assays was reported to be between 0.8 and 0.96 (33). The marker can be assayed both in serum and in gastric juice, but the correlation between the two sets of values in patients with gastric cancer is low (20). CA72-4 is characterized by high tumor specificity and elevated levels are rarely seen in benign conditions.

CA72-4 is a useful marker for monitoring the course and therapeutic response of carcinomas of the stomach. The sensitivity has been reported to 30–40 % for gastric cancer, which has been considered low (19,20). When this assay is combined with CEA and CA19-9, the sensitivity increases to 64% (19). The specificity for gastric cancer for CA72-4 is high, and values up to 100% have been reported (19). At recurrent gastric cancer, CA72-4 was reported to be the most useful of the three markers, with a sensitivity of 43% at a specificity of 95% (21). This marker also has a special role for monitoring ovarian mucinous carcinomas when CA125 is of limited value.

SUMMARY

Three serum tumor markers, CA74-2, CEA, and CA19-9, are of value in monitoring of gastric cancer after surgical resection or other treatment modalities. However, since the sensitivity for gastric cancer of each marker is comparatively low when used individually (i.e., 20–40%), the markers should be used in combination, which raises the sensitivity to more acceptable levels. None of the markers can be used for screening purposes. CEA shows some promise as a target for therapy and localization of CEA+ gastric cancer. Research should be focused on finding new markers for gastric cancer.

REFERENCES

1. Black RJ, Bray F, Ferlay J, Parkin DM. Cancer incidence and mortality in the European Union: cancer registry data and estimates of national incidence for 1990. Eur J Cancer 1997;33:1075–1107.
2. Sturgeon C, Aronsson AC, Hansson LO, Klapdor R, van Dalen A. European Group on Tumor Markers. Anticancer Res 1999;19: 2785–2820.
3. Gold P, Freedman SO. Specific carcinoembryonic antigens of the human digestive system. J Exp Med 1965;122:467–481.
4. Hammarström S. The carcinoembryonic antigen (CEA) family: ctructures, suggested functions, and expression in normal and malignant tissues. Sem Cancer Biol 1999;9:67–81.
5. Beauchemin N, Draber P, Dveksler G, et al. Redefined nomenclature for members of the carcinoembryonic antigen family. Exp Cell Res 1999;252:243–249.
6. Hammarström S, Olsen A, Teglund S, Baranov V. The nature and expression of the human CEA family. In: Stanners C, ed. Cell adhesion and communication mediated by the CEA family: basic and clinical perspectives. Amsterdam: Harwood Academic Publishers, 1997:1–30.
7. Prall F, Nollau P, Neumaier M, Haubeck HD, Drzeniek Z, Helmchen U, et al. CD66a (BGP), an adhesion molecule of the carcinoembryonic antigen family, is expressed in epithelium, endothelium, and myeloid cells in a wide range of normal human tissues. J Histochem Cytochem 1996;44:35–41.
8. Nap M, Mollgard K, Burtin P, Fleuren GJ. Immunohistochemistry of carcinoembryonic antigen in the embryo, fetus, and adult. Tumor Biol 1988;9:145–153.
9. Nap M, Hammarström ML, Börmer O, Hammarström S, Wagener C, Handt S, et al. Specificity and affinity of monoclonal antibodies against carcinoembryonic antigen. Cancer Res 1992;52:2329–2339
10. Baranov V, Yeung MMW, Hammarström S. Expression of carcinoembryonic antigen and nonspecific cross-reacting 50 kDa antigen in human normal and cancerous colon mucosa: comparative ultrastructural study with monoclonal antibodies. Cancer Res 1994;54:3305–3314.
11. Frängsmyr L, Baranov V, Hammarström S. Four carcinoembryonic antigen (CEA) subfamily members, CEA, NCA, BGP and CGM2, selectively expressed in the normal human colonic epithe-

lium are integral components of the fuzzy coat. Tumor Biol 1999;20:277–292.
12. Kinugasa T, Kuroki M, Takeo H, Matsuo Y, Ohshima K, Yamashita Y, et al. Expression of four CEA family antigens (CEA, NCA, BGP and CGM2) in normal and cancerous gastric epithelial cells: up-regulation of BGP and CGM2 in carcinomas. Int J Cancer 1998;76:148–153.
13. Kodera Y, Isobe K, Yamauchi M, Satta T, Hasegawa T, Oikawa S, et al. Expression of carcinoembryonic antigen (CEA) and nonspecific cross-reacting antigen (NCA) in gastrointestinal cancer: the correlation with degree of differentiation. Brit J Cancer 1993;68:130–136.
14. Palmqvist R, Engarås B, Lindmark G, Hallmans G, Nilsson O, Hammarström S, Hafström L. Can CEA and CA242 be used for colorectal cancer screening? Results from a prospective cohort study. Europ J Cancer. Submitted 2002.
15. Tas F, Faruk Aykan N, Aydiner A, Yasasever V, Topuz E. Measurement of serum CA 19-9 may be more valuable than CEA in prediction of recurrence in patients with gastric cancer. Am J Clin Oncol 2001;24:148–149.
16. Marrelli D, Pinto E, De Stefano A, Farnetani M, Garosi L, Roviello F. Clinical utility of CEA, CA 19-9, and CA 72-4 in the follow-up of patients with resectable gastric cancer. Am J Surg 2001;181:16–19.
17. Ishigami S, Natsugoe S, Hokita S, Che X, Tokuda K, Nakajo A, et al. Clinical importance of preoperative carcinoembryonic antigen and carbohydrateantigen 19-9 levels in gastric cancer. J Clin Gastroenterol 2001;32:41–44.
18. Gaspar MJ, Arribas I, Coca MC, Diez-Alonso M. Prognostic value of carcinoembryonic antigen, CA 19-9 and CA 72-4 in gastric carcinoma. Tumor Biol 2001;22:318–322.
19. Lopez JB, Royan GP, Lakhwani MN, Mahadaven M, Timor J. CA 72-4 compared with CEA and CA 19-9 as a marker of some gastrointestinal malignancies. Int J Biol Markers 1999;14:172–177.
20. Tocchi A, Costa G, Lepre L, Liotta G, Mazzoni G, Cianetti A, Vannini P. The role of serum and gastric juice levels of carcinoembryonic antigen, CA19.9, and CA72.4 in patients with gastric cancer. J Cancer Res Clin Oncol 1998; 124:450–455.
21. Gartner U, Scheulen ME, Conradt C, Wiefelsputz J, Kruck P, Aghabi E, Delbruck H. Value of tumor-associated antigens CA 72-4 vs. CEA and CA 19-9 in the follow-up after stomach cancer. Dtsch Med Wochenschr 1998;123: 69–73.
22. Naketa B, Chung KH, Muguruma K, Yamashita Y, Inoue T, Matsuoka T, et al. Changes in tumor marker levels as a predictor of chemotherapeutic effect in patients with gastric cancer. Cancer 1998;83:19–24.
23. Haruno M, Kuroki M, Matsunga K, Takata J, Karube Y, Senba T, et al. Tumor-specific accumulation of 125I-labeled mouse-human chimeric anti-CEA antibody in xenografted human cancer model demonstrated by whole-body autoradiography and immunostaining. Nucl Med Biol 1996;23:821–826.
24. Karube Y, Katsuno K, Takata J, Matsunaga K, Haruno M, Kuroki M, et al. Radioimmunoscintigraphy using technetium 99m-labeled parental mouse and mouse-human chimeric antibodies to carcinoembryonic antigen in athymic nude mice bearing tumor. Nucl Med Biol 1996;23:753–759.
25. Karube Y, Katsuno K, Ito S, Matsunaga K, Takata J, Kuroki M, et al. Tumor scintigraphy by the method for subtracting initial image with technetium-99m labeled antibody. Ann Nucl Med 1999;13: 407–413.
26. Khare PD, Shao-Xi L, Kuroki M, Hirose Y, Arakawa F, Nakamura K, et al. Specifically targeted killing of carcinoembryonic antigen (CEA)- expressing cells by a retroviral vector displaying single-chain variable fragmented antibody to CEA and carrying the gene for inducible nitric oxide synthase. Cancer Res 2001;61: 370–375.
27. Yonemura Y, Endou Y, Fujimura T, Fushida S, Bandou E, Kinoshita K, et al. Diagnostic value of preoperative RT-PCR based screening method to detect carcinoembryonic antigen-expressing free cancer cells in the peritoneal cavity from patients with gastric cancer. ANZ J Surg 2001;71:521–528.
28. Koprowski H, Steplewski Z, Mitchell K, Herlyn M, Herlyn D, Fuhrer P. Colorectal carcinoma antigens detected by hybridoma antibodies. Somatic Cell Genet 1979;5:957–971.
29. Rye PD, Bovin NV, Vlasova EV, Molodyk AA, Baryshnikov A, Kreutz FT, et al. Summary report on the ISOBM TD-6 workshop: analysis of 20 monoclonal antibodies against Sialyl Lewis a and related antigens. Montreux, Switzerland; September 19–24, 1997. Tumor Biol 1998;19:390–420.
30. Isshiki S, Togayachi A, Kudo T, Nishihara S, Watanabe M, Kubota T, et al. Cloning, expression, and characterization of a novel UDP-galactose:beta-N-acetylglucosamine beta1,3-galactosyltransferase (beta3Gal-T5) responsible for synthesis of type 1 chain in colorectal and pancreatic epithelia and tumor cells derived therefrom. J Biol Chem 1999; 274:12499–12507.
31. Ychou M, Duffour J, Kramar A, Gourgou S, Grenier J. Clinical significance and prognostic value of CA72-4 compared with CEA and CA19-9 in patients with gastric cancer. Dis Markers 2000;16: 105–110.
32. Muraro R, Kuroki M, Wunderlich D, Poole D.J, Colcher D, Thor A, et al. Generation and characterization of B72.3 2nd-generation monoclonal-antibodies reactive with the tumor-associated glycoprotein 72 antigen. Cancer Res 1988;48:4588–4596.
33. Filella X, Friese S, Roth HJ, Nussbaum S, Wehnl B. Technical performance of the Elecsys CA 72-4 test—development and field study. Anticancer Res. 2000;20:5229–5232.

Part Three
Genomic and Proteomic Approaches for Biomarker Discovery

Chapter 32

Microarray Technology in Cancer

Paul C. Park, Ben Beheshti, and Jeremy A. Squire

Tumorigenesis is a complex process that involves alterations at the genomic, transcript, and protein levels. The central paradigm in cancer research is to identify these molecular alterations and to characterize their effects on the tumor phenotype. There are several major challenges hindering this task. First, given that there are an estimated 31,000 protein-coding genes in the human genome (1), just to identify the aberrations in all the genes and their respective products is an ambitious undertaking. Secondly, not all the molecular alterations in a tumor are directly relevant to cancer progression. Therefore, the critical molecular changes that drive the process must be sorted out from the secondary or serendipitous ones and correlated to the clinical end points. Finally, most of the key genes exert their effect in concert with other genes, as a part of complex, interacting molecular pathways. To ascribe functions to these genes, therefore, requires analysis of the interaction of their products in numerous different combinations. Clearly, such a task would be too enormous to be handled by the traditional "gene-by-gene" molecular techniques.

Over the past few years, microarrays have been introduced as a high-throughput platform for simultaneous analysis of many genes or gene products in a parallel manner. The underlying principle of this approach is to represent a large number of genes that are linked to bioinformatics databases, on a solid surface, and to screen with the query samples. This method has been adapted to accommodate the genomic DNA and cDNA as well as the proteins. The end result of such survey is a comprehensive, global view of the genome, transcriptome, and the proteome, respectively. This chapter will highlight the key advances in microarray technology, and their impact on cancer biology.

GENOMIC PROFILING USING SNP ARRAYS

It is estimated that in the human genome, single nucleotide polymorphisms (SNP) occur at a frequency of approximately one in 1,000 bases (2,3). To date, the SNP database has accumulated over a million entries and is likely to grow. These polymorphisms can affect the coding sequences as well as the transcriptional regulation and splicing, and may serve as markers defining the susceptibility to various forms of cancer or resistance to therapeutic regimens (4,5). Moreover, loss of heterozygosity (LOH) of chromosomal regions bearing mutated tumor suppressor genes is a key event in the evolution of epithelial and mesenchymal tumors. Global patterns of LOH can be understood through allelotyping of tumors with polymorphic genetic markers.

Genotyping based on such large numbers of permutations, however, requires a system that can handle parallel screening of a large set of possibilities (6,7). SNP arrays consist of known oligonucleotides that act as allele-specific targets, arrayed at high density on glass surfaces by combinatorial light directed *in situ* synthesis (8). When hybridized with labeled, PCR-amplified DNA samples, perfect matches hybridize more strongly and produce more intense fluorescence than mismatched spots. Although the sensitivity of this method is debatable, it has been suggested that heterozygous base pair polymorphisms, mutations, insertions, and deletions can be detected by this approach (9–11).

Of interest to cancer genomics, the end point of this technology is the capacity for genome-wide screening using high-density SNP arrays for simultaneous monitoring of tens of thousands of genetic variations. This information may yield valuable linkage relationships for complex heritable patterns in familial cancers. To this end, a recent work by Favis et al. employed SNP arrays modeled after the founder mutations in the Ashkenazi Jewish population to detect small insertions and deletions in BRCA1 and BRCA2 genes (12). Furthermore, Lindblad-Toh et al. genotyped 1500 loci using a high-density SNP array to derive a global profile of LOH in human small cell lung cancer (13). These results illustrate the potential for microarray analysis in the routine identification of SNPs in the context of both clinical diagnosis and population studies.

ARRAY-BASED CGH FOR SURVEY OF THE GENOME

Comparative genomic hybridization (CGH) to metaphase chromosome targets (14,15) has emerged in recent years as a dominant tool for detecting genomic markers in the cytogenetically more complex tumor types (reviewed in 16,17). The unique advantage of chromosome CGH is its capacity to screen the entire genome for copy number changes. However, because the target DNA within the chromosome is highly condensed and supercoiled, the resolution for determining copy number changes is limited to 10 Mb for copy losses (14) and to 2 Mb for gains, depending on the amplicon size and copy number (14,18). This resolution, while capable of providing a starting point for positional cloning studies, will still encompass too many genes to derive any focused information regarding the biological significance of imbalances. Moreover, more subtle changes will likely be missed by this method, making this an unreliable tool for routine screening of tumor markers.

Recently a novel strategy has emerged that couples CGH with the microarray technology. Instead of using metaphase chromosomes, CGH is applied to arrayed sequences of genomic DNA bound to glass slides and probed with genomes of interest. The arrays are constructed from a tiling path of genomic clones that cover chromosomal loci of interest (e.g., see the MapViewer resource at the National Center for Biotechnology Information: http://www.ncbi.nlm.nih.gov/), or are obtained commercially (e.g., GenoSensor System™ at http://www.vysis.com). With sufficient representation on the microarray, this system significantly increases resolution for localizing regions of imbalance. Notably, the first high-density whole genome microarray (approximately 2000 BAC clones) was recently introduced (19) and demonstrated its ability to precisely delineate genome-wide segmental aneuploidy breakpoints in tumor cells.

To date, several groups have published results that demonstrate the utility of array CGH in cancer biology (19–27). For example, Pinkel et al. (21) screened DNA arrays and detected genomic imbalances within a sub-band of chromosome 20 in breast cancer that had failed to be observed using chromosome CGH. Also, by mapping the position of amplicon boundaries within cytoband 20q13.2 at high resolution, Albertson et al. localized *CYP24* within the minimal amplified region, identifying it as a new candidate oncogene in breast cancer (22). In another study, CGH was carried out on high resolution arrays constructed from BACs, PACs, and cosmid clones along a 7Mb tiling path encompassing the *NF2* locus on chromosome 22 (23). This system was sufficiently sensitive to detect single copy losses and homozygous deletions in neurofibromatosis type 2 patients, making it a reliable tool for screening patient samples. Moreover, refinements made by Daigo et al. to screen arrays using genome amplified by DOP-PCR from laser-capture microdissected specimens make this method amenable to screening limited archival materials (24,28).

High resolution CGH has also been carried out on cDNA arrays, normally employed in expression screening, for examining genomic copy number imbalances. Despite the fact that the cDNA targets are considerably less complex structurally, the hybridization with the genomic probes seems to be sufficiently sensitive to detect low levels of amplification (29). In fact, the authors report that *MYCN* amplifications of 5-fold and greater were readily detected by this method, even in samples that were significantly contaminated with normal genome (29).

The advantage of increased resolution provided by cDNA array CGH was recently demonstrated by screening for *MYCN* (chromosome region 2p24) amplification status in neuroblastoma patients and cell lines (30). In this study, analysis of high-density 19200 feature microarrays revealed the co-amplification of the oncogene *MEIS1* (31) with *MYCN* in the cell line IMR32, and further identified novel gene amplifications in the cell line and the patient samples. Similarly, Pei et al. employed the increased resolving power of cDNA array CGH to delineate the amplicon boundaries in pediatric carcinomas (32).

Perhaps the greatest advantage of cDNA arrays is that duplicate arrays may be used in parallel to provide a comprehensive overview of both expression and gene copy number change in the same tissue (33). In a report by Pollack et al., CGH was carried out on 3360 feature cDNA microarrays to detect copy number gains and single deletion losses in breast tumors and cell lines. Interrogation of the transcriptome of the same samples, using a duplicate cDNA array, revealed that not all amplified genes were overexpressed, nor were most highly overexpressed genes amplified. A subset of the genes, however, including *ERBB2*, was observed to be both amplified and overexpressed. Similarly, the effects of amplification of the 17q23 region in breast cancer cell lines have also been examined by specifically analyzing the expression of the 156 genes localized in that region using cDNA array (34). With the increasing availability of a variety of cDNA microarrays representing different clone sets, this emerging platform promises to provide comprehensive information regarding the interaction between the genome and the transcriptome changes in cancer.

EXPRESSION PROFILING WITH MICROARRAYS

Tumorigenesis involves changes in the expression of many genes. In the past, profiling these expression changes was a formidable challenge. Quantitative methods such as Northern blotting typically require large amounts of RNA and are suited only for gene-by-gene analysis. More global, comparative profiling of the entire transcriptome using molecular techniques such as SAGE or RDA analysis, on the other hand, is very time consuming. These labor-intensive methods are not suitable for analyzing large number of samples, and are thus impractical for identifying the consensus events associated with tumor progression.

Recently cDNA microarrays have emerged as an accepted method for surveying of thousands of genes in a parallel fashion with relatively small amount of material. The relative ease with which these surveys can be performed makes this approach ideal for high-throughput analysis of sufficient number of patient or experimental samples for discovery of novel class and molecular pathways in cancer.

The expression arrays consist of oligonucleotides or cDNA derived from expressed sequence tags (ESTs), spotted in an orderly fashion on a nylon membrane or glass surface. With the more advanced arrayers, the density of the spots can reach into the tens of thousands within a surface area that is suitable for a single experiment. Moreover, the newer generations of commercially available arrays contain well-characterized, non-redundant clone sets, which focus on the genes involved in specific cellular functions or pathways. These featured spots serve as the targets for hybridization with the transcriptome of the query sample, and the signal intensity for each spot is taken to represent the abundance of that particular gene product within the transcriptome.

Currently, two strategies are widely used for expression profiling. The first method uses multiple replicate arrays for separately screening the RNA samples to be compared, typically with radioactively labeled cDNA probes derived from tumor and normal RNA. For this approach, the hybridization of the cDNA probes of each sample occurs independently, and the expression profiling is achieved by quantifying and comparing the signal intensities of each individual gene among the arrays. The quality of replication of the arrays is therefore crucial in this strategy, in that the quantity of each target spotted is equal from array to array. For this reason, this approach is typically restricted to commercial sources, where a strict quality control is in place. In addition, the radioactive probe, while being sensitive, produces signals that do not localize tightly over the target spot, and hence the arrays cannot be spotted at high density. Within these restrictions, these low-density arrays are useful for a limited survey of the overall expression changes in cancer. For example, El-Rifai et al. compared the expression levels of 1200 cancer-related genes in gastric carcinoma samples against normal gastric epithelial cells using Atlas Human Cancer 1.2k arrays (35). This array found 38 genes to be differentially expressed, with up to sixteen-fold range of over- or underexpression in carcinoma. Similarly, malignant and normal prostate epithelium was compared using membrane-based, broad coverage cDNA array (36). This study reported that of the panel of 588 genes represented on the array, 87 exhibited significant differential expression with respect to the normal tissue. It is noteworthy, however, that a similar comparison between malignant and normal prostate epithelium by Chaib et al. yielded a remarkably different result, with only 15 of the 588 genes showing significant changes in expression levels (37). Furthermore, the latter study reported that the level of over- or underexpression from the array analysis were inconsistent with the results of the confirmatory RT-PCR and Northern blot analysis. It is unlikely that this striking discrepancy in results is solely due to the sample variability, and suggests insufficiencies in the microarray technique itself.

An alternate method, which is quickly becoming the standard for expression profiling, employs paired comparisons of the normal and tumor transcriptome to the same array. Specifically, cDNA probes are generated by reverse transcription of the normal and tumor total RNA samples in the presence of Cy3- or Cy5-conjugated dNTPs, and competitively hybridized in equal concentration against the targets on the array. The results are usually interpreted based on the fluorescence intensity ratios of the two signal colors, and therefore this approach circumvents the problems associated with technical, batch-to-batch inconsistencies in the arraying procedures. Furthermore, because the fluorescent signals localize well over the spots with minimal spatial dispersion, even at very high intensities, this technique can accommodate high-density arrays with thousands of features on a single microscope slide.

The high-density arrays provide a more comprehensive insight about global changes in the transcriptome, and are thus ideal tools for novel class discovery in cancer (38). In fact, just within the past few years, several types of cancer, including breast cancer, melanoma, and serous ovarian carcinoma, have been subtyped based on the transcription profiles (39–41). In addition, Miyazato et al. used oligonucleotide arrays to identify markers to differentiate myelodysplastic syndrome from de novo acute myeloid leukemia (42). As these authors pointed out, it is foreseeable that these molecular taxonomy schemes will have a significant impact on various clinical aspects of cancer, such as disease stratification, prognostication, and management strategies. For example, work by Golub et al. defined a class prediction algorithm for distinction of leukemia into acute myeloid and lymphoid based on the expression profile (43). More recently, an "invasive profile," based on panel of 27 genes that correlate with aggressive phenotype, was defined in breast cancer using high-density cDNA microarrays (44). Similarly, screening of lung adenocarcinoma cell lines with 9600 feature EST arrays found that approximately 2.9% of the featured genes, particularly those associated with cell adhesion, motility, angiogenesis, and signal transduction, correlated positively with invasive phenotype (45). In another study, Wang et al. investigated the molecular basis for resistance to thymidylate synthase inhibitors in cell lines using 1176 feature cDNA arrays, and found 28 genes to be consistently overexpressed (46).

To date, many studies that use microarrays for class discovery have been exploratory in nature without in-depth analysis of the biological significance of the observed expression changes. A recent report by Kannan et al., however, demonstrates the potential for microarrays in elucidating the functions of specific genes in cancer biology. In this paper, a human cancer cell line that expresses temperature-sensitive murine p53 was screened using oligonucleotide arrays. By profiling the expression at different time points after temperature shift, the investigators dissected the transcriptional program involving 259 genes, regulated by p53 (47).

With the abundance of quantifiable data generated by high-density microarrays, sophisticated statistical methods for handling large data sets, along with bioinformatics, are necessary and integral tools for expression profiling. Several clustering strategies, such as agglomerative algorithm, hierarchical algorithm, and two-way clustering methods have all been used to reduce the large sets of data from high-density microarrays into focused groups of genes or samples (48,49). Other methods including the principal component analysis, Shannon entropy analysis, k-means, and self-organizing maps have also been used to reduce data sets and to identify outliers as the genes with the most dynamic patterns of expression (50–52). The power of these statistical tools is illustrated by the work of Hilsenbeck et al., in which the principal component analysis was applied to identify two genes that underlie tamoxifen resistance from a starting point of 9000 data points consisting of 15 tumors and 600 genes (50). The end point of these analyses is to reduce the quantitative data into trends. It is important to note, however, that the associations of genes or tumors suggested by these trends do not necessarily translate into a single molecular pathway or a tumor class. These trends, rather, provide a vantage point to refine the hypothesis and to further analyze a smaller subset of genes.

PROTEIN ARRAYS FOR FUNCTIONAL ANALYSIS OF THE PROTEOME

Proteins are major biological effector molecules, and are involved in every aspect of cellular structure and function. There are obvious reasons why the functional status of a protein cannot

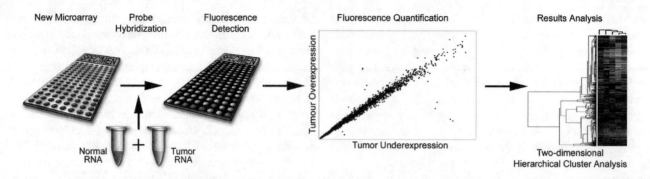

Figure 1 A schematic diagram of expression profiling using a cDNA microarray. A microarray featuring a clone set of interest is competitively hybridized with a probe cocktail consisting of equal amounts of labeled cDNA derived from tumor (green) and the normal (red) tissue. The red-to-green fluorescence intensity ratio is calculated for each spot and represented in a scatter plot. The differential expression of specific genes, and the extent thereof, is identified from the deviation of that data point from the 1:1 fluorescence ratio. The representation of the data in the form of an mXn matrix (where m represents the total number of samples analyzed, columns; and n represents the number of spots on the array, rows) permits clustering the data sets according to the genes that are co-regulated or the phenotypes of the tumors. **Color representation of figure appears on Color Plate 3.**

be accurately predicted from the profiles of its gene and the transcript alone. For example, the rate of translation is not necessarily proportional to the abundance of the transcripts alone, and the functional status of the protein depends to a large extent on post-translational modifications (53). Moreover, because proteins play integral roles in transcription as well as in maintenance of the genome, one cannot draw a simple unidirectional cause-effect relationship from the genome to transcriptome to the proteome. It is therefore necessary to assess the abundance and the functional status of the protein directly, particularly in cancer biology where many of the important gene products exert their effect through regulation of other downstream genes.

Protein arrays are an emerging, relatively novel platform in comparison to the DNA expression arrays. As with the genomic

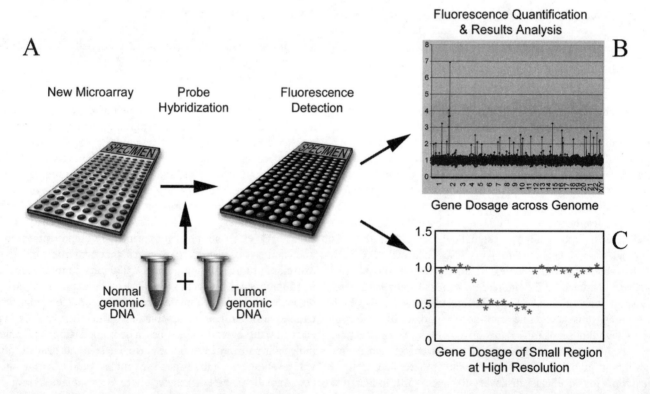

Figure 2 Profiling of the genomic aberrations using a genomic DNA or a cDNA array. (A) The array consists of genomic clones (e.g. BAC, PAC) representing a tiling path along the chromosome regions of interest, or cDNA clones of the genes located therein. Alternatively, clones from representative regions throughout the genome can be arrayed for a global survey of the entire genome at a lower resolution. The genomic DNA from the tumor (green) and normal (red) tissue are differentially labeled and hybridized in equal amounts against the targets on the array. The analysis of the fluorescence intensities for each spot permits the identification of the amplified (higher green:red) or deleted (lower green:red) regions in the tumor. Represented as a plot of fluorescence intensity ratio against the ordered, chromosomal location of the targets, the data set can identify the gene dosage changes at a low (B) or high (C) resolution. **Color representation of figure appears on Color Plate 3.**

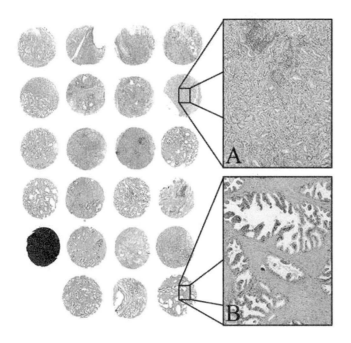

Figure 3 Tissue array of 22 prostate samples containing lesions of varying histological grades. The insets A (prostate tumor of Gleason pattern 4) and B (high-grade prostate intra-epithelial neoplasia) illustrate the architectural preservation of the tissue. This format allows a cell-by-cell analysis of the genome, the transcriptome, or the proteome of multiple samples in a parallel manner. **Color representation of figure appears on Color Plate 4.**

and cDNA arrays, this format allows parallel quantitation of massive number of protein species at once. Moreover, the sensitivity afforded by this technique allows visualization of the more rare, but functionally important, proteins such as transcription regulators, which would be missed by Western blotting. For quantitation of proteins in biological samples, high-density array can be generated from antibodies or oligonucleotide aptamers with known specificities for specific epitopes (54,55). These arrays are probed with labeled proteins from the query samples and analyzed in a similar manner as the DNA expression arrays. A recent report by Huang et al. demonstrated that multiple cytokines could be simultaneously detected from patient sera and conditioned media using this approach (56). With modifications, Belov et al. were able to screen intact cell suspensions using antibody arrays to phenotype leukemia based on the CD antigens (57). Protein arrays can also be generated from a focused panel of functionally important factors such as transcriptional regulators. Such arrays would facilitate the simultaneous analysis of thousands of interactions in a single experiment (58,59). This latter application is particularly promising in elucidating the pathways involved in cancer biology, and will constitute the major effort in the post-genomic era.

TISSUE ARRAYS FOR VALIDATION AND CLINICAL CORRELATION

To date, many studies using microarrays have employed classical molecular techniques to validate the results. While this may be feasible for work with cell lines, clinical samples are often limited in quantity, and cannot be analyzed by methods such as Southern and Northern blots. In addition, tumor tissues usually contain several different cell types. Analysis using bulk extracted material from tissues therefore, frequently suffers from contamination, and often produces diluted results. This problem is well exemplified by prostate tumors, which are often heterogeneous and multi-focal and require analysis at the cell-by-cell resolution (60). Finally, the volume of data poses a major obstacle to a thorough validation of results in a high-density microarray analysis. To confirm the data on any given gene on the array, multiple analyses must be performed on many samples, and this task can quickly range into unmanageable numbers.

Recently, tissue arrays have been introduced as a high-throughput platform for *in situ* detection of molecular changes in large number of clinical samples (34,61,62). These arrays consist of many tissue specimens, each of which is linked to pathological and clinical information. As with the other array formats, tissue arrays permit a large number of clinical samples to be screened in parallel at the DNA, RNA, or protein levels. Moreover, because the tissue morphology is preserved in these arrays, the molecular alterations can be localized at the cell-by-cell, or even at the subcellular resolution. This platform is thus well suited to derive correlations between molecular alterations and clinical information such as the histopathologic grade or other features of the tumor (63).

OTHER APPLICATIONS OF MICROARRAYS IN CANCER BIOLOGY

Despite the enormous advantages offered by the microarrays over the low-throughput methods, profiles of the genome, transcriptome, and the proteome yield only limited information when considered alone. As the data from these analyses continue to increase, there is a mounting need for innovations that link these individual platforms in a seamless manner. To this end, the capacity to profile both the genome and the expression of the same clinical sample with cDNA array will play a significant role in discerning the effect of genomic aberrations in cancer (34). Furthermore, a recently introduced technique known as protein *in situ* immobilization utilizes cell free expression of PCR-generated DNA to produce protein product in one step (64). Similarly, Ziauddin et al. describe a strategy in which lawns of specific protein-expressing colonies of bacteria can be produced by localized transfection of expression vectors arrayed onto a glass surface (65). These approaches will allow the same panel of genes to be interrogated at both the DNA and protein levels in a high-throughput, microarray format.

Another interesting study employed modified chromatin immunoprecipitation to isolate the DNA-binding proteins, which were subsequently labeled and screened against DNA microarrays (66). Using this platform, the investigators were able to not only quantify all the DNA-binding proteins in yeast, but also localize their respective binding sites within the genome. As higher-density, human genomic arrays become available in the future, methods that can integrate the different microarray platforms will become a valuable tool in determining the function of the regulatory proteins in cancer (58).

SUMMARY

Although still in its early stages, microarray technology has already made a considerable impact in cancer biology. With the more global view of the molecular alterations that drive cancer progression, the scope of research has expanded from single genes or gene products to a more comprehensive hypothesis regarding molecular programs or pathways. The existing challenge is to integrate the individual platforms, and to consolidate the emerging data regarding these processes at the genome, transcriptome, and proteome levels.

Acknowledgment

This work was supported by the National Cancer Institute of Canada.

REFERENCES

1. Baltimore D. Our genome unveiled. Nature 2001;409:814–816.
2. Sachidanandam R, Weissman D, Schmidt SC, Kakol JM, Stein LD, Marth G, et al. A map of human genome sequence variation containing 1.42 million single nucleotide polymorphisms. Nature 2001;409:928–933.
3. Venter JC, Adams MD, Myers EW, Li PW, Mural RJ, Sutton GG, et al. The sequence of the human genome. Science 2001;291:1304–1351.
4. Shi MM. Enabling large-scale pharmacogenetic studies by high-throughput mutation detection and genotyping technologies. Clin Chem 2001;47:164–172.
5. Kleyn PW, Vesell ES. Genetic variation as a guide to drug development. Science 1998;281:1820–1821.
6. Hacia JG, Collins FS. Mutational analysis using oligonucleotide microarrays. J Med Genet 1999;36:730–736.
7. Pastinen T, Kurg A, Metspalu A, Peltonen L, Syvanen AC. Minisequencing: a specific tool for DNA analysis and diagnostics on oligonucleotide arrays. Genome Res 1997;7:606–614.
8. Fodor SP, Rava RP, Huang XC, Pease AC, Holmes CP, Adams CL. Multiplexed biochemical assays with biological chips. Nature 1993;364:555–556.
9. Chee M, Yang R, Hubbell E, Berno A, Huang XC, Stern D, et al. Accessing genetic information with high-density DNA arrays. Science 1996;274:610–614.
10. Lipshutz RJ, Fodor SP, Gingeras TR, Lockhart DJ. High-density synthetic oligonucleotide arrays. Nat Genet 1999;21:20–24.
11. Favis R, Day JP, Gerry NP, Phelan C, Narod S, Barany F. Universal DNA array detection of small insertions and deletions in BRCA1 and BRCA2. Nat Biotechnol 2000;18:561–564.
12. Favis R, Barany F. Mutation detection in K-ras, BRCA1, BRCA2, and p53 using PCR/LDR and a universal DNA microarray. Ann N Y Acad Sci 2000;906:39–43.
13. Lindblad-Toh K, Tanenbaum DM, Daly MJ, Winchester E, Lui WO, Villapakkam A, et al. Loss-of-heterozygosity analysis of small-cell lung carcinomas using single-nucleotide polymorphism arrays. Nat Biotechnol 2000;18:1001–1005.
14. Kallioniemi A, Kallioniemi OP, Sudar D, Rutovitz D, Gray JW, Waldman F, et al. Comparative genomic hybridization for molecular cytogenetic analysis of solid tumors. Science 1992;258:818–821.
15. Kallioniemi OP, Kallioniemi A, Sudar D, Rutovitz D, Gray JW, Waldman F, et al. Comparative genomic hybridization: a rapid new method for detecting and mapping DNA amplification in tumors. Semin Cancer Biol 1993;4:41–46.
16. Forozan F, Karhu R, Kononen J, Kallioniemi A, Kallioniemi OP. Genome screening by comparative genomic hybridization. Trends Genet 1997;13:405–409.
17. James LA. Comparative genomic hybridization as a tool in tumor cytogenetics. J Pathol 1999;187:385–395.
18. Parente F, Gaudray P, Carle GF, Turc-Carel C. Experimental assessment of the detection limit of genomic amplification by comparative genomic hybridization CGH. Cytogenet Cell Genet 1997;78:65–68.
19. Cheung VG, Nowak N, Jang W, Kirsch IR, Zhao S, Chen XN, et al. Integration of cytogenetic landmarks into the draft sequence of the human genome. Nature 2001;409:953–958.
20. Solinas-Toldo S, Lampel S, Stilgenbauer S, Nickolenko J, Benner A, Dohner H, et al. Matrix-based comparative genomic hybridization: biochips to screen for genomic imbalances. Genes, Chrom Cancer 1997;20:399–407.
21. Pinkel D, Segraves R, Sudar D, Clark S, Poole I, Kowbel D, et al. High-resolution analysis of DNA copy number variation using comparative genomic hybridization to microarrays. Nature Genet 1998;20:207–211.
22. Albertson DG, Ylstra B, Segraves R, Collins C, Dairkee SH, Kowbel D, et al. Quantitative mapping of amplicon structure by array CGH identifies CYP24 as a candidate oncogene. Nature Genet 2000;25:144–146.
23. Bruder CE, Hirvela C, Tapia-Paez I, Fransson I, Segraves R, Hamilton G, et al. High-resolution deletion analysis of constitutional DNA from neurofibromatosis type 2 (NF2) patients using microarray-CGH. Human Mol Genet 2001;10:271–282.
24. Daigo Y, Chin SF, Gorringe KL, Bobrow LG, Ponder BA, Pharoah PD, et al. Degenerate oligonucleotide primed-polymerase chain reaction-based array comparative genomic hybridization for extensive amplicon profiling of breast cancers: a new approach for the molecular analysis of paraffin-embedded cancer tissue. Amer J Pathol 2001;158:1623–1631.
25. Weber T, Weber RG, Kaulich K, Actor B, Meyer-Puttlitz B, Lampel S, et al. Characteristic chromosomal imbalances in primary central nervous system lymphomas of the diffuse large B-cell type. Brain Pathol 2000;10:73–84.
26. Geschwind DH, Gregg J, Boone K, Karrim J, Pawlikowska-Haddal A, Rao E, et al. Klinefelter's syndrome as a model of anomalous cerebral laterality: testing gene dosage in the X chromosome pseudoautosomal region using a DNA microarray. Dev Genet 1998;23:215–229.
27. Hui AB, Lo KW, Yin XL, Poon WS, Ng HK. Detection of multiple gene amplifications in glioblastoma multi-form using array-based comparative genomic hybridization. Lab Invest 2001;81:717–723.
28. Telenius H, Carter NP, Bebb CE, Nordenskjold M, Ponder BA, Tunnacliffe A. Degenerate oligonucleotide-primed PCR: general amplification of target DNA by a single degenerate primer. Genomics 1992;13:718–725.
29. Heiskanen MA, Bittner ML, Chen Y, Khan J, Adler KE, Trent JM, et al. Detection of gene amplification by genomic hybridization to cDNA microarrays. Cancer Res 2000;60:799–802.
30. Beheshti B, Braude I, Marrano P, Zielenska M, Squire JA. Survey of DNA amplifications in neuroblastoma tumors using cDNA microarrays. (In preparation).

31. Jones TA, Flomen RH, Senger G, Nizetic D, Sheer D. The homeobox gene MEIS1 is amplified in IMR-32 and highly expressed in other neuroblastoma cell lines. Eur J Cancer 2000;36: 2368–2374.
32. Pei J, Beheshti B, Squire JA, Zielenska M. cDNA array CGH analysis of pediatric osteosarcomas identifies regions of amplification on chromosome 17. (In preparation).
33. Pollack JR, Perou CM, Alizadeh AA, Eisen MB, Pergamenschikov A, Williams CF, et al. Genome-wide analysis of DNA copy-number changes using cDNA microarrays. Nature Genet 1999; 23:41–46.
34. Monni O, Barlund M, Mousses S, Kononen J, Sauter G, Heiskanen M, et al. Comprehensive copy number and gene expression profiling of the 17q23 amplicon in human breast cancer. Proc Natl Acad Sci U S A 2001;98:5711–5716.
35. El-Rifai W, Frierson HF, Jr., Harper JC, Powell SM, Knuutila S. Expression profiling of gastric adenocarcinoma using cDNA array. Int J Cancer 2001;92:832–838.
36. Chetcuti A, Margan S, Mann S, Russell P, Handelsman D, Rogers J, et al. Identification of differentially expressed genes in organ-confined prostate cancer by gene expression array. Prostate 2001; 47:132–140.
37. Chaib H, Cockrell EK, Rubin MA, Macoska JA. Profiling and verification of gene expression patterns in normal and malignant human prostate tissues by cDNA microarray analysis. Neoplasia 2001;3:43–52.
38. Zhang S, Day IN, Ye S. Microarray analysis of nicotine-induced changes in gene expression in endothelial cells. Physiol Genomics 2001;5:187–192.
39. Perou CM, Jeffrey SS, van de Rijn M, Rees CA, Eisen MB, Ross DT, et al. Distinctive gene expression patterns in human mammary epithelial cells and breast cancers. Proc Natl Acad Sci USA 1999;96:9212–9217.
40. Bittner M, Meltzer P, Chen Y, Jiang Y, Seftor E, Hendrix M, et al. Molecular classification of cutaneous malignant melanoma by gene expression profiling. Nature 2000;406:536–540.
41. Tapper J, Kettunen E, El-Rifai W, Seppala M, Andersson LC, Knuutila S. Changes in gene expression during progression of ovarian carcinoma. Cancer Genet Cytogenet 2001;128:1–6.
42. Miyazato A, Ueno S, Ohmine K, Ueda M, Yoshida K, Yamashita Y, et al. Identification of myelodysplastic syndrome-specific genes by DNA microarray analysis with purified hematopoietic stem cell fraction. Blood 2001;98:422–427.
43. Golub TR, Slonim DK, Tamayo P, Huard C, Gaasenbeek M, Mesirov JP, et al. Molecular classification of cancer: class discovery and class prediction by gene expression monitoring. Science 1999;286:531–537.
44. Zajchowski DA, Bartholdi MF, Gong Y, Webster L, Liu HL, Munishkin A, et al. Identification of gene expression profiles that predict the aggressive behavior of breast cancer cells. Cancer Res 2001;61:5168–5178.
45. Chen JJ, Peck K, Hong TM, Yang SC, Sher YP, Shih JY, et al. Global analysis of gene expression in invasion by a lung cancer model. Cancer Res 2001;61:5223–5230.
46. Wang W, Marsh S, Cassidy J, McLeod HL. Pharmacogenomic dissection of resistance to thymidylate synthase inhibitors. Cancer Res 2001;61:5505–5510.
47. Kannan K, Kaminski N, Rechavi G, Jakob-Hirsch J, Amariglio N, Givol D. DNA microarray analysis of genes involved in p53-mediated apoptosis: activation of Apaf-1. Oncogene 2001;20: 3449–3455.
48. Alon U, Barkai N, Notterman DA, Gish K, Ybarra S, Mack D, et al. Broad patterns of gene expression revealed by clustering analysis of tumor and normal colon tissues probed by oligonucleotide arrays. Proc Natl Acad Sci USA 1999;96:6745–6750.
49. Eisen MB, Spellman PT, Brown PO, Botstein D. Cluster analysis and display of genome-wide expression patterns. Proc Natl Acad Sci USA 1998;95:14863–14868.
50. Hilsenbeck SG, Friedrichs WE, Schiff R, O'Connell P, Hansen RK, Osborne CK, et al. Statistical analysis of array expression data as applied to the problem of tamoxifen resistance. J Natl Cancer Inst 1999;91:453–459.
51. Tamayo P, Slonim D, Mesirov J, Zhu Q, Kitareewan S, Dmitrovsky E, et al. Interpreting patterns of gene expression with self-organizing maps: methods and application to hematopoietic differentiation. Proc Natl Acad Sci USA 1999;96:2907–2912.
52. Tavazoie S, Hughes JD, Campbell MJ, Cho RJ, Church GM. Systematic determination of genetic network architecture. Nat Genet 1999;22:281–285.
53. Gygi SP, Han DK, Gingras AC, Sonenberg N, Aebersold R. Protein analysis by mass spectrometry and sequence database searching: tools for cancer research in the post-genomic era. Electrophoresis 1999;20:310–319.
54. Eggers M, Bader U, Enders G. Combination of microneutralization and avidity assays: improved diagnosis of recent primary human cytomegalovirus infection in single serum sample of second trimester pregnancy. J Med Virol 2000;60:324–330.
55. Brody EN, Gold L. Aptamers as therapeutic and diagnostic agents. J Biotechnol 2000;74:5–13.
56. Huang RP, Huang R, Fan Y, Lin Y. Simultaneous detection of multiple cytokines from conditioned media and patient's sera by an antibody-based protein array system. Anal Biochem 2001;294: 55–62.
57. Belov L, de la Vega O, dos Remedios CG, Mulligan SP, Christopherson RI. Immunophenotyping of leukemias using a cluster of differentiation antibody microarray. Cancer Res 2001; 61: 4483–4489.
58. Ge H. UPA, a universal protein array system for quantitative detection of protein–protein, protein–DNA, protein–RNA and protein–ligand interactions. Nucleic Acids Res 2000;28:e3.
59. MacBeath G, Schreiber SL. Printing proteins as microarrays for high-throughput function determination. Science 2000;289: 1760–1763.
60. Beheshti B, Vukovic B, Marrano P, Squire JA, Park PC. Resolution of genotypic heterogeneity in prostate tumors using DOP-PCR and CGH on microdissected carcinoma and PIN foci. Cancer Genet Cytogenet (in press 2002).
61. Rimm DL. Impact of microarray technologies on cytopathology. Overview of technologies and commentary on current and future implications for pathologists and cytopathologists. Acta Cytol 2001;45:111–114.
62. Kononen J, Bubendorf L, Kallioniemi A, Barlund M, Schraml P, Leighton S, et al. Tissue microarrays for high-throughput molecular profiling of tumor specimens. Nat Med 1998;4:844–847.
63. Simon R, Nocito A, Hubscher T, Bucher C, Torhorst J, Schraml P, et al. Patterns of Her-2/neu amplification and overexpression in primary and metastatic breast cancer. J Natl Cancer Inst 2001; 93:1141–1146.
64. He M, Taussig MJ. Single-step generation of protein arrays from DNA by cell-free expression and in situ immobilization (PISA method). Nucleic Acids Res 2001;29:E73–73.
65. Ziauddin J, Sabatini DM. Microarrays of cells expressing defined cDNAs. Nature 2001;411:107–110.
66. Ren B, Robert F, Wyrick JJ, Aparicio O, Jennings EG, Simon I, et al. Genome-wide location and function of DNA-binding proteins. Science 2000;290:2306–2309.

Chapter 33

Proteomic Approaches to Tumor Marker Discovery

Darryl Palmer-Toy, Scott Kuzdzal, and Daniel W. Chan

The discovery of tumor markers has progressed slowly during the last forty years. The traditional method for tumor marker discovery was to develop monoclonal antibodies against tumor cell extracts. This approach is time consuming and limited; however, new technologies are being developed that will accelerate the discovery process, particularly in the field of proteomics.

Proteomics, the natural successor to genomics, is the study of the protein products of the genes. Proteomics is protein science adapted for industrial scale, high-throughput, and massive parallelism. Facets of proteomics include

- the enumeration of gene expression, protein-by-protein/tissue-by-tissue/disease-by-disease;
- the identification of co- and post-translational modifications not explicitly encoded by the genes;
- the mapping of intermolecular interactions and biochemical networks; and
- the elucidation of three-dimensional structure and structure–activity relationships.

Proteomic techniques include gel electrophoresis and liquid chromatography, mass spectrometry, protein chips, and bioinformatics.

In this chapter we will focus on proteomics as applied to biomarker discovery. We first discuss the nature of proteomics, and then expand upon some of the tools that are used and the principles by which they work. Finally, we describe some successful applications of proteomic approaches to tumor marker discovery.

THE PROTEOME IN ONCOGENESIS

The dynamic spatial and temporal nature of protein expression is in dramatic contrast to the relatively stable and invariant genome of an individual's somatic cells. Protein expression is not only determined by cell lineage, but is influenced by environmental stimuli and the cell's physiologic history and state. Thus, each cell may have its own "proteome."

While the proteome is dynamic and individual proteins may be exported or recycled into constituent amino acids, most proteins are sufficiently stable to accumulate with sustained gene expression. In contrast, mRNA expression (the "transcriptome") steps up more rapidly, but is evanescent, and thus more faithfully mirrors instantaneous gene expression. In mathematical terms:

Proteome = $\int$ (gene expression(t) − protein catabolism and export) dt
Transcriptome = gene expression(t)

This distinction is important, not only because it explains the discrepancies noted experimentally between mRNA and protein expression [1,2], but also because it suggests that the proteome may be less perturbed than the transcriptome by the rigors of tissue collection and processing.

Although only a subset of genes may be expressed in any given cell, the complexity of the proteome is substantially greater than that of the genome. The one-gene-to-one-protein hypothesis has been refuted: one gene can give rise to multiple distinct mRNA transcripts or splice variants. Moreover, the distinct proteins encoded by each transcript are often subjected to co- and post-translational modifications [3,4]. These post-translational processes can alter the protein structure and function. Dozens of distinct chemical moieties can be added, modified, or removed, including carbohydrates, lipids, hydroxyl groups, methyl groups, and phosphates. These changes are constantly occurring. By regulating protein function in this manner, cells can rapidly and transiently activate signaling pathways and metabolic networks more readily than if *de novo* protein synthesis was required.

The modified forms of a given protein represent molecular diversity, that is, microheterogeneity (see Figure 1). Developing analytical methods capable of monitoring these changes is more challenging than simply verifying the expression of a given gene. Yet, most current tumor markers are glycoproteins, so the elucidation of such modifications will be crucial in the development of novel tumor markers.

The term "functional genomics" is sometimes used interchangeably with transcriptomics or proteomics. The functional aspects of proteomics fall into two categories: protein interaction mapping and structural proteomics. Although these areas are essential for the understanding of pathophysiology and pharmaceutical design, they play little role in the development of diagnostic markers and will be discussed only briefly.

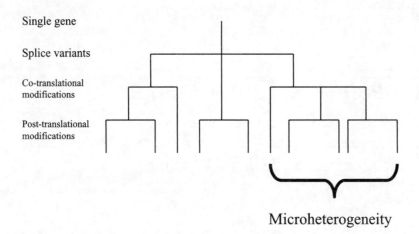

Figure 1 Demise of the one gene — one protein hypothesis.

Protein interaction mapping seeks to identify the myriad of biochemicals that bind to any given protein *in a physiologic context*. Among the tools commonly employed in these studies are yeast two-hybrid systems, co-precipitation, and affinity purification. The great challenge in this work is to overcome non-specific or non-physiologic binding.

Structural proteomics studies commonly utilize X-ray crystallography, nuclear magnetic resonance spectroscopy, circular dichroism, and molecular modeling. Three-dimensional protein structures are essential to determine structure–activity relationships and to understand protein function at the atomic level. Formerly, these studies were the major bottleneck in protein science. Now, these efforts have been brought to industrial scale by groups such as the Protein Structure Factory in Germany, and the Northeast Structural Genomics Consortium in North America. High-resolution structures for novel proteins are emerging on a daily basis. We refer the reader to some excellent reviews of protein interaction mapping (5,6) and structural proteomics (7,8).

TOOLS FOR PROTEOME ANALYSIS
Specimen Procurement

Tissue banks. Resected tumors, not surprisingly, have been the historic wellspring of tumor markers. Flow cytometric profiles and immunohistochemical phenotypes are routinely employed for diagnosing a tumor, identifying its tissue of origin, and sometimes even characterizing prognostic features. But many markers found in tumors or tumor-derived cell lines are dilute or non-existent in the serum, urine, CSF, or paraneoplastic effusions. As the emphasis shifts towards earlier diagnosis and even targeted chemoprevention, such fluids are under increased scrutiny.

Tissue banks are a booming business. As biotech entrepreneurs jump into proteomics, access to a well-curated tissue bank is highly prized. Yet, the homegrown collections upon which many academic researchers have built careers are often not up to the task. Lacking are sufficient clinical information, adequate preservation, and appropriate patient consent. The pillars of an ideal tissue bank are these:

- *Tissue harvested within 30 minutes of resection and snap-frozen in liquid nitrogen to preserve proteins and mRNA*. The tissues should be maintained thereafter at -60 °C to -70 °C. Even at dry ice temperatures some enzymatic activity may persist. Conventional freezers are much too warm. Those with "frost-free" operation actually intermittently cycle above 0 °C, which can reduce tissues to the consistency of a TV dinner.
- *Clinical information essential to specimen utilization*. Diseases, especially cancer, rarely reduce to binary states of present or absent. Tumors vary in type, grade, stage, treatment status, and treatment response. Even the choice of controls depends on the nature of the clinical question: e.g., healthy people, patients with benign conditions that mimic cancer, cancer patients post-successful treatment.
- *Paired sera and/or other bodily fluids for screening studies*. Markers are often easier to initially identify in tumor cells, but the real promise of early detection depends on their identification in easily accessible fluids. Also, some known tumor markers are elevated in the serum, yet are present at normal or reduced levels in tumor cells (e.g. PSA) (9). These, too, need to be aliquoted soon after collection, anonymously coded to link to the frozen tissue, and stored at -70 °C to -80 °C.
- *Linkage to genomic data*. This permits identification of allelic variation more readily than analysis of the proteins themselves, as will be explained below. Transcriptome data are invaluable in providing independent collaboration of gene up-regulation or down-regulation noted in protein expression studies, albeit with the caveats described earlier.
- *IRB approval and explicit patient consent*. Approval and consent have assumed even greater importance in the wake of the more aggressive stance the FDA has taken in recent years. Many investigators are questioning whether they will ever be able to use the collections that they have assembled over the years because they obtained general consent for then-unspecified medical research.

Microdissection. Tissue samples are generally obtained through gross examination and dissection of surgical specimens. Little more could be done to enhance the purity of solid tumor specimens, except for a few researchers with steely nerves and steady hands who would further dissect under the microscope. Recently, laser microdissection technology has put microdissection under direct visualization into the hands of the masses. Three methods are now widely available commercially:

- laser capture microdissection (LCM, Arcturus Corp., Mountain View, CA; *www.arctur.com*);
- laser microdissection (LMD; Leica Mikrosysteme Vertrieb GmbH, Bensheim, Germany; www.leica-microsystems.com/website/lms.nsf); and
- laser microbeam microdissection/laser pressure catapulting (LMM/LPC, P.A.L.M. Microlaser Technologies AG, Bernried, Germany; www.palm-mikrolaser.com)(10–11).

LCM employs an infrared (IR) laser to transiently and focally melt an ethylene vinyl acetate (EVA) thermoplastic film applied to a tissue section (see Figure 2). The user selects cells while observing through an inverted microscope. During the IR laser pulse, the EVA transfer film fuses with the underlying cells, which still adhere when the film is separated from the tissue section. The laser can be focused to melt a spot as small as 7.5 µm, and thousands of cells can be collected from a single frozen section. In most applications, the transfer film, which is mounted on an optically clear plastic cap, is subsequently immersed in a lysis buffer to extract soluble molecules from the captured cells and their microenvironment, and the lysate is used in further analysis. However, MALDI-ToF mass spectra can be collected directly from microdissected cells of interest (12).

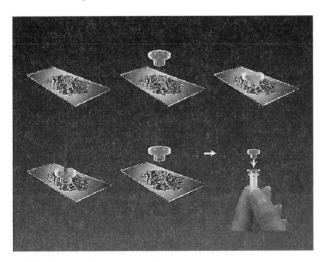

Figure 2 Steps in LCM: (1) User selects cells of interest through an inverted microscope and aligns laser with them. (2) An infrared (IR) laser transiently and focally melts an ethylene vinyl acetate (EVA) thermoplastic film attached to an optically clear plastic cap. The melted plastic fuses with the underlying cells of interest. (3) The cap is removed, with the cells adherent (© Arcturus Engineering, Inc., used with permission). **Color representation of figure appears on Color Plate 4.**

LMM/LPC uses an ultraviolet (UV) laser to literally carve out the cells of interest from surrounding tissue, and then physically project (catapult) them onto a cap by the pressure of the laser light. The catapulted tissue can range from one to several hundred µm in diameter, can be irregular in shape, and can be "touched-up" by laser ablation of unwanted cells. The LMD system is similar, except that an infrared (IR) laser is used to carve out the cells from an inverted slide. The microdissected cells simply drop into a collection vial. IR may have less detrimental effects on the DNA and RNA.

Cell sorters. The purification of hematopoetic tumor cells and other noncohesive tumor cells is considerably easier than the purification of solid tumor cells. Several methods of cell sorting are available; a few of the most common will be described here. In an important distinction to microdissection, these methods can yield viable cell populations.

Flow cytometers use a combination of specific labels to detect the cells of interest and electrostatic deflection of charged droplets for cell selection. The labels can be tagged antibodies to membrane proteins or compounds that directly interact with DNA. Labeled cells initially flow single-file in a liquid medium through a column that traverses the path of a laser beam. As the labeled cell intercepts the laser beam, light is scattered from the cell itself as well as from the labels. These signals determine whether or not a cell will be selected, based upon designated criteria. At the end of the column, high frequency vibrations break the cell stream into individual cell-containing droplets. A charge can be imparted to each droplet. An applied electrostatic field thereby determines the trajectory of the droplet. The deflection method of droplet manipulation is similar to that used in ink-jet printers. Since either a positive or negative charge can be imparted to the cell droplet, it is possible to sort two separate populations from the same sample.

Affinity purification is also widely used for cell sorting. The most common approach involves the covalent attachment of cell marker-specific antibodies to agarose beads, which are then packed into a column. The heterogeneous cell population is poured over the column, and non-adherent cells are washed free with a physiologic buffer. The cells of interest are subsequently eluted by washing the column with a buffer of high salt content. In a newer variant of this technique, the antibodies are linked to paramagnetic beads (Miltenyi Biotec GMBH, Bergisch Gladbach, Germany; http://www.miltenyibiotec.com). The labeled cells of interest are retained by a strong permanent magnet placed around the column. Removing the magnet allows the cells to be eluted. These affinity purification methods are equally applicable to proteins as they are to cells.

Protein Separations

2D-PAGE. Two-dimensional polyacrylamide gel electrophoresis (2D-PAGE) is still the standard way to separate protein mixtures for identification. Proteins are separated first in one direction according to their isoelectric point (pI), and then in a second direction according to their size. The result is an "electrophoretic map." Currently, 2D-PAGE technology can resolve up to 10,000 proteins with 2,000 proteins being somewhat routine (13). The separated proteins can be stably maintained in dried gels indefinitely. The parallelism of the second dimension separation is still unrivaled by other techniques. The proteins within the spots can be identified by immunolabeling (Western Blots) or recovered from the gel and sequenced by various methods.

There are, however, many limitations inherent to this technique. The time and effort involved in producing quality, consistent results is substantial. It is difficult to detect low abundance proteins, insoluble proteins, basic proteins, and either very small or very large proteins. Typically, only a few samples are run at a time, and each 2D gel can take days to prepare. But the recent interest in proteomics has spurred substantial progress in surmounting several of these limitations.

One step forward in the ease and reproducibility of 2-D PAGE has been the development of immobilized pH gradient (IPG) strips for isoelectric focusing (IEF) in the first dimension (14,15). The strips are commercially available, stable for months, and are available in various sizes and pH ranges spanning 7–24 cm and 1–9 pH units respectively. Electronic devices are available for rehydrating and running a dozen of these strips in an automated fashion overnight (Amersham-Pharmacia Biotech, Piscataway, NJ; *www.apbiotech.com*; Bio-Rad Laboratories, Hercules, CA; www.bio-rad.com). Similarly, commercially available units can run 12 large-format second dimension gels in parallel. The use of the 24 cm × 20 cm, one pH unit "zoom gel" effectively increases resolution 48-fold over a typical 7 cm × 10 cm, 7 pH unit "minigel." The gains in sensitivity can be significant if the pH range is chosen to exclude the most abundant proteins. Stains have also improved significantly in sensitivity and linearity, such that protein can routinely be detected over a range of 50 femtomoles to 50 picomoles with fluorescent stains (Molecular Probes, Inc., Eugene, OR; www.probes.com). A listing of 2D-PAGE equipment suppliers is available on line (http://www.the-scientist.com/images/yr2001/pdfs/lab_010402.pdf).

Many researchers also use preliminary fractionation in order to detect the low-abundance proteins and to provide subcellular localization. Newly developed solutions aid in the detection of insoluble proteins (16,17). For separating very large and very small proteins, modifications to the gel composition is often necessary. No one gel or protocol is capable of resolving all proteins.

HPLC and CE. An alternative to 2D gels is emerging in 2D high performance liquid chromatography (HPLC). In some 2D HPLC systems, the first dimension involves a liquid phase IEF separation or ion exchange, in which proteins are separated according to their pI. The second dimension separation by reversed phase HPLC is based on hydrophobicity. Unlike gels, where the proteins must be stained, excised, and then analyzed off-line by mass spectrometry, the proteins in the liquid phase of the HPLC eluent may be collected or introduced directly into online mass spectrometry detectors to determine the molecular weight of the intact proteins. The result is a 3-D mass map based upon pI vs. hydrophobicity vs. molecular weight. Some researchers have reported improved resolution of low mass and basic proteins using this approach (18).

Another variation on this theme involves the initial enzymatic digestion of the entire proteome into constituent peptides, which subsequently are resolved by 1D- or 2D HPLC, and then characterized by online mass spectrometry (19,20). Advances in enzyme immobilization and automation have made it possible to perform enzymatic digestions fairly rapidly using multidimensional LC. The trade-offs of this approach are the improved chromatographic and mass spectrometric resolution and sensitivity for peptides versus the tremendous increase in complexity, as scores of peptides can arise from a single protein. Although this approach reveals many more low abundance proteins than does a 2D gel approach, the relative abundances are obscured. Labeling strategies may help restore this abundance information (21).

The term capillary electrophoresis (CE) covers several modes of separation, all of which utilize electrical forces in capillary tubes for analytical purposes. CE has found applications throughout chemistry, pharmaceuticals, and biotechnology, with separations of both charged and uncharged species ranging in size from metal ions to proteins. The technique offers extremely high separation efficiencies with good reproducibility. Capillary isoelectric focusing (CIEF) as well as size-based separations is possible (22).

Spin columns are another alternative for size exclusion, charge, and affinity-based separation of small samples. The separations lack the resolution of the other methods described, but can be performed on the benchtop in minutes, and with low up-front cost (23,24).

Analysis

Edman degradation. Protein identification is becoming increasingly important because the identity of proteins is impossible to predict from gene sequence alone. Until recently, protein could be identified from gel spots only by electroblotting or eluting the protein or its constituent peptides from the gel, and then subjecting this material to amino acid sequencing via Edman degradation. Automated sequencers capable of picomole sensitivity, and runs of up to 50 amino acids for three proteins a day, are commercially available (Applied Biosystems, Foster City, CA ; www.appliedbiosystems.com). Although mass spectrometric "fingerprinting" strategies have largely replaced sequencing in most proteomic applications, sequencing is still a valuable alternative for identifying proteins from the many species with unsequenced genomes.

Mass spectrometry (MS). MS is playing an ever-increasing role in protein identification because of its specificity and sensitivity. Modern mass spectrometers can measure the molecular mass of both intact proteins and protein degradation products produced by either chemical or enzymatic digestions, and can do so with as little as tens of femtomoles of protein in microliter specimens (25). Mass spectrometers have three basic components: an ion source, an analyzer for sorting ions by mass-to-charge ratio (m/z), and a detector for counting the number of ions in each m/z interval. A list of mass spectrometer suppliers is available online (http://www.the-scientist.com/images/yr2001/pdfs/lab_010820.pdf).

Ion sources. Two ionization modes predominate in protein MS: matrix-assisted laser desorption/ionization (MALDI) and electrospray ionization (ESI). MALDI MS has rapidly emerged as the MS technique of choice for the rapid screening of molecular weights of peptides and proteins from gel spots. Analyte molecules are co-crystallized with an excess of small organic molecules known as the matrix, a process that takes minutes. The matrix serves to absorb the UV or IR laser energy, instantly desorbing and ionizing the analyte into gas phase molecular ions as the matrix decomposes into a plume of free radicals. In general, only singly charged molecular ions are produced and very little fragmentation occurs. This makes the method ideally suited for high molecular weight determinations and complex mixture analysis, even without prior separation or clean-up (26,27).

In ESI MS, a liquid sample is introduced into the spectrometer as a mist of charged droplets. As the droplets pass through a drying gas, solvent evaporates and the charge concentrates on the analyte molecules until the droplet explodes from electrostatic repulsion (see Figure 3). Analyte molecules generally form multiply charged ions, which enhances resolution, but necessitates data deconvolution to arrive at the actual molecular weight. For this reason, complex mixtures are difficult to analyze in this fashion. Fortunately, this ESI is well suited for online MS of chromatographic effluent, so individual analytes can be resolved prior to mass spectrometric analysis.

Mass analyzers. With time-of-flight (ToF) analysis, an electric field is applied to focus and accelerate all ions to a uniform kinetic energy. They then "fly" down an evacuated, field-free flight tube towards a detector. Smaller, more highly charged molecules travel faster than larger ones and masses can be determined by measuring their arrival time at the end of the flight tube. The m/z range of ToF instruments is theoretically infinite, while observation of m/z >100,000 is routine.

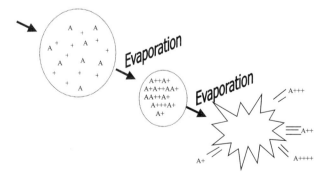

Figure 3 Electrospray microscopic view of electrospray ionization. Charged droplets of analyte molecule "A" pass through a drying gas. The solvent content of the droplet gradually evaporates until electrostatic repulsion causes the droplet to explode, releasing multiply multiply charged ions of A.

Multi-pole mass analyzers form a band pass filter, allowing only ions within a narrow m/z range to follow stable paths through the applied electromagnetic field. The m/z range of multi-pole mass analyzers typically runs to a few thousand, but this is sufficient to characterize proteins if they are highly charged. Multiple multi-pole analyzers are often arranged sequentially to form tandem mass spectrometers. Tandem mass spectrometers have a central collision cell, so that parent ions selected at the first multi-pole can be fragmented by striking gas molecules in the collision cell, and then the fragments can be analyzed by the final multi-pole. This is known as collision-induced dissociation (CID). Fragmentation is also possible on ToF instruments through a process known as post-source decay (PSD). Recently, quadrupole-ToF instruments have achieved great popularity for their high resolution and CID capabilities.

In ion trap MS, a high-frequency electric field is used to confine ions of interest. These ions are then separated and presented to a detector by adjusting the field so as to selectively induce path instability according to their respective mass/charge ratios. Their m/z range is as high as 12,000; this is considerably higher than that typically obtainable on a quadrupole instrument but lower than that achievable on a time-of-flight mass spectrometer (28).

Fourier transform (FT) instruments also trap ions in stable orbits within an electromagnetic field. In contrast to the other forms of MS described, FT detects ions not by having them impact a detector, but by measuring the m/z-dependent characteristic frequency radiated by each ion as they orbit. The m/z range is several thousand, but the real strength of FT-MS is the extreme resolution achieved.

Hybrid approaches. With traditional proteomics, different techniques are used to resolve, identify, quantify and characterize proteins. Attempts are being made to combine many of these steps into a single analysis format for rapid, reproducible, inexpensive screening. Gene chips are the inspiration for many of these approaches, yet the creation of protein chips has proven more challenging. These chips are intended for the rapid screening of complex samples to identify protein biomarkers as well as determine intermolecular interactions between specific proteins.

The complexities associated with creating a single array capable of analyzing every protein has caused protein chip manufacturers to "specialize." These specialties are of three distinct entities, although some overlap exists. The first group primarily uses activated surfaces to capture target proteins and then identify them with a mass spectrometer (e.g., Ciphergen, LumiCyte, Inc., Fremont, CA, www.lumicyte.com). A second group is focused on designing chips that will contain specific capture molecules for binding the target proteins (e.g., BIACore International AB, Uppsala, Sweden; *www.biacore.com*; Graffinity Pharmaceutical Design GMBH, Heidelberg, Germany, *www.graffinity.com*). A hybrid class of companies, (e.g., Luminex Corp., Austin, TX; www.luminexcorp.com) is focused on solution-phase approaches in attempt to avoid many of the problems the chip makers face with surface chemistry.

Ciphergen has developed ProteinChip® arrays to affinity-capture minute quantities of proteins via specific surface chemistries. Array surface chemistries include hydrophobic, hydrophilic, anionic, and cationic surfaces, as well as customizable surface for the binding of specific interacting molecules. Each aluminum array contains eight or more individual, chemically treated spots for sample application and mates with a 96-well "bioprocessor"; this set-up facilitates automated analysis of multiple samples in parallel. Samples are placed on each spot, and unbound material is washed away. Subsequent to sample clean-up, MALDI-ToF analysis is performed. Thus, this hybrid approach is termed Surface-Enhanced Laser Desorption/Ionization (SELDI). LumiCyte also employs SELDI.

BIACore chips start with the user attaching specific proteins of interest. Then complex mixtures of potentially interacting molecules are applied, and the kinetics of binding are monitored using surface plasmon resonance (SPR). Identification of bound ligands occurs with MALDI-ToF analysis of the same chip. Graffinity's Goldfinger' chips take the opposite approach, with immobilized ligands binding proteins in cell lysates and biological fluids. Their chips are also read using SPR.

Another company, Phylos, Inc. (Lexington, MA, www.phylos.com), has developed the Trinectin chip, an array of antibody-like capture proteins for specific target proteins. Capture proteins are developed as RNA–protein fusion molecules. This RNA–protein linkage permits amplification of highly interacting capture protein through PCR. Multiple cellular libraries have been constructed and utilized for protein:protein, protein:drug, and enzyme:substrate interaction mapping. High-affinity capture proteins have been used to create a micro-ELISA type protein affinity chip. This technology can work with multiple detection systems, including MS, fluorescence, and SPR.

Laboratory multi-analyte profiling (Luminex Corp., Austin, TX; www.luminexcorp.com) utilizes IR and optically coded beads that can be decorated with antibodies or other molecules. As each bead passes through a laminar flow system, each bead can be identified, and the binding status of the surface molecule can be determined. Up to 100 distinct bead-based assays can be performed in parallel in a homogeneous format.

Most diseases involve alterations in signaling or metabolic protein pathways. Most therapeutic drugs so far have targeted proteins or are proteins themselves. Thus, a better understanding of functional proteomics is necessary to improve the understanding of pathological processes, as well as to discover new disease-related markers or therapeutics. Hybrigenics (Paris, France; www.hybrigenics.com) has developed PIM (Protein Interaction Maps®) technology. Using genomic DNA from microbial pathogens or cDNA from normal or diseased tissues, Hybrigenics first identifies interacting proteins, and then reconstitutes functional signaling or metabolic pathways through high throughput yeast two-hybrid screening. The modulators (inhibitors or up-regulators) of these interactions area then identified.

Bioinformatics

Bioinformatics is the discipline that encompass all aspects of biological information acquisition, processing, storage, distribution, analysis, and interpretation. The Human Genome Project created immense amounts of data and sparked an interest in relational databases and tools to search them. Functional proteomics has extended the need for new informatics structures. Proteomic data include images of 2-D gels, chromatographs, 3-D molecular structures, and protein interaction maps. Several groups have been established to define and cre-

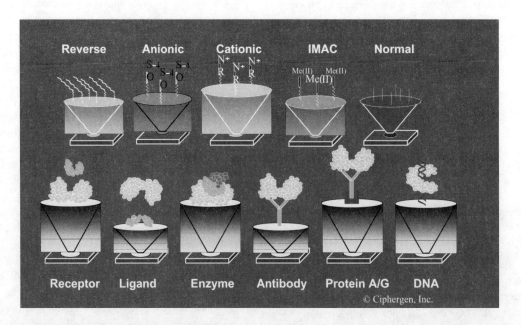

Figure 4 Surface chemistries available for Surface-Enhanced Laser Desorption/Ionization (SELDI) mass spectrometry using ProteinChip® arrays (Ciphergen Biosystems, Inc., used with permission). **Color representation of figure appears on Color Plate 4.**

ate key data models, analytical tools, and research applications for pathways-based discovery, such as the BioPathways Consortium and the National Biotechnology Directorate.

Bioinformatics also creates a need for disciplined cooperation. To make proteomics data available in a format that is easy to mine, steps must be taken to standardize both the collection of data and the compatibility of databases. Whereas research in the past has been performed in individual laboratories using different tools, research of the future will require much greater collaboration.

The use of bioinformatics to integrate and validate genomic data will be addressed more thoroughly elsewhere in this book (Chapter 11). Two bioinformatic-intensive proteomic applications will be discussed at length: peptide mass fingerprinting and protein profiling.

Peptide mass fingerprinting (PMF). PMF is the most commonly used strategy for protein identification by MS (see Figure 5). The protein of interest is usually isolated by cutting a spot or band from a gel. The protein is digested within the gel piece with a proteolytic enzyme (e.g., trypsin) and the mass spectrometer is used to measure masses of the peptides that are eluted. These masses can then be compared with databases of theoretical peptide fragments from known protein or gene sequence libraries. The closest match or matches are obtained by applying an appropriate statistical analysis.

PMF has several limitations. The process of in-gel digestion and peptide elution is inefficient, so only a small fraction of potential proteolytic fragments may be collected, and partial cleavages and unintended chemical modifications can occur. Moreover not every peptide eluted will "fly" in the mass spectrometer. Identification is often made with less than 20% of sequence coverage, but this requires using very stringent mass tolerance during database searching. Mass measurement accuracy is at least 0.1% with an externally calibrated high-quality MALDI-ToF instrument. This provides a mass uncertainty between 1 and 2 Da for a typical tryptic peptide. Accuracy can be increased to 0.01% or better if the spectrum contains a peak of known mass that can be used as an internal calibrant. For the human proteome, even 0.5 Da accuracy results in several thousand candidate peptides for a given mass. The popular PMF analysis software can usually surmount all of these obstacles (e.g. MS-FIT; Profound; PeptIdent).

When accurate mass assignments of peptide fragments do not provide enough information to unambiguously identify a protein, determination of partial amino acid sequences of the peptide fragments, with mass accuracy sufficient to distinguish between the amino acids, adds a much greater degree of specificity and confidence to database searching (29). Partial amino acid sequences can be determined from the tryptic peptides by CID or PSD. Automated commercial instruments (Ettan Amersham-Pharmacia Biotech, Piscataway, NJ; Proteome Works System BioRad, Hercules, CA), provide the means for "beginning-to-end" proteomic analysis. This system integrates sample processing, 2-D PAGE, image acquisition and analysis, spot picking, in-gel digestion, mass spectrometric analysis, and bioinformatics data processing.

Modern mass spectrometers allow the collection of mass spectra of peptides in microseconds. These instruments can analyze thousands of peptides per second. Modern computers can handle the required data acquisition, storage, and database searches. The field of chromatography, however, lacks the desired speed, and will be the rate-limiting step in proteomics (30)

Protein profiling. An important aspect of proteomics is identifying changes in the levels of protein expression in different tissues and cellular states. Variations in protein expression levels may be influenced by and correlated with disease states, treatment, cellular stress, genetic manipulation, or metabolic changes. Protein profiling efforts are underway towards distinguishing the proteins of normal cells from early-stage cancer cells, and more indolent cancer cells from those with high metastatic potential. Obtaining "protein profiles" of various cells in different disease states may provide a better understanding of protein function, and eventually physiology.

Another important emphasis is on profiling bodily fluids in persons afflicted by various diseases. This poses additional challenges as the proteins of interest may be quite dilute, and may not even correlate with the levels in the affected cells. Still, such fluids offer the greatest utility in cancer screening.

Among the significant technical challenges in profiling studies are the immense dynamic range of protein abundances, the inability to unambiguously identify proteins by intact molecular weight, and limits of instrument resolution. Across the range of conventional analytes in serum, concentrations range from mM (e.g., albumin) to sub-pM (e.g., PTH)—ten orders of magnitude! No single analytic approach could effectively address this range of abundances without prefractionation, so biomarker identification must correlate information from several experiments for each sample.

The identification and resolution issues are linked, but not identical. The abundance of C, H, O, N, and S isotopes is sufficient that most proteins will contain a few heavy isotopes on average, but any given molecule may contain from none to several. This creates a "picket fence" pattern split at 1 Da (hydrogen → deuterium) or less that is further split by the microheterogeneity of the protein. Even high-end MALDI-ToF instruments have a resolution >50 ppm, so at molecular weight

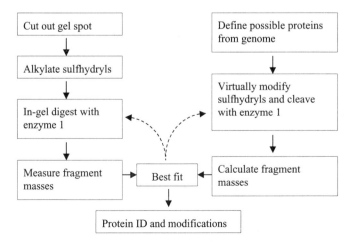

Figure 5 Peptide mass fingerprinting (PMF).

>20,000 Da, this picket fence becomes a broad hump that defies detection of point mutations or changes in glycosylation or phosphorylation. Biomarker identification becomes the recognition of peaks or other gross spectral features.

PROTEOMICS IN ACTION

As a few recent reviews have surveyed the application of proteomics to cancer diagnosis (31–33), we will focus on an example from our own laboratory.

Chronic lymphocytic leukemia (CLL) is the most common form of leukemia in the western hemisphere, accounting for approximately 25–30% of all leukemias. Although the etiology of CLL is unknown, recent laboratory investigations have improved our knowledge of this disorder. CLL is a slow growth of malignant B-lymphocytes that have an extended life span. Patients with CLL may develop serious infections because of reduced numbers of infection-fighting neutrophils.

There is a scarcity of data on protein modifications related to the malignant behavior of hematologic malignancies, including CLL. This is partly due to technical difficulties in the purification and identification of small amounts of protein, which in contrast to nucleic acid, cannot be readily amplified. Voss and coworkers compared the protein expression patterns obtained by two-dimensional gel electrophoresis with clinical features in human B-cell chronic lymphocytic leukemia (34). Proteins capable of distinguishing patient groups with defined chromosomal characteristics were identified.

We applied SELDI to a series of cases of CLL and other lymphoproliferative disorders previously characterized by four-color flow cytometry (35). Whole blood specimens were lysed, extracted with triton X100R, and applied to selective protein chips. Nine cases of typical CLL (CD191, CD201dim, CD51, CD231); two cases of atypical CLL expressing bright CD20 and/or CD79b, but positive for CD5 and CD23; and one case of a CD5-negative B-cell lymphoproliferative disorder were analyzed along with 8 samples of normal peripheral blood and 2 samples of flow-sorted CD19-positive normal B cells.

SELDI MS was used to rapidly determine the molecular weights of sample proteins using as few as 2×10^5 cells. Two SELDI chip surfaces were used: Normal Phase (NP1 and NP2) chips, which represent a hydrophilic general binding surface, and Immobilized Metal Affinity Capture chips, (IMAC) isolating proteins with metal binding residues. Following the application of a sample, the chip surface was washed under selective conditions, and analyzed by SELDI. Aliquots of either normal peripheral blood or flow-sorted CD19+ normal B cells were similarly treated. Numerous protein peaks in the molecular weight region between 1 and 300 kD were observed in both patient samples and normal peripheral blood. However, the comparison of protein profiles of chronic lymphocytic leukemia and normal peripheral blood revealed three unique peaks that were observed exclusively in the leukemic samples. These peaks were located at 11.3, 13.8, and 14.0 kD (see Figure 6).

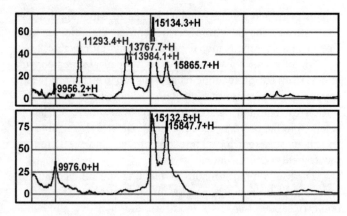

Figure 6 Comparison of protein profiles of CLL patient (top) to normal control patient (bottom). Peaks that represent potential biomarkers are evident at 11.3, 13.8, and 14.0 kD.

Subsequently, the protein profiles of chronic lymphocytic leukemia were compared to those of flow-sorted CD19-positive peripheral blood lymphocytes, which confirmed that the peaks described above were present exclusively in B-cell lymphoproliferative disorders (see Figure 7). Efforts are currently underway to identify these biomarkers.

FUTURE DIRECTIONS

As these exciting proteomic tools advance and improve, new tumor markers will be discovered at a fairly rapid pace. Individual tumor markers will be better than the current tumor markers in terms of clinical sensitivity and specificity. More importantly, a panel or a profile of markers will be used to enhance the sensitivity and specificity for cancer detection at an earlier stage. At this earlier stage of tumor development, removal of the tumor will be more likely to cure the patient or at least increase his/her survival. New tumor markers will provide better predictive value for selecting appropriate therapies. Cancer classifications will change from being based on morphology to being based on genomic or proteomic profiling.

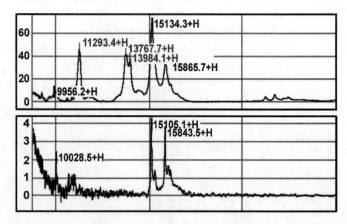

Figure 7 Protein profiles of chronic lymphocytic leukemia (top) and flow-sorted CD19-positive peripheral blood lymphocytes (bottom).

This disease classification will be more accurate and precise. Bioinformatics will be important in integrating tumor marker values and/or profiles with clinical information to achieve better diagnostic outcomes. In addition, new drug targets will be discovered using proteomic techniques. Tumor markers would be used to determine the efficacy and monitoring the use of these new drugs. In summary, significant improvements in the values of tumor markers will lead to the increased use of tumor markers in the detection of cancer and in the selection and monitoring of cancer therapies.

REFERENCES

1. Anderson L and Seilhamer J. A comparison of selected mRNA and protein abundances in human liver. Electrophoresis 1997;18: 533–537.
2. Gygi SP, Rochon Y, Franza BR, Aebersold R. Correlation between protein and mRNA abundance in yeast. Mol Cell Biol 1999;19: 1720–1730.
3. Krishna R, Wold F. Posttranslational modifications. In: Angeletti R, ed. Proteins. San Diego, California: Academic Press, 1998; 126–132.
4. Kivirikko K, Myllyla R, Philajaniemi T. Kivirikko K, Myllyla R, Philajaniemi T. Hydroxylation of proline and lysine residues in collagens and other animal and plant proteins. In: Harding J, Crabbe M, eds. Post-translational modification of proteins. Boca Raton, FL: CRC Press, 1992;1–51.
5. Tucker CL, Gera JF, Uetz P. Towards an understanding of complex protein networks. Trends Cell Biol 2001;11:102–106.
6. Legrain P, Wojcik J, Gauthier JM. Protein–protein interaction maps: a lead towards cellular functions. Trends Genet 2001;17: 346–352.
7. Teichmann SA, Murzin AG, Chothia C. Determination of protein function, evolution, and interactions by structural genomics. Curr Opin Struct Biol 2001;11:354–363.
8. Heinemann U, Frevert J, Hofmann K, Illing G, Maurer C, Oschkinat H, Saenger W. An integrated approach to structural genomics. Prog Biophys Mol Biol 2000;73(5):347–362.
9. Stege RH, Tribukait B, Carlstrom KA, Grande M, Pousette AH. Tissue PSA from fine-needle biopsies of prostatic carcinoma as related to serum PSA, clinical stage, cytological grade, and DNA ploidy. Prostate 1999;38(3):183–188.
10. Emmert-Buck MR, Gillespie JW, Paweletz CP, Ornstein DK, Basrur V, Appella E, Wang QH, Huang J, Hu N, Taylor P, Petricoin EF III. An approach to proteomic analysis of human tumors. Mol Carcinog 2000;27(3):158–165.
11. Schütze K, Lahr G. Identification of expressed genes by laser-mediated manipulation of single cells. Nat Biotechnol 1998; 16(8):737–742.
12. Palmer-Toy DE, Sarracino DA, Sgroi D, LeVangie R, Leopold PE. Direct acquisition of matrix-assisted laser desorption/ionization time-of-flight mass spectra from laser-capture microdissected tissues. Clin Chem 2000;46:1513–1516.
13. Klose, J., Kobalz, U. Two-dimensional electrophoresis of proteins: an updated protocol and implications for a functional analysis of the genome. Electrophoresis 1995;16:1034–1059.
14. Righetti PG, Bossi A. Isoelectric focusing in immobilized pH gradients: recent analytical and preparative developments. Anal Biochem 1997;247:1–10.
15. Gorg A, Obermaier C, Boguth G, Harder A, Scheibe B, Wildgruber R, Weiss W. The current state of two-dimensional electrophoresis with immobilized pH gradients. Electrophoresis 2000;21:1037–1053.
16. Molloy MP, Herbert BR, Walsh BJ, Tyler MI, Traini M, Sanchez JC, Hochstrasser DF, Williams KL, Gooley AA. Extraction of membrane proteins by differential solubilization for separation using two-dimensional gel electrophoresis. Electrophoresis 1998; 19:837–844.
17. Rabilloud T. Use of thiourea to increase the solubility of membrane proteins in two-dimensional electrophoresis. Electrophoresis 1998;19:758 760.
18. Wall DB, Kachman MT, Gong S, Hinderer R, Parus S, Misek DE, Hanash SM, Lubman DM. Isoelectric focusing nonporous RP HPLC: a two-dimensional liquid-phase separation method for mapping of cellular proteins with identification using MALDI-TOF mass spectrometry. Anal Chem 2000;72:1099–1111.
19. Wagner K, Racaityte K, Unger KK, Miliotis T, Edholm LE, Bischoff R, Marko-Varga G. Protein mapping by two-dimensional high performance liquid chromatography. J Chromatogr A 2000;893:293–305.
20. Washburn MP, Wolters D, Yates III JR. Large-scale analysis of the yeast proteome by multi-dimensional protein identification technology. Nat Biotechnol 2001;19:242–247.
21. Gygi SP, Rist B, Gerber SA, Turecek F, Gelb MH, Aebersold R. Quantitative analysis of complex protein mixtures using isotope-coded affinity tags. Nat Biotechnol 1999;17:994–999.
22. Righetti PG, Gelfi C, Conti M. Current trends in capillary isoelectric focusing of proteins. J Chromatogr B Biomed Sci Appl 1997;699:91–104.
23. Moy FJ, Haraki K, Mobilio D, Walker G, Powers R, Tabei K, Tong H, Siegel MM. MS/NMR: a structure-based approach for discovering protein ligands and for drug design by coupling size exclusion chromatography, mass spectrometry, and nuclear magnetic resonance spectroscopy. Anal Chem. 2001;73:571–581.
24. Hoyt PR, Doktycz MJ, Warmack RJ, Allison DP. Spin-column isolation of DNA-protein interactions from complex protein mixtures for AFM imaging. Ultramicroscopy 2001;86:139–143.
25. Yates JR. J. Mass spectrometry and the age of the proteome. Mass Spectrom 1998;33:1–19.
26. Yates JR, Link AJ, Schleitz D. Direct analysis of proteins in mixtures. In: Chapman JR, ed. Methods in molecular biology, vol. 146: Mass spectrometry of proteins and peptides. Totowa, NJ: Humana Press, 2000;17–26.
27. Leopold PE, Palmer-Toy DE, Sarracino DA. A data analysis method to identify complex protein mixtures using MALDI-ToF mass spectroscopy. Protein Science 1999;8:155.
28. Haynes PA, Yates JR. Proteome profiling—pitfalls and progress. Yeast 2000;17:81–87.
29. Cao P, Moini M. Capillary electrophoresis/electrospray ionization high mass accuracy time-of-flight mass spectrometry for protein identification using peptide mapping. Rapid Commun Mass Spectrom 1998;12:864–870.
30. Regnier F, Amini A, Chakraborty A, Geng M, Ji J, et al. Multidimensional chromatography and the signature peptide approach to proteomics. LCGC 2001;19:200–212.
31. Hochstrasser DF. Clinical and biomedical applications of proteomics. In: Wilkins MR, Williams KL, Appel RD, Hochstrasser DF, eds. Proteome research: new frontiers in functional genomics. Berlin: Springer Verlag, 1997;187–219.

32. Alaiya AA, Franzén B, Auer G, Linder S. Cancer proteomics. Electrophoresis 2000;21:1210–1217.
33. Simpson RS, Dorow DS. Cancer proteomics: from signaling networks to tumor markers. Trends Biotech 2001;19:S40–S48.
34. Voss T, Ahorn H, Haberl P, Dohner H, Wilgenbus K. Correlation of clinical data with proteomics profiles in 24 patients with B-cell chronic lymphocytic leukemia. Int J Cancer 2001;91: 180–186.
35. Kuzdzal SA, Silverman BC, Zoltani ZA, Czader M, Borowitz MJ, Chan DW. Identification of biomarkers for chronic lymphocytic leukemia by surface-enhanced laser desorption/ionization mass spectrometry. Clin Chem 2001;47:A137.

Chapter **34**

Tumor Marker Discovery Using Large-Scale DNA Microarray Analysis

Garret M. Hampton, John B. Welsh, and Henry F. Frierson, Jr.

Large-scale expression profiling methods, such as DNA microarray hybridization analysis and serial analysis of gene expression (SAGE), provide new and effective ways to discover and catalog the transcriptional changes that occur in neoplastic cells (see Chapter 32 and Reference *1*). Here, we focus on DNA microarray experiments, and present general approaches that can be used to interrogate these very large datasets to systematically discover genes whose aberrant expression may aid in tumor diagnosis. We highlight the identification of several genes whose expression appears to be consistently elevated in ovarian and prostate carcinomas, and whose protein products may be detectable in the serum of cancer patients. We also describe studies that begin to construct a molecular classification of human cancer that may augment traditional histopathological analyses for more accurate cancer diagnosis.

TUMOR MARKER DISCOVERY

Identification of Candidate Genes by Analysis of Differential Gene Expression

Perhaps the simplest approach toward the systematic identification of potential tumor markers for clinical diagnosis is to uncover those genes whose expression is elevated in a majority of cancers from a specific anatomic site and low or absent in corresponding normal and other adult tissues. For the identification of serologic diagnostic candidates, it is clearly important to seek evidence that the protein product encoded by the candidate gene of interest is secreted or cleaved from the surface of expressing cells, based either on the known function of the protein, or on its sequence characteristics. Genes that are known or suspected to encode secreted proteins can be strongly favored in schemes that rank candidates that have clinically useful potential.

The choice of metrics used to describe a gene's differential expression in tumor tissue depends on the goals of the study. If the goal is to establish that a molecular distinction exists between a group of normal and a group of tumor samples, there is no explicit reason to select genes that are more highly expressed in malignancy and expressed at near-zero levels in normal tissues. Statistically, genes that best distinguish normal from tumor do not necessarily encode potential tumor markers, since many of them are expressed more highly in normal tissue rather than in neoplastic cells.

We have empirically developed an algorithm that identifies candidate marker genes based on their near-uniform overexpression in a set of tumors compared to normal counterpart tissues. In this metric, the expression levels of each gene in the normal (N) and tumor (T) populations are first compared in an unpaired *t*-test. The difference between mean hybridization values (T–N) and the quotient of mean hybridization values (T/N) are then calculated for each gene. Each of these parameters is ranked, with favorable ranks assigned to genes with low *p* scores, high T/N quotients, and high T–N differences; the final agglomerative ranking is based on the sum of these three component ranks (see legend to Figure 1). Although we specifically developed this approach for the analysis of oligonucleotide microarrays, the same general approaches can be used for the analysis of SAGE data and, to an extent, with cDNA microarray data.

In an expression profiling study of ovarian serous papillary adenocarcinoma, the metric described above identified consistent overexpression of several genes including *HE4*, whose product is a secreted protein (*2*), and whose overexpression in ovarian cancer has been previously documented (*3,4*). With one exception, we have found *HE4* to be expressed at levels ~20-fold higher than normal in each of 53 ovarian cancers examined. HE4 was originally isolated from human epididymis, and may play a role in sperm maturation (*5*). The gene is not significantly expressed in a panel of normal adult female tissues (Figure 2). If high and specific expression of *HE4* mRNA in ovarian neoplasms leads to corresponding differential protein expression, HE4 may find use as a serological marker for the diagnosis or monitoring of ovarian cancer.

In a subsequent analysis of the same ovarian tumor RNAs using Affymetrix U95A GeneChips, our hybrid metric for differential expression selected the carcinoma-associated antigen *TACSTD1* as the most highly ranked gene (Figure 1A and 1B). *TACSTD1* is widely expressed in many carcinomas, and has been used as an RT-PCR marker for the detection of micrometastatic breast cancers in peripheral blood and bone (*6*). *HE4* was again highly ranked, as were two other genes encoding secreted proteins, secretory leukocyte protease inhibitor (SLPI) and agrin (AGRN). SLPI is widely expressed

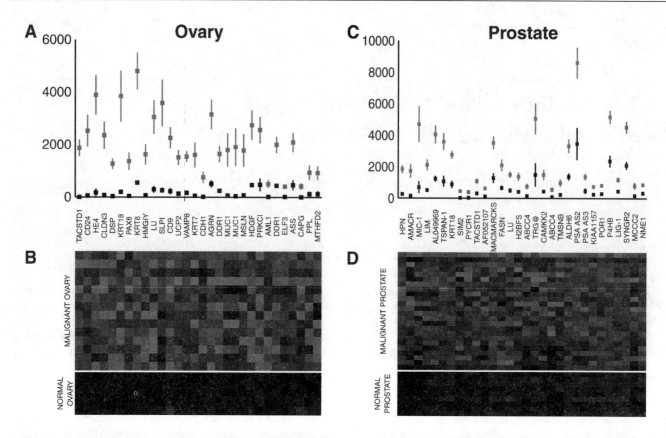

Figure 1 Expression of selected genes in normal and malignant tissue samples from ovary (A and B) and prostate (C and D). Thirty genes from each tissue type were selected for high differential expression in malignant compared to normal counterpart tissue. Ranking is based on a combined score that favors genes with large tumor (T) vs. normal (N) quotients, large T vs. N differences, and small *p* values in an unpaired t test (2). In A and C, the mean and 95% confidence interval for hybridization intensities (ordinate) is shown in a series of 30 genes in malignant (red) and normal (black) samples. In B and D, the expression level of each gene (column) in each normal and malignant sample (row) corresponds to the brightness of each square; high expression levels are shown as relatively bright red squares. **Color representation of figure appears on Color Plate 5.**

in mucous fluids and is elevated in the peritoneal fluid and serum of women with endometriosis (7). The protein may function normally in mucosal defense against infections and in cutaneous wound healing (8). Such evidence of SLPI distribution and function count against it as a potential marker for ovarian cancer diagnosis. Agrin is a glycoprotein secreted from motor neurons, participating in the aggregation of acetylcholine receptors at the neuromuscular junction, and has recently been identified as an antigen expressed by a lung cancer cell line (9). Many of the other genes that were identified in our analysis of serous ovarian carcinomas have also recently been observed using SAGE analysis of a limited number of ovarian tumors, validating their differential expression (3). The authors of the SAGE study highlight several genes whose protein products are secreted from expressing cells including ceruloplasmin, glutathione peroxidase 3, and ApoJ (clusterin). One of these genes, ceruoloplasim, was identified in our analyses of ovarian carcinomas, but not highly ranked by our metric (see Section 1.2, below).

Prostate carcinoma is another neoplasm in which expression profiling has identified genes whose protein products may have importance in clinical diagnosis (10,11). In our study of malignant prostate tissue (12), we ranked genes according to their absolute expression levels as described above. Several genes showed near-zero expression in normal tissues and high expression in most or all of the cancer tissues (Figure 1C and 1D). We highlight two such genes, *MIC-1* and *hepsin*, as especially promising candidate tumor markers.

The secreted protein macrophage inhibitory cytokine 1 (MIC-1) was ranked very highly by our metric for overexpression in malignancy. The transcript for MIC-1 (variably called PLAB, PDF, PTGF-beta, or GDF15) was overexpressed in 21 of 24 prostate cancer tissue samples by microarray analysis, and was confirmed independently by RT-PCR in several randomly selected tumors. MIC-1 belongs to the transforming growth factor-α superfamily of proteins, and its expression is generally low in tissues throughout the human body, with the exception of the placenta in which its role in pregnancy has been investigated. Using a sensitive sandwich ELISA assay, Moore et al. (13) recently demonstrated high levels of the MIC-1 protein in the sera of pregnant women (increasing with gestation), as well as in amniotic fluid. The authors suggest that MIC-1 may suppress the production of maternally derived proinflammatory cytokines within the uterus during pregnancy. Because of the generally restricted tissue expression of MIC-1, and its near-consistent overexpression in prostate cancer samples, this protein can now be investigated as a potential adjunct to PSA in serum tests for prostate cancer.

Several other gene products that were overexpressed in prostate cancer encode transmembrane proteins, which may exist in the serum of cancer patients as proteolytic fragments and have potential as tumor markers. For example, *hepsin*, encoding a type II transmembrane serine protease, was overexpressed in all of the 24 prostate cancers that we examined. A previous study noted its overexpression in ovarian cancer (14), and it has also been found to be uniformly overexpressed in an independent series of prostate cancer tissues (10). On average, *hepsin* is expressed ~7-fold higher in tumors than in normal prostate tissue, and RT-PCR has shown very low or absent expression in normal prostate samples. Expression of hepsin normally occurs in the liver, and to a lesser extent in the kidney and pancreas. The enzyme is similar to the androgen-dependent type II transmembrane-bound serine protease, TMPRSS2, whose expression is high in prostate secretory epithelial cells (15). Through autocatalytic cleavage, the extracellular protease domain of TMPRSS2 is released from prostate cancer cells (16), suggesting that fragments of TMPRSS2 may be detectable in the sera of prostate cancer patients. Autocatalysis has also been reported for hepsin (17), and it is possible that its protease domain is also released into the extracellular space. The value of hepsin as a potential diagnostic marker can be evaluated after the development of antibodies to the extracellular domain of the protein.

Expression of Candidate Diagnostic Markers in Human Tissues

An important consideration in selecting genes for further workup as tumor markers is their expression level in normal human tissues. Ideally, a candidate diagnostic molecule would be entirely specific to the tumor of interest, with low or absent expression in normal counterpart tissue and most normal tissues as well. The development of databases that contain information on the expression of thousands of unique genes in most normal human tissues has been initiated at the Genomics Institute of the Novartis Research Foundation (GNF). These databases, which are publicly available at http://expression.gnf.org, provide a reference for the expression of a large number of genes in most human tissues. As an example of its use, we considered the expression level of 30 genes overexpressed in ovarian cancer (shown in Figure 1) in a panel of 18 normal non-ovarian tissues (Figure 2). Several genes that discriminate well between normal and malignant ovarian tissues are expressed at high levels by many non-ovarian tissues, potentially confounding their use as diagnostics. Although very few genes are entirely specific to malignant ovary, their expression in some normal tissues may be irrelevant (in the case of TACSTD1 expression in testis); in other cases, a potential tumor marker's expression pattern preclude its use as a diagnostic molecule entirely.

Our human tissue database, or other analogous databases, can be used in a more rigorous manner by applying ranking schemes that select against genes whose expression is high in normal tissues. Re-analysis of our ovarian data with additional selective criteria for low expression in non-ovarian tissues iden-

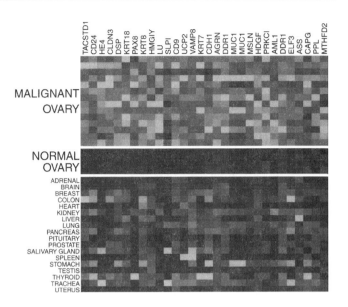

Figure 2 Gene expression in normal and malignant ovarian tissues compared to normal extra-ovarian tissues. Genes (in columns) were ranked for differential expression in malignant (upper rows) and normal (middle rows) ovarian tissues as in Figure 1. Expression levels in a panel of normal tissues (bottom rows) are shown for comparison. **Color representation of figure appears on Color Plate 5.**

tified genes that are highly tissue-specific, but elevated in only a proportion of tumors (Figure 3). These genes are lowly expressed in normal ovary and in a panel of normal tissues, but their elevation in ovarian tumors is not as high or as uniform as the genes depicted in Figure 1A and 1B, suggesting increased specificity at the cost of decreased diagnostic sensitivity.

The decreased sensitivity of individual gene products suggested by Figure 3 is a relative disadvantage; however, elevations in one or more of a panel of gene products may provide better predictive accuracy than elevations of single gene products. For example, it has been noted that carefully chosen com-

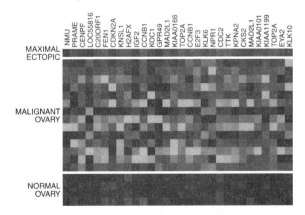

Figure 3 Gene expression in normal and malignant ovarian tissues compared to maximal expression in a panel of normal extra-ovarian tissues. Genes (in columns) were ranked for differential expression in malignant ovarian tissues (middle rows) compared to normal ovarian tissues (bottom rows). Genes whose maximal expression in a panel of normal extra-ovarian tissues was high were penalized in the ranking scheme, resulting in generally low "maximal ectopic" expression (upper row). **Color representation of figure appears on Color Plate 5.**

binations of diagnostic tests for ovarian cancer improves diagnostic sensitivity (18,19). Among the set of genes identified by this approach and shown in Figure 3 are kallikreins 6 and 10 (KLK6 and KLK10), both of which are elevated in serum of some ovarian cancer patients and have been suggested as novel serological biomarkers of this disease (20,21). Elevated expression was also detected from the neuromedin U (NMU) gene, which encodes a secreted neuropeptide, and IGF-2, which is over-expressed in many malignant ovarian tumors (22), and which may protect ovarian cancer cells from apoptosis (23). A combination of serological assays for several of these proteins, including KLK6, KLK10, and HE4, for example, may be useful for detecting serous papillary carcinoma of the ovary. Additional analyses, however, are required to determine whether these potentially diagnostic candidate genes are expressed in other tumor types, or whether they are ovary-specific (see "Molecular Classification of Human Cancer," below).

Similar approaches to those discussed above can be facilitated by public databases. For example, tools within the National Center for Bioinformatics Cancer Genome Anatomy Project (cgap.nci.nih.gov) allow the user to identify genes whose expression is elevated in cancer specimens and low or absent in normal human tissues. This database has been used by others to identify candidate brain tumor markers that were subsequently validated by fluorescent-PCR expression comparison (24), and to identify differentially expressed ESTs from carcinomas that were subsequently validated by RT-PCR (25).

Use of Ancillary Data to Enrich for Secreted Proteins

Thus far, we have highlighted the use of algorithms to rank genes based on their expression in tumors relative to normal tissues, without regard to the encoded protein's function or subcellular localization. As secreted or transmembrane proteins are more likely to appear in the serum than proteins constrained to the intracellular space, we have begun to select genes based on the subcellular localization of their products.

The Gene Ontology (GO) consortium (www.geneontology.org) is a vehicle that describes proteins in terms of their biological role, molecular function, and cellular compartment (26). Compugen (www.cgen.com) assigns vocabulary terms to gene products based on sequence databases, the Medline database, and proprietary software for protein subcellular localization. We have applied the GO annotations to genes on the Affymetrix high-density microarrays, and selected "cellular compartment" terms that imply secretion into the extracellular space. The GO attribute "extracellular," for example, applies to 574 genes represented on the U95a microarray. In this way, we can limit our attention to a much smaller set of genes that likely encode secreted proteins; these genes are then sorted based on their tissue expression levels. Figure 4 shows genes that carry one or more annotations that imply extracellularity and show overexpression in ovarian tumor tissue compared to normal.

As expected, the list of genes shown in Figure 4 is enriched for ones encoding authentic secreted proteins, for example SLPI (secretory leukocyte protease inhibitor), SPP1 (osteopontin),

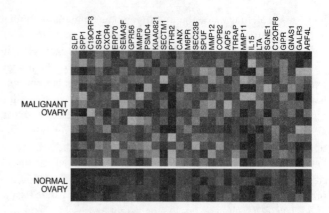

Figure 4 Gene expression in malignant (upper rows) and normal (lower rows) ovarian tissues. Only genes with annotations suggesting extracellularity of their encoded proteins were ranked. Genes were ranked for differential expression as in Figure 1. **Color representation of figure appears on Color Plate 6.**

and SEMA3F (semaphorin). However, not all of the genes encode secreted proteins (such as GPR56 (G-protein coupled receptor-56) and PTHR2 (parathyroid hormone receptor 2), perhaps because the term "extracellular" as applied by the GO consortium refers to only a portion of the encoded molecule. A second observation is that these methods identify very few genes whose expression is convincingly elevated in the majority of tumors; nonetheless, the most highly ranked genes are expressed in very few body tissues and are potentially attractive candidates if they could be used in combination with one another. Third, based on literature reports, annotation-based approaches do not identify all of the proteins that are secreted from expressing cells. The development of bioinformatic approaches to formally evaluate the presence of relevant motifs within the translated amino acid sequences of interrogated genes will be necessary to comprehensively identify genes of interest. At this juncture, we suggest a combination of approaches, such as ranking genes based on body tissue expression, ranking pre-selected genes based on their associated annotations, and considering a combination of both groups as candidate genes.

Functional selection and subsequent profiling of mRNAs that are bound to membrane-associated polysomes is another method to identify secreted or membrane-bound proteins (27). Sedimentation equilibrium or sedimentation velocity allows genes that encode secreted or membrane-associated proteins to be partitioned away from genes that encode cytosolic proteins. Messenger RNAs that copurify with membrane-associated polysomes could be interrogated for the presence or absence of transmembrane domain-encoding regions, further subdividing those genes that encode transmembrane and secreted products. One could then assess the expression of this smaller subset of "secreted" genes in normal and neoplastic tissue.

MOLECULAR CLASSIFICATION OF HUMAN CANCER

Pathologists are often confronted with histologically similar cancers that have different natural histories and require different therapeutic approaches. Several methods supplementing classical histopathological diagnosis, such as immunohistochemistry, RT-PCR, cytogenetics, and fluorescence in situ hybridization, are used to assist in tumor diagnosis, but, at times, some cases remain diagnostically problematic. Molecular classification schemes based on a tumor's profile of expressed genes have begun to be developed, and thus far have been applied in the differential diagnosis of acute myelogenous leukemia (AML) and acute lymphocytic leukemia (ALL) (28), breast tumors with BRCA1 or BRCA2 mutations (29); and most recently to the small round blue cell tumors of childhood (30). Methods that address the fundamental question of which genes best distinguish tumor classes continue to evolve. In a study of AML and ALL, Golub et al. (28) devised methods to assess whether such excesses of genes exist, *a priori*, before attempting to classify the leukemias. Their method relies on neighborhood analysis, in which gene expression for the "true" distinction (i.e., AML versus ALL) is compared to randomly generated groupings. The list of genes useful for the distinction between these two leukemias was measured at the 1% and 5% confidence levels. The authors found ~1,000 of 6,800 genes whose expression correlated with the differences between ALL and AML. Using a weighted correlation method, a subset of as few as 50 of these genes was then used to "vote" for the likely class of leukemia, both in cross-validation studies used to derive the classification method (where one leaves out a sample, re-calculates the predictor gene set in its absence, and then predicts its likely class), as well as in an independent set of "blinded" samples. In both types of analysis, the authors correctly classified ALL and AML in ~70% of cases.

We have used gene expression profiling to construct a classification scheme for the most commonly fatal carcinomas in the United States (31). This classification scheme includes carcinomas of the prostate, female breast, colorectum, lung (adenocarcinoma and squamous cell carcinoma), ovary, pancreas, liver, kidney, gastroesophagus, and bladder/ureter, which together account for ~70% of all cancer-related deaths (32). We selected genes whose expression was uniformly high among carcinomas of a specific anatomic site, and uniformly low among carcinomas of all other anatomic sites or histologic type (termed a "one-versus-all strategy"; Figure 5A). We initially tested the null hypothesis that the expression of genes in one class of tumor is no different from the expression of genes in other classes using a Wilcoxon rank test. The genes in each class that have significant *p*-scores represent those that dispute the null hypothesis. In most tumor classes, we were able to identify many such genes, typically more than 100 per tumor type (Figure 5B). The identification of so many genes per tumor class—even for neoplasms that are biologically expected to be similar, such as gastroesophageal and colorectal tumors—is analogous, in part, to a neighborhood analysis, since the conclusion is that distinctions exist between tumor classes and that these distinctions can be molecularly modeled. Using the sets of statistically ranked genes to "vote" for the class of a blinded tumor by similar methods to those described by Golub et al. (28) resulted in poor classification accuracy. Thus, we sought other supervised methods to re-sort the genes within each tumor class, based on how accurately *each gene* could predict the class of a blinded sample. Support vector machine (SVM) learning algorithms were chosen because they make no assumptions about normal or non-normal behavior of the data sets, and have proven accurate in other independent studies (33, 34). Empirically, cross-validation analyses within the training set of tumors showed that 10 genes per tumor class would be ideal to make the best predictions (a total of 110 genes for 11 tumor classes; Figure 5C; the complete list of genes is available at www.gnf.org/cancer/epican/genes). Table 1 describes the prediction accuracy of our method, both in the presence and absence of a prediction strength score that we implemented to avoid tumor misclassifications (35). Our data show that up to 85% of cases in a blinded study could be accurately predicted above a conservative threshold that minimized the number of misclassified cases (in this test, all "called" classifications were correct, with no misclassifications). It is worth noting that 12 of 75 tumors in the blinded study were metastatic lesions, and in the presence of a conservative threshold for classification, the primary tumor origin was correctly predicted for 9 of 12 cases; in the absence of this threshold, 11 of 12 cases were correctly predicted (Table 2). Remarkably, the use of as few as 11 genes, representing the most accurate classifier gene for each of the 11 tumor classes, resulted in correct classification of 88% of the 75 independent test cases, suggesting their potential importance as markers for tumor diagnosis (Table 3).

Designing a classification system based on tumor class-specific over-expression, rather than on statistical measures of variance within the data (30), was based on the notion that gene expression would be uniform in the majority of carcinomas within a class, and therefore be "diagnostic" of that tumor class. The use of genes whose expression is variable across different tumor types would also include down-regulated genes (30), which are not suited to the development of clinically useful assays. However, we note that he use of statistical methods like principal components analysis, combined with neural network modeling that include down-regulated genes in the analysis, would possibly increase the accuracy of molecular prediction.

The value of a tumor class-specific biostatistical method is apparent upon examination of the genes that constitute the most accurate classifiers. Many genes that we identified are known to be expressed at highly elevated levels in tumors compared to their normal tissue counterparts. Such genes include *MUC-2* and *A33* in colon cancer, the latter of which has been used as an immunotherapeutic target in advanced colorectal carcinomas (36); mammaglobin-1 (*MGB-1*), which has been proposed as highly sensitive diagnostic marker for micrometastatic breast cancer (37); and thyroid transcription factor 1 (*TFF-1*), which has been proposed as a highly accurate marker for the differential diagnosis of lung adenocarcinoma (38). By comparing the expression levels of classifier genes in ovarian tumors to representative samples of normal tissue counterparts, a relatively obvious division was identified between genes that were specific to or elevated in the cancers, and genes that were expressed at essentially the same level in normal and tumor specimens (tissue-specific; Figure 6).

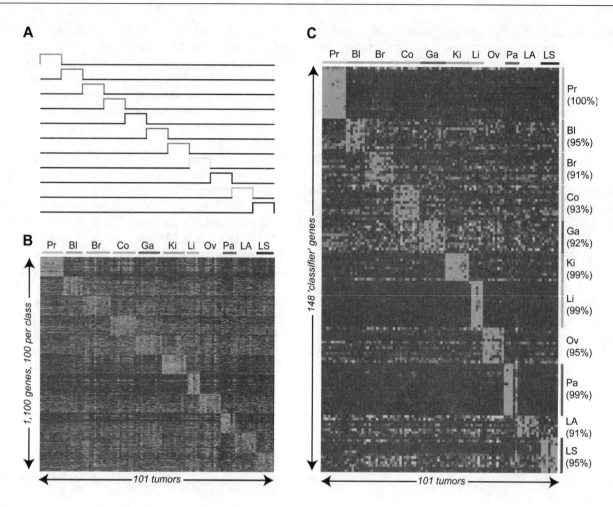

Figure 5 Selection of tumor-specific genes for cancer class prediction. (A) Schematic diagram depicting the idealized expression profile of tumor-specific genes that the method selects as classifiers. The shape of each profile represents genes that are highly expressed in each cancer type relative to all other tumors classes in the training set of tumors. (B) 100 genes per tumor class (1,100 total) with the most significant scores in a Wilcoxon rank sum test for equality were selected as likely candidates for tumor classifiers. Pr—prostate; Bl—bladder; Br—breast; Co—colorectal; Ga—gastroesophageal; Ki—kidney; Li—liver; Ov—ovary; Pa—pancreas; LA—lung adenocarcinomas; LS—lung squamous cell carcinoma. (C) The final refined set of gene classifiers was generated after ranking genes in (B) by SVM/LOOCV accuracy. For clarity, only 8 of 76 predictor genes for lung adenocarcinomas are depicted here. Levels of gene expression (depicted in each row) across all samples (columns) were median-centered and normalized by "Cluster" and output in "Treeview" (45). Red—increased gene expression; blue—decreased expression; black—median level of gene expression. The color intensity is proportional to the hybridization intensity of a gene from its median level across all samples. Reprinted with permission from AACR. **Color representation of figure appears on Color Plate 6.**

Table 1 Accuracy of anatomic class prediction based on a 100-tumor training set

Tumor set	Number of tumors	Dixon confidence threshold			No confidence threshold	
		Correct	Misclassified	No call	Correct	Misclassified
Training set (cross-validation)	100	92 (92%)	2 (2%)	6 (6%)	97 (97%)	3 (3%)
Blinded set	75	64 (85%)	0 (0%)	11 (15%)	71 (95%)	4 (5%)

Note: Two different groups of tumors were predicted using our classification method: 100 tumors comprising the training set (Training set) and a group of 75 tumors (Blinded set). Each sample in the training set was blinded and predicted in a cross-validation study. The blinded set contained samples not included in the training set, the identities of which were unknown during the training and optimization of the method. Reprinted with permission from AACR.

Table 2 Predicting the tumor origin of metastatic lesions

Sample	Prediction	Dixon score	Sample identity
U7	Ovary	0.29	Metastatic serous pap. ca. of the ovary (omentum)
U8	Ovary	0.34	Metastatic serous pap. ca. of the ovary (omentum)
U11	Ovary	0.2	Metastatic serous pap. ca. of the ovary (omentum)
U12	Colon	0.33	Metastatic colon ca. (ovary)
U16	Breast	0.03	Metastatic breast ca. (liver)
U17	Bladder	0.02	Metastatic lung Ad ca. (brain)
U19	Lung SCC	0.36	Metastatic lung SCC ca. (liver)
U40	Prostate	0.54	Metastatic prostate ca. (lymph node)
U41	Prostate	0.47	Metastatic prostate ca. (lymph node)
U42	Colon	0.31	Metatstatic colon ca. (liver)
U43	Colon	0.25	Metatstatic colon ca. (liver)
UX14	Kidney	0.07	Metastatic kidney ca. (colon)

Note: Samples of metastatic carcinomas predicted by the classification method. Metastatic site is in parenthesis. Nine of 12 carcinomas (**bold**) were correctly predicted with high confidence. There are no incorrect predictions with high confidence score. High confidence is defined as above a Dixon score threshold of >0.1. (SCC—squamous cell carcinoma, Ad—adenocarcinoma)

The future use of these classification schemes will be to identify genes whose expression correlates with the clinical characteristics of cancer. The identification of genes whose expression stratifies patients into different prognostic categories or therapeutic options might enable the development of additional immunohistochemical reagents or simple molecular tests that would improve patient management. The construction of custom cancer-specific DNA microarray chips could also be incorporated into the routine histopathological diagnosis of cancer. In the future, histopathological diagnosis, tissue laser microdissection, and gene expression profiling might be the state-of-the-art sequence for cancer diagnosis, prognosis, and treatment strategy.

PRACTICAL CONSIDERATIONS

The observation of differential gene expression in human tumors is an important first step toward the identification of potential markers for diagnosis, whether the intent is to detect the corresponding proteins in the sera of cancer patients, or to detect the proteins by immunohistochemical methods for aid in cancer classification. Several considerations concerning these molecular tools to identify such molecules must be taken into account, however. First, the observation of differential gene expression does not necessarily imply differential expression of the corresponding protein. As yet, there has been no systematic study addressing the concordance between differential gene and differential protein expression. Although several recent studies have shown convincing immunohistochemical validation of differential RNA expression in ovarian (3), prostate (12,39), and bladder carcinomas (40), it will be necessary to systematically evaluate differential protein expression of multiple candidate genes using newly developed antibody reagents and custom-made large-scale tissue microarrays.

The identification of secreted gene products by some of the methods outlined above does not necessarily imply that the proteins will be detectable in the sera of cancer patients. Serum-based diagnostic tests also depend on the stability of the protein target, the association of the protein with other serum proteins, and the presence and extent of post-translational modifications that disrupt or conceal functional epitopes. Any one of these components may hinder the ability to translate these molecular findings into serologically useful reagents.

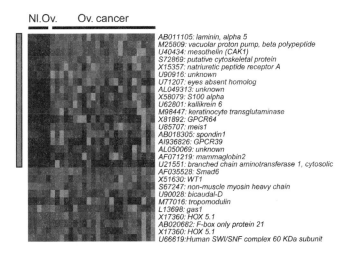

Figure 6 Tumor- and tissue-specific genes as class predictors of ovarian tumors. Shown are the expression levels of 28 highly predictive classifier genes (rows) in five normal (Nl. Ov., left columns) and 24 malignant (Ov. cancer, right columns) samples of ovarian tissue. The green bar indicates 18 of the genes that were significantly ($p < 0.01$ and fold change >3) upregulated in tumors as compared to normal tissues (tumor specificity); expression levels of the other 10 genes were similar in normal and malignant tissue samples (tissue, but not tumor, specificity). The order of genes was first determined using an unpaired, one-tailed t-test to measure the significance of differential expression in normal and tumor tissues, and secondarily by the difference in mean levels of expression. Reprinted with permission from AACR. **Color representation of figure appears on Color Plate 7.**

Table 3 Annotations of selected "predictor" genes

Class	Gene annotation	Gene symbol	Predictive accuracy
Prostate	calcium/calmodulin-dependent protein kinase 1	CAMK1	100
Prostate	Prostate-specific antigen, including alt. splice isoforms	PSA	100
Prostate	Kallikrein 2	KLK2	100
Prostate	T-cell receptor gamma locus	TRG	100
Prostate	transcription factor SIM: lady bird late	LBX1	100
Prostate	prostatic acid phosphatase	ACPP	100
Prostate	six membrane epithelial antigen of the prostate	STEAP	100
Prostate	kinesin family member 5C	KIF5C	100
Prostate	S-adenosylmethionine decarboxylase	AMD1	100
Bladder	uroplakin 2	UPK2	96
Bladder	ralA binding protein 1	RALBP1	96
Bladder	synuclein, gamma	SNGC	96
Bladder	topoisomerase (DNA) II beta (180Kd)	TOP2B	96
Breast	iroquois homeobox protein 5	IRX5	96
Breast	cyclin-dependent kinase inhibitor 1B (p27, Kip1)	CDKN1B	95
Breast	mammaglobin 1	MGB1	92
Colon	caudal type homeo box transcription factor 2	CDX2	97
Colon	caudal type homeo box transcription factor 1	CDX1	95
Colon	solute carrier family 12, member 2	SLC12A2	95
Colon	chloride channel, calcium activated, member 1	CLCA1	94
Colon	glycoprotein A33 (transmembrane)	GPA33	94
Gastric	S-adenosylhomocysteine hydrolase-like 1	AHCYL1	95
Gastric	galectin 7	LGALS7	94
Kidney	endothelial cell-specific molecule 1	ESM1	100
Kidney	glutamyl aminopeptidase (aminopeptidase A)	ENPEP	100
Kidney	PCTAIRE protein kinase 3	PCTK3	100
Liver	complement component 5	C5	100
Liver	vitamin D binding protein	GC	99
Liver	antithrombin, member 1	SERPINC1	99
Liver	kininogen	KNG	99
Ovarian	natriuretic peptide receptor A	NPR1	99
Ovarian	Wilms tumor 1	WT1	99
Ovarian	branched chain aminotransferase 1, cytosolic	BCAT1	98
Ovarian	spondin 1	SPON1	98
Pancreas	carboxyl ester lipase	CEL	100
Pancreas	elastase 3, pancreatic (protease E)	ELA3	100
Pancreas	pancreatic lipase-related protein 2	PNLIPRP2	100
Lung_ad.	thyroid transcription factor 1	TITF1	98
Lung_ad.	Fc fragment of IgE, high affinity I, receptor for; beta polypeptide	MS4A2	94
Lung_ad.	placental protein 14	PAEP	93
Lung_sq	keratin 6A	KRT6A	98
Lung_sq	alcohol dehydrogenase 7	ADH7	96
Lung_sq	p21 (CDKN1A)-activated kinase 2	PAK2	96
Lung_sq	desmoglein 3 (pemphigus vulgaris antigen)	DSG3	96
Lung_sq	tumor protein 63	TP63	96

Note: Shown are the most "predictive" genes for each of 11 different tumor classes. Genes with no annotation or no known function are excluded from the table. The comprehensive list of classifier genes is available from our website at: www.gnf.org/cancer/epican/genes.

Expression profiling techniques also cannot identify putative serum proteins or peptides that are present at elevated levels in the serum as a consequence of other tumor-specific mechanisms. For example, increased serum PSA in men with prostate cancer may depend on increased production within the gland, expansion of the malignant epithelial component, disruption of the normal stromal-epithelial barriers, or encroachment of glands into blood vessels. At the level of transcription, however, PSA is probably not increased in tumor tissue, and may even be decreased relative to the normal prostate (41).

Several of the encoded proteins detected by differential mRNA expression may seem to be unlikely candidates (such as cytokeratins). However, a fragment of CK19 (CYFRA 21-1) is detectable in the serum of patients with non-small-cell lung cancer (NSCLC) (42) [its production from intact cytokeratin 19 may result from increased expression and activity of caspase 3 (43)].

Another example is the serum-soluble fragment of E-cadherin, which is a putative prognostic marker in gastric carcinoma (44).

SUMMARY

Large-scale molecular profiling techniques provide new ways to identify candidate diagnostic markers for the detection and characterization of cancer. Although much validation is needed to assess the extent to which these new techniques are successful in generating clinical reagents, it is already clear that gene expression profiling methods have uncovered a number of potentially important diagnostic molecules. The discovery of genes whose corresponding proteins have been detected at elevated levels in the serum of patients with cancer (e.g., KLK6, KLK10) provides evidence that large-scale hybridization approaches may lead to the discovery of important reagents for cancer detection.

Acknowledgements

We thank our colleagues at the Genomics Institute of the Novartis Research Foundation (GNF) and the University of Virginia for valuable support and discussions. We particularly thank Andrew Su and Drs. John Hogenesch and Michael Cooke for sharing data from the GNF body-map tissue expression database.

REFERENCES

1. Liotta L, Petricoin E. Molecular profiling of human cancer. Nat Rev Genet 2000;1:48–56.
2. Welsh JB, Zarrinkar PP, Sapinoso LM, Kern SG, Behling CA, Monk BJ, et al. Analysis of gene expression profiles in normal and neoplastic ovarian tissue samples identifies candidate molecular markers of epithelial ovarian cancer. Proc Natl Acad Sci USA 2001;98:1176–1181.
3. Hough CD, Sherman-Baust CA, Pizer ES, Montz FJ, Im DD, Rosenshein NB, et al. Large-scale serial analysis of gene expression reveals genes differentially expressed in ovarian cancer. Cancer Res 2000;60:6281–6287.
4. Schummer M, Ng WV, Bumgarner RE, Nelson PS, Schummer B, Bednarski DW, et al. Comparative hybridization of an array of 21,500 ovarian cDNAs for the discovery of genes overexpressed in ovarian carcinomas. Gene 1999;238:375–385.
5. Kirchhoff C, Habben I, Ivell R, Krull N. A major human epididymis-specific cDNA encodes a protein with sequence homology to extracellular proteinase inhibitors. Biol Reprod 1991;45:350–357.
6. Zhong XY, Kaul S, Eichler A, Bastert G. Evaluating GA733-2 mRNA as a marker for the detection of micrometastatic breast cancer in peripheral blood and bone. Arch Gynecol Obstet 1999;263:2–6.
7. Suzumori N, Sato M, Yoneda T, Ozaki Y, Takagi H, Suzumori K. Expression of secretory leukocyte protease inhibitor in women with endometriosis. Fertil Steril 1999;72:857–867.
8. Ashcroft GS, Lei K, Jin W, Longenecker G, Kulkarni AB, Greenwell-Wild T, et al. Secretory leukocyte protease inhibitor mediates non-redundant functions necessary for normal wound healing. Nat Med 2000;6:1147–1153.
9. Benatar M, Blaes F, Johnston I, Wilson K, Vincent A, Beeson D, Lang B. Presynaptic neuronal antigens expressed by a small cell lung carcinoma cell line. J Neuroimmunol 2001;113:153–162.
10. Luo J, Duggan DJ, Chen Y, Sauvageot J, Ewing CM, Bittner ML, et al. Human prostate cancer and benign prostatic hyperplasia: molecular dissection by gene expression profiling. Cancer Res 2001;61:4683–4688.
11. Bull JH, Ellison G, Patel A, Muir G, Walker M, Underwood M, et al. Identification of potential diagnostic markers of prostate cancer and prostatic intraepithelial neoplasia using cDNA microarray. Br J Cancer 2001;84:1512–1519.
12. Welsh JB, Sapinoso LM, Su AI, Kern SG, Wang-Rodriguez J, Moskaluk CA, et al. Analysis of gene expression identifies candidate markers and pharmacological targets in prostate cancer. Cancer Res 2001 (in press).
13. Moore AG, Brown DA, Fairlie WD, Bauskin AR, Brown PK, Munier ML, et al. The transforming growth factor-? superfamily cytokine macrophage inhibitory cytokine-1 is present in high concentrations in the serum of pregnant women. J Clin Endocrinol Metab 2000;85:4781–4788.
14. Tanimoto H, Yan Y, Clarke J, Korourian S, Shigemasa K, Parmley TH, et al. Hepsin, a cell surface serine protease identified in hepatoma cells, is overexpressed in ovarian cancer. Cancer Res 1997;57:2884–2887.
15. Lin B, Ferguson C, White JT, Wang S, Vessella R, True LD, et al. Prostate-localized and androgen-regulated expression of the membrane-bound serine protease TMPRSS2. Cancer Res 1999;59:4180–4184.
16. Afar DE, Vivanco I, Hubert RS, Kuo J, Chen E, Saffran DC, et al. Catalytic cleavage of the androgen-regulated TMPRSS2 protease results in its secretion by prostate and prostate cancer epithelia. Cancer Res 2001;61:1686–1692.
17. Vu T-KH, Liu RW, Haaksma CJ, Tomasek JJ, Howard EW. Identification and cloning of the membrane-associated serine protease, hepsin, from mouse preimplantation embryos. J Biol Chem 1997;272:31315–31320.
18. Robertson DM, Cahir N, Burger HG, Mamers P, McCloud PI, Pettersson K, McGuckin M. Combined inhibin and CA125 assays in the detection of ovarian cancer. Clin Chem 1999;45:651–658.
19. Oehler MK, Sutterlin M, Caffier H. CASA and Ca 125 in diagnosis and follow-up of advanced ovarian cancer. Anticancer Res 1999;19:2513–2518.
20. Luo LY, Bunting P, Scorilas A, Diamandis EP. Human kallikrein 10: a novel tumor marker for ovarian carcinoma? Clin Chim Acta 2001;306:111–118.
21. Diamandis EP, Yousef GM, Soosaipillai AR, Bunting P. Human kallikrein 6 (zyme/protease M/neurosin): a new serum biomarker of ovarian carcinoma. Clin Biochem 2000;33:579–583.
22. Yun K, Kukumoto M, Jinno Y. Monoallelic expression of the insulin-like growth factor-2 gene in ovarian cancer. Am J Pathol 1996;148:1081–1087.
23. Yin DL, Pu L, Pei G. Antisense oligonucleotides to insulin-like growth factor II induces apoptosis in human ovarian cancer AO cell line. Cell Res 1998;8:159–165.
24. Loging WT, Lal A, Siu IM, Loney TL, Wikstrand CJ, Marra MA, et al. Identifying potential tumor markers and antigens by database mining and rapid expression screening. Genome Res 2000;10:1393–1402.
25. Scheurle D, DeYoung MP, Binninger DM, Page H, Jahanzeb M, Narayanan R. Cancer gene discovery using digital differential display. Cancer Res 2000;60:4037–4043.

26. Ashburner M, Ball CA, Blake JA, Botstein D, Butler H, Cherry JM, et al. Gene ontology: tool for the unification of biology. Nat Genet 2000;25:25–29.
27. Diehn M, Eisen MB, Botstein D, Brown PO. Large-scale identification of secreted and membrane-associated gene products using DNA microarrays. Nat Genet 2000;25:58–62.
28. Golub TR, Slonim DK, Tamayo P, Huard C, Gaasenbeek M, Mesirov JP, et al. Molecular classification of cancer: class discovery and class prediction by gene expression monitoring. Science 1999;286:531–537.
29. Hedenfalk I, Duggan D, Chen Y, Radmacher M, Bittner M, Simon R, et al. Gene-expression profiles in hereditary breast cancer. N Engl J Med 2001;344:539–548.
30. Khan J, Wei JS, Ringner M, Saal LH, Ladanyi M, Westermann F, et al. Classification and diagnostic prediction of cancers using gene expression profiling and artificial neural networks. Nat Med 2001;7:673–679.
31. Su AI, Welsh JB, Sapinoso LM, Kern SG, Dimitrov P, Lapp H, Schultz PG, Powell SM, Moskaluk CA, Frierson HF, Jr., Hampton GM. Molecular classification of human carcinomas by use of gene expression signatures.Cancer Res 2001;61:7388–7393.
32. Greenlee RT, Murray T, Bolden S, Wingo PA. Cancer statistics, 2000. CA Cancer J Clin 2000;50:7–33.
33. Furey TS, Cristianini N, Duffy N, Bednarski DW, Schummer M, Haussler D. Support vector machine classification and validation of cancer tissue samples using microarray expression data. Bioinformatics 2000;16:906–914.
34. Chow ML, Moler EJ, Mian IS. Identifying marker genes in transcription profiling data using a mixture of feature relevance experts. Physiol Genomics 2001;5:99–111.
35. Greller LD, Tobin FL. Detecting selective expression of genes and proteins. Genome Res 1999;9:282–296.
36. Tschmelitsch J, Barendswaard E, Williams CJ, Yao TJ, Cohen AM, Old LJ, Welt S. Enhanced anti-tumor activity of combination radioimmunotherapy (131I-labeled monoclonal antibody A33) with chemotherapy (fluorouracil). Cancer Res 1997;57: 2181–2186.
37. Ghossein RA, Carusone L, Bhattacharya S. Molecular detection of micrometastases and circulating tumor cells in melanoma prostatic and breast carcinomas. In vivo 2000;14:237–250.
38. Reis-Filho JS, Carrilho C, Valenti C, Leitao D, Ribeiro CA, Ribeiro SG, Schmitt FC. Is TTF1 a good immunohistochemical marker to distinguish primary from metastatic lung adenocarcinomas? Pathol Res Pract 2000;196:835–840.
39. Waghray A, Schober M, Feroze F, Yao F, Virgin J, Chen YQ. Identification of differentially expressed genes by serial analysis of gene expression in human prostate cancer. Cancer Res 2001; 61:4283–4286.
40. Thykjaer T, Workman C, Kruhoffer M, Demtroder K, Wolf H, Andersen LD, et al. Identification of gene expression patterns in superficial and invasive human bladder cancer. Cancer Res 2001; 61:2492–2499.
41. Magklara A, Scorilas A, Stephan C, Kristiansen GO, Hauptmann S, Jung K, Diamandis EP. Decreased concentrations of prostate-specific antigen and human glandular kallikrein 2 in malignant versus nonmalignant prostatic tissue. Urology 2000;56:527–532.
42. Niklinski J, Furman M, Rapellino M, Chyczewski L, Laudanski J, Oliaro A, Ruffini E. CYFRA 21-1 determination in patients with non-small-cell lung cancer: clinical utility for the detection of recurrences. J Cardiovasc Surg (Torino) 1995;36:501–504.
43. Dohmoto K, Hojo S, Fujita J, Yang Y, Ueda Y, Bandoh S, et al. The role of caspase 3 in producing cytokeratin 19 fragment (CYFRA21-1) in human lung cancer cell lines. Int J Cancer 2001; 91:468–473.
44. Chan AO, Lam SK, Chu KM, Lam CM, Kwok E, Leung SY, et al. Soluble E-cadherin is a valid prognostic marker in gastric carcinoma. Gut 2001;48:808–811.
45. Eisen MB, Spellman PT, Brown PO, Botstein D. Cluster analysis and display of genome-wide expression patterns. Proc Natl Acad Sci USA 1998;95:14863–14868.

Chapter 35

Mining the Cancer Cell's DNA Replication Apparatus for Novel Malignancy Biomarkers

Linda H. Malkas, Pamela E. Bechtel, Jennifer W. Sekowski, Lauren Schnaper, Carla R-V. Lankford, Derek J. Hoelz, Yang Liu, and Robert J. Hickey

Despite extensive research efforts to identify unique molecular markers that indicate the presence of cancer, no characteristic has emerged, to date, that correlates exclusively with malignancy. However, two general hallmarks of malignancy have been recognized: aberrant cell growth and an accumulation of genetic damage.

One process common to both hallmarks is DNA replication. Human cell DNA replication is an exquisitely regulated process. Defects in the mechanisms and/or regulation of DNA synthesis have been correlated with the acquisition of malignancy. In fact, we performed a series of studies demonstrating that a multi-protein DNA replication complex (i.e., the DNA synthesome) isolated from human breast cancer cells has significantly decreased replication fidelity when compared to that of the complex isolated from nonmalignant breast cells, and that several protein components of the DNA synthesome from malignant cells are structurally distinct from that of their nonmalignant cell counterparts.

Using two-dimensional polyacrylamide gel electrophoresis (2D-PAGE), we identified one of these altered components, a novel form of Proliferating Cell Nuclear Antigen (PCNA), in malignant breast cells. PCNA functions in both DNA replication and DNA repair, and is a component of the synthesome. This cancer-specific form of the protein (csPCNA) is not the result of a genetic alteration, but rather appears to result from an alteration in the post-translational modification of the protein in malignant cells. These findings are significant in that it now becomes possible to link changes in the fidelity of DNA replication with the specific alteration of a component of the DNA synthetic apparatus of breast cancer cells. Thus, csPCNA may prove to be a new signature for cancer cells, and it has the potential to serve as a powerful biomarker for malignant disease.

Altered DNA Replication Protein Activity in Cancer Cells

The development of cancer is a multi-step process that is accompanied by alterations in the "normal" patterns of gene expression and the high-level expression of replication errors throughout the cancer cell genome (referred to as RERs or the RER phenotype) (1,2). The process of DNA synthesis in nonmalignant mammalian cells is extraordinarily accurate, with only one nucleotide misincorporation per 10^{10} base pairs replicated per cell division (3,4). In malignant cells, however, there are both an accumulation of genetic mutations and a decrease in replication fidelity. The malignant transformation of normal cells typically proceeds by a sequential mechanism that is oftentimes accompanied by the accumulation of numerous chromosomal alterations (5).

Alterations in the genetic information and chromosomal structure of the cancer cell's genome (during the tumor progression process) suggest that defects in one or more of the cellular processes responsible for maintaining the integrity of the genome may initiate the transformation of the nonmalignant cell. This initiating event may subsequently lead to a cascade of alterations that could include the DNA replication process becoming error-prone. One mechanism by which the replication process could become error-prone points toward the DNA synthetic apparatus altering in some way, enabling it to now actively participate in the mutagenesis process (3). The potential generation of structural alterations in the DNA synthetic apparatus could be mediated by at least two DNA replication-based mutator mechanisms that can contribute to the development of premalignant cells and the progression of these cells to the malignant state.

The first mechanism suggests that the primary amino acid sequence of proteins that function during DNA synthesis might undergo structural changes at positions that are crucial for high-fidelity DNA replication. One example of such a protein is DNA polymerase (6). The amino acid and nucleotide sequence of specific binding domains for engaging the DNA template and deoxyribonucleoside 5'-triphosphates (dNTPs) have been identified (6) and shown through the site-directed mutagenesis of a dNTP binding domain to decrease both the affinity of the DNA polymerase α for nucleotides and lower the fidelity of polymerase α-mediated DNA replication (7).

The second potential mechanism suggests that the function of replication proteins may be altered in malignant cells by the imbalanced expression of specific subunits of these proteins or by aberrant post-translational modification of the proteins. Studies with hepatic DNA polymerase α from mice fed *ad libitum* versus those calorically restricted have shown that there is a decline in the specific activity of DNA polymerase α, and that the chromatographic behavior of the protein differs between the two groups. These observations suggest that alterations in the pattern of gene expression must occur in response to the dietary treatment of these mice (8). Furthermore, the alterations in polymerase function and chromatographic behavior correlate with a reduced DNA synthetic fidelity (8).

Over a quarter century ago, Loeb and his colleagues proposed that cancer cells developed following the alteration of a cell's "normal" phenotype to that of a mutator phenotype. There is now a considerable body of evidence to support this concept; however, only a few published reports compare purified DNA replication proteins from normal and malignant tissues. In these reports, a decrease in the fidelity of DNA polymerase α was observed in human leukemia cells (9) and in rat liver during chemically induced hepatocarcinogenesis (10). Differences in the molecular characteristics and in the binding affinity to DNA and dNTPs were detected when DNA polymerases from two Morris hepatoma cell strains were compared to those from nonmalignant rat liver tissue. These alterations correlated with the degree of dedifferentiation in the hepatomas (11).

Additional evidence to support our suggestion that both the structure and activity of a cell's DNA replication apparatus is altered in tumor cells has been described (12,13). Extracts prepared from malignant human cells were observed to have a four- to five-fold increased level of in vitro SV40 DNA replication activity when compared to that of normal human diploid cells (13). Also, the physiochemical and catalytic properties of DNA polymerases isolated from Novikoff hepatoma cells and normal rat liver indicate that the DNA binding domain of DNA polymerases α, δ, and ε from the hepatoma cells was altered. Evidence for this conclusion came from the observation that the K_m values for these polymerases (which were determined with specific primer templates), are higher than for the polymerases isolated from nonmalignant cells (12). Furthermore, the Stokes' radii, sedimentation, and diffusion coefficients, and frictional coefficient ratios of DNA polymerase α, δ, and ε isolated from the hepatoma cells, deviated significantly from those of the DNA polymerases isolated from the normal liver cells. In addition, the specific DNA polymerase inhibitors aphidicolin, butylphenyl-dGTP, carbonyldiphosphonate, and dideoxy-TTP exhibit significantly lower K_i values for the polymerases isolated from the hepatoma cells (as compared to those isolated from the normal liver cells), indicating that the dNTP binding sites are altered in the polymerases derived from the cancer cells. Popanda et al. (12) concluded that the altered catalytic and molecular properties observed in the hepatoma-derived polymerases result from specific modifications of the proteins by the tumor cells, suggesting that these modifications may be a consequence of the transformation process. These authors also suggested that the structural alterations could lead to a weakening in the binding of nucleotides to the polymerase nucleotide binding domain, which then leads to a lower specificity for nucleotide selection during the base pairing process that occurs during DNA synthesis. This in turn is postulated to increase the mutation rate observed during the progression of the tumor. Our own data are consistent with these observations (see below) and provide further evidence for the alteration of specific components in the DNA synthetic apparatus of tumor cells. Together, these observations provide strong evidence for the hypothesis that molecular changes in the DNA synthetic machinery of tumor cells affect both DNA synthesis and the fidelity of replication in these cells.

In many tumors, including those of breast origin, there is now a strong correlation between high rates of DNA synthesis and poor overall prognoses. Based on the available data, it appears that high levels of breast cancer cell DNA synthesis are associated with an increased probability of lymph node metastases (14–17), and this observation correlates with the extensive accumulation of genetic damage in breast cancer cells. Analyses of thousands of clinical cases indicate that the majority of breast cancer cells are aneuploid (18). Therefore, the observed high rates of DNA synthesis and the accumulation of extensive genetic damage in breast tumors suggest that an alteration(s) in the DNA replication apparatus may at least be partially responsible for the uncontrolled and error-prone DNA synthesis exhibited by the cancer cells.

A DNA Replication-Competent Multi-Protein Complex (DNA Synthesome) Is Present in Mammalian Cells and Tissues

The first successful isolation, extensive purification, and characterization of an intact mammalian cell multi-protein DNA replication complex that is both stable and fully functional *in vitro* have been described (19–28). This replication-competent multi-protein complex has been isolated from a wide variety of human tissues or cultured mammalian cell types, and has been purified approximately 3600-fold using a series of steps that included centrifugation, polyethylene glycol precipitation, ion-exchange chromatography, sucrose density-gradient sedimentation, and native polyacrylamide gel electrophoresis. The complex from human cells has a sedimentation coefficient of 18S in sucrose gradients, and is similar in size to the complex in murine cells (i.e., 17S). It has also been shown that the DNA synthesome migrates as a single discrete protein species in 4% native polyacrylamide gels (26). The integrity of the multi-protein complex was maintained after its treatment with detergents, salt, RNase, DNase, chromatography on anion exchange resins, sedimentation in glycerol and sucrose density gradients, and electrophoresis through native polyacrylamide gels. This result indicated that the association of the replication proteins with one another was independent of nonspecific interaction with other cellular macromolecular components. Most importantly, it was demonstrated that this multi-protein complex was fully competent to replicate DNA in vitro. The human DNA synthesome supported in vitro SV40 DNA synthesis, while the mouse cell complex replicated polyomavirus-origin-containing duplex DNA. This result indicated that all of the cellular activities required for large T-antigen-dependent in vitro papovavirus DNA synthesis were present within the isolated multi-protein form of the DNA polymerase from these cells. Because papovavirus genome replication is extensively dependent on the host cell's DNA synthetic apparatus, our results also indicate that the isolated multi-protein complex mediates not only papovavirus DNA synthesis, but that it must function in mammalian cell DNA replication as well.

The DNA replication proteins identified to co-purify with the synthesome thus far are these: DNA polymerase α, DNA primase, DNA polymerases δ and ε, DNA ligase I, replication protein A (RP-A), replication factor C (RF-C), proliferating cell nuclear antigen (PCNA), poly (ADP) ribose polymerase, and topoisomerases I and II. A DNA helicase activity was also observed to co-purify with the replication-competent multi-protein complex.

A model to represent the mammalian Multi-protein DNA Replication Complex (designated the MRC or DNA synthesome) has been described. This model is based on the observed fractionation, chromatographic, and sedimentation profiles of the individual replication proteins found to co-purify with the complex (Figure 1). The proteins DNA polymerases α, δ, and ε; DNA primase, RF-C, PARP; DNA helicase; DNA ligase I; and topoisomerase II are observed to exclusively co-purify with one another during the isolation of the DNA synthesome. This would suggest that these proteins are "tightly" associated with one another, and it was proposed that these proteins form the "core" of the DNA synthesome. These proteins also function primarily in the elongation phase of DNA synthesis. PCNA, which functions as an accessory factor for DNA polymerase δ, was observed to be more "loosely" associated with the DNA synthesome. This may reflect PCNA's suggested diverse functions in both DNA replication, recombination, and repair. PCNA was represented in the model as a component of the synthesome, but not as a member of the core.

Topoisomerase I and RP-A, together with the helicase activity of the papovavirus large T-antigen, are involved in the initiation events of papovavirus DNA replication. A similar role for the topoisomerase I and RP-A proteins associated with the mammalian DNA synthesome has been proposed. It was observed that topoisomerase I and RP-A, like PCNA, do not "tightly" associate with the DNA synthesome protein members that compose the core. It was therefore proposed that topoisomerase I and RP-A constitute the DNA synthesome's "initiation" component. Together, the core and initiation components constitute the synthesome. Additional evidence was obtained indicating the direct protein-protein interaction of DNA polymerases α and δ, DNA primase, RF-C, and PCNA with each other in the DNA synthesome (22).

To evaluate whether the complex from both malignant and nonmalignant cells and tissues is altered in its function and structure as a result of malignancy, we have begun the proteomic analysis of the synthesome from both malignant and nonmalignant cells. Our data indicate that the DNA replication apparatus of cancer cells is mutagenic, and that this property correlates with the alteration of a specific component of the replication apparatus.

The Synthesome from Malignant Cells Grown in Culture Mediates an Error-Prone DNA Replication Process

To determine whether the DNA replication apparatus of malignant cells carries out error-prone DNA synthesis, as suggested by the mutator phenotype hypothesis, we examined the replication fidelity of the synthesome isolated from malignant and nonmalignant human breast cells grown in culture (29). We purified the synthesome from several malignant human breast cell lines, (MDA-MB468, Hs578T, and MCF7), and from two nonmalignant human breast cell lines, (Hs578Bst and MCF10A), and evaluated the level of fidelity exhibited by these preparations using our forward mutagenesis assay (30). The

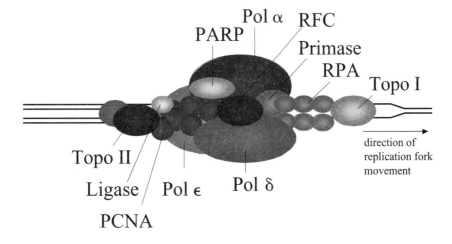

Figure 1 The proposed model for the mammalian DNA synthesome. The mammalian DNA synthesome is composed of DNA polymerases (pol) α, δ, and ε; proliferating cell nuclear antigen (PCNA); primase (primase); replication factor C (RF-C); poly(ADP)ribose polymerase (PARP); replication protein A (RP-A); DNA ligase; and the topoisomerases I and II (Topo I and II). **Color representation of figure appears on Color Plate 7.**

synthesome-driven in vitro DNA replication reactions used a DNA template (pBK-CMV) containing the SV40 origin of replication and a target reporter gene (lacZα) (29). Replication-induced mutations occurring in the target gene resulted in the expression of a nonfunctional β-D-galactosidase enzyme in bacteria transformed with the replicated plasmid. E. coli bacteria expressing the nonfunctional enzyme were detected by the development of colonies expressing a white phenotype, whereas expression of a functional enzyme in the bacteria produced phenotypically blue colonies. By scoring the number of white versus blue colonies a relative replication error frequency was derived. The error frequency was then converted to the number of detectable nucleotide errors per target gene using the formula described by Roberts and Kunkel (31) (see Table 1).

Using this assay we observed that the synthesome derived from MCF7 cells produced 4.4-fold more nucleotide errors in the newly replicated DNA than did the synthesome of the nonmalignant MCF10A cells (Table 1). Similarly, the synthesome isolated from the malignant Hs578T cell line exhibited a 5.7-fold higher DNA replication error frequency when compared to the synthesome derived from its genetically matched counterpart (Hs578Bst) (Table 1). Furthermore, the replication mediated by the synthesome prepared from the estrogen receptor-negative malignant cell line MDA-MB468 was also error-prone (Table 1), and the reduction in fidelity was comparable to that demonstrated by the synthesome from the MCF7 and the Hs578T cell lines (Table 1). Taken together, these data indicate that malignant human breast cells grown in culture contain an error-prone DNA replication apparatus.

Validation that Human Breast Tumors also Contain an Error-Prone DNA Replication Apparatus

To demonstrate that the results of our studies with the synthesome derived from the breast cancer cell lines were representative of the molecular events occurring in human breast tissue, we repeated the forward mutagenesis assay using the synthesome derived from surgically resected malignant and nonmalignant human breast tissue (29). To eliminate the possibility that potential differences in replication fidelity were due to individual genetic variations between patients, we examined the synthesome derived from genetically matched (i.e., from the same patient) malignant and nonmalignant tissue from several different breast cancer patients who had not received any treatment prior to surgical removal of the tumor. We measured the fidelity of replication mediated by the malignant breast tissue synthesome versus that carried out by the synthesome derived from genetically matched nonmalignant breast tissue, and found that the replication fidelity of the synthesome derived from malignant breast tissue was lower than that mediated by the genetically matched nonmalignant breast tissue synthesome. In addition, the level of replication fidelity observed for the synthesome derived from nonmalignant breast tissue was essentially equivalent to that of the synthesome purified from nonmalignant breast cell cultures (e.g., MCF10A), and the fold-mutation frequency of the breast tumor tissue synthesome was similar to that observed for the complex derived from the malignant MCF 7 cell cultures (Table 2). Thus, these data indicate that a distinctly error-prone DNA replication apparatus is not merely a feature of the cultured breast cancer cells, but is a significant characteristic common to all malignant human breast cells.

Nonmalignant Breast Tissue from Cancer Patients Contain a Synthetic Apparatus that Replicates DNA Faithfully

To demonstrate that our measurements of the error frequency of the synthesome derived from nonmalignant breast tissue from cancer patients were truly representative of the normal, healthy breast cell DNA synthetic apparatus, we isolated the synthesome from healthy breast tissue resected during routine breast reduction surgery We also isolated the synthesome from

Table 1 DNA replication fidelity of the synthesome from malignant and nonmalignant cell lines

Source of DNA synthesome	Total number of colonies scored	Number of mutant colonies	Mutant frequency ($\times 10^{-5}$ nucleotides)[a]	Fold mutation frequency[b]
Malignant breast cell lines				
MCF7	6.0×10^4	576	5.15	4.4
Hs578T	6.0×10^4	960	8.65	5.7
MDA-MB468	6.0×10^4	762	6.81	N/A[c]
Nonmalignant breast cell lines				
MCF10A	4.0×10^4	66	1.18	1
Hs578Bst	4.0×10^4	113	1.50	1

[a] Values represent the relative number of errors created per nucleotide of the replicated plasmid. This derivation was based on the following formula described by Roberts and Kunkel (31): number of mutant colonies/total number of transformed colonies − background mutation frequency (number of mutations detected in 5×10^{-8} colonies)/chance of a nucleotide defect within the lacZα gene if the colony expresses a white phenotype (0.5)/number of sites in the target gene (373 base pairs). The lacZα gene comprises 8.25% of the total pBK-CMV plasmid (4518 bp). Each value reported in the table represents the average of at least three individual experiments, and the values did not deviate from the average by more than 5%.

[b] Values represent the fold increase in mutation frequency of the malignant cell synthesome, as compared to its genetically matched nonmalignant cell counterpart.

[c] N/A no genetically matched counterpart available.

Table 2 Fidelity of the DNA replication complex from malignant and nonmalignant tissue samples

Source of the DNA synthesome	Total number of colonies scored	Number of mutant colonies	Mutant frequency ($\times 10^{-5}$ nucleotides)[a]	Fold mutation frequency[b]
Malignant breast tissues				
Tumor A[c] (IDC[d]) [ER−; PR−; Ki-67, 24% (high); 52% (high); p53+]	3.0×10^4	141	2.52	3.6
Tumor B (IDC) [ER+; PR+; diploid; S-phase, 6%]	3.0×10^4	209	3.72	3.8
Tumor C (ILC) [ER+ high, PR−; unknown ploidy; Ki-67, 2% (low); HER2/neu, 42% (high); p53−]	3.4×10^4	122	1.92	2.4
Tumor D (ILC) [ER+ (low); PR+ (high); diploid; S-phase, 7.2% (high)]	3.0×10^4	130	2.35	4.4
Nonmalignant breast tissue[e]				
Tissue A	1.0×10^4	13	0.70	1
Tissue B	1.0×10^4	18	0.96	1
Tissue C	1.0×10^4	15	0.80	1
Tissue D	1.0×10^4	10	0.54	1

[a] Values represent the relative number of errors created per nucleotide of the replicated plasmid. This derivation was based on the following formula described by Roberts and Kunkel (31): number of mutant colonies/total number of transformed colonies − background mutation frequency (number of mutations detected in 5×10^8 colonies)/chance of a nucleotide defect within the lacZα gene if the colony expresses a white phenotype (0.5)/number of sites in the target gene (373 base pairs). The lacZα gene comprises 8.25% of the total pBK-CMV plasmid (4518 bp). Each value reported in the table represents the average of at least three individual experiments, and the values did not deviate from the average by more than 5%.

[b] Values represent the fold increase in mutation frequency of the malignant cell synthesome, as compared to its genetically matched nonmalignant cell counterpart.

[c] Surgically resected female human breast tissue. Genetically matched samples are denoted by corresponding alphanumeric designations (tumor A, tissue A, and so on). Factors such as stage of malignancy, genetics, race, and age were double-blind during data collection.

[d] IDC, infiltrating ductal carcinoma; ILC, infiltrating lobular carcinoma—determined by pathological diagnosis of tumor tissue.

[e] Surgically resected breast reduction tissue from healthy females used to derived synthesome from frozen sample (tissue A) or from primary cultures (primary culture sample).

normal breast epithelial primary cell cultures (29). The observed replication fidelity of the synthesome was comparable when isolated from both the normal breast tissue (i.e., normal 1 and 2) and a normal primary epithelial cell culture (Table 3). This observation confirmed that the synthesome complex from normal cells mediates replication with high fidelity (Table 3), and that the mutation frequency was similar to that observed for the genetically matched, nonmalignant breast tissue synthesome (i.e., Tissues A–D, Table 2). From these data we concluded that the observed fidelity difference between the malignant and nonmalignant breast tissue synthesome preparations derived from the same cancer patient accurately demonstrates that the malignant breast cell DNA synthetic apparatus is significantly more error-prone than the apparatus isolated from normal, disease-free breast tissue.

Error-Prone Replication Is Not Due to Hyperplastic Pathology

To determine that the observed increased mutation frequency of the malignant cell synthesome was not a result of the hyperplastic phenotype of breast cancer cells, we examined the replication fidelity of the synthesome from surgically resected benign breast tissue exhibiting a benign hyperplastic pathology (29). The observed error frequencies for the synthesome isolated from two benign fibroadenomas, a phyllodes tumor, and a sample of ductal epithelial hyperplasia were found to be low and similar to those observed for the nonmalignant and normal (tissue from a non-cancer mammoplasty, not exhibiting any hyperplasia) breast tissue synthesome samples (Table 3). Therefore, the decreased replication fidelity of the malignant breast cell synthesome was not due to the hyperplastic pathology of breast cancer cells, but was a characteristic of the malignant phenotype.

Error-Prone Replication by the Synthesome of Malignant Cells Does Not Correlate with Increased in vitro DNA Synthesis

We examined the DNA replication level mediated by the synthesome from genetically matched malignant and nonmalignant breast tissue in order to demonstrate that the observed increase in the mutation frequency of the purified malignant breast cell replication apparatus was not simply a result of an increase in in vitro DNA synthetic activity (29). Using the SV40 in vitro DNA replication assay, the incorporation of ([α^{32}P]-dCMP) into the nascent daughter DNA molecules was measured, and the level of replication activity reported in Table

Table 3 Fidelity of the DNA replication complex from benign tumor and normal tissue samples

Source of DNA synthesome	Total number of colonies scored	Number of mutant colonies	Mutant frequency ($\times 10^{-5}$ nucleotides)[a]
Benign breast pathology[b]			
Juvenile fibroadenoma	4.0×10^4	13	0.17
Fibroadenoma	4.0×10^4	22	0.30
Benign phyllodes tumor	4.0×10^4	33	0.44
Ductal epithelial hyperplasia without atypia	4.6×10^4	17	0.35
Normal breast tissue and cells[c]			
Normal tissue A	1.0×10^4	12	0.64
Normal tissue B	2.0×10^4	22	0.59
Primary breast cell culture	4.0×10^4	65	0.87

[a] Values represent the relative number of errors created per nucleotide of the replicated plasmid. This derivation was based on the following formula described by Roberts and Kunkel (31): *number of mutant colonies/total number of transformed colonies − background mutation frequency (number of mutations detected in 5×10^8 colonies)/chance of a nucleotide defect within the lacZα gene if the colony expresses a white phenotype (0.5)/number of sites in the target gene (373 base pairs)*. The lacZα gene comprises 8.25% of the total pBK-CMV plasmid (4518 bp). Each value reported in the table represents the average of at least three individual experiments, and the values did not deviate from the average by more than 5%.

[b] Surgically resected female human breast tissue. Factors such as genetics, race, and age were double-blind during data collection.

[c] Surgically resected breast reduction tissue from healthy females used to derived synthesome from frozen tissue sample or from primary cultures.

4. Our results demonstrated that the replication activity of the synthesome isolated from malignant breast tumor tissue was not significantly higher than that observed for the nonmalignant breast tissue complex. These data indicate that the significant decrease in replicative fidelity observed for the malignant cell synthesome does not result from an increase in the in vitro DNA replication activity of the replication complex.

Types of Errors Made by the Synthesome of Breast Cells

We sequenced the target gene (i.e., *lacZα*) contained in the plasmid used as the template in the in vitro DNA replication assay in order to determine the types of mutations created during the replication reaction mediated by the malignant or non-

Table 4 DNA replication activity of the genetically matched malignant and nonmalignant breast DNA synthesome

Source of the DNA synthesome	Units of T-antigen dependent DNA replication activity ($\times 10^{-2}$)[a]	Fold T-antigen dependent replication activity[b]
Malignant human breast cells		
Tumor A[c] (IDC[d])	11.5	0.8
Tumor B (IDC)	11	1.3
Tumor C (ILC)	23.5	2.0
Tumor D (ILC)	12.5	1.0
Average	14.6	1.3
Nonmalignant human breast cells		
Tissue A	15.0	1.0
Tissue B	8.7	1.0
Tissue C	11.5	1.0
Tissue D	11.5	1.0
Average	11.7	1.0

[a] In vitro DNA replication activity assays were performed as described previously (19). Units represent the amount of T-antigen dependent DNA replication *values of the reaction with T-antigen − values of the reaction without T-antigen*). 1 unit = 1 picomole of nascent DNA synthesized/μg of synthesome protein/hour. The values represent the average of two independent experiments. Replication values deviated by less than 3% from the average.

[b] Fold DNA replication activity was calculated by dividing the units of replication observed for the malignant breast cell DNA synthesome by the replication units observed for the DNA synthesome isolated from the genetically matched nonmalignant breast cells. Each value represents the average of at least two experiments. Replication values deviated by less than 3% from the average.

[c] Surgically resected female human breast tissue. Genetically matched samples are denoted by corresponding alphanumeric designations (tumor A, tissue A, and so on). Factors such as stage of malignancy, genetics, race, and age were double-blind during data collection.

[d] IDC, infiltrating ductal carcinoma; ILC, infiltrating lobular carcinoma—determined by pathological diagnosis of tumor tissue.

malignant cell DNA synthesome (29). This target gene was isolated from bacterial colonies transformed with the reaction products from the in vitro DNA replication reaction and exhibiting a white (mutant) phenotype. As a positive control, plasmid DNA isolated from wild-type (dark blue) transformants was purified, sequenced, and compared to the published sequence of the *lacZα* gene (Stratagene). These wild-type *lacZα* sequences were used to identify the nucleotide sequence errors within the target gene sequence. Automated dideoxynucleotide sequencing of the double-stranded *lacZα* gene demonstrated that, while the total number of mutations present in the DNA replication products created by the malignant breast cell synthesome was greater than those formed by the complex from nonmalignant cells (Table 1), there was no significant difference in the types or frequency of mutations found in the replicated DNA products (Table 5). The synthesome from the malignant breast cell cultures and the genetically matched malignant breast tissue samples produced a relatively small percentage of nucleotide insertions (18% ±2%) and single nucleotide deletions (9% ±5%). The bulk of the errors consisted of single point mismatches (73% ±7%). Fewer overall mutations (Table 1 and 2) were produced by the synthesome isolated from the nonmalignant cell cultures and from the genetically matched nonmalignant breast tissue samples. Synthesome preparations from both types of tissue created nearly the same percentage of mutations of each type: 16% ±7% insertions; 9% ±5% deletions; and 75% ±12% single point mismatches (Table 5). It was also observed that there were neither mutational hot spots nor a particular type of mismatch found to be preferentially formed during replication of the *lacZα* gene.

A Specific Component of the Synthesome Is Modified in Malignant Breast Cells Grown in Culture

Based upon the observation that the breast cancer cell synthesome replicated DNA with a lower fidelity than the synthesome from nonmalignant cells, we analyzed the electrophoretic mobility of the components of the DNA synthesome isolated from malignant and nonmalignant cells using two-dimensional polyacrylamide gel electrophoresis (2D-PAGE). We then compared the 2D-PAGE protein patterns to one another in order to determine whether any components of the synthesome from malignant cells were structurally distinct from those of the nonmalignant cell synthesome (32). We isolated the synthesome from four established breast cell lines (the malignant cell lines MCF7, MDA-MB 468, Hs578T, and early passage nonmalignant MCF-10A), as well as from nonmalignant primary breast epithelial cells; resolved the synthesome components from one another using 2D-PAGE gels; and then probed Western blots of these gels using a commercially available antibody that recognized the 36 kDa PCNA polypeptide. A comparison of the mobility of the PCNA component of the MCF10A, MCF7, MDA-MB468, Hs578T, and primary breast cell synthesome (Figure 2) indicated a clear and significant difference in this protein's 2D-PAGE profile for the nonmalignant and malignant cells. The PCNA associated with the synthesome isolated from malignant MCF7 and MDA-MB 468 cells was present in two forms, a basic form and an acidic form (Figure 2A, E), while the PCNA isolated from the malignant Hs578T cells expressed high levels of PCNA having an acidic pI, (Figure 2C), and barely detectable levels of a PCNA isoform having a basic pI.

Table 5 Types of replication errors produced by the breast cell DNA synthesome

Breast Cell Type (source of the synthesome)	Percentage[a] replication-induced errors[b]		
	Nucleotide Insertions	Nucleotide deletions	Nucleotide mismatches
Malignant			
MCF7 (n = 3)	20	10	70
Hs578T (n = 4)	16	5	79
Malignant tumor tissue (n = 3)	20	14	66
Average[c]	18 ± 2%	9 ± 5%	73 ± 7%
Nonmalignant			
MCF10A (n = 3)	13	6	81
Hs578Bst (n = 4)	23	14	63
Nonmalignant tissue (n = 3)	8	4	88
Average[c]	16 ± 7%	9 ± 5%	75 ± 12%

[a] Percentages were derived from the number of nucleotide errors observed in the double-stranded nucleotide sequences of the replicated plasmid isolated from individual mutant bacterial transformant colonies, produced using separate forward mutagenesis assays.

[b] All replication-induced errors were measured by comparing double-stranded nucleotide sequences of the *lacZα* gene of the replicated pBK-CMV template isolated from a mutant (white phenotype) bacterial transformant with that of a wild-type *lacZα* sequence. Mutant transformant colonies were selected from three to four individual forward mutagenesis assays. The sequences from normal transformant colonies (n = 7; blue wild-type phenotype) isolated from forward mutagenesis assays mediated by MCF7, MCF10A, Hs578Bst, and Hs578T, resected breast tumor, and nonmalignant tissue derived DNA synthesome (data not shown) were checked against the published wild-type sequence for *lacZα* and were not found to contain any mutations.

[c] The averages reported were calculated to reflect the number of independent analyses of each cell line sampled and each tumor sampled. The number of each type of error produced during the analysis of each tumor or tissue sample (n = 4) was summed and the average was calculated for each category of nucleotide sequence error.

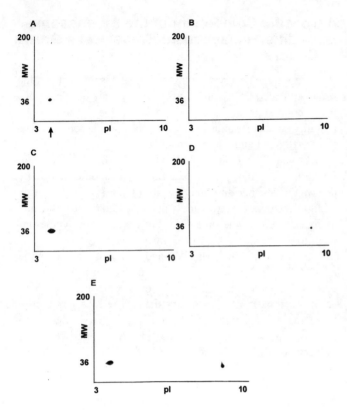

Figure 2 Protein migration of PCNA from human breast cell lines. Thirty micrograms of DNA synthesome protein isolated from four human breast cell lines (MCF7, MDA-MB468, Hs578T, and MCF10A) and nonmalignant primary breast cells were subjected to 2D-PAGE. The resolved polypeptides were transferred to nitrocellulose membranes and analyzed by Western blot with an antibody directed against PCNA. The protein migration patterns shown are *A*, MCF7; *B*, MCF10A; *C*, Hs578T; *D*, nonmalignant primary breast cells; and *E*, MDA-MB468. The arrow points to the form of PCNA that is unique to malignant breast cells. Reprinted with permission from Bechtel PE, Hickey RJ, Schnaper L, Sekowski JW, Long BJ, Freund R, et al. A unique form of proliferating cell nuclear antigen is present in malignant breast cells. Cancer Res 1998;58:3264–3269.

PCNA in nonmalignant MCF10A and primary breast cells was present as a single form that exhibited a basic pI (Figure 2B,D). The acidic form of PCNA was not detectable in the nonmalignant cells. In a separate mixing experiment, 2D-PAGE analyses were performed using samples containing the isolated synthesome from both MCF7 and MCF10A cells. The resulting protein migration pattern showed only one basic form and one acidic form of PCNA (data not shown), indicating that the basic form of PCNA was identical in both the malignant and nonmalignant cells, while the acidic form of PCNA was unique to the malignant cells.

Breast Tumors also Contain the Unique Form of PCNA

To determine whether the synthesome from nonmalignant and malignant breast tissue exhibited the same 2D-PAGE profile for PCNA as was observed in the nonmalignant and malignant breast cell cultures (32), the synthesome was isolated from a virally induced mouse breast tumor (33), six human lobular breast tumors, and four ductal breast tumors. For comparison, the synthesome-associated PCNA isolated from nonmalignant tissue was examined from two sources (breast reduction tissue and genetically matched nonmalignant tissue taken from the patients with malignant breast tumors). The components of the synthesome isolated from these tissues were resolved by 2D-PAGE, and Western blots of the gels were probed with an antibody directed against PCNA. PCNA from malignant mouse and human tumor tissue had a 2D-PAGE profile consistent with that of the malignant cell lines (Figures 3A–D, F). There were two forms of PCNA present, an acidic form and a basic form. Consistent with the 2D-PAGE profile of PCNA from the MCF 10A cells, nonmalignant tissue PCNA was found exclusively in the basic form (Figure 3E).

The Unique Form of PCNA Is Not Proliferation-Dependent

To demonstrate that the appearance of the acidic form of PCNA in these tumors and malignant cell lines was not a proliferation response, but was unique to the malignant breast cell phenotype, we analyzed the 2D-PAGE profile of PCNA isolated from benign proliferative breast tumors and estrogen-stimulated MCF7 cells (32) using a Western blot analysis. We demonstrated that estrogen stimulated the proliferation of MCF7 cells, and that there was clearly an overall increase in the level of PCNA in estrogen-stimulated cells. However, there was no effect on the 2D-PAGE profile for the PCNA peptides present in these cells (Figure 4A, B). Similarly, Western blot analyses of the synthesome isolated from several benign breast tumors resulted in 2D-PAGE profiles for the PCNA that were identical to that of the profile from nonmalignant cells grown in culture and nonmalignant breast tissue (compare Figure 3E and 4C). These data provide compelling evidence demonstrating that the acidic form of PCNA is a characteristic of only malignant breast cells.

Genetic Mutation Is Not Responsible for the Acidic Form of PCNA in Malignant Breast Cells

Total cellular RNA isolated from MCF7 and MCF10A cells was used to clone the cDNA encoding the entire PCNA translation unit from each cell line. Nucleotide sequence analysis of four independent clones encoding the *PCNA* gene derived from MCF7 cells and four independent clones from MCF10A cells indicated that these eight independent clones have an identical nucleotide sequence (32). Furthermore, this nucleotide sequence does not differ from that of the sequence for the *PCNA* gene cloned from the human lymphoma cell line MOLT-4 (34).

SUMMARY

An extensive body of work now supports the contention that the DNA synthesome is essentially the DNA synthetic apparatus of the cell. Furthermore, our conceptualization of the synthesome

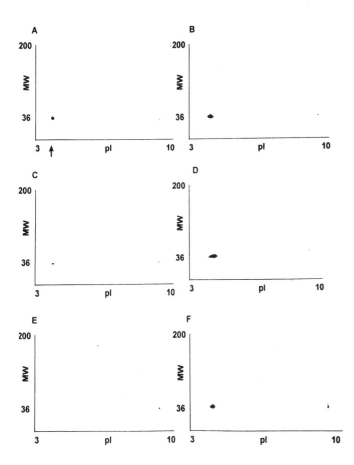

ties of the synthesome in these two cell types, and enable us to determine how regulation of the activity of individual synthesome components differs between malignant and nonmalignant cells. Our own data indicate that the polypeptide structure of several polypeptide components of the synthesome differ between malignant and nonmalignant cells (data not shown). Identification of all of those polypeptides exhibiting differences in structure should enable us to develop an understanding of how the reduction in the fidelity of the DNA synthetic process carried out by malignant cells is linked to these alterations in the structure of synthesome components. Furthermore, application of mass spectroscopic techniques to the structural analysis of these altered components of the synthesome holds the promise of identifying the specific site(s) on these polypeptides that are altered, as well as identifying the type of alteration present. There is also a high probability that these analyses of the synthesome could lead to the identification of new biomarkers for malignancy and improve our understanding and/or the usefulness of existing biomarkers for malignancy (e.g., PCNA).

As an example of the importance of these types of studies, one immediate goal of the structural analysis of the malignant form of PCNA (csPCNA) is to identify the molecular pathways responsible for producing the alteration in the structure of this protein in malignant cells. Once the metabolic pathways involved in differentially modifying PCNA have been identified, strategies for either activating and/or inhibiting key

Figure 3 Protein migration of PCNA from malignant human and mouse breast tissue and nonmalignant human breast tissue. Thirty micrograms of isolated DNA synthesome from malignant human mouse breast tumors and nonmalignant human breast tissue were subjected to 2D-PAGE. The resolved polypeptides were transferred to nitrocellulose membranes and analyzed by Western blot using an antibody directed against PCNA. The resulting protein migration patterns are shown: A and B, human ductal tumor; C and D, human lobular tumor; E, nonmalignant human breast tissue; and F, mouse tumor. The nonmalignant breast tissue (E) is derived from the same source as the lobular tumor in D. The arrow indicates the position of the form of PCNA that is unique to breast cancer cells. Reprinted with permission from Bechtel PE, Hickey RJ, Schnaper L, Sekowski JW, Long BJ, Freund R, et al. A unique form of proliferating cell nuclear antigen is present in malignant breast cells. Cancer Res 1998;58:3264–3269.

presents a testable model that is useful both for identifying specific interactions between individual components of the replication apparatus, and for determining how the activity of the synthesome is regulated in malignant and nonmalignant cells. While much remains to be learned of the precise composition and the mechanism(s) by which the activity of the synthesome are regulated, the identification of all of the components of the synthesome, and their precise stoichiometric relationship to one another, should significantly improve our image of this multi-protein DNA replication complex. Furthermore, kinetic analyses of the activity of individual synthesome components isolated from malignant and nonmalignant cell lines and tissue samples should also improve our understanding of the proper-

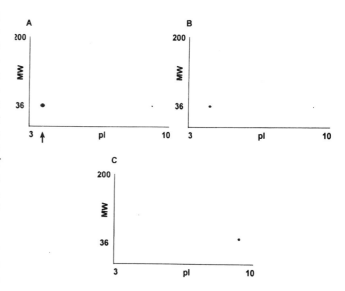

Figure 4 Protein migration pattern of PCNA from 17β-estradiol-treated MCF7 cells (A), control (untreated) MCF7 cells (B), and a benign breast tumor (C). Thirty to sixty micrograms of DNA synthesome isolated from the samples were analyzed by Western blot using an antibody directed against PCNA. The arrow indicates the position of the form of PCNA found exclusively in malignant cells. Reprinted with permission from Bechtel PE, Hickey RJ, Schnaper L, Sekowski JW, Long BJ, Freund R, et al. A unique form of proliferating cell nuclear antigen is present in malignant breast cells. Cancer Res 1998;58:3264–3269.

enzymes within these pathways can be devised. However before these metabolic pathways can be identified and appropriate strategies developed to restore the metabolic imbalance exhibited by malignant cells, it is necessary to identify the site (or domain) within the PCNA polypeptide sequence that differs between nonmalignant and malignant cells.

One implication of identifying this site within the polypeptide is that suitable reagents, such as antibodies, can be developed that specifically recognize this site on the csPCNA polypeptide. Using this reagent it should be possible to improve the histopathological assessment of biopsy material that is now considered of unclear or questionable malignancy. This is because a positive reaction with this reagent will provide a positive identification of the presence of cells with a clear potential for developing a malignant tumor. In addition, a serum test, such as an enzyme-linked immunosorbent assay (ELISA), can be developed around this reagent that will complement existing methodologies for monitoring the remission status of patients who are undergoing treatment for malignancy. The appearance of this csPCNA polypeptide in all malignancies of both solid and hematopoietic origin examined to date (data not shown) suggests that the usefulness of a reagent specifically recognizing the cancer-specific form of PCNA would not be limited to a specific type of cancer. Thus, such a reagent would be a useful tool for monitoring the presence of all types of malignancy, and would enable physicians to alter therapeutic protocols and potentially improve patient outcome sooner than would be possible using existing methodologies.

Finally, by identifying the type of modification sustained by csPCNA that distinguishes it from the form of PCNA expressed in nonmalignant cells, it becomes realistic to speak of targeting very early metabolic events that correlate with malignancy, and potentially drive the malignant transformation process itself. The implications of this statement are many fold, but of key importance to the clinician is the understanding that a cancer-specific therapeutic agent could potentially be developed. Such a therapeutic should not only be specific for the malignant cell, but it could have the potential to halt progression of this type of cell and perhaps reverse the entire transformation process. The potential to reverse the entire transformation process stems from the idea that the change in the structure of the PCNA molecule exhibited by malignant cells is due to post-translational modifications and not mutations. Consequently, any change in the ability of the cell to modify PCNA post-translationally would most likely have global ramifications to the cell, and alterations to the post-translationally modified structure of other proteins within the cell should also be present. The global consequences of altering the structure of numerous cellular proteins would be to affect the overall metabolic and consequently the "normal" phenotypic expression of the cell. Thus, identification of the molecular pathways responsible for altering the expression of PCNA to that of the form of this protein found only in malignant cells undoubtedly holds one of the keys to understanding how the malignant transformation process occurs, and how we might intervene to halt and/or potentially reverse this process using targeted therapeutic approaches.

Acknowledgments

We wish to thank the National Institutes of Health/National Cancer Institute for their generous support in the form of research grants (CA83199, CA57350, CA73060, and CA65754) to LHM and (CA74904) to RJH; the Department of Defense Breast Cancer Research Program for its support of PEB, JWS, and DJH with fellowship awards; and the Vera Bradley Foundation for its generous support of LHM.

REFERENCES

1. Peinado MA, Malkhosyan S, Velazquez A, Perucho M. Isolation and characterization of allelic losses and gains in colorectal tumors by arbitrarily primed polymerase chain reaction. Proc Natl Acad Sci USA 1992; 89:10065–10069.
2. Gleeson CM, Sloan JM, McGuigan JA, Ritchie AJ, Weber JL, Hilary Russell SE. Ubiquitous somatic alterations at microsatellite alleles occur infrequently in Barrett's-associated esophageal adenocarcinoma. Cancer Res 1996;56:259–263.
3. Loeb LA. Mutator phenotype may be required for multistage carcinogenesis. Cancer Res 1991;51:3075–3079.
4. Chu EHY, Boehnke M, Hanash SM, Kuick RD, Lamb BJ, Neel JV, et al. Estimation of mutation rates based on the analysis of polypeptide constituents of cultured human lymphoblastoid cells. Genetics 1988;119:693–703.
5. Nowell PC. Mechanisms of tumor progression. Cancer Res 1986; 46:2203–2207.
6. Wong SW, Wahl AF, Yuan P-M, Arai N, Pearson BE, Arai K, et al. Human DNA polymerase α gene expression is cell proliferation dependent and its primary structure is similar to both prokaryotic and eukaryotic replicative DNA polymerases. EMBO J 1988;7: 37–47.
7. Copeland WC, Lam NK, Wang TS-F. Fidelity studies of human DNA polymerase α. J Biol Chem 1993;268:11041–11049.
8. Srivastava V, Tilley R, Miller S, Hart R, Busbee D. Effects of aging and dietary restriction on DNA polymerases: gene expression, enzyme fidelity, and DNA excision repair. Exp Gerontol 1992;27:593–613.
9. Springgate CF, Loeb L. Mutagenic DNA polymerase in human leukemia cells. Proc Natl Acad Sci USA 1973;70:245–249.
10. Chan JYH, Becker FF. Decreased fidelity of DNA polymerase activity during N-2-fluorenylacetamide hepatocarcinogenesis. Proc Natl Acad Sci USA 1979;76:814–818.
11. Popanda O, Thielmann HW. DNA polymerase α from normal rat liver is different than DNA polymerase α from Morris hepatoma strains. Eur J Biochem 1989;183:5–13.
12. Popanda O, Fox G, Thielmann HW. DNA polymerases alpha, delta and epsilon of Novikoff hepatoma cells differ from those of normal rat liver in physicochemical and catalytic properties. J Mol Med 1995;73:259–268.
13. Boyer JC, Thomas DC, Maher VM, McCormick JJ, Kunkel TA. Fidelity of DNA replication by extracts of normal and malignantly transformed human cells. Cancer Res 1993;53:3270–3275.
14. Meyer JS, Prey MU, Babcock DS, McDivitt RW. Breast carcinoma, cell kinetics, morphology, stage, and host characteristics. A thymidine labeling study. Lab Invest 1986;54:41–51.

15. Kallioniemi O-P, Hietanen T, Mattila J, Lehtinen M, Lauslahti K, Koivula T. Aneuploid DNA content and high S-phase fraction of tumor cells are related to poor prognosis in patients with primary breast cancer. Eur J Cancer Clin Oncol 1987;23: 277–282.
16. Hedley DW, Rugg CA, Gelberg RD. Association of DNA index and S-phase fraction with prognosis of node positive early breast cancer. Cancer Res 1987;47:4729–4735.
17. Klintenberg S, Stal O, Nordenskjold B, Wallgren A, Arvidsson S, Skoog L. Proliferative index, cytosol estrogen receptor, and axillary node status as prognostic predictors in human mammary carcinoma. Breast Cancer Res Treat 1987;7:99–106.
18. Ponten J, Holmberg L, Trichopoulos D, Kallioniemi O-P, Kvale G, Wallgren A, Taylor-Papadimitriou J. Biology and natural history of breast cancer. Int J Cancer 1990;5:5–21.
19. Malkas LH, Hickey RJ, Li CJ, Pederson N, Baril EF. A 21S enzyme complex from HeLa cells that functions in simian virus 40 (SV40) DNA replication in vitro. Biochem 1990;29: 6362–6374.
20. Wu Y, Hickey RJ, Lawlor K, Wills P, Yu F, Ozer H, et al. A 17S multi-protein form of murine cell DNA polymerase mediates polyoma virus DNA replication in vitro. J Cell Biochem 1994;54: 32–46.
21. Applegren N, Hickey RJ, Kleinschmidt AM, Zhou Q, Wills P, Coll J, et al. Further characterization of the human cell multi-protein DNA replication complex. J Cell Biochem 1995;59:91–107.
22. Coll JM, Hickey RJ, Cronkey EA, Jiang H-Y, Schnaper L, Lee MYWT, Vitto L, Syvaoja JE, Malkas LH. Mapping specific protein–protein interactions within the core component of the breast cell DNA synthesome. Oncol Res 1997;9:629–639.
23. Coll JM, Weeks J, Hickey R, Schnaper L, Yue W, Brodie A, Malkas LH. The human breast cell DNA synthesome: its purification from tumor and cell culture. Oncol Res 1996;8: 435–447.
24. Lin S, Hickey R, Malkas L. The biochemical status of the DNA synthesome can distinguish between permanent and temporary cell growth arrest. Cell Growth Differ 1997;8:1359–1369.
25. Wills P, Hickey RJ, Ross D, Cuddy D, Malkas LH. A novel model system for the study of ara-C in vitro. Cancer Chemother Pharmacol 1996;38:366–372.
26. Jiang HY, Hickey RJ, Bechtel PE, Wills PW, Han S, Tom TD, Wei Y, Malkas LH. Bio-Rad whole gel eluter purification of a functional multi-protein DNA replication complex. Bioradiations 1998;102: 18–20.
27. Simbulan CMG, Rosenthal DS, Hilz H, Hickey R, Malkas L, Applegren N, Wu Y, Bers G, Smulson ME. The expression of poly(ADP-ribose) polymerase during differentiation-linked DNA replication reveals that it is a component of the multi-protein DNA replication complex. Biochemistry 1996;35:11622–11633.
28. Simbulan-Rosenthal CM, Rosenthal DS, Boulares AH, Hickey RJ, Malkas LH, Coll JM, Smulson ME. Regulation of the expression or recruitment of components of the DNA synthesome by poly(ADP-ribose) polymerase. Biochemistry 1998;37: 9363–9370.
29. Sekowski JW, Malkas LH, Schnaper L, Bechtel PE, Long BJ, Hickey RJ. Human breast cancer cells contain an error-prone DNA replication apparatus. Cancer Res 1998;58:3259–3263.
30. Sekowski JW, Malkas LH, Y Wei, Hickey RJ. Mercuric ion inhibits the activity and fidelity of the human cell DNA synthesome. Toxicol Appl Pharmacol 1997;145:268–276.
31. Roberts JD, Kunkel TA. Fidelity of a human cell DNA replication complex. Proc Nat Acad Sci USA 1988;85:7064–7068.
32. Bechtel PE, Hickey RJ, Schnaper L, Sekowski JW, Long BJ, Freund R, Liu N, Rodriguez-Valenzuela C, Malkas LH. A unique form of proliferating cell nuclear antigen is present in malignant human breast cells. Cancer Res 1998; 58:3264–3269.
33. Dawe CJ, Freund R, Mandel G, Ballmar-Hofer K, Talmage DA, Benjamin TL. Variations in polyoma virus genotype in relation to tumor induction in mice. Am J Path 1995;127(2):243–261.
34. Almendral J, Huebuch D, Blundell P, MacDonald-Bravo H, Bravo R. Cloning and sequence analysis of the human protein cyclin: homology with DNA binding proteins. Proc Natl Acad Sci USA 1987;84:1575–1579.

Part Four
Some Emerging Tumor Markers

Chapter 36

Adhesion Molecules as Tumor Markers

Subhas Chakrabarty and Herbert A. Fritsche

Cell adhesion to the extracellular matrix (ECM) is a fundamental and distinguishing feature of multi-cellular organisms. Cell matrix adhesion plays a crucial role in maintaining normal tissue architecture, cellular differentiation, and function. All three major cell types—mesenchymal, endothelial, and epithelial—contribute to the production and maintenance of the ECM. How cell-matrix interaction controls such diverse biological processes is not fully understood. It is known, however, that cellular adhesion to the ECM is a dynamic process in which specific and distinct molecules interact to generate the signals required for proper gene expression. For example, interaction of the ECM adhesion molecule laminin with its cell-surface integrin receptor is required for the maintenance of a differentiated mammary epithelial cell function (1).

Because disruption of cell-matrix adhesion is a hallmark of malignant transformation and plays a critical role in tumor progression and subsequent metastasis of tumor cells, ECM adhesion molecules and/or cell-surface receptors for these molecules may offer new opportunities in the search for useful markers for malignant diseases. In this chapter, we discuss the tumor marker potential of the ECM adhesion molecule fibronectin (FN).

FIBRONECTIN (FN)

FN is a large, multifunctional, adhesion glycoprotein present in body fluids, basement membranes, and the ECM. FN participates in a variety of physiologic functions: cell-matrix adhesion, cell migration, cellular differentiation, angiogenesis, homeostasis/thrombosis, wound healing, inflammation, fibrosis, and phagocytosis/opsonization (2). Interaction of ECM FN with its cell-surface integrin receptor initiates signal transduction cascades that lead to gene expression in a tissue-specific manner (1–2).

FN is encoded by a single gene. Its pre-mRNA, however, can be alternately spliced at three different sites, and as many as 20 different spliced FN protein isoforms can be generated (3). The alternate splicing regions of FN are shown in Figure 1. Plasma FN (PFN) is synthesized and secreted by hepatocytes of the liver, while mesenchymal, endothelial, and epithelial cells synthesize and secrete cellular FN (CFN) into the ECM (3). The expression of CFN in cells is transformation-sensitive and is modulated in cellular transformation and in the induction of differentiation or reversal of the transformed phenotype (4–5). CFN contains one or both of the extra domains A and B (EDA

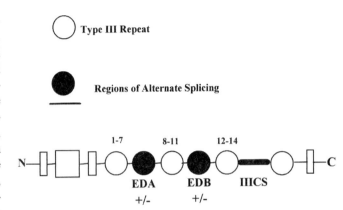

Figure 1 Alternate splicing regions of FN. FN is composed mainly of three types of repeating domains (types I, II, and III). Two type III repeats (their positions depicted by solid black circles, located between type III-7 and 8 and between type III-11 and 12) encoded by a single exon undergo alternate splicing by an exon-skipping mechanism. The exon encoding the IIICS segment also undergoes alternate splicing by exon subdivision giving rise to five variants.

and EDB) while PFN is EDA- and EDB-negative (Figure 1). Both the EDA and EDB domains are spliced out in hepatocytes during synthesis of the matured FN mRNA (Figure 1). However, upon transformation, hepatocellular carcinomas re-express the EDA and EDB domains (6).

Alternately spliced FN isoforms may be expressed in a tissue-specific manner, and the splicing pattern may also be regulated by growth factors, during ontogeny and development and during aging and cellular transformation (3,6,7). It has been hypothesized that different FN isoforms possess different physiologic functions (3), and the EDA and EDB domains are implicated to play a functional role in the malignant behavior of tumor cells. Thus, the development of assays to measure CFN in serum or plasma is a first step in probing the tumor marker potential of tumor cell-associated CFN. The ultimate goal is the development of assays to measure specific malignant disease-associated CFN isoforms in serum or plasma.

CLINICAL APPLICATIONS

We have developed an enzyme-linked immunosorbent assay (ELISA) using a monoclonal antibody directed against the EDA domain of CFN as a first step in determining if there is an increase in EDA immunoreactivity in the sera of patients with malignant diseases. Because upregulated FN expression and secretion by malignant tissues and cells have been reported (8–10), we hypothesize that elevated EDA levels in patients' sera (if any, by comparison with sera from normal individuals) are derived from malignant cells

Figure 2 shows the results of such an assay. Five out of ten normal sera were found to have detectable EDA immunoreactivity, while ten out of ten sera from patients with liver cancer were EDA-positive. The increase in EDA immunoreactivity in eight of these sera were dramatic and of statistical significance. This is not surprising in view of the fact that serum FN is derived from hepatocyes, and hepatocellular carcinomas re-express the EDA and EDB domains of CFN. The high level of EDA immunoreactivity in the sera of liver cancer patients may also illustrate the ease with which FN is released into the circulation; after all, one of the functions of liver is to synthesize and secrete FN into the blood. Eight out of ten sera from colon cancer patients were positive for EDA immunoreactivity and four had significant increases in EDA immunoreactivity over that of normal sera. Five out of ten prostate and nine out of ten lung cancer patient sera were positive for EDA immunoreactivity, and one lung and four prostate sera showed significant increases in EDA immunoreactivity over that of normal sera.

These data show that higher-than-normal EDA immunoreactivity was detectable in the sera of some liver, colon, prostate, and lung cancer patients, with the strongest immunoreactivity observed in liver cancer sera. Thus, EDA immunoreactivity did not appear to be specific for a particular cancer type and appeared to possess a higher sensitivity for liver cancer.

FUTURE DIRECTIONS

Molecular characterization of the alternate splicing profile of CFN from different cancer phenotypes and development of specific antibodies directed to these regions of CFN will be needed to further develop this marker. For example, measuring EDA may not be ideal for prostate cancer if prostate cancer cells express more EDB than EDA. In addition to the EDA and EDB domains, characterization of the splicing profile of the type III connecting segment (IIICS) (Figure 1) region is also needed to determine a complete molecular splicing profile of CFN in different cancer types. Development of quantitative immunoassays using protein standards corresponding to the spliced regions of interest will then be needed to measure accurately the amount of these molecules in serum or plasma in order to fully determine the marker potential of CFN for various malignant diseases.

REFERENCES

1. Roskelly CD, Desprez PY, Bissel MJ. Extracellular matrix dependent tissue-specific gene expression in mammary epithelial cells required both physical and biochemical signal transduction. Proc Natl Acad Sci 1994;91:12378–12382.
2. Johansson S, Svinen S, Wennerberg K, Armulik A, Lohikangas L. Fibronectin–integrin interactions. Frontiers in Biosci 1997;2:126–146.
3. Kornblihtt AR, Pescee CG, Alonso CR, Cramer P, Srebrow A, Werbajh S, Muro AF. The fibronectin gene as a model for splicing and transcription studies (review). FASEB J 1996;10:248–257.
4. Varani J, Chakrabarty S. Changes in the extracellular matrix during transformation and differentiation. In: Orr FW, Buchanan MR, Weiss L (eds.). Microcirculation in cancer metastasis. Boca Raton, FL: CRC Press, 1991:1–22.
5. Huang S, Chakrabarty S. Regulation of fibronectin and laminin receptor expression fibronectin and laminin secretion in human colon cancer cells by transforming growth factor β1. Int J Cancer 1994;57:742–746.
6. Tavian D, De Petro G, Colombi M, Portolani N, Giulini SM, Gardella R, Barlati S. RT- PCR detection of fibronectin EDA+ and EDA–mRNA isoforms: molecular markers for hepatocellular carcinoma. Int J Cancer 1994;56:820–825.
7. Magnuson VL, Young M, Schattenberg DG, Mancini MA, Chen DL, Steffensen B, Klebe RJ. The alternate splicing of fibronectin pre-mRNA is altered during aging and in response to growth factors. J Biol Chem 1991;266:14654–14662.
8. Sonmez H, Suer S, Karaarslan I, Baloglu IT, Kokoglue E. Tissue fibronectin levels of human prostate cancer as a tumor marker. Cancer Biochem Biophys 1995;15:107–110.
9. Suer S, Sonmez H, Karaarslan I, Baloglu IT, Kokoglue E. Tissue sialic acid and fibronectin levels in human prostate cancer. Cancer Letters 1996;99:135–137.
10. Rajagopal S, Navone NM, Troncoso P, Fritsche HA, Chakrabarty S. Modulation of cellular proliferation and production of prostate-specific antigen and matrix adhesion molecules in human prostate carcinoma cells by polypeptide growth factors: comparative analyses of MDA PCa2a with established cell lines. Int J Oncology 1998;12:589–595.

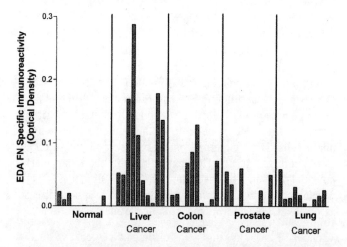

Figure 2 EDA FN specific immunoreactivity in serum by ELISA. Insolubilized polyclonal anti-human FN antibodies were first used to capture total FN in sera. The amount of EDA FN was then determined with a specific monoclonal antibody directed against the EDA domain of FN. EDA immunoreactivity was determined in 10 sera in each of the panels.

Chapter 37

Soluble ErbB Receptors (sEGFR/sErbBs): Serum Biomarkers in Breast and Ovarian Cancer

Jacqueline M. Lafky, Tammy M. Greenwood, Andre T. Baron,

Cecelia H. Boardman, Elsa M. Cora, and Nita J. Maihle

The activation or altered expression of growth-promoting oncogenes is thought to play a critical role in the development and progression of many human cancers. As a consequence, oncogenes and their related protein products are being investigated as potential tumor markers. In this regard, the *ERBB* family of proto-oncogenes is being studied intensely in many types of human carcinomas.

This family of proto-oncogenes encodes four structurally related transmembrane receptors: the epidermal growth factor receptor (EGFR, ErbB1, HER1); ErbB2 (HER2, neu); ErbB3 (HER3); and ErbB4 (HER4). These ErbB receptor tyrosine kinases play important physiologic roles in cell proliferation, differentiation, and survival. Hence, it is not surprising that gene amplification, protein overexpression, and genetic mutations resulting in aberrant ErbB receptor structure and signal transduction have been shown to contribute to the process of malignant transformation.

Numerous investigators have reported *ERBB* gene amplification and/or ErbB receptor overexpression in a variety of human carcinomas, including breast and ovarian cancers. Clinically, *ERBB* oncogene amplification and/or ErbB oncoprotein overexpression in tumors correlate with disease recurrence and poor patient prognosis, as well as with responsiveness to therapy (1,2).

In addition to the full-length transmembrane forms of EGF/ErbB receptors, soluble receptor isoforms (sEGFR/sErbBs) have been identified for all four members of the ErbB family (3). These sErbB proteins contain only the extracellular domain of the receptor and can be generated by either alternate mRNA splicing/processing events or by proteolytic cleavage of the holoreceptor. Alternate mRNA transcripts that encode 60-kDa and 110-kDa sErbB1; 68-kDa and 110-kDa sErbB2; 20-kDa, 45-kDA, 50-kDa, 76-kDa, and 85-kDa sErbB3 isoforms; as well as proteolytic 105-kDa sErbB2 and 120-kDa sErbB4 isoforms, have been identified.

Previous studies have shown that sErbB isoforms decrease cell proliferation both in vitro (4–6) and in vivo (7). The mechanism underlying decreased cell proliferation may involve competitive binding of sErbB isoforms to growth factors (6,8) and/or kinase inhibition via the formation of sErbB and full-length ErbB receptor heterodimers (6,9). Given the important role of ErbB receptors and sErbB isoforms in modulating cell proliferation and transformation, and the ability to quantify serum sErbB using noninvasive immunoassay methods involving minimal risk to patients, sErbB isoforms recently have become a major focus of research aimed at evaluating their clinical utility as cancer biomarkers.

CLINICAL APPLICATION

A number of immunoassays have been developed to quantify sErbB1 and sErbB2, and these assays have been used to study these proteins as potential serum biomarkers in breast (Table 1) and ovarian (Table 2) cancer patients. There are no current immunoassays to measure sErbB3 and sErbB4 isoforms reported in the literature. Although several sErbB1 and sErbB2 immunoassays have been developed, not all have been well characterized, and only a few are commercially available. Of the assays that have been commercialized, the Chiron Diagnostics and Dupont sErbB2 and the Triton Diagnostics/Ciba-Corning Diagnostics sErbB1 and sErbB2 immunoassay kits have been discontinued; the Nichirei Corporation sErbB2 enzyme-linked immunosorbent assay (ELISA) is not available in the United States.

Table 3 lists the sErbB1 and sErbB2 immunoassays that are currently available commercially (as of 2001) in the United States. The two commercial sErbB1 assays are sandwich-type ELISA kits marketed by Oncogene Research Products (San Diego, CA) or OncogeneScience (Cambridge, MA). Three of the four commercially available sErbB2 immunoassays are sandwich type ELISA kits and are distributed by OncogeneScience, Oncogene Research Products, and Bender Med-Systems Diagnostics GmbH (Vienna, Austria). The fourth commercial sErbB2 immunoassay is marketed as a fully automated central laboratory instrument, Bayer Immuno 1™ Immuno-assay System (Bayer Diagnostics, Tarrytown, NY). In addition, according to its web-

Table 1 Summary of serum sErbB immunoassays used in breast cancer studies

sErbB analyzed	Immunoassay used (measurement units)	Reference
sErbB1	Triton Diagnostics ELISA (fmol/mg protein)	Streckfus C, et al. Clin Cancer Res 2000;6:2363.
	ALISA not commercially available (fmol/mL)	Cora EM, et al. Proc Am Assoc Cancer Res 2000;41:640. Perez E, et al. Ann Oncol 2002. In press.
	EIA not commercially available (fmol/mL)	Kumar RR, et al. Hum Antibodies 2001;10:143.
sErbB2	Applied Biotechnology ELISA (HNU/mL) (Later became OncogeneScience, Inc.)	Yasasever V, et al. J Tumor Marker Oncol 1992;7:33.
	Bayer Immuno 1™ Immunoassay System (ng/mL)	Cheung KL, et al. Int J Biol Markers 2000;15:203. Schwartz MK, et al. Int J Biol Markers 2000;15:324. Cook GB, et al. Anticancer Res 2001;21:1465. Esteva FJ, et al. J Clin Oncol 2002;20:1800. Lipton A, et al. J Clin Oncol 2002;20;1467.
	Bender MedSystems Diagnostics ELISA (ng/mL)	Willsher PC, et al. Breast Cancer Res Treat 1996;40:251. Visco V, et al. Am J Pathol 2000;156:1417. Perez E, et al. Ann Oncol 2002. In press.
	Calbiochem ELISA (U/mL)	Streckfus C, et al. Clin Cancer Res 2000;6:2363.
	Chiron Diagnostics ELISA (U/mL)	Luftner D, et al. Int J Biol Markers 1999;14:55. Harris LN, et al. J Clin Oncol 2001;19:1698.
	Nichirei Corporation EIA (ng/mL)	Mori S, et al. Jpn J Cancer Res 1990;81:489. Yu FZ, et al. Rinsho Byori 1991;39:1087. Hosono M, et al. Jpn J Cancer Res 1993;84:147. Sugano K, et al. Gan To Kagaku Ryoho 1994;21:1245. Sugano K, et al. Gan To Kagaku Ryoho 1994;21:1255. Imoto S, et al. Jpn J Clin Oncol 1999;29:336. Chearskul S, et al. J Med Assoc Thai 2000;83:886. Sugano K, et al. Int J Cancer 2000;89:329.
	Oncogene Research Products ELISA (fmol/mL)	Colomer R, et al. Clin Cancer Res 2000;6:2356. Bewick M, et al. Bone Marrow Transplant 2001;27:847.
	OncogeneScience ELISA (HNU/mL)	Carney WP, et al. J Tumor Marker Oncol 1991;6:53. Breuer B, et al. Med Sci Res 1993;21:383. Kath R, et al. Ann Oncol 1993;4:585. Breuer B, et al. Cancer Epidemiol Biomarkers Prev 1994;3:63. Andersen TI, et al. Acta Oncol 1995;34:499. Eskelinen M, et al. Anticancer Res 1997;17:1231. Yamauchi H, et al. J Clin Oncol 1997;15:2518. Breuer B, et al. Breast Cancer Res Treat 1998;49:261. Krajewska B, et al. Int J Occup Med Environ Health 1998;11:343. Kasimir-Bauer S, et al. Breast Cancer Res Treat 2001;69:123 Kasimir-Bauer S, et al. Clin Cancer Res 2001;7:1582
	Triton Diagnostics/Ciba-Corning Diagnostics EIA (U/mL)	Leitzel K, et al. J Clin Oncol 1992;10:1436. Narita T, et al. Breast Cancer Res Treat 1993;24:97. Kynast B, et al. J Cancer Res Clin Oncol 1993;119:249. Wu JT, et al. J Clin Lab Anal 1993;7:31. Fontana X, et al. Anticancer Res 1994;14:2099. Isola JJ, et al. Cancer 1994;73:652. Kandl H, et al. Br J Cancer 1994;70:739. Narita T, et al. Jpn J Clin Oncol 1994;24:74. Watanabe N, et al. Acta Oncol 1994;33:901. Leitzel K, et al. J Clin Oncol 1995;13:1129. Wu JT, et al. J Clin Lab Anal 1995;9:151.

		Molina R, et al. Anticancer Res 1996;16:2295.
		Molina R, et al. Br J Cancer 1996;74:1126.
		Volas GH, et al. Cancer 1996;78:267.
		Esteva-Lorenzo FJ, et al. Acta Oncol 1997;36:651.
		Krainer M, et al. Oncology 1997;54:475.
		Mansour OA, et al. Anticancer Res 1997;17:3101.
		Molina R, et al. Tumour Biol 1997;18:188.
		Molina R, et al. Breast Cancer Res Treat 1998;51:109.
		Molina R, et al. Anticancer Res 1999;19:2551.
	DDIRMA not commercially available (ng/mL)	Pupa SM, et al. Oncogene 1993;8:2917.
	ELISA not commercially available (fmol/mL)	Fehm T, et al. Breast Cancer Res Treat 1997;43:87.
	ELISA not commercially available (fmol/mL)	Fehm T, et al. Oncology 1998;55:33.
	ELISA not commercially available (fmol/mL)	Yasasever V, et al. Clin Biochem 2000;33:315.
	Immunoassay used is unknown	Ohuchi N, et al. Nippon Geka Gakkai Zasshi 1991;92:1530.
		Narita T, et al. Gan to Kagaku Ryoho 1992;19:909.
		Konishi K, et al. Rinsho Byori 1993;41:1108.

ELISA, enzyme-linked immunosorbent assay; ALISA, acridinium-linked immunosorbent assay; EIA, enzyme immunosorbent assay; DDIRMA, double-determinant radioimmunoassay.

site, Bayer Diagnostics is in the process of developing additional HER2/neu assays using their ADVIA Centaur® and ACS:180® automated laboratory platforms (see http://www.bayerdiag.com/products/lab/oncology.html).

Table 3 lists the pertinent characteristics of the sErbB1 and sErbB2 immunoassays commercially available in the United States (i.e., linear range, detection limit, and intra and inter assay coefficients of variance). Comparison of the properties of the commercial versus the noncommercial sErbB immunoassays reveals that different analytical standards, as well as different capture and detection antibodies, are used in these assays. Moreover, some immunoassays report data in absolute values (e.g., µg/mL or ng/mL; fmol/mL), whereas others report results in relative values (e.g., U/mL or HNU/mL). The Oncogene Research Product and Bender MedSystems Diagnostics HER2 ELISAs, for example, use full-length p185 ErbB2 as the standard, whereas the OncogeneScience ELISA uses a recombinant form of p105 sErbB2 as the standard. These analytical standards may differ in their antibody recognition properties and therefore may produce unique dose-response curves, which may result in disparate sErbB concentrations for test samples.

Table 2 Summary of serum sErbB immunoassays used in ovarian cancer studies

sErbB analyzed	Immunoassay used (measurement units)	Reference
sErbB1	ALISA not commercially available (fmol/mL)	Baron AT, et al. Cancer Epidemiol Biomarkers Prev 1999;8:129.
		Boardman CH. Proc Am Assoc Cancer Res 2000;41:730.
		Baron AT, et al. In preparation.
sErbB2	Chiron Diagnostics ELISA (U/mL)	Cheung TH, et al. Gynecol Obstet Invest 1999;48:133.
	DuPont ELISA (HNU/mL)	McKenzie SJ, et al. Cancer 1993;71:3942.
	Nichirei Corporation IRMA (U/mL)	Hosono M, et al. Jpn J Cancer Res 1993;84:147.
	Oncogene Research Products ELISA (fmol/mL)	Yazici H, et al. Cancer Invest 2000;18:110.
	OncogeneScience ELISA (HNU/mL)	Meden H, et al. J Cancer Res Clin Oncol 1994;120:378.
		Meden H, et al. Anticancer Res 1997;17:757.
		Marx D, et al. Anticancer Res 1998;18:2891.
		Abendstein B, et al. Anticancer Res 2000;20:569.
	Triton Diagnostics/Ciba-Corning Diagnostics EIA (U/mL)	Leitzel K, et al. J Clin Oncol 1992;10:1436.
		Wu JT, et al. J Clin Lab Anal 1993;7:31.
		Felip E, et al. Med Clin (Barc) 1995;105:5.
		Wu JT, et al. J Clin Lab Anal 1995;9:151.
		Molina R, et al. Tumour Biol 1997;18:188.

ALISA, acridinium-linked immunosorbent assay; ELISA, enzyme-linked immunosorbent assay; IRMA, immunoradiometric assay; EIA, enzyme immunosorbent assay.

Table 3 Commercially available sErbB immunoassays

Company	Product description (Catalog number)	Performance characteristics	Comments
Bayer Diagnostics (Tarrytown, NY)	Bayer Immuno 1™ Immunoassay System for HER2/neu	Linear range: 0.1–250 µg/L Sensitivity: 0.1 µg/L Intra assay CV[a]: 0.8–1.2% Inter assay CV: 1.1–1.7%	This heterogenous sandwich magnetic separation assay uses an automated central laboratory instrument. This immunoassay system was designed in collaboration with Oncogene Sciences and uses monoclonal antibodies, NB-3 and TA-1. Performance characteristics were obtained from Payne RC, et al. Clin Chem 2000;46:175.
Bender MedSystems™ (MedSystems Diagnostics GmbH, Vienna, Austria)	sp185^{HER2}(c-neu) ELISA[b] (BMS207) sp185^{HER2}(c-neu) Module Set[b] (BMS207MST)	Standard range: 0.16–10 ng/mL Sensitivity: 0.1 ng/mL Intra assay CV: 1.9% Inter assay CV: 5.8%	This ELISA uses two undisclosed monoclonal antibodies. Performance characteristics were obtained from the Bender MedSystems' web site: http://www.bendermedsystems.com.
Oncogene Research Products (A Brand of CN BioSciences, Inc., Darmstadt, Germany)	EGF Receptor ELISA Kit[b] (QIA35)	Assay range: 0–100 fmol/mL Sensitivity: 0.3 fmol/mL Intra assay CV: ~<10.5% Inter assay CV: ~<15%	This EGFR ELISA uses two undisclosed monoclonal antibodies. Performance characteristics were obtained from the CN BioSciences' web site: http://www.cnbi.com.
	c-erbB2/c-neu Rapid Format ELISA[b] (QIA10)	Assay range: 0–3 ng/mL Sensitivity: 0.024 ng/mL Intra assay CV: ~<20% Inter assay CV: ~<9.5%	This HER2/neu ELISA uses two undisclosed monoclonal antibodies. Performance characteristics were obtained from the CN BioSciences' web site: http://www.cnbi.com.
OncogeneScience (Division of Bayer Diagnostics, Tarrytown, NY)	EGFR Microtiter ELISA[b] (OSDI-23-RUO—1 plate/pack) EGFR Microtiter ELISA[b] (OSDI-23M-RUO—5 plates/pack)	Assay range: 0.25–300 ng/mL Sensitivity: 0.25 ng/mL Intra assay CV: Not available Inter assay CV: Not available	This EGFR ELISA uses two undisclosed monoclonal antibodies. Performance characteristics were not available from the web site, but were obtained through personal communication (J. Whitaker, Sales, Marketing and Business Development Manager, OncogeneScience).
	HER-2/neu Microtiter ELISA[c] (OSDI-10—1 plate/pack) HER-2/neu Microtiter ELISA[c] (OSDI-10M—5 plates/pack) HER-2/neu Microtiter ELISA[b] (OSDI-10-RUO—1 plate/pack) HER-2/neu Microtiter ELISA[b] (OSDI-10M-RUO—5 plates/pack)	Analytical range: 0–35 ng/mL Sensitivity: 1.5 ng/mL Intra assay CV: 6.0–10.2% Inter assay CV: 10.4–17.7%	This ELISA was originally developed by Carney WP, et al. J Tumor Marker Oncol 1991; 6:53. The original immunoassay used monoclonal antibodies, NB-3 and TA-1. Performance characteristics were not available from the web site, but were obtained from the OncogeneScience product sheets.

[a] CV, coefficient of variation.
[b] Product sheets indicate for research use only.
[c] Product has been FDA-cleared for in vitro diagnostic use.

The unique attributes of these different immunoassays, including differences between assay antibodies and standards, as well as differences in readout, have made it difficult to directly compare sErbB concentrations between studies, and may explain some of the discrepancies that have been reported for serum sErbB1 and sErbB2 concentrations in breast and ovarian cancer patients (see Tables 1 and 2 for summary). Given the recent discovery of multiple sErbB1 (60-kDa and 110-kDa) and sErbB2 (68-kDa, 105-kDa, and 110-kDa) isoforms, it is also possible that each of these immunoassays may detect a particular subset of sErbB proteins and/or a unique pattern of sErbB isoform complexes (e.g., sErbB isoforms in complex with each other, with growth factors, with serum-binding proteins, etc.).

Given the known complexity of this family of receptor isoforms and the large number of possible permutations of serum complexes that may be generated by various growth factors and serum-binding proteins, one might anticipate that our ability to accurately measure these proteins in serum (and our subsequent interpretation of these measurements) will evolve over time, much as the measurement of the prostate-specific antigen (PSA; "free" vs. "complexed" vs. "total") has evolved over the past decade to the point where it is now clinically useful and reliable (10).

Despite the limitations of the current repertoire of sErbB immunoassays, preliminary studies in this field have identified several potential clinical uses for serum sErbB. These include the utility of these serum biomarkers for identifying individuals at increased cancer risk, detecting preclinical cancer, diagnosing a clinically detectable mass, predicting responsiveness to therapy, monitoring responsiveness to therapy, monitoring disease recurrence, and predicting disease outcome.

In this regard, serum sErbB1 concentrations appear to be significantly lower in ovarian cancer patients (11) whereas serum sErbB2 concentrations appear to be elevated in both breast and ovarian cancer patients (1,12). In ovarian cancer patients, low sErbB1 concentrations are currently being evaluated for risk assessment, as well as for their utility in screening, diagnosing, and monitoring disease recurrence. In breast cancer patients, elevated sErbB2 concentrations have been associated with poor patient prognosis, early disease recurrence, and poor responsiveness to hormonal therapy. Studies to better define the clinical utility of serum sErbB2 concentrations as a prognosticator of breast cancer, and as a predictor of disease recurrence and therapy, are of particular importance and promise.

FUTURE DIRECTIONS

In summary, sErbB isoforms are ideal candidates for the development of serum biomarkers clinically useful in the assessment of disease activity in both breast and ovarian cancer patients. Studies in both breast and ovarian cancer have produced exciting and promising results, and have identified several potential clinical applications for the measurement of both serum sErbB1 and sErbB2. Well-designed prospective clinical trials, cross-sectional studies, case-control studies, and cohort studies are now warranted and will be necessary to (i) identify potential effect modifiers and/or confounders of serum sErbB concentrations; (ii) define normal reference ranges and cut-off values; and (iii) determine test sensitivity, specificity, and positive and negative predictive values.

In addition to population-based studies, laboratory research is needed to develop immunoassays to quantify sErbB3 and sErbB4 isoforms, and to better characterize the sErbB isoforms/sErbB complexes being measured by each immunoassay. Finally, to allow for comparisons between different study populations, we recommend that future immunoassays use a common analytical standard, preferably a purified isoform of sErbB, and report concentrations in mole/volume (i.e., absolute serum values) units of measurement.

Acknowledgements

The authors would like to thank Mr. Jeffrey R. Whittaker (Manager Sales, Marketing and Business Development, OncogeneScience) for personal communication. This work has been supported by NIH grants KO7 CA76170, R21 CA82520, and RO3 CA82091 to ATB; K01 CA73859 to EMC, R01 CA57534 and UO1 CA85133 to NJM; and by the NIH Office of Women's Health Research, Friends You Can Count On, and the Prospect Creek Foundation.

REFERENCES

1. Harris L, Luftner D, Jager W, Robertson JF. c-erbB-2 in serum of patients with breast cancer. Int J Biol Markers 1999;14: 8–15.
2. Mendelsohn J, Baselga J. The EGF receptor family as targets for cancer therapy. Oncogene 2000;19:6550–6565.
3. Maihle NJ, Lafky JM, Baron AT, Boardman CH, Greenwood T, Christensen TA, Reiter JL, Cora EM, Lee H, Suman VJ, Fishman DA, Perez EA, Podratz KC. EGF receptor/ErbB isoforms as serum biomarkers in breast and ovarian cancer. J Clin Ligand Assay (in press).
4. Petch LA, Harris J, Raymond VW, Blasband A, Lee DC, Earp HS. A truncated, secreted form of the epidermal growth factor receptor is encoded by an alternatively spliced transcript in normal rat tissue. Mol Cell Biol 1990;10:2973–2982.
5. Flickinger TW, Maihle NJ, Kung HJ. An alternatively processed mRNA from the avian c-erbB gene encodes a soluble, truncated form of the receptor that can block ligand-dependent transformation. Mol Cell Biol 1992;12:883–893.
6. Lee H, Akita RW, Sliwkowski MX, Maihle NJ. A naturally occurring secreted human ErbB3 receptor isoform inhibits heregulin-stimulated activation of ErbB2, ErbB3, and ErbB4. Cancer Res 2001;61:4467–4473.
7. Nieto-Sampedro M, Broderick JT. A soluble brain molecule related to epidermal growth factor receptor is a mitogen inhibitor for astrocytes. J Neurosci Res 1989;22:28–35.
8. Cadena DL, Gill GN. Expression and purification of the epidermal growth factor receptor extracellular domain utilizing a polycistronic expression system. Protein Expr Purif 1993;4: 177–186.
9. Basu A, Raghunath M, Bishayee S, Das M. Inhibition of tyrosine kinase activity of the epidermal growth factor (EGF) receptor by a truncated receptor form that binds to EGF: role for inter-receptor interaction in kinase regulation. Mol Cell Biol 1989;9: 671–677.
10. Stephan C, Jung K, Lein M, Sinha P, Schnorr D, Loening SA. Molecular forms of prostate-specific antigen and human kallikrein 2 as promising tools for early diagnosis of prostate cancer. Cancer Epidemiol Biomarkers Prev 2000;9:1133–1147.
11. Baron AT, Lafky JM, Boardman CH, Balasubramaniam S, Suman VJ, Podratz KC, Maihle NJ. Serum sErbB1 and epidermal growth factor levels as tumor biomarkers in women with stage III or IV epithelial ovarian cancer. Cancer Epidemiol Biomarkers Prev 1999;8:129–137.
12. Meden H, Kuhn W. Overexpression of the oncogene c-erbB-2 (HER2/neu) in ovarian cancer: a new prognostic factor. Eur J Obstet Gynecol Reprod Biol 1997;71:173–179.

Chapter **38**

A Multiplex Real-Time PCR Assay for the Detection of Mammaglobin and Complementary Transcribed Genes in Breast Cancer

Barbara K. Zehentner, Davin C. Dillon, Yuqiu Jiang, Jiangchun Xu, Steven G. Reed, David H. Persing, and Raymond L. Houghton

Mammaglobin, a homologue of the rabbit uteroglobin and the rat steroid binding protein subunit C3, is a low-molecular-weight, highly glycosylated protein (1,2). It belongs to the uteroglobin family of small, secretory proteins with unclear physiological functions. All five known human family members (Clara cell 10-kDa protein, lipophilins A and B, lacryglobin/ mammaglobin B/lipophilin C, and mammaglobin) are localized on chromosome 11q12.2 in a dense cluster (3). In contrast to its homologues, mammaglobin has been reported to be breast-specific and its expression has been described in 70–80 % of primary and metastatic breast tumor biopsies (1,2,4–6).

Since mammaglobin is not universally expressed in breast cancers, additional markers are necessary to develop a sensitive detection system for malignant breast cancer cells. Genetic subtraction, DNA microarray analysis, and real-time polymerase chain reaction (PCR) have identified three genes—*B305D*, γ-aminobutyrate type A receptor π subunit (*GABAπ*), and *B726P*—as therapeutic and diagnostic target candidates in breast cancer (7,8). The expression profiles of these candidate genes have been shown to complement the expression of mammaglobin in breast cancers.

The novel gene designated as *B305D* (*AP001465.1*) is located on chromosome 21q11.1, c1 region; its corresponding cDNA has been isolated by using differential display PCR technique. B305D is predicted by PSORT, a computer program for the prediction of protein subcellular localization sites from their amino acid sequences, to be a type II membrane protein that contains a series of ankyrin repeats.

GABAπ (*U95367*) is a known gene that complements *B305D* expression in breast cancer. This gene is a member of the $GABA_A$ receptor family and its expression was shown in lung, thymus, and normal prostate tissue at low levels, and in the uterus at high levels (9). The tissue expression profile of *GABAπ* is in contrast to other $GABA_A$ receptors that are typically expressed in neuronal tissues.

B726P cDNA (AL357148) was derived from PCR subtraction and is located on chromosome 10. *B726P* is a novel gene, with mRNA splicing yielding several different putative open reading frames. The identification of one of these splice forms has been described using serological screening of a breast cancer library (10).

Mammaglobin, *B305D*, *GABAπ*, and *B726P* have been shown to be tumor-specific target genes for breast cancer (7). The single expression of any of these candidate genes can only be detected in a certain percentage of breast tumors. However, due to their complementary expression profiles, the four genes could be collectively utilized as diagnostic or prognostic indicators for breast cancer.

CLINICAL APPLICATION

A multiplex real-time PCR assay was established to detect the expression of mammaglobin, *B305D*, *GABAπ*, and *B726P* simultaneously. Specific PCR primers and Taqman probes were used in combination to detect the combined mRNA expression profile of the four target genes in 50 metastatic breast cancer lymph node samples, 27 primary breast tumor samples, and 27 normal lymph node samples.

Total RNA was extracted from liquid nitrogen-frozen tissue samples by homogenization in Trizol® reagent (Gibco BRL, Bethesda, MD) and cDNA was prepared using Oligo dT (Roche Diagnostics, Indianapolis, IN) primer with superscript II reverse transcriptase (Gibco BRL, Bethesda, MD). The expression level of single genes of interest or their combined expression level in the multiplex assay was determined by quantitative real-time PCR. This was performed on the ABI 7700 Prism sequence detection system (Applied Biosystems, Foster City, CA) using 6-carboxy-fluorescein (FAM) -labeled Taqman probes. Actin was used to normalize expression levels. Forty PCR cycles were performed with 0.025 U/μl TaqGold (Applied Biosystems).

The cDNA of 50 pathology-positive metastatic breast cancer lymph node samples and 27 normal or nonrelevant disease lymph node samples was tested. The multiplex assay detected positive expression signals (copy number >2) in all 50 metastatic breast cancer samples whereas non-breast-cancer lymph node specimens were negative (Figure 1).

Real-time PCR was positive for mammaglobin in 40, for *B305D* in 36, for *GABAπ* in 15, and for *B726P* in 22 metastatic breast cancer lymph node specimens (Table 1). All mammaglobin-negative breast cancer lymph node samples were detected positive by a combined expression profile of *B305D* and *GABAπ*. However, *B726P* expression enhanced signal intensity in four out of ten mammaglobin-negative samples.

Additionally, 27 primary breast tumor samples were tested and found to be positive in the multiplex PCR assay. Mammaglobin was overexpressed in 17, *B305D* in 16, *GABAπ* in 10, and *B726P* in 14 specimens (Table 1). The primary tumor samples negative for mammaglobin could be detected by a combination of *B305D* and *GABAπ* in nine cases. One primary breast tumor sample was negative for mammaglobin, *B305D*, and *GABAπ*, but positive for *B726P* expression.

The multiplex real-time PCR assay detected a positive signal for all 50 metastatic lymph nodes and all 27 primary tumor specimens. Two genes in particular, *B305D* and *GABAπ*, added to the diagnostic sensitivity of mammaglobin detection. The detection of *B726P* expression added one primary tumor sample and enhanced the detection sensitivity in samples that expressed other target genes at low levels.

FUTURE DIRECTIONS

The presence of disseminated tumor cells constitutes a source for recurrence of disease. Consequently, lymph node staging is an important diagnostic step to determine appropriate adjuvant therapy. Conventional axillary lymph node dissection or alternatively, the less invasive strategy of sentinel lymph node biopsies (5), is used to detect residual disease and to provide prognostic values for staging and treatment of the disease.

Current approaches to identify nodal micrometastases use staining (hematoxylin or eosin) or immunohistochemical analysis for cytokeratin proteins (10). False-negative results can be obtained by missing small metastatic foci due to inadequate sectioning. Immunohistochemistry can result in false-positive results due to illegitimate expression of cytokeratins (reticulum cells) (10).

RT-PCR could provide a more sensitive technique for tumor cell detection but its application is limited due to the lack of a single specific breast cancer marker. The detection of cytokeratin expression by PCR to identify tumor cells is limited by its specificity and the expression of cytokeratins does not provide additional information useful for prognosis and therapeutic possibilities.

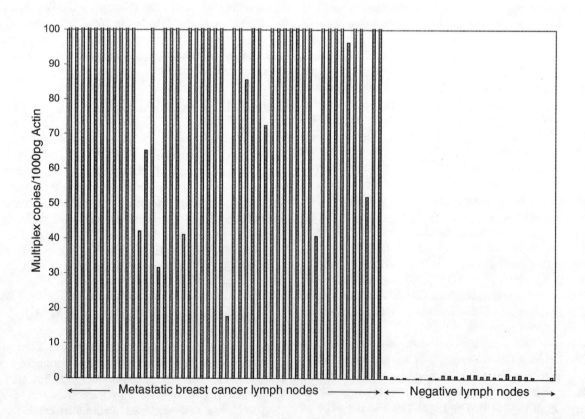

Figure 1 The multiplex real-time PCR assay detected significant combined expression signals for mammaglobin, *B305D*, *GABAπ*, and *B726P* in 50 metastatic breast cancer lymph nodes. Twenty-seven other lymph nodes (24 normal + 2 melanoma + 1 lymphoma) showed no significant expression signals (copies <2).

Table 1 Summary of mammaglobin, GABAπ, B305D, and B726P expression in 50 metastatic breast cancer lymph nodes, 27 primary breast cancer, and 27 normal or nonrelevant disease lymph node samples, respectively

		Breast cancer		Other lymph nodes	
		Metastatic lymph nodes	Primary tumors	Melanoma/ lymphoma	Normal
Mammaglobin		40/50	17/27	0/3	0/24
B305D		36/50	16/27	0/3	0/24
GABAπ		15/50	10/27	0/3	0/24
B726P		22/50	14/27	0/3	0/24
Multiplex assay		50/50	27/27	0/3	0/24
Mammaglobin-negative	B305D	6/10	6/10	0/3	0/24
	GABAπ	8/10	4/10	0/3	0/24
	B726P	2/10	3/10	0/3	0/24
	B305D + GABAπ	10/10	9/10	0/3	0/24

Analysis for residual disease in lymph nodes requires specific, sensitive breast cancer tumor markers with high coverage of the patient population. Breast cancer resembles a heterogeneous disease for which a specific universal tumor marker has not yet been discovered. Several breast tumor markers have been described, but none of them can be found in 100% of the patient population. This report demonstrates an approach to simultaneously use specific complementary markers.

The multimarker assay described here increases the likelihood of cancer detection while minimizing false-positive results. While this study focuses on lymph nodes, this approach could also provide a sensitive detection system for breast cancer cells in bone marrow, peripheral blood, and small-needle biopsy aspirates.

Besides the importance of detecting disseminated tumor cells for prognosis of disease recurrence, their molecular analysis might lead to individualized therapeutic approaches. Similar to current Her-2/neu expression evaluation and consequent application of Herceptin™ therapy, mammaglobin, B305D, GABAπ, and B726P expression analysis might lead to specific immunotherapeutic strategies in the future.

The molecular detection and characterization of disseminated tumor cells in this assay can improve prognostic capabilities and monitoring of disease recurrence, and provide additional criteria to optimize therapy.

Acknowledgements

Primary breast cancer, normal, and tumor lymph node tissue samples were kindly provided by Dr. Elizabeth Repasky (Roswell Park Cancer Institute, Buffalo, NY). Tissue samples were also obtained from the National Disease Research Interchange (NDRI). Lymph node cDNA samples were kindly provided by Dr. Michael Mitas (Medical University of South Carolina, Charleston, SC) and Dr. Timothy P. Fleming (Washington University School of Medicine, St. Louis, MO).

This work was supported in part by NIH grants CA-75794 and CA-86673.

REFERENCES

1. Watson MA, Fleming TP. Mammaglobin, a mammary-specific member of the uteroglobin gene family, is overexpressed in human breast cancer. Cancer Res 1996;56:860–865.
2. Watson MA, Dintzis S, Darrow CM, Voss LE, DiPersio J, Jensen R, et al. Mammaglobin expression in primary, metastatic, and occult breast cancer. Cancer Res 1999;59:3028–3031.
3. Ni J, Klaff-Suske M, Gentz R, Schageman J, Beato M, Klug J. All human genes of the uteroglobin family are localized on chromosome 11q12.2 and form a dense cluster. Ann NY Acad Sci 2000; 923:25–42.
4. Leygue E, Snell L, Dotzlaw H, Hole K, Troup S, Hiller-Hitchcock T, et al. Mammaglobin, a potential marker of breast cancer nodal metastasis. J Pathol 1999;189:28–33.
5. Min CJ, Tafra L, Verbanac KM. Identification of superior markers for polymerase chain reaction detection of breast cancer metastases in sentinel lymph nodes. Cancer Res 1998;58:4581–4584.
6. Fleming TP, Watson MA. Mammaglobin, a breast-specific gene, and its utility as a marker for breast cancer. Ann NY Acad Sci 2000;923:78–89.
7. Houghton RL, Dillon DC, Molesh DA, Zehentner BK, Xu JC, Jiang J, et al. Transcriptional complementarity in breast cancer: application to detection of circulating tumor cells. Molecular Diagnosis 2001;6:79–691.
8. Jiang Y, Harlocker SL, Molesh DA, Dillon DC, Stolk JA, Houghton RL, Repasky EA, Badaro R, Reed SG, Xu JC. Discovery of differentially expressed genes in human breast cancer using substracted cDNA libraries and cDNA microarrays. Oncogene 2002;21:2270–2282.
9. Hedblom E, Kirkness EF. A novel class of $GABA_A$ receptor subunit in tissues of the reproductive system. J Biol Chem 1997;272:15346–15350.
10. Jäger D, Stockert E, Güre AO, Scanlan MJ, Karbach J, Jäger E, et al. Identification of a tissue-specific putative transcription factor in breast tissue by serological screening of a breast cancer library. Cancer Res 2001;61:2055–2061.
11. Köstler WJ, Brodowicz T, Hejna M, Wiltschke C, Zielinski CC. Detection of minimal residual disease in patients with cancer: a review of techniques, clinical implications, and emerging therapeutic consequences. Cancer Detect Prev 2000;24:376–403.

Chapter **39**

Beta-Catenin and Maspin as Tumor Markers

Yong Wen and Mien-Chie Hung

As the understanding of the genetic and molecular basis of human malignancies evolves, specific molecular changes in human cancers are being evaluated as potential molecular markers. If these changes can be validated as tumor markers, they may guide treatment decisions and identify candidates for preventive treatments. In this review, we summarize our recent studies relating to markers of clinical prognosis: β-catenin, an example of a marker of poor prognosis, and maspin, a marker of favorable prognosis.

β-CATENIN AS AN ONCOGENE

β-catenin, originally identified on the basis of its association with cadherin adhesion molecules, is now widely recognized as an essential element of the Wingless-Wnt signaling cascade (1). Wnt signaling stabilizes β-catenin, leading to its accumulation in the cytoplasm and nucleus. In the nucleus, β-catenin associates with T-cell factor (Tcf) and lymphoid enhancer factor (Lef) families of transcriptional factors and regulates the expression of target genes (2–4). APC, together with axin and glycogen synthase kinase (GSK)-3β, binds β-catenin. GSK-3β phosphorylates β-catenin at the N-terminus, targeting it for ubiquitination and degradation by the proteasome complex. Recent studies have demonstrated that APC proteins contain highly conserved and functional nuclear export signals that shuttle β-catenin from the nucleus to the cytoplasm (5,6). Therefore, wild-type APC controls the nuclear accumulation of β-catenin by a combination of nuclear export and cytoplasmic degradation.

In colorectal cancer, and also in melanoma, APC mutations or activating β-catenin mutations increase β-catenin/Tcf-4 complex activity, activating gene expression (7–9). Identification of these functions established the role of β-catenin as an oncogene. Genes that might be targets for transcriptional activation by the β-catenin/Tcf-4 complex relevant to tumorigenesis have been identified recently, including c-myc and cyclin D1 (10,11).

Transgenic mice expressing an oncogenic form of β-catenin in the intestine showed abnormal branched architecture of the villi and an increased proliferation of stem cells (12). This increase in cell proliferation was balanced by increased apoptosis levels in the crypts, and tumor formation was not observed. In contrast, transgenic mice expressing the activated β-catenin in the skin are predisposed to developing skin tumors resembling human pilomatricomas (13). Pilomatricomas are derived from hair matrix cells and in their nucleus they overexpress LEF-1, which is a TCF family member and the β-catenin partner protein (14).

β-CATENIN SIGNALING IN BREAST CANCER

Wnt was first identified as the cellular gene activated by mouse mammary tumor virus (MMTV) integration (15). Several members of the wnt gene family have been identified as activated oncogenes in mouse mammary tumors (16). Expression of wnt-1 oncogene in reconstituted mammary gland induces hyperplasia of mouse mammary epithelium (17). In contrast to the mouse, in which Wnt-1 and Wnt-3 are involved in tumorigenesis, Wnt-2, Wnt-4, Wnt-7b, and Wnt-10b are associated with abnormal proliferation in human breast tissues (18,19). The transformation by Wnt family proteins correlates with the regulation of β-catenin (20). Thus, the stabilization of β-catenin is likely to be the key event in the oncogenicity of the Wnt signal.

β-CATENIN ACTIVATES CYCLIN D1 IN BREAST CANCER

Cyclin D1 plays an important role in regulating the progress of the cell during the G1 phase of the cell cycle. The protein activates the cyclin-dependent kinases (cdks) cdk4 and cdk6, which in turn phosphorylates the retinoblastoma protein (pRb). Recent studies demonstrated that cyclin D1 is one of the targets of β-catenin/Tcf transcriptional activation in breast cancer cells (11,21,22). The cyclin D1 promoter region contains a Tcf-4-binding site (CTTTGATC) located between nucleotides −80 and −73. The promoter activity of cyclin D1 and its production can be upregulated by β-catenin. In breast cancer cell lines, we found a strong correlation between cyclin D1 production and β-catenin/Tcf-4 activity. For example, BT549 and HBL100 cell lines, which expressed almost no detectable cyclin D1, had only background levels of transactivating activity of β-catenin/Tcf-4. In contrast, MCF-7, which expressed the highest level of cyclin D1 protein, had the most significant β-catenin/Tcf-4 activity.

Furthermore, this correlation was also confirmed in breast cancer tissues. We used immunohistochemical staining to assess the expression of cyclin D1 and the subcellular localization of β-catenin, which reflects β-catenin activity. The cadherin-bound form of β-catenin is anchored at the plasma membrane. The transactivation activity of β-catenin is low when it is localized at the plasma membrane. In contrast, non-membrane-bound β-catenin has a major function in transducing the Wnt signal from the cell surface to the nucleus. The accumulation of β-catenin in the cytoplasm and/or the nucleus increases when cells have stabilized β-catenin and therefore, represent the activated β-catenin/Tcf-4 activity. In 123 primary human breast cancer tissues stained, the β-catenin activity and cyclin D1 expression significantly correlated. The stained samples showed either high β-catenin activity with high cyclin D1 expression or low β-catenin activity with negative cyclin D1 staining. Among the 53 cases staining positive for cyclin D1, 49 cases (92%) were positive for β-catenin activity.

Early experimental and clinical studies have suggested that cyclin D1 is involved in transformation and tumor progression. Cyclin D1 mRNA and protein are overexpressed in approximately 50% of primary breast carcinomas; however, CCND1, the gene that encodes cyclin D1, is amplified in only 15–20% of breast cancers. Therefore, cyclin D1 overexpression must result from mechanisms other than gene amplification, such as up-regulation of gene transcription. Our study demonstrated that transactivation by β-catenin may play a substantial role in cyclin D1 overexpression in breast cancer tissues.

β-CATENIN AS A PROGNOSTIC MARKER FOR BREAST CANCER

On the question of whether cyclin D1 is a biological marker in breast cancer, early immunohistochemical prognostic studies produced equivocal results. In our study, we found that both cyclin D1 overexpression and activated β-catenin were associated with a poor prognosis and negatively correlated with patient survival rates (Figure 1).

More importantly, when multivariate analyses for survival rate were performed, activated β-catenin proved a strong prognostic factor that provided predictive information on patient survival rate independent of lymph node metastasis, estrogen receptor and progesterone receptor status, and tumor size.

Cyclin D1 overexpression was also an independent prognostic factor. However, in multivariate analysis of only cyclin D1 expression and β-catenin activity, cyclin D1 was no longer an independent prognostic factor.

These results suggest that activated β-catenin is a more critical player in breast cancer development and that it is directly correlated with poor survival in breast cancer patients. Cyclin D1 overexpression and its prognostic significance could be a consequence of transactivation by β-catenin.

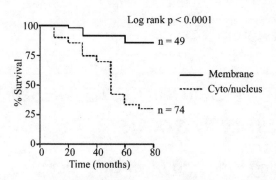

Figure 1 Correlation between activated β-catenin and poor patient survival rate. (Adapted from Lin S-Y, Xia W, Wang JC, Kwong KY, Spohn B, Wen Y, Pestell RG, and Hung M-C. β-catenin, a novel prognostic marker for breast cancer: its roles in cyclin D1 expression and cancer progression. Proc Natl Acad Sci USA 2000;97:4262–4266.)

In contrast to colon cancers, in which defects in the APC gene appear in up to 80% of the cases, mutations in the regulatory regions of β-catenin have been identified in only about 50% of the colon tumors that express wild-type APC. Mutations in the APC gene or the β-catenin gene are less frequent in human breast cancer. APC mutation with associated β-catenin upregulation was reported in only one human breast cancer cell line, DU4475, among 24 human breast cancer cell lines and 3 immortalized human breast epithelial cell lines screened (23). In primary breast tumors, altered APC protein was found in 6% of tumors (24). Although altered β-catenin expression was found in 13–68% of the breast tumors, depending on the individual study, no mutations were observed in the amino-terminal region of the β-catenin gene. β-catenin can be oncogenically activated by direct genetic mutations, by inactivation of the APC tumor suppressor, or by the activation of the wnt-1 signaling pathway.

All three of these mechanisms result in the post-translational stabilization of the β-catenin protein. In this view, the activation of the wnt signaling pathway might contribute to the stabilization of β-catenin in breast cancers. In addition, other cellular defects are probably involved. The detailed mechanisms of the activation of β-catenin warrant further studies. Since β-catenin functions as an oncogene and a marker of poor prognosis, inhibiting the β-catenin signaling pathway may provide a promising approach for breast cancer therapy.

MASPIN: A SERINE PROTEASE INHIBITOR WITH TUMOR SUPPRESSIVE ACTIVITY

Maspin (mammary serine protease inhibitor) is a serine protease inhibitor (serpin) found in mammary epithelial cells (25). It was identified using substractive hybridization and the differential display method. Maspin mRNA is expressed in normal mammary epithelial cell strains, but not in most mammary carcinoma cell lines. The expression of maspin gene is also decreased in human breast cancer tissues and lost in metastatic breast cancer specimens. The differential expression of maspin in normal and carcinoma mammary epithelial cells is regulated at the transcriptional level through the Ets and Ap1 sites in the promoter, which were found inactive in tumor cells (26).

Maspin is located in the cell membrane. Recombinant maspin acts on the cell membrane and inhibits the invasion of human breast cancer and prostate cancer cells by blocking cell mobility (27). In one study, transfection of mammary carcinoma cells with the maspin gene reduced the cells' tumorigenicity and metastasis (25).

FUNCTIONS OF MASPIN

Maspin has been shown to serve as a substrate rather than as an inhibitor for trypsin-like serine proteinases. One study demonstrated that the single-chain tissue plasminogen activator (sctPA) was maspin's target protease (28). Maspin binds to sctPA and has biphasic effects on sctPA, acting as a competitive inhibitor at low concentrations and as a stimulator at higher concentrations. This effect is specific since it has no effect on several other serine proteases, including urokinase-type plasminogen activator, plasmin, chymotrypsin, trypsin, and elastase.

The molecular and biological mechanisms of maspin functions were not well known until recently. Recombinant maspin (rMaspin) reduces the invasive phenotype of MDA-MB-435 cells by altering their integrin profile, particularly alpha 5, which in turn converts these cells to a more benign epithelial phenotype, with less invasive ability (29).

A recent study reported that maspin is an angiogenesis inhibitor (30). Maspin inhibits endothelial cell migration towards bFGF and VEGF in vitro and inhibits corneal neovascularization in vivo. In a xenograft mouse model, systemic treatment with maspin suppressed tumor growth and neovascularization in nude mice. How maspin blocks angiogenesis is not clear yet. The ability to inhibit angiogenesis raises the possibility that maspin may also have therapeutic potential.

In transgenic mice that overexpress maspin in mammary epithelial cells under the control of mammary-specific whey acidic protein (WAP) promoter, mammary gland development during pregnancy is inhibited and apoptosis is induced (31). In WAP-Tag/WAP-maspin bitransgenic mice, maspin has a protective effect on mammary tumor progression, by reducing angiogenesis, increasing apoptosis, and reducing metastasis.

THE REGULATION OF MASPIN EXPRESSION

Maspin expression is regulated by the p53 tumor suppressor pathway (32). Wild-type p53 expression from an adenovirus p53 expression vector induces maspin expression in human prostate cancer cells and breast cancer cells. DNA-damaging agents and cytotoxic drugs induce maspin expression in cells containing the wild-type p53 but not in cells with mutant p53. The maspin promoter is activated when p53 binds directly to the p53-consensus-binding site present in the maspin promoter. Maspin represents a new category of p53-regulated target.

MASPIN: A FAVORABLE PROGNOSTIC MARKER

Maspin is present in the epithelial cells of many human organs, particularly in the myoepithelia of the breast (33). Using an immunohistochemical technique, we found that in 44 cases of oral squamous cell carcinoma (SCC), 66% expressed low to intermediate levels of maspin and 34% expressed high levels (34). In six SCC cell lines from the head and neck we examined, all but one expressed low or no maspin protein. When we compared the clinicopathological features of the oral SCC cases with the maspin expression level, we found that high maspin expression was associated with the absence of lymph node metastasis. More important, higher maspin expression was significantly associated with better rates of overall survival. Our studies suggest that high maspin expression has prognostic value as a favorable marker.

SUMMARY

We conclude that β-catenin activity is an independent marker of poor survival in breast cancer, and maspin is a marker of favorable prognosis in oral squamous cell carcinoma. The studies warrant further investigation of the prognostic value of these markers in other cancer types, and whether they can serve as potential biomarkers for early diagnosis for human cancers.

REFERENCES

1. Gumbiner BM. Signal transduction of beta-catenin, Curr Opin Cell Biol 1995;7:634–640.
2. Behrens J, von Kries J. P, Kuhl M, Bruhn L, Wedlich D, Grosschedl R, and Birchmeier W. Functional interaction of beta-catenin with the transcription factor LEF-1. Nature 1996;382: 638–642.
3. Molenaar M, van de Wetering M, Oosterwegel M, Peterson-Maduro J, Godsave S, Korinek, V, Roose J, Destree O, and Clevers H. XTcf-3 transcription factor mediates beta-catenin-induced axis formation in Xenopus embryos. Cell 1996;86: 391–399.
4. Huber O, Korn R, McLaughlin J, Ohsugi M, Herrmann BG, and Kemler R. Nuclear localization of beta-catenin by interaction with transcription factor LEF-1. Mech Dev 1996;59:3–10.
5. Rosin-Arbesfeld R, Townsley F, and Bienz M. The APC tumor suppressor has a nuclear export function. Nature 2000;406: 1009–1012.
6. Henderson BR. Nuclear-cytoplasmic shuttling of APC regulates beta-catenin subcellular localization and turnover. Nat Cell Biol 2000;2:653–660.
7. Korinek V, Barker N, Morin P. J, van Wichen D, de Weger R, Kinzler KW, Vogelstein B, and Clevers H. Constitutive transcriptional activation by a beta-catenin-Tcf complex in APC$^{-/-}$ colon carcinoma. Science 1997;275:1784–1787.
8. Morin PJ, Sparks, AB, Korinek V, Barker N, Clevers H, Vogelstein B, and Kinzler KW. Activation of beta-catenin-Tcf signaling in colon cancer by mutations in beta-catenin or APC. Science 1997; 275:1787–1790.

9. Rubinfeld B, Robbins P, El-Gamil M, Albert I, Porfiri E, and Polakis P. Stabilization of beta-catenin by genetic defects in melanoma cell lines. Science 1997;275:1790–1792.
10. He TC, Sparks AB, Rago C, Hermeking H, Zawel L, da Costa LT, Morin PJ, Vogelstein B, and Kinzler KW. Identification of c-MYC as a target of the APC pathway. Science 1998;281:1509–1512.
11. Tetsu O and McCormick F. Beta-catenin regulates expression of cyclin D1 in colon carcinoma cells. Nature 1999;398:422–426.
12. Wong MH, Rubinfeld B, and Gordon JI. Effects of forced expression of an NH2-terminal truncated beta-catenin on mouse intestinal epithelial homeostasis. J Cell Biol 1998;141:765–777.
13. Gat U, DasGupta R, Degenstein L, and Fuchs E. De novo hair follicle morphogenesis and hair tumors in mice expressing a truncated beta-catenin in skin. Cell 1998;95:605–614.
14. Chan EF, Gat U, McNiff JM, and Fuchs E. A common human skin tumor is caused by activating mutations in beta-catenin. Nat Genet 1999;21:410–413.
15. Nusse R. and Varmus HE. Many tumors induced by the mouse mammary tumor virus contain a provirus integrated in the same region of the host genome. Cell 1982;31:99–109.
16. Nusse R. The Wnt gene family in tumorigenesis and in normal development. J Steroid Biochem Mol Biol 1992;43:9–12.
17. Edwards PA, Hiby SE, Papkoff J, and Bradbury JM. Hyperplasia of mouse mammary epithelium induced by expression of the Wnt-1 (int-1) oncogene in reconstituted mammary gland. Oncogene 1992;7:2041–2051.
18. Huguet EL, McMahon JA, McMahon AP, Bicknell R, and Harris AL. Differential expression of human Wnt genes 2, 3, 4, and 7B in human breast cell lines and normal and disease states of human breast tissue. Cancer Res 1994;54:2615–2621.
19. Bui TD, Rankin J, Smith K, Huguet EL, Ruben S, Strachan T, Harris AL, and Lindsay, S. A novel human Wnt gene, WNT10B, maps to 12q13 and is expressed in human breast carcinomas. Oncogene 1997;14:1249–1253.
20. Shimizu H, Julius MA, Giarre M, Zheng Z, Brown AM, and Kitajewski J. Transformation by Wnt family proteins correlates with regulation of beta-catenin. Cell Growth Differ 1997;8:1349–1358.
21. Lin SY, Xia W, Wang JC, Kwong KY, Spohn B, Wen Y, Pestell RG, and Hung MC. Beta-catenin, a novel prognostic marker for breast cancer: its roles in cyclin D1 expression and cancer progression. Proc Natl Acad Sci USA 2000;97:4262–4266.
22. Shtutman M, Zhurinsky J, Simcha I, Albanese C, D'Amico M, Pestell R, and Ben-Ze'ev A. The cyclin D1 gene is a target of the beta-catenin/LEF-1 pathway. Proc Natl Acad Sci USA 1999;96:5522–5527.
23. Schlosshauer PW, Brown SA, Eisinger K, Yan Q, Guglielminetti ER, Parsons R, Ellenson LH, and Kitajewski J. APC truncation and increased beta-catenin levels in a human breast cancer cell line. Carcinogenesis 2000;21:1453–1456.
24. Jonsson M, Borg A, Nilbert M, and Andersson T. Involvement of adenomatous polyposis coli (APC)/beta-catenin signaling in human breast cancer. Eur J Cancer 2000;36:242–248.
25. Zou Z, Anisowicz A, Hendrix MJ, Thor A, Neveu M, Sheng S, Rafidi K, Seftor E, and Sager R. Maspin, a serpin with tumor-suppressing activity in human mammary epithelial cells. Science 1994;263:526–529.
26. Zhang M, Maass N, Magit D, and Sager R. Transactivation through Ets and Ap1 transcription sites determines the expression of the tumor-suppressing gene maspin. Cell Growth Differ 1997;8:179–186.
27. Sheng S, Carey J, Sefto, EA, Dias L, Hendrix MJ, and Sager R. Maspin acts at the cell membrane to inhibit invasion and motility of mammary and prostatic cancer cells. Proc Natl Acad Sci USA 1996;93:11669–11674.
28. Sheng S, Truong B, Fredrickson D, Wu R, Pardee AB, and Sager R. Tissue-type plasminogen activator is a target of the tumor suppressor gene maspin. Proc Natl Acad Sci USA 1998;95:499–504.
29. Seftor RE, Seftor EA, Sheng S, Pemberton PA, Sager R, and Hendrix MJ. Maspin suppresses the invasive phenotype of human breast carcinoma. Cancer Res 1998;58:5681–5685.
30. Zhang M, Volpert O, Shi YH, and Bouck N. Maspin is an angiogenesis inhibitor. Nat Med 2000;6:196–199.
31. Zhang M, Shi Y, Magit D, Furth PA, and Sager R. Reduced mammary tumor progression in WAP-TAg/WAP-maspin bitransgenic mice. Oncogene 2000;19:6053–6058.
32. Zou Z, Gao C, Nagaich AK, Connell T, Saito S, Moul, JW, Seth P, Appella E, and Srivastava S. p53 regulates the expression of the tumor suppressor gene maspin. J Biol Chem 2000;275:6051–6054.
33. Pemberton PA, Tipton AR, Pavloff N, Smith J, Erickson JR, Mouchabeck ZM, and Kiefer MC. Maspin is an intracellular serpin that partitions into secretory vesicles and is present at the cell surface. J Histochem Cytochem 1997;45:1697–1706.
34. Xia W, Lau YK, Hu MC, Li L, Johnston DA, Sheng S, El-Naggar A, and Hung MC. High tumoral maspin expression is associated with improved survival of patients with oral squamous cell carcinoma. Oncogene 2000;19:2398–2403.

Chapter 40

TIMP-1 in Colorectal Cancer

Mads Holten-Andersen, Ib Jarle Christensen,
Hans Jørgen Nielsen, and Nils Brünner

A large number of biochemical and cell biological studies have indicated the pivotal role of proteinases in the growth and dissemination of cancer. Most direct evidence comes from studies in which experimental tumors are reduced in growth rate and metastatic potential by systemic treatment with synthetic proteinase inhibitors.

The biological functions of proteinases in cancer progression include activation of latent growth factors or growth factors anchored to the extracellular matrix (ECM), and dissolution of the ECM and basement membranes (BM), thereby governing the migration of cancer cells and cell-to-cell attachment or cell-to-matrix attachment. In addition, fragments formed following proteolytic digestion of the ECM and BM may act as chemokines or angiogenesis-modulating factors.

Several different families of proteinases have been identified: e.g., the matrix metalloproteinases (MMPs), the serine proteinases, and the cystein proteinases. For each of these proteinase families, endogenously produced inhibitors—e.g., tissue inhibitors of metalloproteinases (TIMPs), plasminogen activator inhibitors (PAIs), stefins, and cystatins—are present. The key function of these inhibitors is to regulate ongoing proteolysis in time and space. In addition, some of the proteinases may bind to specific receptors at the cell surface thereby localizing the proteolytic activity to the vicinity of the cells (1).

Since metastatic disease is the principal cause of cancer patient morbidity and mortality, proteins involved in the pathway of tumor invasion and metastasis are attractive as potential diagnostic and prognostic markers. Indeed, proteinases such as urokinase plasminogen activator (uPA), its receptor (uPAR), MMP-2, MMP-9, cathepsin B, cathepsin L have all been associated with cancer patient prognosis (for example, the higher tumor tissue content of these proteins, the shorter survival of the patients). Studies on the levels of uPA in breast cancer tissue extracts have now reached Level of Evidence I, and therefore uPA should be considered as a valid marker for clinical decision making in patients who have primary breast cancer.

Surprisingly, high levels of the proteinase inhibitors are also associated with shorter patient survival. It has been suggested that these inhibitors are responsible for additional activities such as promoting tumor angiogenesis and inhibiting apoptosis; functions that have been demonstrated to be distinct from their proteinase inhibitory action.

In vitro studies have shown that during the process of cell transformation (i.e., when a damaged cell evolves into a malignant cell type), the transformed cells may "turn on" the expression of proteinases and/or their inhibitors. One example is TIMP-1. Similar findings have been reported from studies that compared gene expression between benign and malignant pancreatic and colon lesions. TIMP-1 mRNA was the mRNA species with the highest difference in expression between benign and malignant tissues.

If early-stage tumors release these molecules into the circulation, they might represent potential diagnostic markers. Prostate-specific antigen (PSA), a serine proteinase, is an excellent example of a proteinase that is secreted into the circulation and that carries valuable diagnostic information.

Indeed, many other proteinases, their receptors and inhibitors are secreted from the tumor tissue and find their way into the circulation. Using well-characterized and validated assays such as ELISA, the amount of these molecules can easily be quantitated in serum or plasma or even in urine.

CLINICAL APPLICATION

Colorectal cancer (CRC) is the fourth most frequent cancer in the Western world. Forty to fifty percent of all CRC patients are diagnosed with early-stage disease (Dukes A or Dukes B stage disease) and the majority of these patients are cured by surgery alone. However, 10% of patients with Dukes A and 25–30% with Dukes B will experience recurrent disease following potential curative surgery.

Though all Dukes C patients (60–70% recurrence rate) are offered adjuvant chemotherapy, there is no standard treatment for patients with early-stage disease. Following relapse, the risk of disease-related death is significant. Consequently, the risk of recurrence and subsequent death is closely related to the stage of disease at the time of primary diagnosis. It is therefore reasonable to assume that the survival rate of CRC could be improved if more patients could be diagnosed when their cancer is at an earlier stage. Indeed, recent studies on fecal-occult-blood testing have shown that when the detection of CRC is shifted towards earlier disease stages, CRC-related survival is improved among screened individuals (2).

We have in our laboratory worked intensively with TIMP-1. TIMP-1 is a 28kD molecule that can form tight 1:1 stoichiometric complexes with the activated forms of MMPs, thereby inhibiting the catalytic activity of these enzymes. TIMP-1 is stored in the α-granules of platelets and is released upon platelet activation. In colon cancer, TIMP-1 protein has been localized to the tumor stroma, and high expression of TIMP-1 in these tissues was correlated to poor patient prognosis.

We have developed an ELISA for the quantitation of total TIMP-1 in plasma. The assay has been extensively validated and demonstrated good precision with low intra- and inter-assay coefficients of variation, good recovery, linearity, and unique analytical specificity for TIMP-1 (3). Each of the capture and detection antibodies binds free and MMP-bound TIMP-1. The assay thus detects all forms of TIMP-1 and can be used to measure the total amount of TIMP-1 in plasma.

Using this ELISA, we have shown that healthy individuals (n = 100) have a very narrow range of TIMP-1 concentrations (EDTA plasma: mean 73.5 ± 14.2 µg/L; Citrate plasma: 69.2 ± 13.1 µg/L). No significant differences in total plasma TIMP-1 levels were found between healthy individuals, patients with inflammatory bowel diseases (n = 50), or patients with primary breast cancer (n = 322). In contrast, patients with Dukes D (metastatic or locally but not radically resected disease) colorectal cancer (n = 143) had significantly increased plasma TIMP-1 levels (mean: 240 ± 145 µg/L).

Figure 1 shows box and whiskers plots of EDTA plasma TIMP-1 values in blood donors (n = 100) and in preoperatively sampled EDTA plasma from patients with Dukes D stage colorectal cancer (n = 143). A comparison between the two groups shows a highly significant difference (p < 0.0001). We have recently extended our studies to include patients with Dukes stage A, B, and C disease, and the results obtained so far show that patients with early-stage CRC (Dukes stage A and B disease) also have significantly increased plasma TIMP-1 levels (4). These results are in line with those published by Simpson et al. (5) and Öberg et al. (6). We are currently analyzing a large number of plasma samples obtained from blood donors, patients with non-cancer diseases, patients with cancer diseases of origin other than CRC, and patients with CRC. These results will allow us to validate the specificity and sensitivity of plasma TIMP-1 as a serological marker for early-stage CRC.

Diagnosis of early-stage CRC should make available markers that could separate patients into prognostic groups, e.g., one group consisting of patients most likely to be cured by surgery alone, and another group with a high risk of recurrence and therefore in need of adjuvant treatment. By analyzing preoperative plasma TIMP-1 levels in a cohort of 588 patients with CRC we have shown that the total amount of plasma TIMP-1 is highly significantly associated with patient survival, i.e., higher TIMP-1 levels associate with shorter patient survival (7). The hazard ratio between patients with low vs. patients with high TIMP-1 levels was 3.3 (based on 1 log difference).

Multivariate analysis indicated that TIMP-1 provided highly significant prognostic information (hazard ratio 2.5) independent of Dukes stage, which suggests that TIMP-1 can be used to predict prognosis in the individual Dukes stages regardless of which stage of disease the patient's diagnosis indicates.

The survival curves presented in Figure 2 illustrate the prognostic power of plasma TIMP-1 in patients with Dukes stage A or B colon cancer (n = 156). The patients were divided into two groups based on a clinically relevant cut-point of 75% (plasma TIMP-1 = 193 µg/L)—i.e., approximately 75% of these patients will be alive after 5 years. This cut-off point separates patients into two highly significantly different prognostic groups, low plasma TIMP-1 being associated with better prognosis.

We have also calculated the expected survival for a cohort drawn from the general Danish population and matched with the patients with Dukes stage A or B colon cancer with respect to age and gender (solid line). As shown in Figure 2, the 75% of Dukes stage A or B colon cancer patients with the lowest plasma TIMP-1 levels had a death rate indistinguishable from that expected in the age- and gender-matched cohort.

FUTURE DIRECTIONS

TIMP-1 can exist either in its free form or in complex with MMPs. Using an antibody that reacts exclusively against free TIMP-1 (7), we are currently developing an ELISA for the specific detection of free TIMP-1 in plasma. This assay will enable us to differentially identify the free form of circulating TIMP-1 and assess its diagnostic and prognostic potential. Algorithms to calculate total, free, and complexed TIMP-1 may prove useful in improving the diagnostic and prognostic performance of this serological test.

An alternative approach to increase the clinical value of TIMP-1 is to investigate whether plasma TIMP-1 measurements can be combined with the measurement of other CRC markers. e.g., CEA or CA 19-9.

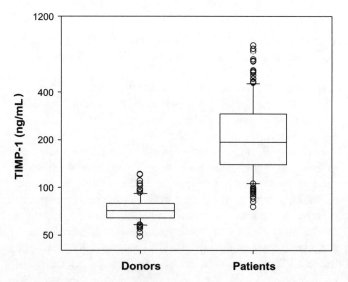

Figure 1 Box and Whiskers plot of plasma TIMP-1 levels (log scale) in healthy controls and in patients with advanced colorectal cancer. Boxes indicate 25th, 50th and 75th percentiles. Whiskers indicate 5th and 95th percentiles.

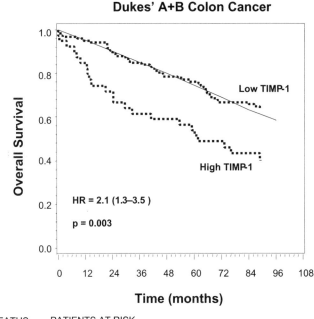

Figure 2 Overall survival of 156 Dukes stage A or B colon cancer patients divided into two groups according to preoperative plasma TIMP-1 values (the lowest 75% TIMP-1 values vs. the highest 25% TIMP-1 values). The solid line represents the survival curve for an age- and sex-matched cohort drawn from the general Danish population.

The number of patients at risk at 0, 24, 48 and 72 months is shown below the figure for each group. In addition, the number of deaths (death from all causes) for each group is shown to the left of the number of patients at risk for each group.

In order to further validate the clinical usefulness of plasma TIMP-1 measurements in the diagnosis of early CRC or in the prognostic stratification of patients with early-stage CRC, studies on independent patient/donor material should be initiated and followed by a meta-analysis and a prospectively planned clinical trial. These studies should also be used to establish clinically relevant scoring for diagnosis and prognosis.

REFERENCES

1. Liotta LA, Steeg,PS, Stetler-Stevenson WG. Cancer metastasis and angiogenesis: an imbalance of positive and negative regulation. Cell 1991;64:327–336.
2. Kronborg O, Fenger C, Olsen, J, Jørgensen OD, Søndergaard O. Randomized study of screening for colorectal cancer with fecal-occult-blood test. Lancet 1996;348:1467–1471.
3. Holten-Andersen MN, Murphy G, Nielsen HJ, Pedersen AN, Christensen IJ, Høyer-Hansen G, et al. Quantitation of TIMP-1 in plasma of healthy blood donors and patients with advanced cancer. Br J Cancer 1999;80:495–503.
4. Holten-Andersen M, Stephens RW, Nielsen HJ, Murphy G, Christensen IJ, Stetler-Stevenson W, Brünner N. High preoperative plasma TIMP-1 levels are associated with short survival of patients with colorectal cancer. Clin Cancer Res 2000;6: 4292–4299.
5. Simpson RA, Hemingway DM, Thompson MM. Plasma TIMP-1—a marker of metastasis in colorectal cancer. Colorectal Disease 2000;2:100–105.
6. Öberg A, Hoyhtya M, Tavelin B, Stenling R, Lindmark G. Limited value of preoperative serum analyses of matrix metalloproteinases (MMP-2, MMP-9) and tissue inhibitors of matrix metalloproteinases (TIMP-1, TIMP-2) in colorectal cancer. Anticancer Res 2000;20:1085–1091.
7. Holten-Andersen M, Christensen IJ, Nielsen HJ, Stephens RW, Jensen V, Nielsen OH, et al. Total levels of tissue inhibitor of metalloproteinases 1 in plasma yield high diagnostic sensitivity and specificity in patients with colorectal cancer. Clin Cancer Res 2002;8:156–164.
8. Holten-Andersen M, Brünner N, Maimonis P, Jensen V, Murphy G, Piironen T. Characterization of monoclonal antibodies to tissue inhibitor of metalloproteinases 1. J Clin Ligand Assay (in press).

Chapter 41

uPA and PAI-1 in Breast Cancer

Manfred Schmitt, Viktor Magdolen, Ute Reuning, and Nadia Harbeck

The majority of breast cancer patients do not die from their primary tumor but from distant metastases. Determination of two tumor-associated proteins linked to tumor invasion and metastasis in primary tumor tissue, uPA and PAI-1, can help to individualize adjuvant therapy decisions in women with primary breast cancer. Several retrospective and prospective studies in different countries (Europe, USA, Asia) have determined that uPA and PAI-1 are present in significantly greater amounts in breast cancer tissue than in normal or benign tissue. Substantial data by these international clinical research groups has been put forward associating elevated levels of uPA and/or PAI-1 protein with shorter disease-free and overall patient survival in node-negative as well as node-positive breast cancer patients (1,2).

Recent data from a prospective German therapy trial are convincing enough to recommend routine testing of these two tumor-associated proteins in order to help determine treatment strategies, especially for node-negative breast cancer patients whose axillary lymph nodes do not show any sign of cancer cells (3). uPA and PAI-1 identify those women with node-negative breast cancer whose risk of disease recurrence is low enough that they may be candidates for being spared the burden of adjuvant chemotherapy. It was also revealed in this study that high-risk node-negative breast cancer patients as defined by increased uPA and/or PAI-1 values do benefit from adjuvant chemotherapy.

Plasminogen activators uPA (urokinase-type plasminogen activator) and tPA (tissue-type plasminogen activator), their inhibitor PAI-1 (plasminogen activator inhibitor type 1), the uPA receptor (CD87), and the serine protease plasmin are key players in a proteolytic cascade involved in physiological and pathophysiological degradation processes of the extracellular matrix. uPA, when bound to its cellular receptor CD87, efficiently converts plasminogen into the broad-spectrum serine protease plasmin; its action on plasminogen is controlled by PAI-1. Plasmin destroys many components of the connective tissue, and in malignancy, the tumor stroma surrounding the tumor cell nests. Major protein components of the extracellular matrix are fibrin, laminin, fibronectin, vitronectin, elastin, and different types of collagen (4).

The plasminogen activation system, also known as the *Fibrinolysis System,* is interfaced with the blood coagulation system. The interplay between the two different blood coagulation pathways and the fibrin clot degrading *Fibrinolysis System* is depicted in Figure 1. The *Contact Factor Pathway* (intrinsic pathway) begins when blood-clotting factors interact with negatively charged biological surfaces that get exposed due to tissue injury. Blood factors involved in the initial phase of contact activation are factor XII, (pre)-kallikrein, and high-molecular weight kininogen (HMWK).

More important under physiological conditions is the second route of blood coagulation, the *Tissue Factor Pathway* (extrinsic pathway). During tissue injury, the subendothelium containing the receptor protein tissue factor is exposed to blood-clotting factors, thereby triggering the second but major blood coagulation cascade. Action of tissue factor is controlled by TFPI (tissue factor pathway inhibitor). At the end of the blood coagulation cascade an insoluble fibrin network is formed by the serine protease thrombin from the plasma protein fibrinogen. Proteolytic action of thrombin is controlled by the inhibitors antithrombin III and heparin cofactor II.

The anticoagulant *Protein C Pathway* (not shown in Figure 1) involves protein C, protein S, and the cell membrane protein thrombomodulin. This pathway targets and inactivates factors Va and VIIIa. Deficiencies in protein C and S can lead to excessive intravascular fibrin clot formation, a cause of thrombosis. Enzymatic action of plasmin on the fibrin clot and on the extracellular matrix is controlled by the inhibitors α2-antiplasmin and α2-macroglobulin. In blood, plasmin degrades fibrin clots thereby releasing fibrin degradation products (FDP) of different molecular sizes. D-dimer is the smallest of the crosslinked FDPs (FXDP). TAFI (thrombin-activated fibrinolysis inhibitor) destroys the catalytic fibrin clot surface thus preventing interaction with tPA.

CLINICAL APPLICATION

Overexpression of the serine protease uPA, its cell surface receptor CD87, and the inhibitor PAI-1 in tumor tissues is a prerequisite for efficient focal proteolysis as well as tumor cell invasion and metastasis (5). After binding of uPA to its receptor CD87, this complex interacts with PAI-1, which then is internalized by the cell, thereby initiating signal transduction, proliferation, adhesion, and migration of the tumor cell. In breast cancer, components of the plasminogen activation system are localized to a varying extent to both tumor cells and host cells.

As uPA and PAI-1 are both strong and statistically independent prognostic factors in breast cancer patients, simultane-

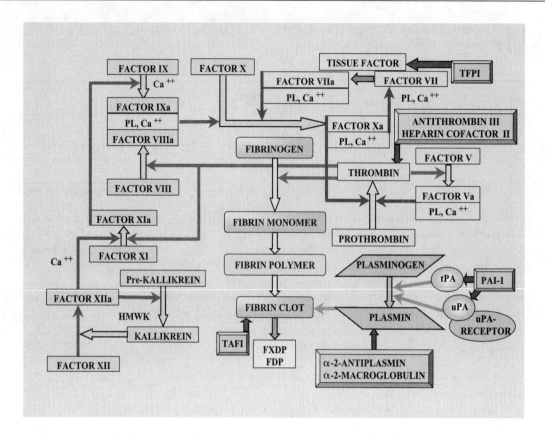

Figure 1 Blood coagulation cascade, fibrin formation, and fibrinolysis. Blood coagulation factors are primarily synthesized by the liver and released into the bloodstream. Usually, coagulation factors are synthesized as proteolytically inactive pro-enzymes, others serve as substrates or co-factors that can be transformed from an activate precursor state to the active form by various stimuli. All of the blood coagulation factors, except the cell membrane-associated tissue factor, are plasma proteins. Blood coagulation is initiated by tissue injury or factors affecting hemostasis.

Two different blood coagulation pathways are shown: the intrinsic pathway, known as *Contact Factor Pathway* (pink), and the extrinsic pathway, also named *Tissue Factor Pathway* (brown). The two pathways are interactive and meet at Factor IX and X, from where they initiate thrombin (green) and fibrin (cyan) formation. As a counterpart to fibrin clot formation, the fibrinolytic system (blue) is activated in a series of enzymatic reactions. It then generates the broad-spectrum serine protease plasmin from the proteolytically inactive plasma protein plasminogen by action of the plasminogen activators tPA (tissue-type plasminogen activator) or uPA (urokinase-type plasminogen activator). Plasmin destroys intravascular fibrin clots and, in addition to other proteins, fibrin contained within the extracellular matrix. Inhibitors are shown in red.

Under physiological conditions, such as wound healing, a critical balance between fibrin formation and fibrin degradation is maintained. In solid malignant tumors, excess production of uPA, and surprisingly of its inhibitor PAI-1, is associated with tumor cell invasion, metastasis, and early death of the cancer patient. (Scheme is based on the information provided by Kolde, H.J, Hemostasis, Pentapharm Ltd., 2001). **Color representation of figure appears on Color Plate 8.**

ous determination of both factors is recommended to yield optimal prognostic information. For this purpose, a small piece of primary tumor tissue (about 100 to 300 mg) is snap-frozen in liquid nitrogen and then pulverized in the frozen state (e.g., by using the Braun Dismembrator device). The tissue powder is suspended in Tris-buffered saline (TBS, pH 8.5), followed by centrifugation to yield the so-called cytosol fraction. A large fraction of uPA and almost all of PAI-1 is contained in this cytosol fraction. Adding 1% of the nonionic detergent Triton X-100 will free additional, membrane-bound uPA and uPA from intracellular stores; additional PAI-1 is not released by this technique (6).

The majority of clinically relevant results on uPA and PAI-1 relating to breast cancer prognosis has been obtained by determining the protein content of these analytes in primary tumor tissue extracts using **e**nzyme-**l**inked **i**mmunosorbent **a**ssays (ELISA). The most frequently used uPA and PAI-1 ELISAs cited in the scientific literature, which also perform well in controlled quality assurance reports, are from American Diagnostica Inc., Greenwich, CT (uPA ELISA: Imubind #894; PAI-1 ELISA: Imubind #821). By convention, the uPA and PAI-1 content in tumor tissue extracts is expressed as ng of the analyte per mg of total tumor tissue protein.

Usually, total tissue protein is determined by the Pierce BCA or the Bradford protein assay (7). For PAI-1, no difference in antigen yield or prognostic impact is found between the cytosol or the detergent extract. For uPA, however, detergent-based extraction yields about twice as much uPA antigen and provides a considerably better assessment of disease-free patient survival than uPA measured in cytosol fractions (6). Therefore, the detergent-based extraction method is recommended.

Using American Diagnostica ELISA formats and Pierce BCA protein determination, the clinical relevance of uPA and

PAI-1 for breast cancer prognosis has been evaluated for more than ten years in a prospective fashion at the Department of Obstetrics and Gynecology of the Technical University of Munich, Germany. As an example, a Kaplan-Meier curve demonstrating the course of the disease (risk of developing disease recurrence expressed as probability of disease-free survival) in relation to uPA and PAI-1 levels in primary tumor tissue extracts is shown for 764 breast cancer patients in Figure 2. Elevated uPA and / or PAI-1 levels indicate poor prognosis; levels of both analytes below the statistically optimized cut-offs of 3 ng uPA and 14 ng PAI-1 per mg of total tumor tissue protein indicate a significantly better prognosis of the patients.

We have developed a technique to quantitatively measure uPA and PAI-1 in small pieces of breast cancer specimens, including fine needle aspirates, core biopsies, and cryostat sections (7). For instance, a few 90 µm-thick cryostat sections provided by the pathologist are sufficient to prepare the tumor tissue extract. The cryostat sections are placed into the vessel of a Downs homogenizer containing 1% of the nonionic detergent Triton X-100 in TBS. After ultracentrifugation, the supernatant serves as the source to determine uPA and PAI-1 antigen content using the standard ELISA technique.

To yield clinically relevant prognostic information, uPA and PAI-1 need to be determined in primary tumor extracts; immunohistochemical assessment is not suited to yield quantitative data. Determination of uPA and PAI-1 in serum or plasma is not recommended. Blood and blood vessel cells express uPA (neutrophils, monocytes) and PAI-1 (platelets, endothelial cells), obscuring the uPA and PAI-1 content set free from tumor cells and released into the blood stream.

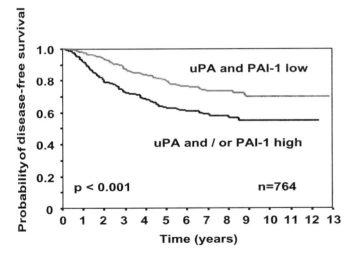

Figure 2 Probability of disease-free survival in primary breast cancer patients as a function of proteolytic factors uPA and PAI-1. Patients with high tumor antigen levels of uPA and/or PAI-1 have a significantly shorter disease-free survival (lower curve) than patients with low levels of both factors (upper curve). Previously optimized and re-evaluated cut-offs of 3 ng uPA and 14 ng PAI-1 per mg tumor tissue extract protein were applied to distinguish between high and low antigen levels of the analytes in the primary tumor (3). Low uPA and PAI-1: n = 415 with 78 relapses vs. high uPA and/or PAI-1: n = 349 with 113 relapses. Median time of follow-up for patients still alive at time of analysis was 56.5 (1–163) months.

FUTURE DIRECTIONS

In the scientific literature, all reports support the prognostic impact of uPA and/or PAI-1 for patients with solid malignant tumors, if measured by ELISA.

In a new collaborative study, researchers within the European Organization for Research and Treatment of Cancer, EORTC, pooled data on 8,377 women treated for primary breast cancer at 18 European institutions between 1978 and 1995 (8). uPA and PAI-1 levels in primary tumor tissue extracts were quantified by ELISA. The prognostic impact of these two factors was determined in multivariate analysis, including established risk factors as age, tumor size, grade, lymph node status, steroid hormone receptor status, and type of adjuvant therapy. uPA and PAI-1 levels were the strongest prognostic factors next to lymph node status, associated with both disease-free and overall survival. This pooled analysis (8) and the recent results of the above mentioned randomized node-negative breast cancer therapy trial (3) yield strong enough evidence to recommend routine uPA/PAI-1 testing in breast cancer, particularly in node-negative patients, in order to help physicians and their patients to determine treatment strategies.

In contrast to most European countries, logistical problems in the United States are still preventing widespread uPA/PAI-1 testing as the ELISA assays require fresh or frozen tissue. In the past, there was no need for US pathologists to freeze tumor tissue for histologic diagnosis due to the availability of immunohistochemistry assays performed on formalin-fixed, paraffin-embedded tissue sections (9). But widespread uPA and PAI-1 testing may now become available even for patients in the USA since the ELISA assays can also be performed on small amounts of frozen tissue such as routine cryosections or core biopsies (7).

The plasminogen activation system in cancer has evolved as an important target for new therapeutic approaches (10). Researchers in academia and in the pharmaceutical industry are currently exploring whether drugs targeting uPA and/or PAI-1 can help treat breast cancer patients. An attractive approach for controlling tumor invasion and metastasis is to inhibit the enzymatic activity of uPA by synthetic inhibitors. This approach already shows promising data in preclinical studies. Other promising approaches aim at interruption of the uPA/uPA-R-interaction by synthetic uPA-derived peptides, antibodies to uPA or CD87, or soluble recombinant CD87 which functions as a scavenger for uPA (10).

REFERENCES

1. Schmitt M, Harbeck N, Thomssen C, Wilhelm O, Magdolen V, Reuning U, et al. Clinical impact of the plasminogen activation system in tumor invasion and metastasis: prognostic relevance and target for therapy. Thromb Haemost 1997;78:285–296.
2. Andreasen PA, Kjöller L, Christensen L, Duffy MJ. The urokinase-type plasminogen activator system in cancer metastasis: a review. Int J Cancer 1997;72:1–22.
3. Jänicke F, Prechtl A, Thomssen C, Harbeck N, Meisner C, Untch M, et al. Randomized adjuvant chemotherapy trial in high-risk, lymph node-negative breast cancer patients identified by

urokinase-type plasminogen activator and plasminogen activator inhibitor type 1. J Natl Cancer Inst 2001;93:913–920.

4. Schmitt M, Harbeck N, Thomssen C, Wilhelm O, Magdolen V, Reuning U, et al. Clinical impact of the plasminogen activation system in tumor invasion and metastasis: prognostic relevance and target for therapy. Thromb Hemost 1997;78:285–296.

5. Bajou K, Noel A, Gerard RD, Masson V, Brünner N, Holst-Hansen C, et al. Absence of host plasminogen activator inhibitor 1 prevents cancer invasion and vascularization. Nature Med 1998; 4:923–928.

6. Jänicke F, Pache L, Schmitt M, Ulm K, Thomssen C, Prechtl A, et al. Both the cytosols and detergent extracts of breast cancer tissues are suited to evaluate the prognostic impact of the urokinase-type plasminogen activator and its inhibitor, plasminogen activator inhibitor type 1. Cancer Res 1994;54:2527–2530.

7. Schmitt M, Lienert S, Prechtel D, Sedlaczek E, Welk A, Reuning U, et al. The urokinase protease system as a target for breast cancer prognosis and therapy: technical considerations. J Clin Ligand Assay Soc; (in press).

8. Look MP, van Putten WLJ, Duffy MJ, Harbeck N, Christensen IJ, Thomssen C, et al. Pooled analysis of prognostic impact of urokinase-type plasminogen activator and its inhibitor PAI-1 in 8377 breast cancer patients. J Natl Cancer Inst 2002;94:116–128.

9. Stephenson, J. Study indicates utility for new breast cancer prognostic markers. JAMA 2001;285:3077–3078.

10. Schmitt M, Wilhelm OG, Reuning U, Krüger A, Harbeck N, Lengyel E, et al. The urokinase plasminogen activator system as a novel target for tumor therapy. Fibrinol & Proteol 2000;14: 114–132.

Chapter 42

Tumor-Associated Trypsin Inhibitor (TATI)

Ulf-Håkan Stenman and Annukka Paju

Tumor-associated trypsin inhibitor (TATI) is a 6 kDa peptide identified in search of tumor-associated peptides in urine of patients with ovarian cancer (1). High concentrations occur in mucinous ovarian cyst fluid, and TATI isolated from this source is identical to pancreatic secretory trypsin inhibitor (PSTI) (2). TATI/PSTI is also called the Kazal inhibitor (3). The name TATI is used in most studies on this peptide as a tumor marker.

STRUCTURE AND FUNCTION

The *TATI* gene is 7.5 kb long. It comprises 4 exons and is located on chromosome 5. The promoter region of the gene contains an interleukin-6 (IL-6) responsive element (4). The mature peptide contains 56 amino acids, having a calculated molecular weight of 6242 and a pI of 5.8 (2). TATI contains three intramolecular disulfide bridges and shows some homology with epidermal growth factor but is not thought to be derived from a common ancestral gene (3).

The physiological function of PSTI/TATI in the pancreas is thought to protect pancreatic cells from destruction induced by inadvertent activation of trypsinogen. In the gastrointestinal (GI) tract, TATI may prevent digestion of the GI mucus. In addition to trypsin, TATI also occurs in seminal plasma and inhibits acrosin. Thus it may play a role in reproduction (5). TATI is an efficient inhibitor of trypsin with a Ki of 0.06 nmol/L, which is much lower than the median concentration in serum, about 2 nmol/L. The affinity for serine protease other than acrosin is 150-fold lower and probably not of physiological significance (6).

TATI acts as an acute phase reactant but the function and origin of TATI in this condition is not known (reviewed in ref. 5). TATI has been found to exert growth factor-like properties in cell culture. It stimulates the growth of human fibroblasts, endothelial cells, and rat pancreatic cancer cells. However, the stimulation of cell growth may be brought about by general inhibition of tryptic activity and thereby degradation of other growth factors (7).

EXPRESSION

TATI is secreted at high concentrations together with trypsinogen from pancreatic acinar cells into pancreatic juice, where it constitutes 0.1–0.8% of total protein (8). TATI is also produced in several extrapancreatic tissues, especially in the gastrointestinal and urogenital tract. It is expressed at high concentrations in mucus-producing cells of the small intestine, colon, and stomach, as well as in the gall bladder, biliary tract, kidney, lung, liver and breast. TATI is also expressed by several cancers, e.g., ovarian, endometrioid, cervical, pancreatic, colorectal, gastric, liver, lung, breast, biliary tract, and gall bladder (reviewed in ref. 5).

Very high concentrations of TATI occur in benign and malignant mucinous ovarian cyst fluid. In the pancreas and in tumors, TATI expression is associated with trypsinogen expression and many tumor cell lines of various origin express both TATI and trypsinogen (9). Expression in hepatoma cells is stimulated by co-culture with mononuclear blood cells, but this does not induce expression in pancreatic cancer cells. Thus the expression is regulated by different mechanisms in different cells (10).

METABOLISM

TATI is cleared from the circulation mainly by renal excretion with a half-life of 6 min (11). Thus serum TATI increases in patients with impaired renal function and very high serum levels occur in patients with severe renal failure (12).

CLINICAL APPLICATIONS
Reference Values

The mean concentration of TATI in serum of healthy subjects is 11 µg/L (reference range 3–21 µg/L) and in urine 25 µg/L (reference range 7–51 µg/L). Somewhat lower levels are obtained by an assay based on monoclonal antibodies (mean concentration 6.9 µg/L and reference range 3.1–16 µg/L) (5). The serum levels remain within this range after total pancreatectomy, suggesting that only part of TATI in circulation of healthy subjects is derived from the pancreas (13). Other potential sources are gastrointestinal mucosa and the liver.

Benign Disease

Patients with severe injury and inflammatory disease have strongly elevated TATI concentrations, suggesting that it may behave as an acute phase protein (12,14). Although this is a limiting factor, it does not invalidate TATI as a tumor marker (15). Comparison between TATI and C-reactive protein (CRP) in patients with pelvic inflammatory disease has shown that TATI levels become elevated only when serum CRP level is clearly elevated, i. e., over 90 mg/L. This shows that a strong acute phase stimulus is required before TATI expression is triggered.

TATI (or rather PSTI) is strongly elevated in pancreatitis, and the elevation correlates with the severity of the disease (16). Recently, mutations in the TATI gene have been found to be associated with chronic pancreatitis. It is thought that the mutations make TATI a less efficient inhibitor and therefore it is less capable of preventing inadvertent trypsin activation and pancreatitis (17).

Increased expression of TATI/PSTI has been observed in the liver of patients with adult onset type II citrullinemia and these patients also have elevated serum levels. It is not clear how this disease, which is caused by deficiency of argininosuccinate synthetase, induces TATI expression (18).

Malignant Disease

The serum and urine levels of TATI are often elevated in patients with various types of cancer (5). The elevation is mainly caused by production in the tumor, but an acute phase reaction induced by tissue destruction associated with cancer invasion can contribute to the elevation of TATI in advanced disease (3). The frequency of elevated serum levels reported in various studies is shown in Table 1 (reviewed in ref. 5).

Ovarian cancer. Elevated serum and urine levels of TATI occur frequently in ovarian cancer and especially in patients with mucinous tumors, which constitute 10–15% of all ovarian cancers. TATI is therefore a complement to CA125, which is the most sensitive marker for other types of ovarian cancer but least sensitive for mucinous tumors. The combined use of TATI and CA125 is useful in differentiating benign and malignant ovarian masses and for monitoring patients with mucinous ovarian cancer (19,20). Expression of TATI is associated with high-grade tumors; an elevated serum TATI level prior to therapy is an independent prognostic factor for adverse outcome in stage III ovarian cancer (21).

Endometrial cancer. A fairly high frequency of elevated TATI levels has been observed in advanced endometrial cancers, but TATI is not a sensitive marker for early disease (5,22).

Cervical cancer. Elevated TATI levels occur in cervical cancer, but the sensitivity of TATI is inferior to SCC antigen and CEA and is therefore not useful in this disease (23).

Pancreatic cancer. The serum concentrations of TATI are elevated in the majority of patients with pancreatic cancer, but the utility of TATI is limited by frequent elevation in patients with pancreatitis and benign hepatobiliary disease. However, if pancreatitis can be excluded, TATI is a very sensitive cancer marker and with a high cut-off (100–200 µg/L), the specificity is also acceptable (see reference 5).

Gastric cancer. About 50% of patients with gastric cancer have increased TATI levels. This is more common in anaplastic than in well-differentiated tumors, which is contrary to the behavior of CEA. Therefore TATI may be a useful complement to CA 19-9 and CEA. Strongly elevated pre-operative serum levels indicate poor prognosis (reviewed in ref. 5).

Hepatoma and biliary cancer. Elevated TATI levels are common in hepatocellular and biliary tract cancer (reviewed in ref. 5). The concentrations in bile are higher in patients with malignant than in those with benign biliary tract disease, suggesting that TATI is produced by the tumor (24). Sensitivity and specificity are similar to those of AFP, and therefore TATI may be useful in AFP-negative patients.

Colorectal cancer. In colorectal cancer, elevated serum levels of TATI are fairly common (5), but TATI is clearly inferior to CEA, and the combined use of TATI and CEA does not substantially improve the diagnostic accuracy (25).

Bladder cancer. TATI has been found to be a more useful marker for bladder cancer than seven other commonly used markers, i.e., TPA, CEA, AFP, hCG, PSA, SCC, and CA 19-9. Thus TATI can be used for monitoring this disease (26). Recently TATI has been found to be a strong prognostic factor for adverse outcome in bladder cancer. An elevated serum TATI is associated with a five-fold higher risk of cancer death than a normal level (Kelloniemi et al., submitted).

Renal cell carcinoma (RCC). TATI has been found to be a more sensitive marker (69%) than CEA, CA 15-3, CA 125, CA 19-9, and ferritin, the sensitivities of which are 5%, 10%, 13%, 5%, 35%, respectively. TATI was considered suitable for monitoring of disease progression after surgery but not for early diagnosis (27). TATI has recently been found to be an independent prognostic factor in RCC (28).

Lung cancer. Elevated TATI levels are fairly common in lung cancer, but this marker is clearly inferior to CEA. In a comparative study of TATI, CEA, CA 50, and NSE as markers for lung cancer screening, the combination of TATI and CEA gave the highest sensitivity (74%) at a specificity level of 90%. However, none of the markers appeared to be useful for screening this disease (29).

Breast cancer. In breast cancer TATI is elevated mainly in advanced disease and is less sensitive than CA 15-3. The combination of TATI with other markers is not useful (30).

Table 1 Frequency of elevated TATI-concentrations in cancer of various types reported in various studies and reviewed in reference 5

Tumor type	Elevated values
Ovarian, all types	23–68%
Mucinous	43–100%
Non-mucinous	23–51%
Endometrial	21–57%
Cervical	11–65%
Lung	20–50%
Breast	24–60%
Esophageal	41–57%
Gastric	42–66%
Colorectal	34–74%
Pancreatic	74–95%
Biliary tract	75–100%
Hepatic	60–83%
Kidney	37–69%
Bladder	22–70%
Thyroid	57%
Head and neck	29–60%
Osteosarcoma	83%

Head and neck cancer. Elevated TATI levels occur in about two-thirds of patients with nasopharyngeal tumors, and changes in the levels reflect the course of the disease. In a comparative study, TATI was found to be superior to Cyfra 21-1 (31). Thus TATI appears to be a useful marker for this disease.

Osteosarcoma. TATI is more often elevated in serum of patients with osteosarcoma (83%) than in those with metastatic bone disease, of whom 33% had elevated levels. However, the utility of TATI is limited by a fairly high frequency of false positive results in non-malignant bone disease (reviewed in ref. 5).

FUTURE DIRECTIONS

The use of TATI as a cancer marker is restricted by the limited availability of commercial assays (but two tests are available in Europe and Asia). As a marker for diagnosis and monitoring, TATI has been found to be most useful in detecting ovarian and bladder cancer, while its use in head and neck, gastric, liver, and pancreatic cancer is promising but requires further study.

The use of markers for prognostic purposes is clinically relevant if it affects treatment decisions. Patients with bladder cancer must be monitored for the rest of their lives, and regular cystoscopies are an essential part of follow-up. It would be of great value if some of these invasive procedures could be replaced by serum determinations of TATI. In ovarian cancer, an elevated TATI level in early-stage disease could help decide whether adjuvant treatment is indicated. Tumor invasion requires activation of a cascade of proteases that mediates invasion by degrading extracellular matrix and basement membrane. Trypsin appears to play a role in this process by activating the urokinase plasmin pathway (32) and matrix metalloproteinases MMP-2 and MMP-9, which degrade type-IV collagen (33). TATI is expressed by tumors that express trypsin, and therefore an elevation of TATI in serum of cancer patients indicates that the tumor expresses trypsin, which is a sign of aggressive disease. This probably explains the prognostic value of TATI in several cancers.

Inhibition of proteases that mediate tumor invasion is a potential method of controlling tumor growth. Several collagenase inhibitors are being evaluated as cancer drugs. The trypsin inhibitor aprotinin, which is isolated from bovine lung tissue, has been used to treat pancreatitis but not for human cancers. Long-term treatment with aprotinin may not be feasible because this 6 kD peptide may be expected to induce immunity. However, if synthetic low-molecular-weight trypsin inhibitors become available and prove to be of use in cancer treatment, determination of TATI might be useful for identification of patients that could benefit from this treatment.

REFERENCES

1. Stenman UH, Huhtala ML, Koistinen R, Seppälä M. Immunochemical demonstration of an ovarian cancer-associated urinary peptide. Int J Cancer 1982;30:53–57.
2. Huhtala ML, Pesonen K, Kalkkinen N, Stenman UH. Purification and characterization of a tumor-associated trypsin inhibitor from the urine of a patient with ovarian cancer. J Biol Chem 1982;257:13713–13716.
3. Stenman UH, Koivunen E, Itkonen O. Biology and function of tumor-associated trypsin inhibitor, TATI. [Review] [51 refs]. Scandinavian Journal of Clinical & Laboratory Investigation Supplement 1991;207:5–9.
4. Ohmachi Y, Murata A, Matsuura N, Yasuda T, Monden M, Mori T, Ogawa M, Matsubara K. Specific expression of the pancreatic-secretory-trypsin-inhibitor (PSTI) gene in hepatocellular carcinoma [published erratum appears in Int J Cancer 1994 Apr 1;57(1):139]. Int J Cancer 1993;55:728–734.
5. Stenman U-H, Koivunen E, Itkonen O, Halila H. Clinical use and biological function of tumor-associated trypsin inhibitor. In: Ballesta A, Torre C, Bombardieri E, Gion M, Molina R, eds. Updating on tumor markers in tissues and biological fluids: basic aspects and clinical applications. Torino, Italy: Edizione Minerva Medica, 1993;351–361.
6. Turpeinen U, Koivunen E, Stenman UH. Reaction of a tumor-associated trypsin inhibitor with serine proteinases associated with coagulation and tumor invasion. Biochem J 1988;254:911–914.
7. Freeman TC, Curry BJ, Calam J, Woodburn JR. Pancreatic secretory trypsin inhibitor stimulates the growth of rat pancreatic carcinoma cells. Gastroenterology 1990;99:1414–1420.
8. Pubols MH, Bartelt DC, Greene LJ. Trypsin inhibitor from human pancreas and pancreatic juice. J Biol Chem 1974;249:2235–2242.
9. Koivunen E, Saksela O, Itkonen O, Osman S, Huhtala ML, Stenman UH. Human colon carcinoma, fibrosarcoma, and leukemia cell lines produce tumor-associated trypsinogen. Int J Cancer 1991;47:592–596.
10. Jönsson P, Linder C, Genell S, Ohlsson K. Extra-pancreatic origin of the pancreatic secretory trypsin inhibitor as an acute-phase reactant. Pancreas 1996;12:303–307.
11. Marks WH, Ohlsson K. Elimination of pancreatic secretory trypsin inhibitor from the circulation. A study in man. Scand J Gastroenterol 1983;18:955–959.
12. Lasson A, Borgström A, Ohlsson K. Elevated pancreatic secretory trypsin inhibitor levels during severe inflammatory disease, renal insufficiency, and after various surgical procedures. Scand J Gastroenterol 1986;21:1275–1280.
13. Halila H, Huhtala ML, Schroder T, Kiviluoto T, Stenman UH. Pancreatic secretory trypsin inhibitor-like immunoreactivity in pancreatectomized patients. Clin Chim Acta 1985;153:209–216.
14. Ogawa M, Matsuda K, Shibata T, Matsuda Y, Ukai T, Ohta M, Mori T. Elevation of serum pancreatic secretory trypsin inhibitor (PSTI) in patients with serious injury. Res Commun Chem Pathol Pharmacol 1985;50:259–266.
15. Paavonen J, Lehtinen M, Lehto M, Laine S, Aine R, Räsänen L, Stenman UH. Concentrations of tumor-associated trypsin inhibitor and C-reactive protein in serum in acute pelvic inflammatory disease. Clin Chem 1989;35:869–871.
16. Eddeland A, Ohlsson K. A radioimmunoassay for measurement of human pancreatic secretory trypsin inhibitor in different body fluids. Hoppe Seylers Z Physiol Chem 1978;359:671–675.
17. Chen JM, Mercier B, Audrezet MP, Ferec C. Mutational analysis of the human pancreatic secretory trypsin inhibitor (PSTI) gene in hereditary and sporadic chronic pancreatitis [letter]. J Med Genet 2000;37:67–69.
18. Kobayashi K, Horiuchi M, Saheki T. Pancreatic secretory trypsin inhibitor as a diagnostic marker for adult-onset type II citrullinemia. Hepatology 1997;25:1160–1165.

19. Halila H, Lehtovirta P, Stenman UH, Seppälä M. CA 125 in the follow-up of patients with ovarian cancer. Acta Obstet Gynecol Scand 1988;67:53–58.
20. Peters-Engl C, Medl M, Ogris E, Leodolter S. Tumor-associated trypsin inhibitor (TATI) and cancer antigen 125 (CA125) in patients with epithelial ovarian cancer. Anticancer Res 1995;15: 2727–2730.
21. Venesmaa P, Stenman UH, Forss M, Leminen A, Lehtovirta P, Vartiainen J, Paavonen J. Pre-operative serum level of tumor-associated trypsin inhibitor and residual tumor size as prognostic indicators in Stage III epithelial ovarian cancer. Br J Obstet Gynaecol 1998;105:508–511.
22. Peters-Engl C, Buxbaum P, Ogris E, Sevelda P, Medl M. TATI (tumor-associated trypsin inhibitor) and cancer antigen 125 (CA 125) in patients with early-stage endometrial cancer. Anticancer Res 1998;18:4635–4639.
23. Pectasides D, Economides N, Bourazanis J, Pozadzizou P, Gogou L, Koutsiouba P, Athanassiou A. Squamous cell carcinoma antigen, tumor-associated trypsin inhibitor, and carcinoembryonic antigen for monitoring cervical cancer. Am J Clin Oncol 1994;17: 307–312.
24. Hedstrom J, Haglund C, Leinonen J, Nordling S, Stenman UH. Trypsinogen-1, -2 and tumor-associated trypsin-inhibitor in bile and biliary tract tissues from patients with biliary tract diseases and pancreatic carcinomas. Scand J Clin Lab Invest 2001;61:111–118.
25. Pasanen P, Eskelinen M, Kulju A, Penttila I, Janatuinen E, Alhava E. Tumor-associated trypsin inhibitor (TATI) in patients with colorectal cancer: a comparison with CEA, CA 50, and CA 242. Scand J Clin Lab Invest 1995;55:119–124.
26. Pectasides D, Bafaloucos D, Antoniou F, Gogou L, Economides N, Varthalitis J, Dimitriades M, Kosmidis P, Athanassiou A. TPA, TATI, CEA, AFP, beta-HCG, PSA, SCC, and CA 19-9 for monitoring transitional cell carcinoma of the bladder. Am J Clin Oncol 1996;19:271–277.
27. Meria P, Toubert ME, Cussenot O, Bassi S, Janssen T, Desgrandchamps F, Cortesse A, Schlageter MH, Teillac P, Le Duc A. Tumor-associated trypsin inhibitor and renal cell carcinoma. Eur Urol 1995;27:223–226.
28. Paju A, J. J, Rasmuson T, Stenman U-H, Ljungberg B. Tumor-associated trypsin inhibitor as a prognostic factor in renal cell carcinoma. J Urol 2000;84:1363–1371.
29. Järvisalo J, Hakama M, Knekt P, Stenman UH, Leino A, Teppo L, Maatela J, Aromaa A. Serum tumor markers CEA, CA 50, TATI, and NSE in lung cancer screening. Cancer 1993;71:1982–1988.
30. Sjöström J, Alfthan H, Joensuu H, Stenman UH, Lundin J, Blomqvist C. Serum tumor markers CA 15-3, TPA, TPS, hCGbeta, and TATI in the monitoring of chemotherapy response in metastatic breast cancer. Scand J Clin Lab Invest 2001;61: 431–441.
31. Goumas PD, Mastronikolis NS, Mastorakou AN, Vassilakos PJ, Nikiforidis GC. Evaluation of TATI and CYFRA 21-1 in patients with head and neck squamous cell carcinoma. ORL J Otorhinolaryngol Relat Spec 1997;59:106–114.
32. Koivunen E, Ristimaki A, Itkonen O, Osman S, Vuento M, Stenman UH. Tumor-associated trypsin participates in cancer cell-mediated degradation of extracellular matrix. Cancer Res 1991;51:2107–2112.
33. Sorsa T, Salo T, Koivunen E, Tyynelä J, Konttinen YT, Bergmann U, Tuuttila A, Niemi E, Teronen O, Heikkila P, Tschesche H, Leinonen J, Osman S, Stenman UH. Activation of type IV procollagenases by human tumor-associated trypsin-2. J Biol Chem 1997;272:21067–21074.

Chapter 43

Estrogen Receptor-β: Role in Breast Cancer

Michael J. Duffy

The estrogen receptor (ER) is a nuclear transcription factor that mediates the actions of the female hormone, estrogen. Assay of this protein is widely used in selecting breast cancers that are likely to respond to hormone therapy. In both early and advanced breast cancer, ER-positive patients are 7–8 times more likely to respond to endocrine therapy than ER-negative patients (for review, see ref. 1). Because of its strong predictive value, expert panels in both the US (American Society of Clinical Oncology) (2) and Europe (European Group on Tumor Markers) (3) have recommended that the ER assay be performed on all patients with breast cancer. Furthermore, a recent US National Cancer Institute Consensus Statement recommended that women whose breast cancer contained steroid hormone receptors, regardless of age, menopausal status, axillary node status, or tumor size, should receive adjuvant hormonal therapy (4). Such therapy was not recommended for women whose breast tumors did not express steroid receptors.

In addition to predicting response to therapy, the ER assay can also provide prognostic information. For the initial four to five years after diagnosis, ER-positive patients generally have a more favorable outcome than those who lack ER (1). However, after about five years, this beneficial effect of ER is reversed as ER-negative patients then have fewer relapses compared to ER-positive patients. Overall, the ER is regarded to be a relatively weak prognostic indicator in breast cancer and of little value in axillary node-negative patients, the subgroup of breast cancer patients for whom new prognostic factors are most urgently required (1).

In 1996, a new ER gene was identified and shown to be expressed in many different tissues including human breast cancer (for review, see ref. 5). This new form of ER was designated ERβ to differentiate it from the original ER, which was renamed ERα. These two forms of ER have similar overall structures, displaying a high degree of homology in the DNA-binding domain (95% amino acid identity), moderate conservation in the ligand-binding domain (55–60% amino acid identity), but considerable diversity at both the amino- and carboxy-terminal regions (5). The genes for the two forms of ER are located on different chromosomes, ERα being found on chromosome 6 while ERβ is present on chromosome 14.

ERα and ERβ exhibit overlapping but also distinct expression patterns. Whereas ERα is the main subtype expressed in uterus, cervix, vagina, and breast tissues, ERβ is found at highest levels in prostate, ovary, testis, spleen, and lung (5). In a number of tissue types, ERα and ERβ are expressed in different cell types. Thus, in the ovary, ERβ is mainly found in the granulosa cells but ERα can also be detected in the theca cells, interstitial gland cells, and germinal epithelium. In the adult rat uterus, ERβ is present only in the glandular epithelium cells whereas ERα is expressed in the luminal and glandular cells as well as the stroma (5).

Although both receptors bind estradiol and anti-estrogens such as tamoxifen and 4-hydroxy-tamoxifen with broadly similar affinities and interact with identical DNA response elements (5), a number of functional differences exist between the two receptors. For example, ERβ binds certain plant estrogens such as genistein with greater affinity than ERα (6). On the other hand, the anti-estrogen raloxifene has a considerably higher affinity for ERα than for ERβ (6). Furthermore, at the activator protein-1(AP1) enhancer element, ERα and ERβ signal in opposite ways. Thus, when bound to ERα, estrogen activates transcription whereas with ERβ, transcription is inhibited (7). These different actions of ERα and ERβ at the AP1 site appear due to the unique sites at both the amino- and carboxy-terminal ends (8). At the AP1 site, tamoxifen activates rather than inhibits both forms of the receptor (7).

Further evidence of different biological functions for the two subtypes of ER can be gleaned from the contrasting phenotypes observed in ER-deficient mice. For ERα-knockout (KO) mice, the most striking phenotype in females includes infertility, lack of pubertal mammary gland development, and excess adipose tissue. In contrast, ERβKO female mice are fertile, but less fertile than control mice. In males, ERαKO mice are also infertile but the ERβKO animals show no obvious phenotype apart from the development of prostatic hyperplasia early in life (5).

The discovery of ERβ raises multiple questions concerning breast cancer (9,10):

- Which form of ER is being measured by the ER assays in routine use?
- Will the measurement of ERβ enhance the predictive and prognostic value of the current ER assays? In particular, can it identify the 50% of ER-positive patients who fail to respond to endocrine therapy?

- Can ERβ provide an insight into the mechanism by which estrogens cause breast cancer?
- Can selective estrogen receptor response modifiers (SERMS) that bind selectively to either ERα or ERβ be developed?

MATERIALS AND METHODS

In this investigation, ERα and ERβ were measured at the mRNA level in 181 primary invasive breast cancers using reverse transcriptase-polymerase chain reaction (RT-PCR) (9,10). ER and progesterone receptor (PR) protein levels were measured by enzyme-linked immunosorbent assay (ELISA) (Abbott Diagnostics, Abbott Park, Illinois, www.abbott.com).

RESULTS

Our main findings are as follows (9,10):

- In the carcinomas, ERβ mRNA was expressed less frequently than ERα (43% vs. 67%; p = 0.0001). Furthermore, ERβ was expressed less frequently in the cancers [compared to the fibroadenomas (p = 0.007)]. In contrast, ERα was found in a similar proportion of cancers and fibroadenomas (Figure 1).
- ERα mRNA levels correlated significantly with ER protein levels as determined by ELISA (r = 0.34, p = 0.001) (Figure 2). In contrast, no significant relationship was found between ERβ mRNA levels and ER protein.
- Significantly higher levels of ER protein were found in cancers containing ERα mRNA than in those without this form of the receptor (p = 0001).
- Significantly higher ER protein levels were present in ERβ-negative cancers than in ERβ-positive samples (p = 0.001).
- ERα mRNA levels correlated weakly with PR protein levels (r = 0.202, p = 0.0087) but ERβ levels showed an inverse relation with PR levels (r = −0.202, p = 0.0127).
- PR protein levels were significantly higher in ERα mRNA-positive cancers than ERα mRNA-negative samples (p = 0.044). However, PR protein levels were lower in ERβ

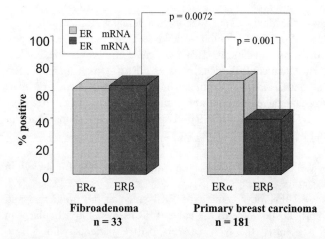

Figure 1 Distribution of ERα and ERβ mRNA in fibroadenomas and breast cancers.

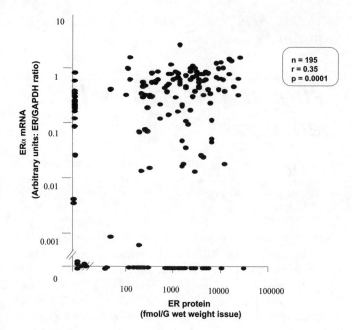

Figure 2 Relationship between ERα mRNA and ER protein.

mRNA-positive samples than ERβ mRNA-negative specimens (p = 0.017).
- Neither ERα nor ERβ mRNA levels correlated significantly with tumor size, tumor grade, axillary nodal status, or patient age.

From these findings, we conclude that ERα and ERβ have different expression patterns in breast cancer. The positive correlation between ERα mRNA and ER protein as determined by a widely used ELISA method suggests that it is detecting mostly the alpha form of ER. Using this ELISA, ERβ is thus unlikely to be detected. Whether ERβ is being detected by the immunohistochemical methods in routine use is likely to depend on the epitope to which the antibody in question is directed against.

It is currently unclear whether ERβ has any predictive or prognostic value in breast cancer. However, our finding of an inverse relationship between ERβ and both ER and PR proteins suggests that the presence of this form of ER may predict resistance rather than sensitivity to tamoxifen. Consistent with this possibility was the recent preliminary report showing higher ERβ levels in tamoxifen-resistant than in tamoxifen-sensitive breast cancers (11).

FUTURE DIRECTIONS

Currently, almost all work carried out on ERβ in breast cancer has been at the mRNA level. Future research should focus on development of specific antibodies against this receptor form for use in both immunohistochemistry and ELISA. Future work should also establish whether ERβ has predictive or prognostic value. Ideally, these studies should be carried out as part of a prospective randomized clinical trial. Finally, ERβ may play a role in breast carcinogenesis. It is of interest that although estrogens have for many years been implicated in breast cancer formation, there is no clear evidence that the classical ER is involved in tumorigenesis. *ERβ* is thus a candidate gene for mediating the carcinogenic effects of estrogen.

REFERENCES

1. Duffy MJ. Prognostic and predictive markers in cancer. J Clin Lig Assay 1999;22:331–334.
2. Anonymous. Clinical practice guidelines for use of tumor in breast and colorectal cancer. J Clin Oncol 1996;14:2843–2877.
3. Molina R, Duffy MJ, Aronsson AC, Lamerz R, Stieber P, van Dalen A. Tumor markers in breast cancer, EGTM recommendations. Anticancer Res 1999;19:2803–2805.
4. National Institute of Health Consensus Development Panel. National Institute of Health Consensus Development Conference Statement: adjuvant therapy for breast cancer, Nov 1–3, 2000. JNCI 2001;93:979–989.
5. Pettersson K, Gustafsson J-K. Role of estrogen receptor beta in estrogen action. Ann Rev Physiol 2001;63:165–192.
6. Kuiper GGJM, Lemmen JG, Carlsson B, Corton JC, Safe SH, van der Saag PT, et al. Interaction of estrogenic chemicals and phytoestrogens with estrogen receptor beta. Endocrinol 1998;139: 4252–4263.
7. Paech K, Webb P, Kuiper GGJM, Nilsson S, Gustaffsson JA, Kusher PJ, et al. Differential ligand activation of estrogen receptors ER-α and ER-β at AP-1 sites. Science 1997;277: 1508–1510.
8. Weatherman RV, Scanlan TS. Unique protein determinants of the subtype-selective ligand responses of the estrogen receptors (ERα and ERβ) at AP-1 sites. J Biol Chem 2001;276:3827–3832.
9. Cullen R, Maguire T, McDermott EW, Hill ADK, O'Higgins N, Duffy MJ. Studies on estrogen receptor-α and β mRNA in breast cancer. Eur J Cancer 2001;37:1118–1122.
10. Cullen R, Maguire T, McDermott E, Hill ADK, O'Higgins N, Duffy MJ. Estrogen receptor-β: role in breast cancer. J Clin Lig (In press).
11. Speirs V, Malone C, Walton DS, Kerin M, Atkin SL. Increased expression of estrogen receptor-β mRNA in tamoxifen-resistant breast cancer patients. Cancer Res 1999;59:5421–5424.

Chapter **44**

Measurement of Tumor-Specific T Cells with MHC Tetramer Technology

Johannes Hampl and Kristine Kuus-Reichel

MHC (major histocompatibility complex) tetramers were first developed by John Altman and Mark Davis in 1996 (1). Since that time, this technology has been used for a number of different clinical and research applications, including monitoring the antigen-specific, T-cell-mediated immune response to different tumors, and cancer vaccine development. The advent of MHC tetramers has allowed the scientific community to characterize and quantitate the immune response with a level of clarity that was previously difficult to achieve. Using tetramers, scientists now have the capability of quantitatively measuring the body's CD8+ T-cell immune response to epitopes within a specific antigen, such as MART-1, in a manner that most accurately represents the in vivo response. To date, MHC tetramers have been used in studying the immune response to multiple types of cancer including breast, prostate, melanoma, colon, lung, and cervical.

MHC tetramers are complexes of four MHC molecules, associated with a specific antigenic peptide and bound to a fluorochrome (Figure 1). MHC tetramers are specific for both a tumor-specific peptide and the subject's human leukocyte antigen (HLA) allele and will therefore bind only to a distinct set of T-cell receptors on a subset of CD8+ T cells, which recognize this combination. By design, MHC tetramers enumerate all peptide-specific, CD8+ T cells regardless of activity or functionality. MHC tetramers enable accurate quantitative analysis of antigen-specific T-cell responses, even for extremely rare events that occur as low as in 0.02–0.10% of CD8+ T cells. An additional mutation in the MHC tetramer minimized non-antigen-specific binding of tetramers to CD8+ cells, further increasing the accuracy of tetramer measurements (2). Tetramers with this mutation show a diminished binding to the general population of CD8+ T cells, but retain peptide-specific binding, thus facilitating the accurate discrimination of rare, antigen-specific CD8+ T cells. MHC tetramers do not damage the integrity of the cells and the sample is therefore available for further analysis to determine functionality and characterize phenotype. Essentially this technology provides a snapshot of the immune response to a specific antigen, as it occurs in vivo, at a particular point in time. Using tetramers, antigen-specific CD8+ cells can also be isolated from human peripheral blood by sorting with a flow cytometer. The isolated cells can be expanded in vitro and used to gather additional information on

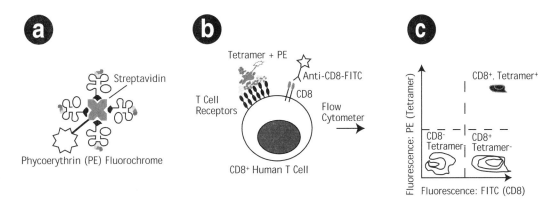

Figure 1 MHC tetramers are complexes of four MHC (major histocompatibility complex) molecules loaded with a specific peptide and bound to a fluorochrome. These complexes bind to a distinct set of T-cell receptors (TCRs) on a subset of CD8+ T cells. Thus, by mixing tetramers with peripheral blood lymphocytes (PBLs) or whole blood and using flow cytometry as a detection system, a count of all T cells that are specific for one peptide and its matched allele is provided, regardless of functionality. (a) Diagram of an MHC tetramer molecule; (b) Binding of MHC tetramer to a CD8+ T cell; (c) Example of data obtained from a flow cytometer showing the discreet CD8+, tetramer-positive T-cell population (upper right quadrant). Reprinted with permission of Cambridge University Press. Julian Hickling (1998). Measuring human T-lymphocyte function. Exp. Rev. Mol. Med. 13 October, http://www-ermm.cbcu.cam.ac.uk/jhc/txt001 jhc.htm.

cell phenotype and for reinfusion into the donor for potential therapeutic purposes.

In addition to applications in cancer, MHC tetramer research has been valuable for the measurement of antigen-specific T cells with a focus on infectious diseases such as human immunodeficiency virus (HIV), Epstein-Barr virus (EBV), cytomegalovirus (CMV), human papilloma virus (HPV), hepatitis C (HCV), and influenza; parasitic infections including malaria; and autoimmune disease. To date, most of the research conducted has been with MHC Class I molecules found on CD8+ T cells. However the development of Class II MHC tetramers, to measure CD4+ T cells, is proceeding rapidly and the introduction of Class II technology promises to further revolutionize immune response measurement.

RATIONALE

Tumor cells express antigens that make them targets of the cellular arm of the immune system, especially MHC Class-I restricted cytotoxic T lymphocytes (CTL). While immunotherapy to battle cancer has been accepted conceptually, clinical success has been limited. Mobilizing immune-competent effector T cells in the fight against cancer is attractive because T cells have the capability to detect and specifically kill tumor cells (3). A detailed understanding of the relationship between the tumor and the immune response against it will be crucial if such efforts are to be successful. The ability to monitor the tumor-specific T-cell repertoire and its functional status will be a key component of this investigation. MHC tetramer technology, with its explicit ability to identify and measure tumor-specific T cell specificities ex vivo, is uniquely suited to give us this much-needed information. The following events need to take place in vivo for an effective anti-tumor T cell response to occur:

1. Expression of tumor-specific antigens.
2. Processing and presentation of tumor antigens with HLA molecules by antigen-presenting cells.
3. Tumor antigen recognition by T cells followed by clonal expansion of the antigen-specific T cell population.
4. Differentiation of tumor-specific T cells into cytotoxic effector cells.

As exemplified in Figure 2, all these steps need to be systematically explored to develop effective tumor therapies.

Expression of Tumor Antigens

Tumor cells may express novel tumor antigens or aberrant quantities of "normal" antigens. Comparison of the gene expression profiles of tumor cells and normal cells can be the first step towards identification of tumor-specific antigens. As such, tumor antigens may not only be gene products carrying a somatic DNA mutation causative of the malignant behavior of the cells (4), but can also be products of "normal" genes that are expressed at much higher levels in tumor cells.

Identification of tumor antigens that can stimulate an immune response is critical for effective vaccination or immunotherapy. Methods including gene expression profiling using DNA arrays and SAGE (Serial Analysis of Gene Expression) can be utilized to identify cancer-associated genes in a comprehensive manner (5).

Processing and Presentation of Tumor Antigens with HLA Molecules

After expression, tumor antigens are processed by antigen-presenting cells (APC), and tumor-specific peptides are presented with MHC molecules on the surface of the APC. Usually, identification of tumor-specific peptides is determined experimentally, but computer algorithms can help identify potential peptide epitopes based on known HLA allele-binding motifs (for more information see reference 5).

While these algorithms can help substantially reduce the numbers of potential epitopes, the existence of these epitopes in vivo should always be verified by bioassays. For example, computer algorithms helped identify a peptide sequence that binds to HLA-A2 within the catalytic domain of human telomerase. T cells that were reactive to this putative tumor antigen were recovered using a synthetic peptide (6). However, this peptide is not naturally produced in sufficient quantities in cells during antigen processing, which raises questions about its utility as cancer vaccine candidate (7). In contrast, a peptide within proteinase 3, called PR1, had been identified through a computer algorithm to bind to HLA-A2, and is upregulated during chronic myelogenous leukemia (8). The existence of PR1-specific T cells in cancer patients has recently been correlated with disease status (9), providing direct evidence that T cells are involved in tumor clearance. A recent review by Schultze and Vonderheide outlines a potential pathway and discusses methods for epitope deduction for the identification of tumor antigens (5).

Tumor Antigen Recognition by T Cells Followed by Clonal Expansion

T cells can recognize a large repertoire of antigenic specificities; the inability to recognize cancer-specific epitopes is not likely to be a limiting factor in the design of cancer immunotherapy. However, many tumor antigens are "self"-antigens; immunoregulatory mechanisms may be in place to limit clonal expansion and/or functional maturation of potentially self-reactive T cells. Thus, it is important to monitor the size of the tumor-specific T-cell repertoire in patients, followed by the assessment of the functional status of these cells if they occur in high frequencies (see below). MHC tetramer is the only technology to unequivocally enumerate the entire population of antigen-specific T cells ex vivo.

Differentiation of tumor specific T cells into cytotoxic effector cells. Once it has been established that an enlarged tumor-specific T-cell population exists in a patient, it is important to ensure that these cells are functionally active, as anergy or ignorance are the default pathways of self-reactive T cells.

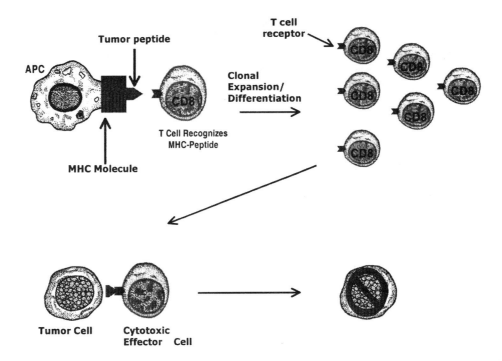

Figure 2 Evolution of the cytotoxic T-cell response. Antigen-presenting cells (APC) process and present tumor-specific antigens on their surface. CD8+ T cells with the appropriate T-cell receptor recognize the peptide/allele-specific MHC complex on the surface of the APC. Tumor peptide-specific, CD8+ T cells proliferate and differentiate into cytotoxic effector cells (CTLs). CTLs kill the tumor cells that express the tumor-specific peptide.

Again, MHC tetramers can help us gain insight into the functional status of the specific repertoire by combining MHC tetramer measurements with multidimensional flow cytometry to detect additional cell surface markers associated with functions (e.g., naïve vs. memory) or with cytokine production. Alternatively, specific T cells can be sorted based on tetramer binding, followed by more classical functional tests such as ^{51}Cr-release assays to directly measure the ability of the CTLs to kill tumor cells. Several current reviews contain lists of known tumor epitopes (10).

If (i) a gene product is abundantly expressed in a relatively specific manner by the tumor, (ii) peptides are generated efficiently from this gene product and presented by HLA molecules on the surface of professional APCs, (iii) T cells specific for this tumor epitope multiply, and (iv) they differentiate into effector cells—then a correlation with a better clinical diagnosis for the cancer patient can be postulated. While direct data do not exist regarding the contribution of the cellular immune system on the prevention of tumor development or the elimination of existing tumors in preclinical stages, it is evident that the immune system is in many cases not capable of controlling tumor progression in later clinical stages. Vaccination or other immunotherapies are being designed to alert the immune system to the danger presented by the tumor and encourage the expansion and maturation of tumor-specific T cells. There is precedence for desirable outcomes of such therapies (9). It is likely that in the near future, novel treatment strategies will be developed that combine classical systemic treatments to reduce tumor burden (chemotherapy, radiation therapy, etc.) in combination with treatments designed to boost the immune response against the tumor for long-lasting benefits to the patient.

FUTURE DIRECTIONS

The ability of MHC tetramer technology to directly enumerate the presence of tumor antigen-specific cytotoxic T cells in peripheral blood samples of cancer patients is a major advance in the monitoring of cancer vaccination and immunotherapy. This technology provides a means of visualizing a cancer patient's status of immunity to his/her own tumor with exquisite sensitivity and specificity.

However, the measurement of the cytotoxic T-cell response represents only a portion of the overall immune response. To truly be able to visualize the ongoing immune response to vaccination or immunotherapy, measurement of helper T cells (CD4+), B cells, and other immunoregulatory cells is required. The ratio and magnitude of the tumor-specific activation and expansion of these cell populations in response to vaccination or immunotherapy will give us critical information on the quality of a patient's immune response. Class II MHC tetramer technology, designed to measure tumor specific CD4+ cells, has been shown to be feasible and is under aggressive development. Assays to measure tumor-specific antibody responses have been developed to a limited degree. Measurement of other potentially tumor-specific regulatory cells, such as natural killer (NK) cells, is also a focus of active research. The ability to accurately and specifically portray the dynamic equilibria and complexity of the human immune response in cancer vaccination and immunotherapy will result in information that will revolutionize effective patient management.

REFERENCES

1. Altman JD, Moss PA, Goulder PJ, Barouch DH, McHeyzer-Williams MG, Bell JI, McMichael AJ, Davis MM. Phenotypic analysis of antigen-specific T lymphocytes. Science 1996;274 (5284):94–96.
2. Bodinier M, Peyrat MA, Tournay C, Davodeau F, Romagne F, Bonneville M, Lang F. Efficient detection and immunomagnetic sorting of T cells using multimers of MHC class I and peptide with reduced CD8 binding. Nat Med 2000;6(6):707–710.
3. Yee C, Riddell SR, Greenberg PD. *In vivo* tracking of tumor-specific T cells. Curr Opin Immunol 2001;13(2):141–146.
4. Baurain JF, Colau D, van Baren N, Landry C, Martelange V, Vikkula M, Boon T, Coulie PG. High frequency of autologous anti-melanoma CTL directed against an antigen generated by a point mutation in a new helicase gene. J Immunol 2000;164(11): 6057–6066.
5. Schultze JL, Vonderheide RH. From cancer genomics to cancer immunotherapy: toward second-generation tumor antigens. Trends Immunol 2001;22(9):516–523.
6. Vonderheide RH, Hahn WC, Schultze JL, Nadler LM. The telomerase catalytic subunit is a widely expressed tumor-associated antigen recognized by cytotoxic T lymphocytes. Immunity 1999; 10(6):673–679.
7. Ayyoub M, Migliaccio M, Guillaume P, Lienard D, Cerottini JC, Romero P, Levy F, Speiser DE, Valmori D. Lack of tumor recognition by hTERT peptide 540-548-specific CD8(+) T cells from melanoma patients reveals inefficient antigen processing. Eur J Immunol 2001;31(9):2642–2651.
8. Molldrem JJ, Clave E, Jiang YZ, Mavroudis D, Raptis A, Hensel N, Agarwala V, Barrett AJ. Cytotoxic T lymphocytes specific for a nonpolymorphic proteinase 3 peptide preferentially inhibit chronic myeloid leukemia colony-forming units. Blood 1997; 90(7):2529–2534.
9. Molldrem JJ, Lee PP, Wang C, Felio K, Kantarjian HM, Champlin RE, Davis MM. Evidence that specific T lymphocytes may participate in the elimination of chronic myelogenous leukemia. Nat Med 2000;6(9):1018–1023.
10. Pittet MJ, Speiser DE, Valmori D, Rimoldi D, Lienard D, Lejeune F, Cerottini JC, Romero P. Ex vivo analysis of tumor antigen-specific CD8+ T cell responses using MHC/peptide tetramers in cancer patients. Int Immunopharmacol 2001;1(7):1235–1247.

Chapter 45

A New Discovery Approach for Hormone-Responsive Genes: PC1 *Prostate Cancer Gene*

Cynthia French and Karen Yamamoto

The progression of chronic and malignant reproductive tissue diseases is dependent largely on the interactions of the endocrine system with both genomic and non-genomic components that structure the environment of the affected tissues. In hormone-driven carcinogenesis, steroid hormone-signaling pathways play an intermediary role between the genetic and physiological state of the whole organism, and the microenvironment of the tumorigenic target tissue (1). Endocrine-responsive cancers include cancers of the prostate (androgens), breast and ovary (estrogens), endometrium (estrogen, progesterone), larynx (androgen), and lymphoid tissues (glucocorticoids, estrogen) (2).

We have focused on identifying steroid hormone-modulated gene expression patterns and subsequent protein modifications in a prototype prostate cancer xenograft model. Development of a human xenograft animal model provides a biologically and clinically relevant hormone model for the isolation of steroid hormone-induced disease genes involved in actual disease. The natural animal model provides the correct hormone milieu of factors such as integrins, stroma, growth factors, and additional hormone breakdown metabolites found to be lacking in many in vitro cell culture systems currently used in the field (3). In the xenograft model, it is the direct cellular contact and signal transduction exchanges between the host tissue and tumor cell lines that promote changes in disease tissue architecture, maintain steroid hormone receptor integrity, and that regulate expression of the malignant phenotype. Using the xenograft model and a differential biosystems screen, a number of genes were identified that are steroid hormone-induced or repressed specifically in human prostate cancer. *PC1* is the first gene isolated using this technology, and its product is expressed specifically in prostate cancers (4).

ISOLATION OF TESTOSTERONE HORMONALLY REGULATED SEQUENCES IN PROSTATE CANCER

LNCaP human prostate tumor cells were propagated in both male and female athymic mice. The tumors, which typically took at least two to three months to develop into palpable masses, showed remarkably different features depending on whether they were propagated in a male or a female environment (5). Tumors that developed in male mice (male-LNCaP) showed extensive vascularization and morphological destruction compared to the highly regular and homogeneous composition of the tumors in females (female-LNCaP). Additionally, the tumors raised in male hosts had gained metastatic potential, whereas no metastases were ever detected in female mice (data not shown).

A male-LNCaP-specific probe was generated by three rounds of subtractive hybridization with female-LNCaP tumor cDNA. This male-LNCaP specific probe was then used to perform a primary screen of a lambda-ZAP-male-LNCaP tumor cDNA library. Positive plaques were subjected to a dual secondary screen, using the male-LNCaP-specific probe and total female-LNCaP tumor cDNA. Clones were considered positive if they hybridized strongly to the "male-specific" probe and weakly to the female probe (Figure 1). The resulting positives were subjected to a tertiary screen in which the clones were "rescued" and their plasmid DNA was subjected to duplicate Southern hybridizations using total male-LNCaP or total female-LNCaP cDNA. The DNA from clones hybridizing more strongly to male-LNCaP sequences was then subjected to Northern analyses. The DNA from one clone, *PC1*, when hybridized to equivalent amounts of RNA from male-LNCaP tumors, female-LNCaP tumors, LNCaP cells, and PC-3 cells, showed an ~10X amplification of a single 4.4 kilobase (kb) mRNA in male-LNCaP tumors (Figure 2).

Sequence Analysis of *PC1*

Initial sequence analysis of clone *PC1* did not reveal any significant open reading frames (ORFs) in either direction. Subsequently, an overlapping clone, PS5-1, was isolated from the male-LNCaP tumor library by hybridization with an oligonucleotide probe encoding 5' sequences contained within the *PC1* insert. Directionality of the *PC1* clone was inferred from the presence of a putative poly-A tail. The complete coding region was determined by sequencing PS5-1, a 5' end cDNA clone derived from an overlapping rapid amplification of cDNA ends-polymerase chain reaction (RACE-PCR).

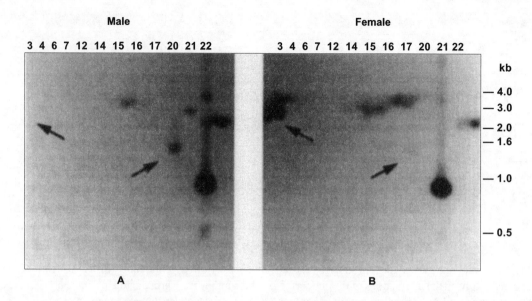

Figure 1 Reverse Southern blot hybridization to male-specific and female probes. Plasmid DNA isolated from subtractive screen candidates were hybridized to either a male-LNCaP-specific probe generated by three rounds of subtractive hybridization with female-LNCaP tumor cDNA (male-specific), panel A; or cDNA from xenografts propagated in a female host (female probes), panel B.

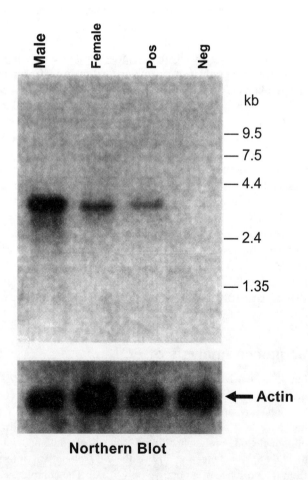

Figure 2 Northern hybridization of *PC1* to RNA derived from either male-LNCaP tumors (Male), female-LNCaP tumors (Female), LNCaP cells (positive control), or androgen-nonresponsive PC3 cells (negative control).

Sequence analysis of the overlapping clones revealed a single 1275 base pair (bp) ORF encoding 425 amino acids, followed by a 2466 bp 3′ untranslated region to which a polyadenylate tail was added. The M_r and pI were calculated to be 48,070 and 8.83, respectively. The predicted amino acid sequence of the C-terminal region of *PC1* contained two copies of a 116-amino acid direct repeat that had 34% identify (41% similarity) with each other. These repeats were found to be homologous to the C2 regulatory domain of calcium-dependent isoforms of protein kinase C (PKC), and to isoforms of synaptotagmin.

PC1 is Human Synaptotagmin IV

PC1 is a member of the synaptotagmin family of genes whose protein products function in vesicle trafficking. Synaptotagmin proteins are characterized by an intravesicular amino terminus, a short transmembrane domain, and a cytosolic domain containing two regions similar to the C2 domain identified in protein kinase C (6). *PC1* expression has been detected by reverse transcriptase (RT)-PCR analysis specifically in blood and tumor biopsies of staged cancer patients; it is not detectable in males or females who are cancer-free. Furthermore, *PC1* is not expressed in normal prostate tissue or in benign prostatic hyperplasia.

Synaptotagmins represent a family of highly conserved, abundant synaptic vesicle proteins that potentially play a role in regulating synaptic vesicle translocation to the presynaptic release site of the plasma membrane (docking) and/or fusion of these two membranes (7). Structurally, synaptotagmin isoforms can be divided into several domains. These include an intravesicular, amino-terminal domain; a single transmembrane domain; and a cytoplasmic, carboxyl-terminal domain that consists of two repeats homologous to the C2 regulatory domain of PKC termed A and B. Homologs of synaptotagmin have shown

Table 1 Expression of *PC1* in prostate carcinoma

Tissue source	*PC1* PCR hybridization
LNCaP Tumor (male)[a]	++
+ DNase	+++
+ RNase	−
Normal Prostate	−
+ DNase	−
+ RNase	−
Prostate Adenocarcinoma[b]	++
+ DNase	+
+ RNase	−
Prostatic Benign Hyperplasia	−
Uterus	−

[a] LNCaP Tumor tissue grown in male athymic mice.
[b] Compilation of analysis from 3 different prostate adenocarcinomas.

PC1-specific bands: +++ very strong hybridization; ++ strong hybridization; + moderate hybridization; − no hybridization.

greater conservation of sequence identity and similarity in the cytoplasmic domain containing the two PKC C2-homologous repeats than in the N-terminal intravesicular or transmembrane domains. A recent publication from the laboratory of Herschman confirms *PC1* is indeed synaptotagmin IV (8). Additional sequence analysis indicates that the two internal repeats of *PC1* are approximately as homologous to each other (34% identity) as to the corresponding region of PKC (identity between 28% and 37% depending on the isoform). As in the other forms of synaptotagmin, the amino acid residues that are identical between the two internal repeats of *PC1* are also conserved between *PC1* and PKC, revealing a core consensus sequence of SDPYV/IK followed by a stretch of basic residues. Additionally, when the internal repeat sequences of *PC1* and *Drosophila* synaptotagmin are aligned with each other and with the C2 regulatory domain of a PKC isoform, each repeat is more highly conserved between synaptotagmins than it is identical with the isoform.

Hydrophobicity plots of the amino acid sequence of *PC1* revealed a single segment, from residues 15–37, of sufficient length and hydrophobicity to constitute a transmembrane domain. Although this domain does not align colinearly with the corresponding domain in the other synaptotagmins, it also displays the unusual transmembrane boundaries reported for other synaptotagmins (9). The amino-terminal border of the putative transmembrane domain is flanked by a proline; the carboxyl-terminus of the domain is flanked by cysteine residues followed by a highly positively charged region.

A Single, Evolution-Conserved *PC1* Gene Localizes to Chromosome 18

Southern blot analyses of *PC1* hybridization to human genomic DNA revealed a non-complex pattern indicating a single copy sequence. Analysis of *PC1* hybridization to genomic DNAs from a panel of phylogenetically distinct species showed that the sequences encoding *PC1* were highly conserved, hybridizing to yeast DNA even under high stringency conditions.

CLINICAL APPLICATIONS: EXPRESSION OF *PC1* IN PROSTATE CARCINOMA AND IN OTHER TISSUES

In order to compare the expression of *PC1* in normal prostate with its expression in prostate adenocarcinomas and benign hyperplasias, *PC1* sequences were specifically amplified from RNA isolated from a number of well-characterized tissue sources by RT-PCR. These products were fractionated, transferred, and hybridized with a *PC1* probe and the level of expression was graded by relative signal intensity of the *PC1*-specific bands (Table 1). *PC1* sequences were only present in the RNAs isolated from prostatic adenocarcinoma samples and were not detectable in samples representing benign hyperplasias. To ensure that the amplified sequences were not due to genomic DNA contaminants, control reactions were performed, adding RNase or DNase prior to the first strand synthesis step.

PC1 expression in additional carcinomas and tissues was investigated by RNA blot analysis (Figure 3). *PC1* expression was not detected in any other prostate or non-prostate carcino-

Table 2 *PC1* mRNA in human cell lines and mammalian tissues—summary of Northern hybridization results for different human cell lines and mammalian tissues

Cell line expression	Tissue source	*PC1*
LNCaP	Prostate adenocarcinoma	+
LNCaP	Male tumors[a]	+
LNCaP	Female tumors[b]	+
PC-3	Prostate carcinoma	−
DU-145	Prostate carcinoma	−
BT-20	Breast carcinoma	−
T-47D	Breast ductal carcinoma	−
BT-474	Breast ductal carcinoma	−
MCF-7	Breast adenocarcinoma	−
SK-BR-3	Breast adenocarcinoma	−
MDA-MB-231	Breast adenocarcinoma	−
LS174T	Colon adenocarcinoma	−
NIH:OVCAR-3	Ovary adenocarcinoma	−
3a5	Hybridoma—SP2/0 fusion myeloma	−
	Placenta, human	+
	Pancreas, human	−
	Pituitary, human	−
	Liver, human	−
	Spleen, human	−
	Brain, human	+
	Heart, human	−
	Skeletal muscle, human	−
	Kidney, human	−
	Pancreas, canine	−
	Pituitary, canine	−
	Spleen, mouse	−
	Rubella (strain M33)	−

[a] LNCaP xenograft tumors propagated in male athymic mice.
[b] LNCaP xenograft tumors propagated in female athymic mice.
+ indicates detectable expression; − absence of detectable expression.

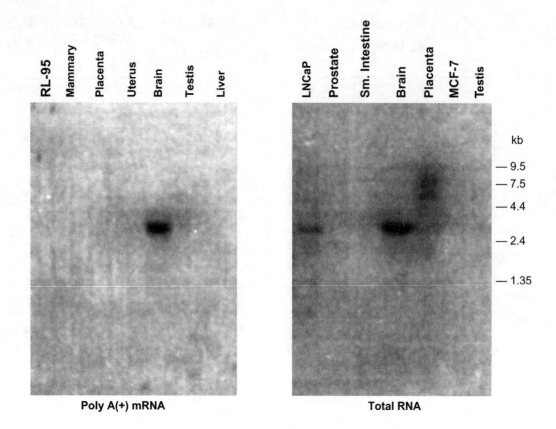

Figure 3 Northern blot analysis of *PC1* cDNA to polyA+ RNA or total RNA isolated from the tissues listed.

ma cell lines besides the LNCaP line, nor was it detected in any other normal tissue except for brain (Table 2). Interestingly, this is precisely the tissue where the synaptotagmin family is expressed, suggesting that LNCaP cells are aberrantly expressing a gene that encodes a protein involved in the regulated secretory pathway.

FUTURE DIRECTIONS: CLINICAL STUDY PROTOCOLS

Several clinical studies using both RT-PCR and immunohistochemical assay approaches for determining the specificity and sensitivity of *PC1* as a prostate cancer clinical marker are being initiated. Both tissue biopsy and blood samples obtained from patient outcome databases are being analyzed and correlated with prostate-specific antigen (PSA) measurements. Initial results suggest that *PC1* correlates with highly aggressive metastatic prostate cancer stages and appears to be a valuable clinical reagent in differentiating benign prostate clinical conditions from prostate cancers.

Additional molecular studies are also underway to investigate the function of *PC1* in tumor biology and the potential role of *PC1* in aggressive prostate cancer disease and progression to androgen independence.

REFERENCES

1. Kodama M, Kodama T. An essay on the nature of hormonal codes involved in the genesis of human neoplasias. Anticancer Res 1994;14:2653–2666.
2. Giovanella BC, Fogh J. The nude mouse in cancer research. Adv Cancer Res 1995;44:70–120.
3. Park C, Bissell M, Barcellos-Hoff M. The influence of the microenvironment on the malignant phenotype. Mol Med Today 2000;6:324–329.
4. French C, Yamamoto K, Scheneider P. Prostate cancer specific marker 2001;US Patent 6,218,523 B1.
5. French C, Yamamoto K. Methods for identifying hormonally modulated genes 1998. PCT WO 98/39661.
6. Berton F, Iborra C, Boudier J, Seager M, Marqueze B. Developmental regulation of synaptotagmin I, II, III, and IV mRNAs in the rat CNS. J Neurosci 1997;17(4):1206–1216.
7. Gersti J. SNARE and SNARE regulators in membrane fusion and exocytosis. Cell Mol Life Sci1999;55:707–734.
8. Ferguson G, Chen X, Korenberg J, Herschman H. The human synaptotagmin IV gene defines an evolutionary break point between syntenic mouse and human chromosome regions and retains ligand inducibility and tissue specificity. J Biol Chem 2000;275(47):36920–36926.
9. Bajjalien S. Synaptic vesicle docking and fusion. Curr Opin Neurobiol1999;9:321–326.

Chapter 46

Kallikreins as Cancer Biomarkers

George M. Yousef and Eleftherios P. Diamandis

Recently, the complete genomic organization of the human tissue kallikrein gene family and the identification of fifteen members, which share significant similarities at both the DNA and amino acid level, have been described (1,2). For some of these members, highly sensitive and specific immunoassays have already been developed. These methods are suitable for measuring these secreted proteins in serum and other biological fluids. In addition to prostate-specific antigen (PSA) and human glandular kallikrein 2 (hK2), which have already found clinical applicability as prostate cancer biomarkers, accumulating evidence indicates that other kallikreins are differentially regulated in different endocrine-related malignancies and are potential new cancer biomarkers.

In this chapter, we will briefly describe the reported utility of kallikrein genes and proteins for diagnosis, prognosis, prediction of therapeutic response, and monitoring of patients with different malignancies.

WHAT IS A KALLIKREIN?

The term "kallikrein" was introduced in the 1930s by Werle and colleagues who found high levels of their original isolates in the pancreas (in Greek, the "Kallikreas"). Later, a functional definition of a "kallikrein" was introduced to describe proteolytic enzymes that can release small vasoactive peptides from high-molecular-weight precursors.

There are two categories of kallikrein enzymes, plasma and tissue. The plasma kallikrein is encoded by a single gene on chromosome 4. This enzyme (a serine protease) releases the vasoactive peptide bradykinin from a high-molecular-weight precursor synthesized in the liver. The tissue kallikreins are a family of genes localized on chromosome 19q13.4 that also encode for serine protease enzymes.

Based on the original definition of kallikreins, which is based on the kininogenase activity of these enzymes, only one

Table 1 Approved new nomenclature for human kallikreins

New gene Symbol[a]	Previous gene Symbol(s)	New protein Symbol	Other protein Names/Symbols
KLK1	KLK1	hK1	Pancreatic/renal kallikrein, hPRK
KLK2	KLK2	hK2	Human glandular kallikrein 1, hGK-1
KLK3	KLK3	hK3	Prostate-specific antigen, PSA
KLK4	PRSS17, KLK-L1, KLK4	hK4	Prostase, KLK-L1 protein, EMSP1
KLK5	KLK-L2	hK5	KLK-L2 protein, HSCTE
KLK6	PRSS9	hK6	Zyme, Protease M, Neurosin
KLK7	PRSS6	hK7	HSCCE
KLK8	PRSS19	hK8	Neuropsin, Ovasin, TADG-14
KLK9	KLK-L3	hK9	KLK-L3 protein
KLK10	PRSSL1, NES1	hK10	NES1 protein
KLK11	PRSS20	hK11	TLSP/Hippostasin
KLK12	KLK-L5	hK12	KLK-L5 protein
KLK13	KLK-L4	hK13	KLK-L4 protein
KLK14	KLK-L6	hK14	KLK-L6 protein
KLK15	—	hK15	Prostinogen

[a] The order of the genes on chromosome 19q13.4 is shown in Figure 1.
KLK, kallikrein; PRK, pancreatic/renal kallikrein; EMSP1, enamel matrix serine proteinase 1; HSCTE, human stratum corneum tryptic enzyme; PSA, prostate-specific antigen; HSCCE, human stratum corneum chymotryptic enzyme; TADG-14, tumor-associated differentially expressed gene-14; NES1, normal epithelial cell-specific 1; TLSP, trypsin-like serine protease; PRSS, protease, serine; PRSSL, protease, serine-like; hGk-1, human glandular kallikrein 1.

of the tissue kallikreins, pancreatic/renal kallikrein (KLK1), fulfills this criterion. Until a few years ago, two other enzymes, human glandular kallikrein 2 and human kallikrein 3 (PSA), were also classified as members of the human tissue kallikrein gene family, based on a number of significant homologies and similarities with the pancreatic/renal kallikrein. More recently, other genes encoding for similar enzymes have also been classified as members of the human kallikrein gene family. This classification is not based on the functional definition, but rather on other criteria, including structural similarities and proximity of map location on chromosome 19q13.4. Based on the newer definition, the number of genes that are included in the human tissue kallikrein gene family has now been increased to 15.

The expansion of the human tissue kallikrein gene family and the identification of new genes has led to the conclusion that this human gene family, originally thought to be much smaller than similar families found in rodents, is now as large as the orthologous families found in rat and mouse (1).

THE HUMAN TISSUE KALLIKREIN GENE FAMILY

A schematic diagram showing the human tissue kallikrein gene locus on chromosome 19q13.4 is shown in Figure 1. All known kallikrein genes map within an approximate 300 kilobase (kb) region and the lengths of the genes, the distances between them as well as the direction of transcription have now been accurately defined (2). Telomerically, from the last kallikrein gene identified (*KLK14*), starts another family of genes, the Siglec gene family. This finding suggests that this area defines the end of the kallikrein gene family and the beginning of the Siglec family of genes. Centromerically from the *KLK1* gene, a novel gene was cloned, named "testicular acid phosphatase" (*ACPT*), which is not a kallikrein and appears to indicate the end of the kallikrein gene family from this end. Thus, it appears that between those two non-kallikrein genes (*ACPT* and *Siglec9*), there are 15 kallikrein genes that are aligned as shown in Figure 1.

The genomic organization of each one of these kallikrein genes is very similar (described in detail in ref. 1). All of these genes and proteins exhibit many other similarities as well. In short, all the genes encode for putative secreted serine proteases and have five coding exons of similar lengths. All genes share significant sequence homologies at both the DNA and amino acid level and many of them are regulated by steroid hormones. Despite these similarities, the tissue expression of these genes differs from one another. Some genes are expressed in one or very few tissues while others are abundantly expressed in most tissues. Detailed tissue expression data can be found elsewhere (1–3).

In order to simplify communication, an international group of scientists working in the field has established uniform nomenclature for the kallikrein genes and encoded proteins. In Table 2, we present the official nomenclature for each one of these genes (as approved by the human gene nomenclature committee) along with names originally assigned by individual

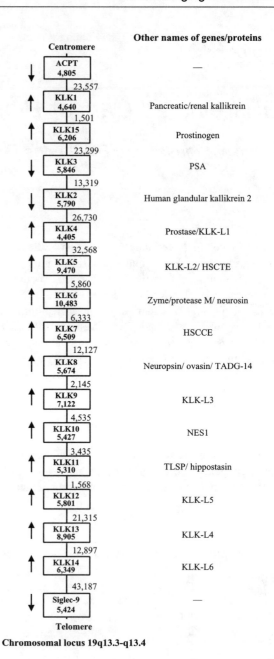

Figure 1 An approximate 300-kb region of contiguous genomic sequence around chromosome 19q13.4. The direction of transcription of each gene is illustrated by *arrows*. *Boxes* represent genes and contain the gene names and their genomic length, in base pairs. Other commonly used names for these genes are also mentioned. Distances between genes in base pairs are shown between *boxes*. The *Siglec* and *ACPT* (testicular acid phosphatase) genes do not belong to the tissue kallikrein gene family. Figure is not drawn to scale. For full gene names, see Table 1 and abbreviation footnote.

investigators (4). In this chapter, the official nomenclature for these genes and proteins is used throughout.

CLINICAL APPLICATIONS

Among all kallikrein genes, at least three have very restricted tissue expression. Prostate-specific antigen (*hK3*), human glan-

Table 2 Clinical application of the kallikrein genes and their encoded proteins as cancer biomarkers

Gene/protein name	Sample used	Method	Application	References
hK3 (PSA) and hK2			Established cancer biomarkers (see Chapter 17)	
KLK4	mRNA from ovarian cancer tissues	RT-PCR[a]	Ovarian cancer prognosis; overexpression of KLK4 in more aggressive cancers (late stage; higher grade; shorter disease-free and overall survival).	5
KLK5	mRNA from ovarian cancer tissues	RT-PCR	Ovarian cancer prognosis; overexpression of KLK5 in more aggressive cancers (late stage; higher grade; shorter disease-free and overall survival).	6
KLK6	mRNA from breast, prostate, and ovarian cancer cell lines and tissues	Northern blot	Higher level of message in some cell lines and tissues. No application specified.	7
	Serum	Immunoassay	Diagnosis and monitoring of ovarian cancer.	8
	Breast cancer cytosols	Immunoassay	Prognosis; association to hormone receptors.	9
	Ovarian cancer cytosols	Immunoassay	Prognosis; higher levels associated with late stage and decreased disease-free and overall patient survival.	Our unpublished data
KLK7	Ovarian cancer RNA and extracts	RT-PCR; Northern blots; Western blots; Immunohistochemistry	Overexpression of KLK7 mRNA and protein in the majority of ovarian tumors.	10
KLK8	mRNA from ovarian cancer tissue	RT-PCR	Prognosis; higher expression is associated with lower grade and improved patient disease-free disease-free and overall survival.	11
KLK9	mRNA from ovarian cancer tissue	RT-PCR	Prognosis; higher expression is associated with early stages and optimal debulking.	12
KLK10	mRNA and extracts from breast cancer tissue and cell lines	Northern blots, Western blots	Down-regulation of KLK10 in cancer cell lines.	13, 14
	Serum	Immunoassay	Diagnosis and monitoring of ovarian cancer.	15
	Breast cancer cytosols	Immunoassay	Prognosis (negatively associated with estrogen and progesterone receptors).	9
	Ovarian cancer cytosols	Immunoassay; Immunohistochemistry	Prognosis; high levels are associated with late stage disease and decreased disease-free and overall patient survival.	16

Table continued on next page

Table 2 *(continued)*

Gene/protein name	Sample used	Method	Application	References
KLK10	Testicular tissue extracts	RT-PCR; immunohistochemistry	Prognosis; down-regulation in cancer in comparison to normal tissues.	17
KLK11	Serum	Immunoassay	Serum level elevated in ovarian and prostate cancer patients	18
KLK12	mRNA from breast cancer	RT-PCR	Down-regulation in a subset of breast tumors.	19
KLK13	mRNA from breast cancer	RT-PCR	Down-regulation in a subset of breast tumors.	20
KLK14	mRNA from breast cancer	RT-PCR	Down-regulation in a subset of breast tumors.	21
KLK15	mRNA from prostatic tissues	RT-PCR	Overexpression in more aggressive forms of prostate cancer.	22

a Reverse transcriptase-polymerase chain reaction.

dular kallikrein (hK2), and prostase (KLK4) are tandemly localized; they are highly expressed in the prostate and to a much lower extent in other tissues. This restricted tissue expression and secretion into biological fluids make them ideal markers for prostatic diseases. A more detailed discussion about hK2 and hK3 as cancer biomarkers is presented in Chapter 17. Among other kallikreins, their tissue expression is more ubiquitous, although some of them are predominantly expressed in only a few tissues (for more details about tissue-specific expression of all kallikrein genes, please refer to our previously published review) (1).

The elevation of serum concentration of these biomarkers in cancer is likely due to the increased vasculature (angiogenesis) of cancerous tissues, the destruction of the glandular architecture of the tissues involved, and the subsequent leakage of these proteins into the general circulation. It is possible that the concentration of other kallikreins may be increased in serum due to gene overexpression, as well as to increased diffusion of these molecules into the general circulation.

Current Application of Kallikrein Analysis

In Table 2, we summarize published data on measurement of kallikrein proteins in biological fluids or tissue extracts for the purpose of disease diagnosis, monitoring, prognosis, or subclassification. Studies related to prognostic and predictive value of kallikrein mRNA analysis in tissues have also been included. It is clear from these data that at least a few kallikreins have already found important clinical applications while some other members show promising potential. The availability of sensitive analytical methods for the remaining kallikreins will allow for their examination as candidate cancer biomarkers.

It is possible that some kallikreins may become valuable therapeutic targets when the involved biological pathways are delineated. For example, the enzymatic activity of these serine proteases may initiate biological events (e.g., tumor invasion, activation of hormones, growth factors, other enzymes, receptors or cytokines, amyloid formation) or terminate them (e.g., inhibition of angiogenesis; inactivation of growth factors, hormones, enzymes, cytokines, or receptors). Once known, these events could be manipulated by enzyme inhibitors or activators for therapeutic purposes. Literature on these issues does not currently exist since the function of most kallikrein enzymes is not known at present.

FUTURE DIRECTIONS

Currently, very few cancer biomarkers have had a major impact in clinical practice; a notable exception is prostate-specific antigen (hK3). One of the reasons for this low impact is that most of the current cancer biomarkers are not tissue- or cancer-specific; they are elevated in benign as well as in malignant diseases of many organs and they lack sensitivity and specificity for early disease diagnosis. For monitoring, the time window from biochemical to clinical relapse is usually short (less than one year) and therapeutic approaches for treating relapsing disease are not generally very successful. It is clear that we need more specific and sensitive cancer biomarkers for early detection and more efficient monitoring of cancer.

It is anticipated, with the completion of the human genome project, that many new analytes will be examined as disease biomarkers. In our opinion, not a single biomarker will be effective for any disease (with some notable exceptions). It is conceivable that a combination of a carefully selected panel of biomarkers will offer the required sensitivity and specificity. The advent of new, miniaturized, multi-parametric testing (e.g., microarray technology) will likely facilitate introduction of multiple tests for each disease, and bioinformatic approaches (e.g., neural networks, pattern recognition, and logistic regression) will bring about the required sensitivity and specificity.

The human kallikrein gene family has already contributed the best-known cancer biomarker (PSA/hK3). Another new biomarker, human glandular kallikrein 2 (hK2), has been tested and it shows promise of being a complementary test. The new information presented here highlights the fact that a few other members of this gene family may have applicability as diagnostic, prognostic, and predictive indicators in various cancers. The availability of reliable analytical methodologies for all members of the kallikrein gene family will facilitate further research. It is conceivable that the kallikrein chip (multi-parametric testing of all kallikreins simultaneously) as well as their combination with other biomarkers may bring about a powerful diagnostic and prognostic multi-parametric procedure.

The challenge over the next 5–10 years is to identify the biological function of these enzymes, their physiological substrates, and the connection of overexpression, underexpression, and mutation of these genes with the pathogenesis of various human diseases, including cancer.

REFERENCES

1. Yousef GM, Diamandis EP. The new human tissue kallikrein gene family: structure, function, and association to disease. Endocr Rev 2001;22:184–204.
2. Yousef GM, Chang A, Scorilas A, Diamandis EP. Genomic organization of the human kallikrein gene family on chromosome 19q13.3-q13.4. Biochem Biophys Res Commun 2000;276:125–133.
3. Harvey TJ, Hooper JD, Myers SA, Stephenson SA, Ashworth LK, Clements JA. Tissue-specific expression patterns and fine mapping of the human kallikrein (KLK) locus on proximal 19q13.4. J Biol Chem 2000;275:37397–37406.
4. Diamandis EP, Yousef GM, Clements J, Ashworth LK, Yoshida S, Egelrud T, Nelson PS, Shiosaka S, Little S, Lilja H, Stenman UH, Rittenhouse HG, Wain H. New nomenclature for the human tissue kallikrein gene family. Clin Chem 2000;46:1855–1858.
5. Obiezu CV, Scorilas A, Katsaros D, Massobrio M, Yousef GM, Fracchioli S, Rigault De La Longrais IA, Arisio R, Diamandis EP. Higher human kallikrein gene 4 (klk4) expression indicates poor prognosis of ovarian cancer patients. Clin Cancer Res 2001;7:2380–2386.
6. Kim H, Scorilas A, Katsaros D, Yousef GM, Massobrio M, Fracchioli S, Piccinno R, Gordini G, Diamandis EP. Human kallikrein gene 5 (KLK5) expression is an indicator of poor prognosis in ovarian cancer. Br J Cancer 2001;84:643–650.
7. Anisowicz A, Sotiropoulou G, Stenman G, Mok SC, Sager R. A novel protease homolog differentially expressed in breast and ovarian cancer. Mol Med 1996;2:624–636.
8. Diamandis EP, Yousef GM, Soosaipillai AR, Bunting P. Human kallikrein 6 (zyme/protease M/neurosin): a new serum biomarker of ovarian carcinoma. Clin Biochem 2000;33:579–583.
9. Luo LY, Diamandis EP, Look MP, Soosaipillai A, Foekens, JA. Higher expression of human kallikrein 10 in breast tissue predicts tamoxifen resistance. Br J Cancer 2002;(in press).
10. Tanimoto H, Underwood LJ, Shigemasa K, Yan Yan MS, Clarke J, Parmley TH, O'Brien TJ. The stratum corneum chymotryptic enzyme that mediates shedding and desquamation of skin cells is highly overexpressed in ovarian tumor cells. Cancer 1999;86:2074–2082.
11. Magklara A, Scorilas A, Katsaros D, Massobrio M, Yousef GM, Fracchioli S, Danese S, Diamandis EP. The human KLK8 (neuropsin/ovasin) gene: identification of two novel splice variants and its prognostic value in ovarian cancer. Clin Cancer Res 2001;7:806–811.
12. Yousef GM, Kyriakopoulou LG, Scorilas A, Fracchioli S, Ghiringhello B, Zarghooni M, Chang A, Diamandis M, Giardina G, Hartwick WJ, Richiardi G, Massobrio M, Diamandis EP, Katsaros D. Quantitative expression of the human kallikrein gene 9 (KLK9) in ovarian cancer: a new independent and favorable prognostic marker. Cancer Res 2001;61:7811–7818.
13. Liu XL, Wazer DE, Watanabe K, Band V. Identification of a novel serine protease-like gene, the expression of which is down-regulated during breast cancer progression. Cancer Res 1996;56:3371–3379.
14. Goyal J, Smith KM, Cowan JM, Wazer DE, Lee SW, Band V. The role for NES1 serine protease as a novel tumor suppressor. Cancer Res 1998;58:4782–4686.
15. Luo L, Bunting P, Scorilas A, Diamandis EP. Human kallikrein 10: a novel tumor marker for ovarian carcinoma? Clin Chim Acta 2001;306:111–118.
16. Luo LY, Katsaros D, Scorilas A, Fracchioli S, Piccinno R, Rigauls de la Longrais IA, Howarth DJ, Diamandis EP. Prognostic value of human kallikrein 10 expression in epithelial ovarian carcinoma. Clin Cancer Res 2001;7:2372–2379.
17. Luo LY, Rajpert-De Meyts ER, Jung K, Diamandis EP. Expression of the normal epithelial cell-specific 1 (NES1; KLK10) candidate tumor suppressor gene in normal and malignant testicular tissue. Br J Cancer 2001;85:220–224.
18. Diamandis EP, Okui A, Mistui S, Luo LY, Soosaipillai A, Grass L, Nakamura T, Howarth DJ, Yamaguchi N. Human kallikrein 11: a new biomarker of prostate and ovarian carcinoma. Cancer Res 2002;62:295–300.
19. Yousef GM, Magklara A, Diamandis EP. KLK12 is a novel serine protease and a new member of the human kallikrein gene family—differential expression in breast cancer. Genomics 2000;69:331–341.
20. Yousef GM, Chang A, Diamandis EP. Identification and characterization of KLK-L4, a new kallikrein-like gene that appears to be down-regulated in breast cancer tissues. J Biol Chem 2000;275:11891–11898.
21. Yousef GM, Magklara A, Chang A, Jung K, Katsaros D, Diamandis EP. Cloning of a new member of the human kallikrein gene family, KLK14, which is down-regulated in different malignancies. Cancer Res 2001;61:3425–3431.
22. Yousef GM, Scorilas A, Jung K, Ashworth LK, Diamandis EP. Molecular cloning of the human kallikrein 15 gene (KLK15). Up-regulation in prostate cancer. J Biol Chem 2001;276:53–61.

Chapter 47

Tumor M2-PK: A Marker of the Tumor Metabolome

Sybille Mazurek, Diana Lüftner, Hans Werner Wechsel, Joachim Schneider, and Erich Eigenbrodt

Analogous to *genome* and *proteome*, the expression *metabolome* was coined to summarize the metabolic network of the cells. The tumor metabolome is generally characterized by a high glycolytic capacity, high phosphometabolite levels, a high channeling of glucose carbons to synthetic processes (such as nucleic acid, phospholipid, and amino acid synthesis), a low (ATP+GTP) : (CTP+UTP) ratio, and a high glutaminolytic capacity (Figure 1) (1,2).

GENERAL ROLE OF TUMOR M2-PK IN THE TUMOR METABOLOME

The key regulator of the metabolic alterations found in tumor cells is the glycolytic isoenzyme pyruvate kinase type M2 that is generally expressed in all proliferating cells and overexpressed in all tumor cells investigated to date (1,2) (*http://www.pubmed.gov*; see nucleotides and tumor pyruvate kinase type M2).

During carcinogenesis a shift in the pyruvate kinase isoenzyme equipment always takes place, such that the tissue-specific isoenzymes disappear (such as M1-PK in muscle and brain, L-PK in liver and kidney, and R-PK in red blood cells), and M2-PK is expressed (1,2).

M2-PK can exist in a highly active tetrameric form with a high affinity to its substrate, phosphoenolpyruvate (PEP), and in a dimeric form with a low PEP affinity. The dimeric form of M2-PK is virtually inactive at cellular PEP concentration. When M2-PK is dimeric, glucose carbons are channeled to synthetic processes, such as nucleic acid, phospholipid, and amino acid synthesis (Figure 1). Furthermore, there is increased conversion of the amino acid glutamine to lactate, which has been termed *glutaminolysis* in analogy to *glycolysis*, to ensure the energy production of the tumor cells. This is due to the lack of pyruvate caused by the inhibition of pyruvate kinase in tumor cells. High levels of the glycolytic phosphometabolite fructose-1,6-P_2 (FBP) and of the amino acid serine induce reassociation from the dimeric to the tetrameric form (Figure 1). Pyruvate kinase catalyzes the transfer of phosphate

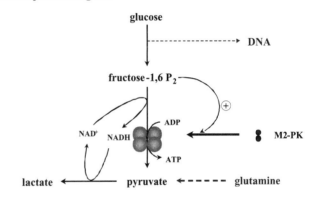

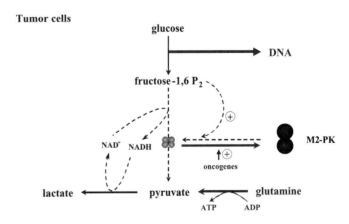

Figure 1 Metabolic scheme for the regulatory role of pyruvate kinase type M2. **Color representation of figure appears on Color Plate 9.**

from PEP to adenosine diphosphate (ADP) or guanosine diphosphate (GDP) under the production of pyruvate and adenosine triphosphate (ATP) or guanosine triphosphate

(GTP), respectively. Thus, within the glycolytic sequence, pyruvate kinase is responsible for net energy production. Consequently, pyruvate kinase controls the ATP:ADP and GTP:GDP ratio and also the adenosine monophosphate (AMP) levels (together with adenylate kinase and 6-phosphofructo-1-kinase) (2). An increase in AMP levels inhibits DNA synthesis and cell proliferation by decreasing nicotinamide adenine dinucleotide (NAD), uridine triphosphate (UTP), and cytidine triphosphate (CTP) synthesis. By this mechanism M2-PK adapts energy-consuming cell proliferation and nutrient supply (1, 2).

In tumor cells a high amount of the less active, dimeric form of M2-PK is always found. Therefore, the dimeric form of M2-PK has been termed Tumor M2-PK (Tu M2-PK) (1).

The ability of Tumor M2-PK to reassociate to the highly active tetrameric form at high FBP and serine concentrations shifts the tumor metabolome from anabolic processes, in which the glucose carbons are channeled to synthetic processes, to energy-producing (catabolic) processes (2). In contrast to mitochondrial respiration, energy production by pyruvate kinase is independent of oxygen supply. Therefore the oscillation of M2-PK between the highly active tetrameric and the less active dimeric form allows tumor cells to proliferate despite the poor vascularization and strong variations in glucose and oxygen supply that are generally found in solid tumors (1). Presumably due to its central role in regulating catabolism and anabolism, M2-PK is directly targeted by certain oncoproteins, such as pp60[v-src] kinase and the E7 oncoprotein of the human papilloma virus type 16 (HPV-16). The pp60[v-src] kinase phosphorylates M2-PK in tyrosine; the HPV-16 E7 oncoprotein directly binds to M2-PK. Both interactions lead to a dimerization of M2-PK and higher FBP and serine levels are necessary to reassociate M2-PK to the tetrameric form (1,2).

QUANTIFICATION OF TUMOR M2-PK

In order to study the central role of pyruvate kinase in cell metabolism, monoclonal antibodies against the different isoenzymes of pyruvate kinase, as well as to the tetrameric and dimeric forms of M2-PK, have been produced. Immunohistological studies of various tumors have revealed a heterogeneous distribution of Tumor M2-PK in the primary tumors, whereas their metastases are characterized by a homogeneously large amount of M2-PK.

An enzyme-linked immunosorbent assay (ELISA) for the determination of Tumor M2-PK in ethylenediaminetetraacetic acid (EDTA)-plasma is available from ScheBo Biotech AG, Giessen, Germany.

In accordance with results from immunohistological staining, the amount of Tumor M2-PK in EDTA-plasma samples from patients with renal cell carcinoma, pancreatic, lung, breast, and colon cancer directly reflected the metastatic state of the tumors (3–9). Therefore, Tumor M2-PK is a strong marker of metastasis, but not an organ-specific marker.

The recommended cut-off value for Tumor M2-PK of 15 U/mL corresponds to a specificity of 90% in a control group with nonmalignant diseases. Investigations in patients with a variety of diseases other than tumors revealed an increase of Tumor M2-PK only in severe inflammation and polytrauma (3,10). This Tumor M2-PK mainly derives from activated granulocytes, which elevate PK levels more than 20-fold after polytrauma (10).

Tumor M2-PK plasma concentration reflects tumor size and growth in various tumor cells and is well correlated with tumor staging (3–9). Increasing Tumor M2-PK plasma concentrations were observed with progressive tumor stages in lung cancer patients (Figure 2). Lung cancer patients in disease stages III or IV had significantly higher Tumor M2-PK concentrations than those in stage I.

Figure 2 shows the high correlation between Tumor M2-PK levels and the staging of different tumors. In lung tumors the sensitivity of Tumor M2-PK is calculated to be 28% in stage I, increasing progressively to 73% in stage IV. A similar correlation between Tumor M2-PK and the Robson score is found for kidney tumors, increasing from 25% in stage I to 71% in stage IV, as well as for gastrointestinal tumors (5–7,9).

However, the sensitivity for nonmetastatic tumors can be strongly improved by the combination of Tumor M2-PK with appropriate "traditional" organ-specific markers. These include carcinoembryonic antigen (CEA) in colorectal cancers; CA19-9 in pancreatic cancer; and CA-72-4 in esophageal and gastric cancers; alpha-fetoprotein (AFP) and human chorionic gonadotropin (HCG) in testicular cancer; and CYFRA 21-1 or neuron-specific enolase (NSE) in lung cancer (2,5,7,9). In patients suffering from silicosis, the use of X-rays for the detection of lung cancer is of limited diagnostic value. Efficiency in pre-invasive diagnosis of suspicious lesions will be improved by using tumor markers in the differential diagnosis between malignant and benign diseases.

Overall, the greatest advantage of Tumor M2-PK as an organ-unspecific marker is that it detects metastatic occurrence and aggressively growing tumors with a sensitivity of 60–70 % by a simple blood measurement.

STUDIES MONITORING THE EFFICACY OF TUMOR THERAPY USING TUMOR M2-PK

Several chemotherapeutic drugs, such as cisplatin, cyclophosphamide, and vinblastine, or modalities such as radiation that target DNA, depress NAD levels and glycolysis (1). These effects take place since poly-(ADP-ribose) polymerase (PARP), the enzyme that is responsible for DNA repair, consumes NAD. The decreased NAD level inhibits glyceraldehyde 3-phosphate dehydrogenase and lactate dehydrogenase, and increases FBP. In normal proliferating cells, these FBP levels are high enough to reassociate the dimeric form of M2-PK to the tetrameric form, which is the opposite of the situation in tumor cells. Therefore, in normal cells, sufficient nucleotide triphosphates

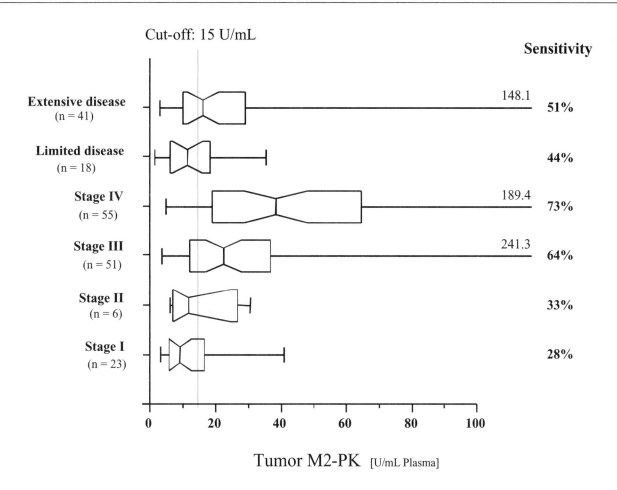

Figure 2 Correlation between Tumor M2-PK plasma concentrations and staging in lung cancer. The whiskers indicate the 25th and 75th percentiles. The center of the notches indicates the median. Lack of overlap indicates significant differences between the groups. Limited disease is compared with extensive disease for small-cell lung cancers. Stages I–IV are presented for all non-small-cell carcinomas. The sensitivity was calculated using the manufacturer's cut-off. **Color representation of figure appears on Color Plate 10.**

(NTPs) are available for DNA repair and the cells survive (Figure 1).

In tumor cells, the increase of FBP levels is not high enough for the tetramerization of M2-PK. Consequently tumor cells are unable to maintain sufficiently high NTP levels for DNA repair and the cells undergo apoptosis (1). The amount of Tumor M2-PK has been demonstrated to increase accordingly in necrotic areas in renal cell carcinomas.

Thus, the measurement of Tumor M2-PK in EDTA plasma samples from tumor patients allows direct monitoring of the energy status of the tumor cells during tumor therapy. Indeed, studies with breast cancer, metastatic renal cancer, and lung cancer patients revealed that the levels of Tumor M2-PK directly reflected the success or failure of the tumor therapy protocol (Figures 3A,B) (3,8,9).

Therefore, the measurement of Tumor M2-PK levels in EDTA plasma samples during tumor therapy promises to be an efficient tool to enable clinicians to apply an individualized, enzyme-guided tumor therapy for each patient (e.g., choice of therapy, dose, and duration).

FUTURE ASPECTS

Tumor M2-PK levels will be compared with glucose uptake by positron emission tomography (PET) in future studies in order to characterize the metabolic status of the tumor and to further individualize tumor therapy based on the individual tumor metabolome (1).

Furthermore, using long-term measurements of Tumor M2-PK levels in EDTA-plasma samples from healthy controls and from high-risk groups (such as smokers or workers with prior exposure to carcinogenic agents), Tumor M2-PK will be tested as a "generalized" marker for the early detection of malignant tumors, both alone and in combination with other markers.

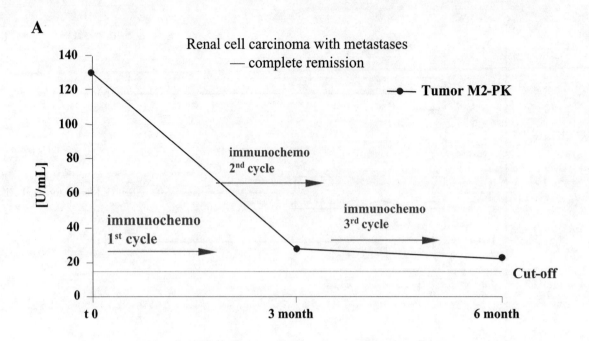

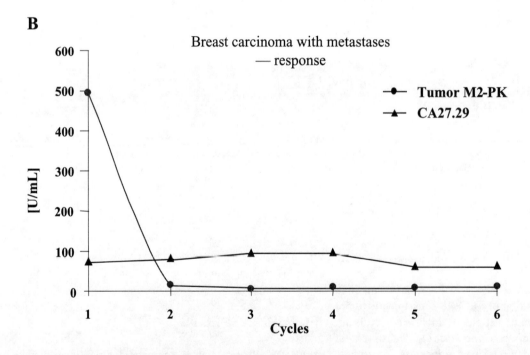

Figure 3 (A) Metastasized renal cell carcinoma: follow up with Tumor M2-PK. Tumor M2-PK levels in a patient with metastatic renal cell cancer (Robson IV) under immunochemotherapy, with complete remission after eight months. Radiological monitoring correlated well with Tumor M2-PK levels. (B) Longitudinal levels of Tumor M2-PK and CA27.29 levels in relation to response. Patient with partial response: elevated baseline level with prompt normalization after the start of chemotherapy. **Color representation of figure appears on Color Plate 11.**

REFERENCES

1. Mazurek S, Boschek CB, Eigenbrodt E. The role of phosphometabolites in cell proliferation, energy metabolism, and tumor therapy. J Bioenerg Biomembr 1997;29:315–330.
2. Mazurek S, Zwerschke W, Jansen-Dürr P, Eigenbrodt E. Metabolic cooperation between different oncogenes during cell transformation: interaction between activated ras and HPV-16 E7. Oncogene 2001;20:6891–6898.
3. Schneider J, Morr H, Velcovsky HG, Weisse G, Eigenbrodt E. Quantitative detection of Tumor M2-pyruvate kinase in plasma of patients with lung cancer in comparison to other lung diseases. Cancer Detec Prev 2000;24:531–535.
4. Hardt PD, Ngoumou BK, Rupp J, Schnell-Kretschmer H, Kloer HU. Tumor M2-pyruvate kinase: a promising tumor marker in the diagnosis of gastro-intestinal cancer. Anticancer Res 2000;20:4965–4968.
5. Schulze G. The tumor marker Tumor M2-PK: an application in the diagnosis of gastrointestinal cancer. Anticancer Res 2000;20:4961–4964.
6. Oremek GM, Sapoutzis N, Kramer W, Bivkeboller R, Jonas D. Value of Tumor M2-PK (Tu M2-PK) in patients with renal carcinoma. Anticancer Res 2000;20:5095–5098.
7. Roigas J, Schulze G, Raytarowski S, Jung K, Schnorr D, Loening SA. Tumor M2 pyruvate kinase in plasma of patients with urologic tumors. Tumor Biol 2001;22:282–285.
8. Lüftner D, Mesterharm J, Akrivakis C, Geppert R, Petrides PE, Wernecke KD, Possinger K. Tumor type M2 pyruvate kinase expression in advanced breast cancer. Anticancer Res 2000;20:5077–5082.
9. Wechsel HW, Petri E, Bichler K-H, Feil G. Marker for renal cell carcinoma (RCC): the dimeric form of pyruvate kinase type M2 (Tu M2-PK). Anticancer Res 1999;19:2583–2590.
10. Oehler R, Weingartmann G, Manhart N, Salzer U, Meissner M, Schlegel W, et al. Polytrauma induces increased expression of pyruvate kinase in neutrophils. Blood 2000;95:1086–1092.

Chapter **48**

Measurement of Hue and Chroma in Assessment of Biomarkers of Colon and Lung Cancer

Peter Horsewood, Michael Evelegh, Norman Marcon, Gerard Cox, and John Miller

The Thomsen-Friedenreich antigen (TF Ag) is defined by the disaccharide sequence, D-galactose-β [1-3]-N-acetyl-D-galactosamine. This sequence occurs on normal mucins in a sialic acid-capped cryptic form but not in the free form. However, during the cancer transformation process, glycosylation patterns are perturbed, and the uncapped TF Ag may become exposed (1).

The antigen has been detected in mucus secretions, on cancer cells, and in the circulation of patients with various carcinomas, and as such, represents a potential pan-specific, tumor-associated antigen (2). While the majority of the investigations detecting the presence of the antigen have been from studies of patients with colon cancer, TF Ag-positive material has been found also in cancers of the lung, breast, ovary, pancreas, prostate, stomach, and uterus. In humans and in animal models, it has been shown that abnormally glycosylated mucins expressing the TF Ag are secreted not only by the colon carcinoma but also from normally appearing mucosa remote from the tumor. Shamsuddin has explained these changes in apparently normal mucosa as occurring through a "field effect" phenomenon (3). Further, since mucus can be readily obtained during a digital rectal examination, this provides a simple and convenient source of samples for investigating the presence of the TF Ag in colon carcinoma. Similarly, spontaneously produced sputum samples provide material for investigating TF Ag in cases of lung cancer. Secretions from other tissues, including cervix, breast, and prostate, should allow screening for cancers at these sites.

Several monoclonal antibodies and various plant lectins, particularly peanut agglutinin, have been used for the histochemical detection of the TF Ag (4). Some of the monoclonal antibodies lack specificity in that they have cross-reactivity to each of the anomeric linkage configurations of the TF Ag. In addition, the lectins have limited utility because they have specificity for other sugar moieties. Galactose oxidase is a copper-containing enzyme that oxidizes the C-6 hydroxyl groups of D-galactose and N-acetyl-D-galactosamine residues to generate aldehyde groups. The enzyme readily oxidizes theses two sugars when present as the TF Ag but not when they are capped with sialic acid residues as they occur in normal mucus. Additionally, the aldehydes that are generated react readily with the colorless Schiff's reagent to produce insoluble, purple/magenta-colored addition products and when used sequentially, these reactions afford a simple and useful method for the detection of the TF Ag. This method was first used by Schulte and Spicer on tracheal gland secretions and later was used on sections taken from colon carcinoma tissue (5,6).

Shamsuddin and Elsayed have developed the method further and tested rectal mucus for the presence of the TF Ag using the galactose oxidase/Schiff's (GOS) reagents. Results from their work indicate that this may be a useful screening method for detecting colon carcinoma (7). The encouraging results from the initial work have been confirmed and extended by others, including one large study of 6,480 asymptomatic subjects in China. A summary of results from these other groups of investigators has been reported (8). However, in all of these GOS assays there is some variability in samples and in staining methods. More importantly, the tests are evaluated visually and the results are therefore subjective.

We have extended the GOS technique further by introducing objective interpretation of the staining and have developed a convenient device for sample handling and processing. We use a small hand-held reflectance spectrophotometer and software to measure the color characteristics of GOS-stained material. These improvements have been incorporated into the ColorectAlert™ (CRA) and LungAlert™ (LA) tests for screening rectal mucus and sputum samples, respectively. The device consists of a plastic slide, bonded onto one end of which is an absorbent glass-fiber membrane and to which either a rectal mucus or sputum sample is applied. The applied samples are allowed to dry and the device and sample are shipped to a laboratory for processing. Following GOS staining, a convenient and permanent visual record of the results is obtained by scanning the samples and color printing the scanned data. Characteristics of the samples are read using a reflectance spectrophotometer linked to a laptop computer equipped with software that records color attributes, including hue and chroma (saturation), along with a spectral curve over the visible range.

These color characteristics allow a controlled and objective interpretation of the staining, and the numerical nature of the output allows statistical comparison of the results. To ensure rectal mucus and sputum sampling has provided sufficient amounts of material, all slides are additionally treated with periodic acid and Schiff's stain after the GOS treatment. This action oxidizes and stains carbohydrate residues of normal and pathologic mucus samples and thereby provides a positive control for mucus application/detection. Hue values were used in the colorectal cancer study since they are relatively independent of the intensity of color staining and this minimizes the variability arising from the amount of mucus obtained by digital rectal sampling. This was confirmed by applying defined amounts of mucin to slides, staining with GOS and showing that hue was essentially constant over a wide range of applied mucin concentrations (25–0.2 mg/mL). Chroma measurements for these mucin samples were directly proportional to the amount of applied mucin.

Clinical trials have been carried out using ColorectAlert on rectal mucus samples collected from patients at St. Michael's Hospital, Toronto, Ontario, and with LungAlert on sputum samples collected from patients at St. Joseph's Hospital, Hamilton, Ontario. The results of these trials indicate the utility of the GOS method when using the simple instrumentation to record and numerically compare results.

CLINICAL APPLICATIONS

Colorectal cancer. Using a clinical diagnosis based on colonoscopy as a gold standard, results were compared for fecal occult blood tests (FOBT) and CRA tests obtained on a study population of 669 patients scheduled for colonoscopy. Approximately one-third of the patients were scheduled for colonoscopy for screening purposes, one-third because of symptoms, and one-third for follow-up of previous procedures. Colonoscopy was completed successfully to the level of the cecum in 97% of the patients but, due to complications, was incomplete in 3%. The population had the following characteristics: mean age, 59 ± 13 years; 53% male; 93% Caucasian; 6% with previous colorectal cancer; 38% with a family history of colorectal cancer. Results of the colonoscopy showed that 3% of the population had colorectal cancer, 36% had polyps, 40% had no pathology, and 21% had other, benign bowel disease (predominantly hemorrhoids). Of those with cancer, 13% were Duke's stage A, 43% Duke's stage B, 25% Duke's stage C, and 19% Duke's stage D.

For individuals without bowel pathology, there was no difference in the CRA value (hue) between males and females and no age-related differences. However, in patients with adenomas or cancer there was a correlation of bowel pathology with CRA value. There was an increase in the number (%) of patients with adenomas and cancers with each quintile of increasing CRA value. Notably, there was no correlation between the CRA quintile and the number of patients having hyperplastic polyps, indicating that the positive relationship was cancer-specific.

These correlations were further illustrated when the pathologic diagnosis was compared to the CRA values (Figure 1).

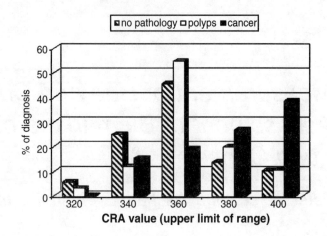

Figure 1 Diagnosis distributed by CRA value. The distribution of the percentage of patients with a particular diagnosis is shown according to the CRA plotted as the upper limit value of the range.

Compared to patients with no bowel pathology and those with polyps, the cancer population showed a steady increase in the number of patients with increasing CRA value (Figure 1). To allow for the best discrimination of cancer patients from normal individuals and those with benign disease, and to determine optimal sensitivity and specificity, a suitable cut-off for the CRA value was required. Samples giving a CRA value below 350 were classed as negative and those giving values greater than 370 were classed as positive. Effective differentiation of those samples that had an intermediate CRA value (350–370) was achieved using an algorithm that accounted for the amount of sample applied to the slide. Those samples that gave an intermediate CRA value were divided into groups that had high or low amounts of applied mucus, based on their staining with periodic acid/Schiff's reagent. Samples that measured in the intermediate CRA range, despite low amounts of mucin, were deemed positive. When all samples were analyzed, 17 of the 26 cancers had a CRA value above 370, 4 cancers had CRA values below 350, and 5 had intermediate values. Of the 5 with intermediate values, 4 were deemed positive after periodic acid/Schiff's analysis.

Thus, the test detected 21 of 26 cancer patients, for a sensitivity of 81%. It is noteworthy that cancers were detected in all regions of the colorectum with equal sensitivity. The overall specificity of the test was 75.1%, but the true specificity of the CRA test may be higher since there is evidence that some of the false-positive group may have had occult disease. Compared to the CRA-negative group, individuals in the false-positive group were more likely to have had a previous cancer at a different site (8.35% vs. 2.5%, p <0.045) and more had a positive FOBT test (59% vs. 38%, p <0.017). The test was more sensitive for the patients receiving colonoscopy for screening purposes and for symptoms than in the population in which colonoscopy was for follow-up of previous cancers (100%, 93.3%, and 50% respectively). This may indicate that the expression of the GOS marker decreases in later stages of the disease. Similar decreases in TF Ag reactivity with disease progression have been observed previously (9). A similar sensitivity was found for the FOBT, but the ColorectAlert test was significantly more specific than FOBT (75.1% vs. 56.5%, χ^2 p <0.001). This improved specificity of the ColorectAlert test could reduce the number of required colonoscopies without compromising sensitivity.

Using two-tier testing, with FOBT as the screening test and CRA as a confirmatory test, the sensitivity was 68.9% and the specificity 87.1%. In this same study, CEA testing was also done; using CEA as a screening test with CRA as a confirmatory test, the sensitivity was 69.2% and the specificity 90.1%. The odds ratio associated with a positive CRA test was 10.7; for FOBT, 5.8; and for CEA, 4.4. For two-tier testing, the best odds ratio (18.4) was achieved using CEA plus CRA tests.

Lung cancer. Seventy-five sputum samples were analyzed in a clinical study using the LungAlert test. The samples were from individuals with cancer (n = 22, mean age 63.9, 54.2% male, 8.3% nonsmokers); benign lung disease (n = 29, mean age 52.1, 50% male, 46.4% nonsmokers); and normal volunteers (n = 24, mean age 35.7, 58.3% male, 62.5% nonsmokers). Sputum was produced spontaneously by all of the cancer patients and 19 of the patients with benign disease but by only two of the normal volunteers. For individuals unable to produce sputum spontaneously it was induced by hypertonic saline inhalation. In this study, the amounts of sputum sample applied to the slides were much more consistent than the amounts of rectal mucus sample applied in the ColorectAlert study, and chroma values rather than hue values were analyzed and compared. An optimized value of chroma that gave the best discrimination was estimated from the receiver-operator characteristics (ROC) curve. Results showed that the assay had an overall sensitivity of 73.3% (17 of the 22 cancers were detected), and while it was most sensitive for those with more advanced disease, it still had a high sensitivity (67%) for stage I and II disease (Figure 2). The overall specificity was 66% but the specificity was higher (76%) for those who produced sputum spontaneously. For those patients with benign lung disease the specificity was 72.4%, with little difference between those who produced sputum spontaneously and those in whom sputum was induced (73.7% and 70% specificity respectively). Specificity in the healthy volunteers was 58.3%.

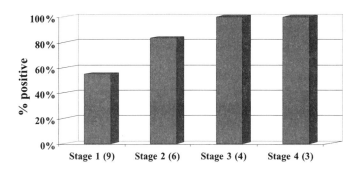

Figure 2 Sensitivity by lung cancer stage. The sensitivity for Lung Alert testing is shown for patients with various stages of lung cancer. The number of patients with a positive test at each stage is shown in brackets.

FUTURE DIRECTIONS

Results from the ColorectAlert testing indicate that it has better specificity than the existing FOBT assays in a high-risk population and these tests will be evaluated in further clinical trials with a low-risk group. These trials will also investigate the effect of bowel preparation before sampling of rectal mucus and the testing of duplicate samples. A larger clinical trial is in progress to confirm and expand the findings of the initial LungAlert study. This trial will also examine a high-risk population (smokers) and additional cancer patients. Sputum samples obtained at intervals after surgery also will be evaluated for GOS reactivity to assess responses to therapy and to assess diagnosis of recurrent cancer.

Clinical studies are also underway for evaluating GOS reactivity in nipple aspirates as a screening method for breast cancer. Future studies are planned for prostate cancer screening using seminal fluid and for cervical cancer using cervical mucus.

REFERENCES

1. Springer GT, Desai PR. Cross-reacting carcinoma-associated antigens with blood group and precursor specificities. Transplant Proc 1977;9:1105–1111.
2. Springer GF. T and Tn, general carcinoma autoantigens. Science 1984;224:1198–1206.
3. Shamsuddin AM, Tyner GT, Guang YY. Common expression of the tumor marker D-galactose-β-[1-3]- N-acetyl-D-galactosamine by different adenocarcinomas: evidence of field effect phenomena. Cancer Res 1995;55:149–152.
4. Hanisch FG, Baldus SE. The Thomsen-Friedenreich (TF) antigen: a critical review on the structural, biosynthetic, and histochemical aspects of a pancarcinoma-associated antigen. Histol Histopathol 1997;12:263–281.
5. Schulte BA, Spicer SS. Light microscopic histochemical detection of sugar residues in secretory glycoproteins of rodent and human tracheal glands with lectin-horseradish peroxidase conjugates and the galactose oxidase-Schiff sequence. J Histochem Cytochem 1987;31:391–403.
6. Elsayed AM, Shamsuddin AM. Detection of altered glycoconjugate in preneoplastic and neoplastic human large intestinal epithelium by galactose oxidase-Schiff sequence. Lab Invest 1987;56:22A.
7. Shamsuddin AM, Elsayed AM. Gal-GalNac: a test for detection of colorectal cancer. Hum Pathol 1988;19:7–10.
8. Shamsuddin AM, Sakamoto K. Carbohydrate tumor marker: basis for a simple test for colorectal cancer. Adv Exp Med Biol 1994;354:83–99.
9. Carter JH, Deddens JA, Pullman JL, Colligan BM, Whiteley LO, Carter HW. Validation of the galactose oxidase-Schiff's reagent sequence for early detection and prognosis in human colorectal adenocarcinoma. Clin Cancer Res 1997;3:1479–1489.

Chapter 49

Heterogeneous Nuclear Ribonucleoprotein A2/B1 as an Early Marker of Preinvasive Lung Cancer

Jordi Tauler, Alfredo Martínez, and James L. Mulshine

Lung cancer is the leading cause of cancer death in the Western world. In the year 2002 in the United States alone, there will be an estimated 169,400 cases of lung cancer and 154,900 deaths (1). Throughout most of the world, even with the best therapeutic approaches, five-year survival is still less than 10%.

The tumors found with the typical detection technique, chest X-ray, have usually spread to other parts of the body. However, those patients diagnosed at an early stage of the disease (stage I) have a five-year survival rate that is much higher than more advanced patients, suggesting that early detection strategies will greatly improve the outcome of this malignancy. About 1 billion cells (10^9) represent 30 cell doublings from the initiation of a cancer from a single cell, thus the carcinogenic process takes about 10–20 years to progress from initiation to detection. This long preclinical history of the tumor provides a great opportunity for detecting lung tumors in early stages.

Obviously, the first step in preventing lung cancer is reducing tobacco consumption, as more than 80% of lung cancer cases result from cigarette smoking. Nevertheless, former smokers maintain an elevated risk of developing lung cancer for almost 15 years, due to persistent bronchial epithelial cell injury.

To obtain a specific marker for those early stage lung cancers, monoclonal antibodies were generated against a whole cell lysate of a non-small-cell lung cancer (NSCLC) cell line. These antibodies were used to screen a sputum specimen archive collected at the Johns Hopkins University. This archive contains preserved sputum samples collected on a yearly basis from a high-risk cohort that was fully followed up to determine eventual diagnosis of lung cancer. The screening, using an immunocytochemical analysis, was focused on the bronchial epithelial cells recovered in sputum. One of the antibodies, 703D4, was able to predict with a 90% accuracy those individuals who would progress to invasive tumors within 2 years (2). Later characterization of 703D4 antigen allowed the purification of a single protein, which was identified as heterogeneous nuclear ribonucleoprotein A2/B1 (hnRNP A2/B1) (3).

The heterogeneous nuclear ribonucleoproteins are a group of RNA-binding proteins involved in different steps of RNA processing such as biogenesis, transport, localization, and metabolism of mRNAs. For instance, an A2-Response Element (A2RE) has been found in the mRNA of myelin basic protein (4). These elements bind to the RNA Recognition Motifs (RRM) of hnRNP A2/B1, which are located at the N-terminal region of the ribonucleoprotein. This class of ribonucleoproteins has also been reported to bind to the telomeres: hnRNP A1 and D are functional single-stranded (ss)DNA-binding proteins that both accelerate telomere elongation and protect the telomere from nuclease digestion. This function has been reported for hnRNP A2/B1 as well (5).

On the other hand, given the important function of hnRNP proteins in the transport of mRNAs from the nucleus to the cytoplasm, the regulation of subcellular localization of hnRNPs must be very precise. It has been shown that hnRNP post-translational modifications such as methylation or phosphorylation could affect their localization. These modifications have been reported for hnRNP A2/B1 in an arginine-glycine-glycine (RGG)-rich domain, near the C-terminus. These RGG motifs are frequently targets for methylation. Moreover, in mammalian cell lines treated with a methyltransferase inhibitor, the expression of hnRNP A2/B1 relocates from the nucleus to the cytoplasm (6). We have reported that in particular breast cancer cell lines, treatment with retinoic acid also resulted in a translocation of hnRNP A2/B1 immunoexpression from the nuclear to the cytoplasmic region (7).

In a recent report, we studied the localization of hnRNP A2/B1 expression and immunoreactivity during the development of the mammalian respiratory system in rodent embryos. We have seen that the expression moved from central to peripheral regions during fetal lung development; however, the expression of this ribonucleoprotein is restricted in mature lung. This study suggests that overexpression of hnRNP A2/B1 during carcinogenesis may represent a recapitulation of ontogenesis, thus making this ribonucleoprotein an oncodevelopmental protein (8).

We have published a preliminary analysis suggesting that hnRNP A2/B1 overexpression may be a good marker for breast cancer. Using a panel of about 150 normal and malignant breast cancer cases, expression was detected in 56.5% of primary invasive breast cancers and only in 9.7% specimens of normal breast tissue. Expression of hnRNP A2/B1 was confirmed by Northern analysis of a panel of breast cancer cell lines (7).

Recent data report novel functions for the ribonucleoprotein family. It has been suggested that hnRNP A1, which is closely related to hnRNP A2/B1, could play a decisive part in the oncogene-regulated splice-silencing complex, which can select between multiple alternatively spliced exons. In this case, hnRNP A1 was silencing the inclusion of exon v5 to prevent the production of an isoform of the cell surface molecule CD44. This form is implicated in tumorigenesis and in tumor progression. Interestingly, this silencing effect may be relieved by co-expression of the oncogenic forms of Ras and Cdc42 through post-translational modifications of hnRNP A1, such as methylation and phosporylation (9). Further work to determine the relevance of that biology to hnRNP A2/B1's potential role in carcinogenesis are underway.

CLINICAL APPLICATION

The use of hnRNP A2/B1 overexpression as a new epithelial marker in the detection of early lung cancer was examined in several cohorts. Five different independent clinical trials have been performed with the antibody 703D4 using sputum samples, representing 8235 patients (2,10,11). These studies have reported an overall sensitivity of about 80–90% and a specificity of 70–85% on the correlation of positive bronchial epithelial cell immunostaining with the eventual development of lung cancer. These results are shown in Table 1.

However, analysis of hnRNP A2/B1 immunoreactivity in serially acquired bronchial biopsies of chronic smokers has demonstrated that 41% of the samples were positive. This high frequency of immunostaining in this context is unlikely to be associated with the eventual development of lung cancer since, historically in this type of cohort, at most 1% of cohort members would progress to lung cancer. This finding contrasts with the high correlation of eventual cancer development in individuals with immunoreactivity found in shed bronchial epithelial cells, and it led us to speculate that the overexpression of hnRNP A2/B1 in exfoliated cells is much more informative than comparable expression in intact bronchial epithelial cells harvested on bronchial biopsy. In fact, the exfoliated cells present in sputum are those that have lost contact with the basement membrane and with neighboring cells. This feature illustrates the ability of these cells to survive in these conditions, which make them good candidates for initiating metastasis. On the other hand, bronchial epithelial cells are exfoliated from carcinogen-initiated sites in the airway long before such an evolving cancer undergoes metastasis and malignant cells enter the bloodstream.

Recent studies have analyzed the correlation between hnRNP A2/B1 overexpression and molecular alterations associated with lung carcinogenesis in phenotypically different epithelial cells of paraffin-embedded pulmonary tissues. The results suggest that the hnRNP A2/B1 immunoreactive cells are clonal in origin. In addition, such areas of immunoreactivity in the airway contain a higher frequency of microsatellite alterations and allelic loss for 14 known markers of genetic instability for lung cancer when compared with cells that did not overexpress hnRNP A2/B1. In addition, a higher number of genetic alterations was associated with a cytoplasmic staining pattern (Figure 1), suggesting that subcellular localization of hnRNP A2/B1 might be critical (12).

This growing body of experimental data suggests that overexpression of hnRNP A2/B1 may be used as an early marker for detecting lung cancer.

FUTURE DIRECTIONS

Overexpression of hnRNP A2/B1 in airway cells should be considered an indication that at least some molecular events consistent with lung carcinogenesis have occurred. Nevertheless, the correlation between hnRNP A2/B1 overexpression and the progression of lung cancer is still unclear. Further experimental work in this interesting area will be required to firmly establish the contribution of hnRNP A2/B1 to the process of lung carcinogenesis and to better understand the molecular biology of hnRNP A2/B1.

Table 1 Results of independent clinical trials performed by immunocytochemical screening with the antibody 703D4 in sputum samples

Study	Population size	Sensitivity	Specificity	Reference
JHU	626	91%	88%	2
JHU	626	64%	88%	2
LCEDWG	595	77%	82%	10
YTC	6285	82%	65%	10
LLP	103	96%	82%	11

JHU, Johns Hopkins University; LCEDWG, Lung Cancer Early Detection Working Group; YTC, Yunnan Tin Corp.; LLP, Liverpool Lung Project.

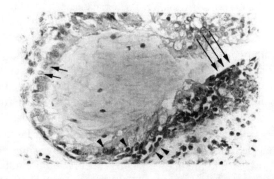

Figure 1 Cross-section profile of a small bronchiole, in which the normal-appearing bronchial epithelial cells (short arrows) are devoid of hnRNP A2/B1 expression, whereas the hyperplastic cells (long arrows) show cytoplasmic hnRNP A2/B1 immunoreactivity. Some of the cells located between the normal and hyperplastic cells display nuclear localization of hnRNP A2/B1 (arrowheads). Reproduced with permission from ref. (12).

REFERENCES

1. Jemal A, Thomas A, Murray T, Thun M. Cancer statistics, 2002. CA Cancer J Clin 2002;52(1):23–47.
2. Tockman MS, Gupta PK, Myers JD, Frost JK, Baylin SB, Gold EB, et al. Sensitive and specific monoclonal antibody recognition of human lung cancer antigen on preserved sputum cells: a new approach to early lung cancer detection. J Clin Oncol 1988;6:1685–1693.
3. Zhou J, Mulshine JL, Unsworth EJ, Scott FM, Avis IM, Vos MD, Treston AM. Purification and characterization of a protein that permits early detection of lung cancer: identification of heterogeneous nuclear ribonucleoprotein-A2/B1 as the antigen for monoclonal antibody 703D4. J Biol Chem 1996;271:10760–10766.
4. Shan J, Moran-Jones K, Munro TP, Kidd GJ, Winzor DJ, Hoek KS, Smith R. Binding of an RNA trafficking response element to heterogeneous nuclear ribonucleoproteins A1 and A2. J Biol Chem 2000;275:38286–38295.
5. Kamma H, Fujimoto M, Fujiwara M, Matsui M, Horiguchi H, Hamasaki M, Satoh H. Interaction of hnRNP A2/B1 isoforms with telomeric ssDNA and the *in vitro* function. Biochem Biophys Res Comm 2001;280:625–630.
6. Nichols RC, Wang XW, Tang J, Hamilton BJ, High FA, Herschman HR, Rigby WFC. The RGG domain in hnRNP A2 affects subcellular localization. Exp Cell Res 2000;256:522–532.
7. Zhou J, Allred DC, Avis I, Martinez A, Vos MD, Smith L, et al. Differential expression of the early lung cancer detection marker, heterogeneous nuclear ribonucleoprotein- A2/B1 (hnRNP-A2/B1) in normal and neoplastic breast cancer. Breast Cancer Res Treat 2001;66:217–224.
8. Montuenga LM, Zhou J, Avis I, Vos M, Martinez A, Cuttitta F, et al. Expression of heterogeneous nuclear ribonucleoprotein A2/B1 changes with critical stages of mammalian lung development. Am J Respir Cell Mol Biol 1998;19:554–562.
9. Matter N, Marx M, Weg-Remers S, Ponta H, Herrlich P, König H. Heterogeneous Ribonucleoprotein A1 is part of an exon-specific splice-silencing complex controlled by oncogenic signaling pathways. J Biol Chem 2000;275:35353–35360.
10. Tockman MS, Mulshine JL, Piantadosi S, Erozan YS, Gupta PK, Ruckdeschel JC, et al. Prospective detection of preclinical lung cancer: results from two studies of hnRNP expression. Clin Cancer Res 1997;3:2237–2246.
11. Fielding P, Turnbull L, Prime W, Walshaw M, Field JK. Heterogeneous nuclear ribonucleoprotein A2/B1 up-regulation in bronchial lavage specimens: a clinical marker of early lung cancer detection. Clin Canc Res 1999;5:4048–4052.
12. Man YG, Martinez A, Avis IM, Hong SH, Cuttitta F, Venzon DJ, Mulshine JL. Phenotypically different cells with heterogeneous nuclear ribonucleoprotein A2/B1 overexpression show similar genetic alterations. Am J Respir Cell Mol Biol 2000;23:636–645.

Chapter 50

Viral Markers RAK in Early Diagnosis and Therapy of Breast, Ovarian, Uterine, and Prostate Cancers

Eva M. Rakowicz-Szulczynska

The extensive hunt for tumor markers, which started after the discovery of monoclonal antibody (MAb) technology, has swallowed millions of dollars but resulted in a relatively low number of clinically useful MAbs directed against tumor antigens. Critical limitations of MAb technology include low specificity due to the expression of the same antigen(s) on several normal cells, and an expression/overexpression of marker proteins or specific epitopes by only some populations of cancer cells. For example, the antigen HER/Neu, which is overexpressed on breast cancer cells, is detectable in no more than 40% of cells within a malignant lesion. Other clinical markers for mammary adenocarcinoma, like CA 15-3, CA 549, CA M26, and CA M29, meet just two desirable criteria: their frequency and degree of expression reflect tumor burden and prognosis, and they may correlate with therapeutic results.

A second class of tumor markers includes the DNA markers, which are mutated, deleted, amplified, or aberrantly expressed in tumor cells as compared to normal cells. Oncogenes, which 20 years ago were believed to have revolutionized cancer detection and treatment, did not result in any breakthrough diagnostic technology. The diagnostic value of *BRCA1* and *BRCA2* genes, highly popularized during recent years, is limited to inherited forms of breast and ovarian cancer and the fact that only one in 800 women carries the mutated *BRCA* genes, while statistically at least 80–100 women of that number will develop breast cancer, limits the role of *BRCA* genes.

Highly specific and sensitive tumor markers were discovered by our laboratory during some combined studies on MAbs directed against human immunodeficiency I (HIV-1) antigens and MAbs directed against cancer. Some HIV-neutralizing antibodies, which were considered beneficial for AIDS patients, highly stimulated growth of breast and cervical cancer cells *in vitro* (1). That unusual sensitivity of cancer cells to anti-HIV-1 antibodies was mediated by HIV-1-like antigens, expressed by cancer cells (1,2). These new cancer antigens, which are completely absent in normal, healthy cells, seem to be encoded by some slow virus, and therefore, provide novel sensitive and specific tumor markers, named Rakowicz markers (RAK). RAK antigens p120, p42, and p25 are randomly expressed by 96–100% of the breast, ovarian, uterine, cervical, and vulvar cancers in women, and prostate and testicular cancers in men, independently of the cancer stage and histological origin (3–6). Another antigen, RAK p160, which seems to represent a precursor of RAK p120 and p42, was found in the blood serum of the majority of cancer patients (6,7).

Antigens RAK p120, p42, and p25 express an epitope GRAF (glycine-arginine-alanine-phenylalanine), which is characteristic for the envelope protein gp120 of HIV-1 (2). Consequently, RAK antigens cross-react with an epitope-specific MAb anti-HIV-1 gp120 while the MAb RAK-BrI, directed against breast cancer, cross-reacts with a non-glycosylated form of the HIV-1 gp120.

The use of the polymerase chain reaction (PCR) primers, derived from the HIV-1 gp41 gene encoding for the transmembrane protein gp41, has revealed a 143 bp long fragment of cancer DNA with 92–96% homology to HIV-1 (3–5). The identified DNA sequences of cancer DNA are absent in healthy tissues, providing a new diagnostic and prognostic marker, named *RAK alpha* gene. DNA sequences of the *RAK alpha* gene, as deposited in the gene bank, exhibit higher homology to HIV-1 than the Simian Immunodeficiency Virus (SIV), which is believed to be the ancestor of HIV. High homology of the cancer virus to HIV suggests that cancer virus and HIV-1 could evolve from one or more common ancestors, or even that HIV could evolve from the cancer virus, which pre-existed in the human population.

The mutated *RAK alpha* genes were found in several benign tumors, suggesting that a benign phenotype of tumor might be associated with the presence of an inactive *RAK alpha* gene, while the malignant phenotype seems to be associated with the presence of the *RAK alpha* gene, encoding an active protein (8). Recent studies indicated that in addition to the exogenous (not inherited) form of the *RAK alpha* gene, endogenous *RAK alpha* gene may be detected in the spermatozoa DNA of some people with familiar history of prostate cancer.

An electron microscopic analysis of the thin sections of breast cancer and cervical cancer cells revealed viral particles, which were immuno-gold-labeled with MAb anti-HIV-1 gp120 and with MAb RAK BrI (5,9). Negatively stained viral particles exhibited a size of 120nm and either an oval or a tail-and-head structure (5). Another type of viral particle was found in ovarian cancer cells, isolated from the malignant ascites of cancer patients (6). The production of viral particles in ovarian cancer cells was associated with formation of the huge, highly vacuolated syncytia, strongly labeled with MAb RAK BrI and MAb anti HIV-1 gp120. MAb anti-gp120 and MAb RAK BrI both inhibited syncytia formation, which suggests that the antigen RAK gp120 may play a similar role in the cell fusion, as gp120 plays in HIV-1-infected cells. Viral particles isolated from ovarian cancer syncytia effectively transformed normal breast cells, suggesting that the identified cancer virus encoding for RAK antigens might, in fact, have a role in the malignant transformation (9). That suggestion was supported by the fact that the anti-sense oligonucleotides directed against *RAK alpha* genes inhibited growth of breast and cervical cancer cells *in vitro*. The studies seem to confirm that the long-postulated breast cancer virus might exist but it should belong to a family of HIV-related slow viruses, instead of the mouse mammary tumor virus (MMTV)-like viruses.

Independently of the viral or human origin, and due to their presence in all breast, gynecological, and prostate cancer cases and their absence in normal healthy tissue, antigens RAK and the *RAK alpha* gene represent unusually specific and sensitive cancer markers.

CLINICAL APPLICATION

The comprehensive Diagnostic System RAK includes PCR-based tests (for the detection of the *RAK alpha* gene) and Western blot tests (developed for the detection of the RAK antigens). MAb RAK BrI may also be used in the ELISA and an immunohistochemical staining of the paraffin-embedded tissues (10).

PCR DETECTION OF THE RAK ALPHA GENE IN THE BLOOD CELL DNA

Tests for Determining Cancer Predisposition

In double blind studies, the presence of *RAK alpha* gene was tested in retrospectively collected blood plasma DNA. Of 153 blood DNA samples, 47 samples were strongly PCR positive, 19 moderately positive, and 11 weakly positive. No amplification bands were detected in the blood DNA isolated from 73 people. After decoding the health history of each person, all strongly positive people were found to be cancer patients (20 breast cancer, 12 ovarian cancer, 7 uterine cancer, and 8 prostate cancer cases). Moderately positive were 19 women with first-degree relatives affected by breast cancer. Weakly positive people of both genders contained in their history first- and second-degree relatives affected by breast or prostate cancer. Weakly positive were also 4 healthy individuals with no cancer history. The *RAK*-negative population included 48 healthy women and 10 healthy men with no familiar cancer history, and 15 healthy people with second-, third-, or fourth-degree relatives affected by cancer.

Although more studies are needed to determine whether the currently healthy but *RAK*-positive people will develop cancer in the future, the fact that all cancer patients were correctly selected by using *RAK-alpha* gene for the screening stresses the importance of the *RAK* gene-test in determining predisposition to cancers of the reproductive organs. Cancer predisposition associated with the presence of *RAK alpha* gene should not, however, be compared with the genetic predisposition associated with the presence of the mutated genes like *BRCA1*, *BRCA2*, etc. Since the *RAK alpha* gene seems to belong to a slow virus, people who have that gene might be rather predestined to develop cancer, similarly as the majority of HIV-positive patients are predestined to develop AIDS, or HTLV-I-infected people are predestined to develop acute leukemia.

ANTIGENS RAK P120, P42, AND P25 AND THE RAK ALPHA GENE IN THE PRE-MALIGNANT AND MALIGNANT TISSUE

Molecular Diagnosis

Table 1 summarizes blind clinical studies of several hundred cancer and normal samples. Tissue classification was provided by a pathologist, using traditional histological evaluation. The results indicated that a well-defined breast, cervical, ovarian, or uterine cancer in women and prostate or testicular cancer in men may be detected equally well by a traditional pathological evaluation, as well as by the PCR detection of the *RAK alpha* gene or *RAK* antigens detection. However, *RAK alpha* gene seems to appear in the pathologically normal tissue adjacent to cancer or in the tissue located at the distance from cancer much sooner than any changes become microscopically visible. PCR positivity of the tissue seems to be followed by the expression of *RAK* antigens; however, there is a well-visible lag period between the appearance of the *RAK alpha* gene and the expression of the *RAK* antigens. *RAK alpha* gene might be, therefore, classified as the earliest molecular marker of the processes that lead to malignancy occurring in histologically normal tissue.

ANALYSIS OF POINT MUTATIONS

Diagnosis of the Benign vs. Malignant Tumors

DNA sequences of the *RAK alpha* genes, PCR amplified in 100% of malignant tumors, in both women and men, exhibited over 90% homology to HIV-1 gp41 and encoded functional peptides (Figure 1). In contrast to malignant tumors, no more than 30–40% of benign tumors in women contained RAK markers. The majority of DNA sequences amplified in benign tumors in women exhibited numerous frame shift mutations and encoded for some truncated or nonsense peptides (8). This finding strongly suggests that benign tumors of the reproductive organs might contain some defective retrovirus, as compared to malignant tumors, all of which seemed to have functional variants of the *RAK alpha* gene. In contrast to benign tumors of ovary, breast, or uterus in women, no point mutations were found in BPH cases. Although more studies are needed,

Table 1 Distribution pattern of RAK antigens and *RAK alpha* gene in the breast and gynecological cancer in women and prostate and testicular cancer in men

Tissue[a]	RAK antigen tested/tested positive	*RAK* gene % positive	Tissue	RAK antigen tested/tested positive	*RAK* gene % positive
WOMEN					
Breast cancer	160/160	100	Ovarian cancer	89/85	100
Breast ADT+[b]	55/55	100	Ovarian ADT+	18/18	100
Breast ADT−[b]	48/18	50	Ovarian ADT−	23/7	59
Breast "normal"[c]	70/7	10	Fallopian tube−	15/1	7
Breast reduction	26/1	5	Fallopian tube ADT	20/5	25
Breast benign tumor	10/1	10	Ovarian benign tumor	35/4	25
Breast fibrocystic disease	35/5	14	Ovary normal	15/1	6
			Vulvar cancer	60/54	98
Breast milk cells	16/0	0	Muscle ADT	30/11	40
Skin ADT	20/8	45	Uterine cancer	64/62	100
Skin normal	10/0	0	Cervical cancer	100/95	100
Lung normal	8/0	0	Cervix ADT+	20/20	100
Cartilage normal	6/0	0	Cervix "normal"	18/2	50
Colon normal	6/0	0	Leiomyoma	55/20	27
Uterine fibroid	18/6	33	Vagina ADT	25/9	36
MEN					
Prostate cancer	50/48	100	Prostate normal	25/1	4
BPH[d]	40/36	95	Skin normal	8/0	0
BPH[e]	40/28	75	Testicular cancer	10/10	100

[a] Tissue type, as defined by the gold standard, traditional pathology.
[b] ADT−, ADT+ Tissue adjacent to cancer, defined as negative and positive, respectively.
[c] "Normal"—histologically normal tissue from cancer-affected organ.
[d] BPH originated from prostate cancer patients.
[e] BPH originated from cancer-free patients.

these findings suggest that BPH may, in fact, potentially lead to cancer.

Very preliminary studies indicated that some women who were diagnosed with benign tumors but contained an "active" type of the *RAK alpha* gene developed malignant cancers after 2–3 years. Analysis of point mutations in the *RAK alpha* gene might, therefore, provide an additional useful tool in diagnosis of benign forms of tumors that may lead to malignancy.

ANTIGEN RAK P160 DETECTION IN THE BLOOD OF CANCER PATIENTS

Activation of the Virus and Early Pre-Malignant Changes

Some early studies (6,7) indicated that the antigen RAK p160 was expressed in the blood serum of the majority of reproductive tract cancer patients, as well as in patients with familiar cancer history. However, the antigen RAK p160 was expressed at different amounts in different patients. For example, high RAK p160 blood level was found in 50% of women with breast tumors or highly advanced fibrocystic diseases. Women with advanced breast cancer who were strongly RAK alpha gene positive and RAK antigen-positive in a tissue, expressed a relatively low amount of the RAK p160 in the blood serum. Since the frame shift mutations were found in the majority of benign tumors, it is very likely that benign tumors express more stable (inactive) RAK p160, while the malignant tumors express fast-processing (biologically active) versions of the p160.

FUTURE DIRECTIONS

RAK markers, which include antigens RAK p160, p120, p42, p25, and the *RAK alpha* gene, surpass the specificity and sensitivity of any existing tumor markers. Moreover, RAK markers seem to provide sensitive tools for the detection of consecutive events occurring during the process of malignancy:

- Presence of the *RAK alpha* gene in the peripheral blood lymphocytes seems to mark cancer predisposition/predestination.
- Activation of the virus seems to be associated with the presence in the blood of the RAK p160 antigen.
- Pre-malignant or malignant changes occurring in the tissue are associated with the appearance of the *RAK alpha* gene in the tissue DNA.
- The presence of RAK p120, p42, and p25 antigens marks the ongoing malignant process.

Based on the accumulated data, it seems that *RAK alpha* genes are encoded by two retroviruses, one endogenous, and another exogenous. *RAK* sequences might integrate together with the virus with blood lymphocytes of some people, similarly as the HIV-1 integrates with T-cell DNA. In such an inactive

BrCA	GCA	GCA	GGA	AGC	ACT	ATG	GGC	GCA	GCG	TCA	TCA
	Ala	Ala	Gly	Ser	Thr	Met	Gly	Ala	Ala	Ser	Ser
	1				5					10	
HIV-1	**Ala**	**Ala**	**Gly**	**Ser**	**Thr**	**Met**	**Gly**	**Ala**	**Ala**	**Ser**	**Met**

ACT	CTC	ACG	GTA	CAG	GCC	AGA	CAC	TAA	TTG	TCT
Thr	Leu	Thr	Val	Gln	Ala	Arg	His	Leu	Leu	Ser
			15					20		
Thr	**Leu**	**Thr**	**Val**	**Gln**	**Ala**	**Arg**	**Gln**	**Leu**	**Leu**	**Ser**

GGT	ATA	GTG	CAA	CAG	CAC	AAC	AAT	TTG	CTG	AGG
Gly	Ile	Val	Gln	Gln	His	Asn	Asn	Leu	Leu	Arg
		25					30			
Gly	**Ile**	**Val**	**Gln**	**Gln**	**Gln**	**Asn**	**Asn**	**Leu**	**Leu**	**Arg**

GCT	ATT	GAT	GCC	CAA	CAT	CAT	CTG	TTG	CAA	CTC
Ala	Ile	<u>Asp</u>	Ala	Gln	His	His	Leu	Leu	Gln	Leu
		35				40				
Ala	**Ile**	**<u>Glu</u>**	**Ala**	**Gln**	**Gln**	**His**	**Leu**	**Leu**	**Gln**	**Leu**

ACA	GTC	TGG
Thr	Val	Trp
45		
Thr	**Val**	**Trp**

Figure 1 DNA sequences of the *RAK alpha* gene and peptides encoded by the open reading frame in a breast cancer patient (BrCA). Amino acid sequences of the HIV-1 gp41 are shown for comparison. One conserved mutation in codon 36, replacing glutamic acid typical for HIV with aspartic acid typical for cancer patients, was conserved in all malignant tumors (5,8,9). Other point mutations varied in different cancer types. In the majority of benign tumors of the breast, ovary, and uterus, one or more frame shift mutations or nonsense mutations encoded for a truncated or nonsense peptide (8).

form, the virus could exist for a long time, even for the whole life of an individual. Growth factors, hormones, carcinogens, or other factors could activate the virus, leading to its relocation in the reproductive organs. The activated virus could start the process of pre-malignant changes that then evolve into malignancy.

Pre-clinical and early clinical studies of several thousands of patients support the high specificity and sensitivity of the diagnostic tests for *RAK*, which is between 96–100%. Consecutive application of these markers would allow preventive cancer treatment. Association of these markers with cancer might also guide the surgeon during surgery. Lack of *RAK* antigens in certain areas of the breast, ovary, uterus, or prostate, if confirmed by negative histology, would strongly support an organ-preserving surgery. If *RAK* antigens were detected in histologically normal tissue of the organ affected by cancer, radical surgery should be recommended.

Antigens *RAK* and the *RAK alpha* gene also represent excellent targets for immunotherapy and anti-sense therapy, as well as for the development of highly specific anti-cancer vaccines. Since *RAK* antigens are absent in normal tissues but are highly expressed by cancer cells, these novel targets might also be effectively used for the targeted drug delivery (2).

Why have *RAK* markers not entered medical practice, even though so many cancer patients die due to the late diagnosis or from cancer recurrence? The answer is simple: in 1917 Rous discovered the first oncogenic retrovirus, which was a sarcoma virus in chicken. He lost all his grants immediately and was left behind the research community for over 50 years, until, at last, a new generation of scientists confirmed his data. That gap between the discovery of the first oncovirus and acceptance of that fact by the research community greatly postponed other studies on oncoviruses and retroviruses in general, which resulted in the epidemics of HIV and HTLV in some regions of the world. Unfortunately, millions of people still have to die of cancer before the *RAK* system will be accepted in cancer diagnosis.

REFERENCES

1. Rakowicz-Szulczynska EM, McIntosh DG, Smith ML. Mechanisms of cancer growth promotion by HIV-I-neutralizing antibodies. Cancer J 1995;8:143–149.
2. Rakowicz-Szulczynska EM., Kaczmarski W, Steimer KS, Durda PJ. Internalized antibodies as a potential tool against retroviral diseases. In: Rakowicz-Szulczynska EM, ed. Nuclear localization

of growth factors and of monoclonal antibodies. Boca Raton, Ann Arbor, London, Tokyo: CRC Press,1993:180–197.
3. Rakowicz-Szulczynska EM, Roszak A, Mackiewicz A, Markowska J, Karczewska A, Snyder W, et al. New protein and PCR markers RAK for diagnosis, prognosis, and surgery guidance for breast cancer. Cancer Lett 1997;112:93–101.
4. Rakowicz-Szulczynska EM, Jackson B, Snyder W. Prostate, breast, and gynecological cancer markers RAK with homology to HIV-1. Cancer Lett 1998;124:213–223.
5. Rakowicz-Szulczynska EM, Jackson B, Szulczynska A, Snyder W, Smith M. HIV-1-like DNA sequences and immunocrossreactive viral particles in breast cancer. Clin Diag Lab Immunol 1998; 5:645–653.
6. Rakowicz-Szulczynska EM, Roszak A, Mackiewicz A, Markowska J, McIntosh DG, Karczewska A, et al. Diagnostic evaluation of cancer antigens RAK I. Cervical and ovarian cancer. Int J Oncol 1996;9:693–699.
7. Rakowicz-Szulczynska EM, McIntosh DG, Perry M.J, Smith ML. Antigen RAK: a new breast cancer diagnostic marker. J Tumor Marker Oncol 1995;10:25–37.
8. Rakowicz-Szulczynska EM. Relevance of the viral gene RAK alpha in diagnosis of malignant vs. nonmalignant tumors of the ovary and the uterus. Clin Diag Lab Immunol 2000;7:360–365.
9. Rakowicz-Szulczynska EM, McIntosh DG, Smith McClure. Giant syncytia and foamy virus-like infection in ovarian carcinoma cells isolated from ascites. Clin Diag Lab Immunol 1999;6: 115–126.
10. Kyriacou KC, Iacovou F, Adamou, A, Hadjisavvas A, Rakowicz-Szulczynska EM. Immunohistochemical vs. molecular detection of markers RAK in breast tissues. Exper Mol Pathol 2000;69: 27–36.

Chapter 51

Plasma EBV DNA as a Marker for Nasopharyngeal Carcinoma and EBV-Related Lymphomas

Philip J. Johnson

Epstein-Barr virus (EBV) is a herpes virus that has a strong and consistent association with nasopharyngeal carcinoma (NPC) (1), a major public health problem throughout southern China. It is also associated with a number of lymphoid malignancies, including the endemic form of Burkitt's lymphoma, in which there is an almost 100% association (2); Hodgkin's disease, predominantly in the mixed cellularity and nodular sclerosing subtypes (2,3); and post-transplant lymphoproliferative disease (PTLD). A large proportion of B-cell lymphomas arising in individuals with the acquired immunodeficiency syndrome (AIDS) are also related to EBV infection (3), as are most cases of nasal natural killer/T-cell (NK/T-cell) lymphoma (4).

Recently, several groups have shown that cell-free tumor-derived DNA can be detected in plasma or serum, and that it can be used for diagnostic purposes (5). Although the presence of EBV DNA in plasma of patients with EBV-related malignancies is now well described, it is the development of a rapid and accurate method for quantification of EBV DNA that has led to its development as a useful tumor marker. This chapter briefly summarizes the potential of this novel molecular marker.

THE ROLE OF PLASMA EBV DNA IN THE DIAGNOSIS AND MANAGEMENT OF NASOPHARYNGEAL CARCINOMA (NPC)

NPC, in its endemic form, is an undifferentiated carcinoma that arises in the back of the nose and rapidly spreads to lymph nodes in the neck before metastasizing widely to lung, liver, and bone. The primary treatment is with radical radiotherapy, which is successful in curing most patients with early-stage disease. However, more than half the patients present with locoregionally advanced disease (UICC stages III and IV), and these cases have high rates of both local recurrence or persistence and distant metastasis after conventional radiotherapy.

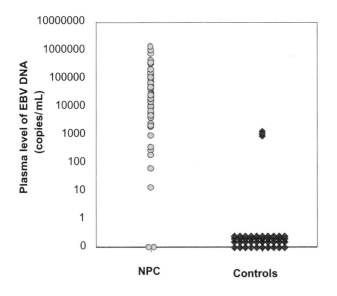

Figure 1 Cell-free EBV-DNA in the plasma of patients with NPC (median value 21,000) and healthy subjects (median value, 0) (7).

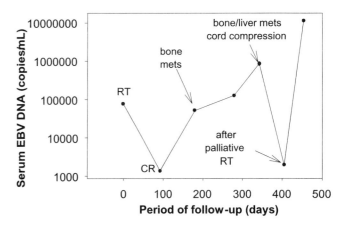

Figure 2 Monitoring response to radiotherapy (RT) with serial EBV DNA estimation. Note that although levels fall dramatically after treatment with RT and response is complete (CR) on clinical grounds, they remain elevated at over 1,000 genome copies/mL. This presages subsequent relapse in bone and liver (9).

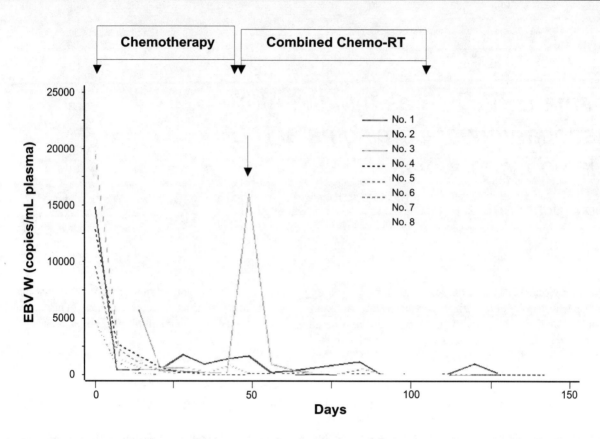

Figure 3 Monitoring response to chemotherapy with serial EBV DNA estimation. Note the rapid decrease in EBV DNA following the initiation of chemotherapy. In the one patient in whom there was a spike of EBV DNA (arrow), radiotherapy was delayed because of toxicity to chemotherapy (10). **Color representation of figure appears on Color Plate 12.**

Cell-free EBV DNA was first detected in the plasma of NPC patients in 1998 (6). Subsequently, using a real-time quantitative PCR assay (toward the *Bam*H1-region of the virus) 96% of patients with NPC were shown to have detectable levels, with a median figure of around 20,000 genome copies/mL. Among a healthy control group, only 7% were positive with a corresponding median figure of zero copies/mL (Figure 1) (7). The long-term outlook for these apparently healthy subjects with raised EBV DNA levels is unknown.

During radiotherapy, levels fall rapidly with a half-life of about 4 hours (8), although there is an initial surge in the first few days of radiotherapy that presumably represents virus released from dying tumor cells (8). Those patients in whom complete remission is obtained achieve very low or even completely negative levels of EBV DNA. In contrast, failure to achieve such low values, or a subsequent rise, is almost always associated with disease relapse (Figure 2) (7,9). NPC is also sensitive to chemotherapy, which is employed in conjunction with radiotherapy for both advanced stage disease and for patients with metastatic disease; again plasma levels of EBV DNA accurately reflect disease progression and response to treatment (Figure 3) (10).

Patients with high levels of EBV DNA have a significantly worse prognosis, even after allowing for disease stage. Thus, for example, while patients with stage IV (advanced disease) have an overall survival rate of around 35%, those with EBV DNA levels of less than 40,000 copies/mL have a five-year survival of about 55% compared to only 20% for those with levels above this cut-off (Figure 4) (11). Overall the relative risk of death from NPC is 1.6 for every 10-fold increase in plasma EBV DNA level.

Precisely how the EBV DNA gains access to the blood, and in what form it circulates, is a topic of intensive current

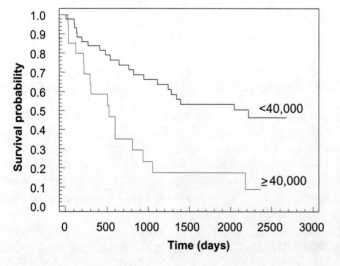

Figure 4 Survival curves for patients with stage IV NPC in relation to EBV DNA levels at presentation. Those with levels below 40,000 genome copies/mL had a significantly better survival than those with values above this figure (11).

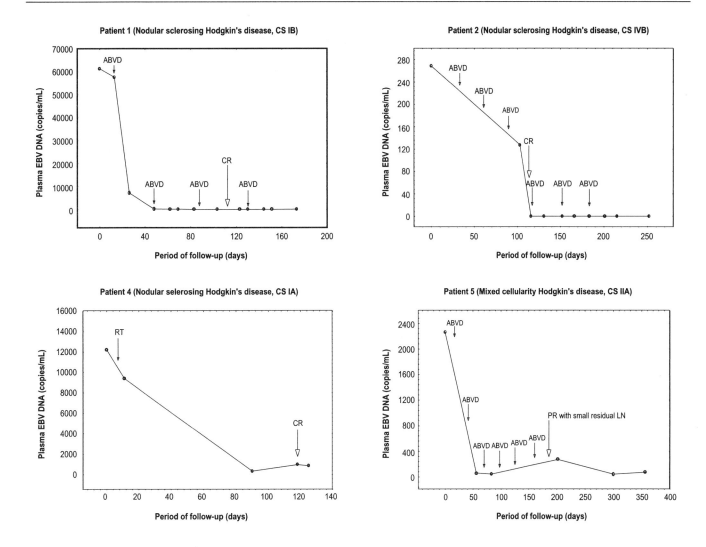

Figure 5 Monitoring response to chemotherapy with serial ENV DNA estimation in patients with Hodgkin's disease. (CR = complete clinical response; PR = partial clinical response; ABVD is a standard combination chemotherapy regimen for Hodgkin's disease; RT = radiotherapy) (18).

research. However, it is clear from a practical point of view that the levels behave as if they reflect tumor burden. The test is therefore rapidly entering routine clinical practice, in areas of the world where NPC is prevalent, for non-invasive monitoring of response to treatment. Whether the test can be used to screen healthy populations for early diagnosis of NPC, and how often raised levels of EBV DNA are detectable in other types of cancer, is also under investigation.

ROLE OF PLASMA DNA IN THE DIAGNOSIS AND MANAGEMENT OF LYMPHOMAS

EBV DNA has been reported to be detectable in the plasma or serum of patients with many EBV-associated lymphoid malignancies, including Hodgkin's disease (12,13); AIDS-related lymphoma (14); and PTLD (12,15). These studies were largely qualitative but, as with NPC, the development of quantitative assays for determining concentrations of circulating EBV DNA (13,16,17) created an opportunity to investigate the use of EBV DNA as a molecular marker.

In the first such study, circulating EBV DNA was detectable in the plasma samples from 12 of 13 patients with Hodgkin's disease, nasal NK/T-cell lymphoma, PTLD, and Burkitt's lymphoma at either diagnosis or recurrence, with a median plasma EBV DNA level of 2,266 copies/mL at presentation (18). In patients with Hodgkin's disease who achieved a complete response, all showed a significant decrease in plasma EBV DNA from their baseline levels to low or undetectable levels during the course of therapy (Figure 5). Patients with nasal NK/T-cell lymphoma who achieved a complete response also demonstrated a reduction of plasma EBV DNA from their baseline concentrations of 181 copies/mL and 8,379 copies/mL to undetectable levels after chemotherapy.

FUTURE DIRECTIONS

It seems likely that plasma EBV DNA estimation will be the first of a growing band of reliable nucleic acid-based molecular markers to enter routine clinical practice. Many questions remain to be answered, however. How does the EBV DNA enter plasma? In what form does the EBV DNA circulate—as random fragments or entire virions? Do the levels of EBV DNA really reflect tumor mass? What is the significance of modestly raised levels of EBV DNA in tumors in which an association with EBV DNA is not normally envisioned, for example, in breast or gastric cancer? Answers to such questions will be needed before this exciting new generation of cancer markers enters clinical practice.

Acknowledgement

The author is indebted to the Kadoorie Charitable Foundations Limited for support of this work.

REFERENCES

1. Rickinson AB, Kieff E. Epstein-Barr virus. In: Fields BN, Knipe DM, Howley PM, eds. Fields Virology, 3rd ed. Philadelphia: Lippincott-Raven Publishers, 1996;2397–2446.
2. Klein G. EBV and B cell lymphomas. In: Medveczky PG, Friedman H, Bendinelli M, eds. Herpes viruses and immunity: infectious agents and pathogenesis. New York: Plenum Press, 1998;163–190.
3. Lyons SF, Liebowitz DN. The roles of human viruses in the pathogenesis of lymphoma. Seminars in Oncology 1998;25:461–475.
4. Chan JK. Natural killer cell neoplasms. Anatomic Pathology 1998;3:77–145.
5. Lo YMD, Chui RWK, Johnson PJ, eds. Circulating nucleic acids in plasma or serum II, Vol. 945. New York: New York Academy of Sciences, 2001.
6. Mutirangura A, Pornthanakasem W, Theamboonlers A, Sriuranpong V, Lertsan-guansinchi P, Yenrudi S, Voravud N, Supiyaphun P, Poovorawan Y. Epstein-Barr viral DNA in serum of patients with nasopharyngeal carcinoma. Clin Cancer Res 1998;4:665–669.
7. Lo YMD, Chan LYS, Lo KW, Leung SF, Zhang J, Chan ATC, Lee JCK, Hjelm HM, Johnson PJ, Huang DP. Quantitative analysis of cell-free Epstein-Barr virus DNA in plasma of patients with nasopharyngeal carcinoma. Cancer Res 1999;59:1188–1191.
8. Lo YMD, Leung SF, Chan LY, Chan AT, Lo KW, Johnson PJ, Huang DP. Kinetics of plasma Epstein-Barr virus DNA during radiation therapy for nasopharyngeal carcinoma. Cancer Res 2000;60:2351–2355.
9. Lo YMD, Chan LYS, Chan ATC, Leung SF, Lo KW, Zhang J, Lee JCK, Hjelm NM, Johnson PJ, Huang DP. Quantitative and temporal correlation between circulating cell-free Epstein-Barr virus DNA and tumor recurrence in nasopharyngeal carcinoma. Cancer Res 1999;59:5452–5455.
10. Chan AT, Lo YM, Chan LY, Lo KW, Leung SF, Huang DP, Johnson PJ. EBV DNA monitoring during chemotherapy for patients with undifferentiated nasopharyngeal carcinoma: a strong predictor of tumor response. Proc ASCO 2001;20:233a.
11. Lo YMD, Chan ATC, Chan LY, Leung SF, Lam CW, Huang DP, Johnson PJ. Molecular prognostication of nasopharyngeal carcinoma by quantitative analysis of circulating Epstein-Barr virus DNA. Cancer Res 2000;60:6878–6881.
12. Fontan J, Bassignot A, Mougin C, Cahn JY, Lab M. Detection of Epstein-Barr virus DNA in serum of transplanted patients: a new diagnostic guide for lymphoproliferative diseases [letter]. Leukemia 1998;12:772.
13. Gallagher A, Armstrong AA, MacKenzie J, Shield L, Khan G, Lake A, Proctor S, Taylor P, Clements GB, Jarrett RF. Detection of Epstein-Barr virus (EBV) genomes in the serum of patients with EBV-associated Hodgkin's disease. Intl J Cancer 1999;84:442–448.
14. Laroche C, Drouet EB, Brousset P, Pain C, Boibieux A. Biron F, Icart J, Denoyel GA, Niveleau A. Measurement by the polymerase chain reaction of the Epstein-Barr virus load in infectious mononucleosis and AIDS-related non-Hodgkin's lymphomas. J Med Virol 1995;46:66–74.
15. Limaye AP, Huang ML, Atienza EE, Ferrenberg JM, Corey L. Detection of Epstein-Barr virus DNA in sera from transplant recipients with lymphoproliferative disorders. J Clin Microbiol 1999;37:1113–1116.
16. Drouet E, Brousset P, Fares F, Icart J, Verniol C, Meggetto F, Schlaifer D, Desmorat-Coat H, Rigal-Huguet F, Niveleau A, Delsol G. High Epstein-Barr virus serum load and elevated titers of anti-ZEBRA antibodies in patients with EBV-harboring tumor cells of Hodgkin's disease. J Med Virol 1999;57:383–389.
17. Stevens SJ, Vervoort MB, van den Brule AJ, Meenhorst PL, Meijer CJ, Middeldorp JM. Monitoring of Epstein-Barr virus DNA load in peripheral blood by quantitative competitive PCR. J Clin Microbiol 1999;37:2852–2857.
18. Lei KIK, Chan LYS, Chan WY, Johnson PJ, Lo YMD. Quantitative analysis of circulating cell-free Epstein-Barr virus DNA levels in patients with EBV-associated lymphoid malignancies. Br J Hematol 2000;111:239–246.

Chapter 52

Circulating Tumor Cells as Cancer Markers: A Sample Preparation and Analysis System

Michael Kagan, David Howard, Teresa Bendele, Chandra Rao, and Leon W.M.M. Terstappen

Circulating tumor cells (CTC) can be detected at extremely low frequencies in the blood of patients with carcinomas (1,2,3,4,5). The number of CTC may represent tumor burden, and changes in CTC numbers could offer a way to evaluate the effectiveness of a given treatment. Assessment of gene and protein expression in CTC offers the potential of determining the presence or absence of therapeutic targets and can be used to guide treatment. To investigate the potential use of CTC in the management of cancer patients, a system that accurately and reliably enumerates and characterizes CTC is needed to perform controlled clinical studies.

CELLSPOTTER™ SYSTEM

The frequency of CTC is often below 1 CTC/mL of blood, and the laborious manual sample preparation and complex analysis methods involved in detecting the presence of CTC often lead to erroneous results. To overcome these limitations, a semi-automated system was developed that minimizes variability and provide more consistent analytical results. The system consists of a semi-automated sample preparation system, an analysis chamber, a magnetic mounting device, and a semi-automated four-color fluorescence microscope system.

SEMI-AUTOMATED SAMPLE PREPARATION SYSTEM

The system is designed to process 7.5 mL of blood and is described in detail elsewhere (6). Epithelial cells are identified from the background of hematopoeitic cells by monoclonal antibodies specific for the epithelial cell adhesion molecule (EpCAM) that is broadly expressed on cells of epithelial cell origin but not on cells of hematopoeitic origin (7).

To reduce the volume and the number of hematopoeitic cells, EpCAM-labeled magnetic nanoparticles are incubated with the blood sample. The cells labeled with the nanoparticles are separated from the non-labeled cells by magnetic means. To reduce differences in capture efficiency of epithelial cells related to differences in EpCAM antigen density, we apply a process referred to as controlled aggregation to increase the magnetic loading of the cells independent of antigen density (8). Reagent additions are performed manually and the system performs the steps that are most prone to human error, such as sample aspiration and movement of sample in and out of the magnetic field. When sample volume is reduced to 200 µL, the magnetically captured cells are fluorescently labeled to differentiate between hematopoeitic and epithelial cells.

The nucleic acid-specific dye DAPI (4,6-diamidino-2-phenylindole) is used to visualize the nucleus. A monoclonal antibody that recognizes keratins 4,6,8,10,13, and 18, conjugated to Phycoerythrin (CK-PE), is used to visualize the cytoplasm of epithelial cells. A monoclonal that recognizes CD45 conjugated to Allophycocyanin (CD45-APC) is used to identify leukocytes. The latter enables the identification of leukocytes that non-specifically bind to cytokeratin, thereby increasing the specificity.

After incubation, the system aspirates and discards the excess staining reagents. The tube is moved out of the magnet and the cells are resuspended. The system transfers more than 99% of the sample into the analysis chamber that is present in a magnetic yoke assembly that holds the chamber between two magnets.

INTERNAL CONTROL

To monitor the accuracy of the procedure, approximately 1,000 internal control cells can be added to the blood before processing. These control cells, derived from the breast cancer tumor cell-line SKBR-3, are stabilized and uniquely labeled with the fluorescent membrane dye DiOC16(3) to permit differentiation from endogenous tumor cells. The control cells express EpCAM and cytokeratin and are captured by the EpCAM magnetic nanoparticles and stained with CK-PE. The percent recovery of added control cells provides an indicator of total reagents and system performance for each specimen, unlike external controls that can detect only systematic errors.

ANALYSIS CHAMBER

The analysis chamber is a disposable device containing 320 µL of sample. The chamber is designed such that it can be closed without air bubble formation and the complete sample can be analyzed. Magnetically labeled cells and free magnetic nanoparticles contained within the chamber move to the upper surface of the chamber under the influence of the magnetic field gradient.

The magnetic mounting device contains two magnets held by a yoke and present on both sides of the chamber. The magnets are designed such that they move the nanoparticles and cells to the viewing surface of the chamber and distribute them evenly over the surface to permit viewing through a microscope objective that has a working distance of 4 mm. The spacing between the magnets allows full viewing of the sample chamber.

DATA ACQUISITION

A fluorescence microscope equipped with a 10X (0.45NA) objective and a computer-controlled CCD camera, X,Y,Z stage and 4-filter cube exchanger, is used for data acquisition. The 80.2 mm² viewing surface of the chamber is scanned for objects stained with DAPI, DiOC16(3), CK-PE, and CD45-APC. The combination of the objective and digital camera results in the acquisition of 560 images (4 × 140) to cover the complete chamber surface.

Before image acquisition, the image acquisition region (X,Y plane) is determined. Using the light emitted by the nucleic acid stain of the cells, iterative determination of the focus at five locations in the chamber is made to determine the focus at each position (Z plane). The CellSpotter™ acquisition program acquires and logs all the images from a sample into a directory.

DATA ANALYSIS

An algorithm is applied to all of the images acquired from a sample to search for locations that stain for DAPI, DiOC16(3), and CK-PE. If the staining area is consistent with that of a control cell (DiOC16(3)+,CK-PE+), the software assigns this location (box) to a control cell. The data analysis software tabulates the number of control cells found in a sample. If the staining area is consistent with that of a potential tumor cell (DAPI+, DiOC16(3)-, CK-PE+), the software stores the location of these areas in a database.

Figure 1 (A,B,C and D) shows a boxed area within the Cytokeratin-PE, DAPI, CD45-APC, and control (DiOC16(3)) images obtained after processing a 7.5-mL blood sample from a patient with breast cancer. In the Cytokeratin-PE image, two round objects are discerned; in the corresponding DAPI image, two cell nuclei are present that correspond to the two objects. Just outside the boxed area is a third nucleus that corresponds to a leukocyte (the corresponding CD45-APC image showed staining). Two other cells did not stain with CD45-APC or DiOC16(3) and confirmed the epithelial cell origin. The relatively large nucleus (large with respect to the cytoplasm) suggests that the cells are tumor cells.

Thumbnail images of each object are presented in a user interface from which the user can determine the presence of

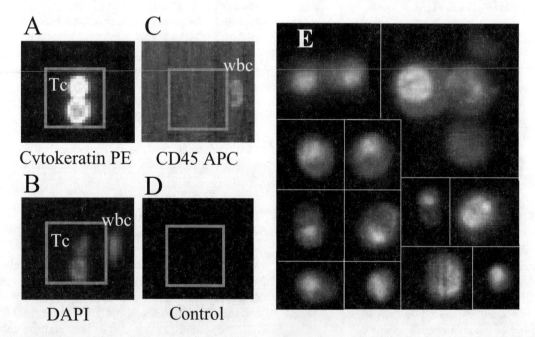

Figure 1 Identification of circulating tumor cells (CTC) by CellSpotter™.
The software identified a location in the Cellspotter™ chamber as potentially containing a CTC. The Cytokeratin-PE, DAPI, CD45-APC, and Control [DiOC16(3)] staining of this location is shown in Panels A, B, C, and D respectively, and the suspect area is indicated by the yellow box. A cluster of two tumor cells (Tc) and one white blood cell (wbc) can be discerned. Panel E shows twelve composites of the cytokeratin staining (green) and the nuclear staining (purple) of tumor cells identified in peripheral blood of breast cancer patients. **Color representation of figure appears on Color Plate 12.**

tumor cells. Figure 1 Panel E shows composites of the cytokeratin staining (green) and the nuclear staining (purple) of tumor cells identified in breast cancer patients. Note the large differences in size and the presence of tumor cell clusters.

SYSTEM PERFORMANCE

The linearity and sensitivity of the system were tested by spiking control cells (n=1000) and 0, 10, 50, 100, 150, and 200 cells of the tumor cell line SKBR-3 in 7.5-mL aliquots of blood from five different donors. The recovery of control was used to demonstrate that the samples were properly processed.

Figure 2 shows the correlation between the number of tumor cells spiked into 7.5 mL of blood and the number of tumor cells detected after sample processing. The correlation between the number of cells spiked and the number of cells recovered was $r^2 = 0.99$ with a slope of 0.83 and an intercept of 1.4, indicating a tumor cell recovery of 83% that is independent of the level of tumor cells spiked. The data demonstrate that the processed blood volume determines the limit of sensitivity.

FUTURE DIRECTIONS

The CellSpotter™ system was developed to accurately and reliably enumerate and characterize CTC so that controlled clinical studies could be performed. The system processes 7.5 mL of blood and places a 320-μL sample containing immunomagnetically enriched and fluorescently labeled epithelial-derived tumor cells in an analysis chamber. The analysis chamber is placed in a magnet device that distributes magnetically labeled cells over the top surface of the chamber for analysis by a semi-automated four-color fluorescent microscope system. The system applies an algorithm on captured images to enumerate an internal control and identify all objects that potentially classify as tumor cell based on size and immunophenotype. Thumbnails of all objects that potentially classify as tumor cells are presented in the user interface, from which the user can make the ultimate judgment. In processing the blood of normal donors and cancer patients, the internal control showed consistent and reproducible results between systems and operators (6). Sample preparation performed by the system clearly outperformed the manual preparation of blood samples as demonstrated by a higher recovery of tumor cells and better reproducibility (6). Data from spiking experiments demonstrated an excellent linearity and sensitivity.

The CellSpotter™ system can now be used to probe if CTC in a clinical laboratory setting can confirm the CTC data reported in various research studies (1–5). The number of CTC as measured by the CellSpotter™ system may represent tumor burden, and changes in the CTC numbers could offer a way to evaluate the effectiveness of a given treatment.

The feature that clearly distinguishes tumor serum markers from CTC enumeration is the ability to assess gene and protein expression in CTC. This offers the potential of performing a "real-time biopsy" of the tumor and can be used to determine the presence or absence of therapeutic targets, thereby potentially guiding treatment. An example of such an application is the assessment of Her2 expression on CTC to determine whether and when treatment with Herceptin is indicated during the course of the disease (9).

Detection of CTC in purportedly healthy individuals may represent an advance in the early detection of cancer. If such early detection is possible, a "non-invasive" biopsy of a solid tumor can be performed by a blood test.

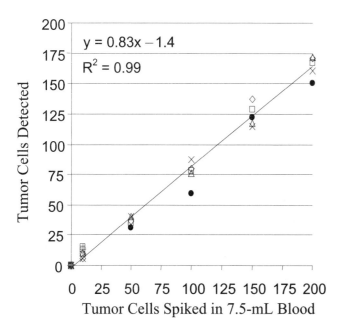

Figure 2 Sensitivity and linearity of the CellSpotter system. After spiking 1,000 control cells and 0, 10, 50, 100, 150, and 200 SKBR-3 cells in 7.5-mL aliquots of blood from five different donors (horizontal axes), the blood samples were processed and CTC were enumerated with the CellSpotter system (vertical axes). $R^2 = 0.99$ is the correlation coefficient and the equation $y = 0.83x - 1.4$ shows a CTC recovery of 83%.

REFERENCES

1. Myerowitz RL, Edwards PA, Sartiano GP. Carcinocythemia (carcinoma cell leukemia) due to metastatic carcinoma of the breast. Cancer 1977;40:3107–3111.
2. Brugger W, Bross K, Glatt M, Weber F, Mertelsmann R, Kanz L. Mobilization of tumor cells and hematopoietic progenitor cells into peripheral blood of patients with solid tumors. Blood 1994; 83:636–640.
3. Moss TJ, To LB, Pantel K. Evaluation of grafts for occult tumor cells. J Hematotherapy 1994;3:163–164.
4. Racila E, Euhus D, Weiss AJ, Rao C, McConnell J, Terstappen LWMM, Uhr JW. Detection and characterization of carcinoma cells in the blood. Proc Natl Acad Sci 1998;95:4589–4594.
5. Moreno JG, O'Hara SM, Gross S, Doyle G, Fritschke H, Gomella LG, Terstappen LWMM. Changes in circulating carcinoma cells in metastatic prostate cancer patients correlate with disease status. Urology 2001;58:386–392.

6. Kagan M, Howard D, Bendele T, Mayes J, Silvia J, Repollet M, Doyle J, Allard J, Tu N, Bui T, Russell T, Rao C, Hermann M, Rutner H, Terstappen LWMM. A sample preparation and analysis system for identification of circulating tumor cells. J Clin Lig Assay (in press).

7. Stahel RA, Gilks WR, Lehmann HP, Schenker T. Third international workshop on lung tumor and differentiation antigens: overview of the results of the central analysis. Int J Cancer Suppl 1994;8:6–26.

8. Liberi PA, Rao CG, Terstappen LWMM. Optimization of ferrofluids and protocols for the enrichment of breast tumor cells in blood. J Magnetism and Magnetic Materials 2001;225: 301–307.

9. Walker TM, Hayes DF, Gross S, Repollet M, Laurich M, Doyle G, Terstappen LWMM. Detection of HER-2/neu cell membrane receptor on circulating tumor cells in patients with advanced breast cancer. Proc AACR 2001;42:11–12.

Chapter 53

Cell Dielectric Properties as Diagnostic Markers for Tumor Cell Isolation

Peter R.C. Gascoyne

Our research addresses the creation of diagnostic systems for combined sample preparation and detection of molecular markers. The goal is to develop integrated fluidic devices able to sort, isolate, and burst target cells from clinically relevant samples and to execute molecular marker assays on them rapidly and automatically at the point of care. It is expected that these devices will offer the advantages of small-size, low-sample-volume requirements, and the potential for mass production at low cost. Such systems will be applicable to reusable systems and disposable medical devices alike.

In order to make such devices possible, the first step is to concentrate and isolate potential tumor cells from a specimen so that they may be analyzed by molecular methods. We will assume that the specimen is collected in suspension (e.g., a blood sample, lavage, nipple aspirate, etc.) or can be prepared as such (e.g., disrupted lymph node biopsy, fine needle aspiration biopsy, trypsinized solid biopsy, etc.). In order to achieve concentration and isolation of the target suspect tumor cells, it is necessary to recognize them via some marker and, in addition, to provide a differential physical force that separates them from normal cells. Here we describe the application of the technique of dielectrophoresis (DEP) to both of these problems.

To understand how DEP can help isolate tumor cells, it is helpful to consider the most common marker for cancer detection used today, namely the identification of atypical cell morphologies via a slide read by a pathologist or a laser-scanning cytometer. Upon transformation, cells exhibit a variety of morphological changes that may include altered cell diameter, unusual peripheral membrane structure, aberrant internal membrane structure, and modified nuclear appearance. All of these changes observed by the pathologist's eye give rise to changes in other physical properties of the cell. DEP is a method that can exploit changes in cell dielectric properties to create a force that can be used to physically move cells (1). For example, two cells of identical size and density can be moved by DEP in opposite directions (2) or, if desired, in the same direction with different forces, if they have different dielectric properties. It is not unreasonable to state that if the pathologist can identify a morphological difference between two cells, especially in their size or cytoplasmic membrane organization, then DEP can likely separate them under appropriate conditions.

The basis for cell separation by DEP is the movement, in an applied alternating electrical field, of ions around and within cells up to biological membranes that bar further ion movement (3). Interestingly, although the physical theory of DEP is complicated (4), the apparatus required to exploit it is extremely simple—suggesting possibilities for inexpensive and disposable applications.

Figure 1A illustrates some of the main characteristics of a cell that control its DEP properties. These include cell volume, total plasma membrane area (see Figure 2B), the endoplasmic reticulum if it is well developed, the nuclear size if it is a reasonably large proportion of total cell size, cytoplasmic ion content, and ion mobility in the cytoplasm (which may be affected by protein content and cytoplasmic structure) (5). Lastly, atypical membranes that are porous to ions also lead to modified DEP responses (6). Ion species in different compartments of the cell take different amounts of time to respond to an applied electrical field and this leads to cellular DEP responses that are highly dependent on the frequency of the AC electrical field.

To summarize, cellular morphology and composition lead to a DEP frequency response that is characteristic of the cell, providing a "fingerprint" that can be used as a marker for that cell type. The fingerprint for a given cell type has been termed the "dielectric phenotype" (7). Figure 1C shows a DEP "fingerprint" for an MDA-MB-435 human breast cancer cell and compares it to peripheral blood monocytes, T-lymphocytes, and erythrocytes. By choosing appropriate working frequencies, the forces experienced by the different cell types can be exploited to differentially manipulate them within the suspending medium without the need to process them with dyes, stains, or other markers.

CLINICAL APPLICATIONS

There are several ways in which DEP may be applied to isolate a target population of cells. One method attempted by several groups is to use DEP simply to trap one cell type while releasing others (2); however, this method only works effectively if there are very large differences in the DEP responses (and hence in the cell morphologies) of the cells to be separated. To exploit DEP both as a means to detect tumor cells and to separate them from complex mixtures of normal cells with the high-

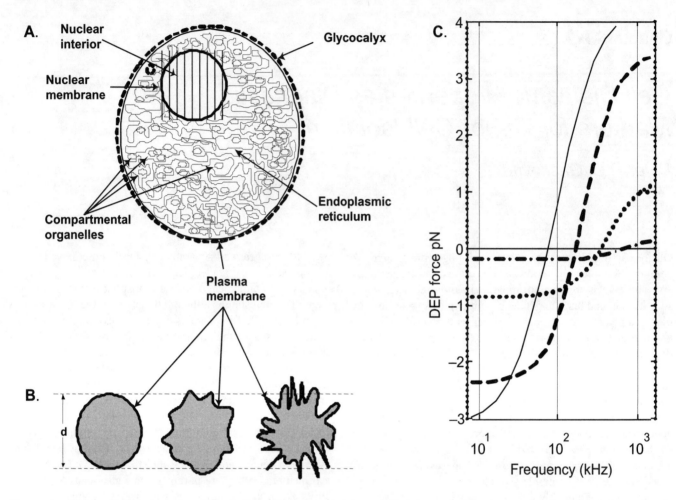

Figure 1 (A) Morphological aspects of mammalian cells that may influence their dielectrophoretic responses. Cell volume and cytoplasmic membrane area are dominant factors. Despite having the same diameter, d, the cells diagrammed in (B) would have hugely different DEP responses because of the differences in the total cytoplasmic membrane areas. Different DEP frequency responses corresponding to different cell dielectric phenotypes are shown in (C) for (——) MDA-MB-435 cultured breast tumor cells, (— —) peripheral monocytes, (. . . .) peripheral T-lymphocytes, and (— · — ·) erythrocytes.

est possible discrimination, we have developed a method called DEP-FFF or "dielectrophoretic field-flow-fractionation" (8; see Figure 2A). In this approach, fluid flows through a flat chamber (for example, 450-mm length, 35-mm width, and 0.4-mm height) and spontaneously sets up a so-called laminar flow profile in the chamber whereby fluid velocity increases from zero at the floor and ceiling to a maximum at the center. An array of electrodes on the chamber floor is used to provide a DEP force that lifts cells into the flow stream to a height where the DEP and sedimentation forces balance. The height at which this balance occurs depends on the cell dielectric properties, so that cell types with different dielectric properties or different densities reach different heights.

Because the velocity of the fluid depends on the height in the flow profile, the cells at different equilibrium heights are carried through at different speeds. Therefore, a mixture of cells injected into one end of the chamber will be separated into fractions as it travels to the other end. DEP provides exquisite sensitivity to small differences in cell dielectric properties and, with complex cell mixtures, the electrical signal to the electrode can be switched through a sequence of frequencies and voltages dur-

ing the separation process to provide the highest discrimination for each fraction as it moves through the chamber (8).

We have applied DEP-FFF to cell differential analysis of normal blood and for other cell separation problems including, as is of most relevance here, the separation of cancer cells from normal cells. Figure 2B, for example, shows the separation of MDA-MD-435 cells from CD34+ cells (9). With the exception of leukemia cells isolated from blood in residual samples, our work with transformed cells has so far been with cell lines. This has allowed us to demonstrate that the expression of just a single oncogene (*src* or *mos*) for a few hours is sufficient to allow cell changes to be discriminated and cells to be separated by DEP.

We have examined nine cultured tumor lines including seven breast tumor and two colon cancer lines. The dielectric phenotypes of all of these cell types are clearly distinguishable from those of all peripheral blood cell subpopulations, and we can separate all of them from blood. Furthermore, in cases where the cell models allow, we have shown it is possible to separate transformed cells from identical cells that have been treated to suppress oncogene expression. This suggests that DEP offers a potentially powerful method for concentrating and

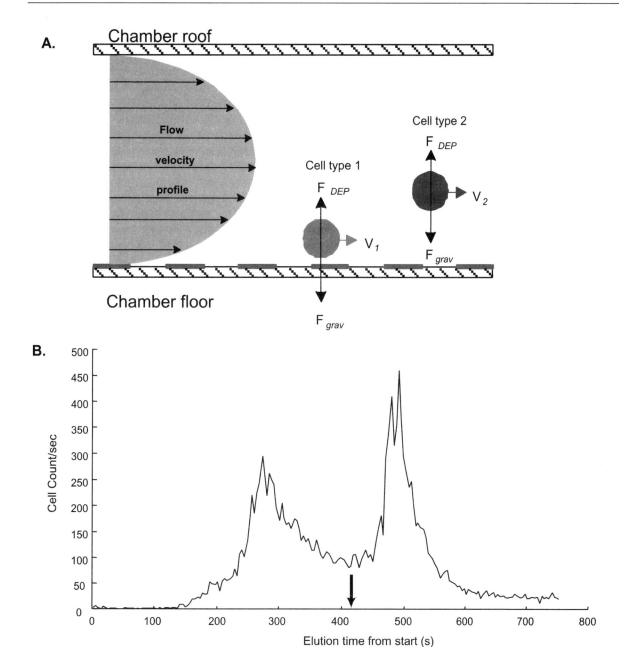

Figure 2 (A) Side view of a DEP-FFF chamber showing the flow velocity profile that forms spontaneously when fluid flow is present. The DEP force provided from electrodes on the chamber floor is shown levitating two cells with different dielectric properties to different heights where they are carried by the flow stream at different speeds. A typical elution profile is shown in (B) for the separation of mobilized (peripheral blood) CD34+ cells from MDA-MB-435 cultured breast cancer cells. The CD34+ cells eluted first, then the electrical field frequency was changed at the time shown by the arrow to release the tumor cells from the chamber. Similar single-stage separations have been achieved for different cultured tumor cell types and all of the peripheral blood subtypes and attainable purities in all cases exceeded 99.7%.

isolating tumor cells from peripheral blood, is likely to work for separating tumor cells from suspended lymph node cell populations, and may allow transformed cells to be isolated from their normal cells of origin.

There are three significant advantages in using DEP to these ends. First, the chambers for cell separations are quite simple and are readily scalable and stackable, making it possible to sort perhaps millions of cells per second. This makes the technology applicable to investigating circulating metastatic cells and residual disease. Second, the basis for the cell separation is cell morphology; there is no requirement to stain or label cells in any way in order to facilitate cell separation by DEP. Third, the method can interface directly with microfluidic molecular analysis methods being widely developed.

FUTURE DIRECTIONS

We are working in three ways to improve this analytical technology to make it suitable for tumor detection in clinical applications.

First, we are initiating two collaborations to investigate clinical samples. Obviously it is important, if DEP is to become an effective method in the clinic, that the types of DEP response differences observed between cultured tumor cell lines, normal cells, and blood cell subpopulations are also observed *in vivo*. However, given that pathologists exploit differences in cell morphology as the basis for identification of transformed cells and can differentiate them from normal and blood cells, we feel confident that corresponding DEP response differences will be found in clinical specimens.

Second, cell surface markers are becoming important in the characterization of some cancers and are being used as the basis for immunomagnetic isolation and subsequent identification of some tumor cell types. It is a relatively trivial extension to add magnetic capabilities to the DEP-FFF method so as to allow cells to be sorted according to the *concentration* of surface markers that they carry in addition to their dielectric properties (10). This represents an advance over traditional magnetically activated cell sorting, which traps cells that possess greater than an arbitrary threshold concentration of surface markers. MAG-DEP-FFF adds the capability to pinpoint cell subpopulations that have an anomalous concentration of surface markers even in the presence of normal cells that carry a different concentration of the same markers. We have already demonstrated this capability for blood cells and are extending it to tumor cell populations.

Third, as already indicated, it is our long-term goal to use DEP as the first stage of an integrated diagnostic device that is able to achieve molecular analysis of isolated cell subpopulations. Accomplishing this requires an intermediate stage that can liberate, isolate, and purify the target molecules followed by a stage that accomplishes the analysis. For molecular targeting and clean-up, we have developed a family of addressable bead carriers that can be moved and identified by DEP. Each bead type in the family has a unique dielectric signature and will be used as the carrier for a unique molecular probe. The cell isolate from the sample will be burst in the presence of a cocktail of multiple bead types, making it possible to isolate many molecular targets simultaneously from a single sample. Interfering debris and molecules will be washed free while the beads are immobilized by a strong attractive DEP force. Finally, the unique dielectric properties of the beads will allow the different target molecules captured from the cell isolates to be tracked as they are subjected to molecular analysis.

REFERENCES

1. Pohl HA. Dielectrophoresis. Cambridge, UK: Cambridge University Press, 1978.
2. Becker FF, Wang X-B, Huang Y, Pethig R, Vykoukal J, Gascoyne PRC. Separation of human breast cancer cells from blood by differential dielectric affinity. Proc Natl Acad Sci USA 1995;29: 860–864.
3. Wang X-B, Huang Y, Gascoyne PRC, Becker FF, Hölzel R, Pethig R. Changes in Friend murine erythroleukemia cell membranes during induced differentiation determined by electrorotation. Biochim Biophys Acta 1994;1193:330–344.
4. Wang X-B, Hughes MP, Huang Y, Becker FF, Gascoyne PRC. Non-uniform distributions of magnitude and phase of AC electric fields determine dielectrophoretic forces. Biochim Biophys Acta 1995;1243:185–194.
5. Huang Y, Wang X-B, Becker FF, Gascoyne PRC. Membrane changes associated with the temperature-sensitive p85 gas-mos-dependent transformation of rat kidney cells as determined by dielectrophoresis and electrorotation. Biochimica Biophysica Acta 1996;1282:76–84.
6. Gascoyne P, Mahidol C, Ruchirawat M, Satayavivad J, Watcharasit P, Becker F. Microsample preparation by dielectrophoresis: isolation of malaria. Lab-on-a-Chip 2002 (in press).
7. Gascoyne PRC, Wang X-B, Huang Y, Becker FF. Dielectrophoretic separation of cancer cells from blood. IEEE Transactions on Industry Applications 1997;33:670–678.
8. Wang X-B, Vykoukal J, Becker FF, Gascoyne PRC. Separation of polystyrene microbeads using dielectrophoretic/gravitational field-flow-fractionation. Biophys J 1998;74:2689–2701.
9. Huang Y, Yang J, Wang X-B, Becker FF, Gascoyne PRC. Cutting-edge communication: the removal of human breast cancer cells from hematopoietic CD34+ stem cells by dielectrophoretic field-flow-fractionation. J Hematother Stem Cell Res 1999;8: 481–490.
10. Gascoyne PRC, Becker FF, Vykoukal J. Methods and apparatus for combined magnetophoretic and dielectrophoretic manipulation of analyte mixtures. World Intellectual Property Organization WO 01/96857 A2.

Chapter 54

Apoptosis and Apoptosis-Related Genes in Cancer

Andreas Scorilas

Apoptosis is the programmed cell death that occurs when the cell is exposed to physiological or toxic death stimuli. The morphological features of apoptosis include cell shrinkage, DNA condensation and fragmentation, membrane blebbing and division of the cell to apoptotic bodies, which are subsequently engulfed by neighboring cells or phagocytes.

THEORY

This type of programmed cell death exists in all multicellular organisms and plays an indispensable role in a variety of physiological procedures by eliminating unwanted cells. For example, during embryonic development and morphogenesis, apoptosis is instrumental as the organism acquires its normal shape after the deletion of the excessive cells. A balance between cell proliferation and programmed cell death promotes tissue homeostasis, as cell death helps the organism to maintain its homeostasis in that it opposes the procedure of cell division (1).

When the cell is exposed to external death signals, the apoptotic mechanism is mediated via a number of specific proteins, termed death receptors (2). These receptors are localized at the cell surface and are responsible for the receipt and transmission of the external apoptotic signal to the intracellular environment. They are members of the tumor necrosis factor (TNF) receptor superfamily, thus they contain highly conserved extracellular cysteine rich domains (2). Additionally, they bear highly conserved cytosolic domains (death domains) that enables them to gain access to specific adapter proteins and transmit the death signal to the apoptotic cascade.

The two best-studied apoptotic pathways involve the receptors TNFR1 (or p55 or CD120a) and FAS (or Apo1 or CD95). The association between the receptor and its ligand (TNF-alpha- and FAS-ligand respectively) results in the homotrimerization of the former, and the subsequent recruitment of the respective cytosolic adapter proteins, which share similar death domains, termed death effector domains or DEDs. TRADD is the adapter for TNFR1 receptor and FADD for FAS (3). The formation of the last complex activates the caspase initiators, which in turn induces a proteolytic cascade resulting in cell execution.

CASPASES

Caspases are the mammalian homologues of CED-3, the protein that is responsible for the execution of apoptosis in *Caenorhabditis elegans* (4). They are cysteine proteases that recognize specific tetrapeptides and cleave sites following aspartic acid residues in the position P1 of their substrates. The first member of this family, caspase-1, is highly homologous to CED-3 interleukin-1β-converting enzyme (ICE) (4).

To date, 14 different caspases have been isolated from mammalian cells (5), not all of them involved in apoptosis. According to their specificity, the family of caspases has been subdivided into three groups. Group I contains the members that recognize the sequence WEHD (caspases-1,-4,-5). The proteins of this category are mainly involved in inflammatory effects and not in apoptosis. Group II includes the effector caspases (caspases-2,-3,-7 and CED-3) whose physiological role is the disruption of cytosolic or nuclear proteins that are essential for DNA repair, DNA replication, RNA splicing, cell division, and cytoskeletal structure. They recognize the tetrapeptide DEXD in their substrates. Group III consists of the enzymes that digest proteins bearing the tetrapeptide (I/L/E)EXD (caspases-6,-8,-9). These are the proteins that receive the death signal and initiate the executioner program. They are called initiator caspases and they act upstream of the executioner proteins.

Caspases are initially translated to zymogens that remain inactive in the living cell (5). These precursors become activated via cleavage by upstream caspases or via autocatalysis. They contain an amino (NH_2) terminal region with at least four residues that are necessary for cleavage and activation. Furthermore, they bear a long and a small domain. When the cell is exposed to an apoptotic stimulus, the enzyme undergoes proteolysis and the two domains separate each other and form a heterodimer. Finally, two of them compose the active tetramer. Initiator caspases are larger molecules because they contain an additional region used for association to their activators (6).

PROTEINS THAT REGULATE CASPASE ACTIVITY

Inhibitor of Apoptosis Proteins (IAPs)

The first inhibitor of apoptosis was discovered in baculovirus and afterwards in *Drosophila melanogaster*. To date, a family of these inhibitors that are highly conserved from insect to human have been identified. All the members of the family share a conserved domain of about 70 amino acid residues known as BIR (bacilovirus IAP repeat) (7). All IAPs contain at least one BIR domain, while some members display some additional regions such as the RING zinc finger domain on their carboxy-terminus.

IAPs are involved in all apoptosis-related diseases but the mechanism by which IAPs mediate apoptosis remains elusive. However, it has been demonstrated that the human protein x-IAP directly inhibits the caspases 3 and 7. On the other hand, IAPs can also be cleaved by caspases. Additionally, there is evidence that x-IAP, c-IAP1, and c-IAP2 can block the activation of pro-caspase 9, but they cannot do the same for pro-caspase-8 (8).

Proteins of the BCL-2 Family

The mammalian counterpart of *Caenorhabditis elegans* CED-9 is BCL-2. BCL-2 was first discovered as a proto-oncogene at the chromosomal breakpoint t(14;18) of B-cell lymphomas. Its overexpression causes tumorigenesis via inhibition of apoptosis rather than stimulation of cell division. To date, more than twenty proteins with high homology to BCL-2 have been identified in human tissues; however only a portion of them display anti-apoptotic activity. Thus, the members of this family are categorized into two subgroups (9).

The first one consists of the anti-apoptotic members that share high structural and functional homology with BCL-2 protein, such as BCL-X, BCL-W, MCL-1, BOO/DIVA, BCL-B and A1/BFL-1 (10,11). The second group includes proteins that share less homology to BCL-2 and display pro-apoptotic activity, such as BAX, BAK, BOK/MTD, BAD, BID, HRK, BIM/BOD, BIK/NBK, BNIP3, NIX/BNIP3L, BLK, BCL-Rambo, BCL-G (10,11). The new members of the BCL-2 gene family—BTF (12), MAP-1 (13), and BCL-2L12 (14)—have been recently identified.

The structural homology among the members of the family is already known. Up to four regions with high sequence homology to the family's founder, called BHs (BH1, BH2, BH3, BH4), are common to the members of the family. These domains correspond to an alpha-helical configuration. The BH1 and BH2 domains are present in all anti-apoptotic proteins, while the BH3 domain is present in the pro-apoptotic members of the family. However, BH3 domains have been identified in some anti-apoptotic proteins such as BCL-2 and BCL-X(L). The BH4 domain appears to be present in the N-terminal domain of the anti-apoptotic BCL-2, BCL-X, and BCL-W proteins and its function is not clear as yet (9).

Mutagenesis and deletion analysis studies revealed that BH domains are required for function, as well as for heterodimerization among the family members. Indeed, the relevant interactions between the death-promoting and death-inhibiting proteins determine the cell's susceptibility to the various apoptotic stimuli (15).

APOPTOSIS-RELATED GENES AS TUMOR BIOMARKERS

The BCL-2 Gene

BCL-2 was first discovered in the t(14;18) chromosomal translocations in non-Hodgkin's follicular B-cell lymphomas, where it contributes to tumorigenesis by preventing cell death rather than causing cell proliferation (16). Overexpression of BCL-2 also takes place in a variety of types of human tumors, including cancers of the prostate, colon, lung, breast, and skin. In some types of cancer this up-regulation can be used as a remarkable prognostic marker (17–19). In lymphoma cells, the anti-apoptotic function of the BCL-2 protein, and therefore its involvement in carcinogenesis, is partly regulated by the phosphorylation/dephosphorylation of the protein. Many chemotherapeutic drugs have been designed to fight tumor progression by down-regulating the production of the protein in tumor cells. Okadaic acid and/or arsenic treatment of leukemia cells provoke the downregulation of the BCL-2 gene. Alternatively, overexpression of the BCL-2 gene is associated with resistance to chemotherapeutic and irradiation treatment. High levels of the BCL-2 protein in acute myeloid leukemia cells result in poor response of the tumor to chemotherapeutic agents (20).

The BAX Gene

BAX is a tumor suppressor, such that in healthy cells, its function promotes the apoptotic death of the excessive or damaging cells, contributing to the tissue homeostasis. However, in malignant incidents the concentration of this protein in cancer cells is reduced. Since the tumor-suppressing activity of BAX is displayed in coordination with its gene regulator p53, BAX defects must be associated with p53 defects. Indeed, p53-deficient mice present abated BAX levels and develop T-cell lymphoma (21). In most cases of cancer the reduced concentrations of BAX are accompanied by mutations in the p53 gene.

A missense mutation in codon 273 of the p53 gene can dramatically decrease the BAX levels in the cell (22). In breast cancer, mutational analysis of the BAX and p53 gene did identify mutations of the p53 gene but no mutations of BAX except for a G → A polymorphism at exon 6, position 552, in all individuals (23). In lung cancers, BAX is localized in the nucleus, and this positional translocation must be the tumor-causing effect. However, mutational analysis of the gene in lung cancers revealed the presence of only the same silent point mutation in codon 184 (TCG → TCA) and some intronic mutations that do not affect the transmembrane domain of the protein (24). Frameshift mutations of BAX gene have been detected in T-cells of acute lymphoblastic leukemia and in endometrium. There are two characteristic missense mutations in codon 169 (Thr → Ala or Thr → Met) in gastrointestinal cancers. These mutations are functional and therefore they inhibit the pro-apoptotic activity of the protein contributing to carcinogenesis (25).

A splicing variant of BAX gene, BAX-sigma (lacking amino acids 159 to 171 compared to BAX-alpha), is widely expressed in human cancer pro-myelocytic cells and in a variety of other human cancer cell lines (26). Chemotherapeutic treatment aims at up-regulation of the BAX gene to block tumor progression. For example, all the anthracycline group of chemotherapeutic agents fight cancer via the enhancement of BAX expression (27). The potent tumor-suppressing activity of this protein is now used for therapeutic purposes. Transfected adenoviral systems that overexpress the BAX protein are used to infect the target tumors in many types of cancer such as prostate and ovarian cancer and gliomas.

The BCL-X Gene

BCL-X is involved in various cancers. The gene undergoes alternative splicing and to date three different splicing variants have been identified. BCL-X(S) derives from splicing of the second exon while the large protein BCL-X(L) encodes the exons 2,3. These two proteins display striking functional and expressional differences. Thus, while the large transcript BCL-X(L) is anti-apoptotic and it is expressed mainly in long-lived cells, such as the cells of the nervous system, the smaller protein BCL-X(S) is expressed in cells with high rate of turnover such as the cells of immune system; it provokes apoptosis via binding to the hydrophobic pocket of BCL-2 or BCL-X(L) to inhibit their anti-apoptotic activity. Another splicing variant called BCL-X gamma has been found to be connected to the T-cell receptors (28).

BCL-X gene is widely detected in a variety of human malignancies, including lymphoma and colon, breast, and ovarian cancer (29). Human acute T lymphocytic leukemia (ATLL) is developed after infection by the human T lymphotropic virus type I (HTLV-I) and II (HTLV-II). The Tax1 and Tax2 transactivators of HTLV-I and II increase the transcription of BCL-X(L) and therefore are responsible for the development of the disease (30). In breast carcinoma cells, the excessive concentration of BCL-X(L) and BCL-2 inhibits the protective action of the tumor necrosis factor (TNF) (31). The down-regulation of BCL-X(L) is in close relationship with c-myb expression and represents a useful prognostic marker in colorectal carcinoma (32).

The BAK Gene

BAK is down-regulated in cancerous conditions. Missence mutations in BAK gene can explain this down-regulation in a proportion of gastrointestinal malignancies (33). Proteolytic degradation of BAK is associated with some other types of malignancies. Indeed, the main course for the development of skin cancer is the proteolytic degradation of BAK by the human papillovirus (HPV) protein E6 (34). Thus, the protein is unable to respond to UV, resulting in the death of damaged cells. Like BAX, adenoviral-mediated overexpression of BAK can be used as a treatment for the targeted malignant cells (35,36).

RECENTLY IDENTIFIED APOPTOSIS-RELATED GENES IN CANCER

BCL-2L12, a new member of the BCL-2 gene family of apoptosis-regulating genes, has recently been identified (14). The novel gene encodes a BCL-2-like proline rich protein. Proline-rich sites have been shown to interact with Src homology region 3 (SH3) domains of several tyrosine kinases, mediating their oncogenic potential. This new gene maps to chromosome 19q13.3 and is located between the IRF3 and PRMT1/HRMT1L2 genes, close to the R-ras gene. BCL-2L12 was found to bind the BCL-X(L) protein and to be expressed mainly in breast, thymus, prostate, fetal liver, colon, placenta, pancreas, small intestine, spinal cord, kidney, bone marrow, and, to a lesser extent, in many other tissues. One splice variant of the BCL-2L12, which is primarily expressed in skeletal muscle, has also been identified. Preliminary results show that BCL-2L12 variants are expressed in normal breast and testis, but their expression is highly variable in breast and testicular cancer tissues (14).

BAD (BCL-X(L)/BCL-2 associated death promoter) is a pro-apoptotic protein that has been initially detected because of its propensity to interact with the anti apoptotic proteins BCL-X(L) and BCL-2. BAD is regulated via phosphorylation/dephosphorylation, the dephosphorylated form being the active form. Only the dephosphorylated form of the molecule can mediate apoptosis via interaction with BCL-X(L). The lack of BAD/BCL-2 heterodimerization in colorectal and other types of cancer is due to its hyperphosphorylation, which was observed in a variety of malignant cell lines (37). Since the phosphorylated form of the protein is sequestered in the cytosol as a complex with the 14-3-3 protein, it is unable to prevent the tissues from excessive growth.

BCL-W is an anti-apoptotic molecule widely expressed in all tissues. Since BCL-W contains the conserved domains 1–4, it can interact with other proteins of the family to modulate apoptosis. BCL-W co-immunoprecipitates with BAX, BAD, BAK, and BIK (38). BCL-W triggers cell survival, preventing the release of cytochrome c. Its gene locates on human chromosome 14q11. Recently it has been shown that the proto-oncogene c-met modulates the expression of BCL-W, inhibiting apoptotic death in colorectal cancer (39).

A1/BFL-1, an anti-apoptotic protein, displays a high degree of similarity to the BH1 and BH2 domains. A1/BFL-1 suppresses apoptosis that is induced by the p53 tumor suppressor. The gene is also up-regulated by the Epstein-Barr virus LMP-1 and promotes the proliferation of lymphoma cells (40). Furthermore, the protein co-operates with *ela* oncogene in epithelial cells causing carcinogenesis. There is evidence of the involvement of A1/BFL-1 in stomach cancer development, hemopoietic malignancies, and melanoma (41).

The use of biomarkers as a tool to predict induction of apoptosis allows identification of biological signs that may indicate increased risk for disease (Table 1). The common methods

Table 1 Apoptosis-related genes in cancer

Gene	Activity of protein	Prognostic value	Reference
BCL-2	Anti-apoptotic	Unfavorable prognostic marker in various cancers	16–20
BAX	Pro-apoptotic	Favorable prognostic marker in various cancers	21–27
BCL-X	Anti-apoptotic	Unfavorable prognostic marker in lymphoma, colorectal, breast, and ovarian cancer.	28–32
BAK	Pro-apoptotic	Down-regulated in gastrointestinal malignancies	33–36
BAD	Pro-apoptotic	Down-regulated in colorectal cancer	10, 37
BCL-W	Anti-apoptotic	Inhibits the apoptotic death in colorectal cancer	39
A1/BFL-1	Anti-apoptotic	Up-regulated in stomach cancer, hemopoietic malignancies, and melanoma	40–41

used to monitor DNA fragmentation and cell morphology as markers of apoptosis have numerous advantages and disadvantages. Growing knowledge of the signaling events that occur during cell death has established the caspases and their regulating proteins as the central cause of apoptosis. Direct monitoring of apoptotic gene events as markers of apoptosis offers advantages over existing assay methods. Recently, several new marker antibodies have been developed that detect proteins of the apoptotic gene family. The clinical use of these molecules for cancer diagnosis, prognosis, monitoring, chemoprevention, and gene therapy targets may be anticipated in the near future.

REFERENCES

1. Saikumar P, Dong Z, Mikhailov V, Denton M, Weinberg JM, Venkatachalam MA. Apoptosis: definition, mechanisms, and relevance to disease. Am J Med 1999;107:489–506.
2. Gruss HJ, Dower SK. Tumor necrosis factor ligand superfamily: involvement in the pathology of malignant lymphomas. Blood 1995;85:3378–3404.
3. Chinnaiyan AM, O'Rourke K, Tewari M, Dixit VM. FADD, a novel death-domain-containing protein, interacts with the death domain of Fas and initiates apoptosis. Cell 1995;81:505–512.
4. Yuan J, Shaham S, Ledoux S, Ellis HM, Horvitz HR. The C. elegans cell death gene ced-3 encodes a protein similar to mammalian interleukin-1 beta-converting enzyme. Cell 1993;75:641–652.
5. Thornberry NA, Lazebnik Y. Caspases: enemies within. Science 1998;281:1312–1316.
6. Wilson KP, Black JA, Thomson JA, Kim EE, Griffith JP, Navia MA, Murcko MA, Chambers SP, Aldape RA, Raybuck SA, et al. Structure and mechanism of interleukin-1 beta-converting enzyme. Nature 1994;370:270–275.
7. Miller LK. An exegesis of IAPs: salvation and surprises from BIR motifs. Trends Cell Biol 1999;9:323–328.
8. Deveraux QL, Roy N, Stennicke HR, Van Arsdale T, Zhou Q, Srinivasula SM, Alnemri ES, Salvesen GS, Reed JC. IAPs block apoptotic events induced by caspase-8 and cytochrome c by direct inhibition of distinct caspases. Embo J 1998;17:2215–2223.
9. Reed JC. Mechanisms of apoptosis. Am J Pathol 2000;157:1415–1430.
10. Mullauer L, Gruber P, Sebinger D, Buch J, Wohlfart S, Chott A. Mutations in apoptosis genes: a pathogenetic factor for human disease. Mutat Res 2001;488:211–231.
11. Evan GI, Vousden KH. Proliferation, cell cycle, and apoptosis in cancer. Nature 2001;411:342–348.
12. Gharavi AG, Yan Y, Scolari F, Schena FP, Frasca GM, Ghiggeri GM, Cooper K, Amoroso A, Viola BF, Battini G, Caridi G, Canova C, Farhi A, Subramanian V, Nelson-Williams C, Woodford S, Julian BA, Wyatt RJ, Lifton RP. IgA nephropathy, the most common cause of glomerulonephritis, is linked to 6q22–23. Nat Genet 2000;26:354–347.
13. Tan KO, Tan KM, Chan SL, Yee KS, Bevort M, Ang KC, Yu VC. MAP-1, a novel pro-apoptotic protein containing a BH3-like motif that associates with Bax through its Bcl-2 homology domains. J Biol Chem 2001;276:2802–2807.
14. Scorilas A, Kyriakopoulou L, Yousef GM, Ashworth LK, Kwamie A, Diamandis EP. Molecular cloning, physical mapping, and expression analysis of a novel gene, BCL-2L12, encoding a proline-rich protein with a highly conserved BH2 domain of the Bcl-2 family. Genomics 2001;72:217–221.
15. Oltvai ZN, Korsmeyer SJ. Checkpoints of dueling dimers foil death wishes. Cell 1994;79:189–192.
16. Katsumata M, Siegel RM, Louie DC, Miyashita T, Tsujimoto Y, Nowell PC, Greene MI, Reed JC. Differential effects of Bcl-2 on T and B cells in transgenic mice. Proc Natl Acad Sci USA 1992;89:11376–11380.
17. Fontanini G, Vignati S, Bigini D, Mussi A, Lucchi M, Angeletti CA, Basolo F, Bevilacqua G. Bcl-2 protein: a prognostic factor inversely correlated to p53 in non-small-cell lung cancer. Br J Cancer 1995;71:1003–1007.
18. Ramsay JA, From L, Kahn HJ. Bcl-2 protein expression in melanocytic neoplasms of the skin. Mod Pathol 1995;8:150–154.
19. Laudanski J, Chyczewski L, Niklinska WE, Kretowska M, Furman M, Sawicki B, Niklinski J. Expression of bcl-2 protein in non-small-cell lung cancer: correlation with clinicopathology and patient survival. Neoplasma 1999;46:25–30.
20. Campos L, Rouault JP, Sabido O, Oriol P, Roubi N, Vasselon C, Archimbaud E, Magaud JP, Guyotat D. High expression of bcl-2 protein in acute myeloid leukemia cells is associated with poor response to chemotherapy. Blood 1993;81:3091–3096.
21. Knudson CM, Johnson GM, Lin Y, Korsmeyer SJ. Bax accelerates tumorigenesis in p53-deficient mice. Cancer Res 2001;61:659–665.
22. Kaneuchi M, Yamashita T, Shindoh M, Segawa K, Takahashi S, Furuta I, Fujimoto S, Fujinaga K. Induction of apoptosis by the p53-273L (Arg→Leu) mutant in HSC3 cells without transactivation of p21Waf1/Cip1/Sdi1 and bax. Mol Carcinog 1999;26:44–52.

23. Sturm I, Papadopoulos S, Hillebrand T, Benter T, Luck HJ, Wolff G, Dorken B, Daniel PT. Impaired BAX protein expression in breast cancer: mutational analysis of the BAX and the p53 gene. Int J Cancer 2000;87:517–521.
24. Salah-eldin A, Inoue S, Tsuda M, Matsuura A. Abnormal intracellular localization of bax with a normal membrane anchor domain in human lung cancer cell lines. Jpn J Cancer Res 2000; 91:1269–1277.
25. Gil J, Yamamoto H, Zapata JM, Reed JC, Perucho M. Impairment of the pro-apoptotic activity of bax by missense mutations found in gastrointestinal cancers. Cancer Res 1999;59:2034–2037.
26. Schmitt E, Paquet C, Beauchemin M, Dever-Bertrand J, Bertrand R. Characterization of bax-sigma, a cell-death-inducing isoform of bax. Biochem Biophys Res Commun 2000;270:868–879.
27. Lu Y, Yagi T. Apoptosis of human tumor cells by chemotherapeutic anthracyclines is enhanced by bax overexpression. J Radiat Res (Tokyo) 1999;40:263–272.
28. Yang XF, Weber GF, Cantor H. A novel Bcl-x isoform connected to the T-cell receptor regulates apoptosis in T cells. Immunity 1997;7:629–639.
29. MacCarthy-Morrogh L, Wood L, Brimmell M, Johnson PW, Packham G. Identification of a novel human BCL-X promoter and exon. Oncogene 2000;19:5534–5538.
30. Nicot C, Mahieux R, Takemoto S, Franchini G. Bcl-X(L) is up-regulated by HTLV-I and HTLV-II in vitro and in ex vivo ATLL samples. Blood 2000;96:275–281.
31. Jaattela M, Benedict M, Tewari M, Shayman JA, Dixit VM. Bcl-x and Bcl-2 inhibit TNF and Fas-induced apoptosis and activation of phospholipase A2 in breast carcinoma cells. Oncogene 1995; 10:2297–2305.
32. Biroccio A, Benassi B, D'Agnano I, D'Angelo C, Buglioni S, Mottolese M, Ricciotti A, Citro G, Cosimelli M, Ramsay RG, Calabretta B, Zupi G. c-Myb and Bcl-x overexpression predicts poor prognosis in colorectal cancer: clinical and experimental findings. Am J Pathol 2001;158:1289–1299.
33. Kondo S, Shinomura Y, Miyazaki Y, Kiyohara T, Tsutsui S, Kitamura S, Nagasawa Y, Nakahara M, Kanayama S, Matsuzawa Y. Mutations of the bak gene in human gastric and colorectal cancers. Cancer Res 2000;60:4328-4330.
34. Jackson S, Harwood C, Thomas M, Banks L, Storey A. Role of bak in UV-induced apoptosis in skin cancer and abrogation by HPV E6 proteins. Genes Dev 2000;14:3065–3073.
35. Pataer A, Fang B, Yu R, Kagawa S, Hunt KK, McDonnell TJ, Roth JA, Swisher SG. Adenoviral bak overexpression mediates caspase-dependent tumor killing. Cancer Res 2000;60:788–792.
36. Pearson AS, Spitz FR, Swisher SG, Kataoka M, Sarkiss MG, Meyn RE, McDonnell TJ, Cristiano RJ, Roth JA. Up-regulation of the pro-apoptotic mediators bax and bak after adenovirus-mediated p53 gene transfer in lung cancer cells. Clin Cancer Res 2000; 6:887–890.
37. Kitada S, Krajewska M, Zhang X, Scudiero D, Zapata JM, Wang HG, Shabaik A, Tudor G, Krajewski S, Myers TG, Johnson GS, Sausville EA, Reed JC. Expression and location of pro-apoptotic Bcl-2 family protein BAD in normal human tissues and tumor cell lines. Am J Pathol 1998;152:51–61.
38. Holmgreen SP, Huang DC, Adams JM, Cory S. Survival activity of Bcl-2 homologs Bcl-w and A1 only partially correlates with their ability to bind pro-apoptotic family members. Cell Death Differ 1999;6:525–532.
39. Kitamura S, Kondo S, Shinomura Y, Kanayama S, Miyazaki Y, Kiyohara T, Hiraoka S, Matsuzawa Y. Met/HGF receptor modulates bcl-w expression and inhibits apoptosis in human colorectal cancers. Br J Cancer 2000;83:668–673.
40. D'Souza B, Rowe M, Walls D. The bfl-1 gene is transcriptionally upregulated by the Epstein-Barr virus LMP1, and its expression promotes the survival of a Burkitt's lymphoma cell line. J Virol 2000;74:6652–6658.
41. Kenny JJ, Knobloch TJ, Augustus M, Carter KC, Rosen CA, Lang JC. GRS, a novel member of the Bcl-2 gene family, is highly expressed in multiple cancer cell lines and in normal leukocytes. Oncogene 1997;14:997–1001.

Chapter 55

Telomerase

Evi Lianidou

In recent years, research on the role of telomerase in human carcinogenesis has grown exponentially. Today, a very strong association between telomerase activation and malignancy has been established, making this enzyme one of the most promising tumor markers and targets for cancer therapy (1).

Telomeres are specialized structures, found at the termini of eukaryotic chromosomes, that are composed of hexameric nucleotide repeats and associated proteins. Telomeres are essential for maintaining chromosomal integrity, since they protect against random fusion events and degradation. However, telomeric DNA is lost during each successive cell division because of the inability of the normal DNA replication system to overcome loss of terminal RNA primers. It is believed that such telomere shortening acts as a mitotic clock that records the replicative history and sets a finite life span for normal somatic cells. This continual loss of telomeric sequence eventually reduces the production of viable cells, due to genomic instability. Telomerase activation is the main mechanism presently known that compensates for this telomeric loss (2).

Telomerase is a cellular ribonucleoprotein reverse transcriptase that synthesizes telomeric DNA onto chromosomal ends, using a segment of its own RNA as a template. Two main components are required for core enzymatic activity of telomerase in vitro: human telomerase RNA (hTR), which contains the template for reverse transcription, and human telomerase reverse transcriptase (hTERT), which consists of the enzyme's catalytic subunit. hTR is expressed in both telomerase-negative and telomerase-positive cells and is not a rate-limiting unit of telomerase activity, while on the contrary, expression of the functional hTERT protein is a prerequisite for acquisition of telomerase activity (3).

In humans, telomerase is active during embryonic development but becomes repressed in most somatic cells before or shortly after birth. Germline cells express telomerase while most somatic cells, regardless of their rate of proliferation, undergo a steady rate of telomere loss and do not possess detectable telomerase activity. In contrast, all immortal cells examined to date show no loss of telomere length or sequence with cell division, suggesting that maintainance of a critical telomere length threshold, provided by telomerase activation, is required for cells to escape from replicative senescence and proliferate indefinitely (4).

Many recent studies provide evidence for a direct role of telomerase in early oncogenic transformation. Activation of telomerase is the most common mechanism through which cancer cells stabilize their telomere size and subsequent sustain their infinite growth (4). Moreover, telomerase activation was recently shown to have an additional protective function that allows cell proliferation without requiring net lengthening of telomeres (5). A recent breakthrough—the in vitro malignant transformation of normal human cells—was achieved by reconstitution of telomerase activity (by induction of hTERT gene expression) in combination with other oncogenes (6).

CLINICAL APPLICATIONS

Interest in the potential application of telomerase as a diagnostic and prognostic tumor marker is growing steadily. This stems from the observation that greater than 85% of most human tumors express telomerase activity, whereas most healthy tissues don't, the only exception being germ line cells and activated lymphocytes (7,8).

The development of the sensitive "telomeric repeat amplification protocol" (TRAP) assay by Kim et al. (4), in which the telomerase-synthesized DNA products are amplified by a subsequent polymerase chain reaction (PCR), enabled the wide screening of many clinical samples for the presence of telomerase activity. Recently, the observation that functional hTERT protein is critical for acquisition of telomerase activity has led to the wide application of hTERT mRNA determination through standard RT-PCR procedures for the identification of telomerase-positive samples.

Essentially all major types of cancer have been screened for the presence of telomerase activity and hTERT mRNA in a variety of clinical specimens (7). Determination of telomerase activity or hTERT mRNA can be useful for early detection of cancer, early detection of micrometastasis, and prognosis.

It is now widely accepted that telomerase activity is only present in cells of somatic origin if they have become immortally transformed and are therefore neoplastic, the only exception being activated T-lymphocytes (8). Telomerase activity was recently shown to be a useful tumor marker of breast carcinoma in fine-needle aspirates (FNAs), and the diagnostic accuracy of this assay was found to be equivalent or slightly higher to that of cytology (86% vs. 70%). Detection of telomerase activity should be considered an alert for false-negative results of FNA cytology and may be useful as a diagnostic marker for breast malignancy, especially in samples cytologically undetermined to be malignant (9).

The presence of telomerase activity in the peripheral blood of cancer patients can be an early indication of circulating tumor cells and micrometastasis, since peripheral mononuclear cells from healthy individuals have very low levels of telomerase activity in comparison to tumor cells. This appears to be a sensitive, specific, and noninvasive approach for detecting circulating epithelial cancer cells in patients with metastatic breast cancer and could be of great value in monitoring the cancer cell proliferation during chemotherapy (10).

There are indications that telomerase activity levels might parallel tumor progression and be of prognostic relevance in neuroblastoma (11). Telomerase activity has proved to be a useful marker for the early detection of cancer in specimens obtained by relatively non-invasive procedures such as urine or bladder washings (12). Detection of hTERT mRNA is useful for cytological screening of cervical cancer, since it is expressed in more than 80% of cervical cancers, while it is not expressed in either normal cervical tissues or in normal primary fibroblast cells (13). hTERT mRNA also may be a useful marker for ovarian cancer diagnosis, since it is detected in more than 80% of ovarian tumors, but is not expressed in the normal ovary, in ovarian cysts, or in early stages of ovary malignancies (14).

In general, measurement of telomerase activity or hTERT expression has high potential for discriminating between healthy and tumor cells in a variety of biological specimens such as peripheral blood, tissues, fine-needle aspirates, and urine and bladder washings. This supports future measurements in pancreatic fluid and esophageal brushings; in this way, cancer can be detected in specimens obtained by relatively non-invasive procedures (12).

FUTURE DIRECTIONS

The development of simple, sensitive, and specific analytical methodology for the quantitative determination of telomerase activity and hTERT mRNA is important for the establishment of telomerase as a general tumor marker.

To date, many limitations concerning the quantitative determination of telomerase activity by the electrophoretic and ELISA-based TRAP assays have been reported (15). The analysis of telomerase activity by the TRAP assay requires enzymatically active specimens and RNA analysis conditions at the same time. This requirement poses serious limitations in the handling of many clinical samples on a routine basis and more importantly is highly affected by the presence of protein activity inhibitors, proteases, or RNAses in clinical samples. Moreover, most of the quantitative methods for telomerase activity reported so far make use of DNA internal standards. These may differ significantly in respect to size and sequence from telomerase products and are mostly suitable for the identification of false negative results due to the presence of PCR inhibitors in tissues and not for an absolute quantitative determination of telomerase activity (16–18). Recently, a quantitative luminometric hybridization assay for telomerase activity, based on the use of a specially designed DNA-IS, has been reported (19).

The hTERT mRNA RT-PCR assay is insensitive to the presence of proteases and protein inhibitors. The inclusion of an endogenous control normalizes the hTERT expression for cDNA input and assay affectors. However, in most studies reported so far, determination of hTERT mRNA is based on conventional RT-PCR qualitative electrophoretic methods that are time-consuming and not suitable for a large number of clinical samples. The recent development of semi-automated quantitative RT-PCR assays for the determination of hTERT mRNA, based on the real time PCR methodology, is a very important step towards automation and clinical applications of telomerase assays (12,20). However, even in this case, post-transcriptional regulatory mechanisms controlling the activity of telomerase and especially alternative splicing of hTERT transcripts must be seriously taken into account, so that the amplified region of hTERT mRNA by RT-PCR will include the full active hTERT transcript (21).

SUMMARY

The enhanced analytical sensitivity and specificity of last-generation telomerase assays in combination with studies in a larger number of patients will determine the clinical specificity and sensitivity of this promising universal tumor marker. However, despite the fact that promising correlations between telomerase and cancer have been reported, a further understanding of the dynamics of telomerase and tumorigenesis is needed before a clinically useful profile of telomerase can be established for diagnostic, therapeutic, and prognostic applications.

REFERENCES

1. O' Reilly M, Teichmann SA, Rhodes D. Telomerases. Curr Opin Struct Biol 1999;9:56–65.
2. Campisi J. The biology of replicative senescence. Eur J Cancer 1997;33:703–709.
3. Nakamura T, Gregg MB, et al. Telomerase catalytic subunit homologs from fission yeast and human. Science 1997;277:955–959.
4. Kim NW, Piatyscetc MA, et al. Specific association of human telomerase activity with immortal cells and cancer. Science 1994;266:2011–2015.
5. Zhu J, Wang H, Bishop JM, Blackburn EH. Telomerase extends the lifespan of virus-transformed human cells without net telomere lengthening. Proc Natl Acad Sci USA 1999;96:3723–3728.
6. Hahn WC, Counter CM, Lundberg AS, Beijersbergen RL, Brooks MW, Weinberg RA. Creation of human tumor cells with defined genetic elements. Nature 1999;400:464–468.
7. Shay JW, Bacchetti S. A survey of telomerase activity in human cancer. Eur J Cancer 1997;33:787–791.
8. Liu K, Schoonmaker MM, Levine BL, June JH, Hodes RJ, Weng NP. Constitutive and regulated expression of telomerase reverse transcriptase (hTERT) in human lymphocytes. Proc Natl Acad Sci USA 1999;96:5147–5152.
9. Hiyama E, Saeki T, Hiyama K, Takashima S, Shay JW, et al. Telomerase activity as a marker of breast carcinoma in fine-needle aspirated samples. Cancer 2000;90:235–238.

10. Soria JC, Gauthier LR, Raymond E, Granotie C, Morat L, et al. Molecular detection of telomerase-positive circulating epithelial cells in metastatic breast cancer patients. Clin Cancer Res 1999; 5:971–975.
11. Hiyama E, Hiyama K, Yokoyama T, Matsuura Y, Piatyszek MA, Shay JW. Correlating telomerase activity levels with human neuroblastoma outcomes. Nat Med 1995;1:249–255.
12. de Kok JB, Ruers TJM, van Muijen GNP, van Bokhoven A, Willens HL, Swinkels DW. Real-time quantification of human telomerase reverse transcriptase mRNA in tumors and healthy tissues. Clin Chem 2000;46:313–318.
13. Takakura M, Kyo S, Kanaya T, Tanaka M, Inoue M. Expression of human telomerase subunits and correlation with telomerase activity in cervical cancer. Cancer Res 1998;58:1558–1561.
14. Kyo S, Kanaya T, Takakura M, Tanaka M, et al. Expression of human telomerase subunits in ovarian malignant, borderline, and benign tumors. Int J Cancer 1999;80:804–809.
15. Wu Y, Hruszkewycz A, Delgado R, et al. Limitations on the quantitative determination of telomerase activity by the electrophoretic and ELISA-based TRAP assays. Clin Chim Acta 2000;293:199–212.
16. Kim NW, Wu F. Advances in quantification and characterization of telomerase activity by the telomeric repeat amplification protocol (TRAP). Nucleic Acids Res 1997;25:2595–2597.
17. Hirose M, Hashimote J, et al. New method to measure telomerase activity by transcription-mediated amplification and hybridization protection assay. Clin Chem 1998;44:2446–2452.
18. Nakamura Y, Hirose M. Simple, rapid, quantitative and sensitive detection of telomere repeats in cell lysate by a hybridization protection assay. Clin Chem 1999;45:1718–1724.
19. Kolioliou M, Talieri M, Lianidou ES. Development of a quantitative luminometric hybridization assay for the determination of telomerase activity. Clin Biochem 2001;34:277–284.
20. Bieche I, Nogues C, Paradis V, Olivi M, Bedossa P, et al. Quantification of hTERT gene expression in sporadic breast tumors with a real time reverse transcription polymerase chain reaction assay. Clin Cancer Res 2000;6:452–459.
21. Ulaner GA, Hu JF, Vu TH, Giudice LC, Hoffmann AR. Telomerase activity in human development is regulated by human telomerase reverse transcriptase (hTERT) transcription and by alternate splicing of hTERT transcripts. Cancer Res 1998;58:4168–4172.

Chapter 56

Single Nucleotide Polymorphism (SNP) Genotyping by Probe Melting Curve Analysis

Carl T. Wittwer, Philip S. Bernard, Andrew O. Crockett, Sandra D. Bohling, and Kojo S.J. Elenitoba-Johnson

Cancer is an acquired genetic disease. Often, more than one genetic hit is necessary before a cell escapes control and the clinical phenotype of cancer is recognized. The Cancer Genome Anatomy Project of the National Cancer Institute is one effort to catalog genetic changes related to cancer (1). Many of the responsible sequence alterations are single nucleotide polymorphisms (SNPs). In a SNP, only a single base change occurs, often resulting in an amino acid change or truncation of the translated protein. For example, most cancer-causing mutations in tumor suppressor genes (*p53*, *BRCA1*, and *BRCA2*), and oncogenes (*ras*, *myc*) are SNPs.

Many techniques are available to genotype SNPs. These range from highly parallel analysis on microarrays to rapid turn-around systems for clinical diagnostics. Some of the methods are highly automated and designed for high-throughput analysis (2). The SNP market is extremely competitive and many platforms are available. Yet the simpler the system, the better. Completely automated systems are attractive. Homogeneous methods that do not require liquid transfer after the input of sample DNA are even better. Real-time methods, such as real-time PCR, achieve this level of simplicity (3).

Even when the scope of SNP methods is limited to real-time PCR, there are many options. Most real-time methods use probes, often dual-labeled probes with a fluorescent dye and a quencher. One probe is required for each allele analyzed. This requires either two tubes for each locus, or the two probes are labeled with different reporter dyes that can be discriminated. When an unexpected allele is encountered, errors often occur (4).

An alternative real-time analysis strategy is popular in clinical diagnostics. This method uses melting curve analysis to interrogate genetic polymorphisms such as SNPs. It was first applied to Factor V Leiden (5). A detection probe with only one label is added before amplification; then PCR is performed and a melting curve acquired. The technique can be thought of as a "dynamic" dot blot. Instead of a "static" dot blot (equilibrium hybridization at a single temperature), probe melting is monitored through a range of temperatures by fluorescence. Different alleles melt at different temperatures that can be predicted by thermodynamics (6). Multiple alleles can be distinguished by using only a single color, simplifying the analysis, and compounding the depth of multiplexing possible (7).

The fluorescence of the detection probe is typically augmented by resonance energy transfer (3,5,7). This was first achieved by labeling one primer with a resonance energy transfer acceptor and annealing the detection probe with a fluorescence donor near this primer (5). Today, it is more common to use an "anchor" probe next to the detection probe. The anchor probe is more stable than the detection probe, so that it remains annealed during the melting transition of the detection probe. The anchor probe is labeled with either the donor or acceptor dye. The detection probe is labeled with the complementary dye and covers the region of sequence variation. An example of this adjacent hybridization probe design is shown in Figure 1A.

CLINICAL APPLICATION

Ras is a proto-oncogene family of proteins that is mutated in approximately 30% of human cancers (8). Most mutations are point mutations. In N-ras, codons 12, 13, and 61 are most frequently altered by a single base change. Many different N-ras mutations can be detected and/or distinguished by melting curve analysis with a single mutation probe (9). For example, the melting curve analysis shown in Figure 1 distinguishes 4 different alleles (wild type + 3 mutant sequences) varying at a single base position. Different mismatches often have different stabilities that are easily predicted by nearest-neighbor thermodynamics (6). In general, any variant that destabilizes the probe can be detected. In addition, some but not all destabilizing variants can be distinguished from each other. For example, an unexpected sequence variant that resulted in false-positives with TaqMan probes was distinguished from other alleles by melting temperature when hybridization probes were used (4).

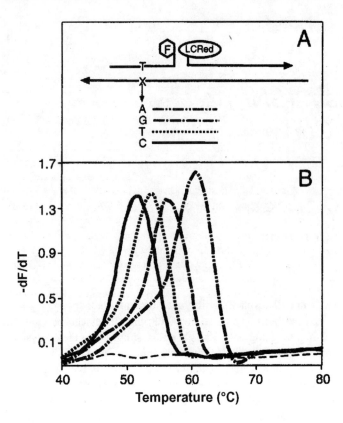

Figure 1 N-ras genotyping by melting curve analysis. (A) Design of adjacent hybridization probes for discrimination of different N-ras mutations. A fluorescein-labeled donor probe includes codons 12 and 13. A more stable "anchor" probe is labeled with LCRed640. When both probes are hybridized, resonance energy transfer occurs between fluorescein (F) and LCRed640, resulting in increased emission of LCRed 640. The PCR template contained 1 of 4 possible bases at position "X." (B) When plotted on a derivative melting curve plot (–dF/dT), each allele appears as a single peak. The perfectly matched allele melted at 60.9 °C, the T:G mismatch at 56.4 °C, the T:T mismatch at 53.8 °C, and the T:C mismatch at 51.5 °C. See (9) for experimental conditions.

In Figure 1, the base changes are homozygous and alleles that differ by about 0.1 °C can be distinguished. However, when an SNP is heterozygous, 50% of each allele is present and the melting curve has two transitions (6). Using standard equipment and software (3,7), heterozygotes produce two clear melting peaks only if their melting temperatures differ by greater than 2–3 °C. For bi-allelic SNPs, probes can always be designed (by choosing the probe strand and the allele match) so that the differences are greater. However, when two alleles are both mismatched to a probe, the peaks may not separate if their melting temperatures are within 2–3 °C. In this case, more sophisticated algorithms are required to identify and quantify the contribution of each allele.

A common problem in molecular oncology is to detect a sequence alteration when it is present in only a small fraction of the tissue. In dilution studies with hybridization probes, melting curves, and custom software, about 1% of a known allele can be detected in the presence of a dominant allele.

Recently, a method that does not require a resonance energy transfer donor for probe melting analysis of SNPs was published (10). Only one probe labeled with fluorescein is necessary for real-time SNP typing. The probes are designed so that fluorescein hybridizes near to one or more deoxyguanosine residues quenching the fluorescence with hybridization. Instead of two dual-labeled or two single-labeled probes, only one fluorescein-labeled probe is necessary for complete typing of a SNP. Typical SNP genotyping by melting curve analysis is shown in Figure 2.

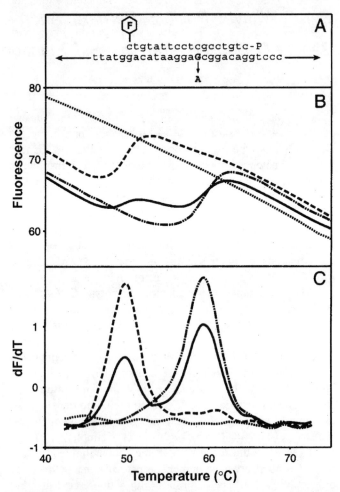

Figure 2 Real-time SNP typing with a simple fluorescein-labeled probe. (A) The 5'-fluorescein-labeled probe was designed so that when hybridization occurs, the fluorescein (F) is approximated to one or more deoxyguanosine residues. The probe is blocked from extension by a 3'-phosphate and covers the SNP, Factor V Leiden. (B) When the probe is hybridized at low temperature, the fluorescein is quenched by deoxyguanosine residues. If the mismatched allele is present, the probe melts at around 50 °C and the fluorescence increases as the influence of the deoxyguanosine is released. An additional increase in fluorescence occurs at about 60 °C if the perfectly matched allele is present. (C) When plotted as a derivative melting curve, each allele corresponds to a peak. All possible genotypes are shown (dash-dot-dot, homozygous wild type; solid, heterozygous Factor V Leiden; dashes, homozygous Factor V Leiden; dots, no template control). Note that the direction of fluorescence change is the opposite of that in Figure 1 (dF/dT vs. –dF/dT). See (10) for experimental details.

FUTURE DIRECTIONS

The ability to follow hybridization over a range of temperatures provides a more robust and accurate assessment of probe:target hybridization than methods that look at only one temperature. Some real-time techniques for SNP analysis are similar to conventional dot blots in that discrimination between different alleles is based on analysis at a single temperature. With the right probes, dynamic hybridization data are readily obtained on today's real-time instruments. This allows multiplexing by melting temperature in addition to dye color. Both color and melting temperature analysis can be combined, providing a two-dimensional matrix for higher-order multiplexing, a virtual "solution array."

Complex enzymatic or resonance energy transfer methods that use dual-labeled probes are not necessary for real-time SNP typing. Single-labeled probes change fluorescence when they hybridize and allow genotyping by melting curve analysis. Depending on the probe, fluorescence may decrease or increase with hybridization. The dexoyguanosine quenching shown in Figure 2 is an example of decreasing fluorescence. In contrast, an increase in fluorescence may occur with a probe that has fluorescein attached to a G residue on the probe (10).

In general, the fluorescence of any labeled probe is expected to change upon hybridization. Today's sensitive instruments can detect these changes. Different dyes in addition to fluorescein can be used for multiplexing. The probe design and experimental conditions (pH, ionic strength) can be modified to change the magnitude and direction of the change in fluorescence that occurs with hybridization.

REFERENCES

1. Riggins GJ, RL Strausberg. Genome and genetic resources from the Cancer Genome Anatomy Project. Hum Mol Genet 2001; 10:663–667.
2. Shi, MM. Enabling large-scale pharmacogenetic studies by high-throughput mutation detection and genotyping technologies. Clin Chem 2001;47:164–172.
3. Wittwer CT, Kusukawa N. Real-time PCR. In: Persing D, Tenover F, Relman D, White T, Tang Y, Versalovic J, and Unger B, eds. Diagnostic molecular microbiology: principles and applications. Washington, DC: ASM Press, 2002 (In press).
4. Teupser D, Rupprecht W, Lohse P, Thiery J. Fluorescence-based detection of the CETP TaqIB polymorphism: false positives with the TaqMan-based exonuclease assay attributable to a previously unknown gene variant. Clin Chem 2001;47:852–857.
5. Lay MJ, Wittwer CT. Real-time fluorescence genotyping of factor V Leiden during rapid cycle PCR. Clin Chem 1997;43: 2262–2267.
6. von Ahsen N, Wittwer CT, Schutz E. Oligonucleotide melting temperatures under PCR conditions: nearest-neighbor corrections for Mg(2+), deoxynucleotide triphosphate, and dimethyl sulfoxide concentrations with comparison to alternative empirical formulas. Clin Chem 2001;47:1956–1961.
7. Wittwer CT, Herrmann MG, Gundry CN, Elenitoba-Johnson KSJ. Real-time multiplex PCR assays. Methods 2002 (In press).
8. Adjei AA. Ras signaling pathway proteins as therapeutic targets. Curr Pharm Des 2001;7:1581–1594.
9. Elenitoba-Johnson KSJ, Bohling SD, Wittwer CT, King TC. Multiplex PCR by multi-color fluorimetry and fluorescence melting curve analysis. Nature Med 2001;7:249–253.
10. Crockett AO, Wittwer CT. Fluorescein-labeled oligonucleotides for real-time PCR: using the inherent quenching of deoxyguanosine nucleotides. Anal Biochem 2001;290:89–97.

Chapter 57

ProGRP Enables Diagnosis of Small-Cell Lung Cancer

Petra Stieber and Ken Yamaguchi

Worldwide, lung cancer is the most frequent and most deadly malignancy, with continuously growing incidence. Despite many efforts to improve diagnosis and therapy, the five-year-survival rate of lung cancer patients increased only to a low extent during the last few decades and is now around 13%.

Prognosis and therapeutic strategy in lung cancer depend mainly on the extension of the tumor and its histological type. Lung cancer is classified as small-cell lung cancer (SCLC), squamous cell carcinoma, primary adenocarcinoma, and large-cell carcinoma (see also Chapter 24). Small-cell lung cancer accounts for 20–25% of the new cases of bronchogenic carcinoma and differs clinically and biologically due to its neuroendocrine differentiation from the other histological types, which behave similarly concerning prognosis and therapy and thus are pooled into one group as non-small-cell lung cancer (NSCLC). Since the incidence of distant metastases at the time of primary diagnosis is high in SCLC—and these tumors are, in contrast to NSCLC, very sensitive to chemotherapeutic reagents and radiotherapy—primary systemic therapy plays an important role in the management of these patients.

Neuroendocrine markers like neuron-specific enolase (NSE), chromogranin A, synaptophysin, and neural cell adhesion molecule (NCAM) are helpful when used in immunohistochemistry to characterize malignant lung tumors (see Chapter 24). The diagnostic accuracy for SCLC is different for each of these molecules. Like NCAM, NSE and synaptophysin are also expressed in non-small-cell lung tumors and other primary tumors, and chromogranin has a higher specificity but a low sensitivity for SCLC. Neuropeptides like bombesin, which is the amphibian counterpart of the mammalian gut hormone gastrin-releasing peptide (GRP), are known to have superior specificity for the lung and to be often produced by cells of SCLC (1). In addition, GRP is thought to stimulate the growth of SCLC cells and to support the metastatic process by cell-to-cell interactions.

When these neuroendocrine molecules and neuropeptides are released in the blood of patients suffering from SCLC they might serve as serum markers of this malignant disease. NSE has been regarded for many years as the marker of first choice for monitoring the course of this disease and also for supporting diagnosis at primary presentation. Chromogranin A and NCAM were found to have a low sensitivity in serum as compared to NSE. Although GRP was described and isolated for the first time in 1978 (2), it was not possible to measure this molecule in blood in a fast and reproducible way due to its extreme instability (its half-life is about two minutes). Therefore, recombinant ProGRP (31-98), a carboxy-terminal region common to three types of previously cloned human ProGRP-molecules, was synthesized; then a radioimmunoassay (3) and finally an ELISA (4) were developed to measure this more stable precursor of GRP in serum.

The first investigations (3–6) revealed ProGRP's high specificity and sensitivity in serum for small-cell lung cancer, although GRP was described to be present in tumor tissue extracts of NSCLC at a frequency of 17%. These findings indicate that ProGRP is valuable in diagnosis of SCLC. To obtain knowledge of the general pattern of release of ProGRP, we investigated this new marker—following the recommendations of the European Group on Tumor Markers (EGTM)—in a broad variety of benign disorders, including influencing factors and malignant diseases other than lung cancer.

CLINICAL APPLICATION

Diagnostic Specificity of ProGRP (Table 1)

Tumor specificity. Values of ProGRP in healthy individuals range from 1–75 pg/mL. The median of our own investigations is around 10 pg/mL and the 95th percentile is about 20 pg/mL.

In benign diseases (n = 500) the medians vary between 10 and 68 pg/mL. We observed the highest single value of 310 pg/mL in a patient with renal failure. This influencing factor has already been described earlier and must be taken into consideration when ProGRP is used for diagnostic purposes in patients suspected of having cancer and suffering from chronic or acute renal failure.

Patients who have benign gynecological disorders (endometriosis, ovarian cysts) have ProGRP values comparable to those in healthy individuals. Benign disorders of the breast (mastopathy, benign tumors, mastitis); lung (tuberculosis, sarcoidosis, chronic obstructive pulmonary disease, hamartoma,

Table 1 Distribution of serum ProGRP in healthy individuals and patients with various benign and malignant diseases, including lung cancer

Group	N=	Mean (pg/mL)	Median (pg/mL)	95th percentile	Range (pg/mL)	Sensitivity at 95% specificity
Healthy individuals	70	10.6	10.3	23	1.0–30	
Ben. lung dis.	186	22.0	18.0	54	1.0–81	
Ben. urol. dis.	51	43.4	31.5	103	1.0–139	
Renal failure	16	87.9	68.0	313	2.0–313	
BPH	49	41.3	36.3	88	3.7–96	
Ben. gyn. dis.	49	10.5	10.6	23	1.0–33	
Ben. gastro. dis.	65	22.5	20.4	52	2.7–119	
Ben. breast dis.	31	24.1	23.9	39	8.2–45	
Autoimmune dis.	30	24.2	22.3	52	7.4–57	
Infectious dis.	23	41.9	31.3	119	9.4–119	
Colorectal cancer	51	18.1	12.9	54	1.0–101	8
Pancreatic cancer	51	12.8	11.7	26	1.0–55	2
Stomach cancer	51	14.6	12.3	38	1.0–58	2
Hepatocell. cancer	50	17.3	12.2	48	1.7–82	6
Breast cancer	53	17.8	15.2	47	1.4–64	6
Ovarian cancer	50	17.9	12.5	35	1.0–102	6
Prostate cancer	51	30.2	29.0	58	5.7–93	2
Bladder cancer	34	28.5	29.1	44	4.1–48	0
Renal cancer	41	27.7	27.5	52	2.3–72	0
Med. thyroid carc.	24	1461	27.7	17939	2–21655	25
All lung cancer	570	340	21.0	1162	1.0–33099	17
NSCLC	450	70	19.0	53	1.0–14432	5
SCLC	120	1353	182	7519	1.0–33099	64

chronic and acute pneumonia, benign pleural effusions, fibrothorax, pleurisy); and autoimmune diseases (without renal involvement) cause only very slightly elevated levels, up to 80 pg/mL. Benign gastrointesinal disorders (liver cirrhosis, acute or chronic hepatitis, primary biliary cirrhosis, cholelithiasis, cholangitis, acute or chronic pancreatitis, pancreatic cysts, gastritis, colitis ulcer, and Crohn's disease); urological diseases (stones, urinary tract infections, bleedings); and infectious diseases (mainly bacterial infections with significant C-reactive protein release before therapy) showed somewhat higher 95th percentiles and reached ProGRP values up to 140 pg/mL.

The respective cut-off values at 95% specificity were calculated as follows: healthy individuals: 23 pg/mL; benign lung disease 54 pg/mL; benign gynecological disease 23 pg/mL; benign gastrointestinal disease 52 pg/mL, benign urological disease 103 pg/mL; benign breast disease 39 pg/mL.

Organ specificity. ProGRP is obviously not released into the circulation by malignant tumors (all at time of primary diagnosis, without therapy) other than lung cancer. The medians of the different groups investigated are almost comparable to the healthy individuals and the highest values reached (about 100 pg/mL) are even lower than those in benign diseases.

But there is one important exception that must be noted: ProGRP might—in rare cases—reach very high levels in medullary thyroid carcinomas. This fact has already been reported in 1984 by Yamaguchi on the basis of tissue investigations (7) and was confirmed by us during routine analysis of ProGRP.

In non-small-cell lung cancer, the median and 95th percentile of ProGRP values is the same as for benign lung diseases, confirming that there is almost no release in these tumors. But in single cases of NSCLC there might be a significant release of ProGRP up to >10,000 pg/mL. One must be aware that the "golden standard" histology is not always 100% correct and depends on the number of sections of the tumor that are examined. In small-cell lung cancer the median (182 pg/mL) and 95th percentile (7,519 pg/mL) are significantly elevated and more than 20% of SCLC patients exhibit serum ProGRP values exceeding 10-fold the cut-off for benign lung diseases.

Diagnostic Sensitivity and Specificity/Sensitivity Profile of ProGRP

Depending on the cut-off value and also on the distribution of tumor stages, ProGRP was described in the literature to possess a sensitivity between 47% and 86% (1,5,6,8–10) for small-cell lung cancer. In our investigations, sensitivity is 64% based on a specificity of 95% for benign lung diseases. The ProGRP release seems not to correlate with tumor stage. ProGRP is already released in low-burden small-cell lung cancer with almost the same high sensitivity as in high-burden disease. The corresponding "false positive" rates in non-small-cell lung cancer are between 0 and 5%.

The overall profile of specificity and sensitivity for all cancers (Figure 1) as compared to the organ-related corresponding

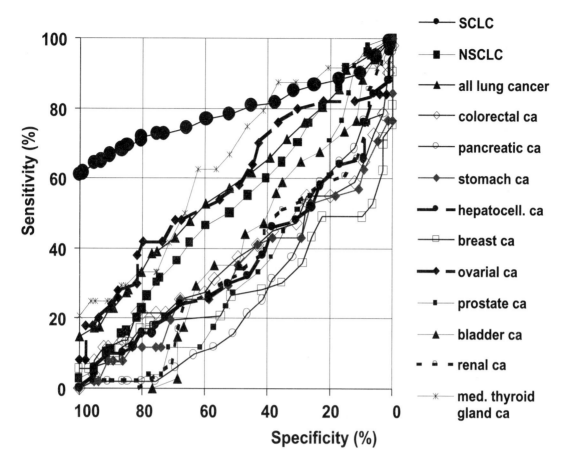

Figure 1 ROC curves for various cancers and their corresponding organ-related benign diseases (N = 1750).

benign diseases shows a high diagnostic capacity for ProGRP in small-cell lung cancer: at a specificity of 100% (for benign lung diseases), a sensitivity of almost 60% for SCLC can be achieved.

The ROC curves for all other investigated cancers demonstrate again the high specificity of ProGRP for small-cell lung cancer and its negligible release by other malignant tumors.

Comparison with Other Tumor Markers

ProGRP as a single marker has a high sensitivity in small-cell lung cancer as compared to benign diseases of the lung. When compared to CEA, CYFRA 21-1, NSE, and chromogranin A, ProGRP proved to be superior, and it has good organ specificity (6,9). The discriminatory value of ProGRP lies in the fact that ProGRP levels and the extent of its release are very low in benign disorders and in malignant tumors other than SCLC (with the exception of medullary thyroid carcinoma).

The sensitivities described by several authors for small-cell lung cancer range from 47% to 86%. These different results depend, at least partly, on the composition of the patient group investigated and also on the different cut-off values used. The diagnostic sensitivity of ProGRP in most publications is higher than NSE (65% vs. 43%) and in a few publications comparable to NSE (47% vs. 45%). Due to the different pathophysiologic roles of ProGRP and NSE, these two analytes have an additive sensitivity of 10–20% in SCLC and play a complementary role in the diagnosis and management of small-cell lung cancer (6,8).

Differentiation of Lung Tumors of Unknown Origin by ProGRP (Figure 2)

In cases where biopsy cannot be performed or histology fails to differentiate between the different types of lung cancer, ProGRP might help. According to our investigations with NSCLC, release of ProGRP is observed in only 3% of patients (NSE up to 26%). Also, in serum of patients with lung metastases due to other primary cancers, there is only a minor ProGRP release of up to 100 pg/mL. In small-cell lung cancer, high serum levels of ProGRP often are observed and can exceed the NSE values considerably. A ProGRP level >500 pg/mL is indicative for primary lung cancer and most probably (99%) of small-cell lung cancer. A ProGRP level >200 pg/mL in primary lung tumors is, regardless of the pathohistological classification, highly suggestive of at least a mixed histology with a small cell component. Lamy et al. confirmed our findings concerning the high diagnostic ability to discriminate between NSCLC and SCLC and found an AUC of 0.97 for ProGRP and 0.95 for NSE (9).

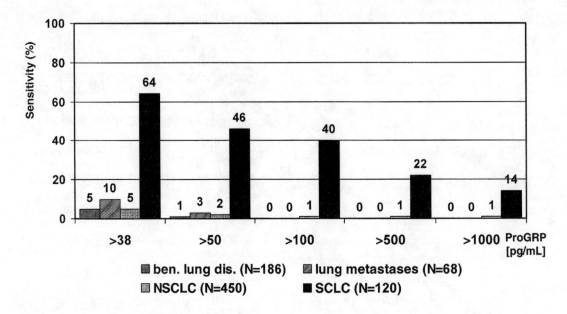

Figure 2 Optimizing the ProGRP cut-off values to reach higher specificity for SCLC.

ProGRP for Monitoring

Few data exist for this important application. In SCLC, recent data report the value of NSE, CEA, and ProGRP in recurrent disease (10). ProGRP, with 74% sensitivity (NSE: 32%, CEA: 56%), achieved the highest detection rate of recurrent disease. It is especially important to note that in none of the patients with elevated ProGRP-levels before primary treatment, ProGRP was negative at the time of recurrent disease (12% NSE and 6% CEA). ProGRP reflected the disease course of patients with SCLC more accurately (67%) than NSE (20%) or CEA (38%). Nevertheless, there was a clear additive effect (79% sensitivity) by combining ProGRP and NSE. The median lead time for the detection of recurrent disease was 35 days for ProGRP; no lead time could be observed for NSE.

FUTURE DIRECTIONS
Confirmation of Results

A meta-analysis of studies on ProGRP is being carried out. In addition, a large prospective international multi-centric trial, performed mainly by members of the lung cancer focus group within the EGTM, is ongoing; its purpose is to validate the profile of specificity and sensitivity of ProGRP in SCLC.

Further Investigations

Investigations on the comparability of the diagnostic efficacy of ProGRP in serum with tissue histology and sputum cytology in patients who have abnormal chest X-ray or CT are also being conducted.

ProGRP analysis could avoid the necessity for potentially dangerous biopsy procedures in severely ill patients and might generally lead to a change in the algorithm to establish final diagnosis of lung cancer. It is important to raise the question as to whether the expression of neuroendocrine molecules in tissue or the release of neuropeptides like ProGRP into the circulation is more relevant for therapeutic decision-making.

Other investigations concern the following:

- *the diagnostic efficacy of ProGRP in combination with other tumor-associated antigens in lung tumors of unknown origin.* Recently, the possible relevance of a pattern of release of several tumor markers into the blood circulation by the tumor of an individual patient became more evident. Comparable to the pattern of expression of various substances in tumor tissue leading to diagnosis and classification of cancer, the release of tumor markers into blood could also have diagnostic value. Although ProGRP is already highly sensitive and specific for small-cell lung cancer, its diagnostic efficiency in the diagnosis of bronchial carcinoma can probably be improved by mathematical evaluation of a tumor marker profile (like CEA, NSE, CYFRA 21-1, and SCCA).
- *the prognostic relevance of ProGRP in early stages (low-burden disease) and its predictive value in advanced stages (high-burden disease)* as compared to clinical parameters as well as to all other analytes that have been previously described to have independent prognostic relevance. These data will be collected mainly during the prospective trial mentioned above.
- *the relevance of ProGRP for reliable assessment of the therapeutic response* in SCLC patients enrolled in randomized studies.
- *the relevance of ProGRP for the early detection of recurrent disease.* As prior investigations have already shown, ProGRP seems to be very sensitive and specific for this indication. However, this modality will only be of value as better second- and third-line therapies for small-cell lung cancer become available.

REFERENCES

1. Yamaguchi K, Abe K, Kamoya T, Adachi I, Taguchi S, Otsubo K, Yanaihura N. Production and molecular size heterogeneity of immunoreactive gastrin-releasing peptide in fetal and adult lungs and primary lung tumors. Cancer Res 1983;43:3932–3939.
2. McDonald TJ, Nilsson G, Vagne M, Ghatei M, Bloom SR, Mutt V. A gastrin-releasing peptide from the porcine non-antral gastric tissue. Gut 1978;19:767–774.
3. Maruno K, Yamaguchi K, Abe K, Suzuki M, Saijo N, Mishima Y, Yanaihara N, Shimosato J. Immunoreactive gastrin-releasing peptide as a specific tumor marker in patients with small-cell lung carcinoma. Cancer Res 1989;49:629–632.
4. Aoyagi K, Miyake Y, Urakami K, Kashiwakuma T, Hasegawa A, Kodama T, Yamaguchi K. Enzyme immunoassay of immunoreactive progastrin-releasing peptide(31-98) as tumor marker for small-cell lung carcinoma: development and evaluation. Clin Chem 1995;41:537–543.
5. Miyake Y, Kodama T, Yamaguchi K. Pro-gastrin-releasing peptide(31-98) is a specific tumor marker in patients with small-cell lung carcinoma. Cancer Res 1994;54:2136–2140.
6. Stieber P, Dienemann H, Schalhorn A, Schmitt UM, Reinmiedl J, Hofmann K, Yamaguchi K. Progastrin-releasing peptide (ProGRP)—a useful marker in small-cell lung carcinomas. Anticancer Res 1999;19:2673–2678.
7. Inaji H, Komoike Y, Motomura K, Higashiyama M, Ohtsuru M, Funai H, Kasugai T, Koyama H. Demonstration and diagnostic significance of pro-gastrin-releasing peptide in medullary thyroid carcinoma. Oncology 2000;59:122–125.
8. Shibayama T, Ueoka H, Nishii K, Kiura K, Tabata M, Miyatake K, Kitajima T, Harada M. Complementary roles of pro-gastrin-releasing peptide (ProGRP) and neuron-specific enolase (NSE) in diagnosis and prognosis of small-cell lung cancer (SCLC). Lung Cancer 2001;32:61–69.
9. Lamy P, Grenier J, Kramar A, Pujol JL. Pro-gastrin-releasing peptide, neuron-specific enolase, and chromogranin A as serum markers of small-cell lung cancer. Lung Cancer. 2000;29: 197–203.
10. Niho S, Nishiwaki Y, Goto K, Ohmatsu H, Matsumoto T, Hojo F, Ohe Y, Kakinuma R, Kodama T. Significance of serum pro-gastrin-releasing peptide as a predictor of relapse of small-cell lung cancer: comparative evaluation with neuron-specific enolase and carcinoembryonic antigen. Lung Cancer 2000;27:159–167.

Index

0⁶-Methyl-guanine-DNA methyltransferase (MGMT), brain tumor marker, 331
1F10 monoclonal antibody, lung cancer marker, 289
5C7 monoclonal antibody, lung cancer marker, 289
5E8 monoclonal antibody, lung cancer marker, 289
6H5MI2C, melanoma marker, 362, 363

A

A1/BFL-1 gene, apoptosis marker, 505–506
A2/B1 ribonucleoprotein (hrNP), 481–482
ABL proto-oncogene, 86
Accuracy, of assays, 67–68
Acid phosphatase, discovery of, 3–4
ACS:180 kit (Bayer), 242, 429
Acute lymphoblastic leukemia (ALL), markers for, 322–323, 325
Acute myeloid leukemia (AML), 323–324
  leukemias with binding factor translocations, 324
  markers for, 322, 325
Acute promyelocytic leukemia (APL), 324, 325
Adenocarcinoma
  lung cancer markers, 55
  lung, predictor markers for, 408
  of the prostate (PCA), 201–202
Adhesion molecules. *See* Cell adhesion molecules
Adrenocorticotrophic hormone (ACTH), carcinoid of the gut, marker for, 343
ADVIA Centaur® (Bayer), 429
AE1/3 antibody, lymph node micrometastases marker, 296
AE1 antibody, bone marrow micrometastases marker, 297
AE3 antibody, bone marrow micrometastases marker, 297
Affymetrix, Inc., 401
Age
  breast cancer risk and, 181
  estrogen/progestin receptor distribution, in breast carcinoma, 38
  prostate cancer and, 201–202
Agrin, ovarian cancer marker, 401–402
AIA-PACK kit (Tosoh), 242
AKT2 protein, ovarian cancer marker, 246
Albumin, hepatocellular carcinoma marker, 115
Aldolase A, hepatocellular carcinoma marker, 275
ALISA, *sErbB* receptors, 427, 429

Alkaline phosphatase (ALP). *See also* Placental alkaline phosphatase (PLAP)
  half-life, 355
  hepatocellular carcinoma marker, 275
  immunohistochemical staining, 27
Alpha-fetoprotein (AFP)
  brain tumor marker, 330
  comparability of results, 65, 66
  discovery of, 4, 270
  gastrointestinal cancer marker, 271
  gene expression, 272
  germ cell tumor marker, 52–53, 57
  half-life, 10, 52–53
  hepatocellular carcinoma marker, 115, 270–273
  international standard, 67–68
  isoforms, 272–273
  reference values, 352
  structure and function of, 270
  testicular cancer marker, 115, 352
  tissue production, 10
Alphavbeta3, melanoma marker, 362, 363
American Cancer Society, prostate cancer early detection, 44, 57
American Diagnostica, Inc., 446–447
American Society of Clinical Oncology (ASCO)
  breast cancer guidelines, 57, 182
  colorectal cancer guidelines, 47–48, 57
  prostate cancer guidelines, 57
  Tumor Marker Utility Grading System (TMUGS), 19–21, 30
AML/ETO1 fusion transcript, leukemia marker, 324, 325
Amplification, proto-oncogenes, 86
Amsterdam criteria, HNPCC, 259–260
Amyloidosis, primary
  classification of, 306
  diagnosis, 307, 316–317
  epidemiology of, 316
  prognosis and treatment, 317
Analytic-specific reagents (ASRs), 29
Androgen receptors
  amplification, 209
  polymorphisms and mutations, 209
  prostate cancer marker, 208–209
  prostatic, 196, 197

Angiogenesis
   in cancer development and progression, 152, 156
   markers for, 185, 362, 366
   prostatic, 197
   targeted therapy and, 157
Anti-analyte antibodies, 72
Anti-Hu antibodies, lung cancer markers, 291
Anti-reagent antibodies, 72, 73–75
Antibodies. *See also* Autoantibodies; Human anti-mouse antibodies (HAMA)
   anti-analyte, 72
   anti-reagent, 72, 73–75
   antineuronal, 291
   erroneous test results, cause of, 36
   heterophilic, 36, 76–77
Antibody specification and standardization, 26–27
α-1-Antichymotrypsin (ACT), prostate cancer staging, 217
Anticoagulants, assay interference, 71
Antigen retrieval, optimal protocol, determining, 26, 27
Antineuronal antibodies, lung cancer markers, 291
Antiproteases
   kallikrein 2 complexes, 206–207
   prostate-specific antigen (PSA) complexes, 204–205
α-1-Antitrypsin, hepatocellular carcinoma marker, 275
AP-2 growth factor, melanoma marker, 362, 367
APC tumor suppressor gene, 84, 88, 295
Apoptosis
   anti-apoptosis markers, 504–505
   bcl-2 gene, breast cancer, 184–185
   definition of, 503
   inhibitor of apoptosis proteins (IAP), 504
   inhibitors, melanoma markers, 362, 365–366
   resistance to, in cancer development and progression, 152
   role, in cancer, 503–506
   targeted therapy and, 157
Applied Biotechnology, 428
Aromatase inhibitors, breast cancer treatment, 183
Artificial neural networks (ANN), 136–138
Aryl sulfatase B, colorectal cancer marker, 257
Assay kits
   CA 125, 242
   circulating tumor cells (CTC), 495–497
   complement factor H (CFH), 282
   epidermal growth factor receptors (EGFR), 430
   HER-2/neu, 430
   nuclear matrix protein 22 (NMP22), 282–283
   plasminogen activation inhibitor (PAI-1), 446–447
   sErbB receptors, 427–429
   Thompson-Friedenreich antigen (TF Ag), 477–479
   urokinase-type plasminogen activator (uPA), 101, 446–447
   validation of, 153
Assays. *See also* Immunoassays; Immunohistochemical assays
   alpha-fetoprotein, 270
   analytic-specific reagents (ASR) in, 29
   cathepsin B, 102
   cathepsin D, 102–103

   circulating tumor cells (CTC), 107–111
   development of, 29–30
   dielectrophoresis (DEP), 499–502
   erroneous test results, cause of, 36
   estrogen receptors, 454
   FDA regulation of, 29
   limitations of, 65–80
   mammaglobulin, 433–435
   matrix metalloproteinases, 103
   pre-market application (PMA) and approval, 29
   progestin receptors, 454
   standardization, need for, 152–153
   telomerase, 509–510
   tissue inhibitors of MMPs (TIMPs), 441–443
Astrocytomas, 329
ATM tumor suppressor gene, 84, 88
Atrial natriuretic peptide (ANP), lung cancer marker, 292
Atypical hyperplasia, breast cancer risk and, 181
Autoantibodies
   assays for, 123–126
   circulating, as markers, 123–131
   ELISA, 123–126
   limitations of, 130
   prognositc, 128
AxSYM kit (Abbott), 242

B

B-cell leukemia, markers for, 116, 321–322, 325
B305 gene, RT-PCR assay, 433–435
B726P gene, RT-PCR assay, 433–435
Bacterial contamination, of samples, 72
Bacterial prostatitis, 200–201
BAD gene, apoptosis marker, 505–506
BAK gene, apoptosis marker, 505–506
Basic fibroblast growth factor (bFGF)
   melanoma marker, 362, 366
   non-Hodgkin's lymphoma marker, 322
BAX gene, apoptosis marker, 157, 185, 504–506
Bayer Diagnostics, 242, 427, 428, 429, 430
BCL-2 gene
   apoptosis marker, 504–506
   lung cancer marker, 293, 294, 301
Bcl-2, melanoma marker, 366
BCL-W gene, apoptosis marker, 505–506
BCL-X gene, apoptosis marker, 157, 185, 505–506
Bcl/Bax/Bcl-x, apoptosis marker, 157, 185
BCR/ABL fusion transcript, leukemia marker, 323, 325
Bence-Jones protein
   discovery of, 3, 4, 65
   in multiple myeloma, 307
   in Waldenström's macroglobulinemia, 315
Bence-Jones proteinuria, 306
Bender Med-Systems Diagnostics GmbH, 427, 428, 430
Benign monoclonal gammopathy, 305, 306
Benign prostatic hyperplasia (BPH), 199–200, 210, 214

Ber-EP-4 antibody
    bone marrow micrometastases marker, 297
    lymph node micrometastases marker, 296
Beta1/beta3, melanoma marker, 362, 363
Bethesda criteria, HNPCC, 259–260
BIACore International AB, 395, 396
Biclonal gammopathies, 306
Biliary cancer, marker for, 450
Biochemical failure, prostate cancer, 223–224
Biochips, market for, 16–17
Bioinformatics
    definition of, 16, 396–397
    historical background, 4
Biological Stain Commission, 28
Biomarker Pattern Software, 16
Bladder cancer
    features of, 281–282
    markers for, 283, 450
    predictor genes for, 408
    prognostic autoantibodies, 128
    RB/p53 tumor suppressor gene pathway, 92–95
    tumor progression, model of, 90–95
BLCA-4, bladder cancer marker, 283
Blood
    kallikrein 2 complexes, 206
    NSCLC, free tumor cells in, 297–298
    prostate-specific antigen (PSA) complexes, 204–205
Blood coagulation factors, 445–447
Blood collection tubes and additives, 70–71
Bone marrow, 298–299
    biopsy, multiple myeloma, 310
    lung cancer micrometastases, 296–299
    multiple myeloma, 306–307
BR -27.29. See CA 27.29
Brain tumors
    markers for, 330–333, 330–334
    metastatic, 333–334
    primary, 329–333
    treatment, 329–330
BRCA1 tumor suppressor gene, 84, 88
    breast cancer risk and, 189
    clinical significance, 190–191
    functions and characteristics, 189
BRCA2 tumor suppressor gene, 84
    breast cancer risk and, 189
    clinical significance, 190–191
    functions and characteristics, 189
Breast cancer
    angiogenesis, markers for, 185
    β-catenin in, 437–438
    BRCA genes, 189–192
    CA 125 monitoring, 129
    CEA monitoring, 129
    cell cycle/cell death markers, 184–185
    DNA marker, cell-free, 116
    epidemiology of, 35–36, 165, 181

    genetics of, 181
    levels of evidence (LOE) categories, 20, 182
    markers for, 37–41, 57, 112, 165–176, 433–435, 437–439, 450, 481–482, 485–488
    metastasis, lymph nodes, 434–435
    metastatic, markers for, 38, 170–175, 185
    node-negative, 154
    predictive markers, 173–174
    predictor genes for, 408
    prognosis, DNA synthesis rates, 412
    prognosis, factors for, 165
    prognostic autoantibodies, 128
    prognostic factors, traditional, 99
    prognostic markers, 100–101, 437–439
    proliferation, markers for, 183
    recurrence, early diagnosis of, 169–171
    RT-PCR assay for markers, 433–435
    sErbB receptor assay kits, 427–429
    specimen collection and preparation, 37–38
    tumor size/nodal development, markers and, 166–167
Breast cancer cells
    DNA replication, error-prone, 413–414
    DNA synthesome, 414–418
    DNA synthesome error types, 416–418
    non-malignant, DNA replication, 414–415
    PCNA alterations, 417–418
    replication altered, 413–414
BTA-stat test (Polymedco), 282
BTA-trak test (Polymedco), 282

C

c-erb B2. See HER-2/neu oncoprotein
c-erbB-2 autoantibody, breast cancer prognosis, 128
c-erbB-2 tumor suppressor gene, 84, 293, 300. See also *sErbB* receptors
c-myc gene, gastrointestinal cancer marker, 254
c-myc protein, melanoma marker, 362, 367
C-reactive protein, monoclonal gammopathy of undetermined significance (MGUS) marker, 312
C3 complement, in semen, 199
CA 125
    assay kits, 242
    breast cancer monitoring, 129
    discovery of, 4
    endometrial cancer marker, 43
    immunoassays, 241–243
    international standard, 67–68
    lung cancer marker, 289–290, 299–300
    non-Hodgkin's lymphoma marker, 322
    ovarian cancer marker, 41–42, 57, 241–244
    pancreatic cancer marker, 267
    as surrogate marker, 157
CA 15-3
    breast cancer marker, 37, 38–39, 57, 165–167
    breast cancer prognosis marker, 165–167, 173–174

CA 15-3 (continued)
  breast cancer recurrence marker, 169–170
  discovery of, 4
  international standard, 67–68
  metastatic breast cancer marker, 170–175
CA 195
  gastrointestinal cancer marker, 254
  pancreatic cancer marker, 267
CA 19.9
  cholestasis and, 70
  colorectal cancer marker, 256
  discovery of, 4
  gastric cancer marker, 376–378
  gastrointestinal cancer marker, 254
  international standard, 67–68
  Intrahepatic cholangiosarcoma marker, 276
  pancreatic cancer marker, 144, 266
CA 242, pancreatic cancer marker, 266–267
CA 27.29, breast cancer marker, 10, 37, 39, 57
CA 494, pancreatic cancer marker, 267
CA 50
  gastrointestinal cancer marker, 254
  pancreatic cancer marker, 266
CA 72-4
  colorectal cancer marker, 256–257
  gastric cancer marker, 376, 378
  gastrointestinal cancer marker, 254
  international standard, 67–68
Calbiochem, 428
Calcitonin, medullary thyroid carcinoma, marker for, 49, 50–51, 57, 345, 346
Calibration, of assays, 67–68
CAM 17.1, pancreatic cancer marker, 267
CAM 5.2 antibody, 296, 297
Campath-1H, 325
Cancer
  cytotoxic therapy for, 151
  definition of, 9
  development of, biological mechanisms, 152
  epidemiology of, 9
  genetic predisposition to, 7
  invasion process, 185
  microarray applications, 383–388
  molecular classification, 404–407
  oncogenes, role of, 83–95
  predictor genes for, 407–409
  predisposition testing, 486
  progression of, biological mechanisms, 152
  tumor suppressor genes, 83–95
Cancer-associated serum antigen (CASA), ovarian cancer marker, 241, 245–246
Cancer cells. See also Circulating tumor cells (CTC)
  altered DNA replication in, 411–412
  apoptosis and, 503–506
  dielectric properties, cell separation and, 499–502
  DNA replication, error-prone, 413–414

Capillary electrophoresis (CE)
  M-protein quantification, 54
  protein separation, 394
Carbohydrate antigens, discovery of, 4
Carcinoembryonic antigen (CEA)
  in body fluids and tissues, 256
  breast cancer marker, 37, 38, 57, 112, 165–167
  breast cancer, metastatic, 170–175
  breast cancer monitoring, 129
  breast cancer prognosis, 165–167, 173–174
  breast cancer recurrence marker, 169–170
  breast tissue levels, 175–176
  colorectal cancer marker, 47–48, 57, 115, 253–256
  discovery of, 4
  gastric cancer marker, 115, 375–377
  gastrointestinal cancer marker, 254
  high-dose hook effect, 77, 79
  international standard, 67–68
  lung cancer, free tumor cell marker, 298, 299–300
  lung cancer marker, 55, 57, 115, 288, 289, 291
  medullary thyroid carcinoma, marker for, 345
  molecular subgroup structures, 375–376
  ovarian cancer marker, 241, 245
  pancreatic cancer marker, 115, 265, 266
  tissue production, 10
Carcinoid syndrome, 342–343
Carcinoid tumors
  classification of, 342
  diagnosis and treatment, 342
  markers for, 49–52, 342–343, 345
Carry-over, in assays, 69–70, 71
Caspases, 503–504
Catecholamines
  neuroblastoma marker, 49, 57
  pheochromocytoma marker, 49, 57
  reference values, 50
β-catenin, assay for, 437–439
β-catenin gene, 437
Cathepsin B
  assays for, 102
  gastrointestinal cancer marker, 254
  metastasis and, 100
  prognostic marker, 102
  structure and function of, 102
Cathepsin D
  breast cancer marker, 40–41, 185
  metastasis and, 100
  prognostic marker, 102
  structure and function of, 102
CBFβ/MYH11 gene rearrangement, leukemia marker, 324, 325
CCND-1/IGH, lymphoma marker, 325
CD23, leukemia marker, 321
CD44
  brain tumor marker, 333
  leukemia marker, 322

lymphoma marker, 322
melanoma marker, 362–363
CD54. *See* Intracellular adhesion molecule (ICAM)
CDKN2A gene, melanoma marker, 368
cDNA
    expression profiling, with microarrays, 385–387
    PCR-based amplification, 110
    synthesis, from mRNA, 109–110
Cell adhesion molecules
    brain tumor markers, 333, 334
    CEACAMS, 375–376
    melanoma markers, 362
    neural cell adhesion molecule (NCAM), 292, 298
    potential tumor markers, 425–426
Cell-map proteomics, 14
Cell sorting, 393
CellSpotter™ system, 495–497
Cervical cancer, markers for, 42–43, 115, 450, 485–488
Chemotherapy, 151. *See also* Therapeutic monitoring
    brain tumors, 329–330
    hepatocellular carcinoma, alpha-fetoprotein (AFP) monitoring, 273–274
    molecular-targeted agents vs., 154–157
    monoclonal gammopathy of undetermined significance (MGUS) treatment, 312–314
    Waldenström's macroglobulinemia, 316
Chiron Diagnostics, 427, 428, 429
Cholangiosarcoma, intrahepatic, 275–276
Cholestasis, CA 19.9 variability, 70
Chorionic gonadotropin (human, hCG)
    brain tumor marker, 330
    carcinoid of the gut, marker for, 343, 345
    cross-reactions to, 72
    forms of, 353–354
    germ cell tumor marker, 52–53, 57
    half-life, 10, 53, 355
    heterophilic antibody misdiagnosis, 76
    international standard, 67–68
    medullary thyroid carcinoma, marker for, 345
    neuroblastoma marker, 345
    nomenclature, 353
    ovarian cancer marker, 241, 246
    pancreatic endocrine tumor marker, 344, 345
    pheochromocytoma marker, 345
    reference values, 354
    stability, heat and, 71
    standards, 353
    testicular cancer marker, 115, 353–354
    testing spectrum, 68
    tissue production, 10
Chromogranin A (CgA)
    carcinoid of the gut, marker for, 343, 345
    lung cancer marker, 292
    medullary thyroid carcinoma, marker for, 345
    neuroblastoma marker, 345, 346
    from neuroendocrine cells, 339–342

    pancreatic endocrine tumor marker, 344, 345
    pheochromocytoma marker, 345–346
Chromogranin B (CgB)
    carcinoid of the gut, marker for, 343, 345
    medullary thyroid carcinoma, marker for, 345
    neuroblastoma marker, 345
    from neuroendocrine cells, 339–342
    pancreatic endocrine tumor marker, 344, 345
    pheochromocytoma marker, 345
Chromogranin-related peptides, 341–342
Chromosomes, loss, in brain tumors, 331
Chronic lymphocytic leukemia (CLL), proteonomics in, 398
Chronic myeloid leukemia (CML), 84, 324, 325
Ciba-Corning Diagnostics, 427, 428–429
Ciphergen Biosystems, Inc., 395
    Biomarker Pattern Software, 16
    ProteinChip® technique, 15, 16, 396
    Surface-Enhanced Laser Desorption/Ionization (SELDI), 15
Circulating autoantibodies, as markers, 123–131
Circulating cell-free DNA, as marker, 114, 116
Circulating tumor cells (CTC). *See also* Cancer cells
    assays for, 107–111, 495–497
    breast cancer diagnosis, 112–113
    epithelial tumor diagnosis, 111
    molecular detection techniques, 107–108
    prostate cancer diagnosis, 111–112
    solid tumor diagnosis, 115
Citric acid, in semen, 198
Classification and Regression Tree (CART), 16, 134–136, 217, 219
Classification systems
    brain tumors, 329
    molecular, for cancer, 404–407
    molecular, for leukemia, 151
    monoclonal gammopathies, 306
    ovarian cancer, 239
    prostate cancer, 202
    prostatitis, 201
    staging, 9
    testicular cancer, 351–352
Clinical Laboratory Improvement Act (CLIA), 29, 33–34
Clinical studies, tamoxifen, for breast cancer, 183
Clinical trials, 143–148
    A2/B1 ribonucleoprotein (hrNP), 482
    assays, concurrent disease, 142, 145–146
    biomarker-oriented vs. disease-oriented, 157–159
    cancer control studies, 143, 148–149
    ColorectAlert™ test, 478–479
    LungAlert™ test, 479
    phases, for biomarker targeted therapy, 157–159
    phases, for tumor marker development, 143–148
    predictive markers, evaluation protocols, 154–157
    prospective screening studies, 143, 147–148
    retrospective, 142–143, 146–147
    standardization, need for, 154–156
    for tumor marker development, 29–30

CN BioSciences, Inc. (OncogeneScience Products), 427, 428, 429, 430
College of American Pathologists (CAP), 25
Colon cancer
    ColorectAlert™ test, 477–479
    markers for, 477–479
    predictor genes for, 408
    tumor progression, model of, 90
Colorectal cancer
    DNA marker, cell-free, 116
    early detection, 47
    epidemiology of, 46, 259
    guidelines for markers, 48
    hereditary nonpolyposis colorectal cancer (HNPCC), 259–262
    markers for, 47–48, 57, 115, 253–257, 441–443, 450
    prognostic autoantibodies, 128
    staging, 254
    TIMP-1 gene, 441–443
ColorectAlert™ test, 477–479
Communications, between staff members, 78
Comparative genomic hybridization (CGH), 15, 383–384
Complement factor H (CFH), bladder cancer marker, 282
Compugen, Inc., 404
Computer modeling, nomograms, 46
Contact factor pathway, 445–447
Contamination, assay results and, 70–71
Cortisol, carcinoid of the gut, marker for, 343
COT proto-oncogene, 86
Creatinine kinase BB (CK-BB), lung cancer marker, 292
Critical difference, 67
Cross-reactions, in assays, 71–73, 206–207
Cryoglobulins, myeloma markers, 54
Cyclin-dependent kinases (CDKs), melanoma markers, 368
Cyclin E, lung cancer marker, 294
Cyclins, 367–368, 437–438
CYFRA 21-1, lung cancer marker, 55–57, 288–289, 291
5-S-Cysteinyldopa (5SCD), melanoma marker, 361–362
Cytokeratin 19 fragment. See CYFRA 21-1
Cytokeratin 19 mRNA, breast cancer marker, 112
Cytokeratins (CK)
    bladder cancer markers, 283
    bone marrow micrometastases marker, 297
    breast cancer markers, 165
    colorectal cancer markers, 115
    endometrial cancer marker, 115
    gastric cancer markers, 115
    lung cancer, free tumor cell markers, 298
    lung cancer markers, 115
    oral cancer marker, 115
    ovarian cancer marker, 115
    pancreatic cancer markers, 115, 265–266
    thyroid carcinoma marker, 115
    urothelial carcinoma marker, 115
Cytokeratins (CK) polyclonal antibody, lymph node micrometastases marker, 296
Cytotoxic T lymphocytes, 457–460
Cytotoxic therapy, for cancer, 151

D

DAPK gene, lung cancer methylation marker, 295
Databases, genomics, 403
Davidson Dye Marking Kit, 38
DCC tumor suppressor gene, 84, 88
Density gradient centrifugation, 108
Des-γ carboxy prothrombin (DCP), hepatocellular carcinoma marker, 275
Diagnosis and diagnostic markers
    amyloidosis, primary, 316–317
    artificial neuron network-based (ANN), 137–138
    bladder cancer, 94
    brain tumors, 330
    breast cancer, 165–167
    hepatocellular carcinoma, 271–272
    historical background, 3–7
    limitations of, 5
    lung cancer, 55–56
    ovarian cancer, 41
    overview, 11
    testicular cancer, 355
    Waldenström's macroglobulinemia, 314–315
Dielectric properties, of cancer cells, 499–502
Dielectrophoresis (DEP), 499–502
Digital rectal examination
    prostate cancer diagnosis, 44, 57, 202–203
    PSA sampling and, 70
Direct RNA isolation, 108
DNA
    cDNA PCR-based amplification, 110
    cDNA synthesis, from mRNA, 109–110
    circulating cell-free, as marker, 114, 116
    *ds*DNA, colorectal cancer prognosis, 128
    Epstein-Barr virus (EBV), 491–494
    methylation markers, 294–295
    replication altered, in cancer cells, 411–412, 413–418
    serological analysis of recombinant cDNA expression libraries (SEREX), 247–248
DNA ligase, DNA synthesome, 413
DNA polymerase, 411–413
DNA synthesome
    breast cancer cells, modification of, 417–418
    error-prone, breast cancer cells, 414–415, 414–418
    non-malignant breast cancer cells, 414–415
    structure and function of, 412–413
    types of errors, breast cancer cells, 416–417
Dopamine
    neuroblastoma marker, 345, 346
    pheochromocytoma marker, 49, 345
    reference values, 50
Drug development, 141
Drug therapy, for cancer. See Chemotherapy

*ds*DNA, colorectal cancer prognosis, 128
DU-PAN 2 monoclonal antibody, 266
DuPont Co., 427, 429

E

E-cadherin, brain tumor marker, 333
Edman degradation, 394
Elastase-1, pancreatic cancer marker, 266
Elecsys 1010/2010 kits (Roche), 242
Electrospray ionization (ES), 395
ELISA
   autoantibodies, 123–126
   sErbB receptors, 427–429
   tissue inhibitors of MMPs (TIMPs), 441–443
Endocrine pancreatic tumors, markers for, 345
Endometrial cancer, markers for, 43, 115, 450
Enzymes
   detection, for immunohistochemical techniques, 27
   radiolabel signal detection variability, 66
Epidermal growth factor receptors (EGFR)
   assay kits, 430
   brain tumor markers, 331–332
   breast cancer marker, 40
   breast cancer markers, 427–431
   colorectal cancer markers, 115
   gastrointestinal cancer markers, 254
   lung cancer, free tumor cell marker, 298
   ovarian cancer markers, 427–431
   tumor growth factor marker, 157
Epinephrine
   neuroblastoma marker, 345
   pheochromocytoma marker, 49, 345–346
   reference values, 50
Epithelial tumors, 110–111
Epstein-Barr virus (EBV) DNA, 491–494
ERBB gene, 427
Erythropoietin, monoclonal gammopathy of undetermined significance (MGUS) treatment, 313
Escherichia coli, assay interference, 77
Esophageal carcinoma, DNA marker, cell-free, 116
Estrogen receptors
   α and β variants, 37
   analytical concerns, 38
   breast cancer markers, 37–38, 57, 453–455
   complexity of, 152, 182–183
   distribution, in breast carcinoma, 38
   reference values, 37
   RT-PCR assay, 454
   status, breast cancer treatment, 182–183
European Group on Tumor Markers (EGTM), 57
   analytical requirements guidelines, 35
   breast cancer marker guidelines, 38, 39–40, 57, 165
   colorectal cancer marker guidelines, 48, 57
   erroneous results, cause of, 36
   germ cell tumor marker guidelines, 52, 53, 57
   lung cancer marker guidelines, 56, 57
   ovarian cancer marker guidelines, 42, 57
   overview, 34
   postanalytical and reporting requirements, 36
   preanalytical requirements guidelines, 34
   prostate cancer, PSA guidelines, 46, 57
Ewing sarcoma, markers for, 115
EWS-FLI, Ewing sarcoma marker, 115
Expression proteonomics, 14
External quality assessment (EQA), 34, 35
Extracellular matrix (ECM)
   adhesion molecules, function of, 425–426
   cathepsin B effect on, 100
   cathepsin D effect on, 100
   dissolution, metastasis and, 99
   matrix metalloproteinases, effect on, 103
   uPA effect on, 100

F

False-positive rate (FPR), 144–147
Familial adenomatous polyposis (FAP, 259
Fas receptor, 362, 365–366, 503
FDFr1-4 proto-oncogene, 86
Federation of Gynecology and Obstetrics (FIGO), ovarian cancer classification, 239
Ferritin, hepatocellular carcinoma marker, 274
FGR proto-oncogene, 86
Fibrinolysis system, 445–447
Fibrinolytic markers, ovarian cancer, 241, 246
Fibronectin (FN), potential tumor marker, 425–426
Follicular lymphoma (FL), 325
Food and Drug Administration (FDA), regulation of tumor marker assays, 29, 33
Formalin, as fixative, 26
Fructose, in semen, 198
α-L-fucosidase, hepatocellular carcinoma marker, 275
Fujirebio Diagnostics RIA (Fujirebio), 242
Functional genomics, 391

G

GABAπ gene, RT-PCR assay, 433–435
GAGE, melanoma marker, 112
β-Galactosidase, immunohistochemical staining, 27
Gastric cancer
   epidemiology of, 375
   markers for, 115, 271, 375–378, 450
   predictor genes for, 408
Gastrin, 343, 345
Gastrin releasing factor (GRF)-omas, 343, 344
Gastrin-releasing polypeptide (GRP), lung cancer marker, 292, 517
Gastrinomas, 343, 344
Gastrointestinal cancer. *See also* Colorectal cancer; Gastric cancer

Gastrointestinal cancer *(continued)*
  carcinoid of the gut, markers for, 49–50
  markers for, 254, 271
  neuroendocrine tumors, 339
  prognostic markers, 101
Gel electrophoresis, 14
Gene expression
  analysis, tumor marker discovery and, 401–403
  apoptosis, 503–506
  estrogen receptors, 453
  maspin, 439
  PC1 gene, 463–463
  profiling, with microarrays, 384–385
  replication errors (RERs), 411–412
  tumor-associated trypsin inhibitor (TATI), 449
  for tumor classification, 6–7, 404–407
Gene expression analysis, 15
Gene Ontology Consortium (GO), 404
Gene therapy, targeted therapy and, 157
Genetic testing and counseling, *BRCA* genes, 190–191
Genetics
  breast cancer risk and, 181
  hereditary nonpolyposis colorectal cancer (HNPCC), 259–261
Genomic imprinting, tumor suppressor genes and, 88
Genomics
  definition of, 15
  methods, 15–16
  microarrays in, 15, 383–388
Genomics Institute, Novartis Research Foundation, 403
Germ cell tumors, 52–53, 57
GIP proto-oncogene, 86
Gleason Grading System, 203
Glial fibrillary acidic protein (GFAP), brain tumor marker, 330
Glucagon, pancreatic endocrine tumor marker, 345
Glucagonomas, 343, 344
Glucose oxidase, immunohistochemical staining, 27
Glucose phosphate isomerase, colorectal cancer marker, 257
Glycoprotein hormones, α subunit
  carcinoid of the gut, marker for, 345
  medullary thyroid carcinoma, marker for, 345
  neuroblastoma marker, 345
  pancreatic endocrine tumor marker, 345
  pheochromocytoma marker, 345
Zn-α-2-Glycoprotein, in semen, 199
Glycosyltransferases
  colorectal cancer marker, 257
  gastrointestinal cancer markers, 254
Graffinity Pharmaceutical Design GmbH, 395
Growth factor oncogenes, 85
Growth factor receptor oncogenes, 86, 183–184
Growth factors
  B-cell leukemia marker, 322
  gastrointestinal cancer markers, 254
  non-Hodgkin's lymphoma marker, 322
  targeted therapy and, 157
Growth hormone, carcinoid of the gut, marker for, 343
Growth hormone releasing hormone (GHRH), carcinoid of the gut, marker for, 343
GSP gene, 84, 86
GT1B, brain tumor marker, 334
γ-GTP isoenzyme, hepatocellular carcinoma marker, 274–275
Guanine nucleotide binding proteins, genetic mutation of, 86
Guidelines, 57
  assay working groups, 34
  breast cancer markers, 39–40, 57, 165
  clinical trial phases, for biomarker targeted therapy, 157–159
  colorectal cancer markers, 47–49, 57
  germ cell tumor markers, 52–53, 57
  immunohistochemistry assays, 27
  lung cancer diagnosis, 300
  lung cancer markers, 56, 57
  multiple myeloma diagnosis, 311
  multiple myeloma markers, 54–55
  myeloma markers, 57
  neuroendocrine tumor markers, 51–52, 57
  ovarian cancer markers, 42, 57
  prostate cancer early detection, 44
  PSA guidelines in prostate cancer, 46, 57
  quality requirements and control, 34–35
  specimen collection and preparation, 13
  for tumor marker development, 29–30
  tumor marker development, 142–149
Gynecological cancer, epidemiology of, 41

H

H-*RAS* gene, 84
Ha-RAS gene, gastrointestinal cancer marker, 254
Hamburg Symposia, 34
HE4 gene, ovarian cancer marker, 401–402
Head and neck tumors, 116, 450
Hepatitis, 271
Hepatocellular carcinoma (HCC), 269
  diagnosis, 271–272
  DNA marker, cell-free, 116
  early detection, 273
  epidemiology of, 269
  fibrolamellar variant, 275
  markers for, 115, 269–274
  predictor genes for, 408
  screening, 273
  staging, 273
Hepatoma, marker for, 450
Hepsin, 403
HER-2/neu oncogene, breast cancer, 183–184
HER-2/neu oncoprotein
  assay kits, 430
  autoantibody detection, 126

Index

breast cancer marker, 37, 40, 57, 154, 165–167
breast cancer, metastatic, marker, 171–175
breast cancer, metastatic, prognosis, 173–174
breast cancer, predictive marker, 174–175
breast cancer prognosis, 165–167, 167–169
ovarian cancer marker, 246
tumor growth factor marker, 157
HER family, of receptors, 183–184
Herceptin®, patient selection, for treatment, 40, 57, 175
Hereditary nonpolyposis colorectal cancer (HNPCC), 259–262
Heterogeneous ribonuclear protein A2/B1, 481–482
Heterophilic antibodies
    assay interference, 76–77
    erroneous test results, cause of, 36
Heterozygosity, loss of, 86–87, 88, 89
High-dose hook effect, 72
    carcinoembryonic antigen (CEA) elevated, 77–78, 79
    erroneous test results, cause of, 36
Hilar cholangiosarcoma, 276
Histamine, carcinoid of the gut, marker for, 343
HLM, lung cancer marker, 115
Homovanillic acid (HVA)
    drug interference with, 50
    neuroblastoma marker, 57, 345, 346
    pheochromocytoma marker, 49, 57, 345–346
    reference values, 49–50
Horseradish peroxidase, immunohistochemical staining, 27
HPLC, protein separation, 394
Human anti-mouse antibodies (HAMA)
    assay interference, 72, 75–76
    assay results variability, 70
    erroneous test results, cause of, 36
Human chorionic gonadotropin. *See* Chorionic gonadotropin (human, hCG)
Human Genome Project, 396
Human papilloma virus (HPV), cervical cancer marker, 115
Human telomerase reverse transcriptase (hTERT), 509–510
Hyaluronic acid (HA), bladder cancer marker, 284
Hyaluronidase, bladder cancer marker, 284
5-Hydroxyindoleacetic acid (5-HIAA)
    carcinoid of the gut, marker for, 49, 50, 343, 345
    drug and food interference with, 51
    reference values, 50
Hypercalcemia, 307
Hyperplasia, DNA replication errors, 415
Hypothalamic-pituitary-gonadal (HPG) axis, prostate function and, 194
Hypothalamus, prostate function and, 194–195

I

IGF2 gene, 85
IGH/BCL-2, lymphoma marker, 325
Immulite kit (DPC), 242
Immuno 1 kit (Bayer), 242
Immuno 1™ Immuno-assay System (Bayer), 427, 428, 430
Immunoassays
    analytical specificity, 68–69
    autoantibodies, 123–126
    CA 125, 241–243
    carry-over, 69–70, 71
    comparability of results, 65–69
    complement factor H (CFH), 282
    cross-reactions in, 71–73
    endogenous interferences, 71–78
    exogenous interferences, 69–71
    interferences in, 69–79
    kallikrein 2 complexes, 206
    linearity, 68
    method robustness, 69–78
    missampling, by automated analyzers, 71
    nonspecific interference in, 72–73
    overview, 13–14
    preanalytical requirements, 70
    precision and reproducibility, 66–67
    prostate-specific antigen (PSA), 205
    radiolabel signal detection variability, 66
    sensitivity and detection limits, 66
    sErbB receptors, 427–429
    standardization, need for, 152–153
    working range, 66
Immunocyt test (Diagno-Cure), 283
Immunoglobulins
    melanoma markers, 362–363
    myeloma markers, 54, 308–310
    in semen, 199
    in Waldenström's macroglobulinemia, 315
Immunohistochemical assays
    interpretation and reporting criteria, 28–29
    lymph node micrometastases, 296
    precision and reproducibility, 28
    quality control and standardization, need for, 25–30
    sensitivity and specificity determination, 27, 28
Immunohistochemistry
    methods and detection enzymes, 27
    quality control and standardization, 27–28
Imprecision, of assays, 66–67
Imubind assays (American Diagnostica), 446–447
Informatics, Inc, ProPeak software, 16
β-Inhibin, in semen, 199
Inhibitor of apoptosis proteins (IAP), 504
INK4 family, melanoma markers, 368
Insulin
    islet cell carcinoma, marker for, 49
    pancreatic endocrine tumor marker, 345
Insulin-like growth factors (IGF)
    carcinoid of the gut, marker for, 343
    prostate cancer marker, 209–210
    prostate function and, 196–197
Insulinomas, 343, 344
INT2 gene, 84

Integrins, melanoma markers, 363
Interference, in assays, 69–79
Interleukin-10 (Il-10)
  leukemia marker, 322
  lymphoma marker, 322
  melanoma marker, 362, 365
Interleukin-2 (Il-2), melanoma marker, 362, 365
Interleukin-6 (Il-6)
  melanoma marker, 362, 365
  monoclonal gammopathy of undetermined significance (MGUS) marker, 312
  non-Hodgkin's lymphoma marker, 322
  ovarian cancer marker, 241, 246
Internal quality control (IQC), 34, 35
International Committee on Harmonization (ICH), 141
Intracellular adhesion molecule (ICAM), melanoma marker, 363
Intrahepatic cholangiosarcoma, 275–276
Ionization, protein analysis, 395

K

K-*ras* gene, 84
  bone marrow micrometastases, 297
  lung cancer marker, 293
  pancreatic cancer marker, 267–268
Kallikrein 2
  nonprostatic sources, 207
  prostate cancer marker, 206–207, 215–216
  prostate cancer staging, 217–218, 220
  in semen, 199
Kallikrein 3. *See* Prostate-specific antigen (PSA)
Kallikreins
  clinical significance, 466–468
  gene family, 466–468
  nomenclature, 465, 467–468
  ovarian cancer markers, 6, 241, 244–245, 404
Ki-67 gene, lung cancer marker, 300, 301
Ki67
  brain tumor marker, 330–331
  melanoma marker, 362, 367
Kidney cancer, 115, 408
Kidney failure, assay results variability, 70
KIP family, melanoma markers, 368
KIT proto-oncogene, 86
Knudson two-hit hypothesis, 88, 89

L

Laboratory Medicine Practice Guidelines (LMPG), 34
Lactate dehydrogenase (LDH)
  colorectal cancer marker, 257
  gastrointestinal cancer marker, 254
  germ cell tumor marker, 52–53, 57
  lung cancer marker, 288, 291–292, 300–301
  melanoma marker, 362, 365
  non-Hodgkin's lymphoma marker, 321, 322
  testicular cancer marker, 354
Laser Capture Microdissection (LCM, Arcturus Corp.), 393
Laser microdissection/laser pressure catapulting (LMM/LPC, P.A.L.M. Microlaser Technologies), 393
Laser Microdissection (LMD, Leica Mikrosysteme Vertrieb GmbH), 393
Leucine aminopeptidase, in semen, 199
Leukemia
  DNA marker, cell-free, 116
  markers for, 321–325
  molecular classification, 151
Level of Evidence Categories, for TMUGS, 20
Linearity, of assays, 68
Liver cirrhosis, 271
Lobular carcinoma in situ (LCIS), breast cancer risk and, 181
Localization, test limitations, 5
Loss of heterozygosity-related alterations, 86–87, 88, 89, 383
LumiCyte, Inc., 395, 396
Luminex Corp., 395, 396
Lung cancer
  bone marrow micrometastases, 296–297
  carcinoids, 343
  diagnostic guidelines, 300
  epidemiology of, 481
  free tumor cell markers, 297–299
  histological classification, 55
  markers for, 55–57, 115, 450, 478–479, 481–482, 517–520
  metastatic, markers for, 295–301
  methylation markers, 294–295
  molecular markers, 292–294
  predictor genes for, 408
  response prediction markers, 299–301
  serum markers, 287–292
  staging, 473
LungAlert™ test, 477, 479
Lymph nodes
  breast cancer metastasis, 434–435
  lung cancer micrometastases, 295–296
  melanoma prognosis, 369
Lymphomas
  Epstein-Barr virus (EBV) DNA, 493–494
  markers for, 321–325, 493–494
Lysophosphatidic acid (LPA), ovarian cancer marker, 245

M

M-proteins, 309
  monoclonal gammopathy of undetermined significance (MGUS), 311
  multiple myeloma markers, 54–55, 307–308
Macrophage inhibitory cytokine 1 (MIC-1), prostate cancer marker, 402–403
MAGE3, melanoma marker, 112
Major histocompatibility complex (MHC) tetramers, T-cell assay, 457–460

Malignant melanoma, 112, 113–114
Mammaglobulin, 112, 433–435
Mammary serine protease inhibitor (maspin), 437, 438–439
Mammograms, 181
Mantle cell lymphoma (MCL), 325
MART1, melanoma marker, 112, 362, 364
Maspin, assay for, 437, 438–439
Mass analyzers, protein analysis, 395
Mass spectrometry (MS)
  historical background, 4
  protein analysis, 394–395
  protein identification, 14–15
MassARRAY™, 16
Matritech Corp., 282–283, 284
Matrix-assisted laser desorption/ionization (MALDI), 395
Matrix metalloproteinases (MMPs). *See also* Tissue inhibitors of MMPs (TIMPs)
  assays for, 103–104
  brain tumor markers, 332, 333–334
  melanoma markers, 362, 366–367
  metastasis and, 100
  prognostic marker, 103
  structure and function of, 103
  table of, 103
MCC tumor suppressor gene, 84, 88
MDR gene, lung cancer marker, 301
Medical Devices Amendment (1976), 33
MedSystems Diagnostics GmbH (Bender MedSystems), 427, 428, 430
Medullary thyroid carcinoma
  etiology and physiology, 346
  markers for, 49–52, 57, 345, 346
Melan-A, melanoma marker, 364
Melanin synthesis pathway, 361–362
Melanoma, 361–369
Melanoma cell adhesion molecule (MCAM), melanoma marker, 362, 363
Melanoma inhibitory activity (MIA) protein, melanoma marker, 362, 368
MEN1 tumor suppressor gene, 84
Menstruation, CA 125, 34
MET proto-oncogene, 86
Metabolome, 471–474
Metanephrins, 345
Metastasis
  biological mechanisms, 152
  brain tumor markers, 333–334
  breast cancer angiogenesis, markers for, 185
  breast cancer markers, 170–175
  definition and steps of, 99
  lung cancer, 295–301
  origin, predicting, 405, 407
  overview, 7
  protease markers, 99–104
  sites, survival and, 170

MIB
  brain tumor marker, 330–331
  melanoma marker, 367
Microarrays
  applications, in cancer biology, 383–388
  comparative genomic hybridization (CGH), 383–384
  gene expression profiling, 384–385
  in genomics, 15, 383–388
  historical background, 4
  protein analysis, 395–396
  ProteinChip® technique, 15
  in proteonomics, 385–387
  SNP, 16
  tissue, for validation and clinical correlation, 387
  in transcriptonomics, 385–387
  in tumor marker discovery, 401–409
Microdissection, in specimen collection and preparation, 393
β2-Microglobulin
  leukemia marker, 321, 322
  monoclonal gammopathy of undetermined significance (MGUS) marker, 312
  non-Hodgkin's lymphoma marker, 321, 322
Microphthalmia transcription factor (MITF), melanoma marker, 362, 367
Microsatellite markers, bladder cancer, 284
β-Microseminoprotein, in semen, 199
MLH gene, 84
MLuC1 antibody, bone marrow micrometastic marker, 299
MN/CA9, kidney cancer marker, 115
MNF116 antibody, lymph node micrometastases marker, 296
Monitoring. *See* Therapeutic monitoring
Monoclonal antibodies. *See also* Trastuzumab
  cross-reactivity to antigens, 68
  historical background, 4
  lung cancer marker, 289
  non-Hodgkin's lymphoma treatment, 325
  pancreatic cancer markers, 266
Monoclonal gammopathies, 53–55, 305–306. *See also* Multiple myeloma
Monoclonal gammopathy of undetermined significance (MGUS), 305, 306, 311–314
MOS proto-oncogene, 86
Mouse Double Minute-2 (MDM) gene, brain tumor marker, 332
mRNA, 107–109, 115
MTS1 gene, 84
Mucin-type (MUC) markers
  autoantibody detection, correlation with, 124–125, 126
  bone marrow micrometastases, 297
  breast cancer, 38, 112, 128, 165, 175
  colorectal cancer, 115
  pancreatic cancer, 266
Multi-Layer Perceptron (MLP) neural network, 136–138
Multidimensional chromatography, 15
Multiparametric analysis, historical background, 4

Multiple endocrine neoplasia (MEN-2), 344
Multiple myeloma
    bone disease, 306–307
    diagnosis, 307–311
    epidemiology of, 305
    etiology and physiology, 305–306
    markers for, 54–55, 307–311
Multivariate models, of diagnosis, 133–138
Mutations
    BRCA genes, 189–190
    in cancer development and progression, 152
    proto-oncogenes, 86, 87
myc proto-oncogene family, 86
    Burkitt lymphoma mutation, 86
    c-myc gene, 254
    gastrointestinal cancer markers, 254
    lung cancer marker, 294
    N-myc gene, 84
Myeloma
    diagnosis and monitoring, 54
    markers for, 54–55, 57
    specimen collection and preparation, 54

N

Nasopharyngeal carcinoma, 491–494
National Academy of Clinical Biochemistry (NACB), 34, 57
    breast cancer marker recommendations, 39–40, 57
    colorectal cancer marker guidelines, 48, 57
    germ cell tumor marker guidelines, 53, 57
    myeloma marker guidelines, 54–55, 57
    neuroendocrine tumor marker guidelines, 51–52, 57
    ovarian cancer marker guidelines, 42, 57
    prostate cancer, PSA guidelines, 46, 57
National Cancer Institute (NCI), Program for the Assessment of Clinical Cancer Tests (PACCT), 29
National Committee for Clinical Laboratory Standards (NCCLS), immunohistochemistry assay guidelines, 27
NCC-LU243 antibody, bone marrow micrometastic marker, 299
NCC-LU246 antibody, bone marrow micrometastic marker, 299
Nephelometry, 54
Neural cell adhesion molecule (NCAM), 292, 298
Neural networks, 4, 136
Neuroblastoma
    etiology and physiology, 346
    markers for, 49–52, 57, 345, 346
Neuroendocrine cells, secretory products, 339, 340
Neuroendocrine markers, lung cancer, 300
Neuroendocrine tumors, 49–52, 57, 339–347
Neurofibromatosis, 345
Neurokinin-A (NKA), carcinoid of the gut, marker for, 343
Neuron-specific enolase (NSE)
    carcinoid of the gut, marker for, 345
    lung cancer marker, 55–57, 288–291, 300–301
    medullary thyroid carcinoma, marker for, 345
    neuroblastoma marker, 345, 346
    pancreatic endocrine tumor marker, 345
    pheochromocytoma marker, 345
Neuropeptide-K (NPK), carcinoid of the gut, marker for, 343, 345
Neuropeptide-Y (NPY), 345
Neurotrophin receptor kinase C, brain tumor marker, 333
NF1 tumor suppressor gene, 88
NF2 tumor suppressor gene, 84, 88
Nichirei Corp., 427, 428, 429
nm23 gene, melanoma marker, 362, 367
Nm23-H1, 322
NMP22 test (Matritech), 282–283, 284
nn23-Hi gene, gastrointestinal cancer marker, 254
Nomograms, 46, 217, 221–223
Non-functioning pancreatic tumors, 343
Non-Hodgkin's lymphoma (NHL)
    markers for, 321–322, 325
    treatment, 325
Non-seminomatous germ cell tumors, markers for, 52–53, 57
Non-small-cell lung cancer (NSCLC)
    bone marrow micrometastases, 296–297
    DNA marker, cell-free, 116
    free tumor cell markers, 297–298
    lymph node micrometastases, 295–296
    markers for, 55–56
    methylation markers, 295
    prognostic autoantibodies, 128
    response prediction markers, 299–300
    serum markers, 287–290
Nonspecific cross-reacting antigen 50/90 (NCA 50/90), lung cancer marker, 289
Nordic Myeloma Study Group, 311
Norepinephrine
    neuroblastoma marker, 345
    pheochromocytoma marker, 49, 345–346
    reference values, 50
Novartis Research Foundation, 403
Nuclear matrix protein 22 (NMP22), bladder cancer marker, 282–283
Nuclear proto-oncogenes, 86
5′-nucleotide phosphodiesterase V (5′-NPD), hepatocellular carcinoma marker, 275

O

Oncogene Research Products, 427, 428, 429, 430
Oncogenes
    alterations, types of, 86
    amplified chromosomal sites, 84
    in cancer development and progression, 152
    cell proliferation control, 83–84
    classification of, 85–86
    discovery of, 4
    functions of, 85–86

identification of, 84–85
proto-oncogenes, 85–86
retroviral, 85
table of, 84
OncogeneScience Products, 427, 428, 429, 430
Oral cancer, markers for, 115
Ornithine decarboxylase, 254, 257
Osteosarcoma, markers for, 450
Ovarian cancer, 128
BRCA genes, 189–192
carcinoma, appearance of, 240
clinical management, 240–241
early detection, 243
epidemiology of, 239
genetic classification of, 405, 407
histologic classification, 239
markers for, 41, 57, 115, 241–246, 450, 486
pathogenesis, 239–240
predictor genes for, 408
screening, 41
sErbB receptor assay kits, 429–430
serous papillary adenocarcinoma, gene expression profiling, 401–403

P

P15Ink4B gene, 84
p16 gene, lung cancer marker, 293
p16/INK4A tumor suppressor gene, 88
p21 gene, lung cancer marker, 301
p21 protein, melanoma marker, 368
p53 autoantibodies, 126
bladder cancer prognosis, 128
breast cancer monitoring, 128–129
breast cancer prognosis, 128
colorectal cancer prognosis, 128
lung cancer marker, 288
lung cancer prognosis, 128
lymph node micrometastases marker, 296
ovarian cancer prognosis, 128
p53 tumor suppressor gene, 84
bladder cancer, 91–95
bone marrow micrometastases, 297
brain tumor marker, 332, 333
breast cancer marker, 184
gastrointestinal cancer marker, 254
lung cancer marker, 292–293, 294, 300, 301
pancreatic cancer marker, 267, 269
pathways, apoptosis marker, 157
Pancreatic cancer
CA 19.9 histograms and ROC curve, 144
diagnosis, 343–344
DNA marker, cell-free, 116
endocrine tumors, 343–346
islet cell carcinoma, markers for, 49–52
markers for, 115, 265–268, 345, 450
predictor genes for, 408
Pancreatic oncofetal antigen (POA), pancreatic cancer marker, 265, 266
Pancreatic polypeptide (PP), 343, 344, 345
PC1 gene, 461–464
Peptide mass fingerprinting (PMF), 397
Peptide YY (PYY), carcinoid of the gut, marker for, 343
Personnel, communications, importance of, 78
Pgp-1. *See* CD44
Phases, of clinical studies
for biomarker targeted therapy, 158
of tumor marker development, 142–149
Pheochromocytoma
etiology and physiology, 344–345
markers for, 49–52, 57, 345–346
Phosphoryl choline, in semen, 198
Phylos, Inc., 396
Pilomatricoma, 437
Pituitary gland, prostate function and, 195
Placental alkaline phosphatase (PLAP). *See also* Alkaline phosphatase (ALP)
brain tumor marker, 330
germ cell tumor marker, 57
half-life, 355
testicular cancer marker, 354–355
Plasmin, substrates, 100
Plasminogen activation inhibitor (PAI-1)
breast cancer marker, 29, 185, 445–447
uPA inhibition, 100
Plasminogen activation system, 445–447
PML-RARα, leukemia marker, 324, 325
Polyacrylamide gel electrophoresis, 2D-PAGE, 393–394
Poly(ADP)ribose polymerase (PARP), DNA synthesome, 413
Polymerase chain reaction (PCR)
circulating tumor cells (CTC), 107–111
digital, ovarian cancer diagnosis, 248–249
mammaglobulin assay, 433–435
Pre-market application (PMA) and approval, 29
Pre-progastrin-releasing peptide (PreProGP), lung cancer, free tumor cell marker, 298
Precancerous lesions, detection, 149
Precision, of assays, 66–67
Preclinical studies, tumor marker development, 142, 143–145
Predictive markers
breast cancer, 173–174
evaluation protocols, 154–157
grading, of clinical utility, 20–22
Predictive value model, in validation, 11–12
Primase, DNA synthesome, 413
Pro-gastrin-releasing peptide (ProGRP)
lung cancer marker, 55–57, 517–520
reference values, 517–518
Probe melting curve analysis, 513–515
Progastrin-releasing peptide (ProGP), lung cancer marker, 288, 289

Progestin receptors
    analytical concerns, 38
    breast cancer markers, 37–38, 57
    distribution, in breast carcinoma, 38
    reference values, 37
    RT-PCR assay, 454
Prognosis and prognostic markers
    alpha-fetoprotein, 273
    amyloidosis, primary, 317
    autoantibody detection, 127–128
    β-catenin, 437–439
    bladder cancer, 94, 284
    breast cancer, 100–101, 165, 167–169, 173–174, 181–186, 437–439, 447
    CA 125, in breast cancer, 244
    cathepsin B, 102
    cathepsin D, 102
    cervical cancer, 115
    colorectal cancer, 115, 255
    gastrointestinal cancer, 101
    germ cell tumors, 52
    grading, of clinical utility, 20–22
    HER-2, in breast cancer, 183–184
    limitations of, 5
    lung cancer, 56, 115, 299–301
    maspin, 437–439
    matrix metalloproteinases, 103
    melanoma, 369
    monoclonal gammopathy of undetermined significance (MGUS), 311–312
    nomograms, 46
    ovarian cancer, 41–42
    overview, 11
    prostate cancer, 45–46
    untreated locoregional breast cancer, 167–168
    uPA as, 99–101
    urothelial carcinoma, 115
    Waldenström's macroglobulinemia, 315–316
Program for the Assessment of Clinical Cancer Tests (PACCT), 29
Proinsulin, pancreatic endocrine tumor marker, 345
Proliferating cell nuclear antigen (PCNA)
    brain tumor marker, 330–331
    in breast cancer cells, 417–418
    DNA synthesome, 413
ProPeak software (Informatics), 16
Prostaglandins, 157, 198
Prostase, in semen, 199
Prostasin, 199, 241, 245
Prostate cancer
    adenocarcinoma of, 201–202
    algorithms and nomograms, 221–223
    androgen sensitive/insensitive, 221–222
    benign vs. malignant, PSA and, 213
    biochemical failure, 223–224
    classification of, 202
    diagnosis and monitoring, 111, 202
    DNA marker, cell-free, 116
    early detection, 44–45, 57, 202–204, 211–214
    gene expression profiling, 402–403
    grading systems, 203
    markers for, 43–46, 57, 112, 204–210, 486–488
    PC1 gene, 461–464
    predictor genes for, 408
    prognosis, 111
    prostate-specific antigen (PSA), 210–211
    screening for, 43–45, 224
    staging, 204, 216–219
    transition zone, 203–204
    WHO grading system, 203
Prostate gland
    anatomy and physiology of, 193–198
    angiogenesis, 197
    disorders of, 199–202, 210–216
    epithelial function regulation, 196
    kallikrein 2 complexes, 206
    secretory products, 198–199
    stromal function regulation, 196–198
    volume, PSA and, 214
Prostate-specific antigen (PSA)
    (-2)pPSA, 214
    androgen ablation and, 221–222
    benign prostatic hyperplasia (BPH), 210
    BPSA, 213
    complexed, in prostate cancer early detection, 213
    discovery of, 4
    free, in prostate cancer early detection, 212–214
    guidelines for use, 46
    half-life, 10
    hK3 gene, 466, 467
    hormonal therapy and, 219–222
    inactive pro-PSA, 205
    intact, 214
    international standard, 67–68
    isoforms, 205–206
    as kallikrein, 467
    measurement of, 205–206
    metabolism and elimination, 205
    nonprostatic sources, 207
    patient management, 45–46
    prostate cancer marker, 43–46, 57, 211–215
    in prostate gland, 193
    radiation therapy and, 222–224
    radical prostatectomy and, 218–219
    reference values, 43
    in semen, 198–199
    in serum, 204–205
    stability of, 206
    staging, prostate cancer, 217, 218
    subfractions, in prostate cancer early detection, 213–214
    as surrogate marker, 157
    total, in prostate cancer early detection, 211–212, 215

transition zone prostate cancer, 204
underexpression of, 6
variability of, 70
Prostate-specific membrane antigen (PSMA)
prostate cancer marker, 112, 207–208
radioimmunoscintigraphy, 208
serum analysis, 208
therapeutic uses, 208
Prostate-specific protein-94, in semen, 199
Prostatic acid phosphatase, 43, 198, 207
Prostatic intraepithelial neoplasia (PIN), 201, 210
Prostatitis, 34, 200–201, 210
Proteases, metastasis, markers for, 99–104
Protein C pathway, 445–447
Protein serine-threonine kinases, genetic mutation of, 86
ProteinChip® technique (Ciphergen Biosystems), 15, 16, 396
Proteins
analytical techniques, 394–398
microarrays, analysis and, 395–396
protein profiling, 397–398
separation and identification, 14–15, 393–394
Proteome
analysis, tools for, 392–396
oncogenesis and, 391–392
protein analysis, 394–396
protein separation techniques, 393–394
Proteonomics
bioinformatics and, 16, 396–398
in chronic lymphocytic leukemia (CLL), 398
methods, 14–15
microarrays in, 385–387
Proto-oncogenes, 85–86
PTEN tumor suppressor gene, 84
PTP tumor suppressor gene, 88
Pyruvate kinase type M2 (M2-PK)
lung cancer marker, 289
quantification of, 472
tumor metabolome, role in, 471–474

Q

Quality assurance and control, in testing
analytical requirements, 34–35
diagnosis, tumor markers and, 3–7
overview, 14
postanalytical and reporting requirements, 35, 36
preanalytical requirements, 34
standardization, need for, 25–30

R

Race/ethnicity
breast cancer risk and, 181
life tables, men, 202
Radioimmunoassay, historical background, 4, 65

Radiolabel signal detection variability, in assays, 66
Radiotherapy
brain tumors, 333
hepatocellular carcinoma, alpha-fetoprotein (AFP), 273–274
monoclonal gammopathy of undetermined significance (MGUS) treatment, 313
nasopharyngeal carcinoma, 491–494
prostate cancer, prostate-specific antigen (PSA), 222–224
RAF1 proto-oncogene, 86
RAK α gene, 485–488
RAK antigens, 485–488
Rakowicz (RAK) antigens, 485–488
Ras FTase, signal transduction marker, 157
RAS proto-oncogene family
function of, 86
gastrointestinal cancer marker, 254
pancreatic cancer marker, 267
probe melting curve analysis, 513–515
RB tumor suppressor gene, 88, 294
bladder cancer, 91–95
inactivation, in bladder cancer, 93
lung cancer marker, 293–294
RB1 tumor suppressor gene, 84
Receiver operating characteristic (ROC) curve, 12, 144, 145–147, 220, 519
Recombinant DNA
oncogene identification, 85
tumor suppressor gene identification, 87
Recurrence
breast cancer markers, 39, 169–171
breast cancer, predictive characteristics, 181
colorectal cancer markers, 255
overview, 10, 11
test limitations, 5
Reference change value (RCV), 67
Reference materials, quality control and standardization, 28
Reference values
alpha-fetoprotein, 270, 271–272
CA 125, in breast cancer, 243
disadvantages of, 154
prostate-specific antigen (PSA), 211–215
in validation, 11
Regression, multivariate logistic, 134–135
Relapse, breast cancer marker, 39
Remission, test limitations, 5
Renal cell carcinoma (RCC), markers for, 450
Replication factor C, DNA synthesome, 413
Replication protein A, DNA synthesome, 413
Reporting requirements, 35, 36
Resistance, to drug therapy, 151
RET gene, 84, 86
Retinoblastoma, model, of tumor suppressor gene function, 87–88
Retinoblastoma (*Rb*) gene, 293–294

Retrospective studies, 142–143, 146–147
Retroviral oncogenes, oncogene identification, 85
Reverse transcriptase polymerase chain reaction (RT-PCR)
　circulating tumor cells (CTC), 107–111
　prostate-specific membrane antigen (PSMA), 208
Rheumatoid factor, 72, 77
Ribonuclear protein A2/B1 (hrNP), 481–482
RNA
　isolation of, 108–109
　mRNA as circulating tumor marker, 107–108, 115
　mRNA isolation of, 108–109
Robustness, of assay method, 69–78

S

S-100 proteins, melanoma markers, 368–369
Saliva, contamination by, 70
Sampling. *See also* Specimen collection and preparation
　cancer control studies, sample size, 148–149
　concurrent disease (clinical trial) assays, sample size, 146
　missampling, by automated analyzers, 71
　prospective screening studies, sample size, 148
　retrospective studies, in marker development, sample size, 146–147
　sample size, in tumor marker development, 145
Sclerosing cholangitis, 276
Screening
　autoantibody detection, 126–127
　bladder cancer, 284
　breast cancer, 181
　hepatocellular carcinoma, 273
　limitations of, 5
　lung cancer, 55–56
　objectives, 141–142
　ovarian cancer, 41
　overview, 11
　precancerous lesion detection, 149
　prospective screening studies, 143, 147–148
　prostate cancer, 43–45, 224
Secretogranins, from neuroendocrine cells, 339–341
Semen, composition of, 198–199
Seminal fluid, 204, 206
Sensitivity and detection limits, of assays
　autoantibodies, 124
　breast cancer markers, 166
　overview, 66
　pro-gastrin-releasing peptide (ProGRP), 518–520
　in tumor marker development, 144–147
Separation techniques, proteins, 393–394
Sequenom, Inc, MassARRAY™, 16
Sequential chromatography, 15
sErbB receptors
　assay kits, 427–431
　breast cancer markers, 427–431
　ovarian cancer markers, 427–431

Serial analysis for gene expression (SAGE), 247, 248
Serological analysis of recombinant cDNA expression libraries (SEREX), 247–248
Serotonin, tissue production, 10
Serum viscosity
　in multiple myeloma, 307
　in Waldenström's macroglobulinemia, 54
Short tandem repeat polymorphism (STRP) analysis, 87
Signal transducer oncogenes, 86
Signal transduction pathway, targeted therapy and, 157
Significance, of test results, 67
Single nucleotide polymorphisms (SNPs)
　definition of, 15–16
　genomic profiling, 383, 513–515
　probe melting curve analysis, 513–515
　technology development, 7
SLP1 gene, ovarian cancer marker, 401–402
Small cell lung cancer (SCLC)
　DNA marker, cell-free, 116
　free tumor cell markers, 299
　markers for, 55–56, 288, 290–292
　methylation markers, 295
　micrometastases in, 298–299
　molecular markers, 294
　response prediction markers, 300–301
Smoking, assay results variability, 70
Somatostatin, 343, 345
Somatostatinomas, 343, 344
SPAN-1 monoclonal antibody, 266
Specificity, of assays
　autoantibodies, 124
　overview, 68–69
　in tumor marker development, 144–147
Specimen carryover, erroneous test results, cause of, 36
Specimen collection and preparation
　assay results variability, 69, 70
　blood collection tubes and additives, 70–71
　blood, for circulating tumor cells (CTC), 108
　breast tissue markers, 37–38
　cell sorting, 393
　collection and purification guidelines, 13
　concurrent disease (clinical trial) assays, 145
　lung cancer markers, 56
　microdissection in, 393
　multiple myeloma, 310
　prostate cancer, 203
　prostate cancer markers, 46
　PSA stability, 206
　quality control and standardization, need for, 25–26
　retrospective studies, in marker development, 146
　standardization, need for, 153
　storage and stability, 70, 71
　tissue banks, for proteome analysis, 392
　tissue fixation, 26
　in tumor marker development, 144
Spermine and spermidine, in semen, 198

Squamous cell carcinoma antigen (SCCA)
    cervical cancer marker, 42–43, 115
    lung cancer marker, 55, 288
    markers for, 287–288
SRC proto-oncogene, 86
Staging
    classification system, 9
    definition of, 9
    gastrointestinal cancer, 254
    hepatocellular carcinoma, 273
    lung cancer, 473
    marker quantification for, 10
    overview, 7, 11
    prostate cancer, 204, 216–219
    test limitations, 5
    testicular cancer, 355
Standardization
    of clinical studies, 154–156
    of specimen collection and storage, 153
    of tumor marker assays, 25–30, 152–153
Standards
    chorionic gonadotropin (human, hCG), 353
    internal, for RT-PCR, 110–111
    for tumor markers, 67–68
Statistical methods
    in bioinformatics, 16
    Multi-Layer Perceptron (MLP) neural network, 136–138
    multivariate models, of diagnosis, 134–135
    neural networks, 136–138
    regression, multivariate logistic, 134–135
    support vector machine (SVM), 136–137
Storage and stability, of samples, 70, 71
Substance P, carcinoid of the gut, marker for, 343, 345
Support vector machine (SVM), 136–137
Suppression, proto-oncogenes, 86
Surface-Enhanced Laser Desorption/Ionization (SELDI), 15, 396
Surrogate markers, 157
Surveillance. *See* Therapeutic monitoring
Survivin, bladder cancer marker, 284
Synaptotagmin IV, 462–463

T

T-cells, 457–460
TA90. *See* Tumor-associated glycoprotein antigen (TA90)
TACSTD1 gene, ovarian cancer marker, 401–402
Tamoxifen, breast cancer treatment, 183
Targeted therapy. *See* Therapeutic targets
Tele-methylimidazoleacetic acid (Melmil)
    medullary thyroid carcinoma, marker for, 345
    pancreatic endocrine tumor marker, 345
Telomerase
    bladder cancer marker, 283
    brain tumor marker, 332–333
    lung cancer marker, 115
    structure and function of, 509
Telomeric Repeat Amplification Protocol (TRAP, Geron), 283, 509
Testes, prostate function and, 195
Testicular cancer
    classification of, 351–352
    diagnosis and staging, 355
    etiology and physiology, 351
    markers for, 115, 351–356
Testosterone, homeostasis, in blood, 195–196
Thalidomide, monoclonal gammopathy of undetermined significance (MGUS) treatment, 313
Therapeutic monitoring, 355–356
    autoantibody detection, 127–128
    bladder cancer, 94–95
    brain tumors, 330
    BRCA genes, 191–192
    breast cancer, 172–173, 191–192
    CA 125, in breast cancer, 244
    colorectal cancer, 48, 255
    germ cell tumors, 52–53
    hepatocellular carcinoma, 273
    lung cancer, 56, 520
    nasopharyngeal carcinoma, 491–494
    ovarian cancer, 41–42, 191–192
    overview, 10, 11
    prostate cancer, 45–46, 219–222
    test limitations, 5
    tumor M2-PK, 472–473
    validation and, 12
Therapeutic response prediction, limitations of, 5
Therapeutic targeting, clinical trial phases for, 143–148
Therapeutic targets
    cell signal systems and, 156–157
    molecular-targeted agents vs. cytotoxic drugs, 154–157
    tumor markers as, 151–160
Thompson-Friedenreich antigen (TF Ag), 477
Thymidine kinase, B-cell leukemia marker, 322
Thyroglobulin (TG), thyroid carcinoma marker, 115
Thyroid carcinoma
    markers for, 115
    medullary, etiology and physiology, 346
    medullary, markers for, 49–52, 57, 345, 346
Time-of-flight (ToF) analysis, 395
Tissue banks, for proteome analysis, 392
Tissue inhibitors of MMPs (TIMPs). *See also* Matrix metalloproteinases (MMPs)
    brain tumor markers, 332, 333–334
    colorectal cancer marker, 441–443
Tissue polypeptide antigen (TPA)
    bladder cancer marker, 283
    hepatocellular carcinoma marker, 275
    lung cancer marker, 288, 289–290, 292
    ovarian cancer marker, 241, 245
    pancreatic cancer marker, 265, 266

Tissue polypeptide specific antigen (TPS), 265–266
TNF-related apoptosis-inducing ligand (TRAIL), melanoma marker, 362, 366
Topo genes, lung cancer markers, 300–301
Topoisomerases, DNA synthesome, 413
TP53 tumor suppressor gene, 88, 89, 93
Transcription factors, genetic mutation of, 86
Transcriptonomics, 15, 385–387
Transferrin, in semen, 199
Translocations, proto-oncogenes, 86
Transrectal ultrasonography, 203
Trastuzumab, patient selection, for treatment, 40, 57, 175
Triton Diagnostics, 427, 428–429
TRK proto-oncogene, 86
Tropomyosin autoantibody, colorectal cancer prognosis, 128
TRP-MET gene, 84
True-positive rate (TPR), 144–147
Truth table, for IHC assays, 28
Tumor-associated glycoprotein antigen (TA90), 362, 364
Tumor-associated trypsin inhibitor (TATI)
   in benign disease, 449–450
   biliary cancer marker, 450
   bladder cancer marker, 450
   breast cancer marker, 450
   cervical cancer marker, 450
   colorectal cancer marker, 450
   endometrial cancer marker, 450
   gastric cancer marker, 450
   head and neck cancer marker, 451
   hepatoma marker, 450
   lung cancer marker, 450
   osteosarcoma marker, 451
   ovarian cancer marker, 241, 245, 450
   pancreatic cancer marker, 266, 450
   reference values, 449
   renal cell carcinoma (RCC) marker, 450
   structure and function of, 449
Tumor classification, gene expression and, 6–7
Tumor growth factors, targeted therapy and, 157
Tumor M2-PK
   lung cancer marker, 289
   quantification of, 472
   tumor metabolome, role in, 471–474
Tumor Marker Utility Grading System (TMUGS), 19–21, 30, 182
Tumor markers, 113–114
   clinical utility of, 19–21, 29–30
   comparability of results, 65–69
   definition of, 9–10, 19, 33
   development of, 29–30, 141–150
   discovery, proteomic approaches, 391–399
   discovery technologies, 6, 401–409
   future of, 16–17
   grading, of clinical utility, 19–21
   guidelines for development, 29–30
   historical background, 3–4
   international standards, 67–68
   limitations of, 5
   multiple, use of, 133–138
   predictive, 20–22, 154–157
   selection and uses, 10, 11
   surrogate, 157
   as therapeutic targets, 151–160
   validation of, 10–12, 29
Tumor necrosis factor receptors (TNFR), 503
Tumor suppressor genes
   in cancer development and progression, 152
   cell proliferation control, 83–84
   cloned, relevant, 88
   discovery of, 4
   function, models of, 87–88
   genomic imprinting and, 88
   identification of, 86–87
   inactivation, in bladder cancer, 92–95
   table of, 84
Tumor volume, estimating, 11
Tumorigenesis
   models of, 89–90
   oncogenes and tumor suppressor genes in, 83–84
   proteome and, 391–392
   pyruvate kinase isoenzymes, 471
Tyrosinase, melanoma marker, 112, 362, 364, 369
Tyrosine kinases, genetic mutation of, 86

U

U95367 gene, RT-PCR assay, 433–435
Unified Maximum Separability Analysis (UMSA), 16
University of Cologne, Germany, 300
Urine tumor markers, bladder cancer and, 282
Urokinase-type plasminogen activator (uPA)
   assays for, 101
   breast cancer marker, 29, 41, 100–101, 185, 445–447
   function of, 99–100
   gastrointestinal cancer marker, 101
   metastasis and, 100
Uroplaktins, urothelial carcinoma markers, 115
Urothelial carcinoma, markers for, 115

V

Validation
   microarrays in, 387
   of tumor markers, 10–12, 29
Vanillylmandelic acid (VMA)
   drug interference with, 50
   neuroblastoma marker, 57, 345, 346
   pheochromocytoma marker, 49, 57, 345–346
   reference values, 49–50
Vascular endothelial growth factor receptor (VEGFR), B-cell leukemia marker, 322

Vascular endothelial growth factor (VEGF)
   blood collection standardization, 153
   in breast cancer, 154
   melanoma marker, 362, 366
Vasoactive intestinal polypeptide (VIP)
   neuroblastoma marker, 345
   pheochromocytoma marker, 345
Vasoactive intestinal polypeptide (VIP)-omas, 343, 344
VHL tumor suppressor gene, 84
Viral markers, 485–488
Vitros kit (Ortho), 242
Von Hippel-Landau gene transcript, kidney cancer marker, 115
Von Hippel-Lindau disease, 344

W

Waldenström's macroglobulinemia, 314–316
   classification of, 306
   diagnosis, 314–315
   epidemiology, etiology, and biology, 314
   markers for, 54–55
   treatment and prognosis, 315–316
Wilms' tumors, 85, 88
Working range, of assays, 66
World Health Organization (WHO)
   brain tumor classification, 329
   ovarian cancer classification, 239
   prostate cancer grading system, 203
WT1 tumor suppressor gene, 84, 88
WT2 tumor suppressor gene, 84

Z

Zinc, in semen, 1986